Bacterial Infections of Humans

Epidemiology and Control

SECOND EDITION

Bacterial Infections of Humans

Epidemiology and Control

SECOND EDITION

Edited by

Alfred S. Evans

John Rodman Paul Professor of Epidemiology, Emeritus
Yale University School of Medicine
New Haven, Connecticut

and

Philip S. Brachman

Emory University School of Public Health
Atlanta, Georgia

PLENUM MEDICAL BOOK COMPANY
New York and London

Library of Congress Cataloging-in-Publication Data

Bacterial infections of humans : epidemiology and control / edited by
  Alfred S. Evans and Philip S. Brachman. -- 2nd ed.
      p.   cm.
  Includes bibliographical references.
  Includes index.
  ISBN 0-306-43343-5
  1. Bacterial diseases--Epidemiology. 2. Bacterial diseases-
-Prevention.   I. Evans, Alfred S., 1917-   . II. Brachman, Philip
S.
  [DNLM: 1. Bacterial Infections--epidemiology. 2. Bacterial
Infections--prevention & control.   WC 200 B131]
  RA644.B32B33 1990
  614.5'7--dc20
  DNLM/DLC
  for Library of Congress   90-14169
                                                        CIP

© 1991 Plenum Publishing Corporation
233 Spring Street, New York, N.Y. 10013

Plenum Medical Book Company is an imprint of Plenum Publishing Corporation

Printed in the United States of America

This edition is dedicated to

Harry A. Feldman, M.D.,
co-editor of the First Edition,

and to our families

Contributors

E. Russell Alexander, Division of Sexually Transmitted Diseases, Center for Prevention Services, Centers for Disease Control, Atlanta, Georgia 30333. *Present address:* Seattle–King County Department of Public Health, Seattle, Washington 98104

Donald Armstrong, Department of Medicine, Memorial Sloan–Kettering Cancer Center, and Cornell University Medical College, New York, New York 10021

Robert S. Baltimore, Departments of Pediatrics and Epidemiology and Public Health, Yale University School of Medicine, New Haven, Connecticut 06510

Abram S. Benenson, Graduate School of Public Health, San Diego State University, San Diego, California 92182

Michael L. Bennish, International Centre for Diarrhoeal Disease Research–Bangladesh, Ohaka, Bangladesh; Departments of Pediatrics and Medicine, Division of Geographic Medicine and Infectious Diseases, New England Medical Center Hospitals, Boston, Massachusetts 02111

Robert E. Black, Department of International Health, School of Hygiene and Public Health, Department of Medicine, Division of Infectious Diseases, School of Medicine, The Johns Hopkins University, Baltimore, Maryland 21205

Martin J. Blaser, Division of Infectious Diseases, Vanderbilt University School of Medicine, Nashville, Tennessee 37232

Philip S. Brachman, Emory University School of Public Health, Atlanta, Georgia 30329

Stephen L. Cochi, Division of Immunization, Center for Prevention Services, Centers for Disease Control, Atlanta, Georgia 30333

George W. Comstock, School of Hygiene and Public Health, The Johns Hopkins University, Baltimore, Maryland 21205

Herbert L. DuPont, Program in Infectious Diseases and Clinical Microbiology, The University of Texas Medical School at Houston, Houston, Texas 77225

Alfred S. Evans, Department of Epidemiology and Public Health, Yale University School of Medicine, New Haven, Connecticut 06510

Solly Faine, Department of Microbiology, Monash University, Melbourne, Australia

Harry A. Feldman,† Department of Preventive Medicine, State University of New York, Upstate Medical Center, Syracuse, New York 13210

Paul Fiset, Department of Microbiology and Immunology, University of Maryland School of Medicine, Baltimore, Maryland 21201

Hjordis M. Foy, Department of Epidemiology, School of Public Health and Community Medicine, University of Washington, Seattle, Washington 98195

David W. Fraser, Office of the President, Swarthmore College, Swarthmore, Pennsylvania 19081

†Deceased.

viii Contributors

Sherwood L. Gorbach, Departments of Clinical Microbiology, Epidemiology, Medicine, Pathology, and Community Health, New England Medical Center and Tufts University School of Medicine, Boston, Massachusetts 02111

Barry M. Gray, Department of Pediatrics, University of Alabama School of Medicine, Birmingham, Alabama 35294

Wendell H. Hall, Research Service, Veterans Administration Medical Center, Minneapolis, and Departments of Medicine and Microbiology, University of Minnesota Medical School, Minneapolis, Minnesota 55455

H. Robert Harrison, Division of Sexually Transmitted Diseases, Center for Prevention Services, Centers for Disease Control, Atlanta, Georgia 30333

Craig W. Hedberg, Acute Disease Epidemiology Section, Minnesota Department of Health, Minneapolis, Minnesota 55440

Walter J. Hierholzer, Jr., Yale University School of Medicine, Department of Hospital Epidemiology and Infection Control, Yale–New Haven Hospital, New Haven, Connecticut 06504

Richard B. Hornick, Medical Education Administration, Orlando Regional Medical Center, Orlando, Florida 32806

Robert R. Jacobson, Clinical Branch, Gillis W. Long Hansen's Disease Center, Carville, Louisiana 70721

Gerald T. Keusch, Department of Medicine, Division of Geographic Medicine and Infectious Diseases, New England Medical Center Hospitals, Boston, Massachusetts 02111

Stephen J. Kraus, Clinical Research Branch, Division of Sexually Transmitted Disease, Center for Prevention Services, Centers for Disease Control, Atlanta, Georgia 30333

Joseph G. Lossick, Clinical Research Branch, Division of Sexually Transmitted Disease, Center for Prevention Services, Centers for Disease Control, Atlanta, Georgia 30333

Kristine L. MacDonald, Acute Disease Epidemiology Section, Minnesota Department of Health, Minneapolis, Minnesota 55440

John J. Mathewson, Program in Infectious Diseases and Clinical Microbiology, The University of Texas Medical School at Houston, Houston, Texas 77225

Edward A. Mortimer, Jr., Departments of Epidemiology and Biostatistics and Pediatrics, Case Western Reserve University School of Medicine, Cleveland, Ohio 44106

Carl William Norden, Infectious Diseases Unit, Department of Medicine, Montefiore Hospital, University of Pittsburgh School of Medicine, Pittsburgh, Pennsylvania 15213

Richard J. O'Brien, Clinical Research Branch, Division of Tuberculosis Control, Center for Prevention Services, Centers for Disease Control, Atlanta, Georgia 30333

Walter A. Orenstein, Division of Immunization, Center for Prevention Services, Centers for Disease Control, Atlanta, Georgia 30333

Michael T. Osterholm, Acute Disease Epidemiology Section, Minnesota Department of Health, Minneapolis, Minnesota 55440

Andrew T. Pavia, Department of Medicine, Division of Infectious Diseases, University of Utah Medical Center, Salt Lake City, Utah 84132

Peter L. Perine, Division of Tropical Public Health, Department of Preventive Medicine, F. Edward Hébert School of Medicine, Uniformed Services University of the Health Sciences, Bethesda, Maryland 20814

Arthur L. Reingold, Department of Biomedical and Environmental Health Sciences, University of California, Berkeley, California 94720

Frederick L. Ruben, Infectious Diseases Unit, Department of Medicine, Montefiore Hospital, University of Pittsburgh School of Medicine, Pittsburgh, Pennsylvania 15213

Michael E. St. Louis, Enteric Diseases Branch, Division of Bacterial Diseases, Center for Infectious Diseases, Centers for Disease Control, Atlanta, Georgia 30333

George P. Schmid, Division of STD/HIV Prevention, Center for Prevention Services, Centers for Disease Control, Atlanta, Georgia 30333

Eugene D. Shapiro, Departments of Pediatrics and Epidemiology and Public Health, Yale University School of Medicine, New Haven, Connecticut 06510

Sally Bryna Slome, Department of International Health, School of Hygiene and Public Health, Department of Medicine, Division of Infectious Diseases, School of Medicine, The Johns Hopkins University, Baltimore, Maryland 21205. *Present address:* Kaiser Permanente Medical Center, Oakland, California 94611

David R. Snydman, Departments of Clinical Microbiology, Epidemiology, Medicine, Pathology, and Community Health, New England Medical Center and Tufts University School of Medicine, Boston, Massachusetts 02111

Robert V. Tauxe, Enteric Diseases Branch, Division of Bacterial Diseases, Center for Infectious Diseases, Centers for Disease Control, Atlanta, Georgia 30333

David N. Taylor, Department of Bacterial Diseases, Walter Reed Army Institute of Research, Washington, D.C. 20307

W. D. Tigertt, *American Journal of Tropical Medicine and Hygiene,* Baltimore, Maryland 21201

Joel I. Ward, Harbor–UCLA Medical Center, UCLA School of Medicine, Torrance, California 90509

Steven G. F. Wassilak, Division of Immunization, Center for Prevention Services, Centers for Disease Control, Atlanta, Georgia 30333

Paul F. Wehrle, Department of Pediatrics, University of Southern California and Los Angeles County–University of Southern California Medical Center, Los Angeles, California 90033

Paul J. Wiesner, Training and Laboratory Program Office, Centers for Disease Control, Atlanta, Georgia 30333. *Present address:* Dekalb County Board of Health, Decatur, Georgia 30030

Theodore E. Woodward, Department of Medicine, University of Maryland School of Medicine, Baltimore, Maryland 21201

Jonathan Zenilman, Division of Sexually Transmitted Diseases, Center for Prevention Services, Centers for Disease Control, Atlanta, Georgia 30333. *Present address:* Division of Infectious Diseases, Johns Hopkins Hospital, Baltimore, Maryland 21205

Marcus J. Zervos, William Beaumont Hospital, Division of Infectious Diseases, Royal Oak, Michigan 48072

Preface to the Second Edition

The objectives of this second edition remain the same as stated in the first edition. Dr. Feldman died January 6, 1985, and Dr. Philip S. Brachman has replaced him as coeditor. All chapters in this book have been updated by the authors, and new chapters have been added on listeriosis, Lyme disease, toxic shock syndrome, and yersiniosis. The summaries below review advances in each chapter since the first edition in 1982, as well as review the new chapters.

I. Introduction and Concepts

Chapter 1: Epidemiological concepts, updated and expanded. The sections on methods, immunization, and immunity have been updated and reviewed. A section on etiological agents involved in different clinical syndromes has been added.

Chapter 2: Surveillance. Disease surveillance is increasingly being recognized as a critical element in the control and prevention of disease. The development of computer software packages and personal computers has made it possible for many public health organizations to improve their surveillance programs by analyzing data in a more timely manner using more sophisticated methodology. Internationally, more countries are developing disease surveillance systems and making the data available to other countries and the World Health Organization. International collaborative surveillance has become an important ally in the control and prevention of disease on a global basis.

II. Acute Bacterial Infections

Chapter 3: Anthrax. Generally, anthrax is not a major public health problem. However, epidemics still occur. A major outbreak occurred in Zimbabwe between 1979 and 1985, in which more than 10,000 human cases of primarily cutaneous disease were reported that resulted from human exposure to anthrax-infected animals or their products. Cases continue to occur, suggesting that an endemic focus has been established. Advances have been made in the development of serological tests for anthrax. The ELISA test is more sensitive than the indirect hemagglutination test. More recently, an electrophoretic–immunoblot method has been developed that is more sensitive than the ELISA test.

Chapter 4: Bacterial food poisoning. Over the past five years there have been some remarkable advances in our understanding of bacterial food poisoning. We now recognize a number of new pathogens that are important contributors to the problem of food poisoning. Many of these are discussed in other chapters but are also mentioned here; for example, *Campylobacter fetus* ss. *jejuni* is one of the most common causes of infectious diarrhea and is predominantly transmitted by the foodborne route. We now recognize a new enteropathogenic form of *E. coli* that produces a toxin. This organism is associated with ingestion of poorly cooked beef and is a relatively common cause of infectious diarrhea. In addition, this pathogen has been epidemiologically implicated with the hemolytic uremic syndrome.

Another pathogen that has recently been recognized as a foodborne pathogen is *Listeria monocytogenes*. We now know that it may be associated with milk and ice cream products, and is not readily killed by pasteurization. New diagnostic modalities employing molecular techniques have been developed.

Chapter 5: Botulism. The epidemiology of botulism in the United States has changed rapidly. Large outbreaks of foodborne botulism associated with restaurants have given substance to long-held concerns about epidemic botulism transmitted by commercially distributed foods. Vehicles of recent outbreaks have increasingly included mishandled fresh foods, such as sauteed onions, meat potpies, and potato salad. These differ from traditional vehicles in that they were not canned, bottled, or otherwise preserved. The recent discovery of infant botulism resulting from the multiplication of *Clostridium botulinum* in the intestine, with *in vivo* production of toxin, was followed by the demonstration that enteric infectious botulism can, on rare occasions, cause botulism in adults. Infant botulism, meanwhile, has become the most common form of botulism in the United States. Also, social changes have given rise to a new group of patients with wound botulism, i.e., drug abusers.

Chapter 6: Brucellosis. The history of the discovery of epidemics of abortions in kennel-raised beagle hounds caused by a new species, *Brucella canis,* is briefly reviewed. Reference is made to 16 infections reported in man. A new diagnostic serological test, the ELISA test, appears to be sensitive and specific for brucellosis. Several epidemics of human brucellosis have been reported recently. Some have occurred in common circumstances, as in workers in abattoirs during the killing of large numbers of infected cattle and pigs. Other, more unusual epidemics have occurred among tourists and urban residents ingesting fresh cheese made from unpasteurized milk from goats or sheep. The prevalence of brucellosis in humans continues to be low in the United States. Elsewhere in the world, human brucellosis remains a serious problem, as in Spain, Italy, north Africa, Iran, India, the USSR, China, and South and Central America. Important new observations are reported concerning the ultrastructural events within fetal chorioallantoic cells of the infected placenta of goats inoculated with *Brucella abortus.*

Chapter 7: *Campylobacter* infections. Many new *Campylobacter* species have been epidemiologically associated with diarrheal disease. A new table describes these species. Many of these new species were found as a result of a newly described method of isolation of *Campylobacter*. More is now known about the worldwide distribution of serotypes. The use of two serotyping systems has shown that, although there are hundreds of different serotypes, there are a few predominant serotypes that are similar throughout the world. *Campylobacter pylori* is a new species that has been associated with type B gastritis and duodenal ulcer. Pathogenesis still remains a clouded subject. While toxigenic and invasive strains have been described, there has not yet been a clear association reported with clinical syndromes. An important study in volunteers has shed light on dose, clinical features, and homologous immunity from *Campylobacter* infections. More is now known about *Campylobacter* in the developing world. *Campylobacter* is hyperendemic in many parts of the developing world. In this setting it is immunity rather than strain variation that determines the outcome of infection. Although chickens have been identified as important vehicles, there still appears to be no practical way to rid flocks of this organism. Treatment with erythromycin has been shown to be efficacious for dysenteric *Campylobacter* infections. The quinolines, such as ciprofloxacin, may also prove useful for this form of the disease; however, most infections are mild and do not require antibiotics.

Chapter 8: Chancroid. Although a common sexually transmitted disease in developing countries, chancroid has for many years been an uncommon and geographically localized disease in the United States. Beginning in Orange County, California, in 1981, however, increasingly numerous outbreaks have established chancroid as a significant sexually transmitted disease and, in 1987, 5047 cases were reported in the United States, the largest number since 1949. Adding to the importance of the numerical rise in cases is the recognition that diseases characterized by genital ulcers are associated with an increased risk of HIV transmission.

Chapter 9: Chlamydial infections. The major additions regarding chlamydial infections concern knowledge gained about infection with *Chlamydia pneumoniae* (TWAR strain). It has been learned that this previously unrecognized organism infects more than a third of most populations studied before 40 years of age, and that the manifestations range from asymptomatic infection, upper respiratory disease (including otitis media), to lower respiratory tract disease (including interstitial pneumonia). The discovery of *C. pneumoniae* infections has helped to clarify some unanswered problems of chlamydial epidemiology. The accumulation of chlamydial antibody in early childhood by a proportion of children, without recognized chlamydial infection, can now be attributed to *C. pneumoniae,* when more discriminating antibody tests are performed.

Additional advances in our knowledge include the recognition of a *C. trachomatis* syndrome of mucopurulent cervicitis in women, accompanied by cervical inflammation, ectopy, and friability, and the experimental demonstration of tubal obstruction in a nonhuman model after repeated salpingeal infection. Also, there is clearer substantiation of *C. trachomatis* as a contributor to the sexually acquired reactive arthritis (SARA) syndrome. This has been accomplished by finding evidence of chlamydial antigen (by microimmunofluorescent techniques) in synovium or synovial fluid cells. Another major advance has been in the field of diagnostic testing. Direct fluorescent antibody smear tests and enzyme immunoassay tests for chlamydial antigen have been developed and are commercially available.

Chapter 10: Cholera. A significant recent finding has been the demonstration of a phase in the life history of cholera vibrios during which they survive in water sources but do not grow in usual laboratory culture media. However, when injected into ileal loops, or fed to volunteers, they revert to their customary biological form, i.e., they are culturable and can produce clinical disease. This stage has great significance from a surveillance point of view; in pond and river waters in Bangladesh, viable vibrios could be detected in concentrations up to 1000 organisms per milliliter, yet none could be recovered by standard isolation techniques. An association between susceptibility to cholera and blood type has been demonstrated; clinical cholera, and the more severe cases of cholera, are much more likely to occur among the type O blood group than those with type AB erythrocytes. From the point of view of prevention, a field trial has been carried out in an endemic area in which a killed whole-cell vaccine, especially when it also contained the B-subunit cholera toxoid, was effective in protecting against infection in children and women when given orally in three doses. In treatment, there is increasing use of cereal starches (e.g., from rice, corn, sorghum, millet) in place of glucose in oral rehydration therapy solutions.

Chapter 11: Diphtheria. Perhaps the most interesting development in diphtheria includes the virtual disappearance of the disease in the United States. Reported cases have varied from five in 1983 to one in 1986, averaging fewer than three per year since 1980. Although the incidence is much less, there is no clear evidence that the virulence or clinical characteristics are different from earlier years when the disease was highly endemic in the United States. Another advance worthy of attention is the recognition of the effectiveness of diphtheria toxoid as a protein conjugate to improve the performance of the polysaccharide vaccines used among young infants. The major challenge for preventive medicine remains the maintenance of immunization programs despite the absence of disease.

Chapter 12: *Escherichia coli* diarrhea. During recent years, enterohemorrhagic *E. coli* was recognized as an important enteropathogen and its pathogenic mechanism began to be elucidated. The development of DNA probe technology to detect diarrheagenic *E. coli* strains will facilitate large-scale field studies and, in turn, better understanding of the prevalence and epidemiology of these organisms. Also, great strides have been made in understanding how the first recognized group of diarrheagenic *E. coli,* enteropathogenic *E. coli,* cause disease.

Chapter 13: Gonococcal infections. Epidemiologically, the incidence of gonorrhea has decreased in the past 10 years, especially among homosexual men, probably due to a behavioral response to the HIV threat. There has been a further definition of the "core groups" for transmission of gonorrhea. Inner-city residents and "crack" cocaine abusers are at highest risk. Pathogenetically, there has been an explosion of recent advances in our knowledge of the genetics of *Neisseria gonorrhoeae*. In particular, the concept of antigenic phase variation has particular implications for the development of an effective vaccine. Probably the most important development since 1982 has been that of antimicrobial resistance. Penicillinase-producing *N. gonorrhoeae* (PPNG) morbidity has increased geometrically, and new forms of antimicrobial resistance have emerged. They include plasmid-mediated tetracycline resistance (TRNG), high-level spectinomycin resistance, and chromosomally mediated resistance to penicillin. The key points of the most recent CDC guidelines on the treatment of gonococcal infections are included.

Chapter 14: *Haemophilus influenzae* type b. There have been many new developments during the past five years. Epidemiological studies have led to a better definition of risk factors for acquisition of invasive Hib disease. The risk of secondary transmission among contacts in household and day-care centers has been elucidated, and has led to recommendations for the use of rifampin prophylaxis to prevent such transmission. We have learned about the T-cell-independent nature of the immune response to Hib capsular polysaccharide (PRP). Methods have been developed to overcome the relatively poor immunogenicity of plain PRP by covalently linking or conjugating a protein carrier antigen to PRP to make a PRP–protein conjugate vaccine. Within the last four years, the first licensed vaccines (first, PRP vaccine, followed by two PRP–protein conjugate vaccines) have become available for use in children 18 months of age or older for the prevention of Hib disease. Compelling evidence for the protective efficacy of anticapsular antibody has come from efficacy studies conducted in Finland with PRP vaccine and a PRP–protein conjugate vaccine. The latter vaccine is one of a group of new second-generation Hib vaccines that have been developed with the ultimate goal of providing an effective vaccine for infants and younger children.

Chapter 15: Legionellosis. The range and taxonomic location of *Legionella* have been expanded with the addition of the 17th species and description of its relationship to the purple sulfur bacteria. The utility of ELISA and radioimmunoassay diagnosis of legionellosis is described. Our knowledge of the role of water as a source of legionellosis has been greatly expanded. Emphasis is placed on the hot water side of potable water systems in hospitals and other institutions, as well as the occasional role of whirlpool baths, grinding fluid, nebulizers, and humidifiers. The role of cell-mediated immunity in legionellosis has been further defined with evidence that activated mononuclear phagocytes inhibit intracellular multiplication of *L. pneumophila*. The section on control and prevention has been updated to reflect the importance of interrupting transmission of *Legionella* from a watery environment to humans. Shutting off machinery that generates aerosols or treating the water with either heat or disinfectant has proved successful in a series of outbreaks.

Chapter 16: Leprosy. There have been major developments in leprosy research that may lead to improvement in control and prevention. Trials have been initiated utilizing a specific vaccine. The cloning and expression of the entire *Mycobacterium leprae* genome in *E. coli* has been accomplished. A successful, widespread implementation of short-term therapy for leprosy has been initiated. An important serological test has been developed for the disease. Considerable progress has been made in defining its immunopathology and genetic factors.

Chapter 17: Leptospirosis. New developments include the characterization of the lipopolysaccharides (LPS) and their role as a protective antigen, the presence of a leptospiral toxin, and bacterial restriction endonuclear DNA typing (BRENDA). A new classification has been proposed based on DNA similarities between species. Serovar-specific and species-specific antigens have been described. New technology for investigation of leptospiral disease has been developed, including monoclonal antibodies, immunoassays, and gene probe techniques. An oral vaccine is being tested in animals. Epidemiologically, serovar *hardjo* has emerged as a worldwide major pathogen; and infections are being increasingly associated with leisure water sports.

Chapter 18: *Listeria monocytogenes* infections. *Listeria monocytogenes* is now recognized as the only human pathogen among a number of species of the genus *Listeria*. The organism is ubiquitous, being found in soil, silage, sewage, and most animals tested. Recently, foodborne outbreaks have been more regularly recognized. There appear to be geographic variations and an increase in incidence in certain parts of the world, but this could reflect keen interest and better reporting.

Chapter 19: Lyme disease. Lyme disease is a tickborne multisystem illness caused by the spirochete *Borrelia burgdorferi*. The disease was first described in 1975 following identification of a cluster of cases in children living in Old Lyme, Connecticut who were diagnosed with juvenile rheumatoid arthritis. The causative organism was not clearly demonstrated until 1983. While fatal cases of Lyme disease are extremely rare, infection with *B. burgdorferi* can be associated with severe systemic manifestations, including arthritis, neurological illness (meningitis, encephalopathy, and radiculoneuritis), and cardiac involvement (endocarditis, endomyocarditis, and pericarditis). Infection with this pathogen can lead to substantial morbidity, particularly if not appropriately diagnosed and treated. Currently, Lyme disease is the most commonly reported tickborne illness in the United States, with over 1000 cases reported annually. Cases of Lyme disease have been reported from more than 30 states in the United States and from at least 21 countries on four continents including Europe, Asia, and Australia. The incidence of Lyme disease appears to be increasing in the United States and elsewhere. However, it is not clear whether the increase in case reports represent a true increase in incidence over time or improved awareness and diagnosis of the condition.

Chapter 20: Meningococcal infections. The epidemic behavior of this organism remains as previously discussed, but serogroups Y and W-135 have emerged as important pathogens and are responsible for a significant proportion of the varied manifestations of invasive meningococcal infections. A new meningococcal vaccine combining the polysaccharide antigens of groups A, C, Y, and W-135 has been shown to be safe and effective, and is now generally the vaccine of choice. Despite considerable investigatory effort, an effective group B meningococcal vaccine has not been marketed. Our understanding of the pathogenesis of meningococcal disease has improved with the discovery of serum complement deficiencies in many sporadic cases, and the detection of blocking antibodies in the sera of affected patients during outbreaks.

Chapter 21: *Mycoplasma pneumoniae*. This organism has now been recovered from many sites outside the respiratory tract including synovial fluid in hypogammaglobulinemic patients with joint symptoms, from blood, and from cerebrospinal fluid in patients with neurological complications. The number of case reports of deaths seems to be increasing. This would not be remarkable except for the fact that few hospitals have the laboratory facilities to diagnose the disease, especially by growing the organism. Thus, the mortality rate may have been underestimated. Most reported deaths are in adults or the elderly. A rapid diagnostic test for the practitioner is not available but a DNA probe is under development. There are numerous serological tests, but since these are not measured against isolation of the organism as the gold standard, it is difficult to tell which one is the best. Specificity is also a concern. Suffice it to say that at present serological tests have severe limitations, particularly when used to diagnose disease of unknown etiology.

Chapter 22: Nosocomial bacterial infections. The final report of the SENIC project has appeared and indicated the potential for a one-third reduction of nosocomial infections with the application of a comprehensive surveillance and control program by trained professionals in acute-care hospitals. Changes in health care financing have modified the case mix and severity of patients in both acute and extended care facilities, while at the same time moving many interventions into the unknown risk area of ambulatory care. As a consequence of infections with HIV and the occurrence of AIDS, there has been an increase in the number of bacterial infections and disease in immunocompromised young adults constituting a new epidemic.

Chapter 23: Pertussis. Evidence recently accumulated increasingly points to young adults and teenagers with waning immunity as a major reservoir for pertussis. The biology of the organism in relation to pathogenesis and immunity is much better understood, though as yet incompletely defined.

Japanese acellular pertussis vaccines appear to be effective in controlling pertussis, at least in older children. However, their efficacy in persons less than 2 years of age is not yet established. In the United States and elsewhere, several candidate acellular vaccines are in various stages of development and evaluation.

Chapter 24: Plague. The number of human plague cases reported annually has continued to decline. The zoonosis persists in well-known foci in the Americas, Africa, and Asia. Pneumonic plague resulting from exposure to a pet cat has been recorded, and the value of early therapy has again been demonstrated. Drug resistance of importance at the clinical level has not been reported. The usefulness of the ELISA test in the recognition of plague antigen in human infections has been demonstrated.

Chapter 25: Pneumococcal infections. The epidemiological behavior of the pneumococcus has not changed materially but there have been significant alterations in our approach to treatment and control. Clusters of cases due to penicillin-resistant pneumococci began to be reported in 1977 from South Africa. Since then, this problem has increased throughout the world and has resulted in intensive surveillance and testing of clinical isolates. Study of resistant strains has improved our understanding of the mode of action of penicillin on the pneumococcus. A 14-serotype pneumococcal vaccine was licensed in 1977 but was not enthusiastically adopted for routine administration for targeted populations, partially due to the inconclusive results of field studies in the United States. Newer studies suggesting reasonable efficacy, the introduction of a 23-serotype vaccine, and the endorsement of several advisory groups should result in a boost in its utilization.

Chapter 26: Q fever. In diagnosis, it has been found that a high Phase I antibody titer rarely develops during the acute disease, and is considered indicative of chronic Q fever, hepatitis, or endocarditis; high Phase I IgA levels are especially indicative of Q fever endocarditis. There still seems to be only one serotype of *Coxiella burnetii*. However, it seems that the LPS of strains isolated from cases of endocarditis is different from that isolated from cases of acute Q fever or from cases of hepatitis. While there is no commercially available vaccine, the Rocky Mountain Laboratory has developed an effective Phase I vaccine, now in use for over 25 years in their laboratory workers with excellent results, provided side reactions are avoided by giving it only to persons who are skin test negative to *Coxiella* antigen. [Recently a Phase I vaccine has been licensed in Australia after extensive field trials in the major abattoirs (B. P. Marmion, personal communication).] The vaccine would also be useful in other laboratory workers who have a high risk of infection, as well as slaughterhouse and dairy workers. The unsolved problems remain as to why persons exposed to large doses of the agent often develop inapparent or subclinical infections, whereas a severe experimental disease can be produced with just one to ten organisms; similarly, the massive recrudescence of infection that occurs during gestation is, inexplicably, without pathological changes or long-term effects on the human infant.

Chapter 27: Rocky Mountain spotted fever. During the past several years there has been a diminution in the number of spotted fever cases in the United States. From a high of 1100–1200 reported cases annually from 1976 to 1983, there was an average of 650 cases annually for the years 1985 and 1988. The cause for this difference is unknown but it suggests possibly a cyclic change of the host–parasite relationship in nature.

RMSF has recently been reported for the first time from the Bronx, New York, and has also been reported from other new geographic areas.

Chapter 28: Salmonellosis: nontyphoidal. An increasing problem of antimicrobial resistance to one antibiotic, chloramphenicol, has been unequivocally linked epidemiologically to the use of this antibiotic in animal foods. Multiply resistant salmonellosis has appeared as an infectious complication of antibiotic therapy of other conditions, which creates a selective environment for these organisms to proliferate in the patient's gastrointestinal tract. Large outbreaks, such as a 1985 outbreak of *S. typhimurium* infections that affected more than 150,000 persons in the Midwest, and a 1984 outbreak of *S. enteritidis* infections spread by supersonic commercial aircraft, show the potential for affecting many people in widespread areas simultaneously when a breakdown in modern food processing occurs. A new mechanism for detecting a vehicle of infection has been demonstrated. In the mid-1980s, *S. enteritidis* appeared in epidemic form in the northeastern United States, and in other countries as well. This epidemic was associated with grade A hen eggs that were infected *in utero*. The most successful measures for controlling salmonellosis have been those limiting spread from animal reservoirs, such as the pasteurization of milk, increasing the cooking temperature of roast beef, and prohibiting the sale of pet turtles. The challenge for the future will be to find other similarly effective control measures for this pleuripotent infectious agent.

Chapter 29: Shigellosis. New data are largely in the studies of virulence and pathogenesis. It is now clear that invasion is a very complex process, controlled by multiple genes present on both chromosomal and plasmid DNA. The many steps from invasion to intracellular multiplication and cell-to-cell spread of *Shigella* involve induced endocytosis in the intestinal epithelial cell, and consequently necessitate reorganization of cytoskeletal, actin, and myosin elements brought about by the presence of the organism and specific gene products. The mechanism by which this happens is not at all clear. Second, the biochemistry of toxins produced by *Shigella* species has been greatly advanced by the discovery of the mechanism of action of Shiga toxin and the identification of the mammalian cell surface toxin receptor as a particular cellular glycolipid. The presence of this receptor on villus but not crypt cells may explain why toxin induces a net secretion in animal models, which may represent the mechanism for the watery diarrhea observed in human infection. Finally, new information is also provided concerning vaccine strategies and the initial evaluation of prototype vaccine strains.

Chapter 30: Staphylococcal infections. Since 1982, many developments have occurred in this field. Toxic shock syndrome is better appreciated, including the link with tampons that are highly absorbent, and its occurrence with wounds, after surgery, and, more recently, after influenza outbreaks. Methicillin-resistant *S. aureus* have become more widespread in the United States, in virtually every state, city, hospital, and nursing home. Finally, *S. epidermidis* has now become recognized as a very formidable pathogen in certain settings, particularly in compromised hosts, whose numbers are every day increasing. The field is becoming ever more complex and the staphylococcus more difficult to control.

Chapter 31: Streptococcal infections. This chapter has been broadened to include all of the major pathogens in this large group of organisms. The group A streptococcus remains the main focus, especially in view of the recent resurgence of acute rheumatic fever throughout the United States. The group B streptococci continue to be among the most important causes of acute perinatal infections. Dental and enteric streptococci, and the enterococci, are now being recognized as major health problems and causes of opportunistic infections. Our knowledge of all these organisms has greatly expanded over the past decade.

Chapter 32: Syphilis. The major recent advances in syphilis include the following: (1) increased recognition that serological screening for syphilis is more effective if targeted to populations at highest risk for infection rather than broadly applied to the general population; (2) elimination of the erythromycin treatment regimen for the treatment of prenatal syphilis; (3) recognition that the prevention of congenital syphilis requires not only prenatal screening for syphilis in endemic areas, but also community efforts to get women at risk for syphilis enrolled in perinatal care early in gestation; (4) marked decrease in syphilis morbidity in homosexual males coincident with the increasing of safe sex practices in this population; (5) recognition that syphilis treatment regimens may need to be intensified in the presence of occult immunodeficiency associated with HIV infection.

Chapter 33: Nonvenereal treponematoses. The Third International Symposium on yaws and other endemic treponematoses was held in Washington, D.C., in April 1984, and was followed by regional meetings in Indonesia in 1985 and in the Congo and Jordan in 1986. New control efforts were recommended for those areas of the world where active foci of disease persist, especially in west Africa, using selective mass penicillin treatment campaigns. Such campaigns have begun in Ghana and several other west African nations, but endemic syphilis is spreading rapidly among the seminomadic peoples of Mali, Niger, and Upper Volta, where the control programs are just being implemented.

Unfortunately, the socioeconomic conditions that facilitate transmission of the endemic treponematoses are increasing in much of Africa, and at a time when more threatening disease problems (malaria, AIDS) have a higher priority. The cutaneous manifestations of yaws appear to be much milder in some populations in South America, Oceania, and Indonesia, which may make the correct diagnosis and treatment difficult. There is no evidence, however, that the pathogenic treponemes are becoming resistant to penicillin.

Chapter 34: Tetanus. The major changes relate to an increased focus on prevention. New sections have been incorporated on wound management and a new schedule recommended by the Expanded Programme on Immunization (EPI) of the World Health Organization to prevent perinatal and neonatal tetanus has been added. The routine schedules for tetanus immunization in the United States, as well as the EPI schedule, which applies primarily to the developing world, are included. New data on tetanus cases in the United States show that almost all cases could have been prevented through routine immunization and appropriate wound management. When one discusses the benefits of immunization, it is important to review the risks. Adverse events following tetanus toxoid administration are now reviewed in a separate section. In addition, the chapter includes updates on the epidemiology of tetanus and neonatal tetanus in the United States, as well as the most recent estimates of worldwide deaths from neonatal tetanus. There is a comprehensive discussion of new data regarding routes for acquiring tetanus in the United States. Finally, the chapter contains increased information on serological tests for tetanus immunity, including the importance of IgG antibodies, a more detailed in-depth discussion of the clinical features of tetanus in children and adults, and details concerning the growing consensus that tetanus toxin is transported to the central nervous system through peripheral nerves.

Chapter 35: Toxic shock syndrome. Since the early studies of toxic shock syndrome (TSS) in 1980 and 1981, major advances in our understanding of the disease have resulted from *in vitro* and *in vivo* laboratory studies of the toxin(s) involved in TSS, the factors that affect toxin production, and the pathophysiological mechanisms that underlie the observed clinical features of the illness. At the same time, further epidemiological studies have verified and elaborated on the findings of earlier studies establishing a link between TSS, menstruation, and tampon use. Similarly, ongoing observation of the clinical settings in which TSS occurs continues to demonstrate that *Staphylococcus aureus* infections at any site can cause TSS in susceptible individuals of both sexes, all ages, and all racial groups.

Chapter 36: Tuberculosis. Of special note is the potential for improved diagnosis by new bacteriological and serological tests, the impact on tuberculosis rates by immigration from high-prevalence areas, and the propensity of HIV infections to reactivate latent infections with *Mycobacterium tuberculosis*.

Chapter 37: Nontuberculous mycobacterial disease. Diseases due to nontuberculous bacteria have assumed greater importance with the occurrence of disseminated *Mycobacterium avium* complex among persons with HIV infection and the apparent increase in nosocomial disease due to rapid-growing mycobacteria. Recent studies of the ecology of *M. avium* suggest that infected aerosols from natural sources play a major role in transmission to man. While new diagnostic techniques have facilitated isolation and speciation of organisms in culture, differentiating between disease and colonization, especially of patients with respiratory isolates, remains problematic. Unfortunately, treatment of these diseases is often difficult and no possibility for prophylaxis exists.

Chapter 38: Tularemia. The incidence increased in the early 1980s, dipped in the mid-1980s, and is again increasing in the late 1980s. The reason for the overall increase in the 1980s as compared to the previous decade is not clear. It may reflect an increase in contact between susceptible individuals and the environment as people increase their use of the country's natural, recreational facilities. There have been several improvements in laboratory diagnostic techniques that have increased the sensitivity of confirming the diagnosis of tularemia, which may also have influenced the increase in reported cases.

Chapter 39: Typhoid fever. Recent laboratory work has shown that the ELISA test is more specific and sensitive than the agglutination test. The biological characteristics of the organism have been further clarified especially concerning the role of Vi-containing strains.

Recent surveillance data reveal some interesting findings concerning typhoid fever in the United States. Travel-related cases are increasing and students represent the single most important group among travelers in regard to developing typhoid fever. Travel within the Western Hemisphere (and outside of the United States) is associated with more cases of typhoid fever than is travel to any other region of the world. Morbidity is higher for domestically acquired cases than for cases associated with foreign travel. Twenty-five percent of all cases of typhoid fever reported in the United States are associated with outbreaks.

The third-generation cephalosporin antibiotics have been shown to be highly effective in treating clinical typhoid fever. Several new vaccines are being field-tested. A highly purified Vi antigen vaccine has been shown to induce protection in 75% of young children.

Chapter 40: *Yersinia enterocolitica* infections. This is a new chapter on an important cause of diarrhea, especially in children. Yersiniosis occurs throughout the world; the highest prevalence rates have been reported from Scandinavian and European countries. There does not seem to be a discernible seasonal pattern though some studies suggest it is more common in the summer months. It causes both enterocolitis and "pseudoappendicitis." The highest incidence of yersiniosis is in children 1 to 4 years of age. In one study, the incidence in children 1 to 2 years of age was 2/1000. The incidence of yersiniosis infection in patients with acute endemic enterocolitis has been reported to range from 0 to 5%. Additionally, *Y. enterocolitica* has been isolated from up to 9% of patients with the appendicitis-like syndrome.

Diagnosis can be made using special laboratory media. Further identification of organisms by serotyping and biotyping is important in epidemiological studies. It has been shown that serotypes vary depending on the geographic origin of the individual organisms.

The organism is primarily spread through contaminated food, water, and from domestic animals. Foodborne outbreaks have been reported due to milk, tofu, and bean sprouts. In the latter two outbreaks, the foods were contaminated by use of contaminated water in preparing these foods. Person-to-person spread of disease has been reported, especially in hospitals.

Summary of Contents

Contents

II. Acute Bacterial Infections

Chapter 3

Anthrax
Philip S. Brachman

Chapter 4

Bacterial Food Poisoning
(Bacillus cereus, Clostridium perfringens, Vibrio parahemolyticus, Staphylococcus aureus, Yersinia enterocolitica)
David R. Snydman and Sherwood L. Gorbach

Chapter 5

Botulism
Michael E. St. Louis

Chapter 6   **Brucellosis**

Wendell H. Hall

Chapter 7   *Campylobacter* **Infections**

David N. Taylor and Martin J. Blaser

Chapter 14

Haemophilus influenzae Type b

Stephen L. Cochi and Joel I. Ward

Chapter 15

Legionellosis

David W. Fraser

Chapter 16

Leprosy

Robert R. Jacobson

Chapter 17

Leptospirosis

Solly Faine

Chapter 18

Listeria monocytogenes Infections

Donald Armstrong

Chapter 19

Lyme Disease

Michael T. Osterholm, Kristine L. MacDonald, and Craig W. Hedberg

Chapter 20

Meningococcal Infections

Robert S. Baltimore and Harry A. Feldman

Chapter 21

Mycoplasma pneumoniae

Hjordis M. Foy

Chapter 25

Pneumococcal Infections
Robert S. Baltimore and Eugene D. Shapiro

Chapter 26

Q Fever
Paul Fiset and Theodore E. Woodward

Chapter 27

Rocky Mountain Spotted Fever
Theodore E. Woodward

Chapter 28

Salmonellosis: Nontyphoidal

Andrew T. Pavia and Robert V. Tauxe

Chapter 29

Shigellosis

Gerald T. Keusch and Michael L. Bennish

Chapter 30

Staphylococcal Infections

Frederick L. Ruben and Carl William Norden

Chapter 31

Streptococcal Infections

Barry M. Gray

Chapter 32

Syphilis

Joseph G. Lossick and Stephen J. Kraus

Bacterial Infections of Humans

Epidemiology and Control

PART I

Introduction and Concepts

CHAPTER 1

Epidemiological Concepts

Alfred S. Evans

1. Introduction

Epidemiology is the study of the determinants and distribution of health and disease in populations.[115] It is a quantitative science concerned with the circumstances under which disease processes occur, the factors that affect their incidence and spread, and the use of this knowledge for prevention and control.[65] It includes the pathogenesis of disease in both the community and the individual. For infectious diseases, one must study the circumstances under which both *infection* and *disease* occur, for these may be different. Infection is the consequence of an encounter of a potentially pathogenic microorganism with a susceptible human host through an appropriate portal of entry. Exposure is the key factor, and the sources of infection lie mostly outside the individual human host, within the environment, or in other infected hosts. Disease represents one of the possible consequences of infection, and the factors important in its development are mostly intrinsic to the host, although the dosage and virulence of the infecting microbe play a role. These intrinsic factors include the age at the time of infection, the portal of entry, the presence or absence of immunity, the vigor of the primary defense system, the efficiency and nature of humoral and cell-mediated immune responses, the genetic makeup of the host, the state of nutrition, the pres-

ence of other diseases, and probably psychosocial influences. In addition to the classic clinical features of disease, host responses include mild or atypical forms, subclinical and inapparent infections, and the carrier state, which may exist in the absence of a detectable host response. While the clinician is primarily concerned with disease, the epidemiologist is interested in both infection and disease. Infection without disease is a common phenomenon, so that a study limited to clinical illness alone would give an incomplete epidemiological picture and would be a poor basis for control and prevention.[68] A full understanding involves the pathogenesis of the process leading to clinical disease both in the community and in the individual.

The concepts of epidemiology in bacterial infections are very similar to those of viral infections as expounded in the companion volume, *Viral Infections of Humans*,[67] so there will be overlap and repetition in this volume. Some of the differences between viral and bacterial infection include the intracellular position of all viruses, the requirement for living tissues for viral multiplication, the ease with which many viruses are spread by respiratory routes or by insect vectors, the relatively high order of immunity following viral infection, the usefulness of serological tests for the diagnosis of most viral infections, and the failure of viral infections to respond to antibiotic therapy. Departments of clinical medicine are becoming more interested in viruses as immunosuppression activates viruses in all age groups, as antiviral therapy emerges, and as clinical immunology units become involved in cell-mediated immunity to viruses. On the other hand, studies of bacterial plasmids and other ge-

Alfred S. Evans · Department of Epidemiology and Public Health, Yale University School of Medicine, New Haven, Connecticut 06510.

netic markers of bacteria give new tools to the epidemiologist, and the development of bacterial polysaccharide vaccines requires evaluation in different populations. Advances in molecular biology and in the development of monoclonal antibodies are resulting in a better understanding of the infectious agent and the host's immune response to it, as well as to improved methods of rapid and specific diagnosis, and to the preparation of better vaccines.

Many concepts and methods of epidemiology apply to both infectious and noninfectious diseases, and there should be no essential dichotomy between the two.[4] In general, epidemiology can be regarded as the development, pathogenesis, and expression of infection and disease in a community in much the same way as clinical medicine is concerned with the development, pathogenesis, and expression in the individual. This book will attempt to cover both these aspects. While the "epidemiology of infectious diseases" has disappeared from the curriculum of many schools of medicine and public health in developed countries, the current epidemic of the immunodeficiency disease AIDS has reawakened interest in the subject. In addition, the emergence of new diseases such as Legionnaires' disease, Lyme disease, and the toxic shock syndrome continues to pose challenges to epidemiologists. In developing countries, infectious diseases are still a major cause of morbidity and mortality, and efforts are in progress to develop training programs in epidemiology and in surveillance in such areas. The global epidemiological program of the Centers for Disease Control is a fine example of this effort. Some of the emerging problems in the epidemiology of infectious diseases have recently been reviewed.[69]

2. Definitions and Methods

2.1. Definitions

A working understanding of the terms commonly used in epidemiology and infectious diseases may be helpful to the student, microbiologist, and clinician unfamiliar with them. They are derived from those in *Viral Infections of Humans*[69] and from the APHA handbook entitled *Control of Communicable Disease in Man*.[8] The book *A Dictionary of Epidemiology*[109] provides a full complement of definitions of the terms used in epidemiology. For convenience, most rates are expressed as the number per 100,000 persons at risk.

Attack rate or case ratio: This ratio expresses incidence rates in population groups during specified time periods or under special circumstances such as in an outbreak or epidemic. It is often expressed as a percent (cases per 100). The *secondary attack rate* is the proportion of persons who develop infection within an appropriate incubation period after exposure to a primary case divided by the number exposed. The groups so exposed are frequently family members or located in an institution.

Carrier: A carrier is a person, animal, or arthropod who harbors a specific infectious agent in the absence of clinical illness with or without a detectable immune response. The carrier state may reflect carriage of the organism in the incubation period before clinical symptoms appear, during an apparent or inapparent infection (healthy or asymptomatic carrier), or following recovery from illness; it may be of short or long duration (chronic carrier), and it may be intermittent or continuous. Carriers may spread the infectious agent to others.

Case-fatality rate: Number of deaths of a specific disease divided by the number of cases × 100.

Cell-mediated immunity (CMI): This term has been used previously to designate immune mechanisms largely dependent on lymphocyte activity and in contrast to "humoral immunity." As T lymphocytes are now recognized as playing an important role in both, the term *T-cell immunity* is being more widely used.

Chemoprophylaxis: Administration of a chemical or antibiotic for the prevention of infection or to prevent the development of disease in a person already infected.

Colonization: Multiplication of an organism on a body surface (e.g., skin, epithelium) without evoking a tissue or immune response.

Communicable period: Time during which a person (or animal) is infectious for another person, animal, or arthropod.

Endemic: This term denotes the constant or usual presence of an infection or disease in a community. A high degree of endemicity is termed *hyperendemic,* and one with a particularly high level of infection beginning early in life and affecting most of the population is called *holoendemic.*

Epidemic: An epidemic or outbreak is said to exist when an unusual number of cases of a disease occur in a given time period and geographic area as compared with the previous experience with that disease in that area. For diseases already present in the community, it is necessary to know the number of existing cases (prevalence) as well as new cases (incidence) to determine whether an increase has occurred. The definition of increases or excess cases is arbitrary and will vary from disease to disease. See Section 3 for further discussion.

Host: A person, animal (including birds), or arthropod on which infectious agents subsist or infect under natural conditions. In this book the term will most often refer to the "human host" unless otherwise stated.

Immunity: The specific resistance to an infectious agent resulting from humoral and local antibodies and from cell-mediated responses constitutes immunity. Immunity may be acquired through natural infection, by active immunization with the agent, by transfer of immune factors via the placenta, or by passive immunization with antibodies from another person or animal. The immune state is relative and not absolute, is governed largely through genetic control, and may be altered by disease- or drug-induced immunosuppression.

Immunodeficiency: A state representing impairment of the immune system of the host that affects its ability to respond to a foreign antigen. This may result from an inherited defect, or an acquired one such as a result of the disease itself, or of immunosuppressive drugs or of an infectious agent that depresses the immune system. The human immunodeficiency viruses (HIV 1 and HIV 2) are the major examples of the latter.

Incidence rate: A ratio of the number of *new* events (specific infection or disease) occurring in a given time period in a given population as the numerator and the number of persons in that population in which the event occurred as the denominator. This is usually stated as cases (or infections) per 1000 or 100,000. This rate may be adjusted for an age- or sex-specific numerator and denominator or any other characteristic of interest. In incidence data, the denominator is often given as the number of susceptibles in the group. Laboratory procedures will be required for numerator data on new *infections,* as measured by isolation of the agent or by antibody rises, or by both. They may also be required to identify those actually at risk in the denominator, i.e., those lacking antibody; other means of refining the denominator would be by eliminating adults in calculating rates of childhood diseases or eliminating those with a valid history of a characteristic disease, such as measles.

Incubation period: The incubation period is the interval between exposure and the appearance of the first detectable sign or symptom of the illness. Ill-defined exposure to a source of infection or exposure to persons without apparent illness may obscure the starting point of the incubation period, and vague, premonitory, or prodromal signs of illness may obscure its termination point. The best estimate is often derived from single exposures of short duration to a clinical case or established source of infection (e.g., air, food, water, arthropod vector) and the development of the first characteristic or classic features of the disease. Experimental infections in volunteers give well-defined incubation periods, but these may not always be the same as under natural conditions. See Section 7 for further discussion.

Index case: This is the index or primary case of an illness in a family, institution, or community that may serve as a source of infection to others.

Infection: Infection represents the deposition, colonization, and multiplication of a microorganism in a host (man, animal, arthropod) and is usually accompanied by an immune response. Infection may occur with or without clinical illness.

Isolation: This is a term applied to the separation of *infected* persons or animals in such places and/or under such conditions as to prevent the direct or indirect spread of the infectious agent to others during the period of communicability. Infection control practice in hospitals has divided isolation into seven categories of which two features are common to all: (1) hand washing after contact with an infected patient or contaminated article and (2) appropriate discarding of contaminated articles (see Section 14.2). However, this is now being replaced by *universal precautions,* which deals with all persons exposed to blood or body fluids (see Section 14.2). *Protective* or *reverse isolation* indicates the biologic protection of a patient with a burn, or cancer, or the immunosuppressed patient against infection from others.

Morbidity rate: An incidence rate in which the numerator includes all persons clinically ill in a defined time and population and the denominator is the population involved or a subunit thereof.

Mortality rate: The same as morbidity rate except the numerator consists of deaths. This may be the total number of deaths in a population group (crude mortality rate) or deaths from a specific disease (disease-specific mortality).

Nosocomial infections: This term refers to infections that develop after entry into a hospital or medical institution and that are not present or incubating at the time of admission or the residual of an infection acquired during a previous admission.

Pathogenicity: The ability of an infectious agent to produce disease in a susceptible host. Some nonpathogenic agents can become pathogenic in an immunocompromised host such as persons infected with HIV.

Prevalence rate: The ratio of the number of persons in a defined population who are affected with the disease at any one time as the numerator and the population at that point as the denominator. If this is based on the frequency of cases at a moment in time, then the term *point prevalence* is used. If it reflects the proportion of persons affected over a longer period, then the term *period prevalence* is employed. Most infectious diseases are acute and short-lived, so that prevalence rates are not commonly used. The use of prevalence rates is more relevant to more protracted illnesses such as subacute bacterial endocarditis, tuberculosis, and leprosy, or to reflect carrier states that may persist for months or years. Prevalence rates reflect incidence times duration of disease. In seroepidemiological usage, the term *prevalence* denotes the presence of antibody, antigen, or other component in the blood.

Quarantine: The restriction of persons or animals exposed to an infected source during the incubation period for that disease to observe if the disease develops in order that other persons will not be exposed during that period.

Reservoir: A person, animal, soil, or other environment in which an infectious agent normally exists and multiplies and which can be a source of infection to other hosts.

Surveillance: For medical uses, surveillance is the systematic collection of data pertaining to the occurrences of specific diseases, the analysis and interpretation of these data, and the dissemination of consolidated and processed information to contributors to the program and other interested persons (see Chapter 2 for detailed discussion). *Serological surveillance* is the identification of current and past infection through measurement of antibody or of antigen in serum from representative samples of the population or other target groups.

Susceptibility: A state in which a person or animal is capable of being infected with a microorganism. The lack of specific protective antibody usually indicates susceptibility to that agent although reactivation or reinfection to some agents may occur in the presence of antibody.

Transmission: Any mechanism by which an infectious agent is spread to another host, including both direct and indirect transmission (see Section 5).

Virulence: A measure of the degree of pathogenicity of an infectious agent as reflected by the severity of the disease produced and/or its ability to invade the tissues of the host.

Zoonosis: An infection or infectious disease transmissible under natural conditions from animals to man. It may be endemic (enzootic) or epidemic (epizootic).

2.2. Methods

Epidemiology can be divided into descriptive, analytical, experimental, and serological epidemiology. The major analytic methods in use are the prospective (cohort) and retrospective (case–control). This section will briefly present these concepts. For more detailed descriptions, textbooks and recent articles of epidemiology are recommended.[103,111–112,115] A textbook on epidemiological methods, such as one recently published that includes examples in infectious disease,[103] is recommended before undertaking an epidemiological study.

2.2.1. Types of Epidemiological Studies. Epidemiological studies may be *descriptive* or *analytical*. Descriptive studies are usually based on available data sources and describe the patterns of disease in population groups according to various demographic features such as age, gender, geographic area, socioeconomic status, occupation, marital status, time of occurrence, and so forth. Such information often suggests clues to the etiology of the condition or to the risk factors involved. Analytical studies are then designed to test the various hypotheses of causation and usually require new data to do so.

Three common analytical methods are employed in pursuing epidemiological studies:

a. Cohort Study. This is the most definitive and expensive type of study and is based on identifying a group or groups of persons (cohorts) who are followed over time for the development of disease (or infection) in the presence or absence of suspected risk factors that are measured at the start of the study. These studies are usually carried out by identifying a cohort at the present time and then following the cohort or cohorts longitudinally over time. This is usually called a *prospective cohort study* or simply a prospective study. In infectious disease epidemiology, it may be possible to identify the persons in the cohort who are susceptible or immune at the start of the study by measuring the presence or absence of antibody in the initial serum specimens. Serial serum samples are then taken in which the appearance of antibody indicates the approximate time at which infection occurs. The occurrence of clinical disease at the same time provides information of the clinical/ subclinical ratio. If the appropriate serum samples are taken and frozen, the actual testing can be delayed to the end of the study.

An alternative method of conducting a cohort study is to identify a group of persons at some time *in the past* who were presumably free of the disease under investigation at that time, as indicated by examining existing records. The cohort is then followed to the present, or even beyond, by measuring the occurrence of infection (by serological tests) or disease in that defined population. This approach is called a *historical cohort study* or a *retrospective cohort study.* Because the case–control study is also retrospective in terms of the time when the observations are made, it must be distinguished from the historical cohort study.

In epidemic investigations, the epidemiological study usually begins after the outbreak is well under way, so that the exposed and unexposed cohort must be identified retrospectively and followed forward from that time. Such was the case in the outbreak of Legionnaire's disease that occurred in Philadelphia in 1976[80] (see Chapter 15). At the time the investigation started, the involved population had already left the hotel for their homes, but the potentially exposed cohort could be identified and followed. Once the ill were identified, it was then possible also to carry out a case–control study of ill versus non-ill to measure various possible risk factors.

b. Case–Control Study. This is sometimes called a *retrospective study* because it studies persons already ill with the disease and compares their characteristics with a control group without the disease for the presence or absence of certain possible risk factors. When a significant difference in the prevalence of a characteristic or risk factor is found, then the possibility of a causal association is suspected. Analysis of an outbreak of giardiasis is a good example.[144] Further studies using the cohort method are then often carried out to add strength to the association. The

case–control study is usually the first type made because it is based on existing data, can be completed in a relatively short time, and is the least expensive. However, it cannot define the true incidence of the disease in relation to the various factors because the denominator at risk is not known.

Some of the advantages and disadvantages of these two types of investigation are given in Table 1. In a case–control study the statistical methods involve the calculation of the relative risk of the prevalence in the ill individual as compared with the control selected. This can be calculated using the format of a fourfold matrix as depicted in Table 2. If the frequency, $a/a + c$, of the characteristic in persons *with* the disease (a/a) in this total group $(a + c)$ is statistically significantly greater than the frequency of the characteristic in those *without* the disease $(b/b + d)$, then an association may exist between the characteristic and the disease. For further details of the mathematical and epidemiological techniques and the biases involved in the selection of cases

Table 1. Some Features of Cohort and Case–Control Studies

Features	Cohort	Case–control
Approach	Identify the subsequent incidence of disease in persons with or without given characteristic(s)	Identify the presence or absence of characteristic(s) in persons with or without a given disease
Starting point	Persons with or without certain characteristics	Ill persons and controls (healthy or with other disease)
Measurement	Incidence of infection or disease or both	Prevalence of characteristic
Type of observation	Serial, longitudinal surveillance of entire group for development of infection or disease or both	Single analysis by interview, records, or a laboratory test of the characteristic in persons with and without disease
Advantages and disadvantages		
Incidence	Can be measured directly	Not measurable directly
Risk	Direct assessment	Indirect assessment
Disease spectrum	Can be measured from infection to mild and severe disease in relation to characteristic(s) and to other diseases	Not measurable; a clinical case is the starting point
Factor(s) or characteristic(s)	Defined before disease develops	Factor(s) defined after disease develops
Bias	Little, usually, since information is recorded before the outcome is known, but problems in ascertainment, diagnosis, and follow-up may create bias	Bias may be present in interviewer, in patient, and in control; data from records may be incomplete
Attrition	Individuals may be lost to observation or refuse to be studied	Cases and controls may die prior to completion of study
Time	Often long period of observation	Can be short
Efficiency	Low except for diseases of high incidence	Comparatively high
Sample size	Large, depending on incidence of the infection or disease	Relatively small

Table 2. Matrix for Calculating Relative Risk Ratios

Characteristic or factor	With disease	Without disease	Total
	Number of persons		
Present	a	b	$a + b$
Absent	c	d	$c + d$
Total	$a + c$	$b + d$	

and controls, readers are referred to recent texts such as *Methods in Observational Epidemiology*.[103]

Methods for calculating significance can be found in standard biostatistical texts. Biases may occur in retrospective studies in the selection of cases, in the selection of controls, and in the elicitation of data by interview or records concerning the characteristics in question in both cases and controls. The selection of cases should ensure that they are representative of all patients with that disease. Ideally, this would assume that all patients with the disease seek medical attention, that the correct diagnosis is made and substantiated, that all medical facilities are canvassed, and that all cases are detected. In practice, these criteria are seldom met, and patients from a single hospital are often studied. This introduces a bias, since certain patients may be excluded from a given hospital because of such factors as age (e.g., no pediatric wards), socioeconomic level, or military or civilian status; the patient or physician may select a given hospital because of nearness, religious affiliation, the physician's privileges, nature of payment, or other considerations. These patients are not representative of all patients with the disease. The presence or absence of the characteristic under study may also influence the selection process for either the case or the control group or both, giving spurious associations.

Biases are common in the selection of controls. Usually, controls should be selected from the same population group (e.g., community hospital) from which the patients are drawn and should be closely comparable to the cases in all known characteristics (age, sex, socioeconomic level, ethnic groups) except the one under study. Random selection from a large group may equalize those differences, but usually *groups* matched for certain variables or *individuals* matched carefully for paired comparisons are selected. In a hospital setting, ill patients with diseases other than those under study are sometimes chosen. Bias may occur if some of these patients have diseases that are influenced by the characteristic in question. To limit this, patients with nonin-

fectious diseases are often chosen in an infectious-disease study. In a community setting, healthy controls may be advantageous. In matching, only those variables known to affect the disease should be selected. Each matching factor included, while controlling the results, eliminates the possibility of evaluating that factor itself.

To avoid bias regarding the presence or absence of a characteristic in the procurement of data by interview or from records, those charged with data collection should not know which is case or control, and the ascertainment should be uniform or standard. Once the data have been obtained, the relative risk associated with a given characteristic is calculated from Table 2 by the cross-product of $a \times d$ divided by $b \times c$. This estimate is based on the assumption that the frequency of the disease in the population is relatively small and that cases and controls are representative of their respective ill and non-ill populations for that disease. Examples of retrospective studies for an infectious disease would include the influence of some characteristic such as genetic makeup (HLA type), smoking, preexisting disease, or socioeconomic level as a risk factor in a given disease. It should be emphasized that a particular risk factor might operate at different levels or at several levels: it might affect exposure and infection, the severity of illness after infection has occurred, the duration of disease, the development of complications, or the case-fatality rate.

The advantages of retrospective or case–control studies as compared with prospective studies (see Table 1) include the relatively small numbers of subjects needed, their relatively high efficiency, and their suitability for diseases of low incidence. Their disadvantages include difficulty in finding the needed information about the characteristic in question, or the inaccuracy of the information; bias in obtaining data; and bias in the selection of cases and controls. The appropriate selection of the control groups is probably the most difficult task. What may seem most suitable to the investigator, his colleagues, or a consulting statistician may not be so viewed by others when the study is submitted for publication. The infectious-disease investigator is therefore urged to acquire epidemiological and statistical skills, or to seek advice from those who have them, before launching any important or experimental investigation of risk factors, a clinical trial, a vaccine evaluation, or other study. A pilot trial to identify problem areas before the real trial is recommended in recognition of Murphy's law that if anything can go wrong, it will.

c. Cross-Sectional or Prevalence Study. This third type of investigation examines the occurrence of disease and of suspected risk factors in population groups at a point in time, or over a relatively short period of time. Prevalence rates among those with and without the exposure are determined and compared. This approach is usually limited to diseases of slow onset and long duration for which medical care is often not sought until the disease has progressed to a relatively advanced stage. Thus, the risk factors present at the start of the disease may be difficult to identify. This method is used for certain chronic diseases, such as osteoarthritis, chronic bronchitis, and some mental disorders[103] but may also be useful in certain infectious diseases such as those occurring in a hospital setting.

The reader should review more detailed descriptions of epidemiological methods such as found in Ref. 103, 112, or 115 before undertaking any type of epidemiological study, as well as consult with a statistician in the planning stage to ensure the validity of the procedures and the adequacy of the number of subjects involved.

2.2.2. Experimental Epidemiology. In infectious diseases, this represents planned experiments designed to control the influence of extraneous factors, among those exposed or not exposed to an etiological factor, preventive measure, or environmental manipulation by the investigator. One example is the planned introduction of an infectious agent in a controlled fashion into a group of animals or volunteers and the analysis of the spread of infection and disease within these groups as compared to a nonexposed group. Such studies offer the most scientifically controlled method of epidemiological study. Unfortunately, many bacterial species or agents may not induce infection or disease in animal models. Certain susceptible animals (marmosets, chimpanzees) may not be available for study or are too expensive. Volunteers are very difficult to utilize in today's ethical, legal, and social environment, and there are good reasons for these restrictions.

2.2.3. Serological Epidemiology. The systematic testing of blood samples from a defined sample of a target population for the presence of antibodies, antigens, genetic markers, specific cell-mediated immunity, and other biological characteristics is called a serological or immunological survey. It constitutes an important epidemiological tool. Serological techniques can: (1) identify the past and current *prevalence* of an infectious agent in a community; (2) identify the *incidence* of infection by seroconversion or a rise in titer in samples obtained at two different times; (3) reveal the ratio of subclinical to clinical infections, when combined with clinical data; (4) determine the need for immunization programs and evaluate their effectiveness as to the presence, level, and quality of antibody produced; its duration; and the degree of protection against disease. Serological techniques are useful in defining the incidence, clinical importance, and spectrum of illness of a new agent

such as *Legionella pneumophila*. The presence of antibody or antitoxin to diphtheria, pertussis, and tetanus, as determined in a serological study, is a good reflection of the level of immunization and public-health practice in a community. This is especially true of tetanus, since antitoxin is acquired almost solely through immunization and rarely, if at all, through natural infection. The use of serological surveys in areas where medical care, diagnostic facilities, and reporting practices are inadequate may provide information essential for the control and evaluation of immunization programs. The uses, advantages, and disadvantages of serological surveillance and seroepidemiology for viral infections are presented in Chapter 2 of the companion book.[67]

Seroepidemiology is more widely applicable to viral than to bacterial diseases because of the wider occurrence of demonstrable antibodies in viral than in bacterial infections and because of the better means to measure them. Nevertheless, these techniques have proved useful in variable degrees for brucellosis, cholera, diphtheria, legionellosis, leptospirosis, *Mycoplasma pneumoniae* infections, pertussis, Q fever, Rocky Mountain spotted fever, syphilis, tetanus, tularemia, and typhoid fever. Specific mention of their applicability will be found in the relevant chapters of this book. The development of monoclonal antibodies and of new diagnostic techniques, such as the enzyme-linked immunosorbent assay (ELISA) and the radioimmunoassay (RIA), permit highly specific, sensitive, and rapid serological diagnoses. Development of sensitive and simple DNA probes may further enhance diagnostic microbiology in the future.

3. Epidemics and Their Investigation

Detailed descriptions of the concepts and methods of epidemic investigation can be found in Ref. 103, a practical guide to field investigation in Ref. 85, and a training guide prepared by the U.S. Centers for Disease Control in Ref. 31. This section will only deal with the highlights of epidemic investigation.

3.1. Pathogenesis of an Outbreak

Three essential requirements for an outbreak of an infectious disease are: (1) the presence or introduction of an infectious agent by an infected human, animal, bird, or arthropod vector, or its occurrence in air, water, food, soil, or other environmental source; (2) an adequate number of susceptibles; and (3) an effective means of contact and transmission between the two. Four circumstances in which epidemics occur can be mentioned: first, when a new group of susceptibles is introduced into a setting where a disease is endemic; second, when a new source of infection is introduced into an area from which the microbial agent has been absent and many susceptibles are therefore present, as in the return of visitors from a foreign country, or the arrival of new immigrants, or the contamination of food, water, or other source of exposure by an agent not normally present; third, when an effective contact is made between a preexisting infection of low endemicity with susceptible persons as a result of changes in social, behavioral, sexual, or cultural practices. Crowding as in a prison camp or institution or exposure of a new portal of entry are examples. A fourth possibility is an increased susceptibility to infection or disease or both through immunosuppression or other factors that influence the host response, such as a preceding viral infection, nutritional disorder, treatment with immunosuppressive drugs, or presence of a chronic disease. The devastating effect of HIV on the immune system has resulted in a worldwide epidemic of enormous and increasing proportions. The virus produces disease in three major ways: (1) it increases susceptibility to a wide variety of microbial agents, many of which are not pathogenic in normal subjects, (2) it leads to the reactivation of latent viral, bacterial, and parasitic agents, and (3) it permits the emergence of malignant or premalignant cells ordinarily held in check by the immune system, which results in the development of certain types of cancer, such as Kaposi's sarcoma and B lymphocytic malignancies. In addition, the virus causes directly an early mono-like illness and a later direct or indirect involvement of the central nervous system, so-called AIDS dementia.

Epidemics or outbreaks are often classified from the standpoint of the source of infection. A *common-source outbreak* may result from exposure of a group of persons to a single source of infection. This could be an exposure to a common source occurring at a single point in time, as in most foodborne outbreaks (point epidemics), and characterized by a sharply defined and limited epidemic curve, often within the incubation period of the disease. It could be exposure on a continued or extended basis, as would be the case from a contaminated water supply or air source, and would result in a drawn-out epidemic curve. In the latter setting, variations in the epidemic curve could result from differences in the dosage and time of occurrence of the microbial contaminant in the common vehicle or in the amount consumed, or they could result from changes in the frequency of exposure of the persons at risk to infection. The secondary spread of certain infectious agents from

human to human in a common-source outbreak will also alter the epidemic curve, often producing a group of scattered cases after the initial epidemic wave subsides; these are called secondary cases and can lead to tertiary cases.

A second type of epidemic spread called *propagated* or *progressive* is due to multiplication and spread of an agent from one host to another. This is most often human-to-human spread, but could involve animal or arthropod intermediates. Here, the epidemic curve depends on the number of susceptibles, the degree of contact with an infected host, the incubation period of the disease, the mechanism of transmission, the portal of entry, and the infectiousness of the causative agent. In either common-source or propagated outbreaks, the epidemic decreases or stops (1) when the number of susceptibles effectively exposed to the source is diminished by natural attrition, by immunization, by antibiotic prophylaxis, or by actual development of the disease itself; (2) when the source of infection is eliminated; or (3) when the means of transmission is interrupted.

3.2. Investigation of an Outbreak

The general strategy in the investigation of an outbreak includes establishing whether an epidemic actually exists, determining its extent, identifying the circumstances under which it occurred (e.g., time, place, person), evaluating its probable mode of spread, and initiating the steps to be taken for its control. Notification to appropriate health authorities should be made and help in epidemic investigation sought, if needed, from appropriate national or state communicable disease agencies; written reports should be made. News releases should be prepared to inform but not unnecessarily alarm the public. The epidemiologist, clinician, and laboratory expert all have roles in the analysis and management of an epidemic. The specific steps in epidemic investigations are presented in Table 3.

3.2.1. Determination of the Presence of an Epidemic. An epidemic or outbreak is usually defined as a substantial increase in the number of cases of a disease in a given period of time for that particular geographic area; e.g., an increase in the number of deaths from influenza and pneumonia that exceeds by 2 standard deviations the average experience for that week over the past 5 years is said to indicate an influenza outbreak.

A clinical diagnosis confirmed by laboratory findings is most important in determining whether a *specific* disease has exceeded the number of previously recorded cases. Unfortunately, a laboratory-proved diagnosis may be difficult or impossible to establish, especially early in an epidemic.

A clinical and epidemiological definition of the key

Table 3. Steps in the Investigation of an Epidemic

1. Determine that an epidemic or outbreak actually exists by comparing with previous data on the disease.
2. Establish an etiological diagnosis if possible; if not, define the condition epidemiologically and clinically. Collect materials for isolation and serological tests, and data from sick and well exposed persons.
3. Investigate the extent of the outbreak by a quick survey of hospitals, physicians, and other sources and its basic epidemiological characteristics in terms of time, place, person, probable method of spread, and the spectrum of clinical illness. Prepare a spot map of cases and an epidemic curve. Call in outside help if needed.
4. Formulate a working hypothesis of the source and manner of spread as a basis for further study.
5. Test the hypothesis by determining infection and illness rates in persons exposed or not exposed to putative source(s) of infection by questionnaire, interview, and laboratory tests. Try to isolate the agent from the putative source(s).
6. Extend epidemiological and laboratory studies to other possible cases or to persons exposed but not ill.
7. Analyze the data and consider possible interpretations.
8. On the basis of the analysis, initiate both short- and long-term control measures.
9. Report the outbreak to appropriate public-health officials.
10. Inform physicians, other health officials, and the public of the nature of the outbreak and the ways to control it.

features of the disease may be needed as a guide to reporting and disease recognition until the etiological agent is identified and appropriate methods are developed for isolation of the agent and/or its serological identification. Recent examples of the use of this type of definition are Legionnaires' disease, toxic shock syndrome, and AIDS. Even when the causative agent is known and laboratory tools for diagnosis are available, the disease may not be reportable, thus making comparison with past experiences impossible. On a practical level, any apparent concentration in time or geographic area of an acute illness of marked severity, or with unique clinical features involving the respiratory, gastrointestinal, skin, or central nervous system, deserves evaluation. In the absence of a specific diagnosis, a simple working definition of a *case* should be established on the basis of available clinical and epidemiological data. It should be concise and clear-cut. The number of such cases should then be determined by a quick telephone or record survey of hospitals, clinics, and appropriate practicing physicians in the area. If the epidemic seems to be widespread, as with influenza, a random telephone survey of homes may give an estimate of the attack rate. The rate of absenteeism from key industries and schools may also help define the magnitude of the outbreak.

3.2.2. Determination of the Circumstances under which the Outbreak Occurred. This often involves two phases: a preliminary assessment based on available data and a more intensive investigation when the situation is better defined.

a. Preliminary Assessment. This is usually based on existing clinical records. In addition to the key clinical features, the age, sex, race, occupation, home and work addresses, unusual behavioral or cultural characteristics, date of onset, recent travel, and functions attended by others in the group in the recent past should be recorded. A time graph is drawn of the epidemic curve by date of onset, and the incubation period is estimated. The time from the onset of the first cases to the peak may give a clue to this, as will unique or single exposures to the presumed source of infection. A spot map may reveal clustering of cases or a relationship to a common source in the environment (food, water, air, insect). The data are analyzed to identify the persons at highest risk or some common denominator of risk and to postulate the most likely means of transmission. Early identification of a common-source outbreak is most important for instituting control measures. This might be a single (point) exposure, as in a food outbreak, or a continued exposure, as in a contaminated water supply. Person-to-person spread, airborne transmission, arthropod-borne spread, and zoonotic disease, especially of domestic animals, should be considered.

Appropriate materials for laboratory investigation should be collected early in the outbreak, such as throat washings, stool specimens or rectal swabs, and an acute-phase serum sample. A public-health or hospital laboratory should be consulted in this endeavor. Since antibody to an infectious agent may already be present in many persons already ill in an outbreak, it may be desirable for baseline antibody levels to collect serum from other unexposed persons or from those incubating the disease, such as other family members or neighbors. A higher geometric mean antibody titer (GMT) to a specific agent in ill compared to unexposed persons implicates that agent in the epidemic. Appropriate samples from the environment (water, food) or from possible vectors (mosquitoes, lice) should also be collected for isolating the agent.

On the basis of this preliminary assessment, a hypothesis of spread may be formulated and recommendations for immediate control and isolation techniques made. Surveillance plans for identifying added cases may be drawn up, the appropriate environmental data assembled (water, milk, food, air), and questionnaires prepared for cases and controls in a fashion permitting easy analysis (marginal punch cards, computer). Standardized forms for foodborne outbreaks are available from state health departments and the Centers for Disease Control (CDC).

b. Intensive Study. This analysis should confirm or negate the hypothesis. The questionnaires prepared for this phase should include all possible circumstances under which the epidemic occurred and be administered to those ill, those exposed but not ill, and a comparable group neither exposed nor ill. Sera and other materials should be collected from these groups for antibody and antigen tests. The completed questionnaires may then be analyzed for comparison of *attack rates* (illness rate) in the three groups and as related to various risk factors. Antibody analysis of sera taken at the time of the outbreak and of those taken 2–3 weeks later may not only confirm the diagnosis but also identify the occurrence of infection without illness in persons who were exposed but did not become ill. It may be possible to identify the specific nature of an ongoing outbreak by comparing the GMT of those patients who are acutely ill with that of other patients already convalescing or by comparing the titer of those not exposed with that of those who are ill. More intensive study of the environment, of insect vectors, and of animal reservoirs may be needed. The analysis should include hypotheses to find the one that best fits the available data.

On the basis of this appraisal, control measures, including immunization programs, and other preventive measures should be initiated. Irrespective of whether the causative agent can be identified or not, the key element is the interruption of the chain of transmission. A written analysis of the epidemic should be given to the appropriate authorities. If no causative agent can be identified, then the acute and convalescent sera and material for antigen identification should be frozen for later study when new etiological agents or laboratory techniques are discovered. A good example of the benefit of this procedure is its use in retroactively identifying several outbreaks of Legionnaires' disease that had occurred prior to the outbreak in 1976 in Philadelphia, from which the organism was first isolated.

3.3. Example of Investigating a Foodborne Outbreak

An outbreak of illness characterized by diarrhea, abdominal cramps, and little or no fever involved 366 college students on February 24, 1966, in a new dormitory complex at the University of Wisconsin.[87] A quick assessment indicated that illness was confined to students who ate in three of six dining halls that served food from a common kitchen to 3000 students. No other dormitories were involved, and the cases were sharply limited in time. The epidemic curve shown in Fig. 1 indicates a peak incubation of 14 h. Stool specimens were obtained both from ill and healthy students and from food handlers. Samples of leftover items of food were not available; however, refrigerated samples of routinely collected food items were found for testing. Food menus for the preceding evening revealed that the three dining halls in which ill students had eaten offered a choice of roast beef with gravy or fish, whereas the other three dining halls had a choice of hamburger or fish; the other food items were common to all six dining halls. On the basis of this preliminary assessment, the hypothesis was formulated that this was a foodborne outbreak due to an agent with an average incubation period of about 14 h (range 10–20 h) that was present in or introduced into one or more of the food items served exclusively in the three dining halls where students became ill. The laboratory was notified of this as a guide to its tests. For more intensive investigation, questionnaires concerning foods eaten, time of onset, and the clinical symptoms were distributed to both sick and well students who ate in the three dining halls. They were returned by 366 ill and 740 well students, representing all the ill and two thirds of the well students. The clinical data indicated that the illness lasted less than 24 h and was characterized mainly by diarrhea; about half the ill students complained of abdominal cramps. Nausea, vomiting, and fever were rare. The average incubation period was too long for a staphylococcal toxin, and the clinical features would be unusual for *Salmonella* or *Shigella*.

An analysis of food items is given in Table 4. The evidence incriminating a food is usually based on the greatest difference in percentage ill between those who ate and those who did not eat a given food. In this outbreak, 69.9% of those who ate beef with gravy became ill as compared to 4.9% who did not eat this item; furthermore, no one who ate beef *without* gravy became ill, thus clearly incriminating gravy as the likely source. The gravy as well as other foods available were negative on aerobic and anaerobic culture. Mouse-inoculation tests for toxin in the gravy were also negative; however, it was not known whether the gravy

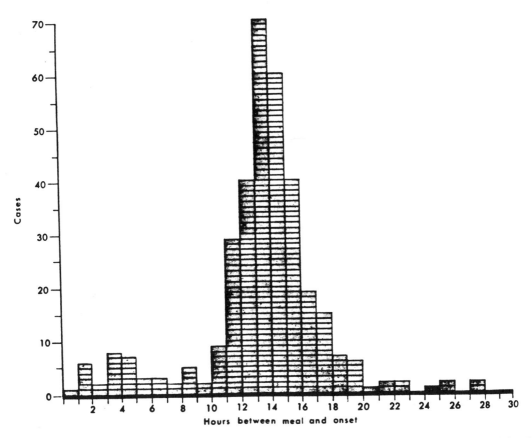

Figure 1. Epidemic curve of outbreak of *Clostridium perfringens* in a food outbreak involving 366 students at the University of Wisconsin. From Helstad *et al.*[87]

sample tested was from the incriminated meal or was set aside from a fresh gravy preparation. Laboratory analysis of fecal samples yielded the answer. Stool specimens from 19 of 20 ill students were positive for heat-resistant *Clostridium perfringens,* as was 1 of 24 stools from food handlers; no stools from 13 healthy students who had not eaten beef with gravy were positive. The organisms were isolated in thioglycollate broth after being heated 1 h in a boiling water bath. It was learned later that approximately 27 gallons of bone beef stock had been kept overnight in the refrigerator in 9-gallon plastic bags, mixed with 7 gallons of fresh beef stock the next day, heated to a rolling boil, and served separately from the roast beef. Apparently, the inadequate heating of a heat-resistant preformed toxin in a very large volume of fluid had failed to destroy it. The control measures instituted were to prohibit future use of leftover

gravy stock and to heat all items in smaller containers. *C. perfringens* food poisoning has an incubation period of 8–22 h with a peak of 10–14 h, closely fitting the outbreak described. In the United States, *C. perfringens* accounted for 10% of 522 foodborne outbreaks of known etiology from 1973 to 1977 but only 3.5% from 1983 to 1986 (CDC, personal communication).

4. Agent

This book deals with microorganisms classified under "Lower protists (Prokaryotic): Bacteria." This grouping includes also: the Chlamydiae (Bedsoniae) and the *Rickettsiae,* which are somewhat smaller than bacteria and are intracellular parasites.[97] *Viruses,* while classed as micro-

Table 4.   Analysis of Attack Rate for Different Foods Eaten in a College Outbreak of Diarrhea[a]

Food item	Ate food			Did not eat food			Difference between ill and non-ill (percent)
	Number	Ill		Number	Ill		
		Number	Percent		Number	Percent	
Fish	391	16	4.1	715	340	47.6	—
Hamburger	188	15	8.0	918	351	38.2	—
Beef							
With gravy	479	335	69.9	627	31	4.9	65.0
Without gravy	48	0	0	1058	366	34.6	—

[a]Derived from Helstad *et al.*[(87)]

organisms, are sharply differentiated from all other cellular forms of life; they consist of a nucleic acid molecule, either DNA or RNA, that is enclosed in a protein coat, or capsid. The principal groups of bacteria are presented in Table 5, which is derived from an "informal classification" presented by Jawetz *et al.*[(97)] in their excellent *Review of Medical Microbiology,* to which readers are referred for discussions of microbiology, immunology, and host–parasite relationships.

The characteristics of microorganisms of epidemiological importance include those concerned with transmission through the environment, the development of infection, and the production of clinical disease. Table 6 summarizes some of these characteristics of eubacteria, which include species pathogenic for humans.

4.1. Characteristics of Organisms That Are Involved in Spread through the Environment

For the spread of infection, a sufficient number of organisms must enter and survive transport through the environment to reach another susceptible host. Resistance to heat, UV light, drying, and chemical agents is important for survival of bacteria in nature. Some organisms such as *Vibrio cholerae* and *Legionella pneumophila* can survive for months in water, even in distilled water; others, such as anthrax bacillus, attain survival through highly resistant spores. Organisms capable of actual multiplication within the environment in soil, plants, food products, milk, and elsewhere have an advantage for survival. The capacity to infect a nonhuman host such as animals or birds, or to be transferred through an insect vector such as the *Rickettsiae,* offers alternative pathways for the persistence and spread of microorganisms.

4.2. Characteristics of Organisms That Are Involved in Production of Infection

Once bacteria have survived transport through the environment or intermediate host to reach a susceptible human host, several features of the bacteria are important in the initiation and development of infection. One is the *infectiousness,* expressed as the ratio: number infected/number susceptible and exposed. A second is *pathogenicity,* a term used to denote the potential for an infectious organism to induce *disease.* It can be expressed quantitatively as: number with disease/number infected. The determinants of pathogenicity include mobile genetic elements such as plasmids, bacteriophages, and transposons.[(138)] After entry, the organism must find appropriate cells on which it can attach or on which it can multiply. Epithelial surfaces provide an appropriate medium for many bacteria. *Mycoplasma pneumoniae* and *Hemophilus influenzae* find attachment sites in the respiratory epithelium, *Neisseria gonorrhoeae* in the urethral epithelium, and many enteric organisms (*Vibrio cholerae, Escherichia coli, Salmonella typhosa, Shigella flexneri*) in intestinal or colonic epithelium. Pathogenic organisms must possess characteristics that protect them against such host defenses as mucus and phagocytic cells. These protective features of the bacteria themselves include polysaccharide capsules (pneumococci, *Klebsiella, Hemophilus*), hyaluronic acid capsules and M proteins (β-hemolytic streptococci), and a surface polypeptide (anthrax bacillus). Certain extracellular enzymes may be important in the establishment of infection and in spread through tissues. These include collagenase (*C. perfringens*), coagulase (staphylococci), hyaluronidases (staphylococci, streptococci, clostridia, pneumococci), streptokinase or fibrinolysin (hemolytic streptococci), and hemolysins and leukocydins (streptococ-

Table 5. Key to Principal Groups of Bacteria Including Species Pathogenic for Humans[a]

Characteristics	Genera
I. Flexible, thin-walled cells with motility conferred by gliding mechanism (gliding bacteria)	
II. Same as I but with motility conferred by axial filament (spirochetes)	*Treponema, Borrelia, Leptospira*
III. Rigid, thick-walled cells, immotile or motility conferred by flagella	
Mycelial (actinomycetes)	*Mycobacterium, Actinomyces, Nocardia, Streptomyces*
Simple unicellular	
Obligate intracellular parasites	*Rickettsia, Coxiella, Chlamydia*
Free-living	
Gram-positive	
Cocci	*Streptococcus, Staphylococcus*
Nonsporulating rods	*Corynebacterium, Listeria, Erysipelothrix*
Sporulating rods	
Obligate aerobes	*Bacillus*
Obligate anaerobes	*Clostridium*
Gram-negative	
Cocci	*Neisseria*
Nonenteric rods	
Spiral forms	*Spirillum*
Straight rods	*Pasteurella, Brucella, Yersinia, Francisella, Haemophilus, Bordetella, Legionella*
Enteric rods	
Facultative anaerobes	*Escherichia* (and related coliforms), *Salmonella, Shigella, Klebsiella, Proteus, Vibrio*
Obligate aerobes	*Pseudomonas*
Obligate anaerobes	*Bacteroides, Fusobacterium*
IV. Lacking cell walls (mycoplasmas)	*Mycoplasma*

[a]Derived from Jawetz *et al.*[97]

ci, staphylococci, clostridia, gram-negative rods), and proteases (*Neisseria,* streptococci) that can hydrolyze immunoglobulins, such as secretory IgA.[97] These surface properties and enzyme production contribute to the *invasiveness* of an organism.

4.3. Characteristics of Organisms That Are Involved in Production of Disease

Disease is a rare consequence of infection. Usually, the presence of microorganisms on various surfaces of the body, their colonization on, or in, diverse epithelial cells, and their multiplication are unattended by signs of clinical disease. As with most viruses, infection without disease is a common outcome. However, since infection is a necessary basis for disease (excepting ingestion of preformed toxin), the attributes of organisms that are involved in infection are also

important in clinical illness (see Section 4.2 and Table 6). The term *virulence* is used as a quantitative expression of the disease-producing potential of a pathogenic organism. Molecular studies of the determinants of virulence include how agents enter epithelial cells, a property that may be carried in different ways. In enterovasive *E. coli* it may be on a large plasmid, whereas for *Yersinia pseudotuberculosis* it is by a small DNA segment of the bacterial chromosome.[138] This property may be exchanged between bacteria, making noninvasive bacteria invasive.

Other molecular studies are directed at the property of bacterial adhesion to mucosal surfaces, an early event in infection. Some organisms may also lose apparent virulence if their structural identity is too close to the host's carbohydrates (for which the term *camouflage strategy* has been suggested). The factors that result in disease in an infected person are also determined by the host, as discussed in

Table 6.   Bacterial Characteristics of Epidemiological Importance[a]

Epidemiological aspects	Bacterial characteristics
1. Features involved in *spread* through the environment	Number of organisms released by infected host
	Resistance to physical agents of environment (e.g., heat, UV, moisture)
	Ability to multiply within the environment
	Ability to infect intermediate host or insect vector
2. Features involved in initiation and development of *infection*	Host range of organisms
	Genetic makeup and antigenic diversity
	Infectivity of organism
	Pathogenicity of organism
	Number of organisms entering host and the portal of entry
	Enzymes involved in spread through tissues
3. Features involved in production of *clinical disease*	Most characteristics under (2)
	Virulence of organism
	Invasiveness of organism
	Production of endo- and exotoxins
	Immunopathological potential

[a] Host attributes are considered in Table 7.

Section 6. Those that relate to the organism are invasiveness, the production of toxins, and the induction of an immune response that usually is beneficial but sometimes is detrimental to the host.

Invasiveness does not always correlate with disease and a widely disseminated organism does not always induce illness, but the wide distribution of a pathogen and its contact with many cells provide the potential amplification of any detrimental host response. That wide dissemination and a large number of organisms, even in the bloodstream, do not inevitably lead to toxemia is exemplified by the minimal host response evoked by large numbers of *Mycobacterium leprae* bacilli in the blood in lepromatous leprosy.

Organisms that produce *endotoxins* or *exotoxins* are likely to produce disease, since most are toxic to cells and evoke inflammatory responses. The exotoxins liberated by many gram-positive bacteria cause local cell and tissue injury; some damage phagocytic cells and thereby facilitate the spread of the organism. Examples include *Clostridium welchii, botulinum,* and *tetani, Corynebacterium diphtheriae, Shigella dysenteriae, Vibrio cholerae, Bacillus anthracis, Bordetella pertussis, Streptococcus pyogenes,* and *Staphylococcus aureus.*[121] Some exotoxins are directly responsible for the characteristic clinical features of the disease, some are antiphagocytic, and some promote spread in tissues. They cause little or no fever in the host.

Endotoxins are an integral part of the cell wall of gram-negative organisms. They are liberated in soluble form both during bacterial growth and presumably during death and disintegration of the organism. Endotoxins are strong immunological adjuvants. They may product fever in man and many other vertebrates; the pyrogenic action is mediated by a product synthesized by monocytes ("endogenous pyrogen") that acts on the thermoregulatory center in the hypothalamus. Other endogenous agents, such as prostaglandins and catecholamines, may also play a role. The lipopolysaccharide (LPS) is the most important component of endotoxin and is composed of a core polysaccharide common to many gram-negative bacteria, an O-specific polysaccharide conferring virulence and serological specificity, and a lipid A portion, mainly responsible for toxicity.[121] The effects of endotoxins appear to be mediated through leukotrienes, prostaglandins, and cachectin/TNF. Cachectin, which is identical to *tumor necrosis factor,*[131] is indistinguishable functionally from lymphotoxin, a product of activated T cells.[138] This protein is produced by macrophages and by T cells in response to bacteria, viruses, and parasites and also occurs during cancers, resulting, in order of increasing dosage, in the following sequence of events: inflammation, cytotoxicity, cachexia, organ failure, irreversible shock, and death. There is a synergism between it and interleukin-1 in this phenomenon. Monoclonal antibody to cachectin/TNF can inhibit these responses and glucosteroids can also prevent endotoxin deaths. The gene for cachectin has been identified, and when put into hamster ovarian cells and then into nude mice results in cachexia. Despite these deleterious effects, cachectin/TNF in small doses appears to be beneficial in serving as a growth factor for macrophages and as a tissue remodeler, a role for which it may have been designed in nature. It is not clear whether all these effects are mediated directly by cachectic/TNF or through mediators released by them. With large doses of endotoxins, there is also an effect that produces vascular collapse and death. Unlike exotoxins, endotoxins are heat-stable and are not fully convertible to protective toxoids. Endotoxins are normally released by many gram-negative bacteria in the intestines of healthy individuals, are presumably absorbed in small amounts, and are degraded by the Kuppfer cells. This occurs without pathological consequences on a continual basis and has a beneficial effect in stimulating the development of the immune system in the immature individual.[121]

Exotoxins are excreted by living cells, are quite unstable to heat, and consist of polypeptides of molecular weights from 10,000 to 900,000. They are highly antigenic and result in high titers of antitoxin which can neutralize the toxin. This antigenic property is useful in immunization with toxins rendered nontoxic by formalin, heat, and other methods. Different toxins produce disease via different mechanisms.[97] *Corynebacterium diphtheriae* toxin results in inhibition of protein synthesis and necrosis of epithelium, heart muscle, kidney, and nerve tissues. The toxin of *Clostridium tetani* reaches the central nervous system by retrograde axon transport where it increases reflex excitation in neurons of the spinal cord by blocking an inhibitor mediator.

Clostridium botulinum exerts its effect on the nervous system by blocking the release of acetylcholine at synapses and neuromuscular junction. Gut organisms, such as *Clostridium difficile,* produce a necrotizing toxin that leads to antibiotic-associated colitis, and that of *Staphylococcus aureus* stimulates neural receptors from which impulses are transmitted to medullary centers controlling gut motility. *Vibrio cholerae* toxin binds to ganglioside receptors on the villi of the small intestine, leading to a large increase in adenylate cyclase and AMP concentrations, and the resulting massive hypersecretion of chloride and water and the impairment of absorption of sodium that characterizes the severe diarrhea and acidosis of cholera. Other toxins, such as that of hemolytic lysogenic streptococci, result in the punctate maculopapular rash of scarlet fever.

The production of clinical disease through immunopathological mechanisms is more important for viral than for bacterial infections, but there are some examples of the latter. In streptococcal infections, antibodies may develop against an unknown component of the organism that is antigenically similar to heart muscle, leading to myocarditis. Immune complexes may also form, deposit in the kidney, and result in glomerulonephritis. In infections due to *Mycoplasma pneumoniae,* the production of "heterophile" antibodies against human O erythrocytes (cold agglutinins) occasionally leads to acute hemolytic anemia. In primary infections by *Mycobacterium tuberculosis,* the pathological picture is dominated by a vigorous and persistent cell-mediated immune response to the invading organism. The inflammatory, pathological, and immunological processes of the host culminating in disease may be detrimental both to the host and to the microorganism. A successful parasite is one that leads to the least host response.

5. Environment

The external environment provides the setting in which the agent and host usually interact and is the usual means of transmission between the two. The effects of the environment on the organism itself are discussed in Section 4.1. The environment also contains the physical and biological mechanisms required for spread. The former includes air, water, and food and the latter animal, bird, and insect vectors and reservoirs. For some bacterial infections, the primary host is not man but some other living creature in the environment. This includes anthrax, brucellosis, leptospirosis, Q fever, bubonic plague, Rocky Mountain spotted fever, salmonellosis, and tularemia. For infections involving insect transmission such as louseborne typhus, Rocky Mountain spotted fever, and bubonic plague, the humidity, temperature, vegetation, and other factors in the environment may play a central role in limiting the occurrence of the infection to well-defined geographic areas favorable to the vector. Through climatic factors, the environment exerts an influence on exposure of the host to microorganisms. Warm weather and tropical climates result in recreational and occupational exposures to water, sewage, swimming pools, wild animals, and insects; they promote spread of skin infections in unclothed persons with abrasions on their skin. Certain organisms grow or survive better in warmer environments, especially enteric organisms. Intestinal infections flourish under such conditions. Inadequate refrigeration leads to foodborne outbreaks. Epidemics of Legionnaires' disease appear to depend on a chain of warm-weather events in a developed country. These include appropriate temperature and humidity for the organism to grow in soil or water, the contamination of a water-cooling tower or air conditioner, and airborne carriage or propulsion of the organism to susceptible humans in an enclosed environment (e.g., hotel, hospital, institution, club); July and August are good months for this. The colder winter months, as well as school seasons in temperate climates of the Northern Hemisphere, bring individuals into close contact in a closed environment, facilitating spread of infections by the respiratory route. This includes bacterial infections of the central nervous system such as the meningococcus, *H. influenzae,* and pneumococcus organisms as well as true respiratory infections such as pertussis, bacterial and mycoplasmal pneumonias, tuberculosis, diphtheria, and streptococcal pharyngitis–tonsillitis. The peak period of different *diseases* varies from one season to another. For example, pertussis and *M. pneumoniae* infections tend to occur most commonly in the fall and streptococcal infections in the spring. In addition, longer-term temporal trends in infection and disease occur within the same environment (as discussed in Chapter 2, Section 8.2). These changes reflect the complex interplay of agent, host, and environment. New strains of the organism, environmental alterations, varying behavioral patterns of the host, and the degree of immunization practice may change the pattern from one season to another.

The particular environmental setting—the place—also influences disease occurrence and its clinical patterns. In hospitals, certain types of skin, wound, and urinary infections are common, and their severity may be enhanced in persons who are already ill with another disease or are receiving immunosuppressive therapy. Antibiotic-resistant organisms are frequent in this setting. In prisons and in institutions for the mentally retarded or ill, low levels of personal hygiene and crowding contribute to the spread of intestinal and skin infections. Exposure in meat-packing and slaughterhouses or tanneries, or travel to developing countries, involves the risk of infection by various bacterial agents within that environment. With regard to children, the day-care center is posing an increasing hazard for them, as well as their parents for certain infectious diseases, especially respiratory and intestinal infections.[3] However, for young children infection is much more common than disease. For example, among 10,860 case contacts of an index case of *H. influenzae* type b infection in day-care centers, none of whom had received rifampin chemoprophylaxis, no clinical *disease* developed over an average 60-day observation period, although the carrier state was common.[123] Thus, rifampin prophylaxis of contacts may be unnecessary in these settings, although some other investigators disagree with this.

6. Host

The occurrence of *infection* depends on exposure to a source of infection and on the susceptibility of the host. The development of *disease* in an infected person depends largely on factors intrinsic to the host, although some properties of the organism itself influence this. Some of the host factors are presented in Table 7. Exposure to a pathogenic organism depends on characteristics of the human host that result in contact with sources of infection within the environment or that promote person-to-person spread. The behavioral pattern of the individual at different ages brings varying types of exposure in different seasons, cultures, and geographic areas. Personal habits such as intravenous drug usage or sexual promiscuity are also determinants of exposure. The family unit comprises an important setting for exposure to, and spread, of infectious agents. The importance of the family has been well documented by Fox.[78] The genetic background, nutritional habits, cultural and behavioral patterns, and level of hygiene within families create common patterns of exposure. The number and age of family members and the degree of crowding within the home also affect the transmissibility of infection. Hospitalization or institutionalization brings new exposures in closed environments. Heightened person-to-person contact and a mixture of susceptibles with infected or infectious individuals (carriers) underlie the increased risk of military recruits, children in day-care centers, and residents of institutions. Streptococcal, meningococcal, *M. pneumoniae,* *H. influenzae* type b, and enteric infections are common in such settings.

Occupational risks involve special types of exposures in certain occupations. The worker in the abattoir or slaughterhouse, meat-packing industry, or even at the butcher block is at risk to brucellosis, tularemia, and various parasitic infections. The sewage and sugar-cane worker and the swine-handler are exposed to leptospirosis, the tannery worker to anthrax, and the hunter to tularemia. The hospital worker is at increased risk to a variety of infectious agents, of which HIV is currently of greatest concern, although the risk is extremely small if universal hospital infection regulations are strictly followed. Hepatitis B infection is also of concern, and HBV vaccine should be given to all hospital staff exposed to blood.

Race does not usually influence *infection* if exposure is equal, but the response to infection may vary, such as the increased severity of tuberculosis in blacks. However, the separation of ethnic origin from other cultural, socioeconomic, behavioral, and genetic differences is often im-

Table 7. Host Factors That Influence Exposure, Infection, and Disease

Factors that influence exposure

Behavioral factors related to age, drug usage, alcohol consumption	Military service
Familial exposure	Occupation
Hospitalization, especially intensive care	Recreation, sports, hobbies
Hygienic habits	Sexual activity: hetero- and homosexual, type and
Institutionalization: nurseries, day care centers, homes for the elderly and mentally retarded, prisons and other closed environments	number of partners
	Socioeconomic level
	Travel, especially to developing countries

Factors that influence infection, and occurrence and severity of disease

Age at the time of infection	Genetic makeup, especially influences on the immune response
Alcoholism	Immune state at time of infection
Anatomic defect	Immunodeficiency: natural, drug-induced, or viral (HIV)
Antibiotic resistance	Mechanism of disease production: inflammatory, immunopathological, or toxic
Antibiotics in tissues	Nutritional status
Coexisting diseases, especially chronic	Receptors for organism on cells needed for attachment or entry of organism
Dosage: amount and virulence of organism to which person is exposed	
Double infection	
Duration of exposure to organism	
Entry portal of organism and presence of trauma at site of implantation	

possible. Recreational pursuits and hobbies influence exposures in both internal and external environments. The homemaker who prepares home preserves improperly may expose the ingestor to botulism; the home gardener or farmer is at risk to tetanus, the outdoorsman to various infections of wild animals. The influence of gender on occupational exposures has become of little importance, since women have entered almost all work areas including military life and many hazardous occupations. On the other hand, pregnancy is attended by special qualitative risks to infection, more commonly viral than bacterial, to which the male is not heir. Differences between sexes in the portal of entry of microorganisms may result in different patterns of infection and disease, as is true in male homosexuals practicing passive rectal intercourse, in which the risk of infection with HIV is greatly increased.

The socioeconomic level of the individual or the community affects the frequency, nature, and age at the time of infection. In developing countries and lower socioeconomic settings, infectious diseases, especially respiratory and enteric, constitute a leading cause of illness and death. The socioeconomic status influences infection and disease through a complex interaction of hygienic practices, environmental contamination, nutritional status, crowding, and exposure to animal and insect vectors.

Travel is an increasingly important risk factor because it may bring individuals into new settings, especially tropical or developing countries. Enteric infections are common hazards, especially toxogenic *E. coli, Campylobacter,* amebiasis, shigellosis typhoid fever, salmonellosis, yersiniosis, and giardiasis. The risk varies according to the country visited and the food or fluid ingested. Dupont *et al.*[57] estimated the risk of diarrhea in American travelers staying an average of 19–21 days in a foreign country in 1970 to be 4.2% in the British Isles and Scandinavia, 5.6% in western England, and 12.1% in countries bordering the Mediterranean. About half the enteric infections of travelers are due to toxigenic *E. coli* (see Chapter 12): other causes are salmonellosis (Chapter 28) and shigellosis (Chapter 29).

Once infection has occurred, a number of factors influence whether clinical disease will develop and determine its severity (Table 7, part 2). The term *clinical illness promotion factor* has been suggested for these influences that result in clinical disease among those infected.[66] Most of these factors are intrinsic to the host, although the dosage, virulence, and antibiotic resistance of the infecting organism play a role (see Section 4), as does the portal of entry. Entry sites that are close to vital organs or that permit easy access to invasion of the bloodstream may result in more severe and complicated infections. Among the host factors, age at the time of infection is an important determinant of the frequency of clinical illness and its clinical features and severity. The presence of chronic diseases or other infections are risk factors. HIV infection greatly enhances the risk of opportunistic infections, of the reactivation of latent agents, and of malignancy. Transmission of infection to the fetus *in utero* may result in fetal death or congenital abnormalities as with *Treponema pallidum*. Infections of the newborn such as those due to *Streptococcus B, Clostridium botulinum,* and *Chlamydia trachomatis* may be severe and fatal. As is true in many viral infections, bacterial infections in childhood are often subclinical and less well localized than in the adult. The concept of "streptococcosis," introduced by Boisvert *et al.*[16] and Powers *et al.*[125] in the 1940s, illustrates this (see Chapter 31). In the newborn infant, respiratory involvement from Group A infections is uncommon, although Group B streptococci may cause sepsis and meningitis. In the age group 6 months to 3 years, Group A infections have insidious development and mild symptoms. In the older infant and preschool child, a nonspecific streptococcal Group A illness may be characterized by low-grade fever, irritability, and nasal discharge, sometimes accompanied by anorexia and vomiting. Clinical diagnosis is difficult. In the school-age child, upper respiratory infections due to Group A predominate, and over half are manifested by the classic features of acute streptococcal pharyngotonsillitis: sore throat, often with tonsillar exudate; pharyngeal edema; dysphagia; enlargement of the anterior cervical nodes; and systemic symptoms (fever, chills, malaise). Another 20% may have milder and less localized illness, and 20% more may have either mild or no illness.

In general, the highest mortality from infection occurs very early in life, when immune defense mechanisms are immature, and in old age when they may be deteriorating. The clinical response to infection may also be more severe in conditions that alter or depress immune defenses. These include preexisting chronic disease, especially of the specific target organ of the infection; occurrence of a viral, parasitic, or other bacterial infection preceding or accompanying the current illness; and the prior use of alcohol, tobacco, or immunosuppressive drugs. The vigor and efficiency of the immune response may alter the host either favorably by control of the infection or unfavorably by certain immunopathological processes. *Genetic traits* influence both susceptibility and disease. Their role in regulating the immune response is an important, but often ill-defined one, in rela-

tion to the occurrence and severity of the clinical disease. Studies have revealed that 61.5% of identical twins had clinical tuberculosis in a family setting as compared with only 18.3% of nonidentical twins or 18.9% of siblings.[101] The *nutritional level* also affects host resistance. Malnutrition (especially severe protein deficiency) adversely affects phagocytosis and other primary defense mechanisms, the development of the thymus, and the efficacy of cell-mediated immunity against infections such as tuberculosis. In general, antibody formation is not impaired. The precise role of nutrition and vitamins in infection and disease is not well understood.

In summary, host factors may be divided into three major stages: (1) those that lead to exposure, (2) those that lead to infection among those effectively exposed, and (3) those that lead to clinical disease among those infected. The concepts of a *clinical illness promotion factor* that leads to clinical illness,[66] and of other, protective factors that result in subclinical, or inapparent illness have recently been discussed.[68] Very little is known about them and they remain an important challenge to epidemiologists, microbiologists, and immunologists.

7. Routes of Transmission

The major routes of transmission of bacterial infections are listed in Table 8 in general order of their importance. Many organisms have several routes. The sequence of spread usually involves the exit of the organism from the infected host; transport through the environment via air, water, food, insect, or animal, with or without bacterial multiplication; and the entry of a sufficient number of viable organisms into an appropriate portal of a susceptible host to initiate infection. For some infectious agents, specific receptors on the cell surface are needed to permit attachment and multiplication of the organism. Table 8 is loosely divided into human, animal–insect, and inanimate sources of infection in order to follow infection from its source to a human host, but the arrangement is sometimes artificial for those infections that exist primarily in other species or for those organisms that can multiply or survive in the natural environment.

7.1. Respiratory or Airborne

Organisms infecting the respiratory tract are either airborne via droplet nuclei or transmitted via droplets that are not considered true airborne transmission. The sources of the organisms carried by the air include infected lesions of

Table 8. Transmission of Bacterial Infections[a]

Route of exit	Route of transmission	Examples	Factors	Route of entry
1. Human source				
1.1. Respiratory	Respiratory droplets or droplet nuclei	Bacterial pneumonias	Close contact or air-borne	Respiratory
	RS and fomites	Diphtheria	Carriers	Respiratory, skin
	Nasal discharges	Leprosy	Household contact	? Skin, respiratory
	RS → droplets	Meningococcus	Crowding, military re-cruits, carriers	Respiratory
	RS → air, fomites	Pertussis	Direct contact	Respiratory
	RS → air	Plague (pneumonic)	Pneumonic case	Respiratory
	RS → droplets	Streptococcal	Close contact, carrier	Respiratory
	RS → droplet nuclei	Tuberculosis	Household contact	Respiratory
1.2. Skin squames	Respiratory, direct contact	Nosocomial bacterial infections	Hospitalization, sur-gery	Nose, respiratory, skin
	Direct contact	Impetigo due to staph and/or strep	Low socioeconomic level, tropics	Skin
	Close contact	Skin diphtheria	War wounds	Skin
		Yaws	Endemic foci	Skin
1.3. Gastrointestinal				
Enteric fevers	Stool → water	Cholera	Water, food, carrier	Mouth
	Stool → food	Salmonellosis	Food, animal contact	Mouth
	Stool → man	Shigellosis	Man-to-man only	Mouth
	Stool → water, food	Typhoid fever	Also food, flies	Mouth
Food poisoning	Food	Staph, *C. perfringens, Salmonella,* strep, *Vibrio para-hemolyticus*	Inadequate refrigera-tion or cooking	
		Botulism	Home canning	Mouth
1.4. Urine	Water (swimming)	Leptospirosis	Infected animals	Skin
	Water	Typhoid fever	Poor sanitation	Oral
1.5. Genital	Sexual contact (hetero- or homo-sexual)	Chancroid	Mostly tropics	Urethra
		Chlamydia	Also carriers	Urethra, rectum
		Gonorrhea	Also carriers	Urethra, rectum
		Syphilis	Moist surfaces	Urethra, placenta
1.6. Placental	Congenital	Syphilis	Up to 4th month of pregnancy	Blood
1.7. Umbilical	Direct contact	Neonatal tetanus	Poor birth hygiene	Cord
2. Animal sources	Infected animal	Anthrax	Tanning	Skin, respiratory
		Tularemia	Skinning, dressing	Skin, eyes
	Bite of tick	Rocky Mt. spotted fever, Lyme disease	Outdoor exposure	Skin
	Rat flea	Bubonic plague	Infected rat	Skin
	Infected placenta via air	Q fever	Cows	Respiratory
3. Inanimate sources	Soil, air, water, food	Tetanus	Wound, childbirth	Skin
		Legionnaires' disease	Warmth, humidity, water coolers, air conditioners, pot-able water supplies	Respiratory

[a]This table is representative only and does not include all organisms. RS, respiratory secretions.

the skin, or droplet nuclei from inanimate sources such as from water cooling towers, as with *Legionella* organisms, or from inanimate sources, the respiratory tract, or oropharynx of infected persons. Their success in reaching a susceptible host depends on the number of organisms present, the particle size, the force with which they are propelled into the environment, the resistance to drying, the temperature and humidity of the air, the presence of air currents, and the distance to the host. Some infections may be carried great distances from their sources, e.g., airborne outbreaks of Q fever, tuberculosis, or Legionnaires' disease. As with viruses, respiratory-transmitted bacterial infections are difficult to control. The dynamics of airborne transmission have been carefully studied by Knight[105] and his colleagues for viral infections. The size of the aerosol created influences its dispersion distance and the site in the respiratory passages at which the particles are trapped. Particles of 6 μm diameter or more are usually filtered out in the nose, while those of 0.6–6.0 μm are deposited on sites along the upper and lower respiratory tract.

7.2. Gastrointestinal or Oral–Fecal

The oral–fecal route of transmission is a close rival to respiratory spread and there are many sources of infection. A first group is called enteric fevers. Bacterial organisms from ill persons or carriers exit via the gastrointestinal tract to the external milieu for transmission via water, food, or direct contact to another individual. They constitute a major group of bacterial infections. The mouth is the common portal of entry. Some enteric infections involve only a human-to-human cycle, such as cholera, typhoid fever, and shigellosis. Others, such as salmonellosis, *Campylobacter* infections, and yersiniosis, also involve animal hosts. A variety of mechanisms may transmit the organism from the infectious stool to a susceptible person. Cholera is commonly transmitted by water, on occasion by food (as in a food outbreak aboard an airplane[21]), and from oysters in Louisiana.[13] Shigellosis has also been found to be related to an airplane meal.[20] Flies and fomites may carry the organism, but are not regarded as important epidemiologically. Typhoid fever is transmitted by food or water contaminated by the feces or urine from a patient or carrier and sometimes through contaminated shellfish or canned goods. *Salmonella* infections are widely disseminated in nature and infect many domestic animals and birds, providing many potential sources of contamination of food and, less commonly, of water. *Campylobacter fetus* subsp. *jejuni* and *Yersinia enterocolitica* also infect many animals, including domestic ones such as puppies, and can infect exposed

humans through direct contact, or through water, milk, or food. For shigellosis, exposure to an infected human during the acute illness or shortly thereafter is the main source of infection; here, direct or indirect oral–fecal contact is usually more important than water or food. There is no extra-human reservoir of infection.

A second group of gastrointestinal infections is called food poisoning. Here, contamination of food may occur from the feces of an infected person or carrier (food-handler), but other sources of the organism are also common. The animal food source may be infected (i.e., *Salmonella* in chickens), or the organism may be present on the skin of the food-handler (staphylococcus, streptococcus), in the environment (staphylococcus), in the soil (*C. perfringens,* botulism), or in raw seafood (*V. parahemolyticus*).

The transmission of enteric fevers and food poisoning is largely preventable. A good source of water, proper chlorination or boiling, frequent hand-washing, appropriate refrigeration of foods, and thorough cooking are effective ways of interrupting the chain of infection. However, in developing countries and low socioeconomic settings, neither the means nor the education to carry them out may be available. Some may be prevented by immunization. Transmission of enteric infections by homosexual activity is a newly recognized and important problem in this group, and infection in AIDS patients may result not only from a wide variety of usual pathogens such as *E. coli,* but also from organisms usually regarded as commensal and nonpathogenic such as the parasitic infection *Cryptosporidium.*

7.3. Dermal

Bacterial infections of the skin are commonly due to a staphylococcus or streptococcus or to a mixture of the two. They are manifested as boils, carbuncles, impetigo, and erysipelas. They are particularly common in warm and tropical climates and in settings of poor hygiene. Transmission usually occurs person to person from an infected lesion or via squamae. Yaws, a nonvenereal, contagious disease of the skin and bones due to *Treponema pertenue,* is endemic in many tropical areas and is similarly transmitted; effective eradication programs with penicillin sponsored by the World Health Organization (WHO) have been carried out in many countries. Diphtheritic skin infections may also occur, especially in tropical climates, and may contaminate wounds.

7.4. Person-to-Person or Personal Contact

This term indicates spread by close contact or by direct transfer of infected discharges from the respiratory or gastrointestinal tract. Fecal–oral spread falls under this heading. Infections transmitted in his way are discussed in Sections 7.1–7.3.

7.5. Urinary

Urinary spread of infection is not common, but may occur in typhoid fever from an infected person and in leptospirosis from many animal hosts. Water is the common vehicle of transmission.

7.6. Genital or Sexually Transmitted

The term *venereally transmitted* is now being limited to the five classic infections clearly transmitted by sexual intercourse (gonorrhea, syphilis, chancroid, lymphogranuloma venereum, and granuloma inguinale). The new term *sexually transmitted diseases* (STD) is broader, applies to both hetero- and homosexual activity, and encompasses all infections transmitted person to person during sexual activity. In recent years, *Chlamydia trachomatis* has been identified in this group as the cause of almost half of nongonorrheal urethritis (see Section 11.2.6 and Chapter 9), and *Ureaplasma* is under evaluation; enteric infections are of increasing importance in male homosexuals. Among viruses, herpes simplex is an important cause of STD, and hepatitis A and B are common infections of homosexuals. HIV is producing a worldwide epidemic of infection and disease among male homosexuals, their sexual contacts and children, i.v. drug users, and recipients of blood or blood products from which HIV has not been excluded. In Africa, transmission is primarily heterosexual although contaminated needles used medically may also be important.

In homosexuals in the United States, the major risk factor is passive anal intercourse, as well as among prostitutes in endemic areas. The number of different partners also plays a role in settings in which the prevalence of infection is relatively modest. In other areas, in which over 70% of active homosexuals or prostitutes are infected, the number of partners plays a minor role as an encounter with a single partner already carries a very high risk of infection. Heterosexual transmission also occurs from infected homosexuals, i.v. drug users, and hemophiliacs. The efficacy of transmission appears in some studies to be higher from infected males to females than vice versa. Infection of the active, insertive partner is rare unless he has a penile lesion, and transmission by oral sex alone is very unusual unless there is prolonged exposure to an infected partner and/or a mucosal lesion exists. Bacterial infections such as gonorrhea, chlamydial infections, and syphilis are also readily

transmitted among these high-risk groups with or without concomitant transmission of HIV. It is possible that the presence of urethritis from one of these causes may enhance the spread of HIV.

7.7. Perinatal

These infections occur at the time of childbirth. In *congenital* infections, the organism is transmitted *vertically* from an infected mother via the placenta to the fetus. Congenital syphilis, rubella, and toxoplasmosis are examples of this. Infections may occur *horizontally* from an infected cervix to the baby as it passes through the birth canal, as in gonococcal ophthalmia and chlamydial infections. Infections may also be acquired immediately after birth, as exemplified by tetanus neonatorum due to contamination of the newly cut umbilical cord.

7.8. Insect Vectors

Rocky Mountain spotted fever is transmitted by the bite of the tick, which may remain infective for a long time, and the infection is maintained in nature by transovarian and transstadial passage. A mite has been suggested as the means of transmission of rickettsialpox from infected house mice. The transmission of bubonic (sylvatic) plague is through the rat flea (mostly *Xenopsylla cheopis*) from infected wild rodents. *Borrelia burgdorferi*, the cause of Lyme disease, is transmitted by small ixoid ticks, such as the deer tick, *Ixodes dammini*.

7.9. Other

Water- and foodborne diseases are discussed in Section 7.2. Some other sources of infection, other than via a biological host, include organisms commonly present in the environment. Legionnaires' bacillus, anthrax, tetanus, and other spore-forming organisms in the soil might be considered in this category. These may be transmitted by contamination of water, be airborne, or come in direct contact with the skin. Organ transplantation, such as kidney, heart, cornea, or dura mater, does not carry the same risk of bacterial infections as it does for viruses such as HIV, cytomegalovirus, rabies, and slow viruses.

8. Pathogenesis

A section on pathogenesis is included in every chapter of this volume that deals with specific infections. Only a few concepts will be presented here. An excellent little book by Mims[121] entitled *The Pathogenesis of Infectious Disease* should be consulted; much of this discussion was derived from that source. Many recent textbooks on infectious diseases include excellent chapters on pathogenesis, immunology, and other agent–host interactions.[74,91,116]

8.1. Localized or Superficial Infections

Many bacterial infections produce disease through the cells with which they first come in contact in skin or epithelial surfaces and remain limited to that area. Tissue damage results from the direct action of the bacteria, microbial toxins, indirect injury, inflammation, or immunopathological processes. Some bacteria have specific attachment sites on epithelial surfaces (see Section 4.2). Examples of localized infections include diphtheria and streptococcal infection of the throat, gonococcal infections of the conjunctiva or urethra, cholera, and most *Salmonella* infections of the intestine. Many gram-negative bacteria have a limited capacity to invade tissues and tend to remain localized; some are able to invade only in debilitated, malnourished, or immunosuppressed patients. Host antibacterial forces limit the spread of many bacteria. At the subepithelial level, three important defense mechanisms are called into play: (1) tissue fluids; (2) the lymphatic system leading to the lymph nodes; and (3) phagocytic cells (macrophages in tissues and polymorphonuclear cells in the blood). Each of these mechanisms depends on the inflammatory response for its action[121] as manifested by four cardinal signs: *redness* and *warmth* due to vasodilation, *swelling* (vasodilation and exudate), and *pain* (tissue distension, pain mediators). Polymorphonuclear cells enter, as well as macrophages and lymphocytes; exudation occurs. Tissue fluids provide plasma proteins, including immunoglobulins such as IgG, complement, and properdin. The primary mediators of inflammation include histamine, 5-hydroxytryptamine, and kinins. Prostaglandins E and F are thought to play a role in the termination of the response.[121] Microorganisms in peripheral lymphatics are rapidly borne to lymph nodes, where they are exposed to macrophages lining the sinus that act as a bacterial filter. Here, too, polymorphs, serum factors accumulating during inflammation, and the initiation of the immune response limit the infection. The phagocytic cells play a key role in the interaction with the microorganisms, ingesting and killing bacterial invaders. Among the chemoattractant factors for phagocytosis are platelet activating factor, leukotriene B4, C5a, and certain formyl peptides.[138] The details are fully described by Mims,[121] as are the ways in which some bacteria are able to resist or interfere with phagocytic activity. Organisms that escape must still face one or two encounters with the macrophages, as well as other immune mechanisms, before successfully reaching the venous system.

8.2. Systemic Infections

Organisms that escape phagocytic cells and the other local defense mechanisms can spread through the tissues and, more distantly, via the lymphatics and the bloodstream. Some viruses (herpes, HIV, poxviruses, measles), some rickettsiae (*R. rickettsii*, *R. prowazekii*), and some bacteria (*Mycobacterium tuberculosis*, *M. leprae*, *Listeria monocytogenes*, *Brucella* spp., and *Legionella pneumophila*) actually multiply in macrophages. The toxins, enzymes, and surface components of bacteria that protect them against phagocytic destruction and promote *invasiveness* have been mentioned in Section 4. It is not clear what exact role the proteinases, collagenases, lipases, and nucleases produced by bacteria play in the pathogenesis of infection or which ones are related to nutritional and bacterial metabolism.

Lymphatic spread may occur from the lymph node, which serves not only as a focus of phagocytic and immune forces but also, if these fail, as a focus of dissemination. These results occur when the lymph flow rate is high from inflammation of tissues or from exercise of muscles, when the number of bacterial particles exceeds the filtration rate or the defense mechanisms of the node or both, and when phagocytic activity is impaired. In some instances, certain organisms such as *Pasteurella pestis* and brucellosis actually multiply in the lymph node and spread via efferent lymph channels. In other instances, vigorous inflammatory responses localize the infection, and the node becomes a graveyard of dead and damaged bacteria and of tissue cells.

Bloodstream or hematogenous spread is the most effective mechanism for the dissemination of an infection throughout the body. Bacteria may exist free in the plasma (pneumococci, anthrax, *Leptospira*), intracellularly in monocytes (*Listeria*, tubercle and leprosy bacilli, *Brucella*), or in association with polymorphonuclear cells (many pyogenic bacteria). The *bacteremia* may be transient and with little or no systemic response, as follows dental extraction in a healthy person; even a continuous bacteremia may exist with few toxic signs, as in leprosy where the organism exists in large numbers inside blood monocytes. On the other hand, severe systemic manifestations may accompany the presence of large numbers of organisms in the blood such as the pneumococcus, meningococcus, or Group A *Streptococcus pyogenes*. This is called a *septicemia*. Bacteria may succeed in setting up foci of infection in areas where the blood flow is slow enough, or they may establish multiplication in sites previously damaged by disease or injury, such as *Streptococcus viridans* on abnormal heart valves producing subacute bacterial endocarditis; or staphylococci in the traumatized long bones of children may lead to osteomyelitis. Depending on the site of the infection, the liver and lung may receive many organisms during bacterial invasion of the bloodstream. The lung, liver, spleen, and bone marrow may also serve as important foci of dissemination of organisms, as in brucellosis, leptospirosis, and typhoid fever. Rashes accompany the dissemination of many viral and some bacterial infections to the skin. They may result from localization and growth of the organism in small blood vessels producing thrombosis, infarction, and hemorrhage as in the rickettsial diseases, Rocky Mountain spotted fever, and typhus, as well as the petechial and purpuric lesions of meningococcemia. Immunopathological processes involving sensitized lymphocytes, antibodies, and immune complexes play a role in many rashes, especially viral. A bacterial toxin may induce the rash as in scarlet fever. Some organisms such as *Treponema pallidum* in secondary syphilis extravasate from blood vessels and multiply in extravascular tissues. This results in highly infectious lesions that discharge to the exterior. Dissemination of *T. pallidum* to the blood–fetal junction in the placenta during pregnancy may result in infection of the fetus; slow blood flow in the placenta may contribute to this possibility.

Central nervous system (CNS) and meningeal involvement can occur by bloodstream carriage of the organism to the blood–cerebrospinal fluid junctions in the meninges or choroid plexus; from there, passive transport occurs into the flow of fluid from ventricles to subarachnoid spaces and throughout the CNS. Examples of bacteria that traverse this barrier and produce meningitis are the meningococcus, tubercle bacillus, *L. monocytogenes*, and *H. influenzae*. Actual spread along peripheral nerves has been shown for rabies and herpesviruses and is the means of centripetal passage of tetanus toxin.[126]

9. Incubation Period

The period of time from exposure to a source of infection to the first sign or symptoms of clinical illness is called the incubation period (IP). It varies with (1) the nature and dosage of the organism; (2) the portal of entry; (3) the type of the infection (localized or systemic); (4) the mechanism responsible for tissue injury (invasion, toxin, immunopathological process); (5) the immune status of the host,

being prolonged in the presence of partial immunity; and (6) other unknown factors individual to the host. The IP has many uses in epidemiology: (1) it helps define the etiological agent in an epidemic; (2) it helps differentiate common-source from propagated epidemics and to identify the reservoir and/or source of the agent; (3) it delineates the period for which a person exposed to an infection is at risk to development of disease; (4) it assists in identifying the period of infectiousness; (5) it provides a guide to the possible effectiveness of active or passive immunization; and (6) it gives clues to the pathogenesis of the disease.

The IPs of common bacterial diseases are given in Fig. 2. Signs and symptoms due to preformed toxins or associated with food poisoning usually occur within 36 h after ingestion, sometimes as soon as 2–4 h, as in diarrhea due to *Bacillus cereus* or staphylococcal contamination of food. Traveler's diarrhea due to toxigenic *E. coli* has an IP of 12–72 h. Pontiac fever, the term used to describe an acute febrile disease without pneumonia recognized first in a Pontiac, Michigan, health department clinic and due to *Legionella pneumophila*, has a peak IP of 36 h, as compared to a peak IP of 5 days for Legionnaires' disease (pneumonia). It is not known whether this difference is due to a larger number of organisms inhaled in Pontiac fever (unlikely because of the comparative mildness of the disease), to dead organisms, or to some other factor.

Diseases due to direct involvement of epithelial surfaces have relatively short IPs, often under a week, such as streptococcal sore throat, bacterial pneumonias, shigellosis, cholera, gonorrhea, and chancroid. This is not invariably true, since diphtheria and pertussis both tend to have an IP of over a week, sometimes up to 3 weeks, and *M. pneumoniae* pneumonia has an IP of 2–3 weeks. These organisms may be less pathogenic. Diseases with longer incubation periods in the range of 2–3 weeks include systemic infections such as typhoid fever and brucellosis. The IP of syphilis most commonly is 3 weeks, although it may be as short as 10 days. Leprosy has an extremely long IP of 7 months to over 5 years.

10. Immune Response

The immune system involves a complex interaction between B and T lymphocytes and macrophages. Rapid advances are being made in our understanding of the process, and the terminology to describe it is constantly changing. A current review of the basic elements of the human immune system[122] categorizes six tasks for our defense system: encounter, recognition, activation, deployment,

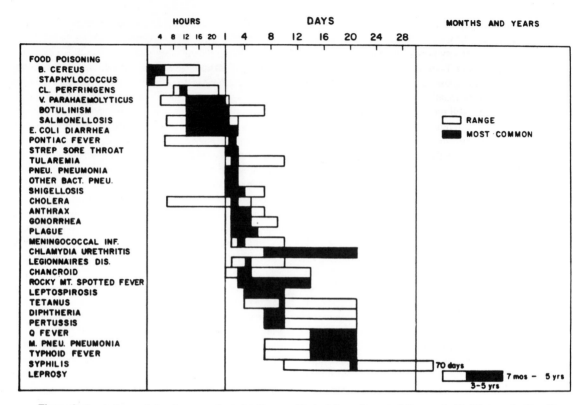

Figure 2. Incubation periods of common bacterial diseases. Derived from *Control of Communicable Diseases in Man.*[8]

discrimination, and regulation. The article provides an excellent description of the overall elements of the immune system. The description that now follows should be regarded as a simplistic and abbreviated one. The reader is urged to consult texts on microbiology[97,110,121] and immunology[5,93,130] as well as recent reviews[54,122] for more recent and detailed descriptions.

The immune response can be divided into that involved in antibody production, both humoral and local, and that concerned with cell-mediated immunity. The lymphocytes play a key and overlapping role in both. The B cells are relatively short-lived cells derived from bone marrow and constitute about 20% of the circulating small lymphocytes. They are destined to be active in antibody production after maturation into plasma cells. The T cells are longer-lived cells of thymus derivation that constitute about 60–80% of the small circulating lymphocytes; they play a key role in cellular immunity. Macrophages also play an important role in the immune response, including direct interaction with B and T cells. They process microbial and other antigens and present them to immune-reactive lymphocytes; this activity

is separate from their antimicrobial functions and may involve a separate subpopulation of macrophages. The macrophage also has receptors for IgG and the third component of complement on its surface. In the laboratory, B cells can be recognized by the presence of surface immunoglobulins, constant-fragment (Fc) receptors, and the receptor for C3d and Epstein–Barr virus on the membrane. Each B cell produces only one antibody but when a specific antigen is presented by a macrophage, rapid proliferation of that specific antibody-producing cell occurs. However, once produced, one antibody can unite with different antigens, and one antigen can unite with many antibodies.

The other arm of the immune system are the T lymphocytes, which are processed through the thymus gland where they develop high specificity for antigen recognition. They participate in both cellular and antibody functions. They have been shown to possess a receptor for antigen and for the major histocompatibility complex (MHC). While B-cell receptors can recognize antigen itself, T cells recognize antigen only in molecular association with restriction elements that are coded by the MHC. Several types of T cells have been identified by phenotypic and functional means. The most important are the CD8 or T8 suppressor/cytotoxic T lymphocytes whose activity is restricted by Class I MHC molecules, and the CD4 or T4-positive helper/inducer cells which are restricted by Class II molecules. In addition, there is a group of functionally defined effector lymphocytes that amplify killer cell proliferation (T_a cells), help B-cell proliferation and differentiation (T_h cells), and those cells involved in delayed-type hypersensitivity (T_d cells). Cells involved in cytotoxic activity include those designated as natural killer (NK) cells, human lymphokine-activated killer (LAK) cells, and the CD8, suppressor cell mentioned above. Lymphocytes produce soluble substances called lymphokines.[54] Lymphokines are polypeptide products of activated B and T cells, as well as other cells, which function as molecular signals between immunocompetent cells. Since neither their production nor their effects are restricted to lymphoid cells, the term *cytokine* is now being introduced.[54] No direct causal role has been established for these substances in any disease, although insufficient or excess production may contribute to certain disease states. Their release results from antigen stimulation of surface immunoglobulins on B lymphocytes and of the antigen receptor on T lymphocytes, but the lymphokines produced are independent of the specific stimulating antigen, as well as the histocompatibility antigens on the presenting macrophage. The lymphokines then function in a nonspecific fashion to amplify the immune response. The terminology for naming lymphokines (or cytokines) was changed in 1986 to account for their multiple functions. Once their amino acid sequence is established, they are designated numerically, i.e., as interleukin 1, 2, 3, and 4. For other lymphokines, whose amino acid sequence is not yet known, the name is derived from their biological property or properties, such as colony-stimulating factor (CSF), B-cell stimulating factor,[5] the interferons (α, β, γ), and tumor necrosis factor.[54,131]

The complex interactions of B and T lymphocytes no longer permit clear-cut differentiation into humoral and cell-mediated functions or immunity. Rather, it seems more appropriate to speak of B or T cell lymphocyte functions or immunity.

10.1. Humoral Immunity

Humoral immunity is mediated through the presence of antibody of various immunoglobulin classes in blood and body tissues. There are five immunoglobulin classes—IgM, IgG, IgA, IgD, and IgE—each with a specific biological function.

IgM antibodies comprise about 6% of the total immunoglobulin present in normal tissue and are the first to be synthesized in response to antigen stimulation. They have five times the number of antigen-reactive sites and Fc sites as IgG. These properties greatly enhance their agglutinating and complement fixing activity over that of IgG. Specific IgM antibodies are seen in some gram-negative bacterial and most viral infections. They are large molecules that do not cross the placenta but are the first to develop in the human fetus, appearing about the 12th week of gestation. The presence of IgM-specific antibodies to rubella, cytomegalovirus, toxoplasmosis, syphilis, or other antigens in the newborn infant thus indicates an intrauterine infection. After infancy, if rheumatoid factor (RF) can be excluded as the cause of the reaction, the presence of IgM-specific antibodies reflects a recent natural infection or immunization, since they are usually short-lived. However, it is now recognized that they may increase in repeated exposures, albeit to a lesser degree than IgG. In other instances, the persistence of antigen may stimulate IgM production over a long period. In general, their presence is usually a good indicator of a recent infection. The IgM antibody system exists largely within the bloodstream because of the large size of the molecules. It operates best as an opsonin, facilitating and cooperating with phagocytic activity. It can also immobilize bacteria by agglutination; IgM can lyse the cell walls of some gram-negative bacilli in the presence of complement.

IgG antibodies constitute about 80% of total immunoglobulin, of which 50–60% are in the blood and the rest in extracellular fluids. They are smaller in size than IgM molecules and thus diffuse actively across the placenta via the Fc fragment. They are long-lasting, show good precipitating activity, and are effective in neutralizing toxins. IgG antibodies can bind to bacteria, enhancing the process of phagocytosis, as well as coat target cells, preparing the way for killing. There are four subclasses of human IgG, which differ in some of these biological properties.

IgA antibodies are present in both the circulation and body secretions, the former representing about 13% of total immunoglobulin in the form of serum IgA. These antibodies reflect infection of mucosal surfaces of the body where they are called secretory IgA and constitute a defense mechanism at these locations, as well as in milk. In submucosal tissues the IgA molecules lack a secretory piece and enter the blood via lymphocytes to give increases in serum IgA levels in mucosal infections. Their role in local immunity is discussed in Section 10.2.

IgD antibodies have no known protective function; they are found on the surface of most B cells and may be involved in their maturation and memory.

IgE antibodies are found in minute amounts in normal sera, but increase greatly in persons with allergic reactivity of the antibody-mediated (immediate) type. IgE is produced by plasma cells, especially below respiratory and intestinal epithelia, attaches to mast cells where an antigen may react, releasing histamine and serotonin. Under normal circumstances, IgE acts as the "immunological" gatekeeper, playing on the release of histamine in the delivery of cells to sites of inflammation.

The production of antibody of various classes involves not only B cells but also T cells and macrophages. The T-cell interactions may either promote or suppress antibody production. Lymphocytes of a subclass called *helper* (T_h or CD4) cells promote the maturation of B cells to antibody-producing plasma cells when the T cells are presented with an antigen processed by a macrophage. The T_h cell releases two classes of soluble factors that affect B-cell activity: one is nonspecific and is generated by antigen-specific stimuli; the other is antigen-specific.

A few antibody responses are not dependent on T-cell cooperation, and these are due to T-cell-independent antigens such as pneumococcal polysaccharides and endotoxins. A second subclass of T cells can inhibit antibody production as well as hypersensitivity responses; such cells are called *suppressor* (T_s or CD8) cells. These suppress the immune responses not only to the presenting antigen but also to other antigens. There appear to be two populations of antigen-specific T_s cells. They elaborate different soluble products. One is called an initiating T_s cell and the other an effector T_s cell.[6]

The T-dependent antibody response involves macrophages. In addition to antigen-processing and presentation, macrophages produce at least five nonspecific lymphocyte-activating factors: T-cell-activating factor (TAF), B-cell-activating factor (BAF), thymocyte-differentiating factor (TDF), thymocyte mitogenic protein (TMP), and genetically related factor (GRF).[53] B-cell immune responses are under the control of *structural* genes for the polypeptide chain and immune-response (*Ir*) genes.

The humoral antibody response is thus a complex interaction in which B cells of high specificity mature and proliferate to produce various classes of specific immunoglobulins in response to an antigen in collaboration with specific and nonspecific interactions with certain T cells and macrophages and their soluble products. Antibody thus produced coats bacteria and renders them more susceptible to phagocytosis in the presence of complement. Antibody also neutralizes toxins such as diphtheria and tetanus.

Humoral antibody functions differently at different ages. In the infant, maternal antibodies of the IgG class that cross the placenta and secretory IgA antibodies in the milk protect the infant for about 6 months depending on the quantitative antibody titer in the mother. As this passive protection decreases, exposure to common microorganisms stimulates the immune response, usually without disease, because of the presence of maternal antibody. However, infections for which the mother may not have provided antibodies to the infant may produce devastating disease. As the child encounters other antigens, the total serum antibody rises with a peak at about age 5. In the elderly, humoral immunity, as well as cell- or T-cell-mediated immunity wanes, making them less resistant to both primary and reactivated infections. For example, some elderly persons in institutions are undergoing *primary* tuberculosis infections because of the loss of cell-mediated immunity, and some childhood infections such as *H. influenzae* type b are reappearing. The response to immunizations with various antigens such as hepatitis B, influenza, and perhaps pneumococcal polysaccharide vaccines is less than optimal in some of these persons, and clinical disease may occur.

10.2. Local Immunity

The presence of antigen-specific local antibody of the IgA class on epithelial surfaces is an important first line of defense. This antibody is provided with a secretory piece that transports it and confers on it the name "secretory IgA system." Secretory IgA antibody is present in various seromucous secretions such as tears, saliva, nasal secretions, colostrum, respiratory tract, and intestinal tract. Its highest concentration is in the gut, where it plays an important role in defense against intestinal pathogens. It can be locally synthesized, as shown in cholera and poliomyelitis infections. Stimulation of IgA antibody at local sites in immunization against influenza, poliomyelitis, cholera, and other epithelial pathogens is one reason that live and attenuated preparations are being developed and introduced through natural portals of entry.

A separate circulating system involves IgA-producing cells. An example of this is that B immunoblasts exposed in the gut to an antigen may migrate via lymphatics and the bloodstream to localize in salivary glands, lung, mammary glands, and elsewhere in the intestine, providing a mechanism for local, specific immune responses at these distant sites.

Newer diagnostic techniques permit sensitive detection of specific IgA antibody. The presence of IgA antibodies in the saliva can now be detected by capture radioimmunoassay (RIA) and ELISA, and the antibody level has been found to parallel that of serum.[124]

10.3. Cell-Mediated or T-Cell Immunity

This type of immunity plays a role during infection with certain organisms, in the course of immunity to soluble protein antigens, in the immune response against tumors and transplanted tissues, in contact sensitivity, and in certain autoimmune diseases.[7] Its role in infection is particularly important to organisms that survive or multiply intracellularly and against which humoral immunity is not fully effective, especially against cell-to-cell spread. These include most viruses, many fungi and protozoa, and intracellular bacteria such as *M. tuberculosis, S. typhosa, Brucella abortus,* and *L. monocytogenes.* Delayed hypersensitivity is a classic manifestation of cell-mediated immunity, as exemplified by the skin test for tuberculosis. Bacterial infections of this type tend to be chronic. In tuberculosis, the polymorphonuclear cell can ingest but not degrade the lipid capsule of the organism, which provides transport to deeper tissues. There is only a limited period of parasitism in the polymorphonuclear cells. Macrophages then ingest the organism, and through cell-mediated events, macrophage inhibition factor (MIF) and chemotactic factors are released, enhancing macrophage activity. This may result in granuloma formation, which walls off or localizes the infection. In severe tuberculosis, or in chronic bacterial infections such as leprosy, a state of *anergy* may develop with loss of delayed hypersensitivity to that and other, unrelated antigens. Some viral infections such as measles and infectious mononucleosis also induce a profound state of anergy and a severe depression of sensitized T-cell responses. These effects are probably mediated through the stimulation of T_s-cell activity alluded to in Section 10.1. This suppressor activity has been shown to be present in infectious mononucleosis.[137]

Cellular immunity is mediated largely through specific subclasses of T cells that bind antigen and, in cooperation with macrophages, release lymphokines and other soluble factors that induce a specific inflammatory response leading to elimination of the antigen. T cells are equally specific and sensitive as B cells in recognizing antigens. Some recognize a foreign antigen in association with host Ia antigen on the surface of the presenting macrophage. Once sensitized to a specific antigen, these cells divide, providing a geometrically expanded population of "memory cells" specifically committed to respond again only to that particular antigen. Responding T cells may (1) differentiate and release lymphokines, (2) trigger B cells to make antibody, (3) suppress and control the immune response (T_s cells). Other T cells recognize the foreign antigen only when it is present with histocompatibility antigens on the surface of host cells.

These are the cytotoxic T cells whose powerful action is activated only when in physical contact with host cells that bear the histocompatibility antigens. T lymphocytes produce three glycoproteins that enhance cell-mediated immunity: (1) interleukin 1 activates resting T cells, is a cofactor for hematopoietic growth, induces fever, sleep, ACTH release, neutrophilia, and other acute-phase responses; (2) interleukin 2 acts as a growth factor for activated T cells, induces the synthesis of other lymphokines and activates cytotoxic lymphocytes; and (3) γ-interferon induces Class I, Class II (DR), and other surface antigens on a variety of cells, activates macrophages and endothelial cells against intracellular pathogens, augments or inhibits other lymphokine activities, augments natural killer activity, and inhibits viral replication.[54]

In viral infections, two important specificities have been shown for sensitized "cytotoxic" lymphocytes: first, for the virus and virus-infected cell to which it has been exposed and the antigens which it can recognize on the target-cell surface; second, for the self component coded for in the *H-2* major histocompatibility complex (MHC), and also represented on the target-cell membrane.[146] The virus-specific cytotoxic T cells are restricted by the *K* and *D* regions of *H-2.* These cytotoxic T cells may be beneficial in destroying virus-infected cells, but can also be detrimental if such cells form part of a vital organ. Most of these studies have been made in experimental viral infections in mice, such as lymphocytic choriomeningitis (LCM). Less is known about cytotoxic T cells in bacterial infections, but studies of *L. monocytogenes* infections in mice indicate that dual specificity of such T cells also applies to intracellular bacteria.[142,146]

Primary bacterial infections in which recovery is mainly dependent on cell-mediated immunity include tuberculosis, leprosy, and typhoid fever. Resistance to reinfection in tuberculosis and leprosy, as well as to reactivated or latent infections with tuberculosis, yeast, and the protozoan *Pneumocystis carinii,* are also dependent on cell-mediated immunity.

Three major types of host–parasite interactions are possible for facultative intracellular bacteria, as based on murine models of listeriosis[102]: (1) activation of host cells with high antibacterial potential, such as phagocytes containing bacteria in association with Class II molecules, which are then recognized by helper T cells, resulting in excretion of macrophage-activation factors which can eliminate intracellular bacteria. (2) Lysis of host cells with low antibacterial potential, such as those of nonmyeloid origin, and are associated with Class I molecules. Class I-restricted cytolytic lymphocytes have the potential to recognize and lyse most such infected cells. Class II expression can be induced in certain nonmyeloid cells by interferon. (3) Lysis of host cells with high antibacterial potential such as mononuclear phagocytes, which express both Class I and Class II molecules, and are thus targets for both lymphokine activation as well as cytolytic cells. The release and dissemination of bacteria in this process may be detrimental to the host. The MHC-coded structures involved in effective bacterial response are coded in the *I* region rather than the *K* or *D* region. The selective expression of *I*-region markers on macrophages and certain lymphocytes is compatible with bacterial infections, as compared with the broader range of cells susceptible to viral infection and the ubiquitous cellular expression of *K* or *D*.

Another type of cell important in cellular immunity is the killer (K) cells, which have Fc receptors but no surface immunoglobulins and which are cytotoxic to target cells coated with antibody [antibody-dependent cellular cytotoxicity (ADCC)]. Finally, in addition to B and T cells recognizable by specific surface markers, there are so-called natural killer (NK) cells. These cells do not require sensitization for their generation, occur naturally, and are thought to be involved in nonspecific killing of virally transformed target cells, in allografts, and in tumor rejection. Their role in bacterial infections has not been defined. In summary, four effector-cell types involved in cellular immunity include B and T cells (T_s and T_h), macrophages, K cells, and NK cells. Much remains to be learned of the action and interaction of these cells in host defense against various infections and of many subclasses of T cells.

11. Patterns of Host Response

The clinician usually deals with persons already ill with an infectious disease severe enough for them to seek medical care. The epidemiologist must study not only those clinically ill but also the full range of host responses that follow infection. These can vary *quantitatively* from inapparent infection to severe illness to death in what is called a *biological gradient*. They can also vary *qualitatively* in different signs and symptoms that make up different clinical syndromes.

11.1. Biological Gradient

When a susceptible host is exposed to a source of infection, a wide range of quantitative responses may occur.[68] These are often depicted as an iceberg, as shown in

Fig. 3, with the largest number of responses occurring subclinically, below the waterline of clinical recognition. The right side of Fig. 3 represents the responses of the whole organism. These range subclinically from exposure without successful attachment or multiplication of the bacterial organism, to colonization without tissue injury, to infection that evokes a host immune response but no clinical disease. The existence of these inapparent events can be recognized only by laboratory means such as isolation of the organism or measurement of the immune response. In viral infections, the ratio of inapparent/apparent (subclinical/clinical) infection has been determined through prospective studies correlating the number with an antibody response to the number clinically ill. The occurrence of inapparent infections is also suggested in persons with antibody but no history of clinical disease. Some information has also come from the rate of secondary infection in families with an index case and from volunteer studies. This type of information is not available for most bacterial infections because serological techniques are not as useful and/or widely employed in measuring infection rates, but a few examples may be cited. In leptospirosis, serological tests of persons heavily exposed (veterinarians, abattoir workers) but without known illness have shown an antibody prevalence of 16%. This suggests that only 16 of 100 *exposed* persons have been *infected* as manifested by an antibody response. There are no data for leptospirosis indicating the subclinical/clinical ratio, but of those *clinically* ill, 90% or so have an acute, self-limited illness without jaundice and with good prognosis; the overall case-fatality rate in 791 cases reported to the CDC from 1965 to 1974 was 7.7% (see Chapter 17). In tuberculosis, it was estimated that of the 50,000 clinical cases reported in 1963, 80% came from the 24 million infected in previous years and 20% from persons infected the same year (see Chapter 36).

In summary, a wide range of quantitative and qualitative responses can occur on exposure to a pathogenic organism. The determinants of this pattern lie both in the pathogenicity and virulence of the infecting organism (see Section 4) and in the age, genetic makeup,[146] immune response, portal of entry, and other characteristics of the host (see Section 6).

The left side of Fig. 3 is a simplistic expression of the response to bacterial infection at the cellular level. Cell injury may result from enzymes and other metabolic products of bacteria, from toxins produced by them, from entry and multiplication of the organisms intracellularly as with *M. tuberculosis*, *M. leprae*, *B. abortus*, or as a consequence of the phagocytic and immunological defense mechanisms induced by the infection. Epidemiologically, the message is

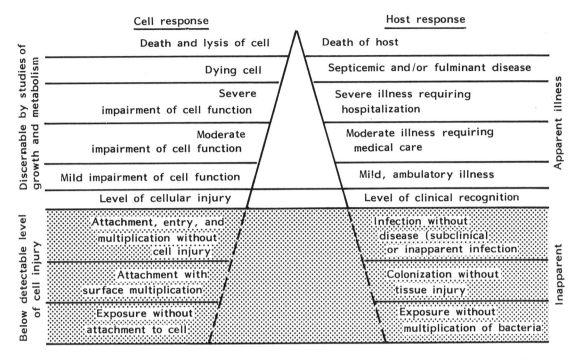

Figure 3. Biological spectrum of response to bacterial infection at the cellular level (*left*) and of the intact host (*right*).

that most organisms do not result in cell dysfunction or death and that the healthy person lives in symbiosis with millions of bacteria.

11.2. Clinical Syndromes

The host can show *qualitative* as well as quantitative differences in response to the same bacterial infection. These qualitative responses are manifested by different clinical syndromes, the patterns of which depend on the portal of entry of the organism, age of the host at the time of infection, immune status, and other factors. This variation is not as great with bacterial infections as with viral infections. Many bacterial infections such as anthrax, cholera, diphtheria, leprosy, pertussis, tetanus, tularemia, and typhoid fever present with fairly characteristic clinical features that vary quantitatively, but not qualitatively, from host to host, and a diagnosis can often be made on clinical grounds alone. Others such as streptococcal infections, leptospirosis, syphilis, and tuberculosis may involve different tissues and organs in different persons, resulting in different clinical presentations depending on the site and age group involved. On the other hand, there are many *clinical syndromes* of diverse cause in which etiological diagnosis is difficult on clinical grounds alone. It is here that epidemiological probabilities will help clinical judgment. Infections of mucosal and serosal surfaces fall into this category because of the limited spectrum of local responses that can result. These can involve the meninges, respiratory tract, intestinal tract, urinary system, and urethra. Invasion of the bloodstream (septicemia) by different bacteria also invokes a common group of signs and symptoms that may be difficult to differentiate etiologically.

This section will present some of the common causes of these clinical syndromes that may vary with the age of the person at the time of infection.

11.2.1. Infections of the CNS. Meningitis is a common clinical syndrome caused by bacteria, viruses, fungi, and protozoa. The clues that suggest bacterial infections are polymorphonuclear leukocytosis in blood and cerebrospinal fluid (CSF) ($500-20,000/mm^3$), low CSF glucose concentrations (usually < 35 mg/100 ml or CSF/serum ratio ≤ 0.5), elevated CSF protein ($80-500$ mg/100 ml), and in about 75%, the presence of bacteria in the Gram-stained smear of a centrifuged sample of CSF. These findings characterize purulent meningitis, but may be altered by treatment with antibiotics so that they resemble nonpurulent bacterial infections, such as *M. tuberculosis* and leptospirosis, or viral meningitis.

The etiological agents that produce meningitis in different age groups will vary some by geographic area, year, and socioeconomic level.

The age-specific incidence per 100,000 of various types of meningitis by age group is presented in Table 9 from an excellent review article on the diagnosis and management of meningitis by Klein *et al.*,[104] which incorporates data from the CDC and a National Surveillance Study by Schlech *et al.*[132] The overall incidence of meningitis is highest in the newborn, drops in the first 2 months of life, and then rises to high levels between 3 and 8 months of life. Based on a National Surveillance Study of 18,642 cases reported from 1973 to 1981, *H. influenzae* accounted overall for 48.3% of the cases, *N. meningitidis* for 19.3%, and *S. pneumoniae* for 13.3%.[132] Rates in males exceeded females (3.3 versus 2.6 per 100,000). By age, the most common causes were as follows: in the newborn, Group B streptococcus and *E. coli;* in infants, *H. influenzae* type b and *N. meningitidis;* in toddlers, similar to the newborn; and in school children and adolescents, *S. pneumoniae, N. meningitidis,* and *H. influenzae* are the major pathogens in the decreased number of cases in that age group. These etiological agents are in general similar to those found in the previous studies of Wehrle[141] in the period 1963–1970, as summarized in the previous edition of this book.[71] In another and earlier analysis of meningitis in the over-40 age group by Benner and Hoeprich,[9] pneumococci accounted for half the cases, and *E. coli,* meningococci, and staphylococci each produced about 10%.

The characteristics of the organisms involved and the patterns of disease can be found in the individual chapters of this book. Suffice it to mention here that in the newborn, most cases of Group B streptococci are due to subtype III and that infection usually arises from vaginal and rectal infections of the mother that can lead to a 40–70% infection rate in the newborn; the K1 antigen of *E. coli* is involved in 75% of neonatal meningitis, and *L. monocytogenes* is becoming increasingly important in meningitis in this age group in several areas of the country.[104] In children beyond the newborn period, head trauma may precede the onset of meningitis and organisms may then enter through the cribiform plate or the paranasal sinuses. Meningitis may also follow neurosurgical procedures or osteomyelitis of the skull or vertebral column.[104]

Acute bacterial meningitis is a medical emergency, and it is most important to establish the identity of the infecting organisms as quickly as possible as a guide to antibiotic therapy. However, until this is done, the data in Table 9 and a Gram-stained smear of the CSF should provide a reasonable basis for initial chemotherapy.

11.2.2. Acute Respiratory Infections. These represent the commonest cause of morbidity in the developed world. Their importance as a cause of both morbidity and mortality in developing countries has recently been recognized and major programs of control have been initiated under the auspices of the World Health Organization. In a comprehensive review of the incidence, causes, and management of these infections in Third World countries, Berman and McIntosh[12] estimate that over 4 million children under the age of 5 die annually of pneumonia, which represents some 30% of the 14.25 million deaths in this age group yearly. For the developed world, the causes of common respiratory diseases are listed in Table 10. Fewer than 10% of acute *upper* respiratory infections (AURIS) are due

Table 9.   Annual Age-Specific Incidence of Meningitis, United States, 1978 to 1981[a]

Age	*Neisseria meningitidis*	*Haemophilus influenzae*	*Streptococcus pneumoniae*	Group B *streptococcus*	*Listeria monocytogenes*	Total meningitis
<1 mo	2.0	6.7	3.5	44.6	7.6	99.5
1–2 mo	9.1	18.6	5.7	10.0	1.3	56.7
3–5 mo	11.5	52.0	11.6	1.4	0.1	83.3
6–8 mo	10.6	65.1	8.0	0.3	0	88.4
9–11 mo	7.9	48.1	4.7	0	0.1	63.3
1–2 yr	3.8	19.0	1.5			25.3
3–4 yr	1.8	3.9	0.5			6.8
5–9 yr	0.7	0.7	0.3			2.0
10–19 yr	0.6	0.1	0.1			1.0

[a]Results are reported as numbers of children with meningitis per 100,000 population. Data were provided by C. V. Broome, Centers for Disease Control, Atlanta, and by Schlech *et al.*[132] From Ref. 104.

Table 10. Bacterial Causes of Acute Respiratory Infections in Different Age Groups[a]

Clinical syndromes	Age group	Bacteria	Estimated contribution to etiology of syndrome
Epiglottitis	9 mo–2 yr	*H. influenzae* type b	90%
Pharyngitis–tonsillitis	Young adult	Group A streptococci	25–30%
Laryngotracheitis	Children	Pertussis	5%
Bronchitis	Children and adults	*M. pneumoniae*	10–15%
Pneumonia 1	< 6 mo	*Chlamydia trachomatis*	30%
2	Young children	*H. influenzae* type b, pneumococci	15–20%
3	Young adults	*M. pneumoniae*	25–50%
4	Adults	Pneumococci	40–45%
5	Older adults	Pneumococci	54%
		H. influenzae type b and untypable	17%
		Klebsiella pneumoniae	8%
6	Superinfection during antibiotic therapy in 18 older adults	*K. pneumoniae*	11%
		S. aureus	33%
		E. coli	11%
		P. mirabilis	17%
		P. aeruginosa	17%

[a]Modified from Fedson and Rusthoven[73] and from Refs. 46, 60, 81, 91, and 133.

to bacteria in either developed or developing countries, although in the latter, infections with *Bordetella pertussis* and *M. pneumoniae* are important in certain settings. The syndrome of epiglottis in children aged 6 months to 2 years (up to age 6), however, is due to a bacterial pathogen, *H. influenzae* type b in about 90% of cases worldwide. This is often a serious and fulminant infection with a high mortality.

The viruses involved in AURIS in both developing and developed countries are respiratory syncytial virus (RSV) in children under 3 years of age, parainfluenza in older children, and coronaviruses, rhinoviruses, and influenza in all ages.

The syndrome of acute pharyngitis and tonsillitis is due to streptococcal infections, mostly Group A, in about one-fourth to one-third of cases, another one-third are due to various viruses, and the remainder are of unidentified cause, although chlamydial infections may play a role in some of these.[70] Streptococcal infections can lead to acute rheumatic fever; this disease had been disappearing rapidly in developed countries until very recently when a recrudescence was reported in several areas of the United States. In developing countries, some 1.2 episodes of rheumatic fever are said to occur for every 1000 untreated streptococcal infections but this, too, seems to be decreasing.[12] *Corynebacterium diphtheriae* is also a cause of exudative tonsillitis in some Third World countries, and a recent outbreak

occurred in Sweden involving 17 cases and 3 deaths despite very high immunization coverage.[127]

Acute *lower* respiratory infections are due mostly to viruses in young children, except for infants, to *M. pneumoniae* and viruses in young adults, and to bacterial pathogens in older adults and the elderly. Prospective studies in community settings of developed countries suggest that five agents—RSV, parainfluenza virus, influenza virus, adenovirus, and *M. pneumoniae*—account for some 80% of acute lower respiratory infections in these population groups.[12]

Common respiratory syndromes in young children such as croup, laryngotracheitis, and bronchiolitis are usually due to viruses, especially RSV and parainfluenza viruses. Diphtheria may also cause a croup syndrome when the toxic membrane involves the larynx. Acute bronchitis may be due to *M. pneumoniae* in 15–16% of older children and young adults.[52] Chronic bronchitis, on the other hand, is largely associated with nontypable *H. influenzae* and pneumococci (*S. pneumoniae*). Pneumonia has varied causes at varied ages. In infancy (under 6 months), about 30% are now recognized as a gradually developing nontoxic illness with cough, pulmonary congestion, rales, and patchy infiltrates on X-ray (see Chapter 9). Chlamydial genital infection of the mother carries a 10–20% risk of pneumonia in her infant.[92] In another study of 205 infants under 3 months old hospitalized with pneumonitis, Brasfield *et al.*[17] identified a causal agent in 70%. *C. trachomatis* was found in 36%, RSV in 23%, cytomegalovirus in 20%, *Pneumocystis carinii* in 17%, and *Ureaplasma urealyticum* in 16%. In *older children,* the causes of pneumonia are roughly one-fourth viral, one-third unknown cause, and the rest bacterial.[46,73] More careful bacteriological culturing techniques have identified a bacterial etiology in 15–50% of this age group: pneomococci (*S. pneumoniae*) are the most common organism and *H. influenzae* next most common; rarely, *Staphylococcus aureus* and Group A streptococci are involved.

A review of the bacteriological aspirates in children with pneumonia from many countries revealed a bacterial agent in 62% of 1029 cases: *H. influenzae* and *S. pneumoniae* accounted for 54% of all isolates while *Staphylococcus aureus* was responsible for 17%.[12] Viral infections were associated with 17–40% of pneumonia in hospitalized children in several developing countries.[12]

The true role of *Chlamydia* and *M. pneumoniae* infections in childhood respiratory infections has not been well studied yet because of technical problems with the laboratory diagnosis, but it seems likely they may play as important a role as in developed countries. In *young adults,* such as college students, etiological studies have shown the main bacterial agent of importance to be *M. pneumoniae,* which accounts for 25–50% of hospitalized cases.[52,72] It has also been shown to be a common infection of military recruits in Argentina, Colombia, and the United States[45,61] and is probably worldwide in military populations. A new chlamydial strain, designated as TWAR (for Taiwan acute respiratory), has recently been shown to be an important pathogen in acute respiratory infections of young adults.[84] It may also play a role in childhood respiratory infections. While this organism has the highest infection rate in younger children, these are usually clinically mild. Even among patients of all ages with *Mycoplasma* pneumonia, only about 2% require hospitalization.[52] The secondary intrafamilial infection rate is high after an index case of *M. pneumoniae* is introduced and involves about 84% of children and 41% of adults.[79] In *adults,* most of the pneumonias are bacterial in origin, of which 50–90% are due to pneumococci (*S. pneumoniae*) in hospitalized patients, as are about 20% in those not requiring hospitalization. *Staphylococcus aureus* and untypable *Haemophilus pneumoniae* account for most of the rest of community-acquired infections[75] and *Legionella pneumophila* is involved in the hospital setting.

Pneumonia accounts for about 10% of all admissions to general hospital wards. The distribution of organisms isolated from 149 cases of primary pneumonia in *older adults* at the Boston City Hospital[135] is shown in Fig. 4. Pneumococci (*S. pneumoniae*) accounted for 53.7% of the cases in older adults, *H. influenzae* for 16.8%, and *K. pneumoniae* for 8.1%. The remaining 21.4% were due to a variety of organisms including double infections in 2.7% and 7.4% of unknown cause. In this series, the average age was 63 years, and 70% were male. In these 149 pneumonia patients, bacteremia was demonstrable in 18 (12%) of which 14 were due to *S. pneumoniae.* In the total series of 149 patients, 14 died of primary pneumonia, 16 of secondary pneumonia, and 5 of other causes for an overall mortality of 23.5%. After the start of antibiotic therapy, a significant increase in organisms in sputum occurred in 88 of 149 (59%). These resulted in 18 secondary pneumonias (of which 16 died) due to the bacteria listed in the lower part of Table 10. There has been a shift in the bacteria involved in primary pneumonia with time; Reimann[128] indicates that 98% were due to pneumococci in 1948 and only 54% in 1969. Increasing percentages are now caused by *H. influenzae, K. pneumoniae,* and gram-negative organisms.

11.2.3. Acute Otitis Media. This common infection in childhood is primarily due to bacteria, including *M. pneumoniae,* which produces a bullous meningitis. About one-third of the cultures of fluid aspirated from the middle ears of patients with acute otitis media are bacteriologically sterile. Viruses are occasionally involved, including RSV, parainfluenza, influenza A, coxsackie, and adenoviruses. Among the bacterial causes of acute suppurative ear infec-

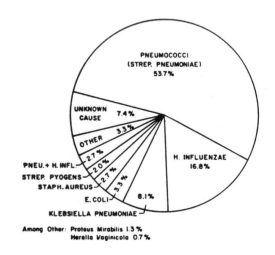

Figure 4. Bacterial causes of primary pneumonia in 149 cases at the Boston City Hospital. From Tillotson and Finland.[135]

tions, the pneumococci (*S. pneumoniae*) predominate and are associated with over 50% of all cases at all ages; *H. influenzae* is an important cause in infancy and sometimes in older children and adults, especially the nontypable strains.[82] *H. influenzae* otitis media may be associated with infectious meningitis, buccal cellulitis, or septicemia. Group A streptococci (*S. pyogenes*) were common agents of acute otitis media in the prepenicillin days, but now are involved in only 10–15% of cases. In a long-term longitudinal study of respiratory infections in young children by Henderson *et al.*[88] prior viral infections were found to increase the relative risk of acute otitis media with effusion (OME) by a factor of 3.9. RSV, influenza A and B, and adenovirus infections conferred the greatest risk. *S. pneumoniae* and *H. influenzae* and/or streptococci were the common organisms in the nasopharynx of patients with OME.

11.2.4. Intestinal Infections and Intoxications. These may be divided into foodborne poisons and intestinal infections. The major features are given in Table 11.

a. Bacterial Food Poisoning. This condition is dealt with in more detail in Chapter 4. The most common causes were reported by Sours and Smith from 1972–1978.[134] In a later analysis of 656 outbreaks reported to CDC in 1982, 222 (34%) were of confirmed cause.[114] In the most recent analysis, published in December 1988 (CDC, personal communication), there were 185 confirmed reported outbreaks from 1983 to 1986, which involved 5776 cases. Bacterial causes accounted for 82.3% of the cases, viruses for 11.5%, chemicals for 4.8%, and parasites for 1.4%. *Salmonella* caused 46.5% of the total cases, *Shigella* 12.2%, and hemolytic streptococci, *Campylobacter, C. perfringens,* and *B. cereus* 3–4% each. It should be emphasized that food outbreaks are greatly underreported.

b. Intestinal Infections (see Table 11). The causes of enteric infections vary with age and geographic area. In this book, they are dealt with under *Campylobacter* (Chapter 7), cholera (Chapter 10), *E. coli* (Chapter 12), salmonellosis (Chapter 28), shigellosis (Chapter 29), typhoid fever (Chapter 39), and yersiniosis (Chapter 40). In children, viruses play a predominant role in some seasons, and the rotaviruses may cause about half the cases of acute diarrhea on a worldwide basis.[51,145] In 378 cases of childhood diarrhea studied by Davidson *et al.*[51] in Australia, rotavirus was identified in 52%, *Salmonella* in 11%, adenovirus in 7%, *E. coli* in 2%, enterovirus in 2%, and *Shigella* species in 1%; no cause could be identified in 25%. Among the bacterial agents in the United States, *E. coli* is responsible for some 15–20% of cases of acute diarrhea in children and *Shigella* for some 10–20% in persons of all

ages.[55,56] In the United States, there were 72,877 isolates of enteric bacteria reported to the CDC in 1978.[28] By 1985 the number of reported cases of enteric infections had increased to 87,241 of which 40.5% were salmonellosis, 19.5% shigellosis, 5.1% amebiasis, and there were 404 cases of typhoid fever.[37] Viral infections, such as those due to rotavirus and Norwalk agent, are not reportable. *E. coli* infections are also not included in the reportable infections, but there was evidence of the importance of enteropathogenic *E. coli* (EPEC) in infancy, where nursery epidemics occurred, and of enterotoxigenic *E. coli* (ETEC) in acute diarrheas of adults who traveled to Mexico, Asia, and Central America. In indigenous populations, ETEC strains have been incriminated primarily in childhood diarrhea in North America, but have been responsible for severe adult diarrhea in Asia and Central America. In the United States, this noninvasive ETEC was associated with over 80% of moderate to severe pediatric diarrheal disease at a major hospital in Chicago.[83]

Campylobacter enteritis is also an increasingly recognized cause of intestinal infections in the United States, Great Britain, and Australia, accounting for some 5–14% of the cases in several large series[8] (see Chapter 7). Outbreaks may also occur, such as the one in Bennington, Vermont, in 1978. The incubation period is 1–4 days. Sources of possible infection include poultry (alive or dressed), dogs, raw milk, and contaminated water. The clinical disease is characterized by watery diarrhea with mucus, blood, or pus, often cramping abdominal pain and fever, and sometimes gross blood in the stools of children. *Yersinia enterocolitica* is another recently recognized cause of acute diarrhea attended by some cramps, fever, and occasionally a rash; the incubation period is 1–3 days. There may be associated mesenteric adenitis, arthritis, and erythema (see Chapter 40).

11.2.5. Acute Urinary-Tract Infections. The most common causes of acute urinary-tract infections as determined in a large study of inpatients and outpatients at six centers are shown in Table 12. In a more recent compilation of etiological agents in hospitalized cases, Andriole[2] found 38% due to *E. coli,* 16.4% due to *P. mirabilis,* 10.1% due to *K. pneumoniae,* and less than 6% each due to other causes.

11.2.6. Sexually Transmitted Diseases. The term *sexually transmitted diseases* (STDs) encompasses the five classic venereal diseases (gonorrhea, syphilis, chancroid, lymphogranuloma venereum, granuloma inguinale) plus newly identified infectious agents (*Chlamydia trachomatis,* herpes simplex, *Ureaplasma*) the transmission of which is associated with sexual activity.[76,86,100,119,120] Hepatitis A and B are also common infections in 30–40% of active

Table 11. Practical Classification of Acute Enteric Diseases: Correlation of Clinical and Epidemiological Characteristics with Specific Causative Agent[a]

| | Signs and symptoms | | | | | | | | | | Epidemiological features | |
| | Upper GI tract | | | Lower GI tract | | | Systemic manifestations | | | | | |
Causative agent	Nausea	Vomiting	Cramps	Diarrhea	Mucus	Blood	Headache	Muscle aches	Fever	Rash	Spread to contacts	Incubation period
I. Poisoning, intoxications, and infections that produce exotoxins												
A. Chemicals (e.g., heavy metals; arsenic, cockroach powder)	++++	++++	++++	0	0	0	0	0	0		0	Minutes
B. Staphylococcal enterotoxin food poisoning	++++	++++	++++	+++	0	0	±	0	0		0	½–7 h
C. *C. perfringens* food poisoning	±	±	+++	+++	0	0	0	0	0		0	9–18 h
D. *V. parahemolyticus* food poisoning	±	+	+++	+++	0	0	±	±	±		0	12–24 h
E. *E. coli* diarrhea, enterotoxic (LT and ST) strains	±	±	+	+++	±	0	0	0	±		?	1–2 days
F. Cholera	±	±	0	++++	+	±	0	(Muscle cramps —late)	±		±–0	1–4 days
G. *B. cereus* (two forms)	++	++	++	±	0	0	0	0	0		0	3–7 h[b]
	+	0	++	++	0	0	0	0	0		0	8–16 h[c]

II. Enteric bacterial and parasitic infections with varying degrees of tissue invasion

A. Bacterial

										Incubation period
1. Salmonellosis	±	+	+++	+	+	+	+	++	±	12–48 h
2. Shigellosis	±	+	+++	++	++	++	++	++++	++	1–5 days
3. E. coli, enteroinvasive strains	±	±	+++	+	±	+	+	++	?	1–3 days
4. Enteric fevers (paratyphoid and typhoid)	+ (variable)	+	+ (variable)	+	+	++++	+++++	+++++	±	5–35 days

B. Parasitic

5. Amebiasis (amebic dysentery)	±	±	++ (chronic)	++	+	+	+	+	0	1–4 weeks
6. Giardiasis	+	+	++ᵈ	0	0	0	0	0	0	7–21 days

C. Recently recognized bacterial enteric infections

7. Yersiniosis (Yersinia enterocolitica)	±	+	++	0	0	±	0	++	?	1–3 daysᵉ
8. Campylobacteriosis (Campylobacter species)	±	±	++	+	+	±	±	++	?	1–3 days

ᵃDerived from Langmuir and Gangarosa.[108]
ᵇEmetic form. Fried rice implicated. Simulates staphylococcal food poisoning.
ᶜSimulates clostridial food poisoning.
ᵈBulky, greasy, malodorous stools.
ᵉDiarrheal form. Often associated with mesenteric adenitis (appendicitis), arthritis, and erythema nodosum.

Table 12.   Distribution of Causes of Urinary Infection in Six Centers[a]

| Organism | With organism (percent) | |
	Inpatients (17,411)	Outpatients (6080)
E. coli	47	64
Proteus mirabilis	21	15
Klebsiella aerogenes	7	4
"Coliformis"	17	9
Gram-positive[b]	8	8
	100	100

[a] From McAllister *et al.*[118]
[b] Included *Streptococcus faecalis, Staphylococcus albus,* and *Staphylococcus reus.*

homosexual males as are many enteric infections. HIV, the cause of AIDS and the AIDS-related complex (ARC), now dominates concern about STDs among homosexuals and more recently among heterosexual contacts and their children. As of July 1989, 100,000 cases of AIDS have been reported in the United States to the CDC, about half of whom have died thus far. In addition, there are many other manifestations of HIV infection that do not fall into the official and reported cases, such as the AIDS-related complex. There are also an estimated 1.5 million HIV-infected persons in the United States of whom some 80% or higher will, over time, develop AIDS or some other manifestation of infection. About two-thirds of AIDS cases are currently homosexual or bisexual persons but the number of i.v. drug-associated cases is slowly rising and exceeding that of homosexuals in New York City and some other urban centers. It is estimated that in 1992, some 80,000 new cases of AIDS and 54,000 deaths will occur, with a cumulative total by then of 365,000.[38] Worldwide, some 377,000 cases have been reported to the World Health Organization and there are an estimated 5 million HIV-infected persons; 1.5 million have been infected in the United States of which about 70% have been homosexuals. About half of the AIDS cases have died. The number of cases in 1991 is estimated at 74,000 with 54,000 deaths.[38]

Many of these newer agents account for as many as or more than the number of genital infections seen in STD clinics or by private physicians than are accounted for by the classic causes. These infections are most common in the 15–30 age group—the time of greatest sexual activity, especially extramarital. They are more commonly diagnosed

in men both because men tend to have more sexual partners than do women (except prostitutes) and because the lesions are more apparent in men. Multiple infections are common in both sexes, and gonorrhea and syphilis should be excluded by appropriate examination in every patient seen with an STD. The changing nature of and the increase in these infections have several causes, including the use of measures other than the condom for contraception, changing practices in heterosexual and homosexual activities, especially involving genital–mouth and genital–anal contact, the importation of infection from Southeast Asia, and increased public confidence in the availability and effectiveness of antibiotic therapy.

The wide spectrum of infections in homosexual males in urban settings poses a special problem for control. The number of cases of gonorrhea reported to the CDC in 1985 was 911,419, a rate of 384.5 per 100,000, and of primary and secondary syphilis 27,131 cases, a rate of 11.5 per 100,000.[37] After a decreasing incidence of syphilis over the previous 5 years, an increase of 23% was reported during early 1987 as compared with 1986. The estimated rate rose to 13.3 per 100,000. These increases were primarily in heterosexuals in Florida, California, and New York City. It is of particular concern because the heterosexual population may be exposed to HIV in these areas and syphilis in AIDS patients has been difficult to treat.[41] In addition, a penile lesion increases the risk of HIV infection. However, there is marked underreporting of both these infections, especially gonorrhea, and many of the newly recognized causes of STD are not reportable at all. Therefore, their true incidence is unknown. An estimate of their relative importance has been obtained by the CDC[98] through an examination of the reason for visits to STD clinics in 12 cities from 1977 to 1985. Of 322,233 visits of men to the clinic, gonorrhea accounted for 22.3% and syphilis for 1.7%.[98] Of 130,320 clinic visits of women, 20.6% were due to gonorrhea, 1.4% to syphilis, and 10.9% to trichomonas vaginitis. Genital herpes represented 2.3% of clinic visits in men and 1.6% in women. Similar data have been reported in Canada.[136]

The increasing importance of chlamydial and herpetic infections deserves emphasis. Chlamydial genital infections include urethritis, acute epididymitis in men, and pelvic inflammatory disease in women; these are discussed in Chapter 9 and in a review.[92] Overall, about half the cases of urethritis in men are nongonococcal, and among male college students, this rises to 80–90%. *C. trachomatis* is responsible for 30–50% of these cases of nongonococcal urethritis (NGU) and is more common in white than in black men and in higher than in lower socioeconomic levels. Its incubation period appears to be longer than that of gonorrhea (GC), and symptoms of urethritis in males may appear 2–3 weeks after penicillin or spectinomycin treatment for GC, involving one-third to two-thirds of these men.[92] Oral therapy of NGU with tetracycline or erythromycin hastens recovery. There is no clinical counterpart of NGU in women who develop chlamydial infections of the cervix with or without cervicitis, but this organism may be involved in up to 30% of pelvic inflammatory diseases in females.[92] The other agents of NGU in men are uncertain, although *Ureaplasma urealyticum* (formerly T-strain *Mycoplasma*) and *Mycoplasma hominis* are important candidates. Because there is no easy, practical method available at present for diagnosis of chlamydial infections, most cases of acute urethritis with overt leukocytic exudate and no *N. gonorrhoeae* on smear are usually treated with tetracycline or erythromycin; a culture confirming the absence of *N. gonorrhoeae* should be made.

For detailed information on STD infections, see Chapter 9 on chlamydial infections, Chapter 13 on gonococcal infections, and Chapter 32 on syphilis.

11.2.7. Hospital Infections. Infections acquired after admission (nosocomial infections) are discussed in detail in Chapter 22. In 1984 there were 26,965 hospital-acquired infections reported from the 51 hospitals participating in the National Nosocomial Infections Surveillance Program of the CDC, which represents a biased sample of all U.S. hospitals.[30,34,94] Of these, 64% were caused by a single pathogen and 20% by multiple pathogens (Fig. 5). No pathogens were found in 6% and no culture was done in 10%. In the 84% of known cause, 86% were due to anaerobic bacteria, 2% to aerobic bacteria, and 8% to fungi. With

regard to the 1970 data from CDC,[18] which were used in the previous edition of this book,[71] the major enteric pathogens were similar: in 1984, *E. coli* (17.8%), *P. aerugenosa* (11.4%), enterococci (10.4%), and *Klebsiella* spp. accounted for almost half of all infections and *S. aureus* contributed 10.3% more. By clinical type, urinary tract infections accounted for 38.5% of hospital-acquired infections, lower respiratory tract infections for 17.8%, surgical wound infections for 16.6%, primary bacteremia for 7.5%, cutaneous infections for 5.8%, and other causes for 13.8%. The overall rate of reported infections, based on the 804,684 patients discharged from the 51 hospitals, was 33.5 infections per 1000 discharges.

12. Diagnosis of Bacterial Infections

Identification of the causal agent is essential to establish the etiology of a bacterial infection and as a guide to selecting appropriate antibiotic therapy. It depends primarily on: (1) microscopic examination of exudates, body fluid, or tissues after staining (Gram stain, acid-fast) or by dark-field examination or immunofluorescent-labeled antibody tests, or by the newer techniques for antigen identification such as counterimmunoelectrophoresis and latex agglutination, as used in respiratory infections[49,140]; (2) appropriate bacteriological culture techniques; (3) serological tests. Serological tests are not as commonly employed as in viral infections because of the ease and rapidity with which the diagnosis can often be established by smear and culture for most bacterial infections. For slow-growing or difficult-

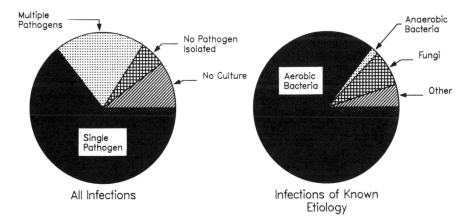

Figure 5. Causes of hospital-acquired infections in 26,965 patients from 51 hospitals reporting to CDC in 1984.[94]

to-culture organisms such as *Legionella pneumophila,* the spirochetes, and the rickettsiae, serological tests are the mainstay of diagnosis. Animal inoculation may be required to identify fastidious organisms and the toxins of certain bacteria, and skin tests may be useful to diagnose infections that show delayed hypersensitivity. This section will briefly review some of these techniques; for more definitive information, see textbooks on laboratory methods,[15,110] medical microbiology,[97] or clinical infectious diseases.[91] An important decision for the physician is the differentiation of bacterial from viral infections on first examination in order to decide on the necessity of antibiotic therapy and as a guide to laboratory tests. This may not always be possible, but the presence of bacterial infections is suggested by the vigor and acuteness of the clinical onset, leukocytosis, and the presence of purulent lesions with polymorphonuclear cells. Nonpurulent responses to bacteria are seen in such diseases as brucellosis, tuberculosis, and typhoid fever.

12.1. Collection of Specimens

The selection of the appropriate site from which to obtain the specimen, its collection prior to antibiotic therapy, and its transport to the laboratory in a manner to preserve the viability of any organisms present are three essential ingredients of successful diagnostic microbiology. The specimen should be taken from the site of the infection or from the body fluid most likely to contain organisms from the infected site. The collection should be made with sterile swabs and collecting units. Cotton applicator swabs are commonly used, but since cotton may be toxic to certain bacteria, a synthetic material such as calcium alginate is preferable. An adequate sample must be obtained to prepare smears and cultures and for special isolation purposes (viruses, fungi). Swabs may be inadequate for this purpose, and the fluid itself, or a washing of it (e.g., throat, nasal, lesion), may be needed for quantitative measurement, as in urine, to determine the number of organisms present. A syringe aspirate is desirable for anaerobic cultures of purulent lesions. Since most large laboratories have special sections for bacterial, viral, fungal, parasitic, and treponemal diagnostic techniques, separate specimens for each microbiological group considered as a possible etiological agent in a given infection should be collected. Special techniques may be needed to avoid contamination by normal flora in needle or surgical aspirations from a lesion or from a transtracheal or transurethral site.

To preserve viability, material from patients may be: (1) inoculated into appropriate transport media directly at the bedside, for which purpose kits are now commercially available; (2) carried to the laboratory for immediate inoculation; (3) preserved in a transport medium that maintains viability, prevents desiccation, and limits overgrowth of other organisms; media containing agar and charcoal are commonly employed (Stuart's transport medium or Arnie's modification thereof). If transport media are used, smears should be prepared separately at the time of collection with a separate swab because the agar in the transport medium makes this difficult. If viruses are suspected, a separate specimen should be collected and immediately frozen in dry ice for transport to the laboratory. Blood samples should be collected aseptically in amounts of 10–15 ml. If shipment to a laboratory is needed, the serum should be separated aseptically and forwarded preferably in the frozen state. Infections of certain sites, or with certain organisms, may require special collection or transport methods or both; these are described in the appropriate individual chapters in this book or in books on bacteriological diagnosis.[15,97,110]

12.2. Requests for Testing

There must be good communication between the physician and the microbiologist. The wide array of specialized laboratory techniques and culture media available makes it necessary that the physician provide guidance based on a clinical and epidemiological assessment of the etiological possibilities. The age, sex, clinical diagnosis (or at least the organ system involved), previous antibiotic therapy, and other pertinent patient information plus the site, time, and date of collection and method of transport to the laboratory of the specimen are helpful data to the laboratory worker in pursuit of the correct techniques to be employed. In return, the clinical microbiologist must provide periodic reports to help the physician in selecting appropriate therapy until the organism is fully identified and its antibiotic sensitivity determined.

12.3. Tests Employed

The details of laboratory methods are beyond the scope of this section, but a few comments will be made; specific techniques are mentioned in each chapter. The importance of a properly obtained and thoroughly examined Gram stain of the exudate or body fluid cannot be overemphasized as a guide to initial therapy. For example, the etiology of some 85% of acute purulent meningitis cases and of many bacterial pneumonias can be identified by smear, especially if capsular swelling occurs in the presence of specific antisera. Simple microscopic examination of an unstained, uncentrifuged specimen of urine that shows bacteria indicates a quantitative bacterial count of 10^4-10^5/ml, and the morphology may point to the proper etiology. The examination of bacteria in fresh preparations, or on culture, after staining with specific, immunofluorescent-labeled antisera provides specific diagnosis of Group A hemolytic streptococci, plague bacillus, and *E. coli;* it has also been useful in identifying the organism in acute meningitis, in cervical gonorrhea, and in primary syphilis.

The rapid detection of antigen in body fluids such as respiratory secretions and in urine is now being accomplished by counterimmunoelectrophoresis and latex agglutination.[49] A number of molecular techniques are now available for both phenotypic and genotypic identification. Those used for epidemiological studies of phenotypic variants include antibiotic resistance patterns (antibiograms), biotyping, bacteriocin production, serotyping, outer membrane protein analysis, phage typing, and multilocus enzyme electrophoresis. The limitations of these techniques are that they do not take genetic exchange or mutations into account, are nonspecific, and are not widely applicable. Genotypic typing methods are used to identify the genetic composition of the organism by study of chromosomal, plasmid, or transposon DNA. They include plasmid profile analysis, restriction endonuclease digestion of plasmids or of chromosomes, DNA–DNA hybridization, and DNA probes. These genotypic methods are simple, rapid, reproducible, and apply to a wide variety of organisms, including bacteria, viruses, and fungi. Their application permits identification of specific patterns of transmission of an organism, differentiation between reinfection and reactivation, and recognition of the geographic distribution of a particular strain. The epidemiology of antibiotic resistance involves (1) R plasmid spread (inter- and intraspecies), (2) strain (clonal) dissemination, and (3) transposition of R genes into R plasmids or chromosomes.

The culture media used will depend on the organisms suspected and whether they are aerobic or anaerobic. Blood agar plates and broth cultures are widely used as a starting point. See individual chapters for specialized media for specific organisms.

Once the organism is isolated, its *antibiotic sensitivity* is usually determined and is useful not only in the selection of the proper antibiotic but also in "fingerprinting" the organism for epidemiological tracing. However, this is not necessary for some organisms that are known to be uniformly sensitive to certain antibiotics or that are uniformly resistant to all but one or two antibiotics. *In vitro* antibiotic testing is not always relevant to a particular infection, especially if the infection is due to mixed organisms. It often does not provide quantitative data or express the effect of an antibiotic on different points in the growth cycle of the organism, and the testing procedure may not include the antibiotic best suited to the clinical situation. The tests must be made on organisms obtained before antibiotic therapy is initiated. Despite these limitations, *in vitro* antibiotic testing is widely employed and is especially useful for organisms prone to develop antibiotic resistance such as staphylococci, enterobacteria, and *M. tuberculosis.*

The *in vitro* tests commonly employed are the disk-diffusion techniques in agar and dilution-sensitivity tests on agar plates or in tubes with nutrient broth. The *disk* procedure is simpler and more rapid, but the zone of inhibition cannot be directly correlated with the concentration of the antibiotic needed to inhibit growth of the organism *in vivo*. Antibiotic resistance to two antibiotics by disk diffusion does not exclude *in vivo* effectiveness of the combination; disk diffusion cannot be used for combinations of antibiotics.

The *dilution* tests provide quantitative data, permitting estimation of the minimal inhibitory concentration (MIC) of the antibiotic as well as the minimal lethal concentration (MLC) necessary for killing, which may differ from the MIC. However, the techniques used for dilution tests vary from laboratory to laboratory; the results are dependent on the size of the inoculum and the broth medium employed. Many laboratories now use automated broth microdilution susceptibility testing, which is rapid and has some economical and procedural advantages over both disk-diffusion and broth macrodilution methods.

As indicated earlier, *serological* tests have limited application for many bacterial infections.[14] However, they are useful for a number of treponemal, leptospiral, and rickettsial infections.[15] Some of the key tests are indicated in Table 13. As with viral diagnostic tests, a fourfold or greater rise in titer is indicative of recent infection. For legionellosis, the titer must reach $1:128$ or higher to be significant because of nonspecificity at lower dilutions; similarly, only cold agglutinin titers of $1:64$ or higher are regarded as diagnostic of *M. pneumoniae* infection, and even then only about 60% of hospitalized *Mycoplasma* pneumonia patients are positive depending on the severity of the infection. The presence of specific IgM antibody is often diagnostic of an acute infection, if demonstrable, as for *Borrelia burgdorferi,* the cause of Lyme disease. For rickettsial infections, both the organism itself and *Proteus* antigens are useful in serological diagnosis. In streptococcal infections, an increase occurs in a group of antienzyme tests but is too late to be useful diagnostically; a high titer is said to place the person at greater risk of developing rheumatic fever. In syphilis, a great variety of serological tests have

Table 13. Some Serological Tests Used in Bacteriological Diagnosis

Disease	Test antigen	Test(s)[a]	Comment
Brucellosis	Organism	Agglutination	Four strains
Legionellosis	Organism	IF	Twenty serotypes
Leptospirosis	Organism	Microagglutination, CF, hemolytic, IFA	Crossings occur; many types
Lyme disease	Organism	ELISA IgG, IgM	Needs standardization
Mycoplasma pneumonia	Organism	IF, TRI, CF	
	O rbc	Cold agglutinins	60% positive
Q fever	Organism	CF, agglutination	
Rickettsialpox	Organism	CF	
Rocky Mountain spotted fever	Soluble antigen	CF	
	Proteus strains	Weil Felix	Ox19+++, Ox2+++
		Agglutination	OxKO
Streptococcosis	Extracellular products	Antistreptolysin O, DNase	Confirm past infection
Syphilis	Nontreponemal	VDRL flocculation test	Presumptive
	Treponemal	Rapid reagent tests	Presumptive
		TPI, CF, FTA-ABS	Specific
Yaws	Same as syphilis	Same as syphilis	Cannot differentiate from syphilis
Tularemia	Organism	Agglutination	Often 1:640 or more
Typhoid fever	O antigen	Widal-agglutination	≤4-fold increase

[a] IF, immunofluorescence; CF, complement fixation; IFA, indirect fluorescent antibody; TRI, tetrazolium-reduction inhibition; VDRL, Venereal Disease Research Laboratory; TPI, treponemal immobilization; FTA-ABS, fluorescent-treponemal-antibody absorption.

been used employing both nontreponemal and treponemal antigens. The VDRL test is most widely employed as an initial test and is highly sensitive and well standardized, but lacks high specificity. The diagnosis can be confirmed by the FTA-Abs test, which is highly specific and available at most state and a few large private laboratories, as well as at the CDC. The TPI test is a highly specific test but requires maintenance of a mobile, live treponemal antigen; it is available at the CDC. Yaws (*T. pertenue*) shares identical reactivities with *T. pallidum* and cannot be differentiated serologically. Typhoid fever results in increases to the H, O, and other antigens of the organism; an increase in O-antigen titer in the absence of recent immunization is indicative of recent infection. In any serological test, both acute and convalescent sera are desirable. There is only one time to take the acute-phase sample—in early illness.

Skin tests may also be useful in diagnosis by demonstration of hypersensitivity to various bacterial antigens. They are commonly employed in tuberculosis, leprosy, nontuberculous mycobacteriosis, brucellosis, and tularemia.

12.4. Interpretation of Tests

The isolation of a bacterial organism from an ill person does not always represent a causal relationship. The organism could reflect: (1) part of the normal flora; (2) a healthy carrier state; (3) contamination during the collection process; (4) a transient microorganism contaminating a body surface; (5) a dual or multiple infection, in which the organism isolated is not the one causing the clinical illness; (6) a laboratory error or mix-up; (7) the true cause of the illness. The factors that point toward a causal relationship are: (1) isolation in pure culture or of only one organism; (2) the presence of large numbers of the same organism; (3) the presence of the organism in direct smear from a lesion; (4) procurement from a site normally free of bacteria; (5) repeated isolation of the same organism; (6) demonstration of an immune response; (7) history of possible recent exposure to the organism in an ill person, in travel, in occupation, or otherwise. The response of the patient to an antibiotic to which the organism is sensitive provides suggestive evidence that the organism caused the disease, but because other organisms are also sensitive to the same antibiotic, this cannot weigh too heavily. Clinical and laboratory judgment plus knowledge of the qualitative and quantitative behavior of human pathogens constitute the best grounds for deciding a causal relationship. It should be remembered that some organisms not usually regarded as pathogenic may cause disease in patients with naturally occurring or drug-induced defects in their immune defenses, or in AIDS and related diseases due to HIV.

On the other hand, the failure to isolate an organism does not exclude a bacterial etiology. Such "false negatives" could result from: (1) prior antibiotic therapy; (2) failure to obtain a specimen from the proper site; (3) collection at the wrong time; (4) a loss of viability during transport to the lab; (5) use of inappropriate media, temperature, gaseous environment, or other conditions for growth of the organism: (6) or failure to hold the culture media for a sufficiently long time, as with certain *Brucella* species.

Serological tests are also subject to misinterpretation. *False-positive* rises can result from cross-reacting antigens, nonspecific inhibitors, double infection with the other organism causing the illness, and antibody response to vaccination rather than to natural infection. *False negatives,* i.e., failure to demonstrate an increase in titer, can occur when the serum specimen is taken too late in illness, two samples are taken too close together to demonstrate a titer rise, the organism is a poor immunogen, the wrong antigen is used in the test, some inhibitor or nonspecificity (as in IF tests) obscures a true rise, or the wrong type of test is used for the timing of the serum specimens. Serological tests are also not available for many bacterial infections. One of the common problems is the interpretation of a high IgG antibody titer in a single specimen. The demonstration of IgM-specific antibody is strong but not absolute evidence of a recent infection; it could result from reactivation. The presence of antibody to a rare infection, or to one not usually present in that area as in a returned traveler, or the history of some recent unusual exposure such as in hunting, a new occupation, or a visit from overseas friends also adds weight to the recency of that infection. Such problems are more common in viral and parasitic infections.

13. Proof of Causation

The classic postulates of causation were suggested by Jakob Henle in 1840,[89] some 40 years before bacteria were discovered, and then further developed by his pupil, Robert

Koch, in 1884 and 1890 after he had isolated *M. tuberculosis*.[106,107] They are presented in Table 14. While fulfillment of these postulates provides strong evidence of a causal association, the failure to fulfill them does not exclude this relationship. Even at the time of presentation in 1890, Koch himself recognized some of these limitations, especially the inability to reproduce some diseases in experimental animals. At that time, this was true of cholera, typhoid fever, diphtheria, leprosy, and relapsing fever, for which Koch felt it necessary to fulfill only the first two postulates. Since then, many other limitations have been recognized[63] as our knowledge of microbiology, epidemiology, and pathogenesis has increased.[62,64] These include recognition of the asymptomatic carrier state, which would invalidate the second postulate if an individual were carrier of organism A and his disease was caused by organism B. The concepts of multiple causation, of inapparent infection, and of the biological gradient of disease are also limitations. The postulates were not generally applicable to viral disease and were first revised to this end by Rivers[129] in 1937, by Huebner[95] in 1957 to include epidemiological concepts, by Evans[58,59] in 1967 to include immunological proof for agents such as EBV and hepatitis virus that could not be propagated in tissue culture, and by Johnson and Gibbs[99] in 1974 for slow viruses that not only failed to grow in culture but also did not produce a measurable immune response. It is clear that all postulates and guidelines of causation are limited by the technology available to prove them and by our knowledge of disease mechanisms at the time.[64] The need for establishing guidelines for causation is ever present in the field of bacteriology, where the causal relationship between parasite and disease must be established for newly recognized diseases such as Lyme disease, Legionnaires' disease, Pittsburgh pneumonia, chlamydial pneumonia and urethritis, infant botulism, enterotoxic *E. coli* diarrhea, toxic shock syndrome, and streptococcal B infections in infancy. New causes for old diseases, new

Table 14. Henle–Koch Postulates[a]

1. Parasite occurs in every case of the disease in question and under circumstances that can account for the pathological changes and clinical cause of the disease
2. Occurs in no other disease as fortuitous and nonpathogenic parasite
3. After being fully isolated from the body and repeatedly grown in pure culture, can induce the disease anew

[a] From Koch,[106,107] translated by Rivers.[129]

diseases from old causes, and new diseases with new causes keep appearing as our techniques for their isolation and identification improve.

14. Control and Prevention

The three major principles of control of infectious diseases are: (1) eliminate or contain the sources of infection; (2) interrupt the chain of transmission; and (3) protect the host against infection or disease or both.

14.1. Environmental Control

The provision of clean and safe air, water, milk, and food; the proper management of sewage and garbage; and the control of insect vectors of disease are regarded as not only essential to health but also a legal right in most countries. The extent to which they are attained depends on the economy, energy resources, political will, and educational level of the country.

14.1.1. Air. While many infectious agents are airborne on particles or droplet nuclei from infected hosts or environmental sources to susceptible subjects, effective control of this means of transmission has been most difficult to achieve. In open environments, it has been impossible to attain, and even in closed environments attempts to sterilize the air by UV light, propylene glycol, filtration, and other chemical aerosols have met with very limited success. At best, control of the air currents generated by air conditioners, water coolers, and fans will help slow down spread of organisms such as *Legionella pneumophila, M. tuberculosis,* and staphylococci. For patient isolation, laminar-flow units have been effective if properly used. The pollution of air by automobiles and industrial sources does not carry a direct risk of infection but may depress host defense mechanisms so that disease develops, as in persons with chronic pulmonary diseases.

14.1.2. Water. Improvement in our water supplies has been one of the major factors in the environmental control of infectious diseases, especially of enteric infections such as *Campylobacter,* yersiniosis, cholera, typhoid fever, amebiasis, and bacillary dysentery. The details of water purification and treatment can be found elsewhere,[117] but involve removal of extraneous materials by filtration, settling, and coagulation, the replenishment of oxygen by aeration, and disinfection by chlorination. Bacteriological and chemical standards for the purity of water have been established and are reinforced by governmental and legal regulations. The presence of *E. coli* in defined numbers per milliliter* is taken as an index of fecal contamination of water. Its absence does not guarantee water safety, since organisms such as hepatitis A virus may escape filtration and chlorination procedures. For the traveler, treatment of water with chlorine-release tablets or a drop of Lugal's iodine solution per quart of water 30 min prior to use, or by boiling for 5 min will decrease the likelihood of acquiring bacterial intestinal infections in developing countries. Should these methods not be available, one can allow the water to run until very hot, collect it, and then use it for drinking water. Bottled water or other beverages are usually safe.

14.1.3. Sewage and Garbage. Sewage water carries fecal material, industrial and chemical products, and other waste products. It must be safely conveyed without human hazard to septic tanks or to reprocessing, filtration, and activated sludge treatment centers, but has not posed a problem of infectious disease. The dumping of untreated sewage into streams, rivers, and the open sea is detrimental to fish and marine life and esthetically distasteful, and impairs recreational use of such waters. It might result in transmission of certain intestinal pathogens via raw seafood to humans, such as the cholera outbreak in Louisiana after ingestion of cooked crabs containing the organism.[13]

The proper disposal of the large amount of garbage, refuse, and other solid waste products produced by our modern society is an increasing challenge to proper land use and modern technology. Direct discharge into the sewage system after grinding and flushing is one method; compactors of garbage and waste material are now available even for home use. If stored and carried elsewhere for disposal, this must be done in closed, stable containers that protect against rats, flies, and other predators. The separation and recycling of certain reuseable products such as glass, bottles, paper, and cans is to be encouraged. Large incinerators for burning garbage and refuse provide a safe but energy-expensive procedure. Landfill sites in communities are increasingly scarce, costly as land values increase, and objected to on esthetic grounds. Disposal of radioactive and other toxic wastes generated by medical, industrial, and energy uses in oceans raises international concern about the long-term food and energy potential of oceans, and land or tank disposal, especially of nuclear wastes, is unacceptable to most communities.

---

*Usually, water is not acceptable for drinking if coliform bacteria exceed 4/100 ml in more than 5% of water samples per month using the membrane-filter technique; samples should be taken at points representative of the distribution system.[117]

14.1.4. Milk and Food. Milk and food must be protected against contamination at their source, during transport and storage, and in their preparation for consumption. Cows must be free from tuberculosis, brucellosis, and Q fever. The milk must be collected under clean conditions, preferably by automated machines that avoid human contamination, and its quality in the raw state and after pasteurization must meet bacteriological standards.* Common pasteurization procedures are heating to 65 °C (149 °F) for 30 min or the high-temperature or flash method at 72 °C (162 °F) for 15 s. The heat inactivation of the enzyme alkaline phosphatase, normally present in milk, provides the basis for the phosphatase test to ensure proper pasteurization. Before, and promptly after, pasteurization, milk must be stored and transported at 5–10 °C (41–50 °F) to storage areas or the consumer. The pasteurization process, even if performed correctly, may not decontaminate some intracellular organisms and those that are cold-tolerant, such as *Listeria.* Milk and other food products may contain antibiotics used in treatment of cattle or for growth promotion and pose a hazard to highly sensitive persons.

Our food supplies must also be properly grown, cultivated, stored, and prepared. In developing and tropical areas, vegetables such as lettuce, and other products grown in soil enriched by human excreta, pose a serious hazard for intestinal infections, and these foods should be avoided by the wary traveler. Human handling during preparation may result in contamination by many bacteria, especially staphylococci, *Salmonella,* and *Shigella.* Thorough cooking immediately prior to eating will reduce the hazard of infection, but may fail to inactivate preformed heat-stable toxins such as *C. perfringens.* Proper refrigeration or freezing of food has been as important as water and sewage management in the reduction of intestinal diseases. It prevents the multiplication of most bacteria and freezing often destroys some parasites such as *Toxoplasma gondii* and *Trichinella spiralis.* However, most organisms or toxins already present at the time of refrigeration or freezing will be preserved in the process and can multiply after thawing and reaching the proper temperature.

14.1.5. Animals and Insect Vectors. Animals provide the source of infection for many of the diseases discussed in this book, such as anthrax, brucellosis, *Campylobacter,* leptospirosis, plague, salmonellosis, tularemia, and yersiniosis. The types of exposure differ: some are occupational (anthrax) or avocational (tularemia), some result from common environmental exposures (leptospirosis, salmonel-

losis), some from close contact with domestic animals (*Campylobacter*) or from contamination of water sources (yersiniosis). Knowledge of these potential sources of infection and of appropriate specific measures to avoid or minimize exposure are needed.

Insect vectors may play a passive or active role in transmission of bacterial infections. Passive transfer of the organisms of cholera, salmonellosis, and typhoid fever by flies and other insects may occur, but does not seem to be of much epidemiological significance. Good food sanitation, proper storage, and screens are useful to prevent such transfer. The active transport of infection involves multiplication in the insect host. Rickettsial infections are commonly transmitted by insect vectors: *Rickettsia rickettsii* of Rocky Mountain spotted fever by wood, dog, and Lone Star ticks; *R. akari* of rickettsialpox by the mouse mite; and *R. prowazekii* of typhus fevers by the body louse (louseborne typhus) or rat flea (murine typhus). *Borrelia burgdorferi,* the spirochete that causes Lyme disease, is transmitted by ticks of the *Ixodid* genus, such as *I. dammini,* the deer tick. The control of many of these insect vectors is very difficult, since they exist widely in nature. Therefore, attention is usually directed at the control or avoidance of the dog, rat, mouse, deer, or other animal hosts on which they usually reside. The body louse is controlled by good personal and clothing hygiene and by delousing procedures (heat and chemical treatment).

14.2. Host Factors

The human host may be protected against infection and disease by quarantine or isolation from the sources of infection, by good personal hygiene, by specific immunization, and by chemoprophylaxis.

14.2.1. Quarantine and Isolation. Quarantine, which began in 1348 as a 30-day period of keeping suspected plague victims aboard ships in Venice from disembarking, has now been rendered largely obsolete by air travel. The WHO now evokes quarantine measures only for plague, yellow fever, and cholera. Smallpox has been officially eradicated from the world for over 13 years so that quarantine regulations are no longer needed. Instead, we now rely on *surveillance* techniques, as discussed in Chapter 2, to provide constant monitoring and analysis of infectious diseases and of other conditions of public-health importance.

Isolation requirements and techniques have also undergone redefinition and reassessment.[10] Varying isolation standards have been developed for various groups of diseases and often depend on state laws or hospital regulations.

---

*Under 200,000 bacteria/ml by standard plate count before pasteurization and under 30,000 bacteria/ml after pasteurization.

Infectious diseases in hospitals have been grouped according to the degree of isolation recommended. Six variables are involved: the need for a private room, gowns, masks, hand-washing, gloves, and the disposition of various articles such as linens, instruments, and dressings that might be contaminated. Hand-washing on entering and leaving the patient's room (and the appropriate disposal of contaminated articles) is a key element of each. Seven levels of categories of isolation or precaution based on the type of disease have been set up by the CDC.[30]

The CDC has issued recommendations for the prevention of HIV transmission in medical care settings.[40] The procedures for control of infection in hospitals are also summarized in a recent Food and Drug Administration bulletin.[77] Since medical history and examination cannot reliably identify all patients with HIV or with other blood-borne pathogens, blood and body-fluid precautions should be consistently used for *all* patients when exposure to such fluids occurs. This approach is called "universal blood and body-fluid precautions" or "universal precautions" and is to be applied to all patients, including those coming into emergency rooms, where there is often risk of such exposures and the status of the patient is usually unknown. The approach also applies to outpatient settings that involve handling of blood or body fluids. Universal precautions would specifically involve the use of "barrier" techniques in which gloves, gowns, protective eyewear, and handwashing would be required for contact with *all* patients, including those in emergency rooms or outpatient settings, when there is exposure to blood or other body fluids. This would apply to the use of gloves when touching blood and body fluids, mucous membranes, or soiled articles or surfaces, and when doing venipunctures or inserting i.v. lines, and to the use of masks in operative or invasive procedures. A mask and eye protection should be worn when there is a possibility of blood or other fluids being splashed onto mucous membranes; gowns are indicated only when splashing is possible. The decision to initiate routine testing or testing of high-risk patients, and of high-risk hospital personnel engaged in invasive or other procedures, is left to physicians or individual institutions. If such testing is carried out, CDC outlines the principles of informed consent and confidentiality involved.[40]

14.2.2. Hygiene. High standards of cleanliness of the individual, the family, the food prepared, and the community contribute to the prevention of infectious diseases. The simple measure of thorough and frequent hand-washing is of the highest importance in protecting the individual against pathogens and in interrupting the spread of organisms to others. It plays an essential role in controlling the spread of infection in hospitals and institutions, in restaurants, and in food processing both in industries and in the home. The promotion, distribution, and proper use of soap and water for personal hygiene in developing countries need greater emphasis. Its use should decrease enteric and respiratory infections.

14.2.3. Immunization. The specific protection of the individual against infection or disease or both is the key to modern preventive practice. It may be either *passive* protection by the transfer of a specific antibody (or antitoxin) from another person or animal immune to it or *active immunization* through induction of antibody by the organism itself or an antigenic derivative of it. An ideal vaccine closely simulates the protection from natural infection; i.e., it produces good humoral, cellular, and local immunity of long duration. Preferably, it should be better than the short-lived or incomplete immunity found in certain infections such as cholera or shigellosis. It should be in a form of administration and at a cost acceptable to the public. The cost of the vaccine and any side effects should be less than those of the natural disease prevented by it. These ideals are most closely met by well-attenuated live vaccines, or antigenic derivatives thereof. The live bacterial vaccines include bacillus Calmette–Guérin (BCG) for tuberculosis and tularemia vaccine. BCG is little used in the United States and contradictory evidence exists as to its efficacy, but the best conducted trials of BCG have shown a high order of efficacy against the more serious manifestations of infection such as miliary tuberculosis and meningitis, which occur in very young children in developing countries.[47] Tularemia vaccine is used in rather small, high-risk groups. Most bacterial vaccines are formalin-, acetone-, or phenol-killed organisms or an antigenic derivative such as the capsular polysaccharides of the meningococcus and pneumococcus, the toxoids of diphtheria and tetanus, or the protein antigens of anthrax.

Newer vaccine preparations for many bacterial diseases are under development such as those for cholera, *H. influenzae* type b, pertussis, shigellosis, and typhoid fever. For example, recent field trials of a new oral cholera vaccine[48] and a Vi capsular polysaccharide for typhoid fever[1] show encouraging results. The use of conjugated polysaccharide vaccines improves their antigenicity, permitting them to be used in young children. Someday, timed-release biodegradable polymers may permit pulsed release of vaccines, such as tetanus, thus permitting a single shot to be effective, and avoid the loss now occurring in women and children who do not return to complete the multiple doses required for most killed vaccines. The Institute of Medicine of the U.S. National Academy of Sciences has published a comprehensive evaluation of vaccine priorities for both developed and developing countries based on their feasibility, cost, need, effectiveness, acceptability, side reactions, and other factors.[96] Among the five top priorities for developed countries there is only one bacterial vaccine, *H. influenzae* type b; the rest are viral agents (HBV, influenza, RSV, and V-Z). In developing countries, three bacterial vaccines are included in the top five: *S. pneumoniae, S. typhi, Shigella* spp. The other two are against malaria and rotavirus infections.

Despite the need for these improved vaccines, it is clear that our available vaccines are not being sufficiently utilized in either developed or developing countries. In Third World countries, WHO's Expanded Program in Immunization is making an enormous effort to vaccinate the young children of the world against six targeted diseases using DPT, polio, measles, and BCG vaccines. Important progress is being made but the 50% coverage figure is just being attained in most areas as of 1989, and Asia and the Far East lag far behind. Other organizations are now joining in this effort as part of a "Child Survival Program" and there is a focus on "growth, oral rehydration therapy, breast feeding, and immunization" (GOBI). In the United States, the recommendation by states that all children be immunized before being allowed into school has greatly expanded coverage in this country, although success in the elimination of measles remains elusive. To correct this, immunization at 9 months is recommended in certain urban settings, and a second dose is given on school entry. However, in our adult population there are serious deficits in immunization status, especially among the elderly.[41] For example, recent serosurveys indicate that 49–66% of persons 60 years or over lack reliable protective levels of circulating antitoxin against tetanus, and 41–84% lack adequate protection against diphtheria. Tetanus is a completely preventable disease and persons over 50 account for 70% of reported cases, so special emphasis must be placed on this age group for tetanus boosters, or an initial series, if not previously vaccinated. Pneumococcal vaccine is also badly underutilized as indicated by the fact that less than 10% of the higher risk groups have been vaccinated.[41] A similar lack of protection of our adult population exists against many viral diseases, especially influenza, measles, mumps, rubella, and hepatitis B.

In general, live vaccines are contraindicated in immunosuppressed patients. Recent studies suggest, however, that the benefits of measles, mumps, and rubella vaccines outweigh the risks to children with AIDS, at least in developing countries.

The WHO thus recommends use of standard EPI vaccines in persons with symptomatic or asymptomatic HIV infections,[143] but suggests that inactivated poliomyelitis vaccine (IPV) be considered as an alternative to oral polio vaccine (OPV). Some complications have arisen with BCG vaccine in such immunosuppressed children, and its use should be suspended in unimmunized individuals with symptomatic AIDS in countries where the other targeted diseases remain serious risks; in asymptomatic HIV-infected individuals, in areas where the risk of tuberculosis is high, BCG is recommended at birth or soon thereafter. Guidelines should be consulted for updated recommendations as data are often incomplete. Separate needles are required to avoid the possibility of parenteral transmission of HIV (and HBV). The jet gun should not be used in immunization programs, except in an epidemic emergency, until further data are available on the possible risks associated with its use.

The common preparations available for passive and active immunization against bacterial infections are listed in Table 15 along with their usage as recommended by the Public Health Service Advisory Committee on Immunization Practices,[23] including recent changes.[22,24–27] Information for international travelers,[44] as well as the uses and limitations of each vaccine, will be found in the appropriate chapters of this book. A brief summary follows.

a. Anthrax. Give the alum-concentrated cell-free vaccine only to high-risk occupational exposures such as persons working with imported goat hair, wool, and hides (sheep and goats) and laboratory workers regularly exposed to this organism. A booster dose is needed yearly.

b. Botulism. Only passive immunization is available consisting of horse serum with anti-A, B, and E toxins and used for persons strongly suspected of botulism or when disease is first diagnosed. The role in infant botulism is not yet clear but probably useful. Trivalent antitoxin is available on a 24-h basis from the CDC in Atlanta. There is a 10–15% risk of adverse reactions (anaphylaxis, serum sickness). Give 8–32 ml according to CDC instructions depending on the age of the patient and the severity of illness; effective toxoid is also available from the CDC for laboratory workers and other exposed personnel.

c. Cholera. This vaccine offers rather poor protection (± 50%) over a short period (3–6 months); the transmission of infection is not prevented.[24] The WHO does not recommend immunization for persons going to or coming from cholera-infected areas, and the United States does not require it. In endemic areas, it may divert funds from more effective control measures. However, certain countries affected or threatened by cholera still require it. One dose of vaccine certified on an International Certificate of Vaccina-

Table 15.   Common Bacterial Vaccines

Name	Type	Recommended for:	Age	Dose and time	Route	Booster	Other
1. Anthrax	Active (from CDC)	High-risk occupational workers	Adult	0.5 ml q 3 wk × 3, then q 6 mo × 3	s.c.	Yearly	—
2. Botulism	Active toxoid (from CDC)	Laboratory and other high-risk workers	Adult	Follow schedule advised by CDC	—	—	—
	Passive (horse serum) (Lederle)	After known exposure or at first diagnosis—use trivalent unless toxin type is known	Any	After testing for sensitivity, follow schedule on package	—	—	—
3. Cholera	Active (inactivated)	Not routinely recommended with current vaccines, but may be required by some countries	Any	In adults, 0.5 ml × 2, 3–6 wk apart, with booster at 6 mo	s.c.	—	—
4. Diphtheria–tetanus–pertussis (DPT)	DPT active	Primary vaccination for all children up to 6 yr	6 wk–6 yr	Usually 0.5 ml (see package insert) at 2, 4, 6, and 15 mo and at 4–6 yr; then adult Td at 14–16 yr and q 10 yr	i.m.	After initial series, q 10 yr	—
	Td for adults	For children ≥ 6 yr not immunized in infancy	6 yr	0.5 ml × 2, 2 mo apart, then 3rd dose 6–12 mo later	i.m.	q 10 yr, or q 5 yr if at high risk	—
5. Diphtheria	Passive (horse serum)	Asymptomatic, unimmunized household contacts	< 6 yr	600,000 U	i.m.	—	Test for sensitivity to horse serum
			≥ 6 yr	1,200,000 U plus penicillin and diphtheria toxoid	i.m.	—	—

Chapter 1 • Epidemiological Concepts **49**

Disease	Type	Recipients/Indications	Age	Dose	Route	Booster	Remarks
6. Meningococcus, groups A and C	Active A, C, or combined (polysaccharide)	Military recruits (A and C); residents of or travelers to epidemic area (monospecific); household contacts of cases (monospecific)	For group A: ≥ 3 mo; for group C: ≥ 2 yr	50 mg of each type, one dose only with protection ≥ 2 yr	s.c.	—	No type B vaccine
7. Plague	Active (inactivated)	Only laboratory and field ≥ 10 yr workers exposed to organism	≥ 10 yr	0.5 ml × 2 at ≥ 4-wk intervals, then 0.2 ml × 3, 4–12 wk after second dose	i.m.	Under continual exposure, give about q 6 mo × 2, then 1–2 yr; smaller dose in children	—
8. Tetanus	Active (Td)	See under DPT (4), for primary immunization, in persons with wounds with no, uncertain, or incomplete series.	< 6 yr ≥ 6 yr	DPT: one dose followed by complete series Td: one dose, then series	i.m.	10 yr 10 yr	Add TIG in tetanus-prone wounds
	Passive (TIG)	In persons with tetanus-prone or neglected wounds with no, incomplete, or uncertain primary immunization. Use in wounds neglected > 24 hr irrespective of previous full immunization	Any	250–500 U TIG using separate syringe and site from toxoid	i.m.		See Chapter 34, Table I
9. Typhoid	Active (inactivated)	Household contacts of cases or carriers; travelers to high-risk areas; laboratory workers with organism	> 10 yr	0.5 ml × 2, ≥ 4 wk apart	s.c.	0.5 ml s.c. or 0.1 ml i.d. q 3 yr if exposed continually	—
			≤ 10 yr	0.25 ml × 2, ≥ 4 wk apart	s.c.	0.25 ml s.c. or 0.1 ml i.d. q 3 yr if exposed continually	—

tion will satisfy most such countries and is valid for 6 months. The vaccine requirements for yellow fever, and the malaria risk, are given country by country in "Health Information for International Travel," published by the CDC in a supplement to the MMWR.[44]

d. Diphtheria–Pertussis–Tetanus (DPT) Vaccine (see Table 16). Primary immunization with DPT vaccine is given to children 6 weeks through 6 years of age, according to the manufacturer's dosage, on four occasions i.m.: three doses at 4- to 8-week intervals and a fourth dose about a year later, plus one at 4 through 6 years. For schoolchildren and adults, give three doses of the adult preparation (Td) containing only tetanus and diphtheria toxoid. The second dose is given 4–8 weeks after the first and the third dose 6–12 months after the second. *Booster dose:* Give in a single i.m. injection to children age 3–6 years on entry into school, and to all persons older than this, give a booster every 10 years. Local Arthus-type reactions and sometimes systemic immune complex reactions (serum sickness) may occur in hyperimmunized adults. These may be attended by severe head, muscle, and joint aches and fever of about 24-h duration. Corticosteroids may be given orally over 3–5 days, for symptomatic relief. Diphtheria *antitoxin* should be given to

asymptomatic, unimmunized contacts in whom close clinical surveillance is not possible, plus penicillin (600,000 U of the benzathine form or, if sensitive, a 7-day course of erythromycin) and injection of diphtheria toxoid. If close clinical surveillance *is* possible, the antitoxin can be omitted. A human hyperimmune pertussis serum for exposed persons is also available, but its value is uncertain.[33]

e. Haemophilus influenzae Type b Vaccine. This infection is an important cause of meningitis in children, particularly those under the age of 5, and is now being recognized as important in older persons whose immunity has waned (see Chapter 14). Previously, a polysaccharide vaccine was recommended for children at age 24 months. Now a more immunogenic capsular polysaccharide vaccine has been linked to diphtheria toxoid (conjugate vaccine) and is recommended for use in all children at age 18 months.[43] Until more information is available on the duration of immunity, revaccination is not currently recommended for children receiving vaccine at 18 months. Preliminary field trials in Finland of the vaccine in a three-dose schedule given to infants 3 to 6 months of age suggest an 87% efficacy in preventing *Haemophilus b* disease. However, variable results have been obtained in different trials in the

Table 16.   New Recommended Schedule for Active Immunization of Normal Infants and Children[a]

Recommended age[b]	Vaccine(s)[c]	Comments
2 months	DPT-1,[d] OPV-1[e]	Can be given earlier in areas of high endemicity
4 months	DPT-2, OPV-2	6-week to 2-month interval desired between OPV doses to avoid interference
6 months	DPT-3	An additional dose of OPV at this time is optional for use in areas with a high risk of polio exposure
15 months[f]	MMR,[g] DPT-4, OPV-3	Completion of primary series of DPT and OPV
24 months	HbPV[h]	Can be given at 18–23 months for children in groups that are thought to be at increased risk of disease, e.g., day-care-center attendees
4–6 years[i]	DPT-5, OPV-4	Preferably at or before school entry
14–16 years	Td[j]	Repeat every 10 years throughout life

[a] See Ref. 35 for the recommended immunization schedules for infants and children up to their seventh birthday not immunized at the recommended time in early infancy and for persons 7 years of age or older.

[b] These recommended ages should not be construed as absolute, i.e., 2 months can be 6–10 weeks, etc.

[c] For all products used, consult manufacturer's package enclosure for instructions for storage, handling, and administration. Immunobiologics prepared by different manufacturers may vary, and those of the same manufacturer may change from time to time. The package insert should be followed for a specific product.

[d] DPT, diphtheria and tetanus toxoids and pertussis vaccine adsorbed.

[e] OPV, poliovirus vaccine live oral; contains poliovirus strains Types 1, 2, and 3.

[f] Provided at least 6 months has elapsed since DPT-3 or, if fewer than three DPTs have been received, at least 5 weeks since last dose of DPT or OPV. MMR vaccine should not be delayed just to allow simultaneous administration with DPT and OPV. Administering MMR at 15 months and DPT-4 and OPV-3 at 18 months continues to be an acceptable alternative.

[g] MMR, measles, mumps, and rubella virus vaccine, live.

[h] HbPV, Hemophilus b polysaccharide vaccine.

[i] Up to the seventh birthday.

[j] Td, tetanus and diptheria toxoids adsorbed (for adult use)—contains the same dose of tetanus toxoid as DPT or DT and a reduced dose of diphtheria toxoid.

United States in this young age group and further studies are needed before this use in infants can be recommended in the United States.

f. Meningococcal Infections. Meningococcal infections can result in epidemics but, in U.S. civilians, most commonly occur as single cases or localized clusters, with a third of the cases occurring in persons 20 years of age or over. Two polysaccharide vaccines are currently available in the United States: a bivalent A–C and a quadrivalent vaccine containing A, C, Y, and W-135 polysaccharides. A single dose of each is adequate to induce serospecific immunity.[32] Routine vaccination is not recommended in the United States because of the relatively low risk of infection and because a good Group B antigen is not available. Vaccine usage is recommended as an adjunct to antibiotic chemoprophylaxis for household and other close contacts of persons with meningococcal disease due to serotypes A, C, Y, and W-135. The quadrivalent vaccine is recommended for travelers to endemic areas. The duration of protection is unclear. Side reactions are infrequent and mild, but the safety for pregnant women has not been established. Because of the high risk in military recruits, they have received meningococcal vaccine on entering the services since the early 1970s. Currently, they receive Groups A, C, Y, and W-135.

g. Plague. The vaccine consists of formalin-inactivated organisms; its efficacy has not been critically evaluated. It should be given only to high-risk groups such as field and laboratory personnel exposed to the organism, and possibly to workers in plague enzootic or endemic rural areas where avoidance of rodents, fleas, and wild rabbits is not feasible (agricultural advisors, Peace Corps volunteers, or military personnel on maneuvers).[26] The schedule (Table 15) consists of five injections with dosage varying with age. In the face of continued exposure, single booster doses at about 6-month intervals are given for two doses, then at 1- to 2-year intervals. Local reactions are common, sterile abscesses are rare, and systemic reactions (fever, headache, and malaise) may occur on repeated injections.

h. Pneumococcal Infections. The estimated annual incidence of pneumococcal pneumonia in the United States is 68 to 260 cases per 100,000 population and of bacteremia, 7–25 per 100,000.[32] Mortality is highest in patients with bacteremia, meningitis, underlying medical conditions, and those over 60 years of age. The currently available pneumococcal polysaccharide vaccine contains purified capsular materials from 23 types of *Streptococcus pneumoniae,* which together account for 87% of recent bacteremic pneumonia in the United States. The vaccine is particularly recommended for three groups: (1) adults with

chronic diseases, especially of the cardiovascular or pulmonary system; (2) adults with chronic illnesses specifically associated with an increased risk of pneumococcal infection or its complications (splenic dysfunction, Hodgkin's disease, multiple myeloma, cirrhosis, alcoholism, renal failure, CSF leaks, and in immunosuppressed patients); (3) older adults, especially those 65 years of age and over who are healthy. Vaccination is recommended for hospitalized patients in these high-risk groups before discharge. A single dose is recommended without a booster. Mild side reactions consisting of erythema and of pain at the site of injection occur in about half the recipients. Medicare helps pay the cost in these designated groups. Pneumococcal infections are also a problem in young children in developing countries, so that there is increasing interest in the use of the vaccine in these groups.

i. Tetanus. See DPT (Section *d*) for routine immunization. For wound management, tetanus–diphtheria (Td) adult-type, or tetanus toxoid (TT) only, is used alone or in combination with tetanus immune globulin (TIG) in doses of 250 U (in separate site and syringe) depending on the severity of the wound and the history of prior immunization as shown in Table 17.[22]

Moderate to severe local and systemic reactions may occur in some hyperimmune adults receiving booster doses or for wound prophylaxis.

j. Typhoid. Active, dried typhoid vaccine has been 70–90% effective in controlled trials. However, in the United States, its use is limited to persons with exposure to

Table 17. Summary Guide to Tetanus Prophylaxis in Routine Wound Management, 1985[a]

History of adsorbed tetanus toxoid	Clean, minor wounds		All other wounds[b]	
	Td[c]	TIG	Td[c]	TIG
Unknown or < 3 doses	Yes	No	Yes	Yes
≥ 3 doses[d]	No[e]	No	No[f]	No

[a] From Ref. 39.
[b] Such as, but not limited to, wounds contaminated with dirt, feces, soil, saliva, etc.; puncture wounds; avulsions; and wounds resulting from missiles, crushing, burns, and frostbite.
[c] For children < 7 years of age; DPT (DT, if pertussis vaccine is contraindicated) is preferred to tetanus toxoid alone. For persons ≥ 7 years of age, Td is preferred to tetanus toxoid alone.
[d] If only 3 doses of *fluid* toxoid have been received, then a fourth dose of toxoid, preferably an adsorbed toxoid, should be given.
[e] Yes, if more than 10 years since last dose.
[f] Yes, if more than 5 years since last dose.

a documented carrier and to travelers to, or workers in, areas where typhoid is known to occur.[25] Its combined use with paratyphoid A is no longer recommended, nor is it useful in common-source outbreaks or as a prophylactic after floods or natural disasters. If it is used, two doses are given s.c. at 4-week or longer intervals in dosages of 0.5 ml for persons over 10 years old and 0.25 ml for children 10 years old or less; under continued exposure, booster doses of the same dosage s.c. or 0.1 ml i.d. are given every 3 years. Local and systemic reactions lasting 1–2 days are common.

14.2.4. Antibiotic Prophylaxis. The success of preventing natural infection or disease or both with antibiotic prophylaxis depends on the sensitivity of the organism to the drug employed, whether single or multiple bacterial species are involved, the timing of administration in relation to infection, and the ability of the drug to reach effective concentrations in body sites before the organism is present. It has been employed in persons at high risk after known exposure in epidemics (meningococcus), in household contacts of cases (e.g., streptococcus, meningococcus, tuber-

culosis), and in sexual partners (gonococcus, syphilis) one of whom is infected. It has been employed *after* infection is diagnosed to prevent further spread or to limit complications (tuberculosis, rheumatic fever) or to limit the duration of the carrier state. The major limitations have been the development of antibiotic resistance, multiple organisms causing the disease, and poor patient compliance for long-term prophylaxis. Any mass prophylactic program aimed at a large group, especially a closed population, over a long term sets the stage for the development of resistance in the organism of interest as well as other circulating organisms. Antibiotic prophylaxis has met with debatable success when the bacterial sensitivity is not high, if the antibiotic is inhibitory but not bactericidal, if multiple organisms are involved (especially gram-negative), and if the risk of infection is relatively low, as in clean surgical operations. For greater detail, see books on clinical infectious diseases[91] or reviews[139] as well as specific chapters in this book.

Table 18 lists some uses of antibiotic prophylaxis. The most successful are the prevention of recurrent streptococcal *infections* in persons with rheumatic heart disease and

Table 18. Prophylactic Uses of Antibiotics*a*

Condition	Chapter (section) in this volume	Persons at risk	Antibiotic	Dose/time
Diphtheria	11(9)	Carriers of toxigenic strains	Penicillin or erythromycin	Full dose over 7–10 days
Gonorrhea	13(9)	Persons sexually exposed to infection	Penicillin	Full dosage as for treatment
Meningococcal meningitis	20(9)	Intimate contacts of cases or in closed outbreaks	Sulfadiazene for sensitive organisms	1 g adults or 0.5 g children q 12 h × 4 doses
			Rifampin	10 mg/kg per day for 4 days
Strep and rheumatic fever	31(9)	Rheumatic heart disease patients (prevention of rheumatic fever)	Penicillin (benzathine), i.m.	1.2 million U/mo
		Sometimes family contacts of strep cases	Penicillin, oral	200,000–250,000 U daily
Surgical infections	22(9.2.8)	Certain surgical patients*b*	Dependent on site of operation	
Syphilis	32(9)	Known exposures ("epidemiological treatment")	Penicillin	Same as treatment
Tuberculosis	36(9.3)	Recent skin test positives Contacts of cases Healed Tb patients; never-treated Tb cases	INH	Adults 5 mg/kg per day for 12 mo

*a*See also Refs. 11 and 90.
*b*C-V, C-section and vaginal hysterectomy, prophylactic hip, certain intestinal, biliary, CNS.

the prevention of *disease* in persons with infections due to *M. tuberculosis*, especially recent infections. Antibiotic prophylaxis with rifampin or minocycline is advocated for family or close contacts of patients with meningococcal meningitis, but adverse vestibular reactions to the latter drug have been reported. "Epidemiological treatment" after known sexual exposure to gonorrhea or syphilis is effective, but requires a full therapeutic regime. Prevention of infection after surgery and burns is advocated in selected situations and operations along guidelines drawn up by the Veterans Administration[139] (see Chapter 22, Section 9.2.8). Patients whose immune status is compromised by steroids, irradiation, alkylating and antimetabolic agents, and other immunosuppressive drugs are at high risk to certain bacterial, fungal, and viral organisms, including some that are not normally pathogenic, but no antimicrobial prophylaxis has been effective. They may be placed in protective isolation (see Section 14.2.1) and closely watched and antibiotic therapy instituted if infection occurs. A possible exception to the ineffectiveness of antibiotics in preventing infections is the prophylactic use of isoniazid (INH) in immunosuppressed patients with inactive tuberculosis. Antibiotics or other prophylactic measures for prevention of traveler's diarrhea are no longer recommended because of the development of antibiotic resistance, doubtful effectiveness, or side reactions.[50]

15. References

1. ACHARA I. L., LOWE, C. V., THAPPA, R., GURUBACHARZA, L. L., SHRESTHA, M. B., CADOZ, M., SCHULZ, D., ARMAND, J., BRYLA, D. A., TROLLFORS, B., CRANSTON, J. P., SCHNEERSON, R., AND ROBBINS, J. B., Prevention of typhoid fever in Nepal with Vi capsular polysaccharide of *Salmonella typhii*. A preliminary report, *N. Engl. J. Med.* **317**:1101–1104 (1987).
2. ANDRIOLE, V. T., Pyelonephritis, in: *Infectious Diseases*, 4th ed. (P. D. HOEPRICH AND M. C. JORDAN, eds.), pp. 578–590, Harper & Row, New York, 1989.
3. ARONSEN, S. S., AND OSTERHOLM, M., Infectious disease in child day care: Management and prevention. Summary of the symposium and recommendations, *Rev. Infect. Dis.* **8**:672–679 (1986).
4. BARRETT-CONNOR, E., Infectious and chronic disease epidemiology: Separate and unequal? *Am. J. Epidemiol.* **109**:245–249 (1979). 249 (1979).
5. BELLANTI, J. A. (ed.), *Immunology*, Saunders, Philadelphia, 1978.
6. BENACERRAF, B., Suppressor T cells and suppressor factor, *Hosp. Pract.* **13(4)**:65–75 (1978).
7. BENACERRAF, B., AND UNANUE, E. R. *Textbook of Immunology*, Williams & Wilkins, Baltimore, 1979.
8. BENENSON, A. S. (ed.) *Control of Communicable Diseases in Man*, 14th ed., American Public Health Association, Washington, D.C., 1985.
9. BENNER, E. J., AND HOEPRICH, P. D., Acute bacterial meningitis, in: *Infectious Diseases* (P. D. Hoeprich, ed.), pp. 931–944, Harper & Row, New York, 1972.
10. BENNETT, J. V., AND BRACHMAN, P. S. (eds.), *Hospital Infections*, 2nd ed., Little, Brown, Boston, 1986.
11. BERGER, S. A., HAZELH, N., AND WEITZMAN, S., Prophylactic antibiotic in surgical procedures, *Surg. Gynecol. Obstet.* **146**:469–475 (1978).
12. BERMAN, S., AND MCINTOSH, K., Selective primary health care: Strategies for control of disease in the developing world. XXI. Acute respiratory infections, *Rev. Infect. Dis.* **7**:674–691 (1985).
13. BLAKE, P. A., ALLEGRA, D. T., SNYDER, J. D., BARNETT, T. J., McFARLAND, L., CARAWAY, C. T., FEELEY, J. C., CRAIG, J. P., LEE, J. V., PUHR, N. D., AND FELDMAN, R. A., Cholera—A possible endemic focus in the United States, *N. Engl. J. Med.* **302**:305–309 (1980)
14. BLAKE, P. J., AND PEREZ, R. C., *Applied Immunological Concepts*, Appleton–Century–Crofts, New York, 1978.
15. BODILY, H. L., UPDYKE, E. L., AND MASON, J. O. (eds.), *Diagnostic Procedures for Bacterial, Mycotic, and Parasitic Infections*, American Public Health Association, New York, 1970.
16. BOISVERT, P. L., DARROW, D. C., POWERS, G. F., AND TRASK, J. D., Streptococcus in children, *Am. J. Dis. Child.* **64**:516–538 (1942).
17. BRASFIELD, D. A., STAGNO, S., WHITLEY, R. J., CLOUD, G., CASSELL, G., AND TELLER, R. E., Infant pneumonitis associated with cytomegalovirus, *Chlamydia, Pneumophilia*, and *Ureaplasma*. Follow up, *Pediatrics* **79**:76–83 (1982).
18. Centers for Disease Control, *68 National Nosocomial Infections, Study and Hospitals*, 1970.
19. Centers for Disease Control, Isolation techniques for use in hospitals, PHS Publ. No. 2054, 1970.
20. Centers for Disease Control, Shigellosis related to an airplane meal, *Morbid. Mortal. Weekly Rep.* **20**:397–402 (1971).
21. Centers for Disease Control, Cholera, *Morbid. Mortal. Weekly Rep.* **21**:392 (1972).
22. Centers for Disease Control, Diphtheria and tetanus toxoids and pertussis vaccine, *Morbid. Mortal. Weekly Rep.* **26**:401–407 (1977).
23. Centers for Disease Control, Selected recommendations of the Public Health Service Advisory Committee on Immunization Practices: Collected recommendations on routine childhood vaccines, *Morbid. Mortal. Weekly Rep.* **26**:401–402, 407, 444 (1977).
24. Centers for Disease Control, Cholera vaccine, *Morbid. Mortal. Weekly Rep.* **27**:173–174 (1978).

25. Centers for Disease Control, Typhoid vaccine, *Morbid. Mortal. Weekly Rep.* **27**:231–233 (1978).

26. Centers for Disease Control, Plague vaccine, *Morbid. Mortal. Weekly Rep.* **27**:255–258 (1978).

27. Centers for Disease Control, Meningococcal polysaccharide vaccines, *Morbid. Mortal. Weekly Rep.* **27**:327–329 (1978).

28. Centers for Disease Control, Reported morbidity and mortality in the United States, 1978, *Morbid. Mortal. Weekly Rep. (Suppl.)* **27(54)**:1–94 (1979).

29. Centers for Disease Control, Nonreported sexually transmissible diseases—United States, *Morbid. Mortal. Weekly Rep.* **28**:61–63 (1979).

30. Centers for Disease Control, National nosocomial infections study report 1977 (Nov. 1979).

31. Centers for Disease Control, Investigation of disease outbreaks, principles of epidemiology, *Homestudy Course 3030-G,* Manual 6, pp. 1–79 (1979).

32. Centers for Disease Control, ACIP recommendations, *Morbid. Mortal. Weekly Rep.* **32**:1–17 (1983).

33. Centers for Disease Control, Supplementary statement of contraindications to receipt of pertussis vaccine, *Morbid. Mortal. Weekly Rep.* **33**:169–171 (1984).

34. Centers for Disease Control, Nosocomial infection surveillance, 1983, CDC Surveillance Summaries, *Morbid. Mortal. Weekly Rep.* **33**:1ss–32ss (1984).

35. Centers for Disease Control, New recommended schedule for active immunization of normal infants and children, *Morbid. Mortal. Weekly Rep.* **35**:577–579 (1986).

36. Centers for Disease Control, Annual summary 1984, *Morbid. Mortal. Weekly Rep.* **33**:1–135 (1986).

37. Centers for Disease Control, Summary of notifiable diseases, United States 1985, *Morbid. Mortal. Weekly Rep.* **34**:1–21 (1987).

38. Centers for Disease Control, AIDS Information Unit, Personal communication (Oct. 22, 1987).

39. Centers for Disease Control, Tetanus—United States, 1985–1986, *Morbid. Mortal. Weekly Rep.* **36**:477–481 (1987).

40. Centers for Disease Control, Public Health Service guidelines for counseling and antibody testing to prevent HIV infection and AIDS, *Morbid. Mortal. Weekly Rep.* **36**:509–515 (1987).

41. Centers for Disease Control, Summary of the second national community forum on adult immunization, *Morbid. Mortal. Weekly Rep.* **36**:677–680 (1987).

42. Centers for Disease Control, Increase in primary and secondary syphilis in the United States, *Morbid. Mortal. Weekly Rep.* **36**:393–396 (1987).

43. Centers for Disease Control, Update. Prevention of *Hemophilus influenzae* type B disease, *Morbid. Mortal. Weekly Rep.* **37**:13–16 (1988).

44. Centers for Disease Control, Health information for international travel, 1989, HHS Publ. No. (CDC) 89-8280.

45. Chanock, R. M., Fox, H. H., James, W. D., Gutekunst, R. R., White, R. J., and Senterfit, L. B., Epidemiology of *M. pneumoniae* infection in military recruits, *Ann. N.Y. Acad. Sci.* **143**:484–496 (1967).

46. Cho, C. T., and Dudding, B. A., *Pediatric-Infectious Diseases,* Medical Examination Publishing, Garden City. N.Y., 1978.

47. Clemens, J. D., Choung, J., and Feinstein, A., The BCG controversy: A methodological and statistical reappraisal, *J. Am. Med. Assoc.* **249**:2362–2369 (1983).

48. Clemens, J. D., Sack, D. A., Harris, J. R., Chakraborty, J., Khan, M. R., Stanton, B. F., Kay, B. A., Khan, M. U., Yunis, M., Atkinson, W., Svennerholm, A.-M., and Holmgren, J., Field trial of oral cholera vaccine in Bangladesh, *Lancet* **2**:124–127 (1986).

49. Congeni, B. L., and Nankervis, G. A., Diagnosis of pneumonia by counterimmunoelectrophoresis of respiratory secretions, *Am. J. Dis. Child.* **132**:684–687 (1978).

50. Consensus Development Conference Panel, Consensus development statement, *Rev. Infect. Dis.* **1**:S227–S233 (1986).

51. Davidson, G. P., Bishop, R. F., Townley, R. R. W., Holmes, I. H., and Ruck, B. J., Importance of a new virus in acute sporadic enteritis in children, *Lancet* **1**:242–246 (1975).

52. Denny, F. W., Clyde, W. A., Jr., and Glezen, W. P., *Mycoplasma pneumoniae* disease: Clinical spectrum, pathophysiology, epidemiology, and control, *J. Infect., Dis.* **123**:74–92 (1971).

53. Diamantstein, T., Oppenheim, J. J., Unanue, E. R., Wood, D. D., Handschumacher, R. E., Rosenstreich, D. L., and Waksman, B. H., Nonspecific "lymphocyte activating" factors produced by macrophages, *Clin. Immunol. Immunopathol.* **14**:264–267 (1979).

54. Dinarello, C. A., and Mier, J. W., Lymphokines, *N. Engl. J. Med.* **317**:940–945 (1987).

55. Drachman, R. H., Acute infectious gastroenteritis, *Pediatr. Clin. North Am.* **25**:711–741 (1978).

56. Dupont, H. L., enteropathogenic organism, new etiologic agent and concepts of disease, *Med. Clin. North Am.* **62**:945–960 (1978).

57. Dupont, H. L., Sullivan, P., Evans, D. G., Pickering, L. K., Evans, D. J., Vollet, J. J., Ericsson, C. D., Ackerman, P. B., and Tjoa, W. S., Prevention of traveler's diarrhea (emporiatric enteritis), *J. Am. Med. Assoc.* **243**:237–271 (1980).

58. Evans, A. S., Clinical syndromes in adults caused by respiratory infection, *Med. Clin. North Am.* **51**:803–818 (1967).

59. Evans, A. S., New discoveries in infectious mononucleosis, *Mod. Med.* **42**:18–24 (1974).

60. Evans, A. S., Diagnosis and prevention of common respiratory infections, *Hosp. Med.* **10**:31–41 (1974).

61. Evans, A. S., Serologic studies of acute respiratory infections in military personnel, *Yale J. Biol. Med.* **48**:201–209 (1975).

62. Evans, A. S., Causation and disease: The Henle–Koch postulates revisited, *Yale J. Biol. Med.* **49**:175–195 (1976).

63. EVANS, A. S., Limitation of Koch's postulates [letter to the editor], *Lancet* **2:**1277–1278 (1977).
64. EVANS, A. S., Causation and disease: A chronological journey, *Am. J. Epidemiol.* **108:**249–258 (1978).
65. EVANS, A. S., Re: Definitions of epidemiology [letter], *Am. J. Epidemiol.* **109:**379–381 (1979).
66. EVANS, A. S., The clinical illness promotion factor: A third ingredient, *Yale J. Biol. Med.* **55:**193–199 (1982).
67. EVANS, A. S. (ed.), *Viral Infections of Humans: Epidemiology and Control,* 3rd ed., Plenum Medical, New York, 1989.
68. EVANS, A. S., Subclinical epidemiology. The First Harry A. Feldman Memorial Lecture, *Am. J. Epidemiol.* **125:**545–555 (1987).
69. EVANS, A. S., AND BRACHMAN, P. S., Emerging issues in infectious disease epidemiology, *J. Chronic Dis.* **39:**1105–1124 (1986).
70. EVANS, A. S., AND DICK, E. C., Acute pharyngitis, tonsillitis in University of Wisconsin students, *J. Am. Med. Assoc.* **190:**699–708 (1964).
71. EVANS, A. S., AND FELDMAN, H. A. (eds.), *Bacterial Infections of Humans: Epidemiology and Control,* Plenum Medical, New York, 1982.
72. EVANS, A. S., ALLEN, V., AND SUELTMANN, S., *Mycoplasma pneumoniae* infections in University of Wisconsin students, *Am. Rev. Respir. Dis.* **96:**237–244 (1967).
73. FEDSON, D. S., AND RUSTHOVEN, J., Acute lower respiratory disease, *Primary Care* **6:**13–41 (1979).
74. FEIGIN, R. D., AND CHERRY, J. D. (eds.), *Textbook of Pediatric Infectious Diseases,* 2nd ed., Saunders, Philadelphia, 1987.
75. FEKETY, F. R., JR., CALDWELL, J., AND GUMP, D., Bacteria, viruses, and mycoplasmas in acute pneumonia in adults, *Am. Rev. Respir. Dis.* **104:**499–507 (1971).
76. FIUMARA, N. J., The sexually transmissible diseases, *Dis. Mon.* **25:**3–38 (1978).
77. Food and Drug Administration, HIV precautions for health care professionals, *FDA Bull.* **17:**16–17 (1987).
78. FOX, J. P., AND HALL, C. E., Viruses in Families: Surveillance as a Key to Epidemiology of Virus Infections. PSG Pub. Co. Littleton, Mass., 1980.
79. FOY, H. M., GRAYSTON, J. T., KENNY, G. E., ALEXANDER, E. R., AND McMAHAN, R., Epidemiology of *Mycoplasma pneumoniae* infection in families, *J. Am. Med. Assoc.* **197:**859–866 (1966).
80. FRASER, D. W., TSAI, T. R., ORENSTEIN, W., PARKIN, W. E., BEECHAM, H. J., SHARRAR, R. G., HARRIS, J., MALLISON, G. F., MARTIN, S. M., McDADE, J. E., SHEPARD, C. C., BRACHMANN, P. B., and the field investigation team, Legionnaire's disease—Description of an epidemic of pneumonia, *N. Engl. J. Med.* **297:**1189–1197 (1977).
81. GLEZEN, W. P., CLYDE, W. A., SENIOR, R. J., SCHEAFFER, C. I., AND DENNY, F. W., Group A streptococci, mycoplasmas, and viruses associated with acute pharyngitis, *J. Am. Med. Assoc.* **202:**455–460 (1967).
82. GLORIG, A., AND GER, K. S., *Otitis Media,* Thomas, Springfield, Ill., 1972.
83. GORBACH, S. L., AND KHURANA, C. M., Toxigenic *Escherichia coli:* A cause of infantile diarrhea in Chicago, *N. Engl. J. Med.* **287:**791–797 (1971).
84. GRAYSTON, J. T., KUO, C. C., WANG, S. P., AND ALTMAN, J., A new *Chlamydia psittace* strain, TWAR, isolated in acute respiratory tract infections, *N. Engl. J. Med.* **315:**161–168 (1986).
85. GREGG, M. B., The principles of epidemic field investigation, in: *Oxford Textbook of Public Health,* Volume 3 (A. Chappie, W. W. Holland, R. Detels, and G. Knox, eds.), pp. 284–297, Oxford University Press, London, 1985.
86. HANDSFIELD, H. H., Gonorrhea and non-gonococcal urethritis: Recent advances, *Med. Clin. North Am.* **62:**925–943 (1978).
87. HELSTAD, A. G., MANDEL, A. D., AND EVANS, A. S., Thermostable *Clostridium perfringens* as cause of food poisoning outbreak, *Public Health Rep.* **82:**157–161 (1967).
88. HENDERSON, F. L., COLLIER, A. M., SANYAL, M. A., WATKINS, J. M., FAIRCLOUGH, D. L., CLYDE, W. A., JR., AND DENNY, F. W., A longitudinal study of respiratory viruses and bacteria in the etiology of acute otitis media with effusion, *N. Engl. J. Med.* **306:**1377–1383 (1982).
89. HENLE, J., *On Miasmata and Contagie,* Johns Hopkins Press, Baltimore, 1938 (translated and with an introduction by G. ROSEN).
90. HOEPRICH, P. D., Chemoprophylaxis of infectious diseases, in: *Infectious Diseases,* 2nd ed. (P. D. HOEPRICH, ed.), pp. 190–206, Harper & Row, New York, 1977.
91. HOEPRICH, P. D. (ed.), *Infectious Diseases,* 3rd ed., Harper & Row, New York, 1983.
92. HOLMES, K. K., AND STAMM, W. E., Chlamydial genital infections: A growing problem, *Hosp. Pract.* **14:**105–117 (1979).
93. HOOD, L. E., WEISSMAN, I. L., AND WOOD, W. B., *Immunology,* 2nd ed., Benjamin/Cummings, Reading, Mass., 1984.
94. HORAN, T. C., WHITE, J. W., JARVIS, W. R., EMORI, T. G., CULVER, D. H., MUNN, V. P., THORNSBERRY, C., OLSON, S. R., AND HUGHES, J. M., Nosocomial infection surveillance, 1984, *Morbid. Mortal. Weekly Rep.* **35:**17ss–29ss (1986).
95. HUEBNER, R. J., The virologist's dilemma, *Ann. N.Y. Acad. Sci.* **67:**430–445 (1957).
96. Institute of Medicine, National Academy of Sciences, *New Vaccine Development, Establishment of Priorities,* National Academy of Sciences, Washington, D.C., 1985.
97. JAWETZ, E., MELNICK, J. L., AND ADELBERG, E. A., *Review of Medical Microbiology,* 17th ed., Lange, Los Altos, Calif., 1987.
98. JENKINS, W. D., Division of Sexually Transmitted Diseases, Centers for Disease Control, Personal communication (March 1986).

99. JOHNSON, R. T., AND GIBBS, C. J., JR., Editorial: Koch's postulates and slow infections of the nervous system, *Arch. Neurol.* **30**:36–38 (1974).

100. JUPA, J. E., Venereal disease, *Primary Care* **6**:113–126 (1979).

101. KALLMAN, F. J., AND REISMAN, D., Twin studies on the significance of genetic factors in tuberculosis, *Am. Rev. Tuberc.* **47**:549–574 (1943).

102. KAUFMAN, S. H. E., Possible role of helper and cytolytic T lymphocytes in antibacterial defense. Conclusions based on a murine model of listeriosis, *Rev. Infect. Dis.* **9**(Suppl. 5):S650–S659 (1987).

103. KELSEY, J., DOUGLAS, W. D., JR., AND EVANS, A. S., *Methods in Observational Epidemiology,* Oxford University Press, London, 1986.

104. KLEIN, J. O., FEIGIN, R. D., AND McCRACKEN, G. H., JR., Report of the task force on diagnosis and management of meningitis, *Pediatrics* **78**(Suppl., Part 2):956–989 (1986).

105. KNIGHT, V. (ed.), *Viral and Mycoplasma Infections of the Respiratory Tract,* Lea & Febiger, Philadelphia, 1973.

106. KOCH, R., Die Aetiologie der Tuberculose, *Berl. Klin. Wochenschr.* **19**:221–230 (1882).

107. KOCH, R., Ueber bacteriologische Forschung, in: *Verh. X Int. Med. Congr.,* p. 35, Verlag von August Hirschwald, Berlin, 1892.

108. LANGMUIR, A. D., AND GANGAROSA, E. J., Practical outline of major forms of enteric disease, Presented at the IEA Regional Scientific Meeting on Enteric Infections, Alexandria, Egypt (1978).

109. LAST, J. M., *A Dictionary of Epidemiology,* Oxford Medical Publications, 2nd ed., New York, 1989.

110. LENNETTE, E. H., BALOWE, A., HAUSLER, W. J., AND SHADOMY, J., (eds.), *Manual of Clinical Microbiology,* 4th ed., American Society for Clinical Microbiology, Bethesda, 1985.

111. LILIENFELD, A. M., The epidemiologic method in cancer research, *J. Chronic Dis.* **8**:647–654 (1958).

112. LILIENFELD, A. M., AND LILIENFELD, D. E., *Fundamentals of Epidemiology,* 2nd ed., Oxford University Press, London, 1982.

113. LILIENFELD, D. E., Definitions of epidemiology, *Am. J. Epidemiol.* **107**:87–90 (1978).

114. MACDONALD, K. L., AND GRIFFIN, D. M., Foodborne disease outbreaks, annual summary, 1982, *Morbid. Mortal. Weekly Rep.* **35**:7ss–16ss (1986).

115. MACMAHON, B., AND PUGH, T. F., *Epidemiology: Principles and Methods,* Little, Brown, Boston, 1970.

116. MANDELL, G. L., DOUGLAS, R. G., JR., AND BENNETT, J. E. (eds.), *Principles and Practice of Infectious Diseases,* 2nd ed., Wiley, New York, 1985.

117. MAXY, K. G., ROSENEAU, M. J., AND LAST, J. M., (eds.), *Public Health and Preventive Medicine,* 12th ed., Appleton–Century–Crofts, New York, 1986.

118. McALLISTER, T. A., PERCIVAL, A., ALEXANDER, J. G., BOYCE, J. M. H., DULAKE, C., AND WORMALD, P. J., Multi-centric study of sensitivities or urinary tract pathogens, *Postgrad. Med. J. (Sept. Suppl.)* **47**:7–14 (1971).

119. McCORMACK, W. M., Sexually transmissible diseases, *Postgrad. Med.* **58**:179–186 (1975).

120. McCORMACK, W. M., Viral, fungal, parasitic, and other sexually transmitted infections, *Forum Infect.* **4**:3–22 (1977).

121. MIMS, C. A., *The Pathogenesis of Infectious Disease,* 3rd ed., Academic Press/Grune & Stratton, New York, 1987.

122. NOSSAL, G. J. V., The basic components of the immune system, *N. Engl. J. Med.* **316**:1320–1325 (1987).

123. OSTERHOLM, M. T., PIERSON, L. M., WHITE, K. E., LIBBY, T. A., KURITSKY, J. N., AND McCOLLOUGH, J. G., The risk of *Hemophilus influenzae* type B disease among children in daycare: Results of a two-year statewide prospective surveillance and contact survey, *N. Engl. J. Med.* **316**:1–5 (1987).

124. PARRY, J. V., PERRY, K. R., AND MORTIMER, P. P., Sensitive assays for viral antibodies in saliva: An alternative to tests on serum, *Lancet* **2**:72–75 (1987).

125. POWERS, G. F., AND BOISVERT, P. L., Age as a factor in streptococcus, *J. Pediatr.* **25**:481–509 (1944).

126. PRICE, D. L., Tetanus toxin: Direct evidence for retrograde intraaxonal transport, *Science* **188**:945–947 (1975).

127. RAPPULE, R., PERGUNI, M., AND FALSEN, E., Molecular epidemiology of the 1984–1986 outbreak of diphtheria in Sweden, *N. Engl. J. Med.* **318**:12–14 (1988).

128. REIMANN, H. M., *The Pneumonias,* Green, St. Louis, 1971.

129. RIVERS, T. M., Viruses and Koch's postulates, *J. Bacteriol.* **33**:1–12 (1937).

130. ROIT, I. M., *Essential Immunology,* 2nd ed., Blackwell, Oxford, 1974.

131. RUDDLE, N., Tumor necrosis factor and related cytotoxins, *Immunol. Today* **8**:129–130 (1987).

132. SCHLECH, W. F., WARD, J. I., BAND, J. D., HIGHTOWER, A., FRASER, D., AND BROOME, C., Bacterial meningitis in the United States, 1978 through 1981, The National Bacterial Meningitis Surveillance Study, *J. Am. Med. Assoc.* **253**:1749–1754 (1985).

133. SETO, D. W. Y., AND HELLER, R. M., Acute respiratory infections, *Pediatr. Clin. North Am.* **21**:683–709 (1974).

134. SOURS, H. E., AND SMITH, D. G., Outbreaks of foodborne diseases in the United States, 1972–1978, *J. Infect. Dis.* **141**:122–125 (1980).

135. TILLOTSON, J. R., AND FINLAND, M., Bacterial colonization and clinical superinfection of the respiratory tract complicating antibiotic treatment of pneumonia, *J. Infect. Dis.* **119**:597–624 (1969).

136. TODD, M. J., Sexually transmitted diseases in Canada in 1985, *Can. Med. Assoc. J.* **136**:849–851 (1985).

137. TOSATO, G., MAGRATH, I., KOSKI, I., DOOLEY, N., AND BLAESE, M., Activation of suppressor T cells during Epstein–Barr-virus-induced infectious mononucleosis, *N. Engl. J. Med.* **301**:1133–1137 (1979).

138. URBASCHEK, B., AND URBASCHEK, R., Introduction and sum-

mary. Perspectives on bacterial pathogenesis and host defense, *Rev. Infect. Dis.* **9:**(Suppl. 5):S431–S436 (1987).

139. Veterans Administration Ad Hoc Interdisciplinary Advisory Committee on Antimicrobial Drug Usage (C. KUNIN, chairman), Audit of antimicrobial usage: Prophylaxis in surgery, *J. Am. Med. Assoc.* **237:**1003–1008 (1977).

140. WARD, J. I., CLEGG, H. W., WASSERMAN, R., ROSENBERG, G., AND SIBER, G. R., *Hemophilus influenzae* pneumonia. A prospective study demonstrating the utility of latex agglutination for diagnosis, *Pediatr. Res.* **15:**124 (Abstr. 1088) (1981).

141. WEHRLE, P. F., Meningitis, in: *Communicable and Infectious Diseases* (F. H. TOP, SR., AND P. F. WEHRLE, eds.), pp. 436–453, Mosby, St. Louis, 1976.

142. WING, E. J., AND REMINGTON, J. S., Cell-mediated immunity and its role in resistance to infection (medical progress), *West. J. Med.* **126:**14–31 (1977).

143. World Health Organization, Special Program on AIDS and Expanded Program in Immunization. Joint statement. Consultation on human immunodeficiency virus and routine childhood immunizations, *WHO Weekly Epidemiol. Rec.* **62:**297–299 (1988).

144. WRIGHT, R. A., SPENCER, H. C., BRODSKY, R. E., AND VERNON, T. M., Giardiasis in Colorado. An epidemiologic study, *Am. J. Epidemiol.* **105:**330–356 (1977).

145. YOLKEN, R. H., WYATT, R. G., ZISSIS, G., BRANDT, C. D., RODRIGUEZ, W. J., KIM, H. W., PARROTT, R. H., URRUTIA, J. J., MATA, L., GREENBERG, H. B., KAPIKIAN, A. Z., AND CHANOCK, R. M., Epidemiology of human rotavirus types 1 and 2 as studied by enzyme-linked immunosorbent assay, *N. Engl. J. Med.* **299:**1156–1161 (1978).

146. ZINKERNAGEL, R. M., Major transplantation antigens in host responses to infection, *Hosp. Pract.* **13:**83–92 (1978).

16. Suggested Reading

BENENSON, A. S. (ed.), *Control of Communicable Diseases in Man,* 13th ed., American Public Health Association, Washington, D.C., 1981.

EVANS, A. S. (ed.), *Viral Infections of Humans: Epidemiology and Control,* 3rd ed., Plenum Medical, New York, 1989.

FEIGIN, R. D., AND CHERRY, J. D. (eds.), *Textbook of Pediatric Infectious Diseases,* 2nd ed., Saunders, Philadelphia, 1987.

HENNEKENS, C. H., AND BURING, J. L., *Epidemiology in Medicine,* Little, Brown, Boston, 1987.

HOEPRICH, P. D. AND JORDAN, M. C. (eds.), *Infectious Diseases,* 4th ed., Harper & Row, New York, 1989.

JAWETZ, E., MELNICK, J. L., AND ADELBERG, E. A., *Review of Medical Microbiology,* 17th ed., Lange, Los Altos, Calif. 1987.

KELSEY, J., THOMPSON, W. D., AND EVANS, A. S., *Methods in Observational Epidemiology,* Oxford University Press, London, 1986.

MANDELL, G. L., DOUGLAS, R. G., JR., AND BENNETT, J. E. (eds.), *Principles and Practice of Infectious Diseases,* Volumes 1 and 2, Wiley, New York, 2nd ed., 1985.

MIMS, C. A., *The Pathogenesis of Infectious Disease,* 3rd ed., Academic Press/Grune & Stratton, New York, 1987.

WEHRLE, P. F., AND TOP, F. H., SR., *Communicable and Infectious Diseases,* 9th ed., Mosby, St. Louis, 1981.

CHAPTER 2

Surveillance

Philip S. Brachman

1. Introduction

The term *surveillance,* derived from the French word meaning "to watch over," may be defined as a system of close observation of all aspects of the occurrence and distribution of a given disease through the systematic collection, tabulation, analysis, and dissemination of all relevant data pertaining to that disease. Although the methodology of surveillance is basically descriptive, its function is more than merely collective and archival. Surveillance must be dynamic, current, purposeful, and result in a public health action. This action frequently results in the establishment of a new or the reinforcement of an existing public health policy. It is fundamental to prompt and effective control and prevention of disease. Traditionally, surveillance was first applied to the acute communicable diseases beginning in the early 1950s.[14] The term has been rapidly expanded since then, to embrace not only a wide variety of noninfectious diseases but also other health-related events such as environmental hazards, injuries, immunizations, the distribution of biological products, and health-care delivery.

2. History

William Farr, of the General Registrar's Office of England and Wales, is credited with initiating disease surveillance in the mid-1800s. He collected, collated, and analyzed vital statistical data and distributed reports to appropriate health personnel as well as to the public.[20] The

collection of national morbidity data was initiated in 1878 when Congress authorized the Public Health Service (PHS) to collect reports of the occurrence of the quarantinable diseases, that is, cholera, plague, smallpox, and yellow fever. In 1893, Congress passed an act stating that weekly health information should be collected from all state and municipal authorities. In 1902, in an attempt to develop uniformity, the Surgeon General of the PHS was directed to provide forms for collecting, compiling, and publishing surveillance data. In 1913, the state and territorial health authorities recommended that every state send weekly telegraphic summaries reporting the occurrence of selected diseases to the PHS. All states were reporting the occurrences of disease by 1925. In 1949, when the National Office of Vital Statistics (NOVS) was established in the PHS, the communicable-disease-reporting function (morbidity reporting) was merged with the national mortality registration and reporting functions that were the primary responsibility of the NOVS. Until the early 1950s, the communicable-disease reports were published weekly in the official journal *Public Health Reports.* When this journal became a monthly publication, the NOVS issued a separate weekly bulletin, the *Morbidity and Mortality Weekly Report* (MMWR), that was distributed to state health officers, state epidemiologists, county and city health officers, and others including persons who requested its receipt. In July 1960, the responsibility for receiving morbidity reports from the states and larger cities and the issuing of the MMWR was transferred from Washington to the Communicable Disease Center [now called the Centers for Disease Control (CDC)] in Atlanta.

Actually, the application of the term *surveillance* to the watchfulness over a nationally important communicable disease (malaria) was begun in 1946 by the CDC[1] in part

Philip S. Brachman   Emory   University   School of Public Health, Atlanta, Georgia 30329.

to monitor veterans who were returning from endemic areas. The application of critical epidemiological evaluation to the former rather crude reports revealed that malaria had ceased to be an indigenous disease. Endemic spread of infection had ceased some years before through control of the vector.

In 1955, following the outbreak of killed vaccine-related poliomyelitis (the so-called "Cutter Incident"), a national surveillance of poliomyelitis was directed by the Surgeon General as an essential step toward a solution of this national disaster.[15]

In 1957, influenza was placed under surveillance because of the impending pandemic of Asian influenza for which a comprehensive national program of widespread immunization and education of doctors and hospitals to meet such a possible disaster was undertaken by the Surgeon General. The influenza surveillance program has continued, and one of its essential functions is to provide information to guide manufacturers in the preparation of influenza vaccine as concerns its antigenic composition and the amount of vaccine to produce. In 1961, because of the increasing public-health concern with salmonellosis, a special *Salmonella* surveillance program was developed in conjunction with the states to define the problem better so that appropriate control and prevention measures could be instituted.

At present, the occurrence of 42 diseases is reported weekly, and that of 7 other diseases is reported annually by state health departments, to the CDC. Additionally, 7 other diseases are reported by either special case-reporting forms or line-listing forms submitted either monthly or annually. These reports are published in the MMWR and are summarized annually in the MMWR *Annual Summary*.[6] These lists are reviewed annually by the state and territorial epidemiologists and changed as indicated by the occurrence of the diseases. Additionally, more intensive surveillance is maintained over selected diseases by means of special surveillance efforts to develop more specific data concerning these diseases. Selected chronic conditions are also under similar surveillance.

National disease surveillance programs are maintained by most countries in the world. The methods used to obtain reports, the diseases reported, the analyses, and the type and frequency of reports vary, but the value and importance of surveillance is universally recognized. The World Health Organization (WHO) maintains surveillance on the quarantinable diseases (cholera, plague, and yellow fever) as well as other selected diseases. The most recent disease to come under worldwide surveillance is AIDS. WHO prepares weekly reports as well as other reports summarizing these data.

3. Use of Surveillance

A surveillance program can be designed to produce a variety of output data depending on the purpose of the program. It can portray the natural history of the disease, including a description of the occurrence of the disease by time, place, and person. Surveillance data should describe the background (or sporadic, endemic, or ongoing) level of the disease, as well as changes in the occurrence of the disease as modified by nonrecurring events such as epidemics or a hyperendemic situation. Surveillance can be used to monitor changes in the agent, such as antibiotic resistance of gonococci.

Analysis of surveillance data can help to establish priorities for developing or allocating appropriate health resources for approaching a problem. Surveillance can also be used to confirm a hypothesis or indicate the need for further study or additional data.

Analysis of surveillance data can lead to the development and/or institution of control and/or prevention measures such as chemotherapy, chemoprophylaxis, new resources or resource allocation (e.g., people, equipment, or monies), or additional training for persons involved in control and prevention activities. Surveillance can be used to evaluate the effectiveness of newly instituted control and/or prevention measures. Surveillance data are also important in forecasting or predicting the future pattern of the occurrence of a disease.

In this chapter, surveillance is discussed primarily as it involves bacterial infectious diseases. Surveillance techniques for other infectious diseases differ little, though there may be some variation in the data-collection procedures.

4. Data Sources

WHO in 1968 codified the term *surveillance* on a truly global basis.[23] Ten "elements" or distinguishable sources of data were identified; one or any combination of the ten can be used to support a disease-specific surveillance program. The sources used to develop the surveillance data depend on the disease itself, the methods used for identifying the disease, the goals of the program, the personnel and material resources available, the population involved, and the characteristics of the disease's occurrence. One source of data can be used regularly and other methods utilized as necessary to improve the sensitivity and/or specificity of the data depicting the occurrence of the disease.

4.1. Mortality Data

Mortality registration has been used the longest, but it is useful only for diseases that are associated with fatalities. If the case-fatality ratio is too low, mortality statistics may not provide an accurate assessment of the occurrence of the disease. If mortality rate data are accurate and if the proportion of deaths to cases is known from past studies, then the number of deaths can provide an estimate of the actual number of cases that have occurred.

Unfortunately, there is wide variation in the accuracy with which death certificates are filled out. Additionally, the disease under surveillance may have been a contributory cause of death and may not be noted on the death certificate. Also, there is a time lag in reporting deaths, so that a surveillance program based on mortality registration has an inherent delay of from weeks to months.

An example of the use of mortality data for surveillance is the collection of pneumonia and influenza weekly mortality reports from 121 American cities.[5] These data are used to describe weekly pneumonia and influenza activity. Another example occurred in the 1960s during an investigation of shigellosis in rural areas in Central America where there was no ongoing surveillance program.[10] The only available reports of any of the cases were listings of deaths that were routinely noted in "vital statistics" books maintained in the communities. By noting the recording of deaths and by knowing the case-fatality ratio, it was possible to develop information concerning the occurrence of cases of shigellosis.

4.2. Morbidity Data

The second source of surveillance data and the one most commonly used is that of morbidity or case reporting. This is a prompt, simple, and relatively accurate system that is dependent on the reporting of cases of the diseases under surveillance. Reporting the occurrence of disease is the responsibility of the patient's physician. He or she may delegate this responsibility to someone else such as a nurse, clerk, or administrator. Cases may be reported by the physician calling the health department or vice versa, or they may be reported each day or each week on a special form sent by mail. Copies of laboratory reports may also be submitted to the public-health authorities. The techniques of reporting are described in greater detail in Section 6.

4.3. Individual Case Reports

Individual case investigation is more likely to be performed with rare diseases or unusual cases of a more common disease. For diseases of high frequency, investigating individual cases is usually neither practical nor necessary, but may be conducted as a check on the validity of morbidity or mortality reporting. As a disease decreases in incidence, individual case investigation may be of increasing importance to determine why the case occurred and to further direct control and prevention measures. If the disease is approaching control (or eradication) status, then intensive investigation of each reported case is important. This was dramatically demonstrated in the smallpox-eradication program.[23]

4.4. Epidemic Reporting

The fourth source of surveillance data is the reporting of epidemics. Frequently, there is quantitative improvement of reporting when clusters of cases occur. Thus, single cases of shigellosis or salmonellosis may not be individually reported, but if there is an epidemic, then all cases that are part of the epidemic may be reported.

4.5. Epidemic Field Investigation

Epidemic field investigations may uncover more cases of the disease than would have been reported without the investigation. In the outbreak of salmonellosis in Riverside, California, in 1965, several hundred cases were initially reported; however, following a field investigation, 16,000 cases were estimated to have occurred.[17] The decision to investigate an epidemic will be based on the specific disease, the seriousness of the outbreak, the extent of the problem, the anticipated need for more specific information concerning the occurrence of the epidemic, availability of resources, research potential, and possibly political pressures.

4.6. Laboratory Reporting

The laboratory is essential in identifying and confirming pathogens. Although many diseases can be adequately described clinically, there are others for which laboratory identification of the etiological agent is essential for accuracy. For example, gastroenteritis may be caused by various organisms; it is frequently not possible to be certain of the etiology on the basis of clinical and epidemiological data alone, and thus it is necessary to incorporate laboratory testing before the etiological agent can be identified. The accuracy of the *Salmonella* and *Shigella* surveillance programs in the United States is dependent on laboratory testing.

In addition to disease identification, the laboratory can also provide important information concerning specific characteristics of microorganisms. For example, the antigenic characteristics of influenza strains are important, since significant changes in the prevalent strain will necessitate changes in formulation of vaccine to be used before the next influenza season. Identifying the serotype of salmonellae isolated from different patients may be necessary in order to associate different isolates as part of a single outbreak. Careful attention to antibiotic-sensitivity patterns can indicate a change in the epidemiological pattern of the disease or be a forewarning of an impending upsurge in the occurrence of the disease. This has been seen in the increasing frequency with which antibiotic-resistant gonococci are being identified and the spread of methicillin-resistant *Staphylococcus aureus*[21] within and between hospitals. A variety of molecular tools are now available that provide highly specific identification of a strain or substrain of an organism. Methods for both phenotypic and genotyping are now used, including DNA probes, to follow the spread of an organism in an outbreak and to differentiate between exogenous reinfection and endogenous reactivation. Unfortunately, these new techniques are performed only in highly specialized laboratories such as the CDC or in research institutions.

The serology laboratory also contributes to surveillance by identifying and/or confirming the presence of a specific disease. Usually, two serum specimens are obtained from each individual, one during the acute phase and one during the convalescent phase of illness, to demonstrate a significant change (usually fourfold) in titer. However, if only a single serum specimen is obtained, the occurrence of a specific disease may be suggested if the antibody titer to that disease is elevated beyond a certain value or by the presence of IgM antibody. Also, if elevated titers are found in serum specimens from a group of patients who had similar illnesses, then these single specimens can be of assistance in making the diagnosis (see Chapter 1).

4.7. Surveys

Surveys can provide information concerning the prevalence of disease. Clinical surveys may include questions related to the occurrence of a disease, physical examination such as spleen surveys to identify patients with malaria, or diagnostic tests such as skin tests to determine the prevalence of histoplasmosis or tuberculosis. In some countries, blood-smear surveys may be used in surveillance for malaria. Other types of surveys include household surveys, such

as the National Health Interview Survey, which includes 55,000 households surveyed annually; cluster surveys, such as used in evaluating immunization programs by WHO; and telephone surveys, which can be used to estimate the magnitude of an outbreak of a disease.

Serological tests for certain bacterial, rickettsial, and treponemal infections carried out on a representative sample of a population can provide prevalence data for different age, sex, and geographic segments of the group tested. Incidence data can be obtained by demonstrating the appearance or rise in antibody titer to a given infection in two serum specimens spaced in time such as the start and end of an epidemic, military service, or a college year; the occurrence of recent infection can also be demonstrated in a single specimen by determining the presence of specific IgM antibody for that infectious agent or by testing for an antibody type of short duration such as certain complement-fixing antibodies. The uses of seroepidemiology are presented in more detail in the companion book on viral infections.[9]

4.8. Animal Reservoir and Vector Distribution

Animal-reservoir and vector-distribution studies are important in maintaining surveillance of zoonotic and arthropod-borne diseases. Information about rabies in animal reservoirs in a specific geographic area can be important in making a decision concerning the need to treat a human exposed to an unidentified animal. The knowledge that tularemia is occurring in animals or that ticks infected with *Francisella tularensis* are present in an area would support reports of suspect cases of tularemia in humans. Similar studies are in progress to define the distribution of Lyme disease, which is caused by *Borrelia burgdorferi* whose vector is one of several Ixodid ticks. Knowledge about the occurrence of plague in prairie dogs or rodents can be important in evaluating surveillance data concerning possible cases of human plague.

4.9. Biologics and Drug Distribution

The utilization of biologics and drugs for treatment or prophylaxis of a disease may be used to monitor disease occurrence. For example, in an outbreak of diarrheal disease, the increasing sales of antidiarrhea medications by pharmacies serve to corroborate the occurrence of disease. Similarly, an increase in requests for immune serum globulin can be a clue to the occurrence of cases of viral hepatitis.

4.10. Demographic and Environmental Data

Demographic and environmental data are necessary in order to analyze disease-occurrence data effectively. Such data may include age, sex, occupation, residence, or other personal information. Incidence rates cannot be determined until denominator data concerning the population are available. For example, when an increase in the number of isolations of *Salmonella eastbourne* was noted, an analysis of cases by age showed a significant number of cases among young children.[8] This fact was an important clue in leading the investigators to identify chocolate candy as the vehicle of infection.

4.11. News Media

Another useful source of surveillance information is public information gathered through the news media. It is not uncommon for the occurrence of a disease, and especially an epidemic, to be first noted by the news media. Additionally, the news media can perform an important role in alerting the public to the occurrence of a disease outbreak and thus stimulate the reporting of cases that otherwise might not have been diagnosed or reported. In an outbreak of botulism associated with a restaurant in a western state, radio reports alerted a patron of the restaurant to the possibility of exposure after the patron had returned to his home several hundred miles from the restaurant.[3] At the time he heard the radio report, he was experiencing some symptoms. Accordingly, he sought medical assistance, botulism was diagnosed, he was successfully treated, and thus another case was reported.

5. Routine Surveillance

As previously indicated, routine surveillance of a specific disease will not include all the data sources discussed above. The methods that provide the most accurate information collected in a practical and efficient manner that satisfies the objectives of the surveillance program should be utilized. If more information is needed concerning occurrence of the disease, then additional sources of information can be incorporated into the surveillance system.

The need for completeness of reporting varies according to the incidence of the disease under surveillance. For those diseases that either normally do not occur in an area or occur at a very low incidence, it is essential, for control purposes, that all cases that occur be reported. Examples (in the United States) include plague, yellow fever, poliomyelitis, and human rabies.

On the other hand, to maintain surveillance on diseases that commonly occur, it is not critical for all cases to be reported. In the United States, it is estimated that only 1% of cases of salmonellosis, 10% of cases of measles, and 15–20% of cases of viral hepatitis are reported. The fact that all cases are not reported should not reduce the effectiveness of surveillance, since it is generally the trends of disease occurrence that are important in the implementation of control and prevention measures. Changes in the trend should reflect real changes in the occurrence of disease and not changes reflecting a variation in the methods of surveillance. If the methods of obtaining the surveillance data have not changed significantly during a period of time, and the data collected are a representative sampling of the cases that have occurred, then these data should be suitable for determining the trend of the disease. However, a change in the methods used to collect the surveillance data, followed by a change in the reported occurrence of the disease, may be falsely interpreted as a change in the incidence of the disease. An example of this artifact could have occurred in the national *Shigella* surveillance program that was initiated in 1964 with routine reporting from 17 states. Several years later, the remaining states began reporting their isolates; the sudden increase in reported cases could have been misinterpreted if attention had not been given to the mechanics of the surveillance program.[2] Similar artifacts in surveillance data have occurred in the national AIDS surveillance program. As the definition of a case of AIDS has been modified to accommodate new knowledge concerning the clinical manifestations of the disease, the overall surveillance data have reflected these changes.

To validate surveillance data, various methods have been used. These include: (1) physicians in the reporting area can be called and asked if they reported all cases of the disease among the patients within a specific time period, (2) hospital records can be checked by means of a prevalence study to see that all notifiable diseases have been reported, (3) laboratory reports from hospital and public health laboratories for a given disease can be compared to the cases reported to the health department.

6. Reporting

In general, detailed individual case data are not necessarily useful in surveillance programs. It is the analysis of collective data that provides meaningful information. If more specific case information is necessary, then individual cases can be traced back and additional data obtained.

The quality of a surveillance program is as good as the quality of the data collected. In morbidity reporting, an integral component is the person who has the responsibility for reporting the occurrence of the disease. Most frequently, this is the person who has medical responsibility for the patient, and usually that person is a physician. This responsibility may be delegated to someone else, such as the physician's nurse or, in a hospital, the house staff or the administrator. In reporting cases of any disease, confidentiality of the patient must be respected and maintained.

Within a community, cases are reported to the local health authority, such as a city health department. At regular intervals, usually weekly, these cases will be reported to the state health department. In the United States the weekly totals and selected individual case data will be reported to the CDC. Computers have been introduced into the surveillance system at various levels.[11] All state health departments report their data to the CDC via computers. Computer reporting by health-care physicians has been initiated in France.[21]

6.1. Motivation

The diligence with which cases are reported reflects the motivation of the person responsible for reporting. Physicians frequently do not wish to assume this responsibility because of the constraints on their time and the low priority they give to reporting. There needs to be some motivation developed for reporting other than that related to disease-reporting laws. Motivation may result from being a participant in a public-health project or from professional or personal gain. A report summarizing the surveillance data (see Section 9) may be motivational (as well as educational) so that the reporter does recognize that there is some action resulting from disease-reporting. Motivation may also be derived from knowledge that surveillance data can support the development of effective control and prevention programs with a decreased incidence in the occurrence of disease.

Reporting may be stimulated by the availability of a physician epidemiologist who can provide assistance to the reporting physician on request. Another source of motivation may be that the reporting of surveillance data results in important clinical and therapeutic data being made available to the practitioner. For example, the recent increase in antibiotic-resistant strains of *Neisseria* gonococci reported through the CDC's surveillance program is important information for practicing physicians to have when they see a patient, make a clinical diagnosis of gonorrhea, and want to initiate therapy immediately. This example of the application of surveillance data to the practice of medicine can serve to motivate physicians to participate in surveillance activities.

Disease-reporting can also be stimulated by making specific therapeutic drugs available to the physician on notification of the occurrence of a specific disease. In some communities, reports of hepatitis A result in serum immune globulin being made available for prophylactic use. A report of a case of botulism may lead public-health authorities to make trivalent botulinum antitoxin available. Reports of certain tropical parasitic diseases make it possible for physicians to obtain certain therapeutic drugs from the CDC not otherwise available. For example, the availability of a drug exclusively from the CDC to treat cases of *Pneumocystis carinii* pneumonia led to recognition of the occurrence of a new disease, AIDS, in 1981.[7]

A reward system for reporting can be used. The reward can be publicity given to the reporting physicians by listing their names in the surveillance report or in a scientific paper summarizing the surveillance data. A monetary reward system has also been used, with an annual payment or a specific amount of money being given for each report submitted.

However, health officials must recognize the negative effect of a reporting mechanism that is too complex or that demands excessive expenditure of time on the part of the reporter. If reporting of cases brings adverse publicity to the patient, physician, hospital, or community, surveillance will be inhibited. Adverse publicity that leads to a loss of money or to legal action against the reporter or hospital also has a negative effect on the reporting of disease. Some countries choose not to report quarantinable diseases to the WHO because of the knowledge that publicity concerning the occurrence of those diseases may have an adverse effect on the movement of people and goods across their borders.

6.2. Ease of Reporting

To stimulate reporting, the mechanisms must be simple and yet compatible with an effective and sensitive surveillance system. There must be a relatively easy mechanism by which cases can be reported to the public-health authorities. However, the information being requested must provide adequate data for developing a meaningful and practical control and prevention program. It is important to request only data that meet the objectives of the surveillance program. If superfluous data are requested and collected but not used, the reporter will question the surveillance effort, and support for the program will decline.

6.3. Case Definition

It is important in developing a surveillance program that specific case definitions be developed and publicized so that those persons participating can accurately report cases. The definition must be simple, acceptable, and understandable and not incorporate diagnostic criteria that are difficult to comprehend; if laboratory test results are part of the definition, they must be readily available and inexpensive and not demand a great deal of the patient. It is also important to consider whether only confirmed cases should be reported or whether reporting should also include presumptive or suspect cases of the disease; if so, the definitions of these categories must be acceptable and publicized.

6.4. Passive Reporting

Surveillance reporting may be passive or active. Passive surveillance is the routine reporting in which case reports are initiated by the reporter. Preprinted postcards or stamped envelopes routinely supplied to the reporter can be used to report the requested surveillance data. These cards can be mailed individually or at weekly or monthly intervals, summarizing all cases seen during that time interval; negative reports, i.e., the lack of occurrence of cases, can also be requested. Some states divide the reportable diseases into those commonly seen and those only rarely seen. The reporting official is asked to provide a negative report if no cases of the common diseases are seen and to fill out the form for a rare disease only when a case is actually seen. The reporting form can be a general form suitable for a number of diseases or a specific form used only for a single disease. Special forms can be developed if more detailed data are desired.

Reporting to the local public-health office may be done by telephone. The report may be taken by a clerk during working hours or taped if phoned in outside working hours. The tape can be subsequently transcribed by a clerk, who can call the physician if more data are required. To stimulate reporting from throughout an area such as an entire state, a toll-free telephone system can be established. It has been demonstrated that the availability of an automatic telephone-answering service for use at any time has stimulated reporting of disease by physicians.

6.5. Active Reporting

An active surveillance system can be instituted to improve the opportunities to obtain surveillance data; it can be used for routine surveillance or be an integral part of a special surveillance program established to monitor a specific disease such as during an epidemic. In active surveillance, the reporter is contacted at regular intervals and specifically asked about the occurrence of the disease(s) under surveillance. Thus, there is an active attempt by public-health officials to obtain disease-occurrence information from the reporter. The introduction of an active surveillance system may greatly increase the number of reported cases of a given disease and may even simulate an outbreak. The users of the surveillance data must be thoroughly informed of such changes in surveillance methods and an interpretation of the increase discussed in an editorial comment.

6.6. Sentinel Physician Reporting

A system that can be used for either active or passive surveillance is known as a sentinel physician reporting system. Depending on the size of the community, the degree of reporting desired, and the disease(s) under surveillance, the sentinel physicians may be a sample drawn from all practicing physicians or from among certain specialists who are more likely to see cases of the disease under surveillance. If a patient with the disease under surveillance may be seen by any physician, then the sample should be drawn from among all practicing physicians; however, if a childhood disease is under surveillance, then pediatricians and family practitioners would be the group from which the sample is drawn. The same sentinel physicians can be requested to report regularly, or alternating sentinel physicians can be selected to report weekly or monthly.

6.7. Laboratory Surveillance

Disease surveillance can also be maintained by regular monitoring of laboratory reports for the identification of organisms etiological for diseases under surveillance. This system may be of secondary importance in that it serves to confirm a clinical diagnosis, or it may be of primary importance in identifying the etiology that was suspected by the clinician. For example, a case of pulmonary tuberculosis can be fairly accurately diagnosed on the basis of history and clinical evidence, including radiographs and a positive skin test. Identification of the organism in sputum confirms the diagnosis. However, with some diseases such as salmonellosis or shigellosis, accurate diagnosis is frequently dependent on the laboratory identification of the etiological agent. In diseases in which the laboratory plays a key role in identifying the etiological agent, it is important to use the appropriate media necessary for this identification. For example, in maintaining surveillance for *Vibrio cholerae* in the United States, it is necessary to use special plating media such as thiosulfate–citrate–bile salt–sucrose (TCBS) agar if the organism is to be identified. Another example is that of recognition of the importance of *Yersinia enterocolitica*. When 3 weeks of cold maintenance was required for culturing the organism, very few cases of diarrhea due to this organism were identified. With the introduction of a new culture medium (CIN) that eliminated cold storage, rapid identification became possible and cases are now being identified in routine laboratories.

6.8. Hospital Surveillance

Surveillance can also be maintained by using hospital records (inpatient or outpatient) to detect either hospital-acquired or community-acquired infections. The records can be abstracted by specially trained enumerators or by record-room personnel. (See Section 7.7 for further discussion of hospital surveillance.)

6.9. Absenteeism Surveillance

Other methods of obtaining surveillance information depend on the specific disease. For diseases with high morbidity, an effective surveillance program can be developed by noting absenteeism from school or industry, depending on the ages of the involved population. All absenteeism during the period under surveillance may not reflect cases of the disease, so that further information may be needed, such as the rate of absenteeism due to other causes. Sickness-benefit or insurance claims can also be utilized to develop surveillance data.

7. Special Surveillance

Special surveillance efforts can be established when the rate of occurrence of a disease increases either as part of the expected trend of that disease (periodic or seasonal increase) or as an unusual increase (epidemic). Special surveillance programs can also be developed in relation to the identification of a new disease entity, to provide disease data for research or investigation projects, to define the population among whom special prevention measures can be instituted, such as vaccination, and also to evaluate control and prevention measures. Once the immediate need for a special surveillance system has been accomplished, either the system should be stopped or a regular surveillance program for that disease should be developed. In 1981, when the first cases of AIDS were reported, a special surveillance program was initiated. Once the national importance of surveillance data was identified, a regular surveillance program was established. All states now routinely report cases of AIDS to the CDC as part of the weekly surveillance program.

7.1. Influenza

Surveillance information concerning influenza is normally developed from the regular weekly reporting by 121 American cities of deaths from pneumonia and influenza. Reports of outbreaks of respiratory disease and reports of virus isolation from laboratories doing routine diagnostic work also provide surveillance data. To complement this system, at the beginning of the anticipated influenza season, additional surveillance activities are initiated to improve our knowledge concerning the occurrence of the disease.[4] Reports of absenteeism are solicited from selected industries and schools, since increased absenteeism may be one indication of increased influenza activity. Virus laboratories are encouraged to process additional specimens from patients with symptoms of respiratory diseases, in order to increase the opportunity of isolating influenza viruses, and subsequently to report the results to public-health authorities. New rapid laboratory methods now facilitate recognition. These special surveillance activities are helpful in increasing the sensitivity of surveillance for influenza.

7.2. Gastroenteritis

During an outbreak of a gastrointestinal illness, such as salmonellosis, special surveillance efforts of a particularly high-risk group can be introduced to improve the information developed concerning the occurrence of the disease. This may include morbidity-reporting, laboratory surveillance, case-reporting, or field investigations. Only with these extra data may it be possible to recommend the most appropriate control and prevention measures.

7.3. Guillain–Barré Syndrome

During the swine-flu vaccination program (1976), the reported occurrence of Guillain–Barré syndrome among vaccinated persons resulted in the development of a separate surveillance effort involving special reports from neurologists.[18]

7.4. Reye Syndrome

To develop information concerning the possible association of Reye syndrome with influenza, special surveillance activities and reporting forms were established for use by pediatricians and neurologists, who were more likely than other physicians to see patients with Reye syndrome.[14]

7.5. Infant Botulism

When the first reports of infant botulism were published, it was apparent that a previously unrecognized public-health problem needed defining. Accordingly, a special attempt at developing surveillance data was initiated by alerting public-health officials as well as pathologists, pediatricians, and laboratories to the disease entity.[12] A special reporting form was developed so that pertinent information could be obtained on each case. These special efforts have resulted in the reporting of additional cases and the accumulation of important epidemiological data that have provided leads to the epidemiology of the disease. Cases of this disease are now reported as part of the routine surveillance program in the United States.

7.6. Legionnaires' Disease

When this disease was first identified, there were many unsolicited reports of possible cases. In an effort to standardize these data to define the clinical entity better and to develop more useful epidemiological data, a special surveillance reporting form was developed and a specific definition of a case of Legionnaires' disease was publicized.[19] This resulted in important, new data being uncovered concerning this newly described disease entity. Also cases of this disease continue to be reported as part of the routine national surveillance program.

7.7. Hospital Infections

Because of the increasing problem of hospital-acquired infections (nosocomial infections), special surveillance efforts have been developed within hospitals to accumulate data that might be useful for instituting procedures to control and prevent nosocomial infections.[13] Of prime importance to these surveillance programs has been the development of infection control committees with many responsibilities, one of which is to supervise a nosocomial-infection surveillance program. Special personnel are usually dedicated to this activity. Surveillance data can be collected by various techniques including individual reports from physicians or floor nurses, ward rounds by the infection-control nurse, and regular review of the laboratory and pathology records. During ward rounds, the infection-control nurse seeks clues to infection by asking physicians and nurses whether any of their patients have infections and noting which patients have elevated temperatures, are receiving chemotherapeutic agents, or are in isolation. The outpatient department and the employee health service can also be kept under surveillance, since infections noted in these areas may reflect infections among inpatients. All these sources of nosocomial-infection surveillance data may not be incorporated in the routine surveillance program at the same time. Also, surveillance may be targeted at specific high-risk patients, areas, or procedures. As with general surveillance programs, the methods incorporated should reflect the specific needs of the program. Community-acquired infections may also be brought under surveillance as an addition to the hospital-infection surveillance program. The surveillance and recognition of hospital infections are dealt with in further detail in Chapter 22.

7.8. High-Risk Population

A special surveillance program can be introduced to identify the high-risk population who will derive the greatest benefit from a particular prevention measure. For example, this has been useful for both meningococcal and pneumococcal disease in which specific, effective vaccines have been developed and are now recommended for use among specific highly susceptible populations.

7.9. Other

Other special surveillance techniques can be incorporated to handle specific problems. If there is concern regarding foodborne diseases, then in addition to the routine reporting of cases and outbreaks, surveillance of potentially contaminated foods can be instituted by utilizing laboratory culturing of foods routinely supplied from commercial sources. Surveillance of human carriers of certain pathogenic organisms such as staphylococci or salmonella can be initiated if there is concern about the occurrence of disease transmitted by asymptomatic carriers.

8. Data Analysis

Once the data have been collected, they must be collated and analyzed at regular intervals. The analysis can be simple or complex depending on the needs of the surveillance program, time constraints, how the data are to be used, and the personnel and facilities available. As surveillance becomes more complex and as more data are handled, computerization of the data may be desirable and necessary. As previously stated, surveillance data can be entered directly into the computer by the reporting office instead of being handled by one or more intermediate individuals. There are software programs available that can analyze the surveillance data and prepare figures summarizing these analyses. National and international computer networks are being developed that will permit rapid analysis and interpretation of data that will help in recognition of national and international epidemics and map the spread of disease. These systems also allow the rapid and broad dissemination of reports.

8.1. Frequency of Review

The frequency, type, and complexity of the analyses are dependent on the use of the summary data. A routine surveillance program may require analyses at monthly intervals; in epidemic circumstances, it may be necessary to review the surveillance data at more frequent intervals, such as weekly or even daily.

The data should be analyzed according to time, place, and person.

8.2. Time

When characterizing the data by time, there are four trends to consider. The first is the *secular* trend, which refers to the occurrence of the disease over a prolonged period of time such as years. The secular trend of diphtheria is one of gradually decreasing incidence (Fig. 1). The decreasing secular trend of an infectious disease is usually the result of specific and nonspecific immunity and improved hygiene (personal and community) among the involved population.

The *periodic* trend, which is the second time trend to consider, refers to the temporary variations from the secular trend. For example, in considering pertussis, periodic increases in incidence approximately every 5 years can be seen on the background of the overall secular trend of decreasing incidence of the disease (Fig. 2). The periodic trends represent variations in the level of immunity to the etiological agent as reflected either by natural infection or vaccination of the population or by changes in the antigenic composition of the agent.

The third trend is that of the *annual* variation, which frequently represents seasonal patterns. For example, foodborne diseases are associated with seasonal increases in the late summer and fall that may represent the influence of the ambient temperature on the ability of organisms to multiply in or on their reservoirs and sources, resulting in an increased concentration of organisms for potential contact

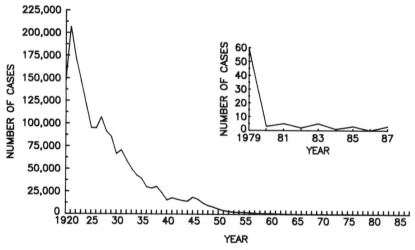

Figure 1. Diphtheria: reported cases, United States, 1920–1987.

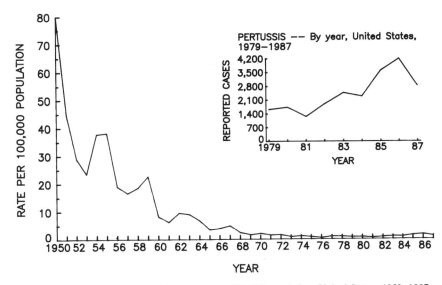

Figure 2. Pertussis: reported incidence rates per 100,000 population, United States, 1950–1987.

with susceptible hosts. Additionally, the frequency of picnics and the lack of refrigeration add to the increased opportunity for small doses of agents to multiply to infectious doses. *Salmonella* surveillance data reflect annual trends (Fig. 3).

The fourth time trend is that of the *epidemic* occurrence of the disease. If not noted earlier, an epidemic may be discovered by analyzing surveillance data. This has been seen when cases related to a common source are scattered over several health jurisdictions. For example, a *Salmonella*-contaminated food may result in the occurrence of cases over the distribution route of the food; the individual cases may not serve to alert any one health jurisdiction, but the collection of multiple cases may be distinct enough to be identified as an epidemic. Thus, surveillance can serve as an early warning system for epidemics.

When surveillance data are analyzed for time trends, it is necessary to compare these data with data collected over past years, to accurately interpret the current pattern of the occurrence of disease. Otherwise, changes in the occurrence of the disease may not be definable as being either normal or unusual variations.

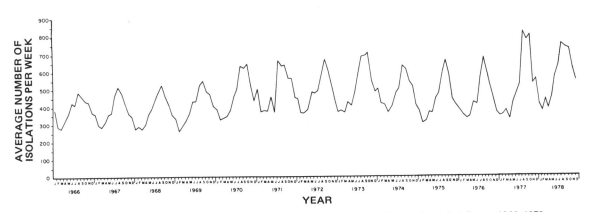

Figure 3. Salmonella: surveillance-program-reported isolations from humans by month, United States, 1966–1978.

8.3. Place

Analyzing data by place refers both to the geographic location of the source and reservoir of the organism and to the location of the patient at the time infection occurred and at the time of onset of clinical disease. The development of effective control and prevention measures depends on carefully defining each of these areas. Control measures directed at the site where the host came into contact with the agent can lead to control of additional similar cases immediately related to the initial case, but may not prevent future cases if there are multiple sources of the organism that can be brought into contact with other susceptible hosts. For example, if a food is contaminated with *Salmonella* in the factory where it is prepared and the exposure of the host occurs in a restaurant serving that food, then closing the restaurant will not prevent cases from occurring in association with another restaurant that also obtained contaminated food from the same factory. Prevention of future cases can be accomplished by eradicating the source of contamination, in this instance at the food-processing plant.

8.4. Person

Person factors to be defined in analyzing the surveillance data may include age, sex, nationality, level of immunity, nutrition, life-style (such as sexual practices and i.v. drug use), socioeconomic status, travel history, hobbies, and occupation. The evaluation of these factors is important in further describing the occurrence of disease. For example, age-specific attack rates can be important in determining where control and prevention measures should be directed. Occupation may give a clue as to where intervention measures need to be directed. For example, in evaluating cases of brucellosis, knowing that abattoir personnel who work on the kill floors are at a higher risk of developing disease than personnel in other areas of the plant indicates where control measures need to be directed. The identification of those at highest risk to HIV is needed to direct initial control programs at these groups and at the specific methods of transmission within them.

Data analysis will usually suggest the best point for intervention. Occasionally, additional data may need to be gathered by additional surveillance activities or by special investigations.

9. Reports

Appropriate reports should be prepared and distributed to those individuals who participate in the surveillance program as well as those who have a responsibility for preventive action. The purpose of the surveillance report is to communicate with people, to disseminate information, to educate the reader, and to direct, stimulate, and motivate the persons responsible for action. Reports can also be useful in bringing recognition of contributors to the collection of surveillance data. The report should not only summarize the surveillance data but also provide an interpretation of the analyses. Control and prevention measures can be discussed. Surveillance reports can also serve to alert the reader to impending problems, newer methods of control and prevention, current investigations, and new information developed from research or field investigations.

Reports are usually prepared at regular intervals such as weekly, monthly, quarterly, or annually. The frequency should reflect the interest in the data as well as the need for distribution of the data as related to control and prevention actions. During an epidemic, the immediate dissemination of data may be critical to the institution of appropriate control measures; thus, daily or weekly reports may be indicated. It may be appropriate to distribute foodborne-disease-surveillance reports at weekly or monthly intervals during the summer and fall months due to the increased incidence of disease at these periods and then reduce the frequency of reports during the remainder of the year. Special reports can be distributed as necessary; if rapid dissemination of the information is important, it can be distributed by fast mail, telegram, telephone, or computer. Rapid dissemination of information over a wide area may be of such critical importance that use of the public news media should be considered.

In the United States, almost all state health departments prepare and distribute at weekly or monthly intervals comprehensive surveillance reports that summarize their disease-surveillance data. The national surveillance data are summarized by the CDC at varying intervals depending on the disease and its frequency. Those diseases reported weekly are summarized in the MMWR; other diseases are summarized in specialty surveillance reports that are distributed at regular intervals, from monthly to annually. Characteristic of many of the CDC surveillance reports and especially of the MMWR is the interpretation of surveillance data and an editorial comment that are integral parts of the report. These reports are available to anyone who would like to receive them. World surveillance data are collected, summarized, and distributed by the WHO in a weekly report.

10. Evaluation

Once a surveillance program has been developed and has been in operation for a period of time, it should be reviewed and evaluated. Thacker and Berkelman[20] discuss the quality of a program and describe seven attributes of a surveillance program that should be evaluated: sensitivity, specificity and predictive value positive, representativeness, timeliness, simplicity, flexibility, and acceptability. Another factor that may be considered is the cost of a program, though conducting a cost–benefit analysis is difficult.

11. Limitations of Surveillance

Surveillance of disease is dependent on a series of events that if not followed may prevent the case from being reported. The events include that the disease be severe enough, that medical attention is sought and if sought, must be available; laboratory diagnostic facilities may be necessary and should be available; the health care provider or his/her representative must report the case; the respective health department must have adequate resources and direction to support the surveillance program. Any alterations in these events may change the apparent pattern of disease. The consistency and stability of the occurrence of these events is vital to the development of reliable surveillance data. In addition to recognition of clinical cases, there may be many infected persons with mild or subclinical illnesses that are not noted in the routine surveillance system. For these cases to be noted, laboratory studies of the distribution of the organism or the antibody to it are required.

12. References

1. ANDREWS, J. M., QUINBY, G. E., AND LANGMUIR, A. D., Malaria eradication in the United States, *Am. J. Public Health* **40**:1405–1411 (1950).
2. Centers for Disease Control, *Shigella Surveillance Rep.* **13**:2 (1966).
3. Centers for Disease Control, Botulism, *Morbid. Mortal. Weekly Rep.* **25**(17):137 (1976).
4. Centers for Disease Control, *National Influenza Immunization Program-13, Influenza Surveillance Manual* (July 1976).
5. Centers for Disease Control, *Influenza Surveillance Rep.* **91** (July 1977).
6. Centers for Disease Control, *Morbid. Mortal. Weekly Rep., Annual Summary* (1978).
7. Centers for Disease Control, AIDS, *Morbid. Mortal. Weekly Rep.* **30**:250 (1981).
8. CRAVEN, P. S., BAINE, W. B., MACKEL, D. C., BARKER, W. H., GANGAROSA, E. J., GOLDFIELD, M., ROSENFELD, J., ALTMAN, R., LACHAPELLE, G., DAVIES, J. W., AND SWANSON, R. C., International outbreak of *Salmonella eastbourne*
9. EVANS, A. S., Surveillance and seroepidemiology, in: *Viral Infections of Humans: Epidemiology and Control,* 3rd ed. (A. S. EVANS, ed.), pp. 51–73, Plenum Medical, New York, 1989.
10. GANGAROSA, E. J., MATA, L. J., PERERA, D. R., RELLER, L. B., AND MORRIS, C. M., Shiga bacillus dysentery in Central America, in: *Uses of Epidemiology in Planning Health Services,* Proceedings of the Sixth International Scientific Meeting, International Epidemiological Association (A. M. DAVIES, ed.), pp. 259–267, Savremena Administracija, Belgrade, 1973.
11. GRAITCER, P. L., AND BURTON, A. H., The epidemiologic surveillance project: A computer-based system for disease surveillance, *Am. J. Prev. Med.* **3**:123–127 (1987).
12. GUNN, R. A., Epidemiologic characteristics of infant botulism in the United States, 1975–1978, *Rev. Infect. Dis.* **1**:642–646 (1979).
13. HALEY, R. W., ABER, R. C., AND BENNETT, J. V., Surveillance of nosocomial infections, in: *Hospital Infections,* 2nd ed. (J. V. BENNETT AND P. S. BRACHMAN, eds.), pp. 51–71, Little, Brown, Boston, 1986.
14. LANGMUIR, A. D., The surveillance of communicable diseases of national importance, *N. Engl. J. Med.* **268**:182–192 (1963).
15. NATHANSON, N., AND LANGMUIR, A. D., The Cutter incident, *Am. J. Hyg.* **78**:16–81 (1964).
16. NELSON, D. B., SULLIVAN-BOLYAI, J. Z., MARKS, J. S., MORENS, D. M., SCHONBERGER, L. B., and the Ohio State Department of Health Reye's Syndrome Investigation Group, Reye syndrome: An epidemiologic assessment based on national surveillance 1977–1978 and a population based study in Ohio 1973–1977, in: *Reye's Syndrome II* (J. F. CROCKER, ed.), pp. 33–46, Grune & Stratton, New York, 1979.
17. Riverside County Health Department, California State Department of Public Health, Centers for Disease Control, National Center for Urban and Industrial Health: A waterborne epidemic of salmonellosis in Riverside, California, 1965—Epidemiologic aspects, *Am. J. Epidemiol.* **99**:33–48 (1970).
18. SCHONBERGER, L. B., BREGMAN, D. J., SULLIVAN-BOLYAI, J. Z., KEENLYSIDE, R. A., ZIEGLER, D. W., RETAILLIAU, H. F., EDDINS, D. L., AND BRYAN, J. A., Guillain–Barré syndrome following vaccination in the national influenza immunization program, United States, 1976–1977, *Am. J. Epidemiol.* **110**:105–123 (1979).
19. STORCH, G., BAINE, W. B., FRASER, D. W., BROOME, C. V., CLEGG, H. W., II, COHEN, B. D., SHEPARD, C. C., AND BENNETT, J. V., Sporadic community-acquired Legionnaires' disease in the United States, *Ann. Intern. Med.* **90**:596–600 (1979).
20. THACKER, S. B., AND BERKELMAN, R. L., Public health surveillance in the United States, *Epidemiol. Rev.* **10**:164–190 (1988).
21. VALLERON, A. J., BOUVET, E., GARNERIN, P., MENARES, J., HEARD, I., LETRAIT, S., AND LEFAUCHEUX, J., A com-

infection traced to contaminated chocolate, *Lancet* **1**:788–793 (1975).

puter network for the surveillance of communicable diseases: The French connection, *Am. J. Public Health* **76:**1289–1292 (1986).

22. WEINSTEIN, R. A., Multiply resistant strains: Epidemiology and control, in: *Hospital Infections,* 2nd ed. (J. V. BENNETT AND P. S. BRACHMAN, eds.), p. 163, Little, Brown, Boston, 1986.

23. World Health Organization, The surveillance of communicable diseases, *WHO Chronicle* **22**(10)**:**439–444 (1968).

Acute Bacterial Infections

CHAPTER 3

Anthrax

Philip S. Brachman

1. Introduction

Anthrax, a zoonotic disease of herbivorous animals transmissible from animals to man, occurs primarily in three forms: cutaneous, inhalation, and gastrointestinal. Meningitis and septicemia occur but are secondary to one of the primary forms; occasionally, cases of anthrax meningitis are reported in which a primary focus is not identified. The etiological agent is *Bacillus anthracis*, a gram-positive organism that in its spore form can persist in nature for prolonged periods, possibly years. The incidence of anthrax has decreased over the past 60 years, so that currently, human cases are seen only occasionally in the United States, where reporting is probably fairly accurate. Synonyms for anthrax include charbon, malignant pustule, Siberian ulcer, malignant edema, woolsorters' disease, and ragpickers' disease.

2. Historical Background

The earliest known description of anthrax is found in the book of Genesis; the fifth plague (1491 B.C.), which appears to have been anthrax, was described as killing the Egyptians' cattle. There are descriptions of anthrax involving both animals and humans in the early literature of the Hindus and Greeks. Virgil described anthrax during the Roman Empire (70–19 B.C.). In the 17th century, a pandemic referred to as "the black bane" swept through Europe causing approximately 60,000 human deaths and many animal deaths. An association between human anthrax and contact with clothing made from wool and hides was reported.

Philip S. Brachman · Emory University School of Public Health, Atlanta, Georgia 30329.

In 1752, Moret more specifically characterized the disease in man, calling it "the malignant pustle." In 1780, Chabert described the disease in animals. The contagious nature of anthrax was noted in 1823 by Barthelemy. The first microscopic description of the organism was written by Delafond in 1838, and the organism was first described in infected animals in 1849 by Pollender. Pasteur discussed anthrax in some of his earlier writings on his germ theory of disease. In 1876, Koch used *B. anthracis* in developing his postulates concerning the relationships between bacteria and the diseases they cause. Greenfield developed an attenuated animal spore vaccine in 1880.[20,29,30] Pasteur, responding to a serious problem with anthrax in the French livestock industry, developed and field tested in sheep his attenuated spore vaccine in 1881. In 1939, Sterne reported his development of an animal vaccine that is a spore suspension of an avirulent, noncapsulated live strain.[27] This is the animal vaccine currently recommended for use.

Anthrax in the United States was first reported among animals in Louisiana in the early 1700s. Subsequently, sporadic animal cases have been reported from throughout the United States, and epizootics have been reported from the southern portion of the Great Plains states and the northeastern part of the country. The first human case was reported in a cattle tender in Kentucky in 1824.

Occupational anthrax occurred in the mid-1800s in England, where it was known as woolsorters' disease,[20] and in Germany, where it was known as ragpickers' disease. Ragpickers' disease occurred in individuals who handled rags that had been woven from contaminated animal fibers. The increasing problem of woolsorters' disease in England led to the development of a government inquiry committee that correctly identified the problem as being related to imported animal fibers contaminated with *B. anthracis*.[2]

75

Subsequently, in 1921, a formaldehyde disinfecting station was built by the government in Liverpool.[32] All "dangerous" imported wools and goat hairs were first washed in formaldehyde baths, which successfully reduced contamination of the animal fibers with *B. anthracis*. The occurrence of inhalation anthrax was drastically reduced, so that only sporadic cases have been reported in England since 1922. The disinfecting station continued to operate until the mid-1970s, by which time the danger had been reduced to such a level that further disinfection with formaldehyde was not deemed necessary or economical.

In the United States, human anthrax cases have been reported from most of the states. Initially, cases were related to animal contact and reflected areas with enzootic and epizootic anthrax, primarily involving cattle and occasionally sheep and horses. As the United States became industrialized, human cases associated with the textile and tanning industries occurred with increasing frequency. In the early 1900s, these cases primarily occurred in the northeastern states. In the 1950s, cases began to occur in southeastern states, reflecting the movement of the industry.

In the 1920s, the annual number of cases reported in the United States ranged from 100 to 200 cases; in the 1950s, from 20 to 50 cases each year; in the 1970s, from 0 to 6 cases each year; and in the 1980s, from 0 to 1 case each year. This decrease is the result of the use of a human cell-free anthrax vaccine among high-risk industrial groups, decreased utilization of imported potentially contaminated animal products, improved hygiene in industry, and improved animal husbandry. The incidence of animal anthrax has likewise decreased so that only occasional cases are reported and epizootics have not been reported for a number of years. This reduction is the result of improved animal husbandry and the appropriate utilization of animal anthrax vaccine.

3. Methodology

3.1. Sources of Mortality and Morbidity Data

In the United States, data on human anthrax are collected in individual states through the routine surveillance system. Usually, individual case data are obtained by use of special case-reporting forms and investigations. These data are then reported by means of the morbidity and mortality reporting system to the Centers for Disease Control (CDC). Epidemic information and, at times, individual case data are reported to the CDC by telephone. Years ago, the reporting of anthrax was spotty; however, as health-care providers have accepted their responsibilities to notify public-health

officials about the occurrence of reportable disease, overall surveillance has improved. Additionally, as the incidence of the disease has decreased and the use of the laboratory in assisting in diagnosing the disease has increased, reporting has become more complete.

Data concerning anthrax in animals are obtained through federal and state departments of agriculture or public health or both.

Worldwide data on anthrax are available from the World Health Organization (WHO) and the Food and Agriculture Organization. However, not all countries maintain adequate surveillance programs for infectious diseases, and thus all do not have data available on cases of human or animal anthrax. Especially deficient will be reports of anthrax associated with rural areas, i.e., animal-associated cases, because of the generally poorer reporting of diseases from rural areas. Another source of data is the scientific literature in which a report of a case or an epidemic of anthrax may be published, even though it was not officially reported to the country's central health authority. Additionally, reports of epidemics in the scientific literature may give the actual number of cases of the disease that occurred, whereas the number reported to the health authorities may only include those cases confirmed in the laboratory.

3.2. Surveys

Population surveys are not practical due to the low incidence of the disease. Serological surveys are not generally useful for obtaining information on anthrax, except in epidemic or epizootic investigations, because of limitations of the laboratory procedure. However, they may also be useful in ascertaining immunity levels in human and livestock populations.

3.3. Laboratory Diagnosis

3.3.1. Isolation and Identification. Swabs from lesions, vesicular fluid, or blood may be examined for the presence of *B. anthracis*.[17] *B. anthracis* is a gram-positive, nonmotile, hemolytic, spore-forming bacillus (1–1.3 × 3–10 μm) that grows on ordinary laboratory media at 37°C, producing round, grayish-white, convex colonies having comma-shaped outshootings with a ground-glass appearance that measure 2–5 mm in diameter. Colonies first appear approximately 8–12 h after inoculation of the agar and show the typical characteristics 24–36 h after inoculation. When an inoculated loop is drawn through the colony, tenacity is demonstrated; the disturbed part of the colony will be drawn perpendicular to the agar and will remain in

this position, resembling beaten egg white. Microscopic examination (such as by Gram stain) of growth from artificial media shows long parallel chains of organisms with square ends, referred to as "boxcars." Spore stains will reveal central or paracentral spores in *B. anthracis* organisms that have incubated at least 24 h. Material from a fresh lesion will show shorter chains with single or two to four organisms in a row with slightly rounded ends. Direct fluorescent-antibody staining may also be used to identify the organisms from vesicular fluid cultures or from tissues.[13]

A bacteriophage designated gamma phage may be used to confirm the identification of *B. anthracis*.[10] Subcutaneous or intraperitoneal inoculation of guinea pigs, mice, or rabbits with agar-grown cells suspended in saline may be useful in differentiating *B. anthracis* from other gram-positive bacilli. *B. anthracis* will cause death from 24 to 72 h after inoculation, and the animal will show evidence of general toxicity and multiple organ hemorrhages. Animals inoculated subcutaneously demonstrate subcutaneous gelatinous, hemorrhagic edema in addition to general toxemia. Broth-grown cultures must not be used because nonspecific death can result.

Tissue from autopsied patients should be cultured and microscopically examined.

3.3.2. Serological and Immunological Diagnostic Methods. The virulence of *B. anthracis* is determined by the presence of three components—edema toxin, lethal toxin, and capsular material. To exert their effect within cells, both toxins require participation of a common transport protein, called protective antigen. The capsule material contains poly-D-glutamic acid, which helps protect the bacillus from ingestion by phagocytes. Production of the toxic factors is regulated by one plasmid and that of the capsular material by a second plasmid.

Initially, an agar-gel precipitation assay and then an indirect microhemagglutination test were developed to identify antibody against the protective antigen.[11] However, these tests lacked sensitivity. An ELISA has been developed that is more sensitive. It measures antibodies to the lethal and edema factors and the protective antigen. A fourfold rise in titer or a single titer of greater than 1 : 32 is indicative of current or recent infection or acquired immunity.[16,21] Additionally, an electrophoretic-immunotransblot test has been developed that measures antibody to the protective antigen and the lethal factor.[21]

3.3.3. Pathology. Autopsy material, commonly from the mediastinal structures, lymph nodes, spleen, and liver, should be examined for organisms and pathological changes.

The most significant findings at autopsy are those seen in patients who have died of inhalation anthrax. The classic finding is that of hemorrhagic mediastinitis with enlarged, hemorrhagic lymphadenitis. There may be inflammation of the pleura and some pleural effusion. Acute splenitis may also be seen. Some patients may have hemorrhagic meningitis, and in one patient, hemorrhages were seen in the gastrointestinal tract.

In deaths due to gastrointestinal anthrax, there typically is hemorrhagic enteritis with congestion, thickening, and edema of the intestinal walls. Mucosal ulcers with necrosis may be seen in the terminal ileum and cecum. The regional lymph nodes are enlarged, edematous, and hemorrhagic with some necrosis. There may be acute splenitis. Peritonitis with ascitic fluid is present.

4. Biological Characteristics of the Organism

The resistance of the spore form of *B. anthracis* to physical and chemical agents is reflected in the persistence of the organism in the inanimate environment. Organisms have been demonstrated to persist for years in factories in which the environment became contaminated during the processing of contaminated imported materials of animal origin. Accordingly, they may serve as the source of infection for people who work in the area. Special efforts are required to decontaminate this environment; one method is to use paraformaldehyde vapor, which is successful in killing *B. anthracis* spores. In the laboratory, surfaces may be decontaminated with either 5% hypochlorite or 5% phenol (carbolic acid); instruments and other equipment may be autoclaved.

B. anthracis may also persist in certain types of soil for years.[18] Alluvial soil with a pH greater than 6.0 is best suited for survival of *B. anthracis*. Persistence of the organism in soil plus environmental conditions such as climatic variations, i.e., flooding and drought, and close grazing of animals are associated with outbreaks of animal anthrax. Areas that are repeatedly the sites of animal anthrax are known as anthrax districts. One such area is the lower Mississippi River valley area, from which sporadic outbreaks of animal anthrax have been reported at irregular intervals for years.

5. Descriptive Epidemiology

5.1. Prevalence and Incidence

In 1958, Glassman,[14] using reports from the WHO, estimated the annual worldwide incidence of human anthrax

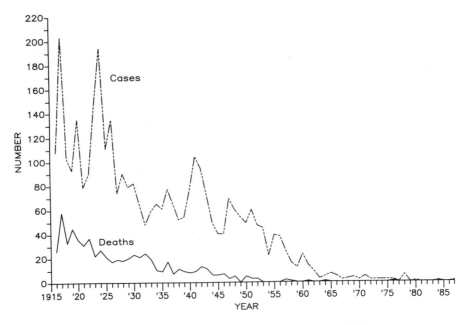

Figure 1. Anthrax in man in the United States, 1916–1987.

to be from 20,000 to 100,000 cases. The most recent data from the WHO[33] are for 1981—3200 cases from 43 countries, which undoubtedly is an underestimate. Animal anthrax remains an endemic problem in various Asiatic, African, South American, and Caribbean countries. In countries with a significant animal-anthrax problem, there is probably a related human-anthrax problem. However, since the reporting of diseases from rural areas is sporadic, these data are not generally available. Industrial anthrax infections are related to the processing of animal products such as goat hair, wool, skins and hides, and dried bones. Industrial countries that process these materials will have industrially related cases at a rate inversely proportional to the level of development of appropriate hygienic measures directed at reducing the threat of anthrax.

In the United States, the annual number of cases of human anthrax decreased from an average of 127 for the years 1916–1925, to 44 cases for 1948–1957, to 9.6 cases for 1958–1967, to 2.4 cases for 1968–1977, and to 0.9 case for 1978–1987 (see Fig. 1).

Approximately 95% of anthrax cases in the United States are cutaneous and 5% are inhalation; confirmed cases of gastrointestinal anthrax have not been reported in the United States and rarely have been reported in other coun-

tries. From 1955 through 1987, 233 cases of anthrax were reported in the United States; 222 cases were cutaneous (21 of which were at unknown sites) and 11 were inhalation. Of the 201 cutaneous cases for which the sites of infection were reported, the majority occurred on the exposed part of the body, with 51% on the arms, 27% on the head and neck, 5% on the trunk, and 3% on the legs (see Table 1).

It is estimated that approximately 20% of untreated cases of cutaneous anthrax will result in death. Of the 222 cutaneous cases that have been reported in the United States since 1955, 11 have been fatal. Inhalation anthrax is almost always fatal; since 1900, 16 of the 18 cases reported in the United States have resulted in death.

In the few reports available, the mortality from gastrointestinal anthrax has usually ranged from 25% to 60%.

5.2. Epidemic Behavior and Contagiousness

The first reports of inhalation anthrax (woolsorters' disease) in England in the late 1800s and early 1900s included clusters of cases associated with the sorting of certain lots of imported goat hair, frequently mohair.[3] In the United States, occasional epidemics occurred in industrial settings, probably related to the processing of batches of

Table 1. Sites of 233 Anthrax Infections, United States, 1955–1987

Sites	Infections	Known cutaneous distribution	
		Number	Percent
Cutaneous	201		
Arms		118	51
Head and neck		64	27
Trunk		11	5
Legs		8	3
Unknown	21		9
Inhalation	11		5

highly contaminated imported animal fibers, particularly goat hair. These epidemics were primarily of cutaneous anthrax.

The largest epidemic reported in the United States occurred in 1957 and involved employees in a goat-hair-processing plant.[24] Among the 600 employees over a 10-week period, there were 9 cases of anthrax: 4 cases of cutaneous anthrax and 5 of inhalation anthrax. None of the patients with cutaneous anthrax died, but 4 of the 5 with the inhalation form died. Epidemiological investigations related the cases to a particular contaminated batch of goat hair imported from Pakistan.[6] More than 50% of samples from this particular batch were culture-positive for *B. anthracis*. A detailed examination of production records revealed that each of the patients had direct contact with this particular lot of goat hair during an appropriate period before the onset of disease.

Human-to-human transmission of anthrax has not been confirmed. Industrial infections result from exposure to the organisms in the industrial environment, from contact with organisms either in the materials actually being processed or in the environment that has been contaminated by previously processed materials. Those employees who work in the earliest processing stages, in which the materials and the environment are more heavily contaminated with *B. anthracis*, are at greater risk of contracting anthrax than those who work with the materials at later stages in the manufacturing cycle. Occasional cases occur in persons who have direct or indirect contact with *B. anthracis* in a laboratory setting.

Agricultural cases occur in veterinarians and others who have direct contact with animals that have died of anthrax. There have been cases of human disease associated with epizootics of anthrax in cattle. The largest reported agricultural outbreak occurred in Zimbabwe with more than 10,000 cases reported between 1979 and 1985.[15] The peak number of cases, more than 6000, were reported to have occurred between October 1979 and March 1980. Endemic cases continue to occur in the involved area. The majority of patients had cutaneous infections located primarily on the exposed parts of the body; some gastrointestinal cases have been reported. Domestic cattle deaths were also noted. The humans were infected from contact with the diseased animals or by handling their carcasses during butchering or burial; the source of infection for the animals was not reported. Routine animal vaccination had not been practiced.

An outbreak of human anthrax occurred in north central Russia in 1979 in which the government health authorities reported the source of infection was contaminated meat (personal communication). There were 96 cases—79 of gastrointestinal anthrax and 17 of cutaneous anthrax.

5.3. Geographic Distribution

Cases are distributed according to their association with an agricultural or industrial source of infection. From 1920 to 1954, more than 50% of all cases in the United States occurred in Pennsylvania, New York, New Jersey, Massachusetts, and New Hampshire, the location of industries that processed animal hair, hide, and bone.[5] Subsequently, industrial cases began to be reported from other states, such as North Carolina and South Carolina, as companies moved southward. In more recent years, cases have not shown a geographic localization, reflecting the decrease in industry-related cases and the low endemicity of agriculture-related cases.

Agricultural cases are distributed in rural areas associated with outbreaks in animals and primarily occur in the previously discussed anthrax districts. Some of these districts are located in Louisiana, Mississippi, and South Dakota.[18] Epizootics usually involve dairy cattle, but sheep and horses may also be involved.

5.4. Temporal Distribution

Industrial cases occur throughout the year without any seasonal pattern. Animal-related cases occur primarily in the spring and summer, the seasons when animal anthrax cases occur with the greatest frequency.

5.5. Age

The age distribution of cases reflects the age of the individuals who work in the involved industry or come in contact with infected carcasses. Primarily, these persons are 20–60 years of age. Occasional cases have been reported in children one of whose parents worked in a factory in which *B. anthracis*-contaminated materials were processed; it has been hypothesized that *B. anthracis* organisms were transported into the home on the parent's clothing.

5.6. Sex

The predominance of males reflects the sex distribution of the people who work in the involved industries or have contact with infected carcasses.

5.7. Race

No distinctive racial patterns are found among persons with anthrax.

5.8. Occupation

Anthrax cases may be divided into two major categories: those associated with an industrial setting and those associated with an agricultural setting (see Table 2). However, some cases occur in people who live in urban areas in which the source of infection is unknown; in these cases, the source is assumed to be industrial. In addition, a few laboratory-associated cases have been seen.

Industrial cases occur in individuals who work in industries in which animal products, usually imported, are

Table 2.   Source of Infection in 233 Cases of Human Anthrax, United States, 1955–1987

Source	Number
Industrial	
Goat hair	113
Wool	34
Goat skins	16
Meat	3
Bone	4
Unknown	12
Agricultural	
Animal	41
Vaccine (animal)	2
Unknown	8

processed.[5,31] In the United States, this primarily involves workers in goat-hair- and wool-processing industries. Goat hair is imported primarily from Asiatic, Middle Eastern, and African countries in bales weighing 200–250 lb each. The hair is processed into yarn used in preparing interlinings for men's suit coats and also into a felt material used as underpads for carpets, insulation for pipes, saddle pads, and washers. The wools that have been implicated in cases of anthrax are imported from the same areas of the world and are primarily the coarser wools used in carpets as distinct from the finer wools used in clothing. Occasionally, however, anthrax has been associated with fine cashmere wool.

Anthrax has also been associated with the tanning industry and has resulted from contact with imported skins and hides. In addition, cases have been associated with the bone-meal-processing industry, in which dried bones are imported for preparing bone meal for fertilizer, animal-food supplements, or gelatin. The dried bones are usually gathered from animal grazing areas and are from animals that have died of unknown causes. However, bones may also be obtained from slaughtering or rendering plants.

There have been cases in which the source of infection has been domestic animal products. For example, in 1924, a number of persons developed cutaneous anthrax following their contact with hides from animals that died during an epizootic of anthrax.

Occasional cases have been reported among persons who have had contact with horsehair and pig bristles that are used in brushes, such as shaving brushes or hairbrushes. The number of cases associated with contaminated imported shaving brushes was significantly reduced in the 1920s by the enactment of laws requiring that these brushes be shown by culture to be free of *B. anthracis* organisms when imported into the country. In recent years, the use of animal fibers has decreased as synthetic materials have been used in increasing quantities. Accordingly, this risk of anthrax is negligible.

Agricultural cases have occurred in individuals who came into contact with sick or dead animals in rural areas. Primarily, these cases have involved cattle owners, veterinarians, and veterinary assistants who have had contact with animals, for example while performing autopsies on infected carcasses. Another route of infection is by ingestion of raw or undercooked infected meat from an infected carcass. A few cases have resulted from the accidental self-injection of animal spore vaccine into a finger or hand.

Agricultural cases have also occurred in individuals who used fertilizer or animal feed that contained contaminated bone meal. One particular epidemic related to feed supplement for pigs involved 846 cases in pigs, with some cases in persons who had contact with the pigs.[26]

Occasional cases have occurred in individuals who have had no known contact with industrial or agricultural sources. Usually, their cases are thought to have been caused by environmental contamination such as in the case of a housewife who lived near a tannery and died of inhalation anthrax. Another case occurred in an individual who every day walked by the receiving room door of a tannery where contaminated hides were processed.[7] It was shown that air could have flowed from the receiving area out into the street, where the individual could have inhaled an infecting dose of airborne *B. anthracis* organisms.

Several cases have occurred in persons whose contact has been in laboratories in which strains of *B. anthracis* have been handled.[4] Two of these cases were fatal inhalation cases.

5.9. Cases Related to Commercial Products

An occasional case has occurred in an individual after contact with a commercial product prepared from animal materials. Examples of cutaneous anthrax include contact with imported souvenir drums with drumheads made of goatskin[12] and a case in which the source of infection was most likely a newly purchased woolen coat. A fatal case of inhalation anthrax in a home weaver followed contact with imported yarn that contained animal fibers.[28]

5.10. Socioeconomic and Other Factors

Socioeconomic or other factors do not contribute significantly to development of anthrax infections. Among some people in certain societies, economic problems may lead to individuals salvaging the meat, hair, or hides from carcasses of animals that died from anthrax, which would increase their risk of developing an anthrax infection.

6. Mechanisms and Routes of Transmission

B. anthracis organisms are primarily transported by the contact or the airborne routes. Organisms can also be transmitted by a common vehicle, food (meat), though this is rare. Vectors (flies) have been reported to transmit organisms, although the actual relationship to subsequent disease has not been proven.

Contact spread is primarily by indirect contact, although direct contact and droplets may also be routes of transmission, and results in cutaneous lesions, most frequently on the exposed parts of the body. Direct contact spread occurs when a susceptible host has direct contact with an animal that is infected with *B. anthracis,* such as a veterinarian who autopsies an animal the tissues of which are contaminated with the organism. Organisms may enter the body through a preexisting skin wound or may be accidentally injected by a sharp bone spicule or a knife.

Meat from an animal that died from anthrax could be infected and could serve as a source of infection if eaten undercooked.

Indirect contact spread accounts for the majority of cutaneous industrial cases. The source of infection is either the animal products being processed or the environment that has been contaminated by animal products previously processed. Rarely, the finished product may be the source. By this route, organisms enter the skin through a preexisting wound, a new wound, or the mucous membranes (i.e., conjunctivae). Goat-hair fibers may be flung from the manufacturing equipment like projectiles and enter the skin like needles, depositing *B. anthracis* organisms in the subcutaneous tissue.

Aerosols containing *B. anthracis* spores may be created by agitation of the hair or wool either when the bales are being opened and the fibers initially handled or as the fibers are being processed by the machinery. These aerosols may travel more than several feet, which represents airborne transmission. Particles less than 5 μm in diameter, if inhaled, may reach the terminal alveoli of the lungs and cause inhalation anthrax (see Section 7.1.2). Infectious aerosols may also be created by the reaerosolization of particles previously deposited in the environment.

The air in several goat-hair-processing plants has been sampled, and significant levels of airborne *B. anthracis* spores have been identified. For example, studies in a goat-hair-processing plant in the Northeast in 1958 demonstrated that "510 spores in particles 5 microns and less in size may be inhaled [by workers] in 8 hours without inducing infection."[14] In a similar mill in a southern state, 91 primates (cynomolgus monkeys) were exposed during a series of experiments to the air in the dustiest part of the mill.[9] They had an anthrax mortality rate of 10–25% from a calculated inhalation dose of 1000–5000 *B. anthracis* organisms accumulated over 3–5 days.

Animals become infected by ingestion of contaminated soil or feed. Some rural areas are associated with sporadic cases or outbreaks of animal anthrax. The soils in these areas are most frequently in the neutral pH range and are alluvial or loessal soils. Soil becomes contaminated from the discharges or carcasses of dead animals. Soil can also become contaminated from use of contaminated fertilizer or feed. It is reported that the spores may remain infectious in nature for many years, though this has never been scientifically proven. There is evidence to suggest that in some areas *B. anthracis* organisms can be considered as part of the endogenous soil flora. With certain climatic conditions, the spores germinate and multiply, resulting in an increase in the number of infectious organisms that could be ingested by susceptible grazing animals.

Insect vectors, such as horseflies, have been reported to transmit *B. anthracis* by means of mechanical transfer of *B. anthracis* organisms from contaminated foci to individuals or animals. Outbreaks of animal anthrax have been reported to result from transmission of *B. anthracis* by horseflies from an infected animal to a second animal. However, there is no scientific documentation, including field studies during an epizootic, that this potential method of transmission has any practical significance.

7. Pathogenesis and Immunity

7.1. Pathogenesis

7.1.1. Cutaneous Anthrax. The incubation period is from 3 to 10 days, most commonly 5–7 days. Spores deposited beneath the skin germinate, and the resulting vegetative forms multiply and produce a toxin. The local lesion results from the action of the toxin on the surrounding tissue, which causes tissue necrosis. This leads to the development of a scar at the site of the lesion. The toxin or organisms or both may be distributed throughout the body by the vascular system, causing systemic symptoms and signs of toxicity or bacteremia. Occasionally, organisms are picked up by the lymphatic system, resulting in lymphangitis and lymphadenopathy.

7.1.2. Inhalation Anthrax. The incubation period is from 1 to 5 days, usually 3–4 days. *B. anthracis*-bearing particles less than 5 μm in size are inhaled and, if they reach the terminal alveoli, are deposited on the alveolar membranes, where they can be ingested by alveolar macrophages, carried across the membranes to the regional lymph nodes, and deposited. Spores will then germinate, multiply, and produce toxin. The toxin, in turn, destroys tissue and subsequently causes necrosis and hemorrhage. The classic picture at death is very distinctive. Examination of the mediastinal area reveals hemorrhagic mediastinitis with varied degrees of destruction of the normal architecture.[1] While the pathological changes are limited to the mediastinal area, there may be secondary involvement of the pulmonary tissue. Toxin may be distributed throughout the body, resulting in systemic symptoms and signs. Orga-

nisms may also be picked up by the vascular system, resulting in bacteremia and septicemia.

7.1.3. Gastrointestinal Anthrax. The incubation period is commonly 3–7 days. There are two clinical presentations following ingestion of *B. anthracis*-contaminated food: abdominal and oropharyngeal.

In the abdominal form, spores are ingested, absorbed through the intestinal mucosa, and deposited in regional lymph nodes; here, they germinate, and the vegetative cells multiply, producing toxin. A lesion caused by the action of the toxin may develop within the mucosa of the gastrointestinal tract, resembling cutaneous anthrax. The lesions are frequently described in the cecum and adjacent areas of the bowel. Some reports have described lesions in the large bowel, and rarely in the duodenum.[22] Alternatively, lymphadenitis or lymphadenopathy may occur. Hemorrhagic areas may develop within the mesentery as well as in the gastrointestinal tract.

In the oropharyngeal form, organisms are transported through the oral mucosa to the cervical lymph nodes, where they germinate, multiply, and produce toxin. The result may be edema and tissue necrosis in the cervical area. There is a report from Thailand as well as several other countries of the development of an inflammatory lesion resembling a cutaneous lesion in the oral cavity involving the posterior wall, the hard palate, or the tonsils.[25]

7.2. Immunity

Apparently, once having had a cutaneous lesion, an individual develops some degree of immunity against another infection. There have been no well-confirmed second cases of cutaneous anthrax in individuals who have had a confirmed first case. However, there have been several reports of two cutaneous anthrax infections in the same individual, but in each of these reports, either one or both of the cases of anthrax have not been well documented.

Extensive serological studies have not been conducted. However, in one study, Norman *et al.*[23] studied 72 unvaccinated employees in a goat-hair-processing mill, none of whom had a history of an anthrax infection. Of the 72, 11 demonstrated a positive titer (precipitation-inhibition test), suggesting previous subclinical infection.

Detailed data concerning immunity following inhalation anthrax are not available because of the rarity of this form of the disease and the high fatality rate. In studies of the several persons who have recovered during the past 25 years, low levels of antibodies were detected following recovery from the clinical disease.

8. Patterns of Host Response

8.1. Clinical Features

8.1.1. Cutaneous Anthrax. Typically, cutaneous anthrax occurs on the exposed parts of the body. The lesion begins innocuously with a small papule that the patient may first notice because of pruritus. The papule develops after several days into a small vesicle or, occasionally, into several vesicles that then coalesce to form a ring. This area may be surrounded by a small ring of erythema and possibly some edema. The pruritus may continue, but there is no pain unless secondary infection or a significant degree of local edema is present. A small dark area can be seen beneath the center of the vesicle, or in the central area if a ring of vesicles has formed. Eventually, the vesicle or vesicular ring ruptures, discharging a clear fluid and revealing a depressed black necrotic central area known as an eschar. After 1–2 weeks, the lesion dries, and the eschar begins to loosen and shortly thereafter separates, revealing a permanent scar.

The lesion is usually 1–3 cm in diameter and remains round and regular. Occasionally, a lesion may be larger and irregularly shaped. There may be regional lymphangitis and lymphadenopathy and some systemic symptoms such as a slight low-grade fever, malaise, and headache. Antibiotic therapy will not change the natural progression of the lesion itself; however, it will decrease or inhibit development of edema and systemic symptoms.

Occasionally, the cutaneous reaction is severe and is characterized by significant local and spreading edema associated with blebs, bullae, induration, chills, and fever. This type of reaction is referred to as malignant edema. Whether malignant edema results from increased pathogenicity or dosage of the organism or because of host factors is unknown.

Lesions in specific body sites occasionally result in more severe local reactions. Several cases have been seen of anthrax involving tissue surrounding the eye in which extensive edema spread over the entire face and extended to the neck and upper thorax. In one such patient, edema involved his entire face and extended down to the upper part of the thorax. In this instance, the spread of the toxin resulted in an extensive cutaneous lesion with necrosis of both eyelids. Plastic surgery was necessary to repair the tissue damage of the eyelids and surrounding tissue.

Infrequently, meningitis may develop as a complication of cutaneous anthrax (see Section 8.1.4).

8.1.2. Inhalation Anthrax. This form shows a biphasic clinical pattern with a benign initial phase followed by an acute, severe second phase that is almost always fatal. The initial phase begins as a nonspecific illness consisting of malaise, fatigue, myalgia, mild fever, nonproductive cough, and, occasionally, a sensation of precordial oppression. Findings of the physical examination are essentially within normal limits except that rhonchi may be present. The illness may resemble a mild upper-respiratory-tract infection such as a cold or the "flu." After 2–4 days, the patient may show signs of improvement. However, there is then the sudden onset of severe respiratory distress with dyspnea, cyanosis, respiratory stridor, and profuse diaphoresis. In several cases, subcutaneous edema of the chest and neck has been described. The pulse, respiratory rate, and temperature become elevated. Physical examination reveals moist, crepitant rales over the lungs and possibly evidence of pleural effusion. Shock may develop. X-ray examination of the chest may reveal widening of the mediastinum and pleural effusion. Septicemia and meningitis may develop. Death occurs in most persons with inhalation anthrax within 24 h after the onset of the acute phase.

8.1.3. Gastrointestinal Anthrax. There are two clinical presentations for disease resulting from ingestion of *B. anthracis,* intestinal and oropharyngeal.

The symptoms of intestinal anthrax are initially nonspecific and include nausea, vomiting, anorexia, and fever. With progression of the disease, abdominal pain, hematemesis, and bloody diarrhea develop. Ascites may be present. Occasionally, the symptoms and signs resemble an acute surgical abdomen, which in some cases has resulted in surgery. With further progression, toxemia develops with shock, cyanosis, and death. The time from onset of symptoms to death has most frequently varied from 2 to 5 days. In a recent outbreak reported from Russia, the average time from onset of symptoms to death was noted to be less than 2 days (personal communication). In oropharyngeal anthrax (also referred to as cervical anthrax), patients have experienced fever, submandibular edema, cervical lymphadenopathy, and anorexia. Some reports describe the presence of acute inflammatory lesions in the oral cavity and/or oropharynx. The mortality rate for gastrointestinal anthrax has been reported to vary from 25% to 60%.

8.1.4. Other Forms. Meningitis, seen in less than 5% of anthrax cases, may be a complication of any of the three forms of primary anthrax infection. Rarely, meningitis is reported without a known primary site of infection. Symptoms of meningeal anthrax develop 1 to several days after the onset of the primary lesion and are similar to those associated with hemorrhagic meningitis. Death, if it occurs, usually does so in 1–6 days after onset of disease.

Septicemia is only rarely seen in patients with cutaneous lesions; it is more commonly seen in patients with inhalation and gastrointestinal anthrax.

8.2. Diagnosis

Of importance in considering a diagnosis of anthrax is a source of exposure to the infectious agent. Only rarely have cases occurred for which the source of infection could not be identified.

Cutaneous anthrax should be suspected when an individual describes a painless, pruritic papule, usually on an exposed part of the body. Vesicular fluid should reveal *B. anthracis* organisms microscopically and on culture. The differential diagnosis should include contagious pustular dermatitis (ecthyma contagiosum or orf), milker's nodule, plague, staphylococcal disease, and tularemia.

The initial symptoms of inhalation anthrax are non-specific and resemble those of an upper-respiratory-tract infection. Characteristically, with the sudden development of the acute phase, there is severe respiratory distress, and radiographic examination of the chest should reveal widening of the mediastinum, a typical occurrence with inhalation anthrax. The acute phase resembles diseases that result in respiratory failure and shock.

In gastrointestinal anthrax, the patient presents with signs and symptoms of gastroenteritis. Organisms may be demonstrable in vomitus and feces from the infected individual. The differential diagnosis includes diseases that cause moderately severe gastroenteritis, such as shigellosis and *Yersinia* gastroenteritis. In the cervical form, the signs and symptoms might suggest pharyngitis, such as seen with streptococcal infections.

In anthrax meningitis, there should be a primary site of infection. CSF should contain *B. anthracis*. In septicemia, blood cultures should be positive for *B. anthracis*.

The diagnosis may be confirmed serologically by demonstrating a fourfold change in titer in acute- and convalescent-phase serum specimens collected 4 weeks apart. The ELISA test is more sensitive than the microhemagglutination test.[16,21] A single titer of 1 : 32 in the former or of 1 : 8 in the latter is indicative of a positive specimen. Another sensitive test, an electrophoretic immunotransblot method, may also be used.[21]

9. Control and Prevention

9.1. General Concepts

Restrictions on the importation of contaminated animal products would significantly decrease the risk of anthrax in the United States. Also, improving animal husbandry so that anthrax is no longer a significant infection among animals in countries from which the animal products are imported could reduce the rate of contamination of imported products. However, these improvements may be very difficult to accomplish. The next line of defense would be disinfecting the animal products either before they are imported or when they enter the United States. Washing with formaldehyde, as was done at the Liverpool Disinfection Station in England for many years, could be used; other methods that could be instituted are ethylene oxide treatment, irradiation, or autoclaving. However, because imported animal products enter the United States through a variety of ports, and due to complexities of these decontamination procedures, development of a central facility in which to process the imported materials would be very difficult.

In the United States, improvements in industrial hygiene have been of some benefit in reducing the exposure of the worker to infectious materials and aerosols. The most important are use of dust-collecting equipment during the initial processing cycle and institution of effective environmental-cleanup procedures.

Employees should be educated about the disease and the recommendations for working in a contaminated environment and for reducing the risk of developing the disease. Medical consultation services should be available to the employees. Adequate cleanup facilities and clothes-changing areas should be available so that workers do not wear their contaminated clothes home.

It should be noted that the risk of industrial infection has been reduced significantly over the past years as the use of imported animal products has been reduced because of changing business conditions and the increased use of synthetic materials (and the use of human vaccine; see Section 9.3).

Gastrointestinal anthrax can be prevented by forbidding the sale for consumption of meat from sick animals or animals that have died from disease. Depending on the circumstances, it may be important to alert individuals who may come in contact with contaminated meat about the disease and about the need to cook all meats thoroughly.

All cases or suspected cases of anthrax should be reported to local public-health officials so that appropriate epidemiological investigations can be conducted. Additional cases in humans or animals may be prevented by the prompt reporting and investigation of circumstances surrounding every case.

In the United States, agricultural anthrax is not a significant problem. This reflects the high standards of animal husbandry practiced in this country. Animals that graze in areas known as anthrax districts should be vaccinated annually with the Sterne strain animal vaccine. All animals suspected of dying from anthrax should be examined microbiologically; blood or tissue smears can be examined microscopically, and cultures can be set up from these same materials. All animals that have died with a confirmed diagnosis of anthrax should be thoroughly burned and the remaining bones and other materials buried deeply. Animals that die with a suspected diagnosis of anthrax should be cultured; this can be done by removing the dependent ear and culturing the cut end. The carcass should then be handled as outlined above. If incineration is not possible, then the carcass should be covered with lime and buried at least 6 ft deep to discourage its being uncovered by scavenging animals.

9.2. Antibiotic Prophylaxis and Chemotherapeutics

Prophylactic antibiotics or chemotherapeutic agents are not used for anthrax except in two situations. If an individual has been inoculated with live spore animal anthrax vaccine, prophylactic penicillin should be given. Additionally, prophylactic antibiotics should be considered if a person is known to have eaten contaminated meat. In these instances, prophylaxis is given to kill any *B. anthracis* organisms that may have been inoculated or ingested and thus prevent the production of toxin. When prophylactic antibiotics are given, the patient should be kept under surveillance for 10 days after initial therapy.

9.3. Immunization

There is an effective anthrax vaccine that was field tested in employees of four different textile mills in the United States, which demonstrated an effectiveness of 92.5%.[8,33] This vaccine should be used for all employees who may be exposed to contaminated materials or environment. Additionally, anyone who comes into a mill processing *B. anthracis*-contaminated materials should also be vaccinated. Currently, the vaccine is given parenterally with three doses given at 2-week intervals followed by three booster inoculations at 6-month intervals and then annual booster inoculations. Veterinarians and other persons who, because of their occupation, have potential contact with anthrax should also be immunized with the human anthrax vaccine. The human vaccine is commercially available. Those interested should contact the Bureau of Disease Control and Laboratory Services, Michigan Department of Public Health, P. O. Box 30035, 3500 N. Logan Street, Lansing, Michigan 48909.

10. References

1. ALBRINK, W. S., BROOKS, S. M., BIRON, R. E., AND KOPEL, M., Human inhalation anthrax, a report of three fatal cases, *Am. J. Pathol.* **36:**457–472 (1960).
2. Anthrax Investigations Board (Bradford & District) First Annual Report (1906), pp. 3–4.
3. BELL, J. H., Anthrax: Its relation to the wool industry, in: *Dangerous Trades* (T. OLIVER, ed.), pp. 634–643, London Button, London, 1902.
4. BRACHMAN, P. S., Inhalation anthrax, *Ann. N.Y. Acad. Sci.* **353:**83–93 (1980).
5. BRACHMAN, P. S., AND FEKETY, F. R., Industrial anthrax, *Ann. N.Y. Acad. Sci.* **70:**574–584 (1958).
6. BRACHMAN, P. S., PLOTKIN, S. A., BUMFORD, F. H., AND ATCHISON, M. A., An epidemic of inhalation anthrax. II. Epidemiologic investigations, *Am. J. Hyg.* **72:**6–23 (1960).
7. BRACHMAN, P. S., PAGANO, J. S., AND ALBRINK, W. S., Two cases of fatal inhalation anthrax, one associated with sarcoidosis, *N. Engl. J. Med.* **265:**203–208 (1961).
8. BRACHMAN, P. S., GOLD, H., PLOTKIN, S. A., FEKETY, F. R., WERRIN, M., AND INGRAHAM, N. R., Field evaluation of human anthrax vaccine, *Am. J. Public Health* **52:**632–645 (1962).
9. BRACHMAN, P. S., KAUFMANN, A. F., AND DALLDORF, F. G., Industrial inhalation anthrax, *Bacteriol. Rev.* **30:**646–657 (1966).
10. BROWN, E. R., AND CHERRY, W. B., Specific identification of *Bacillus anthracis* by means of a variant bacteriophage, *J. Infect. Dis.* **96:**34–39 (1955).
11. BUCHANAN, T. M., FEELEY, J. C., HAYES, P. S. AND BRACHMAN, P. S., Anthrax indirect microhemagglutination test, *J. Immunol.* **107:**1631–1636 (1971).
12. Centers for Disease Control, Cutaneous anthrax acquired from imported Haitian drums, Florida, *Morbid. Mortal. Weekly Rep.* **23:**142, 147 (1974).
13. CHERRY, W. B., AND FREEMAN, E. M., Staining bacterial smears with fluorescent antibody. V. The rapid identification of *Bacillus anthracis* in culture and in human and murine tissues, *Zentralbl. Bakteriol. Parasitenkd. Infektionskr. Hyg. Abt. 1 Orig.* **175:**582–597 (1959).
14. DAHLGREN, C. M., BUCHANAN, L. M., DECKER, H. M., FREED, S. W., PHILLIPS, C. R., AND BRACHMAN, P. S., *Bacillus anthracis* aerosols in a goat hair processing mill, *Am. J. Hyg.* **72:**24–31 (1960).
15. DAVIES, J. C. A., A major epidemic of anthrax in Zimbabwe, *Cent. Afr. J. Med.* Part 1 **28:**291–298 (1982), Part 2 **29:**8–12 (1983), Part 3 **31:**176–180 (1985).
16. EZZELL, J. W., AND ABSHIRE, T. G., Immunological analysis of cell-associated antigens of *Bacillus anthracis*, *Infect. Immun.* **56:**349–356 (1988).
17. FEELEY, J. C., AND BRACHMAN, P. S., *Bacillus anthracis*, in: *Manual of Clinical Microbiology*, 2nd ed.(E. H. LENNETTE, E. H. SPAULDING, AND J. P. TRUANT, eds.), pp. 143–147, American Society for Microbiology, Washington, D.C., 1974.

18. Fox, M., Kaufmann, A. F., Zendel, S. A., Kolb, R. C., Songy, C. G., Jr., Cangelosis, D. A., and Fuller, C. E., Anthrax in Louisiana, 1971: Epizootiologic study, *J. Am. Vet. Med. Assoc.* **163:**446–451 (1973).

19. Glassman, H. N., World incidence of anthrax in man, *Public Health Rep.* **73:**22 (1958).

20. Laforce, F. M., Woolsorters' disease, England, *Bull. N.Y. Acad. Med.* **54:**956–963 (1978).

21. Little, S. F., and Knudson, G. B., Comparative efficacy of *Bacillus anthracis* live spore vaccine and protective antigen vaccine against anthrax in the guinea pig, *Infect. Immun.* **52:**509–512 (1986).

22. Nalin, D. R., Sultana, B., Sahunja, R., Islam, A. K., Rahim, M. A., Islam, M., Costa, B. S., Mawla, N., and Greenough, W. B., Survival of a patient with intestinal anthrax, *Am. J. Med.* **62:**130–132 (1977).

23. Norman, P. S., Ray, J. G., Brachman, P. S., Plotkin, S. A., and Pagano, J. S., Serological testings for anthrax antibodies in workers in a goat hair processing mill, *Am. J. Hyg.* **72:**32–37 (1960).

24. Plotkin, S. A., Brachman, P. S., Utell, M., Bumford, F. H., and Atchison, M. M., An epidemic of inhalation anthrax: The first in the twentieth century. I. Clinical features, *Am. J. Med.* **29:**992–1001 (1960).

25. Sirisantha, T., Navacharoen, N., Tharavichitkul, P., Sirisanthana, V., and Brown, A. E., Outbreak of oral–oropharyngeal anthrax: An unusual manifestation of human infection with *Bacillus anthracis*, *Am. J. Trop. Med. Hyg.* **33:**144–150 (1984).

26. Stein, C. D., and Stoner, M. G., Anthrax in livestock during the first quarter of 1952 with special reference to outbreaks in swine in the mid-west, *Vet. Med.* **47:**274–279 (1952).

27. Sterne, M., The use of anthrax vaccines prepared from avirulent (uncapsulated) variants of *Bacillus anthracis*, *Onderstepoort J. Vet. Sci. Anim. Ind.* **13:**307–312 (1939).

28. Suffin, S. C., Karnes, W. H., and Kaufmann, A. F., Inhalation anthrax in a home craftsman, *Hum. Pathol.* **9:**594–597 (1978).

29. Tigertt, W. D., Personal communication.

30. Wilson, G., The Brown Animal Sanatory Institution, *J. Hyg.* **82:**337–352 (1979).

31. Wolff, A. H., and Heimann, H., Industrial anthrax in the United States: An epidemiologic study, *Am. J. Hyg.* **53:**80–109 (1951).

32. Wool disinfection and anthrax: A year's working of the model station, *Lancet* **2:**1295–1296 (1922).

33. *World Health Statistics Annual, 1980–1981, Infectious Diseases: Cases,* World Health Organization, Geneva, 1981.

34. Wright, J. G., Green, T. W., and Kanode, R. G., Jr., Studies on immunity and anthrax. V. Immunizing activity of alum-precipitated protective antigen, *J. Immunol.* **73:**387 (1954).

11. Suggested Reading

Brachman, P. S., Anthrax, in: *Infectious Diseases,* 4th ed. (P. D. Hoeprich, ed.), pp. 1007–1013, Harper & Row, New York, 1989.

Dutz, W., and Kohout, E., Anthrax, *Pathol. Ann.* **6:**209–248 (1971).

Fox, M. D., Kaufmann, A. F., Zendel, S. A., Kolb, R. C., Songy, C. G., Jr., Cangelosis, D. A., and Fuller, C. E., Anthrax in Louisiana, 1971: Epizootiologic study, *J. Am. Vet. Med. Assoc.* **163:**446–451 (1973).

Lincoln, R. E., Walker, J. S., Klein, F., and Haines, B. W., Anthrax, *Adv. Vet. Sci.* **9:**327–368 (1964).

Van Ness, G. B., Ecology of anthrax, *Science* **172:**1303–1307 (1971).

Bacterial Food Poisoning

(*Bacillus cereus, Clostridium perfringens, Vibrio parahemolyticus, Staphylococcus aureus, Yersinia enterocolitica*)

David R. Snydman and Sherwood L. Gorbach

1. Introduction

Bacterial food poisoning is defined as an illness caused by the consumption of food contaminated with bacteria or bacterial toxins. Food poisoning can also be related to parasites (e.g., trichinosis), viruses (e.g., hepatitis), and chemicals (e.g., mushrooms), but these considerations are not within the scope of this chapter. Food poisoning due to bacteria constitutes approximately two-thirds of the food poisoning outbreaks in the United States for which an etiology can be determined.[10,24,25] However, it should be noted that only 36% of such outbreaks fulfill the criteria for confirmed etiology (see below).

David R. Snydman and Sherwood L. Gorbach Departments of Clinical Microbiology, Epidemiology, Medicine, Pathology, and Community Health, New England Medical Center and Tufts University School of Medicine, Boston, Massachusetts 02111.

The major recognized etiologies of bacterial food poisoning are limited to 12 bacteria, i.e., *Bacillus cereus, Clostridium perfringens, Vibrio parahemolyticus, Staphylococcus aureus, Clostridium botulinum, Vibrio cholerae,* toxigenic *Escherichia coli, Salmonella, Shigella, Campylobacter, Yersinia,* and *Brucella*. The first four are considered in Sections 5–8 of this chapter. Foodborne illness due to *C. botulinum* is discussed in Chapter 5; to *V. cholerae* in Chapter 10; to toxigenic *E. coli* in Chapter 12; to *Salmonella* in Chapters 28 and 39; to *Shigella* in Chapter 29; to *Campylobacter fetus* subsp. *jejuni* in Chapter 7[68,122]; to *Yersinia enterocolitica* in Chapter 40; and to *Brucella* in Chapter 6. Other agents such as streptococci, Arizona species, and *Listeria* have infrequently been implicated as agents in foodborne illness in the United States; however, the latter bacteria are being increasingly recognized as agents of food poisoning (see Chapter 18).

Foodborne illness is a significant public-health problem. It is a major cause of morbidity and an infrequent cause of mortality in the United States. In the 4-year period 1983–1986, there were 785 confirmed outbreaks due to all known causes reported in the United States.[25] Although the number of ill people reported to health authorities was 45,013, surveillance suggests that the true scope of infection related to food poisoning is probably 10–100 times more frequent.[1]

For most public-health authorities, a foodborne disease outbreak is defined by two criteria: (1) two or more persons experience a similar illness, usually gastrointestinal, after ingestion of a common food; and (2) epidemiological analysis implicates food as the source of the illness. There are certain exceptions to this definition. For example, one case of botulism or chemical poisoning constitutes an outbreak for epidemiological investigation and control purposes.

Reported foodborne outbreaks generally are divided into two categories: (1) laboratory-confirmed, i.e., outbreaks in which evidence of a specific etiological agent is obtained and specific laboratory criteria are met (see Sections 5.6.3, 6.6.3, 7.6.3, 8.6.3, 9.1, and 9.2); and (2) undetermined, i.e., outbreaks in which epidemiological evidence implicates a food source, but adequate laboratory confirmation is not obtained.

2. Historical Background

Our understanding of foodborne illness is still in its infancy. About 50 years ago, state and territorial health officers in the United States, concerned about high morbidity and mortality rates caused by typhoid fever and infantile diarrhea, recommended that cases of enteric fever be investigated and reported. In 1923, the United States Public Health Service (PHS) published summaries of outbreaks of gastrointestinal illness attributed to milk. Outbreaks caused by all foods were added in 1938. These activities were instrumental in the enactment of public-health measures that have decreased the incidence of enteric disease.

In 1961, the Centers for Disease Control (CDC) assumed responsibility for publishing and collecting reports on foodborne illness. The current system of surveillance of foodborne disease began in 1966 by incorporating into an annual summary all reports of enteric disease outbreaks in the United States attributed to microbial contamination of food.

3. Methodology

The two federal regulatory agencies that have major responsibility for food protection, the Food and Drug Admin-

istration (FDA) and the U.S. Department of Agriculture (USDA), report episodes of foodborne illness to the CDC and to state and local health departments. Likewise, the local and state agencies investigate complaints by consumers and physicians and initiate epidemiological investigations. Reports of all positive investigations are customarily forwarded to the CDC. On special request, the CDC will participate in an investigation, especially if the outbreak is unusually large or involves products that move by interstate commerce.

3.1. Sources of Mortality Data

Mortality data, with the possible exception of botulism, are most assuredly underreported. Foodborne illness may not be appreciated as a contributing factor in an elderly or debilitated person, especially when death is not immediate. In fact, even in those foodborne outbreaks that are recognized and investigated by health authorities, information on death is not reported in 30% of the incidents.

One hundred twenty-four deaths in the 4 years 1983–1986 were attributed to food: 37 (30%) of these deaths were due to *Salmonella*, 8 (6%) to *C. botulinum*, 4 (3%) to *E. coli*, 3 (2%) to streptococci, 2 (2%) to *C. perfringens*, 2 (2%) to *Shigella*, and 56 (45%) to other bacteria. Chemicals accounted for 8 deaths (6%), viruses for 1 (1%), and parasites for 1 (1%). However, some of the difficulties in laboratory diagnosis of *V. parahemolyticus* and *B. cereus* may obscure any relationship between those organisms and mortality. Because foodborne illnesses are generally mild, mortality figures in no way reflect morbidity data.

3.2. Sources of Morbidity Data

The information reported to health departments and the PHS has many limitations. Many people do not recognize that they are involved in a foodborne outbreak unless they are part of a large group that is affected. Therefore, health authorities usually hear about large outbreaks related to group activities such as church picnics or to confined populations such as schools and institutions. Small outbreaks related to families or to commercial products consumed locally are overlooked.

The likelihood of outbreaks coming to the attention of health authorities is extremely variable and depends to a large extent on consumer awareness and physician interest. Large intra- and interstate outbreaks may skew the data considerably, as will outbreaks of serious illness such as botulism. Various local health authorities have differing interests and expertise in investigating foodborne illness, and this, too, may prejudice the data.

Finally, the problems of transport and bacteriological

Table 1. Confirmed Bacterial Foodborne Disease Outbreaks, Cases, and Deaths, 1983–1986, United States, as Reported to CDC[a]

	1983 Outbreaks	1983 Cases	1984 Outbreaks	1984 Cases	1985 Outbreaks	1985 Cases	1986 Outbreaks	1986 Cases	Total Outbreaks	Total Cases	Distribution (%) Outbreaks	Distribution (%) Cases	Total deaths
B. cereus	0	0	0	0	7	42	5	190	12	232	2.3	0.6	0
Brucella	1	29	3	23	1	9	0	0	5	61	1.0	0.1	1
Campylobacter	8	162	4	125	9	174	4	227	25	688	4.8	1.7	1
C. botulinum	12	45	11	16	17	33	21	26	61	120	11.8	0.3	8
C. perfringens	5	353	8	882	6	1,016	3	202	22	2,453	4.2	5.9	2
E. coli	3	157	2	76	1	370	1	37	7	640	1.4	1.6	4
Salmonella	72	2427	77	4407	79	19,660	63	2696	291	29,190	56.2	70.8	37
Shigella	7	1993	9	470	5	216	11	706	32	3,385	6.2	8.2	2
S. aureus	14	1257	12	1213	13	407	7	250	46	3,127	8.9	7.6	0
Streptococcus Group A	1	535	2	83	1	12	2	248	6	878	1.2	2.1	0
Streptococcus	1	16	0	0	0	0	1	69	2	85	0.4	0.2	3
Vibrio cholerae	1	1	0	0	0	0	1	5	2	6	0.4	0	0
V. parahemolyticus	0	0	0	0	0	0	1	2	1	2	0.2	0	0
Other bacteria	2	87	1	103	1	86	2	98	6	374	1.0	0.9	56
Total	127	7062	129	7398	140	22,025	122	4756	518	41,241	100	100	114

[a] From CDC Surveillance Reports, 1983–1986.

Table 2. Average Number of Cases per Outbreak of Known Bacterial Foodborne Disease by Etiology, 1983–1986[a]

	Outbreaks	Cases	Cases per outbreak
B. cereus	12	232	19
Brucella	5	61	12
Campylobacter	25	688	28
C. botulinum	61	120	2
C. perfringens	22	2,453	112
E. coli	7	640	91
Salmonella	291	29,190	100
Shigella	32	3,385	106
S. aureus	46	3,127	68
Streptococcus Group A	6	878	146
Streptococcus	2	85	43
Vibrio cholerae	2	6	3
V. parahemolyticus	1	2	2
Total	512	40,867	80

[a]From CDC Surveillance Reports, 1983–1986.

culture restrict recognition of certain foodborne illness. Outbreaks of *B. cereus, V. parahemolyticus,* and *Y. enterocolitica* are confirmed less frequently because of the laboratory expertise required. In contrast, *C. perfringens* is relatively easily recognized in the laboratory, but the organism may be lost in transport or the specimen not be cultured anaerobically.

Another variable that may skew the morbidity data is the length of the incubation period. Organisms causing illnesses with a short incubation period, such as *S. aureus,* may be more easily recognized as a common-source problem than those associated with a longer incubation period.

4. Etiological Patterns

Recognizing the significant problems in reporting and the potential errors in the data, let us look at the surveillance data for the United States. From 1983 to 1986, 518 outbreaks affecting 41,241 people were reported to CDC (Table 1).[25] *Salmonella* predominated, accounting for 71% of the cases. This may be due to the awareness of the public and physicians and the relatively large number of cases associated with common-source outbreaks of *Salmonella* which attracts the attention of public-health personnel. The next most frequent cause of foodborne disease cases was *Shigella* with 8.2%, *Staphylococcus aureus* with 7.6%, and *C. perfringens* with 5.9%. *Salmonella* also accounted for the greatest number of outbreaks with 56%, followed by *C. botulinum* with 12%, *S. aureus* with 9%, *Shigella* with 6%, *Campylobacter* with 5%, and *C. perfringens* with 4%.

The largest number of cases per outbreak was seen with *Streptococcus* Group A with an average of 146 cases per outbreak (Table 2); however, there were only 6 outbreaks, with 1 outbreak accounting for 535 cases. The second largest average number of cases per outbreak was seen with *C. perfringens* with 112 cases per outbreak; then *Shigella* with 106 cases per outbreak and *Salmonella* with 100 per outbreak. Though there were 61 outbreaks due to *C. botulinum,* there were only an average of 2 cases associated with each outbreak.

There are several pathogens that are rarely reported, namely, *V. parahemolyticus* and *Y. enterocolitica,* that have been well studied in other parts of the world.[104] Their contribution to foodborne diarrheal illness in the United States has only recently been recognized, and recovery from stool or food requires special laboratory procedures.

It is important to note that etiological patterns may

Table 3. Comparison among the United States, England and Wales, and Japan of the Most Common Foodborne Disease Outbreaks Reported from 1968 to 1972[a]

Organism or disease	United States		England and Wales		Japan	
	Number of outbreaks	Percentage of known etiology	Number of outbreaks	Percentage of known etiology	Number of outbreaks	Percentage of known etiology
S. aureus	208	28.5	96	2.8	891	28.5
Salmonellosis	185	25.4	3149	91.8	414	13.3
C. perfringens	102	14.0	187	5.4	—	—
V. parahemolyticus	9	1.2	1	< 0.1	1679	53.8
B. cereus	6	0.8	6	0.2	—	—

[a]Adapted from Bryan.[17]

vary throughout the world. These patterns are dependent on many factors, such as food preferences, physician and public awareness, and laboratory capabilities. Table 3 lists a comparison of five bacterial agents recognized in outbreaks in three areas of the world: the United States, England and Wales, and Japan.[18] In the United States, *S. aureus* and salmonellosis are the most common agents involved in foodborne outbreaks, representing over 50% of these outbreaks. In contrast, salmonellosis is implicated in over 90% of the recognized foodborne illness in England and Wales. *C. perfringens* is a frequently reported pathogen in both the United States and England. Japan, on the other hand, has very different etiological patterns, probably related to many of the aforementioned factors. *V. parahemolyticus* gastroenteritis, first described in that country, is the dominant pathogen in foodborne outbreaks and represents over 50% of the reported outbreaks. These associations generally reflect the different staples in diets around the world. *S. aureus* and salmonellosis are not uncommon there; however, there are no reports of *C. perfringens*. Clearly, some of these differences represent ascertainment bias; however, there is little doubt that different patterns exist in different regions of the world.

With this background, let us turn to a consideration of the specific agents *B. cereus*, *C. perfringens*, *V. parahemolyticus*, *S. aureus*, and *Y. enterocolitica*. A summary of the agents, common vehicles, symptoms, signs, and types of specimens necessary for confirmation is provided in Table 4.

5. *Bacillus cereus*

5.1. Historical Background

One of the first outbreaks implicating an aerobic spore-forming organism was described by Lubenau[76] in 1906, in which 300 inmates of a sanitorium developed a diarrheal illness from meatballs contaminated with an organism labeled *Bacillus peptonificans*. This isolate closely resembled what is today considered typical of *B. cereus*. Other European investigators cited aerobic spore-forming bacilli similar to *B. cereus* in food poisoning involving vanilla sauce, jellied meat dishes, and boiled beef.[52,95–97,100] Most reports classified the *Bacillus* organism as a member of the *subtilis–mesentericus* group or as an "anthracoid" bacillus.

It is now generally recognized that the classic description of the illness caused by *B. cereus* was made by Hauge,[52] who in 1955 described four Norwegian outbreaks involving 600 people. Interestingly, the vehicle in all

four outbreaks appeared to be a vanilla sauce. Samples of sauce in each instance contained *B. cereus* in concentrations of greater than 10^6 per ml. The patients suffered from a diarrheal illness that was profuse and watery, and associated with abdominal pain and nausea, but rarely with vomiting. Fever was distinctly uncommon, and all symptoms usually abated within 12 h. The incubation period in these outbreaks was about 10 h.

Hauge demonstrated in himself that vanilla sauce inoculated with a strain of *B. cereus* that had been isolated from an outbreak of gastrointestinal illness and allowed to incubate for 24 h would cause severe abdominal pain and diarrhea 13 h after consumption. He was able to culture *B. cereus* from his stool as well. Similar experiments performed in his laboratory with other volunteers substantiated his findings.[52]

Since the early 1950s, most reports of *B. cereus* foodborne illness have come from European countries, particularly the Netherlands and Hungary.[95–97,100] The first well-documented outbreak of gastrointestinal disease in the United States was reported by Midura *et al.*[87] in 1970. In 1974, another form of *B. cereus* food poisoning was recognized that invariably involved fried rice.[91] This illness was distinctly different from those previously described, in that the incubation period was shorter, ranging from 1 to 6 h, and the illness was primarily vomiting (although some patients had diarrhea). Although this condition closely resembled staphylococcal food poisoning, *B. cereus* was recovered from the fried rice. This report heralded the realization that this organism may be responsible for two distinct foodborne syndromes.

5.2. Biological Characteristics of the Organism

B. cereus is a gram-positive, catalase-positive, aerobic spore-forming rod. Although many deviant strains exist, as a species *B. cereus* strains are able to utilize glucose, fructose, and trehalose. There is no metabolism of xylose, arabinose, galactose, sorbose, sorbitol, mannitol, or dulcitol.[47] The production of acetylmethylcarbinol and the reduction of nitrate are characteristic, but some strains fail to manifest these reactions. Starch positivity and gelatin liquefaction are characteristic. Most strains are β-hemolytic.[47] *B. cereus* is differentiated from *B. anthracis* on the basis of resistance to gamma phage, negative fluorescent-antibody test, lack of animal pathogenicity, and presence of β-hemolysis.[47] For a more detailed discussion of the biochemical properties of these organisms, the reader is referred to the review by Goepfert *et al.*[47]

Strains of *B. cereus* produce several extracellular tox-

Table 4.   Characteristics of Bacterial Food Poisoning

Organism	Common vehicles	Median incubation period, h (range)	Toxin, primary in pathogenesis	Clinical features[a]	Median duration, days (range)	Secondary attack rates	Sources of diagnostic material	Laboratory diagnosis
B. cereus (Section 5)	Fried rice, vanilla sauce, cream	2 (1–16)	Heat-stable	V, C, D (33%)	0.4 (0.2–0.5)	—	Vomitus, stool, or food	>10⁵ colonies on peptone–beef extract egg-yolk agar; need controls for stool analysis (may be normal flora), serotyping
	Vanilla sauce, meatballs, boiled beef, barbecued chicken	9 (6–14)	Heat-labile	D, C, V	1 (1–2)	—		
C. perfringens (Section 6)	Beef, turkey, chicken	12 (8–22)	Heat-labile	D, C (N, V, F rare)	1 (0.3–3)	—	Stool or rectal swab; food, food-contact surfaces	Egg-yolk-free tryptose–sulfite–cycloserine agar; Hobbs or bacteriocin typing
V. parahemolyticus (Section 7)	Seafood, rarely salt water or salted vegetables	12 (2–48)	?	D, C, N, V, H, F (25%), B (rare)	3 (2–10)	—	Stool or rectal swab; food, food-contact surfaces; seawater	Thiosulfate–citrate–bile salt agar (TCBS); test for Kanagawa phenomenon (see text), serotyping
S. aureus (Section 8)	Ham, pork, canned beef, cream-filled pastry	3 (1–6)	Heat-stable	V, N, C, D, F (rare)	1 (0.3–1.5)	—	Stool, vomitus; food or food-contact surfaces; nasal, hand, purulent lesion from food preparer	Egg yolk–tellurite–glycine–pyruvate agar or mannitol salt; phage type isolates; enterotoxin testing
Y. enterocolitica	Chocolate or	? 72 (2–144)	Heat-stable	F, C, D, V,	7 (2–30)	20%	Stool from food	Cold enrichment;

Organism	Food	Incubation (hr)	Toxin	Symptoms[a]	Days (range)	%	Specimen/preparer	Media; serotyping, serology
(Section 9.1)	raw milk, pork	(see text)						
Listeria monocytogenes (Section 9.2)	Milk, raw vegetables	?	?	D, F, C, N, V, blood	?	10%	Stool	Cold enrichment, nutrient broth potassium thiocyanate and naladixic acid
C. fetus subsp. *jejuni* (Chapter 7)	Milk, chicken, pet animals	? 48 (24–240)	?	D, F, C, B, H, M, N, V	7 (2–30)	25%	Stool or rectal swab	Brucella-Agar Base with vancomycin, polymyxin, and trimethoprim grown in reduced oxygen
E. coli (Chapter 12)	Salads, beef	24 (8–44)	Heat-labile / Heat-stable / Verotoxin	D, C, N, H, F, M / F, M, D, C / B, C, F, hemolytic–uremic syndrome	3 (1–4)	0	Stool or rectal swab from patients	MacConkey media; *E. coli* must be tested for toxin production (see Chapter 12); serotyping
Salmonella (Chapter 28)	Eggs, meat, poultry	24 (5–72)	—	D, C, N, V, F, H, B (rare), enteric fever	3 (0.5–14)	30–50%	Stool or rectal swab from patients and food-preparation workers; raw food	*Salmonella–Shigella* (SS), deoxycholate–citrate, Hektoen enteric, or xylose–lysine–deoxycholate; phage typing for *S. typhimurium*
Shigella (Chapter 29)	Milk, salads (potato, tuna, turkey)	24 (7–168)	—	C, F, D, B, H, N, V	3 (0.5–14)	40–60%	Stool or rectal swab from patients and food workers; food	Same media as above; colicin typing

[a] B, bloody diarrhea; C, crampy abdominal pain; D, diarrhea; F, fever; H, headache; M, myalgias; N, nausea; V, vomiting.

ins that may contribute to their virulence. Spira and Goepfert[120] found an enterotoxin that produces fluid accumulation in rabbit ileal loops, alters vascular permeability in the skin of rabbits, and kills mice when injected intravenously. This toxin is distinct from the factors that cause hemolysis and egg-yolk turbidity previously described with *B. cereus*. The enterotoxin does not bind tightly to the rabbit ileal-loop receptor site, since elution by washing with saline destroys its activity. Furthermore, homologous antiserum introduced into the loop 10 min after enterotoxin neutralizes its action. This toxin is highly sensitive to heat (destroyed at 56°C in 5 min) and trypsin.[120]

Studies by Turnbull[135] have shown that the diarrheogenic enterotoxin can stimulate the adenylate cyclase–cyclic AMP (cAMP) system in intestinal epithelial cells. Cultures of the strain that elaborate this enterotoxin cause diarrhea when fed to rhesus monkeys.[135]

A second presumptive toxin has been isolated from a strain of *B. cereus* implicated in an outbreak of vomiting-type illness. Cell-free culture filtrates from this strain do not produce fluid accumulation in rabbit ileal loops, do not stimulate the adenylate cyclase–cAMP system, and produce only vomiting when fed to rhesus monkeys. This "vomiting" toxin is heat-stable.[85]

A third toxin has been suggested, a "pyogenic toxin," that was isolated from an organism that caused a necrotic brain abscess. This toxin caused severe necrosis of intestinal mucosa in rabbit ileum.[136]

There is some suggestion that the diarrheogenic toxin may be plasmid- or phage-mediated, since some strains previously positive in the rabbit ileal-loop assay had lost the ability to elicit fluid accumulation.[132]

B. cereus organisms produce lecithinase, phospholipases, and a hemolysin. These substances appear to have no role in the pathogenesis of the food-poisoning syndromes. Most strains of *B. cereus* also have a β-lactamase and are resistant to penicillin. Drug resistance in these organisms has not been important as an epidemiological factor in the transmission or pathogenesis of disease.

5.3. Descriptive Epidemiology

5.3.1. Prevalence and Incidence. Recognition of *B. cereus* food poisoning in the United States did not occur until 1970.

From 1983 to 1986, there were 12 outbreaks (2.3% of all confirmed bacterial foodborne outbreaks) affecting 232 people (0.6% of persons involved in bacterial foodborne outbreaks) (see Tables 1 and 2). This illustrates either an increase in awareness of this pathogen or an increase in contamination of foodstuffs with this pathogen.

Data from other countries are just as sparse. In contrast, an investigative interest has been fostered in Hungary by Nikodemusz,[96] and *B. cereus* ranked as the third most common pathogen in food poisoning from 1960 to 1966; the organism was responsible for 4.4% of all outbreaks and 11.4% of affected individuals.

5.3.2. Epidemic Behavior and Contagiousness. In the original description by Hauge,[52] 82% of individuals who ate the incriminated meal were affected. Of the 19 who were not ill, 11 had not eaten the dessert (implicated vehicle), and 8 had eaten only a small quantity. Other reported outbreaks have indicated attack rates from 50 to 75%. [37,87,100,114] In the reported vomiting-type outbreaks, virtually all individuals who consumed the contaminated fried rice became ill. There is no risk of secondary cases, since heavy contamination of the implicated vehicle is required.

The median incubation period for most diarrheal outbreaks reported in the United States is 9 h (range 6–14 h). The median incubation period of outbreaks of emetic illness is 2 h (range 2–3 h).

5.3.3. Geographic, Temporal, Age, Sex, Racial, and Occupational Distribution. *B. cereus* food poisoning has not shown any geographic or temporal distribution. There has been a suggestion by Bodnar[13] that affected children may become more severely ill than adults and require hospitalization. There does not appear to be any sexual, racial, or occupational predisposition.

5.3.4. Occurrence in Different Settings. Most reports of diarrheal illness have taken place in institutional settings (schools, hospitals, and others). This is probably a reporting artifact, since foodborne outbreaks are more easily recognized in confined populations.

5.3.5. Other Factors. The clear-cut association between the vomiting syndrome and fried rice deserves emphasis. All three reports of outbreaks of vomiting in the United States.[132] and the report by Mortimer and McCann[91] of five outbreaks in Great Britain implicated fried rice as the vehicle. The diarrheal illness, however, has been caused by boiled beef, sausage, chicken soup, vanilla sauce, and puddings.[37,47,91]

5.4. Mechanisms and Routes of Transmission

B. cereus is found in about 25% of many foodstuffs sampled, including cream, pudding, meat, spices, dry potatoes, dry milk, spaghetti sauces, and rice.[45,71] Contamination of the food product generally occurs prior to cooking. If the food is prepared in such a manner that the temperature is maintained at 30–50°C, vegetative cell growth will occur. Spores can survive extreme temperatures, and when allowed to cool relatively slowly, they will germinate and multiply.[46] There is no evidence that human carriage of the organism or other means of contamination play a role in transmission. It is not known whether the ingested organisms multiply and make toxin *in vivo* or whether a preformed toxin is present in food.

Illness characterized by vomiting as the major finding can be attributed to the common practice in Chinese restaurants of allowing large portions of boiled rice to drain unrefrigerated to avoid clumping. The flash frying in the final preparation of the fried rice does not produce enough heat to destroy the preformed heat-stable toxin. Interestingly, a study from England found that almost 90% of uncooked rice contained *B. cereus*, although the level of contamination in rice and the other food products generally was low ($< 10^5$ colony-forming units/g).[45,46]

5.5. Pathogenesis and Immunity

5.5.1. Pathogenesis. *B. cereus* food poisoning appears to be toxin-mediated in both the diarrheal form and the emetic form.[132] The presumptive enterotoxin responsible for the diarrheal illness is heat-labile; it acts like certain other enterotoxins, by stimulating adenylate cyclase. The exact site at which this toxin works has not been determined.

Whether the diarrheogenic, heat-labile enterotoxin is actually ingested or produced *in vivo* is not known; there are, however, several pieces of evidence to suggest that the latter mechanism may be operative. The incubation period in the diarrheal illness is too long for preformed toxin, and a large inoculum ($> 10^6$) is required to cause illness, suggesting a requirement for intestinal colonization.

The emetic illness is presumptively caused by preformed toxin that is heat-stable. The short incubation period and high attack rate provide support for this pathogenic mechanism.

5.5.2. Immunity. Our knowledge of immunity to either of these syndromes is largely uncharted. Antiserum to the enterotoxin introduced into the rabbit ileal-loop model along with the toxin can prevent fluid accumulation; no careful studies in humans have been performed. There are many serotypes of *B. cereus*, but it is not known whether the various enterotoxins have immune cross-reactivity.

5.6. Patterns of Host Response

5.6.1. Clinical Features. The initial report by Hauge[52] described the diarrheal illness of *B. cereus*, and his findings are consistent with what we know today. Illness is characterized by diarrhea (96%), abdominal cramps

(75%), and vomiting (23%). Fever is uncommon. The duration of illness has ranged from 20 to 36 h, with a median of 24 h.[52,132]

The emetic form of the illness has the predominant symptoms of vomiting (100%) and abdominal cramps (100%). Diarrhea is present in only one-third of affected individuals.[132] The duration of this illness has ranged from 8 to 10 h, with a median of 9 h. In both types of illness, the disease is usually mild and self-limited (Table 4).

5.6.2. Diagnosis. The diagnosis of *B. cereus* food poisoning should be considered in any individual who has diarrhea without fever in association with lower abdominal cramps. The incubation period varies from 6 to 14 h. The easiest way to make the diagnosis is by culture of the incriminated food product. The disease caused by *C. perfringens* is so similar to that of *B. cereus* that they cannot be differentiated clinically or epidemiologically; culture methods are required.

5.6.3. Laboratory Diagnosis. *B. cereus* can be cultured on blood agar, grown aerobically at 37°C. Some workers have employed a peptone–beef extract egg-yolk agar containing lithium chloride and polymyxin B as selective agents[71]; typical colonies are surrounded by an opaque zone. Others have utilized mannitol in the egg yolk–polymyxin medium and have advocated incubation at 35–37°C for 24 h. To distinguish *B. cereus* from other *Bacillus* species, the sporangium of sporulating cells is examined for swelling (which is not characteristic of *B. cereus*) and for the presence of a parasporal body characteristic of *B. thuringiensis*.[45] Differentiation of *B. cereus* from *B. anthracis* was described in Section 5.2, and should not be a problem since the clinical syndromes are dissimilar.

The diagnosis can be made by the isolation of 10^5 or more *B. cereus*/g from the incriminated food item. *B. cereus* can sometimes be found in the stools of healthy persons; therefore, isolation of the organism from feces may not be suitable confirmation unless negative stool cultures are obtained from an appropriate control group. Studies of enterotoxin production by the ligated rabbit-ileal loop or adenylate cyclase assays are available only in research laboratories. There is no simple assay available for the emetic toxin.

Some investigators have demonstrated that isolates of *B. cereus* from vomiting outbreaks frequently produce acid from salicin. The significance of this finding is not understood at this time.[101]

5.6.4. Microbiological Serological Studies. Taylor and Gilbert[131] established a provisional serotyping schema by preparing agglutinating antisera against the flagellar (H) antigen of 18 strains isolated from various foodstuffs implicated in foodborne outbreaks around the world. There was no cross-absorption. Three serotypes (types 1, 3, and 5) were involved in 31 of 34 (91%) outbreaks of food poisoning investigated. All the outbreaks investigated in this report were attributed to cooked rice, yet types 1, 3, and 5 were present in only 8% of random samples of uncooked rice.

The studies from this same laboratory have been extended to include samples from a larger number of outbreaks. In 35 of 61 outbreaks of vomiting illness, food or clinical specimens or both yielded only type 1. Type 1 and other serotypes were implicated in 7 other episodes. In 14 more outbreaks, types 3, 4, 5, and 8, or mixtures, were isolated.[45] In contrast, serotype 1 was isolated from only 2 of 9 diarrhea-type outbreaks, but 2, 6, 8, 9, 10, and 12 were responsible for 1 outbreak each. These investigators also examined 400 random food samples. Typable strains could be found in 45% of uncooked rice, 47% of boiled or fried rice, 27% of milk and cream, and 37% of cooked meat and poultry. Type 1 was predominant in the latter three categories of food examined, whereas type 17 was most common in uncooked rice.

The results of the serotyping studies suggest that separate serotypes are associated with distinct syndromes. However, there are no data to link toxin production with serotype. The fact that toxin production may be phage- or plasmid-mediated (as alluded to in Section 5.2) could confuse the epidemiological importance of these serotypic findings.

6. Clostridium perfringens

6.1. Historical Background

C. perfringens was first recognized and confirmed in the United States as a foodborne pathogen in 1945 by McClung,[81] who studied four outbreaks of diarrhea related to the consumption of chickens steamed 24 h prior to consumption. *C. perfringens* was isolated from the cooked chickens. Prior to this discovery, workers in Europe had also recognized that gravy contaminated with anaerobic spore-forming bacilli, including *C. perfringens,* had caused gastrointestinal illness in children.[72,81]

Shortly after McClung's discovery, filtrates from strains of *C. perfringens* were administered by mouth to human subjects. Cramps and diarrhea occurred in some individuals, but the incubation period was short, 45–80 min.[48] Living cultures induced cramps and bloating in 4 h and diarrhea several hours thereafter. Hobbs *et al.*[59] elegantly confirmed these results and outlined the epidemiological features of the disease in Great Britain in 1953.

The other major discovery in the late 1940s was the

outbreak of a severe and often lethal intestinal disease labeled enteritis necroticans or "Darmbrand" that affected over 400 people in Germany[148]; this outbreak was similar to others described later in New Guinea and termed "pigbel"[92] (see Section 6.3.7). Both conditions were due to *C. perfringens.* The strains were originally thought to be a new type, type F; however, today they are classified as variants of type C.[116]

Up to this time, all foodborne outbreaks were felt to be due to heat-resistant *C. perfringens.* Several investigators in the late 1960s confirmed that nonhemolytic and β-hemolytic, heat-sensitive strains could cause food poisoning.[127]

Investigations in the late 1960s and early 1970s provided convincing evidence that the pathogenesis of *C. perfringens* food poisoning is due to enterotoxin production while cells are sporulating. Furthermore, enterotoxin can be demonstrated in *C. perfringens* types A, C, and D. The toxins of types A and C are quite similar with regard to physicochemical properties.

6.2. Biological Characteristics of the Organism

Clostridia are gram-positive, spore-forming obligate anaerobes. Although all species grow better under anaerobic conditions, *C. perfringens* is remarkably aerotolerant and may survive exposure to oxygen for as long as 72 h.

Presumptive identification of *C. perfringens* can be accomplished by the presence of colonies on either rabbit, human, or sheep blood agar plates in which a double zone of hemolysis is present (the inner zone is complete and the outer zone is usually incomplete). Subculture to an egg-yolk agar with *C. perfringens* antitoxin present on one half of the plate is used to support the presumptive identification, since no zone of precipitation develops on the side with antitoxin. *C. paraperfringens* is the only other *Clostridium* species that will produce this reaction, and this species is not usually encountered in clinical material. It having been stated that this organism classically produces a double zone of hemolysis, it must be noted that most strains of *C. perfringens* that cause food poisoning are α- or nonhemolytic.[57] It was once thought that most food-poisoning strains were heat-resistant; however, numerous outbreaks from heat-sensitive strains have been reported.[127] Therefore, temperature resistance of hemolysis cannot be used as an identifying criterion.

C. perfringens is characterized by oval, subterminal spores that are only rarely seen in clinical material. This species is unique among the commonly encountered pathogenic clostridia in its ability to ferment sucrose. Carbohydrate metabolism is associated with inordinate gas production, forming the basis of another useful laboratory test known as "stormy fermentation." *C. perfringens* is also unique among clostridial species in being nonmotile and producing sulfide and nitrite. Although other rare species are able to produce these reactions, they cannot liquefy gelatin. Thus, these tests are the most useful ones in determining the species. The variety of fermentation metabolites that characterize the clostridial species is beyond the scope of this chapter, and the reader should consult Maclennan[77] for more details.

C. perfringens is known to produce 12 toxins that are active in tissues, as well as several enterotoxins. [53,77,116,139] The species has been divided into five types, A–E, on the basis of the four major toxins, alpha, beta, epsilon, and iota. All species produce α-toxin, which is a phospholipase C (lecithinase) that splits lecithin into phosphorylcholine and diglyceride. The inhibition of this activity by antitoxin is the basis of the egg-yolk test described above.

Diarrheal disease is caused by a heat-labile, protein enterotoxin with a molecular weight of approximately 34,000. This toxin is nondialyzable, precipitated by ammonium sulfate, antigenic, and inactivated by pronase but not by trypsin, lipase, or amylase.[121] Duncan[35] and colleagues have shown that the toxin is a structural component of the spore coat and is formed during sporulation. It can be shown to cause fluid accumulation in the rabbit ileal-loop model.[124] Although both cholera vibrios and *C. perfringens* produce enterotoxins, the clostridial toxin differs from cholera toxin in the following respects: Clostridial enterotoxin has its maximum activity in the ileum and has minimal activity in the duodenum, just opposite to that of cholera toxin. Clostridial enterotoxin inhibits glucose transport, damages the intestinal epithelium, and causes protein loss into the intestinal lumen, all of which are not observed with cholera toxin.[83]

An enterotoxin has been isolated from strains of *C. perfringens* type C implicated in the "pig-bel" syndrome in New Guinea in the 1950s. This enterotoxin seems to be quite similar if not identical to the one described from type A strains.[115,116] Prior to the discovery of this toxin, the pathological events had been ascribed to the β-toxin, since antitoxin titers were formed in patients who survived their illness.[92] Whether this toxin or the β-toxin is responsible for the whole syndrome described in New Guinea and Germany is unknown.

In addition, an enterotoxin production has been demonstrated in strains of *C. perfringens* type D. The toxin has not been totally purified, but appears to be immunologically identical to the type A toxin.[139]

The proof that *C. perfringens* enterotoxin can produce diarrheal illness was confirmed by feeding cell-free filtrates to volunteers. Of 15 persons who consumed filtrates from toxin-producing strains, 4 developed diarrhea, whereas none of 16 persons fed filtrates from toxin-negative strains developed illness. The incubation period for illness in these volunteers was 2–2.5 h. Similar results have been obtained in experimental animals.[36,124]

6.3. Descriptive Epidemiology

6.3.1. Prevalence and Incidence. *C. perfringens* food poisoning has accounted for 22 outbreaks in the 4 years 1983–1986, involving 2453 cases. During this 4-year period, *C. perfringens* was associated with about 4% of the outbreaks and 6% of all cases (see Table 1). It is the fifth most common cause of outbreaks and the fourth most common etiology of cases. Similar figures were reported from England and Wales in 1969–1970.[57] Since this diagnosis is often difficult to establish, one must assume that these cases represent a small fraction of actual cases in the United States.

6.3.2. Epidemic Behavior and Contagiousness. Epidemics of *C. perfringens* are usually characterized by high attack rates with a large number of affected individuals[75]; the median number of affected individuals per outbreak was 112 for the years 1983–1986 (see Table 2). Similar figures are reported from Great Britain.[57–59] There is no risk of secondary transmission.

The incubation period in most outbreaks varies between 8 and 14 h (median 12 h), but can be as long as 22 h.

6.3.3. Geographic, Age, Sex, Racial, and Occupational Distribution. Since the organism is widespread in nature, there is no geographic clustering associated with this organism. Outbreaks have been recorded throughout the United States, Europe, and Japan. No age, sex, racial, or occupational predilections are known.

6.3.4. Temporal Distribution. For reasons that are not clear, more cases of *C. perfringens* food poisoning are reported in the fall and winter months.[75] The nadir of reported cases is in the summer, in marked contrast to outbreaks of *Salmonella* and staphylococcal food poisoning. It may be that the kinds of foods usually implicated, such as stews, are eaten less frequently in the summer.

6.3.5. Occurrence in Different Settings. Outbreaks due to this organism are most frequently reported from institutions or large gatherings. The pathogenesis of infection requires that a meat or fish dish be precooked and then reheated to be served. The association with large gatherings may be a reporting artifact, since only such groups may recognize the outbreak as food poisoning.

6.3.6. Nutritional Factors. Beef, turkey, and chicken are the most frequent vehicles of infection with *C. per-*

fringens. The organism is ubiquitous, usually in the gastrointestinal tract or in soil. One survey in the United States found *C. perfringens* in 16% of samples of meat, poultry, and fish.[123] In Japan, outbreaks have been associated with "fried fish paste."

6.3.7. Enteritis Necroticans. This illness deserves to be considered separately, since there are some epidemiological features that distinguish it from *C. perfringens* type A food poisoning.[92] The incidence of pig-bel in New Guinea was roughly 500/100,000[92]; this compares to rates of 11 and 35/100,000 for Darmbrand in Germany in 1947.[148] The German outbreaks had peak seasonal incidence from July to September, while the New Guinea illness peaked in the middle 6 months of the calendar year. Attack rates in New Guinea were highest in the 0- to 10-year age group whereas in Germany most cases occurred in the 4th, 5th, and 6th decades. A clear male preponderance of cases existed in New Guinea, whereas a preponderance of cases in females was present in Germany.

Outbreaks of pig-bel have been clearly related to orgiastic consumption of pig in prolonged native feasts. The pig is improperly cooked, and large quantities are consumed over 3 or 4 days.[92]

6.4. Mechanisms and Routes of Transmission

C. perfringens is a ubiquitous organism that constitutes part of the human and animal fecal flora and can be isolated from soil. When only heat-resistant strains have been sought, contamination of raw meat such as pork, beef, veal, and mutton has varied between 1.5 and 42.7%.[57] McKillop found about 2% heat-resistant strains in raw meat, fish, and poultry; hemolytic strains were present in 72% and non-hemolytic strains in 18% of samples.[84]

The usual mechanism of transmission is intrinsic contamination of a food product, which when prepared incorrectly causes multiplication of the organism to a level that produces disease when ingested.

There has been some suggestion by Hobbs *et al.* [59] that blowflies may play a role in the transmission of the organism. She and her colleagues isolated heat-resistant *C. perfringens* from many batches of blowflies, including flies from a butcher's shop, a fried-fish shop, and a slaughterhouse. Another potential source of contamination is fecal contamination from the hands of food handlers, since fecal carriage of clostridia is common in man.[51]

In most instances, intrinsic contamination of the food product has been assumed; cross-contamination from kitchen supplies, blowflies, or fecal carriers is probably an unimportant mode of spread.

6.5. Pathogenesis and Immunity

6.5.1. Pathogenesis. Almost every outbreak is associated with roasted, boiled, stewed, or steamed meats or poultry as the vehicle of infection. Usually, the meat is cooked in bulk, with the result that heat gain and internal temperature are not sufficient to kill the spores.[129] The implicated food invariably undergoes a period of inadequate cooling, at which time the redox potential of the food is in a reduced state that allows the spores to germinate. This usually happens below 50°C. Unless the food is reheated to a very high temperature, it will contain many viable organisms, which can produce enterotoxin. In fact, heat treatment may enhance enterotoxin production.[138]

The role that "heat-sensitive" strains play in *C. perfringens* food poisoning has only recently been appreciated. As Sutton and Hobbs [127] pointed out, these so-called heat-sensitive strains are in fact more resistant than the classic β-hemolytic strains of *C. perfringens,* being able to survive 100°C for 10 min.

Once the organisms endure the initial heating, they must be ingested in large quantities to cause disease. It also appears that older cultures are more readily able to withstand the acid pH of the stomach than younger cultures.[128] Therefore, food that has been allowed to cool for some period of time may be a better medium to produce disease.

Some workers have estimated that as many as 5×10^8 organisms/g food are required to produce illness. Volunteer experiments have generally utilized at least 10^8 organisms to achieve an attack rate of 50%.[32]

Once ingested, the organism proliferates in the intestine, sporulates, and produces its enterotoxin. Although consumption of both cell-free filtrates and purified enterotoxin can cause illness, it is generally felt that toxin production occurs *in vivo.*[36,117,124] Occasionally, enterotoxin has been demonstrated in food; however, the food generally is not palatable when it has reached that state.[43]

Toxin production in the intestine has a number of effects, including salt and water secretion into the lumen and increased intestinal motility.[126] In addition, the clostridial toxin inhibits glucose transport, damages the intestinal epithelium, and causes protein loss into the intestinal lumen.[82,83]

Recently, *C. perfringens* enterotoxin has been demonstrated in the stools of affected individuals, both by reverse passive hemagglutination and by counterimmunoelectrophoresis.[34,93,117] Both latex agglutination and ELISA have demonstrated *C. perfringens* enterotoxin in stools.[6,80] In one study using a sandwich ELISA, 77% of stools from affected individuals were toxin-positive within the first 2 days of disease onset. However, toxin detection declined considerably after the second day.[80] These methods are still experimental but may soon become clinically applicable. Enterotoxin activity disappears quickly from the stool, but it can be measured easily in the serum.[34,93]

6.5.2. Immunity. Immunity is not well understood. In one study, 65% of Americans and 84% of Brazilians had antienterotoxin activity in serum.[140] The significance of this finding is unknown. No outbreaks have been studied by these methods in which blood was available prior to the outbreaks so that antienterotoxin immunity could be assessed. In animal studies, enterotoxin antiserum can block the action of the toxin on ligated rabbit loops. It has been suggested, however, that the presence of antibody in serum has little or no effect on toxin activity in the intestine.[93,117]

The role of immunity in enteritis necroticans is also unknown. The high attack rates in children in New Guinea, coupled with their high mortality and a high prevalence of anti-β-toxin in the blood of older individuals, suggest that immunity may determine the extent of infection and the outcome.[92]

6.6. Patterns of Host Response

6.6.1. Clinical Features. *C. perfringens* food poisoning is characterized by watery diarrhea and severe, crampy abdominal pain, usually without vomiting, beginning 8–24 h after the incriminated meal. Fever, chills, headache, or other signs of infection usually are not present (Table 4).

The illness is of short duration, 24 h or less. Rare fatalities have been recorded in debilitated or hospitalized patients who are victims of clostridial food poisoning.[133]

Enteritis necroticans is a much more severe, necrotizing disease of the small intestine with a high mortality. After a 24-h incubation period, illness ensues with intense abdominal pain, bloody diarrhea, vomiting, and shock. The mortality rate in this illness is about 40%, usually due to intestinal perforation.

6.6.2. Diagnosis. The diagnosis of *C. perfringens* food poisoning should be considered in any diarrheal illness characterized by abdominal pain and moderate to severe diarrhea, *unaccompanied* by fever or chills. There are usually many other individuals involved in the outbreak, and the suspect food is beef or chicken that has been stewed, roasted, or boiled earlier and then allowed to sit without proper refrigeration. The incubation period is 8–14 h; occasional outbreaks have incubation periods of 5–6 h or as long as 22 h.

B. cereus food poisoning can have a very similar presentation and can be ruled out only by bacteriological study. Enterotoxigenic E. *coli* can also present in this fashion (see Chapter 12 for discussion), although low-grade fever may be present. *Vibrio cholerae* has more profuse diarrhea, which helps differentiate it from clostridial intoxication. *Salmonella* infection usually has accompanying fever, a longer incubation period, and systemic signs.

Enteritis necroticans has not been reported in many years. The association of bloody diarrhea with a preceding feast of partially cooked pig should be enough of a clue to the diagnosis. "Darmbrand" was related to consumption of rancid meat in postwar Germany and has disappeared.

6.6.3. Laboratory Diagnosis. The major laboratory criterion for diagnosis is the isolation of the same organism from epidemiologically incriminated food and from the stools of ill individuals. If no food specimens are available, the isolation of organisms with the same serotype in the stools of most ill individuals, and not in the stools of suitable controls, would suffice for the diagnosis. In the absence of either of the aforementioned findings, a culture of the incriminated food containing 10^5 organisms or greater is suggestive.

The recommended culture medium is the egg-yolk-free tryptose–sulfite–cycloserine agar. It allows sulfite-reducing clostridia to form black colonies and inhibits other facultative anaerobes.[54,55] Colonies can then be selected for nitrate production, motility, and liquefaction of gelatin.[54] Heat resistance is no longer considered a characteristic of food-poisoning strains, and this test is not necessary.

Since *C. perfringens* can be isolated from normal stools, it is helpful to utilize the serotyping schema established by Hobbs and co-workers.[57–59] About 20 different serotypes have been established. In outbreaks, the same serotype of *C. perfringens* should be recovered from the cases. Demonstration of the same serotype in the incriminated food adds confirmation.

Bacteriocin typing has been applied to *C. perfringens,* and a provisional typing schema has been established.[78,143] The recent demonstration of enterotoxin in stools of affected individuals may provide a powerful new tool for the investigation of an outbreak.[34,93,117,138]

7. *Vibrio parahemolyticus*

7.1. Historical Background

V. parahemolyticus was first recognized as a potential foodborne pathogen by Fujino and co-workers[40,41] when it was isolated from autopsy materials collected in relation to a food-poisoning outbreak. The organism was considered to be a member of the genus *Pasteurella,* and the species *Pasteurella parahemolytica* was suggested. Over the next decade, many other outbreaks in Japan incriminated a pleomorphic, halophilic, hemolytic gram-negative organism similar to the one described by Fujino[41] and variously named *Pasteurella parahemolytica, Pseudomonas enteritis,* and *Oceanomonas parahemolytica.* The vehicles in these outbreaks were usually raw fish, shellfish, and cucumbers in brine. Extensive taxonomic studies in the laboratories of Sakazaki and Fujino revealed that the organisms in question belonged to the genus *Vibrio,* and the new species designation *V. parahemolyticus* was officially adopted. [42]

Volunteer-feeding experiments in Japan in the 1960s supplied further evidence of the pathogenicity of this organism.[106] Kato made the next major advance when he observed that strains isolated from ill humans caused hemolysis on Wagatsuma's blood agar, whereas strains obtained from routine food samples lacked this characteristic.[86] It was suggested that this trait correlated with pathogenicity. Indeed, this was borne out in volunteer studies, since only hemolytic strains were pathogenic in humans. This phenomenon has been termed the "Kanagawa phenomenon."

Japanese workers, using various culture media with a high salt content, showed that *V. parahemolyticus* accounts for between 50 and 70% of reported foodborne disease in Japan during the summer months.[104] The use of similar media with high salt content, employed for isolation of *V. cholerae,* revealed that *V. parahemolyticus* is widespread throughout Southeast Asia. It has also been implicated in outbreaks in the United States and Great Britain.[2,26,31,63]

7.2. Biological Characteristics of the Organism

V. parahemolyticus is a gram-negative, straight or curved rod, which is pleomorphic, halophilic, and facultatively anaerobic. These organisms are part of the genus *Vibrio,* which includes *V. cholerae* and *V. alginolyticus.* All vibrios are oxidase-positive and catalase-positive and ferment glucose without gas, and all are highly motile with a single, polar flagellum. In addition, this genus can produce acid from mannitol and has positive lysine and ornithine decarboxylase reactions but negative arginine dihydrolase activity. *V. parahemolyticus* can be differentiated from *V. cholerae* by failure to ferment sucrose, failure to agglutinate in cholera O group antiserum, organic acid fermentations, and ability to grow in high-salt medium (7.5%). *V. parahemolyticus* can be differentiated from *V. alginolyticus* by the latter's ability to ferment sucrose and tolerate higher salt concentrations and by a positive Voges–Proskauer reaction.

Antigenic studies have been carried out with *V. parahemolyticus.* There are 11 O antigens, 5 K antigens, and 1 H antigen. These serological determinants have not proven of value in epidemiological studies.

V. parahemolyticus isolates produce a number of distinct hemolysins, the most significant of which appears to be the one responsible for the "Kanagawa phenomenon." This phenomenon is named for the prefecture in Japan where it was discovered and is based on the hemolysis of human or rabbit red blood cells.[70]

Extensive studies have been undertaken in Japan to demonstrate that Kanagawa-positive isolates are pathogenic and Kanagawa-negative isolates are nonpathogenic. Of isolates from patients, 96% are Kanagawa-positive, compared to only 1% of isolates from the marine environment. Furthermore, in volunteer studies, Kanagawa-positive strains produced infection, whereas as many as 10^9 Kanagawa-negative organisms failed to do so in 15 volunteers.[106]

Apart from studies of the Kanagawa phenomenon, the evocation of pathogenic mechanisms in *V. parahemolyticus* has centered on isolation of hemolysins and evaluation of enterotoxins in several animal models.[69,137] Honda *et al.*[61,62] have characterized a soluble hemolysin as a protein of molecular weight 42,000 with an isoelectric point at pH 4.2. This toxin is lethal for mice, as little as 5 µg i.p. causing death in 1 min. Using very large quantities of concentrated hemolysin, Zen-Yoji *et al.*[149,151] have demonstrated a positive ileal-loop assay in rabbits; the quantity of toxin employed (200–500 µg) was much greater than that for *V. cholerae* enterotoxin.[61,62] Twedt and Brown[137] have reported that sterile, cell-wall preparations of Kanagawa-positive strains grown in brain–heart infusion (BHI) broth cause dilatation in rabbit ileal loops. Others have found a cytotoxic effect on HeLa cells by live *V. parahemolyticus* of both Kanagawa-positive and -negative types.[21] A Kanagawa-negative isolate from a blue crab has been found to produce an exotoxin with characteristics of an enterotoxin; i.e., it is capable of causing diarrhea when force-fed to mice, is lethal on i.p. injection into mice, and causes a positive skin permeability test in rabbit skin.[118] Since this toxin did not cause fluid accumulation in the rabbit ileal loop, there is still some question that it is an "enterotoxin."

The significance of these various toxic bacterial products in the pathogenesis of *V. parahemolyticus* gastroenteritis remains uncertain. In fact, Johnson and Calia[64] noted that broth filtrates of *V. parahemolyticus* produced positive ileal loops only when concentrated 10-fold by lyophilization; this method produces a 20% NaCl concentration, which by itself is capable of causing positive ileal loops.

Furthermore, several investigators have demonstrated an invasive ability for *V. parahemolyticus*. Calia's laboratory demonstrated bloodstream invasion of suckling rabbits following oral challenge with *V. parahemolyticus*.[19] Histological studies of rabbit ileal-loop tissue following exposure to broth cultures have shown evidence of bacterial invasion of the mucosa accompanied by severe inflammation.[107,110,146,147] Of additional interest is that in an intraduodenal dog inoculation model, variants of *V. parahemolyticus* that were Kanagawa-positive but lacked the K antigen could not produce enteritis.[104] This is reminiscent of the K88 antigen required for colonization of toxigenic *E. coli* in the intestine of pigs.[103] It is clear that more studies are required to clarify the quagmire of toxins, hemolysins, and invasive properties associated with this organism.

Antibiotic resistance has not been an important factor in transmission or pathogenesis of this organism.

7.3. Descriptive Epidemiology

7.3.1. Prevalence and Incidence. It is difficult to assess the real incidence of food poisoning due to *V. parahemolyticus* in the United States. In the four years 1983–1986, there was one outbreak affecting two individuals (see Table 1). In Japan, the incidence of *V. parahemolyticus* food poisoning comprises as much as 60% of all individuals with bacterial food poisoning. The incidence or prevalence in other parts of the world is unknown.

7.3.2. Epidemic Behavior and Contagiousness. The attack rates in epidemics reported in the United States have varied between 24 and 86% of exposed individuals and the number of affected individuals from 6 to 600.[2] There have been no secondary cases reported in either the United States or Japan, although 2 individuals with long incubation periods (96 h) may have been secondary cases in one outbreak.[3,4] The median incubation period for most outbreaks has been 13–23 h; the range has been quite variable, from 4 to 48 h (excluding the 2 cases with incubation periods of 96 h).[4]

7.3.3. Geographic and Temporal Distribution. There has been a striking association of *V. parahemolyticus* infection in the United States with coastal states. Most outbreaks have occurred in Maryland, but Massachusetts, Louisiana, New Jersey, Texas, and Washington have all reported outbreaks.[2] In addition, there have been several epidemics on cruise ships.[73]

Although most outbreaks of *V. parahemolyticus* gastroenteritis have been recorded in Japan, many other countries in Southeast Asia, as well as Australia and Great Britain, have documented this infection. The organism is ubiquitous in marine waters and can be found on the United States coastline, in Canada, Great Britain, the Netherlands, and virtually all of Southeast Asia.[5,65–67,134]

The vast majority of reported cases have occurred during the warm months (June–October).[2,104]

7.3.4. Nutritional Factors. The first outbreak reported in Japan was due to boiled sardines,[41] and all subsequent cases have been associated with saltwater fish or seawater.[104] Occasionally, salted vegetables, contaminated from salt water or a knife that had been used to prepare fish, are responsible for an outbreak. In the United States, outbreaks have been related to crabs (both steamed and processed), shrimp (both cooked and uncooked), and oysters.

7.3.5. Age, Sex, Race, Occupation, and Other Factors. There are no known associations with age, sex, race, or occupation in the epidemics thus far investigated.

7.4. Mechanisms and Routes of Transmission

There are several different ways by which food may become contaminated with a sufficient number of organisms to cause illness in humans. Seafood naturally contaminated with a small number of *V. parahemolyticus* may be kept at an improper holding temperature and become heavily contaminated. Likewise, seafood already contaminated may be cooked at an inadequate time or temperature, or both, to kill the organism. *V. parahemolyticus* has a generation time of 12 min and thus can accumulate to millions of organisms in a few hours.[65] Finally, cooked or clean seafood may be washed with contaminated salt water and become contaminated after preparation. The latter mechanism has been described in several outbreaks aboard cruise ships.[73]

The final common pathway in most outbreaks appears to be a hiatus of several hours without adequate refrigeration at an inadequate holding temperature.

7.5. Pathogenesis and Immunity

7.5.1. Pathogenesis. The exact mechanisms of pathogenesis have not been clearly defined. Reported data suggest that the minimal infective dose is approximately 10^5 organisms.[108] In addition, an inverse relationship between the size of the inoculum and the length of the incubation period has been established.[104] As described in Section 7.2, the strains of *V. parahemolyticus* recovered from infected individuals are Kanagawa-positive, whereas most but not all, isolates in the environment are Kanagawa-negative.[104] Broth cultures from diarrheal stools given to volunteers and accidental ingestion in the laboratory provide adequate evidence that the organism can be pathogenic. Strains that are Kanagawa-negative do not produce illness in volunteers even when inocula as large as 10^9 are tried.[104,109]

The role of toxins in this disease is unclear. A significant proportion of patients have fever and chills and an occasional patient has a dysenteric syndrome; these findings suggest that the organism has some invasive properties aside from toxin production. Animal studies have confirmed this hypothesis (see Section 7.2).

7.5.2. Immunity. Multiple serotypes can be isolated from a patient's stools, and frequently more than one strain is isolated from an incriminated food.[105] However, it is not known whether infection results in immunity or whether any given serotype confers immunity homologously or heterologously.

The fortuitous occurrence of three epidemics during one shipboard cruise provided evidence that immunity does not develop in a short time span.[73] In one of the epidemics, *V. parahemolyticus* infection was confirmed; the similarity of symptoms in the other two epidemics plus the incrimination of seafood as the vehicle suggested that this microorganism was involved in the other outbreaks as well, although bacteriological data were unavailable. Many passengers had multiple episodes of diarrhea; attack rates in those people ill during the first epidemic who subsequently were exposed by eating the incriminated vehicle in the second epidemic were not different from attack rates in individuals not exposed in the first outbreak. Thus, immunity apparently did not develop.

Fluorescent-antibody methods have been developed to identify circulating antibody in the blood and to identify organisms in food. These techniques show that antihemolysin titers develop in 5–10 days in very ill patients.[88] However, such assays are not generally available and have not been used extensively.

7.6. Patterns of Host Response

7.6.1. Clinical Features. There was some variation in signs and symptoms observed in eight laboratory-confirmed outbreaks in the United States (Table 4). Explosive watery diarrhea was the cardinal manifestation in over 90% of cases. Abdominal cramps, nausea, vomiting, and headache were common. Fever and chills occurred in approximately 25% of cases. Clinically, this illness resembles that produced by nontyphoidal salmonellosis. However, in one epidemic case in the United States, a bloody dysenteric syndrome was observed with fecal leukocytes and superficial ulcerations on sigmoidoscopic examination; a small percentage of cases on a recent cruise-ship outbreak also reported bloody diarrhea.[14,73]

The duration of illness has generally been mild, with a median of 3 days (range 2 h to 10 days). There have been no deaths in the 1000 cases reported in the United States. This has generally been the experience in Japan, although in the first outbreak reported by Fujino, 20 of 272 ill individuals died.[41]

The diarrhea is usually not profuse like that of *V. cholerae*. Yet, in one outbreak in Great Britain, hypotension and shock occurred in three of five cases.[99] The spectrum of disease is apparently quite varied.

As many as 7% of persons preparing seafood in the summertime may become infected.[104] Subclinical cases have been demonstrated in fewer than 1% of healthy individuals, and have not been detected in the winter, suggesting that the carrier state is probably transient. Individuals do not continue to harbor the organism in their stools once symptoms have disappeared.

V. parahemolyticus can occasionally cause wound infections. Most cases in the United States have been related to trauma associated with a marine environment. Their pathogenic significance has been difficult to assess, since these organisms have been part of a mixed bacterial flora.

There have been two reports of bloodstream infections due to *V. parahemolyticus*. Both cases were accompanied by severe systemic infection with hypotension and a disseminated rash. One patient had been clamming in New England; the other had eaten raw oysters in Florida. Recently, it has been reported that these cases were in fact not due to *V. parahemolyticus*, but were caused by lactose-positive, halophilic vibrios of a different taxonomic group.[12]

7.6.2. Diagnosis. *V. parahemolyticus* should be considered in any outbreak of diarrheal illness related to seafood occurring in the warm months. The occurrence of mild but explosive watery diarrhea with or without dysentery (bloody, mucoid stools) in association with abdominal cramps, nausea, vomiting, and headache is most characteristic. Although the clinical features and incubation period are not sufficiently distinct to allow a diagnosis, the epidemiological features should arouse one's suspicion as to causation. All the United States outbreaks have thus far been limited to coastal states, but there have been outbreaks in other parts of the world related to air travel or contaminated food.

Since the same symptoms can occur in nontyphoidal salmonellosis, this disease must be ruled out. In the very rare patient with a dysenteric-like illness, shigellosis must be included in the differential diagnosis. The occasional patient with profuse diarrhea may raise the question of cholera or toxigenic *E. coli*; appropriate laboratory techniques should be employed to make these diagnoses. One must also consider *C. perfringens* in cases where diarrhea is the predominant symptom, although this organism is associated with a shorter incubation period. It is apparent that a medical practitioner confronted with a sporadic case of diarrhea would find it most difficult to make a diagnosis on clinical grounds.

7.6.3. Laboratory Diagnosis. Rectal swabs or stool specimens should be streaked onto thiosulfate–citrate–bile salts agar (TCBS) or bromothymol blue–Teepol (BTB–Teepol) agar plates and incubated at 35–37°C for 18–24 h.[38] Recent studies have shown mannitol–salt agar to be an acceptable alternative medium.[20] Prior enrichment by briefly incubating the specimen in 1% peptone water containing 3% NaCl may increase the number of positive isolations. If transport or direct inoculation is delayed, Cary–Blair transport medium may be used.[94]

Colonies of *V. parahemolyticus* appear round, 2–3 mm in diameter, and bluish-green on any of the aforementioned media; colonies of *V. alginolyticus* are larger and yellow because of sucrose fermentation.[38]

The confirmed isolates of *V. parahemolyticus* from food, vomitus, or stool should be tested for hemolysis of human or rabbit red blood cells on Wagatsuma's agar (Kanagawa phenomenon). Since this test is delicate, appropriate controls should be employed. It is frequently very difficult to find Kanagawa-positive isolates in the incriminated food vehicle, despite the abundance of Kanagawa-positive isolates in stools of affected individuals. A positive isolation in stool is usually sufficient for bacteriological confirmation.

The value of serotyping is unclear. Frequently, many serotypes are found in the incriminated food, and different serotypes are found in the patient's stool. Immunoserological diagnosis has not been practical and is unproven.

8. *Staphylococcus aureus*

8.1. Historical Background

Although Dack modestly credited others for the discovery of staphylococcal food poisoning, he and his coworkers were the first to prove that this illness was due to toxin production by *S. aureus*.[29] They performed classic experiments in volunteers, demonstrating that culture filtrates of staphylococci isolated from a cream-filled sponge cake that had been the implicated vehicle in a foodborne outbreak could cause gastroenteritis.[28] After these reports had appeared, staphylococcal food poisoning became widely appreciated, so that today it is the second most common agent implicated in foodborne disease.

The work on the enterotoxins produced by *S. aureus* has been fundamental to our understanding of this syndrome. Dolman and Wilson[33] established that antibody to the enterotoxin could be made, and Surgalla *et al.*[126] showed 15 years later that there was more than one immunological type. Since these discoveries, Casman, Bergdoll, and others have characterized the physicochemical properties of these enterotoxins and have established that there are five types: A, B, C, D, and E.[9,22,23,89]

8.2. Biological Characteristics of the Organism

Staphylococci are members of the family Micrococcaceae, which includes the two species *S. aureus* and *S. epidermidis*. These organisms are gram-positive, nonencapsulated, nonmotile, non-spore-forming cocci that usually appear in grapelike clusters, hence the name. They are aerobic and facultatively anaerobic, may be β-hemolytic and catalase-positive, and ferment glucose. *S. aureus*, which is the usual pathogen in foodborne and other diseases, forms acid from mannitol and produces coagulase. *S. epidermidis* is rarely pathogenic and does not produce coagulase or ferment mannitol.

There are a variety of toxic substances produced by *S. aureus* that are hemolytic, leukocytic, dermonecrotic, and lethal to animals.[1] All *S. aureus*, by definition, produce a coagulase that causes coagulation of plasma; it is both free and bound to the cell wall. *S. aureus* also produces a fibrinolysin, hyaluronidase, deoxyribonuclease, and various lipases. Many of these substances are physiologically important for the other manifestations of staphylococcal infections; they are, however, beyond the scope of this chapter, and the reader is referred to more detailed reviews in the volume edited by Cohen[27] for consideration of these toxins, and to Chapter 30 of this book.

These coagulase-positive strains of staphylococci that produce an enterotoxin are the ones involved in the food-poisoning syndrome. Five immunologically distinct enterotoxins have been discovered, termed A, B, C, D, and E.[44] These enterotoxins are heat-resistant, single polypeptide chains that contain large quantities of lysine, aspartic and glutamic acids, and tyrosine. They range in molecular weight from 28,366 to 34,700.[126] The precise mechanism of action is not known; however, when tested in a rat intestinal-loop model, net transport of water and solutes occurs.[125]

The demonstration that toxic substances alone could reproduce staphylococcal poisoning was accomplished by Dack and co-workers in experiments alluded to in Section 8.1. It has been estimated that from 1 to 25 μg can cause illness in man (assuming that 100 g of contaminated food is consumed). The emetic dose for monkeys is between 5 and 10 μg.

8.3. Descriptive Epidemiology

8.3.1. Prevalence and Incidence. *S. aureus* was the second most common agent implicated in bacterial food poisoning in the years 1983–1986. There were 46 reported outbreaks affecting 3127 people. Prior to 1973, staphylococci were the most commonly recognized etiology. The median number of cases per outbreak for outbreaks between 1983 and 1986 was 68 (Table 2).

8.3.2. Epidemic Behavior and Contagiousness. Staphylococcal foodborne outbreaks are characterized by explosive onset between 1 and 6 h after consumption of a contaminated vehicle (median 3 h). Attack rates are usually quite high, since very small quantities of enterotoxin can cause illness. In outbreaks involving single families and uniform doses of enterotoxin, virtually 100% of individuals are affected.[28] Secondary cases are not of concern in this type of food poisoning.

8.3.3. Geographic Distribution. There is no geographic clustering of cases, since outbreaks are related to food contamination from human staphylococcal carriers.

8.3.4. Temporal Distribution. Outbreaks from staphylococci can occur at any time of the year, but most outbreaks are reported during the warm-weather months.

8.3.5. Age, Sex, Race, and Occupation. There are no age, sexual, racial, or occupational characteristics that are peculiar to staphylococcal food poisoning.

8.3.6. Occurrence in Different Settings. Staphylococci are carried by so many people that almost any food-preparation setting can be involved. Most reported outbreaks are from large gatherings, i.e., schools, group picnics, clubs, and restaurants.

8.3.7. Other Factors. Many different foods have been implicated in staphylococcal food poisoning. There are, however, some foods that are frequently implicated: ham, canned beef, pork, or any salted meat, and cream-filled cakes or pastries such as cream puffs. Potato and macaroni salads are occasionally involved. Foods that have a high salt content (ham) or sugar content (custard) selectively favor the growth of staphylococci.

8.4. Mechanisms and Routes of Transmission

With the exception of milk and dairy products, in which staphylococci may be present because of shedding through an infected site in the cow, the single most important source of staphylococcal contamination in foods is man. The primary habitats for *S. aureus* are the mucous membranes of the nasopharynx and skin of man and animals.

Human carriage of staphylococci varies with the population being studied. Most normal individuals outside the hospital have carriage rates of 30–50%. Once in hospitals, both patients and nursing personnel approach carriage rates of 60–70%.[145] The most frequent site of carriage is the nose, and the next most frequent site in one study was the hand.[145]

Foods that are involved in outbreaks have usually been cut, sliced, grated, mixed, or ground by workers who are carriers of enterotoxin-producing strains of staphylococci.[89] Even though many animals and animal carcasses are contaminated before processing, competitive growth from other flora usually contains the slower-growing staphylococci. Therefore, the primary mechanism of transmission is from the food handler to the food product.

8.5. Pathogenesis and Immunity

8.5.1. Pathogenesis. There are three prerequisites for staphylococcal food poisoning to occur: (1) contamination of a food with enterotoxin-producing staphylococci; (2) a food that has suitable growth requirements for the organism; and (3) appropriate time and temperature for the organism to multiply.

Once the organism has the opportunity to multiply, enterotoxin can be produced. Enterotoxin B, the most highly purified preparation, is produced during the latter part of the exponential phase of growth.[8]

Enterotoxins A, B, C, D, and E have all been implicated in outbreaks of staphylococcal food poisoning in the United States and the United Kingdom. Most implicated strains produce A or A and D.[44,60] Of 120 strains of staphylococci isolated from food-poisoning outbreaks, 113 (94%) produced enterotoxin.[44] Interestingly, 7 strains did not produce toxin; of these, 5 were tested, and all culture filtrates produced an emetic response in monkeys suggestive of another as yet unidentified toxin.[44]

In 31 outbreaks in the United Kingdom, 19 foods (of 36 tested) had detectable amounts of enterotoxin in amounts varying between 0.01 and 0.25 μg/g food.[44] The emetic dose of enterotoxin A or B for man has been estimated to be between 1 and 25 μg (assuming 100 g of food is consumed). The emetic dose in monkeys is between 5 and 10 μg.

8.5.2. Immunity. It is not clear whether immunity develops in this illness. Although attack rates are not usually 100% in outbreaks, many individuals may not consume the enterotoxin or enough of the implicated vehicle. In outbreaks where small groups are involved in which everyone consumes the implicated food, attack rates are very high (80–100%). Early attempts to "immunize" man or develop "tolerance" to toxin were not successful when broth filtrates of toxin-producing staphylococci were administered per os.[30]

Clearly, individuals have differing sensitivity to enterotoxin; in one investigation using volunteers, as little as 0.5 ml of a filtrate could cause illness in one person, whereas 13 ml administered to another individual caused no symptoms. Whether this is a case of immunity or physicochemical sensitivity of a receptor site is not clear. Whether immunity from one toxin confers cross-immunity to others has not been determined.

8.6. Patterns of Host Response

8.6.1. Clinical Features. The symptoms of staphylococcal food poisoning are primarily profuse vomiting, nausea, and abdominal cramps, often followed by diarrhea. In severe cases, blood may be observed in the vomitus or stool. Rarely, hypotension and marked prostration occur. Fatalities are unusual, and recovery is complete in 24–48 h.[144] Fever is not a common accompaniment, but may be present if dehydration is severe (Table 4).

8.6.2. Diagnosis. Staphylococcal food intoxication should be considered in anyone who presents with severe vomiting, nausea, cramps, and some diarrhea. A history of ingesting meats of high salt or protein content may be helpful. Usually, the best epidemiological clue is the short incubation period (1–7 h). Of the bacterial foodborne diseases, only *B. cereus* has a similar presenting illness with a short incubation period, of which the emetic form is so closely allied with fried rice as to allow an easy distinction.

8.6.3. Laboratory Diagnosis. The diagnosis can be confirmed by culturing the epidemiologically incriminated food, the skin or nose of the food handler, or occasionally the vomitus or stools of affected individuals. Any *S. aureus* recovered can be phage-typed to prove that the isolated strains are identical in the several samples.[1]

The medium most frequently used to isolate staphylococci is an egg yolk–tellurite–glycine–pyruvate agar. Coagulase-positive staphylococci produce a zone of clearing in egg-yolk emulsion and reduce tellurite salt to tellurium, causing the staphylococci to form black colonies. Mannitol as the sole or major source of carbon in the medium, along with a high NaCl content, can also be used in a selective medium. It should be mentioned that occasional strains of coagulase-negative staphylococci are capable of

producing enterotoxin and have been involved in food-poisoning outbreaks.[16]

Detection of staphylococcal enterotoxin is the ultimate means of making a diagnosis when this test becomes more generally available. Several methods have been developed, including immunofluorescence, hemagglutination, and gel techniques.[102] Recently, radioimmunoassay and enzyme-linked immunoassay have been developed.[111] The latter can detect nanogram quantities of enterotoxin. These tests must still be considered research tools.

9. Other Bacterial Foodborne Pathogens

Many other bacterial agents have been implicated infrequently in foodborne epidemics.

9.1. *Yersinia enterocolitica*

Y. enterocolitica is a non-lactose-fermenting, urease-producing gram-negative rod that can be distinguished from *Y. pestis* by its motility at 25°C and its urease production and from *Y. pseudotuberculosis* by its fermentation of sucrose and positive Voges–Proskauer reaction at 25°C. There are 17 serotypes and 5 biotypes[90] (see Chapter 40).

Isolates from a foodborne epidemic of gastroenteritis have been shown to produce a heat-stable, methanol-soluble enterotoxin when the organism is incubated at 25°C, but not at 37°C.[15] Furthermore, some of these same isolates were able to penetrate guinea pig conjunctival epithelium (Sereny test).[15] Interestingly, this tissue-invasive property appears to be plasmid-mediated.[152] Therefore, these strains show both invasive and toxigenic properties, yet their inability to produce toxin at 37°C questions the role toxin production plays *in vivo*. Further studies will be required to sort out the merits of these pathogenic properties.

Serological analysis has been helpful in evaluating some epidemics; however, antibodies that cross-react with *Brucella abortus* and *Y. enterocolitica*, serotype 9, and a lack of available antisera have limited the usefulness of this technique.[119]

Y. enterocolitica gastroenteritis has been reported more frequently in the Scandinavian countries than in the United States. Several epidemics related to the consumption of contaminated milk have been described in the United States and Canada.[11] The organism can be found in stream water, and it has been isolated from many animals including puppies, cows, chickens, pigs, and others. One epidemic in the United States implicated sick puppies as the source.[50]

The suspicion exists that animals, either as pets or food sources, infect humans.

A recent prospective study of gastroenteritis among children in Montreal has shown *Y. enterocolitica* to be the second most frequent bacterial pathogen (2.8% isolation rate), *Salmonella* being the most frequent pathogen isolated (4.4% of isolation rate).[79] Isolation was most frequent in the summer and fall in contrast to other reports in which *Y. enterocolitica* was isolated more frequently in the winter.[141] Secondary cases in families occurred in about 20% of exposed individuals; the risk for children was four times that for adults. Person-to-person transmission was likely, although common-source exposure could not be ruled out. No chronic carrier state was identified in these subjects; however, individuals can excrete the organism for prolonged periods of time (up to 3 months) after the cessation of diarrhea. Other studies have demonstrated asymptomatic excretors of the organism.[150] Common food or animal sources could not be identified from this study; however, the concurrent isolation of both *Y. enterocolitica* and *Salmonella* from several families does suggest an animal source.

Neither the mechanisms nor the routes of transmission for *Y. enterocolitica* are understood. The pathogenesis of this disease has undergone recent study, and there would appear to be both invasive and toxin-producing properties involved. The presence of fecal leukocytes in some patients suggests that tissue invasion is of primary importance. Furthermore, tissue invasion from *Y. enterocolitica* can be so severe as to mimic appendicitis.[142] In addition, a volunteer study has shown that a large inoculum, 3.5×10^9 organisms, is required to produce infection.[130] Toxin production may be important in the pathogenesis of the gastroenteritis, but from evidence accumulated thus far, tissue invasion would appear to be foremost.

The spectrum of clinical symptoms exhibited by *Y. enterocolitica* infection can be varied. The series from Montreal revealed that almost all cases had diarrhea as their presenting complaint (98%). Other symptoms included fever (68%), crampy abdominal pain (65%), and vomiting (39%). Other epidemiological investigations have shown that fever and severe abdominal pain are the most frequent symptoms.[11,79] The right-lower-quadrant pain may mimic appendicitis. Diarrhea was present in only about 50% of cases in this investigation. Other syndromes seen with *Y. enterocolitica* infection include Reiter's syndrome and erythema nodosum. In one outbreak, pharyngitis was present in several individuals.

The diagnosis of *Y. enterocolitica* infection should be entertained in any individual with fever, severe abdominal pain, and diarrhea. Because of the other unusual manifestations, such as Reiter's syndrome and erythema nodosum, associated with *Y. enterocolitica* infection, one must consider this entity in any patient with diarrhea and skin rash or arthritis. The differential diagnosis includes other bacterial pathogens such as *Salmonella, Shigella, Campylobacter,* and *V. parahemolyticus.* Differentiation from these can be made bacteriologically, especially with the use of the cold-enrichment technique.[98] Serological analysis has been helpful in some epidemic investigations.[49]

Most strains of *Y. enterocolitica* are susceptible *in vitro* to trimethoprim–sulfamethoxazole, ampicillin, tetracycline, chloramphenicol, and aminoglycosides; however, efficacy of these agents in the gastroenteritis syndrome remains to be demonstrated.

9.2. *Listeria monocytogenes*

Listeria is becoming increasingly recognized as a foodborne pathogen[112,113] (see Chapter 18). The organism is a gram-positive, motile rod that is relatively heat resistant. It is widely distributed in nature, found in the intestinal tract of various animals and humans, and in sewage, soil, and water.[7,113]

The syndromes usually associated with *Listeria* infection include meningitis, bacteremia, and focal metastatic disease. A complete discussion of *Listeria* may be found in Chapter 18. The organism has the propensity to affect either adults who are immunosuppressed or those who are pregnant.[7] Nosocomial outbreaks have become increasingly recognized.[56]

Contaminated cole slaw, both raw and pasteurized milk, and processed cheese have been implicated in epidemic listeriosis.[39,56,112] The sources for sporadic infections are less well understood.

9.3. Arizona

The organism Arizona is a motile, gram-negative rod closely related to *Salmonella.* It has been implicated in outbreaks of gastroenteritis and enteric fever. Vehicles include contaminated eggs or poultry. Because of similarities to *Salmonella,* contaminated animal products should be considered the usual vehicle.

The symptoms of Arizona infection are also similar to those of salmonellosis. Gastroenteritis, enteric fever, bacteremia, and localized infection have been described. Usually 24–48 h after ingestion of a contaminated food, symptoms develop. Fever, headache, nausea, vomiting, abdominal pain, and watery diarrhea may occur. Marked prostration may develop and symptoms may persist for several days. Prevention and therapy are similar to those methods found useful for salmonellosis.

10. Control and Prevention

10.1. General Concepts

The common theme that ties all foodborne illnesses together is the presence of an improper food-handling procedure prior to food consumption.

In a review of those factors responsible for foodborne outbreaks in the United States over a 15-year period, Bryan has shown that inadequate refrigeration is the single most frequent factor implicated in foodborne outbreaks (Table 5). Usually, more than one factor is associated with an outbreak, so that inadequate refrigeration, advance preparation of food without adequate storage, and improper reheating or cooling are usually present to one degree or another. To a lesser degree, contaminated equipment, cross-contamination, and food-preparation personnel with poor personal hygiene may contribute to outbreaks. Contaminated raw ingredients are frequently part of the process as well. The ubiquity of *B. cereus* and *C. perfringens* makes it mandatory that food be cooked properly and, when stored, cooled properly. The same can be said for *V. parahemolyticus*, since this organism is present in many seafoods; the mishandling of these foods is what usually enables the organism to multiply to the level of pathogenic contamination. The failure to refrigerate food properly is the major problem in staphylococcal disease, the only difference being the con-

tamination of the food by a carrier at some point prior to service.[17] It becomes obvious that control must be based on inhibiting bacterial growth, preventing contamination after preparation, and killing potential pathogens with cooking. In general, foods should be heated to internal temperatures of 165°F, but lower temperatures for longer periods of time may be equally effective. Once cooked or processed, foods must be kept at temperatures of 40°F or below.

Although these control measures are standard, many places where food preparation takes place do not abide by these guidelines. It is through diligent efforts by public-health officials that reported outbreaks are investigated and food-preparation techniques corrected. Therefore, recognition and reporting of foodborne illness become instrumental to the control of the problem. Education of the public, nurses, physicians, and eating establishments is crucial to the control of foodborne illness. Carriage of most of the organisms considered in this chapter is not a problem, with the exception of staphylococci. Since staphylococcal carriage is a necessary step to the development of staphylococcal foodborne illness, education of food handlers to watch for boils and pustules should be emphasized.

10.2. Antibiotics and Chemotherapeutics

Since these illnesses are self-limited and for the most part toxin-mediated, antibiotics play no role in either therapy or prophylaxis. Fluid replacement is the major consideration in all these illnesses.

10.3. Immunization

In general, immunization has not been attempted in these diseases. The immunogenicity of many of the toxins described has not been totally defined, and the populations at risk are so vast that immunization may not be practical. A recent interesting report using a clostridial toxoid prepared from type C cultures in New Guinea suggests the prevention of "pig-bel" in children.[74] However, that study suffers from inadequate case definition that is reflected in the control group, where the mortality was less than 1%. Thus, the disease process studied by these investigators was not the classic pig-bel syndrome and remains to be confirmed.

11. Unresolved Problems

The largest unresolved problem in this group of illnesses is determining the pathogens that make up the other

Table 5. Factors That Contributed to Foodborne Disease Outbreaks in the United States from 1961 to 1976[a]

Factor	Implicated (percent)[b]
Inadequate refrigeration	47
Food prepared too far in advance of service	21
Infected person with poor personal hygiene	21
Inadequate cooking	16
Inadequate holding temperature	16
Inadequate reheating	12
Contaminated raw ingredient	11
Cross-contamination	7
Dirty equipment	7

[a]From Bryan.[17]
[b]Percentages total more than 100% because more than one factor may contribute to a foodborne outbreak.

70% of presumed bacterial foodborne disease. Granting that some of these outbreaks may be due to the known pathogens, there are surely other pathogens awaiting recognition. The recent recognition of *Y. enterocolitica* and *Campylobacter fetus* attests to the vast array of pathogens awaiting discovery.

Another serious problem is underreporting. An increased awareness of foodborne illness and recognition of outbreaks is necessary to eliminate many of the food-processing problems.

With regard to the pathogens specified in this chapter, many unresolved problems have been cited. One may well ask about staphylococcal disease: Are there other toxins involved? What role does immunity play? What is the physiological basis for toxin action? Is toxin production plasmid-mediated, as some have suggested, or chromosomally mediated?

V. parahemolyticus still involves many unanswered questions. Most health departments and physicians have no understanding of the disease, and therefore its true incidence is not known. The mechanism of pathogenicity remains to be resolved, as well as the relationship of these pathogenic mechanisms to the "Kanagawa phenomenon."

B. cereus is another newcomer with two or more presumptive toxins that need to be more clearly defined. Since its recognition in the United States has been almost nil, the public-health importance of this organism must be assessed. Again, basic physiological mechanisms involved in the pathogenesis should be defined and the suggested role of phage- or plasmid-mediated toxigenesis explored.

The complex toxins of *C. perfringens* remain to be explored. Recent work has focused on the potential for plasmid-mediated toxin production in this species. Inherent in the understanding of all the mechanisms of action in these pathogens is the hope that these tools will provide easier diagnostic tools that are readily applicable. Furthermore, the potential for vaccines against these toxins exists, since most have been shown to be immunogenic.

12. References

1. ANGELOTTI, R., Staphylococcal intoxications, in: *Foodborne Infections and Intoxications* (H. REIMANN, ed.), pp. 359–393, Academic Press, New York, 1969.
2. BARKER, W. H., JR., *Vibrio parahaemolyticus* outbreaks in the United States, *Lancet* 1:551–554 (1974).
3. BARKER, W. H., JR., AND GANGAROSA, E. J., Food poisoning due to *Vibrio parahaemolyticus, Annu. Rev. Med.* 25:75–81 (1974).
4. BARKER, W. H. JR., MACKOWIAK, P. A., FISHBEIN, M., MORRIS, G. K., D'ALFONSO, J. A., HAUSER, G. H., AND FELSENFELD, O., *Vibrio parahaemolyticus* gastroenteritis outbreak in Covington, Louisiana in August, 1972, *Am. J. Epidemiol.* 100:316–323 (1974).
5. BARROW, G. I., AND MILLER, D. C., *Vibrio parahaemolyticus:* A potential pathogen from marine sources in Britain, *Lancet* 1:485–486 (1972).
6. BARTHOLOMEW, B. A., STRINGER, M. F., WATSON, G. N., AND GILBERT, R. J., Development and application of an enzyme linked immunosorbent assay for *Clostridium perfringens* type A enterotoxin, *J. Clin. Pathol.* 38:222–228 (1985).
7. BARZA, M., Listeriosis and milk, *N. Engl. J. Med.* 312:438–440 (1985).
8. BERGDOLL, M. S., BORJA, C. R., AND AVENA, R. M., Identification of a new enterotoxin as enterotoxin C, *J. Bacteriol.* 90:1481–1485 (1965).
9. BERGDOLL, M. S., CZOP, J. K., AND GOULD, S. S., Enterotoxin synthesis by the staphylococci, *Ann. N.Y. Acad. Sci.* 236:307–316 (1974).
10. BLACK, R. E., COX, R. C., AND HOROWITZ, M. A., Outbreaks of foodborne disease in the United States, 1975, *J. Infect. Dis.* 137:213–218 (1978).
11. BLACK, R. E., JACKSON, R. J., TSAI, T., MEDVESKY, M., SHAYEGANI, M., FEELEY, J. C., MACLEOD, K. I. E., AND WAKELEE, A. M., Epidemic *Yersinia enterocolitica* infection due to contaminated chocolate milk, *N. Engl. J. Med.* 298:76–79 (1978).
12. BLAKE, P. A., MERSON, M. H., WEAVER, R. E., HOLLIS, D. G., AND HEUBLEIN, P. C., Disease caused by a marine vibrio, clinical characteristics and epidemiology, *N. Engl. J. Med.* 300:1–5 (1979).
13. BODNAR, S., Über durch *Bacillus cereus* verursachte Lebensmittelvergiftungen, *Z. Gesamte Hyg.* 8:368–372 (1962).
14. BOLEN, J. L., ZAMISKA, S. A., AND GREENOUGH, W. B., III, Clinical features in enteritis due to *Vibrio parahaemolyticus, Am. J. Med.* 57:638–642 (1974).
15. BOYCE, J. M., EVANS, D. J., JR., EVANS, D. G., AND DU-PONT, H. L., Production of heat-stable, methanolsoluble enterotoxin by *Yersinia enterocolitica, Infect. Immun.* 25:532–537 (1979).
16. BRECKINRIDGE, J. C., AND BERGDOLL, M. S., Outbreak of foodborne gastroenteritis due to a coagulase-negative enterotoxin-producing staphylococcus, *N. Engl. J. Med.* 284:541–543 (1971).
17. BRYAN, F. L., Emerging foodborne diseases, *J. Milk Food Technol.* 35:618–625 (1972).
18. BRYAN, F. L., Epidemiology of foodborne diseases, in: *Foodborne Infections and Intoxications* (H. REIMANN AND F. L. BRYAN, eds.), pp. 3–69, Academic Press, New York, 1979.

19. CALIA, F. M., AND JOHNSON, D. E., Bacteremia in suckling rabbits after oral challenge with *Vibrio parahaemolyticus, Infect. Immun.* **11**:1222–1225 (1975).

20. CARRUTHERS, M. M., Cytotoxicity of *Vibrio parahaemolyticus* in HeLa cell culture, *J. Infect. Dis.* **132**:555–560 (1975).

21. CARRUTHERS, M. M., AND KABAT, W. J., Isolation of *Vibrio parahaemolyticus* from fecal specimens on mannitol salt agar, *J. Clin. Microbiol.* **4**:175–179 (1976).

22. CASMAN, E. P., AND BENNETT, R. W., Detection of staphylococcal enterotoxin in food, *Appl. Microbiol.* **13**:181–189 (1965).

23. CASMAN, E. P., BENNETT, R. W., DORSEY, A. E., AND ISSA, J. A., Identification of a fourth staphylococcal enterotoxin, enterotoxin D, *J. Bacteriol.* **94**:1875–1882 (1967).

24. Centers for Disease Control, *Foodborne Surveillance,* 1982 (issued September 1985).

25. Centers for Disease Control, *Foodborne Disease Outbreaks 1983–1986* (personal communication).

26. CHATTERJEE, B. D., NEOGY, K. N., AND GORBACH, S. L., Study of *Vibrio parahaemolyticus* from cases of diarrhoea in Calcutta, *Indian J. Med. Res.* **58**:234–238 (1970).

27. COHEN, J. V. (ed.), *The Staphylococci,* Wiley–Interscience, New York, 1972.

28. DACK, G. M., Staphylococcus food poisoning, in: *Food Poisoning* (G. M. DACK, ed.), pp. 109–158, University of Chicago Press, Chicago, 1956.

29. DACK, G. M., CARY, W. E., WOOLPERT, O., AND WIGGERS, H., An outbreak of food poisoning proved to be due to a yellow hemolytic Staphylococcus, *J. Prev. Med.* **4**:167–175 (1930).

30. DACK, G. M., JORDAN, E. O., AND WOOLPERT, O., Attempts to immunize human volunteers with Staphylococcus filtrates that are toxic to man when swallowed, *J. Prev. Med.* **5**:151–159 (1931).

31. DADISMAN, T. A., JR., NELSON, R., MOLENDA, J. R., AND GARBER, H. J., *Vibrio parahaemolyticus* gastroenteritis in Maryland. I. Clinical and epidemiologic aspects, *Am. J. Epidemiol.* **96**:414–426 (1973).

32. DISCHE, F. E., AND ELEK, S. D., Experimental food-poisoning by *Clostridium welchii, Lancet* **2**:71–74 (1957).

33. DOLMAN, C. E., AND WILSON, R. J., Experiments with staphylococcal enterotoxin, *J. Immunol.* **35**:13–30 (1938).

34. DOWELL, V. R., JR., TORRES-ANJEL, M. J., RIEMANN, H. P., MERSON, M., WHALEY, D., AND DARLAND, G., A new criterion for implicating *Clostridium perfringens* as the cause of food poisoning, *Rev. Latinoam. Microbiol.* **17**:137–142 (1975).

35. DUNCAN, C. L., Time of enterotoxin formation and release during sporulation of *Clostridium perfringens* type A, *J. Bacteriol.* **113**:932–936 (1973).

36. DUNCAN, C. L., AND STRONG, D. H., *Clostridium perfringens* type A food poisoning. I. Response of the rabbit ileum as an indication of enteropathogenicity of strains of *Clostridium perfringens* in monkeys, *Infect. Immun.* **3**:167–170 (1971).

37. Epidemiology: Food poisoning associated with *Bacillus cereus, Br. Med. J.* **1**:189 (1972).

38. FEELEY, J. C., AND BALOWS, A., Vibrio, in: *Manual of Clinical Microbiology* (E. H. LENNETTE, E. H. SPAULDING, AND J. P. TRUANT, eds.), pp. 238–245, American Society for Microbiology, Washington, D.C., 1974.

39. FLEMING, D. W., COCHIS, L., MacDONALD, K. L., BRONDUM, J., HAYES, P. S., PLIKAYTIS, B. D., HOLMES, M. B., AUDURIER, A., BROOME, C. V., AND REINGOLD, L., Pasteurized milk as a vehicle of infection in an outbreak of listeriosis, *N. Engl. J. Med.* **312**:404–407 (1985).

40. FUJINO, T., Discovery of *Vibrio parahaemolyticus,* in: *International Symposium on Vibrio parahaemolyticus* (T. FUJINO, G. SAKAGUCHI, R. SAKAZAKI, AND Y. TAKEDA, eds.), pp. 1–4, Saikon, Tokyo, 1974.

41. FUJINO, T., OKUNO, Y., NAHADA, D., AOYAMA, A., FUKAI, K., MUKAI, T., AND UENO, T., On the bacteriological examination of Shirasu-food poisoning, *Med. J. Osaka Univ.* **4**:299–304 (1953).

42. FUJINO, T., SAKAZAKI, R., AND TAMURA, K., Designation of the type strain of *Vibrio parahaemolyticus* and description of 200 strains of the species, *Int. J. Syst. Bacteriol.* **24**:447–499 (1974).

43. GENIGEORGIS, C., AND RIEMANN, H., *Clostridium perfringens* toxicity, Paper presented to the 6th International Symposium of the World Association of Veterinary Food Hygienists, Elsinor, Denmark, August 1973.

44. GILBERT, R. J., Staphylococcal food poisoning and botulism, *Postgrad. Med. J.* **50**:603–611 (1974).

45. GILBERT, R. J., AND PARRY, J. M., Serotypes of *Bacillus cereus* from outbreaks of food poisoning and from routine foods, *J. Hyg.* **78**:69–74 (1977).

46. GILBERT, R. J., STRINGER, M. F., AND PEACE, T. C., The survival and growth of *Bacillus cereus* in boiled and fried rice in relation to outbreaks of food poisoning, *J. Hyg.* **73**:433–444 (1974).

47. GOEPFERT, J. M., SPIRA, W. M., AND KIM, H. U., *Bacillus cereus:* Food poisoning organism: A review, *J. Milk Food Technol.* **35**:213–227 (1972).

48. GRAVITS, L., AND GILMORE, J. D., Project I-756, Report No. 2, Naval Medical Research Institute, Bethesda (1946).

49. GUERRANT, R. L., LAHITA, R. G., WINN, W. C., AND ROBERTS, R. B., Campylobacteriosis in man: Pathogenic mechanisms and review of 91 bloodstream infections, *Am. J. Med.* **65**:584–592 (1978).

50. GUTMAN, L. T., OTTESEN, E. A., QUAN, T. J., NOCE, P. S., AND KATZ, S. L., An inter-familial outbreak of *Yersinia enterocolitica* enteritis, *N. Engl. J. Med.* **288**:1372–1377 (1973).

51. HALL, H. E., AND HAUSER, G. H., Examination of feces from food handlers for Salmonellae, Shigellae, enteropathogenic *Escherichia coli,* and *Clostridium perfringens, Appl. Microbiol.* **14**:928–933 (1966).

52. HAUGE, S., Food poisoning caused by aerobic spore-forming bacilli, *J. Appl. Bacteriol.* **18**:591–595 (1955).

53. HAUSCHILD, A. H. W., Food poisoning by *Clostridium perfringens, Can. Inst. Food Sci. Technol. J.* **6:**106–110 (1973).

54. HAUSCHILD, A. H. W., Criteria and procedures for implicating *Clostridium perfringens* in foodborne outbreaks, *Can. J. Public Health* **66:**388–392 (1975).

55. HAUSCHILD, A. H. W., AND HILSHEIMER, R., Evaluation and modifications of media for enumeration of *Clostridium perfringens, Appl. Microbiol.* **27:**78–82 (1974).

56. HO, J. L., SHANDS, K. N., FRIEDLAND, G., ECKIND, P., AND FRASER, D. W., A multi-hospital outbreak of type 4b *Listeria monocytogenes* infections, *Arch. Intern. Med.* **146:**520–524 (1986).

57. HOBBS, B. C., *Clostridium perfringens* and *Bacillus cereus* infections, in: *Foodborne Infections and Intoxications* (H. REIMANN, ed.), pp. 131–171, Academic Press, New York, 1969.

58. HOBBS, B. C., *Clostridium welchii* and *Bacillus cereus* infection and intoxication, *Postgrad. Med. J.* **50:**597–602 (1974).

59. HOBBS, B. C., SMITH, M. E., OAKLEY, C. L., WARRACK, G. H., AND CRUICKSHANK, J. C., *Clostridium welchii* food poisoning, *J. Hyg.* **51:**75–101 (1953).

60. HOLMBERG, S. D., AND BLAKE, P. A., Staphylococcal food poisoning in the United States. New facts and old misconceptions, *J. Am. Med. Assoc.* **25:**487–489 (1984).

61. HONDA, T., GOSHIMA, K., TAKEDA, Y., SUGINO, Y., AND MIWATANI, T., Demonstration of the cardiotoxicity of the thermostable direct hemolysin (lethal toxin) produced by *Vibrio parahaemolyticus, Infect. Immun.* **13:**163–171 (1976).

62. HONDA, T., TAGA, S., TAKEDA, T., HASIBUA, M. A., TAKEDA, Y., AND MIWATANI, T., Identification of a lethal toxin with the thermostable direct hemolysin produced by *Vibrio parahaemolyticus* and some physicochemical properties of the purified toxin, *Infect. Immun.* **13:**133–139 (1976).

63. HOOPER, W. L., BARROW, G. I., AND MCNAB, D. J. N., *Vibrio parahaemolyticus* food poisoning in Britain, *Lancet* **1:**1100–1102 (1974).

64. JOHNSON, D. E., AND CALIA, F. M., False-positive rabbit ileal loop reactions attributed to *Vibrio parahaemolyticus* broth filtrates, *J. Infect. Dis.* **133:**436–440 (1976).

65. JOHNSON, H. C., BARROSS, J. A., AND LISTON, J., *Vibrio parahaemolyticus* and its importance in seafood hygiene, *J. Am. Vet. Med. Assoc.* **159:**1470–1473 (1971).

66. KAMPELMACHER, E. H., VAN NOORLE JANSEN, L. M., MOSSEL, D. A. A., AND GROEN, F. J., A survey of the occurrence of *Vibrio parahaemolyticus* and *V. alginolyticus* on mussels and oysters and in estuarine waters in the Netherlands, *J. Appl. Bacteriol.* **35:**431–438 (1972).

67. KANEKO, T., AND COLWELL, R. R., Ecology of *Vibrio parahaemolyticus* in Chesapeake Bay, *J. Bacteriol.* **113:**24–32 (1973).

68. KARMALI, M. A., AND FLEMING, P. C., *Campylobacter* enteritis in children, *J. Pediatr.* **94:**527–533 (1979).

69. KASAI, G. J., Studies on the pathogenicity of *Vibrio parahaemolyticus, Southeast Asian J. Trop. Med. Public Health* **2:**168–173 (1971).

70. KATO, T., OBARA, Y., ICHINOSE, H., YAMAI, S., NAGASHIMA, K., AND SAKAZAKI, R., Hemolytic activity and toxicity of *Vibrio parahaemolyticus, Jpn. J. Bacteriol.* **21:**442–443 (1966).

71. KIM, H. U., AND GOEPFERT, J. M., Occurrence of *Bacillus cereus* in selected dry food products, *J. Milk Food Technol.* **34:**12–15 (1971).

72. KNOX, K., AND MACDONALD, E. K., Outbreak of food poisoning in certain Leicester institutions, *Med. Off.* **69:**21–24 (1943).

73. LAWRENCE, D. N., BLAKE, P. A., YASHUK, J. C., WELLS, J. G., CREECH, W. B., AND HUGHES, J. H., *Vibrio parahaemolyticus* gastroenteritis outbreaks aboard two cruise ships, *Am. J. Epidemiol.* **109:**71–80 (1979).

74. LAWRENCE, G., SHANN, F., FREESTONE, D. S., AND WALKER, P. D., Prevention of necrotising enteritis in Papua New Guinea by active immunization, *Lancet* **1:**227–229 (1979).

75. LOEWENSTEIN, M. S., Epidemiology of *Clostridium perfringens* food poisoning, *N. Engl. J. Med.* **286:**1026–1028 (1972).

76. LUBENAU, C., *Bacillus peptonificans* als Erreger einer Gastroenteritis-Epidemic, *Zentralbl. Bakteriol. Parasitenkd. Infektionskr. Hyg. Abt. 1 Orig.* **40:**433–437 (1906).

77. MACLENNAN, J. D., The histotoxic clostridial infections of man, *Bacteriol. Rev.* **26:**177–276 (1962).

78. MAHONEY, D. E., AND SWANTEE, C. A., Bacteriocin typing of *Clostridium perfringens* in human feces, *J. Clin. Microbiol.* **7:**307–309 (1978).

79. MARKS, M. I., PAI, C. H., LAFLEUR, L., LACKMAN, L., AND HAMMERBERG, O., *Yersinia enterocolitica* gastroenteritis: A prospective study of clinical, bacteriologic, and epidemiologic features, *J. Pediatr.* **96:**26–31 (1980).

80. MCCLANE, B. A., AND SNYDER, J. T., Development and preliminary slide latex agglutination assay for detection of *Clostridium perfringens* type A enterotoxin, *J. Immunol. Methods* **100:**731–736 (1987).

81. MCCLUNG, L. S., Human food poisoning due to growth of *Clostridium perfringens* (*Cl. welchii*) in freshly cooked chicken: A preliminary note, *J. Bacteriol.* **50:**229–233 (1945).

82. MCDONEL, J. L., *In vivo* effects of *Clostridium perfringens* enteropathogenic factors on the rat ileum, *Infect. Immun.* **10:**1156–1162 (1974).

83. MCDONEL, J. L., AND DUNCAN, C. L., Regional localization of activity of *Clostridium perfringens* type A enterotoxin in the rabbit ileum, jejunum, and duodenum, *J. Infect. Dis.* **136:**661–666 (1977).

84. MCKILLOP, E. J., Bacterial contamination of hospital food with special reference to *Clostridium welchii* food poisoning, *J. Hyg.* **57:**31–46 (1959).

85. MELLING, J., CAPEL, B. J., TURNBULL, P. C. B., AND GILBERT, R. J., Identification of a novel enterotoxigenic activity associated with *Bacillus cereus, J. Clin. Pathol.* **29:**938–940 (1976).

86. MIYAMOTO, Y., KATO, T., OBARA, Y., AKIYAMA, S., TAK-

IZAWA, K., AND YAMAI, S., *In vitro* hemolytic characteristic of *Vibrio parahaemolyticus:* Its close correlation with human pathogenicity, *J. Bacteriol.* **100:**1147–1149 (1969).

87. MIDURA, T., GERBER, M., WOOD, R., AND LEONARD, A. R., Outbreak of food poisoning caused by *Bacillus cereus, Public Health Rep.* **85:**45–48 (1970).

88. MINATANI, T., AND TAKEDA, Y., Clinical features of food poisoning due to *Vibrio parahaemolyticus,* in: *Vibrio parahaemolyticus: A Causative Bacterium of Food Poisoning,* pp. 104–109, Saikon, Tokyo, 1976.

89. MINOR, T. E., AND MARCH, E. H., *Staphylococcus aureus* and staphylococcal food poisoning, *J. Milk Food Technol.* **34:**21–29, 77–83, 227–241 (1972); **35:**447–476 (1973).

90. MORRIS, G. K., AND FEELEY, J. C., *Yersinia enterocolitica:* A review of its role in food hygiene, *Bull. WHO* **54:**79–85 (1976).

91. MORTIMER, P. R., AND MCCANN, G., Food poisoning episodes associated with *Bacillus cereus* in fried rice, *Lancet* **1:**1043–1045 (1974).

92. MURRELL, T. G. C., EGERTON, J. R., RAMPLING, A., SAMELS, J., AND WALKER, P. D., The ecology and epidemiology of the pig-bel syndrome in man in New Guinea, *J. Hyg.* **64:**375–396 (1966).

93. NAIK, H. S., AND DUNCAN, C. L., Detection of *Clostridium perfringens* enterotoxin in human fecal samples and antienterotoxin in sera, *J. Clin. Microbiol.* **7:**337–340 (1978).

94. NEUMANN, D. A., BENENSON, M. W., HUBSTER, E., AND THI NHU TUAN, N., Cary–Blair, a transport medium for *Vibrio parahaemolyticus, Am. J. Clin. Pathol.* **57:**33–34 (1972).

95. NIKODEMUSZ, I., *Bacillus cereus* als Ursache von Lebensmittel Vergiftungen, *Z. Hyg.* **145:**335–338 (1958).

96. NIKODEMUSZ, I., Die Atiologie der Lebensmittelvergiftungen in Ungarn in der Jahren 1960 bis 1966, *Z. Hyg.* **155:**204–208 (1968).

97. NIKODEMUSZ, I., AND CZABA, K., Die Bedeutung der aeroben Sporenbildnes bei Lebensmittelvergiftungen, *Z. Hyg.* **146:**156–160 (1959).

98. PAI, C. H., SORGER, S., LAFLEUR, L., LACKMAN, L., AND MARKS, M. L., Efficacy of cold enrichment techniques for recovery of *Yersinia enterocolitica* from human stools, *J. Clin. Microbiol.* **9:**712–715 (1979).

99. PEFFERS, A. S. R., BAILEY, J., BARROW, G. I., AND HOBBS, B. C., *Vibrio parahaemolyticus* gastroenteritis and international air travel, *Lancet* **1:**143–145 (1973).

100. PORTNOY, B. L., GOEPFERT, J. M., AND HARMON, S. M., An outbreak of *Bacillus cereus* food poisoning resulting from contaminated vegetable sprouts, *Am. J. Epidemiol.* **103:**589–594 (1976).

101. RAEVUORI, M., KIUTAMO, T., AND NISKANEN, A., Comparative studies of *Bacillus cereus* strains isolated from various foods and food poisoning outbreaks, *Acta Vet. Scand.* **18:**397–407 (1977).

102. REISER, R., CONAWAY, D., AND BERGDOLL, M. S., Detection of staphylococcal enterotoxin in foods, *Appl. Microbiol.* **27:**83–85 (1974).

103. SACK, R. B., Human diarrheal disease caused by enterotoxigenic *Escherichia coli, Annu. Rev. Microbiol.* **29:**333–353 (1975).

104. SAKAZAKI, R., Halophilic vibrio infections, in: *Foodborne Infections and Intoxications* (H. REIMANN, ed.), pp. 115–119, Academic Press, New York, 1969.

105. SAKAZAKI, R., IWANAMI, S., AND TAMURA, K., Studies on the enteropathogenic, facultatively halophilic bacteria, *Vibrio parahaemolyticus.* II. Serological characteristics, *Jpn. J. Med. Sci. Biol.* **21:**313–324 (1968).

106. SAKAZAKI, R., TAMURA, K., KATO, T., OBARA, Y., YAMAI, S., AND HOBO, K., Studies on the enteropathogenic facultatively halophilic bacteria, *Vibrio parahaemolyticus.* III. Enteropathogenicity, *Jpn. J. Med. Sci. Biol.* **21:**325–331 (1968).

107. SAKAZAKI, R., TAMURA, R. S., KURATA, A. N., GOHDA, A., AND KAZUNO, Y., Enteropathogenic activity of *Vibrio parahaemolyticus,* in: *International Symposium on Vibrio parahaemolyticus* (T. FUJINO, G. SAKAGUCHI, R. SAKAZAKI, AND Y. TAKEDA, eds.), pp. 231–235, Saikon, Tokyo, 1974.

108. SANYAL, S. C., AND SEN, P. C., Human volunteer study on the pathogenicity of *Vibrio parahaemolyticus,* in: *International Symposium on Vibrio parahaemolyticus* (T. FUJINO, G. SAKAGUCHI, R. SAKAZAKI, AND Y. TAKEDA, eds.), pp. 227–230, Saikon, Tokyo, 1974.

109. SANYAL, S., SIL, J., AND SAKAZAKI, R., Laboratory infection by *Vibrio parahaemolyticus, J. Med. Microbiol.* **6:**121–122 (1973).

110. SASAKI, S., GHODA, A., AND YAHAGI, H., Early features of infection in ligated loops of the rabbit small intestine inoculated with *Shigella flexneri* 3a, enteropathogenic *E. coli, Escherichia coli* and *Vibrio parahaemolyticus,* The first report: Variation of bacterial population size in ligated loops after inoculation, *Keio J. Med.* **16:**101–117 (1967).

111. SAUNDERS, G. C., AND BARTLETT, M. L., Double-antibody solid-phase enzyme immunoassay for the detection of staphylococcal enterotoxin A, *Appl. Environ. Microbiol.* **34:**518–522 (1977).

112. SCH'.ECH, W. F., III, New perspectives on the gastrointestinal mode of transmission of invasive *Listeria monocytogenes* infection, *J. Clin. Invest Med.* **7:**321–324 (1984).

113. SCHLECH, W. F., III, LAVIGNE, P. M., BORTOLUSSI, R. A., ALLEN, A. C., HALDANE, E. V., WORT, A. J., HIGHTOWER, A. W., JOHNSON, S. E., KING, S., NICHOLLS, E. S., AND BROOME, C. V., Epidemic listeriosis—Evidence for transmission by food, *N. Engl. J. Med.* **308:**203–206 (1983).

114. SCHMITT, N., BOWMER, E. J., AND WILLOUGHBY, B. A., Food poisoning outbreak attributed to *Bacillus cereus, Can. J. Public Health* **67:**418–422 (1976).

115. SKJELKVÅLE, R., AND DUNCAN, C. L., Enterotoxin formation by different toxigenic types of *Clostridium perfringens, Infect. Immun.* **11:**563–575 (1975).

116. SKJELKVÅLE, R., AND DUNCAN, C. L., Characterization of

enterotoxin purified from *Clostridium perfringens* type C, *Infect. Immun.* **11:**1061–1068 (1975).

117. SKJELKVÅLE, R., AND UEMURA, T., Experimental diarrhoea in human volunteers following oral administration of *Clostridium perfringens* enterotoxin, *J. Appl. Bacteriol.* **43:**281–286 (1977).

118. SOCHARD, M. R., AND COLWELL, R. R., Toxin isolation from a Kanagawa-phenomenon negative strain of *Vibrio parahaemolyticus, Microbiol. Immunol.* **21:**243–254 (1977).

119. SONNENWIRTH, A. C., *Yersinia,* in: *Manual of Clinical Microbiology* (E. H. LENNETTE, E. H. SPAULDING, AND J. P. TRUANT, eds.), pp. 238–245, American Society for Microbiology, Washington, D.C., 1974.

120. SPIRA, W. M., AND GOEPFERT, J. M., Biological characteristics of an enterotoxin produced by *Bacillus cereus, Can. J. Microbiol.* **21:**1236–1246 (1975).

121. STARK, R. L., AND DUNCAN, C. L., Biological characteristics of *Clostridium perfringens* Type A enterotoxin, *Infect. Immun.* **4:**89–96 (1971).

122. STEELE, T. W., AND MCDERMOTT, S., Campylobacter enteritis in South Australia, *Med. J. Aust.* **2:**404–406 (1978).

123. STRONG, D. H., CANADA, J. C., AND GRIFFITHS, B. B., Incidence of *Clostridium perfringens* in American food, *Appl. Microbiol.* **11:**42–44 (1963).

124. STRONG, D. H., DUNCAN, C. L., AND PERNA, G., *Clostridium perfringens* type A food poisoning, *Infect. Immun.* **3:**171–178 (1971).

125. SULLIVAN, R., AND ASANO, T., Effects of staphylococcal enterotoxin B on intestinal transport in the rat, *Am. J. Physiol.* **222:**1793–1799 (1971).

126. SURGALLA, M. J., BERGDOLL, M. S., AND DACK, G. M., Use of antigen–antibody reaction in agar to follow the progress of fractionation of antigenic mixtures: Application to purification of staphylococcal enterotoxin, *J. Immunol.* **72:**398–402 (1954).

127. SUTTON, R. G. A., AND HOBBS, B. C., Food poisoning caused by heat-sensitive *Clostridium welchii:* A report of five recent outbreaks, *J. Hyg.* **66:**135–146 (1965).

128. SUTTON, R. G. A., AND HOBBS, B. C., Resistance of vegetative cells of *Clostridium welchii* to low pH, *J. Med. Microbiol.* **4:**529–543 (1971).

129. SUTTON, R. G. A., KENDALL, M., AND HOBBS, B. C., The effect of two methods of cooking and cooling on *Clostridium welchii* and other bacteria in meat, *J. Hyg.* **70:**415–424 (1972).

130. SZITA, J., KALI, M., AND REDEY, B., Incidence of *Yersinia enterocolitica* infection in Hungary: Observations on the laboratory diagnosis of yersiniosis, in: *Contributions to Microbiology and Immunology,* Vol. 2, *Yersinia, Pasteurella and Francisella* (S. WINBLAD, ed.), pp. 106–110, Karger, Basel, 1973.

131. TAYLOR, A. J., AND GILBERT, R. J., *Bacillus cereus* food poisoning: A provisional serotyping scheme, *J. Med. Microbiol.* **8:**543–550 (1975).

132. TERRANOVA, W., AND BLAKE, P. A., *Bacillus cereus* food poisoning, *N. Engl. J. Med.* **298:**143–144 (1978).

133. THOMAS, M., NOAH, N. D., MALE, G. E., STRINGER, M. F., KENDALL, M., GILBERT, R. J., JONES, P. H., AND PHILLIPS, K. D., Hospital outbreak of *Clostridium perfringens* food poisoning, *Lancet* **1:**1046–1048 (1977).

134. THOMSON, W. K., AND TRENHOLM, D. A., The isolation of *Vibrio parahaemolyticus* and related halophilic bacteria from Canadian Atlantic shellfish, *Can. J. Microbiol.* **17:**545–549 (1970).

135. TURNBULL, P. C. B., Studies on the production of enterotoxins by *Bacillus cereus, J. Clin. Pathol.* **29:**941–948 (1976).

136. TURNBULL, P. C. B., NOTTINGHAM, J. F., AND GHOSH, A. C., A severe necrotic enterotoxin produced by certain food, food poisoning and other clinical isolates of *Bacillus cereus, Br. J. Exp. Pathol.* **58:**273–280 (1977).

137. TWEDT, R. M., AND BROWN, D. F., Toxicity of *Vibrio parahaemolyticus,* in: *Microbiology 1974* (D. SCHLESSINGER, ed.), pp. 241–245, American Society for Microbiology, Washington, D.C., 1975.

138. UEMURA, T., Incidence of enterotoxigenic *Clostridium perfringens* in healthy humans in relation to the enhancement of enterotoxin production by heat treatment. *J. Appl. Bacteriol.* **44:**411–419 (1978).

139. UEMURA, T., AND SKJELKVÅLE, R., An enterotoxin produced by *Clostridium perfringens* type D: Purification by affinity chromatography, *Acta Pathol. Microbiol. Scand.* **84:**414–420 (1976).

140. UEMURA, T., GENIGEORGIS, C., RIEMANN, H. P., AND FRANTI, C. E., Antibody against *Clostridium perfringens* type A enterotoxin in human sera, *Infect. Immun.* **9:**470–471 (1974).

141. VANDEPITTE, J., WAUTERS, G., AND ISEBAERT, A., Epidemiology of *Yersinia enterocolitica* infections in Belgium, in: *Contributions to Microbiology and Immunology,* Vol. 2, *Yersinia, Pasteurella and Francisella* (S. WINBLAD, ed.), pp. 111–119, Karger, Basel, 1973.

142. VANTRAPPEN, G., AGG, H. O., PONETTE, E., GEBOES, K., AND BERTRAND, P., *Yersinia* enteritis and enterocolitis: Gastroenterological aspects, *Gastroenterology* **72:**220–224 (1977).

143. WATSON, G. N., The assessment and application of a bacteriocin typing scheme for *Clostridium perfringens, J. Hyg.* **94:**69–79 (1985).

144. WEED, L. A., MICHAEL, A. C., AND HARGER, R. A., Fatal staphylococcus intoxication from goat milk, *Am. J. Public Health* **33:**1314–1318 (1943).

145. WILLIAMS, R. E. O., Healthy carriage of *Staphylococcus aureus:* Its prevalence and importance, *Bacteriol Rev.* **27:**56–71 (1963).

146. YAHAGI, H., Early features of infection in ligated loops of the rabbit small intestine inoculated with *Shigella flexneri* 3a, enteropathogenic *E. coli, Escherichia coli* and *Vibrio parahaemolyticus,* The second report: Gross appearance and his-

tologic findings of ligated loops after inoculation, *Keio J. Med.* **16:**133–145 (1967).

147. YAHAGI, H., GHODA, A., AND SASAKI, S., Early features of infection in ligated loops of the rabbit small intestine inoculated with *Shigella flexneri* 3a, enteropathogenic *E. coli, Escherichia coli* and *Vibrio parahaemolyticus,* The third report: Study of bacterial invasiveness with the fluorescent antibody technique, *Keio J. Med.* **16:**119–131 (1967).

148. ZEISSLER, J., AND RASSFELD-STERNBERG, L., Enteritis necroticans due to *Clostridium welchii* type F, *Br. Med. J.* **1:**267–270 (1949).

149. ZEN-YOJI, H., HITOKOTO, H., MOROZUMI, S., AND LE CLAIR, R. A., Purification and characterization of a hemolysin produced by *Vibrio parahaemolyticus, J. Infect. Dis.* **123:**665–667 (1971).

150. ZEN-YOJI, H., MARUYAMA, T., SAKAI, S., KIMURA, S., MIZUNO, T., AND MOMOSE, T., An outbreak of enteritis due to *Yersinia enterocolitica* occurring at a junior high school, *Jpn. J. Microbiol.* **17:**220–222 (1973).

151. ZEN-YOJI, H., KUDOH, Y., IGARASKI, H., OHTA, K., AND FUKAI, K., Purification and identification of enteropathogenic toxins "a" and "a¹" produced by *Vibrio parahaemolyticus* and their biological and pathological activities in: *International Symposium on Vibrio parahaemolyticus* (T. FUJINO, G. SAKAGUCHI, R. SAKAZAKI, AND Y. TAKEDA, eds.), pp. 237–243, Saikon, Tokyo, 1974.

152. ZINK, D. L., FEELEY, J. C., WELLS, J. G., VANDERZANT, C., VICKERY, J. C., ROOF, W. D., AND O'DONOVAN, G. A., Plasmid-mediated tissue invasiveness in *Yersinia enterocolitica, Nature* **283:**224–226 (1980).

13. Suggested Reading

Centers for Disease Control, *Foodborne and Waterborne Disease Outbreaks Annual Summary, 1975* (issued September 1976).

DACK, G. M. (ed.), *Food Poisoning,* University of Chicago Press, Chicago, 1956.

HOBBS, B. C., AND CHRISTIAN, J. H. B. (eds.), *The Microbiological Safety of Food,* Academic Press, New York, 1973.

FUJINO, T., SAKAGUCHI, G., SAKAZAKI, R., AND TAKEDA, Y. (eds.), *International Symposium on Vibrio parahaemolyticus,* Saikon, Tokyo, 1974.

REIMANN, H., AND BRYAN, F. L. (eds.), *Foodborne Infections and Intoxications,* 2nd ed., Academic Press, New York, 1979.

CHAPTER 5

Botulism

Michael E. St. Louis

1. Introduction

Botulism is a neuroparalytic illness resulting from the action of a potent toxin produced by the organism *Clostridium botulinum*. Foodborne botulism, although rare, may kill rapidly, and contaminated products may expose many persons. Foodborne botulism therefore represents a medical and a public health emergency that places a premium on rapid, effective communication between clinicians and public health officials.

There are four clinically and epidemiologically distinct botulism syndromes. Foodborne botulism results from the ingestion of food contaminated with preformed toxin. Wound botulism is caused by organisms that multiply and produce toxin in a soil-contaminated wound. Infant botulism is due to the endogenous production of toxin by germinating spores of *C. botulinum* in the intestine of the infant. Adult enteric infectious botulism, due to colonization by *C. botulinum* of the adult gut, has recently been confirmed as a fourth botulism syndrome.

The seven types of *C. botulinum* (A–G) are distinguished by the antigenic characteristics of the neurotoxins they produce. Types A, B, E, and, in rare cases, F cause disease in humans. Types C and D cause disease in birds and mammals. Type G, identified in 1970, has not yet been confirmed as a cause of illness in humans or animals. Important epidemiologic features and some clinical characteristics distinguish the types of botulism that cause human illness.

Michael E. St. Louis · Enteric Diseases Branch, Division of Bacterial Diseases, Center for Infectious Diseases, Centers for Disease Control, Atlanta, Georgia 30333.

2. Historical Background

In the late 18th century, a syndrome characterized by muscle weakness and respiratory failure linked to eating "blood sausage" was described and termed "sausage poisoning."[73] Similar outbreaks related to sausage, other meats, and fish were reported in Germany, Scandinavia, and Russia. In time, the syndrome became known as "botulism" after "botulus," the Latin word for sausage.

In 1897, Van Ermengem [135] detected the potent neurotoxin in a ham implicated in an outbreak of botulism and isolated an organism that produced the toxin and grew only in the absence of oxygen. In a series of pioneering microbiologic experiments, he determined: (1) that foodborne botulism is not an infection, but rather an intoxication caused by a toxin produced in the food by the bacterium; (2) that the bacterium will not produce toxin in food if the salt concentration is high enough; (3) that the toxin is heat-labile; (4) that the toxin when ingested with the contaminated food is resistant to acid and proteolytic enzymes; and (5) that not all animal species are affected equally by ingested toxin.

In 1904, Landman first identified a nonmeat product (home-canned beans) as the cause of an outbreak of botulism.[79] During and shortly after World War I, the practice of home-canning vegetables increased markedly, as did the number of cases of botulism. Dr. K. F. Meyer made major contributions to the understanding of botulism during these years, studying the distribution of spores in soil in the United States and Europe, characterizing the epidemiology of botulism transmitted by home-canned vegetables and fruits, and even identifying a new type of *C. botulinum*. In the mid-1940s, with the increased availability of refrigeration and the widespread application of improved preserva-

115

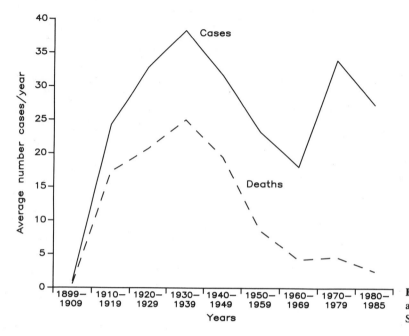

Figure 1. Average annual number of cases and deaths from foodborne botulism, United States, 1899–1985.

tion methods both in the home and by industry, the incidence of botulism began a decline that continued until recent years, when the occurrence of large restaurant-associated outbreaks caused the incidence to rise again (Fig. 1).

Although it had been noted earlier that the toxins of the Van Ermengem and the Landman strains were serologically distinct,[80] it was in 1919 that the first two type designations (A and B) were established.[15,16] The types were based on strains isolated in the United States and could not be related to the earlier European strains since the latter were no longer available for study. *C. botulinum* types C and D were discovered in relation to outbreaks of botulism in domestic birds and animals.[11,99] *C. botulinum* type E was first isolated in 1936 from fish implicated in a botulism outbreak.[55] *C. botulinum* type F was first isolated and recognized as a cause of human botulism in 1960.[105] In 1970, *C. botulinum* type G was isolated from soil in Argentina, but has not yet been confirmed as a cause of botulism.[52]

3. Methodology

3.1. Surveillance

The Centers for Disease Control (CDC) maintains surveillance of botulism in the United States. The sources of

morbidity and mortality surveillance data include: (1) state, territorial, and local health departments (botulism is a reportable disease in most states); (2) the Food and Drug Administration, which becomes involved if the implicated food item is commercially produced or distributed or both; (3) the U.S. Department of Agriculture, which becomes involved if the contaminated food item is derived from meat, poultry, or eggs; (4) clinicians who contact CDC for consultation, laboratory support, or antitoxin; and (5) the manufacturers of antitoxin, who are sometimes contacted initially by a patient's physician.

CDC provides epidemiologic consultation and laboratory diagnostic services to state health departments in suspected botulism cases. In addition, because CDC authorizes the use of all botulism antitoxin administered in the United States, nearly all diagnosed cases of botulism and deaths from botulism are eventually reported to CDC. Underreporting of botulism results mainly when cases are misdiagnosed (as, for example, myasthenia gravis, Guillain–Barré syndrome, or stroke). Mild cases of botulism may escape diagnosis because of a lack of overt neurologic findings,[130] and even severe cases resulting in death may be diagnosed only after death, if at all.[8,65] Misdiagnosis of botulism is an important public health problem because lack of recognition precludes epidemiologic investigation and prevention of subsequent cases due to the same contaminated foods.[65,126]

3.2. Laboratory Diagnosis

Since botulism results from the action of a toxin, the most definitive laboratory confirmation of the disease is the demonstration of the toxin itself in clinical specimens (serum, wound, tissue, or feces) or foods.[23] Isolation of *C. botulinum* spores from foods or wounds supports the diagnosis of botulism but may not be definitive, as the organism may be present in foods or wounds without producing toxin. On the other hand, isolation of *C. botulinum* from human feces is extremely rare except in persons suspected of having botulism, and may be considered strong evidence supporting the diagnosis.[1,39] Botulism may also result from foods in which the responsible organisms have died but the toxin has persisted.

The mouse inoculation assay is currently the most sensitive, specific, and commonly used method for detecting botulinal toxin.[23,59] A standard volume of the test specimen (e.g., an aliquot of serum or extract of feces) is injected into the peritoneum of test mice and from this site is absorbed into the bloodstream. The same volume of test specimen is combined with polyvalent botulinal antitoxin (antitoxin against type A, B, C, D, E, and F toxin) and injected into the peritoneum of control mice. The presence of botulinal toxin is considered proven only if the mice that were inoculated with only the test specimen die while those protected by botulinal antitoxin suffer no ill effects. Death of the control mice demonstrates that some factor capable of killing mice was present in the specimen that was not neutralized by botulinal antitoxin; deaths in the corresponding test mice therefore cannot be attributed to botulism. Further neutralization assays with monovalent (usually types A, B, and E) antitoxins can demonstrate the specific type of toxin present. To increase the specificity of the laboratory diagnosis, experienced laboratory workers also learn to recognize the clinical manifestations of botulism in the mouse. It is therefore important that this specialized assay be conducted in reference laboratories that perform the test frequently enough to maintain expertise.

By definition, the mouse inoculation assay can detect as little as one mouse lethal dose (the lowest dilution of the test specimen that kills 100% of injected mice) of botulinal toxin. One mouse lethal dose is equivalent to approximately 20 pg botulinal toxin. In one instance, an oral human lethal dose of type E toxin was calculated as 500,000 mouse lethal doses.[35] The mouse inoculation assay does, however, have drawbacks. Although positive results may be reported within 24 h, final results are not available until 96 h after inoculation. Also, although the neutralization procedure ensures the specificity of the test, nonspecific toxicity may decrease the sensitivity of the assay by masking the presence of botulinal toxin.

In the attempt to develop more rapid screening tests for the presence of botulinal toxin, several *in vitro* assays have been developed. These include radioimmunoassay,[14] immunofluorescence,[53,85,101] gas chromatography,[93] immunodiffusion,[97,102,136] passive hemagglutination,[71,115] and enzyme-linked immunosorption assay.[123] Nevertheless, because of the extraordinary biologic potency of botulinal toxins, the mouse inoculation assay remains substantially more sensitive and more specific than other tests yet developed. Also, signs of botulism can be observed in mice inoculated with positive samples. Another positive feature of the mouse assay is its ability to detect any type of botulinal toxin rather than being limited to a particular antigenic type. Thus, only the mouse assay would be capable of demonstrating the action of a new type of botulinal toxin that is antigenically distinct from those currently recognized.

C. botulinum may be isolated using a spore-selection technique in enrichment culture.[38] Suspensions of the clinical or environmental specimens are prepared and heated at 80°C for 10 min or treated with 100% ethanol to kill nonsporing organisms. A standard volume of this material is injected into chopped-meat enrichment media, and the tubes are incubated anaerobically. Maximum toxin production occurs in 3–5 days in pure cultures; the optimum time may be longer in specimen cultures. If no toxin is demonstrated in the original sample, toxicity tests are performed on the enrichment culture supernatant before subculturing on egg-yolk and blood agar. The plates are incubated anaerobically for 48 h. Colonies showing the lipase reaction (an irridescent sheen) are then chosen and injected into tubes of chopped-meat–dextrose–starch medium. After incubation at 30°C, the identity of the pure culture can be established by toxicity and neutralization tests and conventional biochemical procedures.[38]

4. Biological Characteristics of the Organism

C. botulinum is not a single species but rather a group of culturally distinct organisms that are alike only in that they are clostridia and produce antigenically distinct neurotoxins with a similar pharmacologic action. *C. botulinum* organisms are straight to slightly curved, gram-positive (in young cultures), motile, anaerobic rods, 0.5–2.0 μm in width by 1.6–22.0 μm in length, with oval, subterminal spores.[20] Certain strains of *C. sporogenes* and *C. novyi* are indistinguishable by culture and by DNA homology, but are nontoxigenic. In recent years, cases of infant botulism due to other species of clostridia, *C. barati*[58] and *C. butyricum*,[7] have further strained the taxonomic classification of botulism-causing organisms. The seven types of *C. botulinum* (A–G) are distinguished by immunologically distinct types of toxin. *C. botulinum* organisms have also been divided into proteolytic (type A and some strains of types B and F) and nonproteolytic (type E and some strains of types B and F), depending on the ability of the strains to hydrolyze complex proteins.

The specific cultural and biochemical characteristics of *C. botulinum* are described elsewhere.[20,32,124] Because of the practical importance of temperature, salt concentration, and pH in the preservation of foods, the effects of these factors on the growth of *C. botulinum* have been thoroughly investigated. All strains of *C. botulinum* are mesophilic, although some nonproteolytic strains have been noted to grow at temperatures as low as 3°C.[111] The organism will generally not grow in an acid environment (pH < 4.6) or in foods with a high salt content. Temperature, pH, and salt content are interrelated factors; lowering the pH or raising the salt concentration increases the minimum temperature at which spores will germinate or vegetative cells will begin to grow.[9]

The ability of *C. botulinum* to cause food poisoning in humans is directly related to the production of heat-resistant spores that survive preservation methods that kill nonsporulating organisms. The heat resistance of spores varies from type to type and even from strain to strain within each type; although some strains will not survive at 80°C, spores of many strains require temperatures above boiling to ensure destruction.[70,113,119] The thermal resistance of spores also increases with higher pH and lower salt content of the medium in which the spores are suspended.[141] In general, type A and proteolytic type B spores are more heat-resistant than type E and nonproteolytic type B spores. Spores are also susceptible to some types and degrees of radiation.[44,112,113] Nitrites are effective as well in preventing growth from spores that germinate[110] and are used commercially in semiprocessed meats.

C. botulinum types C and D have bacteriophages that are associated with toxicity. Nonlysogenic, nontoxigenic mutants have been obtained by "curing" them of their phages. These mutants can be made lysogenic and toxigenic again by infection with phages obtained from other lysogenic strains.[42,43] Hence, the ability of *C. botulinum* types C and D to produce toxin seems to depend on the presence of specific bacteriophages. No association between bacteriophages and toxicity has been found,

however, for type A, B, E, and F strains of *C. botulinum*. The association between lysogenization by phage and toxin production has been noted with *Corynebacterium diphtheriae*. The genetic information for the production of neurotoxin by *Clostridium tetani*, however, appears to be located in a plasmid.[40]

Toxin is released from *C. botulinum* organisms only after lysis of the cells. The lytic enzymes responsible for this autolysis are located in the cell wall. More than one such bacteriolysin has been identified, and at least some appear to be group-specific.[103]

5. Descriptive Epidemiology

5.1. Foodborne Botulism

Botulism has been reported from all parts of the world, although the causative strains of *C. botulinum*, the characteristic food vehicles responsible for botulism, and even the resulting patterns of clinical illness may vary widely among regions. Botulism in continental Europe is almost exclusively type B disease and is predominantly caused by eating home-cured hams. The resulting illness is relatively mild and slowly progressive compared with botulism in the United States.[118] Most outbreaks in Canada and Japan are type E botulism associated with the consumption of preserved seafood.[62,68] In China, home-fermented bean curd is the most common vehicle of botulism poisoning, with the causative strains a mixture of types A and B.[82,122] Case-fatality ratios are substantially higher for type A than for type B botulism in the United States[23] but are marginally higher for type B than for type A botulism in China.[122]

In the United States between 1899 and 1985, 875 outbreaks of foodborne botulism involving 2195 persons were reported. The mean annual incidence of reported foodborne botulism in the United States in 1976 through 1985 was 0.16 case per 1,000,000 persons. Generally, the northern and western states in the contiguous United States have had higher rates of foodborne botulism than the southern and eastern states. Alaska had the most cases (59) between 1976 and 1985 and had by far the highest rate of reported botulism (14.6 cases per 1,000,000 population).

Since botulism in adults most commonly results from eating improperly preserved home-canned (or home-bottled) foods, outbreaks usually occur in family groups and affect small groups of people. In recent years, however, novel vehicles of foodborne botulism have been reported. These differ in being "fresh" rather than preserved, and include potato salad,[91,117] baked potatoes,[24] sautéed onions,[86] commercial potpies,[18] turkey loaves,[24] and beef stew.[24] In each case, these unpreserved foods were prepared by ordinary cooking procedures (which do not kill *C. botulinum* spores) and then stored for many hours to days under relatively anaerobic conditions (e.g., baked potatoes in foil, sautéed onions under melted butter) at temperatures warm enough to encourage the outgrowth of spores and production of toxin but not hot enough to destroy the heat-labile toxin. The foods were then eaten without having been thoroughly reheated.

Food that is commercially prepared or distributed may cause illness in a large number of persons who may be spread over a wide geographic area.[117,126] Since 1976, large outbreaks of botulism have increasingly occurred in association with foods served in restaurants; although such outbreaks constituted only 4% of botulism outbreaks in 1976 through 1984, they accounted for 42% of all cases of botulism.[88] Such large outbreaks of botulism often result in extraordinary economic costs as well as extensive morbidity.[90,92]

Although foodborne botulism affects all age groups, it occurs mainly in persons aged 30–60 years.[12,51,54,66] This age distribution may reflect that of persons who eat home-canned foods. Although it has been hypothesized that younger persons may be less susceptible to botulism, recent evidence indicates that the lower case-fatality ratios for the younger age groups are due to fewer complications during intensive respiratory support rather than to inherent resistance to the effects of botulinal toxin.[67,130] The disease

occurs with nearly equal frequency in men and women. No clear time trend is evident in the incidence of foodborne botulism (Fig. 1).

Corresponding to the distribution of botulinal spores in soil samples,[125] 92% of botulism outbreaks that have occurred in the western United States (excluding Alaska) since 1950 were type A, whereas 57% of outbreaks east of the Mississippi River were due to type B and only 37% were due to type A. In Alaska, approximately 70% of outbreaks were of type E botulism; outbreaks in Alaska have uniformly been due to fermented or otherwise preserved fish or aquatic mammals.[41,137]

5.2. Infant Botulism

Infant botulism is the most common form of botulism reported in the United States. It is epidemiologically distinct from foodborne botulism, representing the effect not of ingestion of toxin preformed in contaminated foods, but of colonization (infection) of the intestine by spores of *C. botulinum*, with subsequent *in vivo* toxin production.[3] Although infant botulism was first described in 1976,[100,109] earlierdd cases have been identified retrospectively, and its detection only in recent years probably reflects advances in diagnostic capabilities rather than the emergence of a new clinical syndrome. Cases have been reported in the United States, Canada, Great Britain, Australia, Czechoslovakia, Sweden, Italy, and Japan.

In the United States, 571 cases were reported from 41

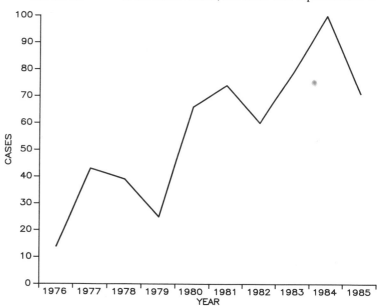

Figure 2. Cases of infant botulism reported to the Centers for Disease Control, United States, 1976–1985.

states to the CDC between 1976 and 1985 (Fig. 2). Since reporting began to stabilize in 1980, the average annual incidence of reported infant botulism in the United States has been approximately 2.1/100,000 live births. Since 1980, 50% of all infant botulism cases have been reported from California, although the incidence is highest in Hawaii and Delaware (13.0 and 10.5 per 100,000 live births), perhaps reflecting better diagnosis and reporting in those states.

The illness is confirmed by demonstrating botulinal toxin in and isolating *C. botulinum* from the infant's stool. Toxin may be detected in serum (13% of tested infants), more often in type A cases (36%) than in type B cases (2%).[60] In the United States, 48% of infant botulism cases were caused by type A *C. botulinum* and 52% by type B. One U.S. case was associated with type F toxin,[58] and two cases in Italy were associated with type E toxin.[7] Infant botulism is first seen most commonly in the second month of life (Fig. 3) and occurs somewhat earlier in cases of type B disease (median: 9 weeks) than in cases of type A disease (median: 11 weeks). There is no race or sex predilection and no apparent pattern of seasonal variation.

The characteristics of infant botulism cases have been clarified in recent years. Infants hospitalized with the disease tend to have had higher birthweights than other infants, and their mothers tend to be white, older, and better educated than mothers in the general population. Affected infants are also more commonly breast-fed[84,107]; breastfeeding is associated with an older age at onset in type B cases.[107] Clustering of cases of infant botulism has been

noted in some suburban areas in the eastern United States and in small towns and rural areas of apparent high incidence of infant botulism in the West.[69,83,132]

Evidence of infant botulism was detected in several cases of sudden infant death syndrome (SIDS) in California.[4] The similar age distribution of infant botulism and SIDS contributed to the hypothesis that unrecognized infant botulism might be an important cause of SIDS. However, despite extensive investigations, no case of SIDS in the United States outside of California has yet been confirmed as a case of infant botulism. In addition, descriptive characteristics of SIDS patients, who tend to be black and have a history of low birthweight, and less well educated mothers living in large cities, differ sharply from those of infant botulism cases.[107]

5.3. Wound Botulism

Wound botulism is a rare disease resulting from the outgrowth of *C. botulinum* spores from a contaminated wound with *in vivo* toxin production. Between 1943, when the syndrome was first recognized,[33] and 1985, 36 cases of wound botulism were reported in the United States. Of 25 laboratory-confirmed cases in the United States, 17 were type A, 7 type B, and 1 a mixture of type A and type B organisms.[59] The median age of the patients was 21 years (range, 6–44 years); 81% were male. The wounds were usually deep and contained avascular areas; many patients had compound fractures, and four had extensive crush inju-

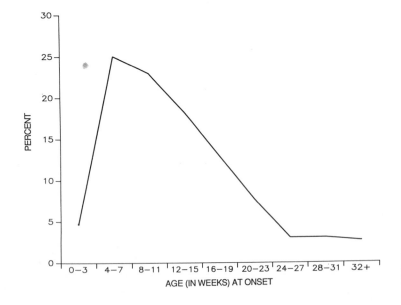

Figure 3. Age distribution (in weeks) of infant botulism cases reported to the Centers for Disease Control, United States, 1975–1985.

ries of the hand. The median incubation period in cases of trauma was 7 days (range: 4–21 days).[96] Since 1980, several wound botulism cases have occurred in persons who abuse drugs; these were associated either with needle puncture sites or with nasal or sinus lesions due to chronic cocaine sniffing.[87] In such cases, as in traditional wound botulism cases, the wounds may not be obvious or grossly infected.

5.4. Adult Enteric Infectious Botulism

Isolated cases of adult botulism in which extensive investigation failed to implicate a specific food as the cause of the disease have been recorded by the CDC since 1978 as cases of "undetermined origin" rather than of foodborne botulism. Although there has been speculation on the matter since the 1920s, careful investigation has now demonstrated that some of these cases are caused by colonization of the gastrointestinal tract by *C. botulinum* with *in vivo* production of toxin, analogous to the pathogenesis of infant botulism.[27,95] Support for the diagnosis of adult enteric infectious botulism is provided by the demonstration of the prolonged excretion of toxin and *C. botulinum* in the stool, and by the demonstration of spores of *C. botulinum* but not preformed toxin in suspect foods. In some adult cases of botulism strongly suspected of representing enteric infection, the patients had preceding gastrointestinal surgery or illnesses—such as inflammatory bowel disease—that may have predisposed them to enteric colonization.[95] No other specific risk factors have been identified.

6. Mechanisms and Routes of Transmission

6.1. Foodborne Botulism

Foodborne botulism is caused by consuming improperly preserved food in which spores of *C. botulinum* have germinated and organisms have grown and produced toxin. Home-processed foods accounted for 94% of foodborne botulism outbreaks in the continental United States in the past decade. Mass-processed commercial foods accounted for only 6% of outbreaks and 4% of cases. Even the large, restaurant-associated outbreaks of recent years have generally been caused by foods either home-canned in the restaurant[63,130] or otherwise mishandled or improperly handled or stored,[86,126] rather than by defective commercially canned products.

Temperatures obtainable only with a pressure cooker are usually necessary to kill *C. botulinum* spores. Boiling

Table 1. Vehicles of Foodborne Botulism in the United States, 1899–1977 (1961 Cases) and 1978–1985 (235 Cases)

Vehicle	% of total cases	
	1899–1977	1978–1985
Unknown	65.5	3.0
Identified	34.5	97.0
Vegetables	57.0	64.0
Fish/aquatic animals	15.6	19.3
Fruits	11.0	0.9
Condiments	8.7	10.1
Meat/dairy	7.5	5.7

alone does not kill the spores of proteolytic strains, but does kill competing organisms and creates an anaerobic environment that will support the growth of *C. botulinum* once the spores germinate. The toxin itself is heat-labile; heating to 80°C for 10 min is sufficient to destroy the toxin. However, some home-canned foods are not cooked before being eaten, and those that are cooked may not be subjected to sufficient heat to destroy all the toxin present.

Although the epidemiologic investigation of outbreaks has improved and the vehicles of botulism outbreaks have been more frequently identified in recent years, the proportional contribution of different types of food to cases of foodborne botulism has remained relatively stable (Table 1). Vegetables, especially those of more neutral pH such as asparagus, green beans, peppers, and mushrooms, are responsible for most type A and type B outbreaks. Spores may survive when either hot-pack or cold-pack canning methods are used [134]; cold-pack canning is acceptable only for certain fruits because of their high acidity or sugar content, which inhibit outgrowth of *C. botulinum* spores. Type E outbreaks are most often caused by products derived from fish and marine mammals. For example, many type E outbreaks in Alaska are associated with "muktuk" and "stink eggs," in which whale blubber or fish eggs are fermented in an anaerobic milieu, allowing the outgrowth of *C. botulinum* organisms.[137]

6.2. Infant, Wound, and Adult Enteric Infectious Botulism

In contrast to foodborne botulism, which is an intoxication, infant, wound, and adult enteric infectious botulism result from infection with or colonization by *C. botulinum*. This organism is widely distributed in nature and can easily be ingested with foods[74,98,125] or contaminate a traumatic wound.[89,114] The low frequency of *C. botulinum* infections despite the ubiquity of the organism in nature suggests that host factors are prominent in the epidemiology of these infectious forms of botulism.

Infant botulism results after colonization of the infant intestine.[72,100] In a prototypical case, type B organisms, but no toxin, were isolated from honey fed to an infant with infant botulism whose fecal specimens contained type B organisms and toxin. Family members who ate some of the same honey did not become ill. In several studies, more than 20% of affected infants had ingested honey before the onset of botulism.[5,28,107] In several such instances, *C. botulinum* spores of the same type were cultured from honey in the same households.

However, since most infants with infant botulism have had no honey exposure, the risk factors and vehicles of transmission of *C. botulinum* for the majority of cases remain unclear. A survey of foods commonly fed to infants revealed *C. botulinum* in specimens of corn syrup as well as honey, but in no other tested category of foods.[74] In other studies, the same types of *C. botulinum* that caused disease were isolated from soil in an infant's yard and from vacuum cleaner dust; investigators have also frequently noted environmental conditions that might expose infants directly to environmental sources of *C. botulinum* spores, such as a shared crib, dusty or windy locales, nearby building construction, or outdoor activities.[69,132] These exposures have not, however, been evaluated by controlled studies. Infants hospitalized with botulism have also more typically been breast-fed than have control infants.[6,84,140] Breast-feeding is known to affect the fecal flora differently than formula feeding; in mice, the fecal flora have been shown to be an important susceptibility factor in challenge experiments with *C. botulinum* type A spores.[139]

Wound botulism, like tetanus, gas gangrene, and other clostridial diseases, can result from soil contamination of a wound.[96] However, the rarity of wound botulism despite the wide distribution of the organism in the environment raises many questions regarding its pathogenesis: are many wounds contaminated but few suitable for proliferation of the organism? Or is wound contamination with *C. botulinum* without signs of botulism truly uncommon? Data are scarce. Part of the problem is the difficulty in obtaining adequate anaerobic cultures and in differentiating *C. sporogenes* (a common wound isolate) from *C. botulinum*. In addition, the factors involved in spore germination, growth, and toxin production in tissues or *in vivo* systems have not been well studied. In wound botulism associated with chronic drug abuse, it is unclear if drugs or needles are

vehicles for transmission of spores or are instead only associated with host factors for colonization, such as depressed immunity or chronically inflamed mucous membrane or skin lesions.[87]

In cases of adult botulism in which enteric infections were proven or suspected, vehicles have included canned cream of coconut[27] and blackberry preserves,[21] in each of which *C. botulinum* organisms of the appropriate type were detected. In a case strongly suggestive of this syndrome, a healthy, 27-year-old asymptomatic consumer of blood sausage was shown to have intestinal carriage of *C. botulinum* 19 days after an outbreak attributed to the sausage, but did not develop clinical symptoms and botulinal toxemia until 47 days after the outbreak.[94] The limited data about enteric infectious botulism in adults do not suggest that the vehicles of transmission are categorically different from those of traditional foodborne botulism due to preformed toxin.

7. Pathogenesis

Incubation periods for foodborne botulism are similar for each toxin type. They are reported to be as short as 6 h or as long as 10 days,[126] but generally the time between toxin ingestion and onset of symptoms ranges from 18 to 36 h.[37] The incubation periods for wound botulism (4–14 days) are longer than those usually seen in cases of foodborne botulism and presumably reflect the time required for the multiplication of *C. botulinum* in the wound and the release of toxin. The incubation period has not been determined for cases of infant botulism. It has been shown that those individuals with shorter incubation periods—apparently those who ingest and/or absorb larger amounts of toxin—have more severe disease and a graver prognosis.[86,129,130]

Botulinal toxin is absorbed into the bloodstream from the gastrointestinal tract or from a wound and is transported via lymphatics and blood to cholinergic neuromuscular junctions. Here the toxin is fixed at and then internalized into the presynaptic nerve ending. It subsequently blocks the release of the neurotransmitter acetylcholine by binding to its release site at the neuronal membrane.[73,127] Evidence suggests that this binding is irreversible[57,127]; hence, functional recovery occurs only with the regeneration of neuronal fibrils and the reestablishment of the neuromuscular junction. This may explain why muscular weakness persists in many individuals for weeks or more after toxin has been eliminated from the intestine and bloodstream and why in severely affected individuals recovery may take many months to years or may never completely occur.[25,78,90]

Botulinal toxin affects acetylcholine release only at peripheral sites; the central nervous system is not affected. Whether this is because botulinal toxin does not cross the blood–brain barrier or because botulinal toxin does not bind to acetylcholine release sites in the central nervous system is not known. Both the autonomic and voluntary motor activities of the cranial nerves seem to be uniquely susceptible to the effects of botulinal toxin. The cranial nerves are nearly always affected earlier and to a greater degree than are the nerves to the peripheral and respiratory muscles. Certain cranial nerves seem to be more sensitive to one botulinal toxin type than to others. Pupillary paralysis, for example, is apparently more commonly noted in type A botulism than in type B botulism.[25,67,125] Correspondingly, distinctions in the effect of type A and B toxin on laboratory preparations of the neuromuscular junction have been observed.[120] Although the reason for this is not clear, molecular differences between toxin types that account for immunological distinction might, through stearic interactions, also result in disparate binding capabilities at neuromuscular junctions.

Botulinal toxin is so potent that the lethal dose is far below that required to induce an antibody response. Hence, immunity from natural intoxication does not occur.[77,116] Whether continuous exposure to low levels of toxin produced by organisms that have colonized the intestine (infant botulism) or a wound (wound botulism) may lead to significant antibody production has not been determined.

Animal models of infant botulism have yielded insight into mechanisms of intestinal colonization and *in vivo* growth of *C. botulinum*. Successful intraintestinal colonization by *C. botulinum* spores inoculated into the stomachs of infant mice is strongly age-dependent, peaking at 7 to 13 days old, a period during which the enteric microbial flora are in transition.[128] Although normal adult mice are highly resistant to colonization, germ-free adult mice may develop botulism after ingesting as few as ten spores,[104] and antimicrobial treatment of normal adult mice dramatically lowers the dose of ingested spores necessary to yield intraluminal outgrowth and production of toxin.[17,138] In mice, therefore, enteric infection is limited to a narrow age range in infancy and to occurrence in adults who have undergone a manipulation of the normal intestinal microbial flora. It is possible that anatomical variations, stasis, or constipation due to mechanical or motility factors, or some combination of these contribute to the creation of an environment favorable to the growth of the organism.

Factors other than just the physical production of toxin in the gut may also contribute to the expression of clinical illness. *C. botulinum* organisms and toxin have been recovered from the feces of human infants more than 8 weeks after the onset of botulism, and the peak excretion of toxin may not occur until several weeks after the illness has already begun to resolve.

8. Patterns of Host Response

8.1. Clinical Features

The clinical syndrome of botulism is dominated by the neurological symptoms and signs resulting from a toxin-induced blockade of the voluntary motor and autonomic cholinergic junctions and is essentially quite similar for each syndrome and toxin type.[3,25,67,72,78,96,100,140] The ingestion of other bacteria and their toxins in the improperly preserved food accounts for the abdominal pain, nausea and vomiting, and diarrhea that often precede or accompany the neurologic symptoms of foodborne botulism. Dryness of the mouth, inability to focus to a near point (prompting the patient to complain of "blurred vision"), and diplopia are usually the earliest neurologic complaints. If the disease is mild, no other symptoms may develop and the initial symptoms will gradually resolve. The individual with mild botulism may not come to medical attention. In more severe cases, however, these initial complaints may be followed by dysphonia, dysarthria, dysphagia, and peripheral-muscle weakness. If illness is severe, respiratory muscles are involved, leading to ventilatory failure and death unless supportive care is provided. Patients have required ventilatory support for up to 7 months before the return of muscular function, although a 2- to 8-week duration of ventilatory support is more common.[67] Death occurs in 5–10% of cases of foodborne botulism; early deaths result from a failure to recognize the severity of disease or from pulmonary or systemic infections, whereas deaths after 2 weeks are from the complications of long-term mechanical ventilatory management or respirator malfunction.[67]

Perhaps because infants are not able to complain about the early effects of botulinal intoxication, the neurologic dysfunction associated with infant botulism often seems to develop suddenly. The major manifestations are poor feeding, diminished suckling and crying ability, neck and peripheral weakness (the infants are often admitted as "floppy babies"), and ventilatory failure.[3,84,140] Constipation is also often seen in infants with botulism and, in some, has preceded by many days the onset of neurologic abnormalities. Loss of facial expression, extraocular muscle paralysis, dilated pupils, and depression of deep tendon reflexes have been reported more frequently with type B than with type A infant botulism.[140] Treatment with aminoglycoside antimicrobials may potentiate neuromuscular weakness in infant botulism[81] and has been associated with an increased likelihood of needing mechanical ventilation.[140] The median length of hospital stay in cases of infant botulism is 27 days (range, 2–150 days).[140] Fewer than 2% of reported cases of infant botulism result in death.

8.2. Diagnosis

Botulism is probably substantially underdiagnosed. The diagnosis is not difficult when it is strongly suspected, as in the setting of a large outbreak. However, since cases of botulism most often occur singly, the diagnosis may pose a more perplexing problem. Findings from many outbreaks involving more than one person have suggested that early cases are commonly misdiagnosed and may only be diagnosed retrospectively after death, after the subsequent clustering of cases of botulism-like illness finally alerts public health personnel to the occurrence of an outbreak of botulism[8,65,77]; other cases are undoubtedly missed entirely. Entire outbreaks may even go undetected despite severe illness in patients; for example, one outbreak was recognized retrospectively only after a second cluster of cases occurred due to the same vehicle.[126]

Botulism should be suspected in any adult with a history of gastrointestinal, autonomic (e.g., dry mouth, difficulty focusing), and cranial-nerve (diplopia, dysarthria, dysphagia) dysfunction or in any infant with poor feeding; diminished sucking and crying ability; neck- and peripheral-muscle weakness; and/or ventilatory distress.[23,37] The demonstration of bilateral cranial-nerve findings and the documentation of neurologic progression (peripheral-muscle weakness, ventilatory compromise) increase the level of suspicion. The diagnosis is even more likely if an adult patient has recently eaten home-canned foods or if family members are similarly ill, or both. If the typical clinical syndrome is present and no food item can be pinpointed as a means of transmission, a contaminated wound should be sought. If the typical syndrome is seen and a wound is identified, the wound should be explored and specimens taken for culture and toxicity testing even if the wound appears clean.

The differential diagnosis includes myasthenia gravis, stroke, Guillain–Barré syndrome, bacterial and chemical food poisoning, tick paralysis, chemical intoxication (e.g., from carbon monoxide, barium carbonate, methyl chloride, methyl alcohol, organic phosphorus compound, or atro-

pine), mushroom poisoning, medication reactions (e.g., from antibiotics such as neomycin, streptomycin, kanamycin, or gentamicin), poliomyelitis, diphtheria, and psychiatric illness. In infant botulism, sepsis (especially meningitis), electrolyte–mineral imbalance, metabolic encephalopathy, Reye syndrome, Werdnig–Hoffman disease, congenital myopathy, and Leigh disease should also be considered.

Routine laboratory studies are not helpful in confirming the clinical suspicion of botulism. Serum electrolytes, renal and liver function tests, complete blood tests, urinalysis, and electrocardiograms will all be normal unless secondary complications occur. A normal cerebrospinal fluid (CSF) examination helps differentiate botulism from Guillain–Barré syndrome, although a slightly elevated CSF protein level is occasionally seen with botulism.[67] Normal neuroradiologic studies, such as computed tomographic scans or magnetic resonance imaging, help to rule out stroke, another condition commonly confused with botulism.[77,126]

Electromyography (EMG) can be very helpful in distinguishing botulism from myasthenia gravis and Guillain–Barré syndrome, diseases that botulism often mimics closely. A characteristic EMG pattern observed in adult patients with botulism has been well described.[25,26,57,76] A low-amplitude response to a single stimulus, a decremental trend in amplitude of the elicited action potentials to repetitive low-frequency stimulation (2–5 Hz), and an incremental trend (facilitation) to rapid repetitive stimulation (20–50 Hz) may be seen. However, rapid repetitive stimulation is much more sensitive and specific for botulism than is low-frequency stimulation.[126] EMGs should be performed on clinically involved muscles; positive results may be obtained from only one muscle even though many are weak.

The most prominent EMG finding in infant botulism is the same as that in adults: an incremental response to rapid repetitive stimulation.[30] However, another EMG pattern has been described as characteristic of infant botulism.[29] This is the pattern of "brief duration, small amplitude, overly abundant (for the amount of power being exerted)" motor unit action potentials, termed "BSAP" by Engel.[45] Polyphasicity may also be part of this pattern. It is not unusual to find either a BAP pattern (if the motor unit potentials are only brief) or an SAP pattern (if the motor unit potentials are only small) in patients who have typical BSAP findings in other parts of a muscle or in other muscles.

Toxicity testing of serum specimens, culture of tissues debrided from a wound, and toxicity testing plus culture of stool specimens or epidemiologically incriminated foods or both are the best methods for confirming the diagnosis of botulism.[23,39] Previous laboratory experience has shown that tests for botulinal toxin in serum or stool specimens are positive in about 35% of clinically diagnosed cases. If both specimens are examined for toxin, about 45% of the cases are confirmed. When positive stool culture results are added, the confirmation rate increases to 72%. However, in any given situation, these tests may not be helpful; large outbreaks have occurred in which all[22] or a very large percentage[130] of specimens have yielded negative results. In addition, laboratory results may not be reported until many hours or days after the specimens are received. The administration of antitoxin is the only specific therapy available for botulism, and evidence suggests that it is effective only if given very early in the course of neurologic dysfunction.[108,129] Hence, the diagnosis of this illness cannot await the results of studies that may be long delayed and be confirmatory only in some cases. The diagnosis should be made on the basis of the history and physical findings.

9. Prevention, Control, and Treatment

9.1. Prevention and Control

The prevention of foodborne botulism depends on destroying all *C. botulinum* spores in food as it is preserved or creating a milieu in the preserved foods that will not allow the growth of any organisms that survive preservation procedures. This requires careful home canning and commercial canning techniques. Several private and government agencies (e.g., the U.S. Department of Agriculture) provide information on the proper methods of home canning. Although the heat resistance of *C. botulinum* spores is quite variable, cooking at 121°C (250°F) or higher is usually sufficient to destroy all spores.[70,113,119] These temperatures can be achieved only in a pressure cooker. Boiling alone may kill competitive organisms and create an anaerobic environment highly favorable to the growth of *C. botulinum*. Boiling is sufficient for fruits and certain vegetables because their high sugar content will not support the growth of *C. botulinum*.[9] Until recently, tomatoes were thought to be an extremely low-risk food because of their acidity. Recent cases of botulism have, however, been caused by contaminated foods that contained tomatoes (such as spaghetti sauce) and by tomato juice.[12,66] These cases have been attributed to the low-acidity tomatoes that are now being bred for increased "sweetness."

Home-canned foods that are contaminated with proteolytic *C. botulinum* organisms or concurrently contaminated with other anaerobic or aerobic organisms will spoil. Foods that look or smell spoiled should not be tasted. Foods contaminated by nonproteolytic strains of *C. botulinum* (and sometimes proteolytic strains as well) may not appear spoiled. Food items suspected of having transmitted botulism should be refrigerated and saved for culture and toxin testing. Although *C. botulinum* spores are resistant to heat, botulinal toxins are heat-labile and are readily destroyed by boiling. Thorough boiling of home-canned foods is an added safeguard against botulism.

Commercial canners use a variety of methods to prevent the growth of *C. botulinum*. Commercial canners[46-48] routinely heat foods to 120°C for 3 min, and often acidify high-risk, low-acid foods such as peppers to inhibit the growth of *C. botulinum*. Semipreserved meat products (e.g., hot dogs and luncheon meats) have nitrites added for similar reasons. Systems for killing spores in foods by radiation are also under investigation. *C. botulinum* is a gas-producing organism, and its growth inside a can may produce enough gas to make the can bulge or swell. More common causes of bulging include overpacking by the manufacturer, gas caused by interaction of the contents and the metal container, or contamination by some other organisms due to a fractured seal. Nevertheless, swollen, bulging cans or cans with spoiled contents should be reported to local health authorities or to the FDA.

Physicians also have an important role in the control of botulism. All suspect cases should be reported to state or local health authorities or directly to CDC in Atlanta (telephone 404-639-2888); it is important that this be done quickly and efficiently, especially if the suspected vehicle is a commercial product. If the diagnosis is suspected, then a search for other cases (initially by identifying those who shared the implicated food) should be immediately undertaken.

Because the mechanism of transmission for infant botulism has not been totally defined, control measures are not available. Controlled epidemiologic studies will be required to develop the necessary data. Since honey is the one identified source of *C. botulinum* spores for susceptible infants and since it is not essential for good infant nutrition, it is recommended that honey not be fed to infants under age 1.[72] The prevention of wound botulism depends on the thorough cleansing and debridement of wounds, especially those of any depth or that are contaminated by soil.

Although antibiotic prophylaxis will not protect against foodborne botulism, since this results from ingestion of preformed toxin, administration of an oral penicillin or a nonabsorbable antibiotic might prove useful in preventing the occurrence or shortening the course of infant botulism. On the other hand, antibiotic-induced lysis of *C. botulinum* organisms might result in the release and subsequent absorption of increased amounts of toxin as is suggested by the higher rate of respiratory failure in infants with infant botulism who have been treated with aminoglycoside antibiotics.[140] Antibiotic prophylaxis for a contaminated wound is indicated for reasons other than the prevention of botulism and cannot substitute for thorough cleansing and debridement. Wound botulism has occurred in patients undergoing treatment with antibiotics that are effective against *C. botulinum* in *in vitro* tests.

Botulinal toxoid is available and effective for active immunization.[19,49,50] However, because of the rarity of botulism in the general population and the side effects of imunization, toxoid administration is recommended only for laboratory personnel working directly with the organism and the toxin. The toxoid is available from CDC.

9.2. Treatment

The mainstays of treatment of foodborne and wound botulism are as follows: (1) administration of botulinal antitoxin in an attempt to prevent neurologic progression of a moderate, slowly progressive illness or to shorten the duration of ventilatory failure in those with a severe, rapidly progressive illness; and (2) careful monitoring of respiratory vital capacity and aggressive respiratory care for those with ventilatory insufficiency.

Antitoxin therapy is more effective if undertaken early in the course of illness.[108,129] This is not surprising when one considers that equine antitoxin neutralizes only toxin molecules yet unbound to nerve endings.[127] If passive immunization is indicated, trivalent equine antitoxin (anti-A, -B, and -E in combination) is recommended and is available free to patients from CDC through state health departments. Most cases (more than 80%) of adult botulism in the United States are treated with antitoxin, while few of the affected infants have been given the product[106] because of early observations that serum toxin was not detected in such cases. Administration of two vials of trivalent botulism antitoxin by the intravenous or intramuscular route results in serum levels of type A, B, and E antibodies capable of neutralizing serum toxin concentrations manyfold in excess of those reported for botulism patients; the circulating antitoxins have a half-life of 5 to 8 days.[61] However, treatment is not without risk, as approximately 9.0% of persons treated experience hypersensitivity reactions.[13] It is therefore extremely important that physicians recognize botulism as early in its course as possible, and yet not mistake other neurologic syndromes for botulism.

10. Unresolved Problems

Much is now known concerning the epidemiologic and clinical aspects of adult forms of botulism. The most prominent persisting problem may be the low index of suspicion for botulism among clinicians who are unlikely to diagnose even one case in a career. The development of laboratory tests more rapid than, but equally as sensitive and specific as, the mouse neutralization assay would be helpful in diagnosing and treating this illness, but is unlikely to take place soon. The development of an antitoxin derived from human serum or by DNA hybridization techniques could provide an approach to antitoxin therapy that is safer (because less likely to cause hypersensitivity reactions than equine antitoxin) and perhaps less expensive. Although the clinical spectrum of illness and descriptive epidemiology of infant botulism have been well characterized in the few years since its discovery, specific risk factors and vehicles of transmission remain obscure for most cases. Controlled epidemiologic studies are needed to further clarify ways of preventing this important source of childhood morbidity. The recent demonstration in some adults of a pathogenic mechanism similar to that of infant botulism blurs somewhat the distinction between adult and infant forms of the disease, and may initiate reconsideration of pathogenesis and treatment in both groups. Finally, the recent discovery of clostridia other than *C. botulinum* that may produce botulinal toxin has further aggravated the taxonomic inconsistencies in this group of organisms, and may finally precipitate a taxonomic reclassification of botulinogenic organisms.

11. References

1. ARNON, S. S., Infant botulism, in: *Clostridia in Gastrointestinal Disease* (S. P. BORRIELLO, ed.), pp. 39–57, CRC Press, Boca Raton, 1985.
2. ARNON, S. S., AND CHIN, J., The clinical spectrum of infant botulism, *Rev. Infect. Dis.* **1**:614–621 (1979).
3. ARNON, S. S., MIDURA, T. F., AND CLAY, S. A., Infant botulism: Epidemiological, clinical, and laboratory aspects, *J. Am. Med. Assoc.* **237**:1946–1951 (1977).
4. ARNON, S. S., MIDURA, T. F., DAMUS, K., WOO, R. M., AND CHIN, J., Intestinal infection and toxin production by *Clostridium botulinum* as one cause of sudden infant death syndrome, *Lancet* **1**:1273–1277 (1978).
5. ARNON, S. S., MIDURA, T. F., AND DAMUS, K., Honey and other environmental risk factors for infant botulism, *J. Pediatr.* **94**:331–336 (1979).

6. ARNON, S. S., DAMUS, K., THOMPSON, B., MIDURA, T. F., AND CHIN, J., Protective role of human milk against sudden death from infant botulism, *J. Pediatr.* **100:**568–573 (1982).

7. AURELI, P., FENICIA, L., PASOLINI, B., GIAFRANCESCHI, M., MCCROSKEY, L. M., AND HATHEWAY, C. L., Two cases of type E infant botulism caused by neurotoxigenic *Clostridium butyricum* in Italy, *J. Infect. Dis.* **154:**207–211 (1986).

8. BADHEY, H., CLERI, D. J., D'AMATO, R. F., VERNALEO, J. R., VEINNI, V., TESSLER, J., WALLMAN, A. A., MASTELLONE, A. J., GIULIANI, M., AND HOCHSTEIN, L., Two fatal cases of type E adult food-borne botulism with early symptoms and terminal neurologic signs, *J. Clin. Microbiol.* **23:**616–618 (1986).

9. BAIRD-PARKER, A. C., AND FREAME, B., Combined effect of water activity, pH, and temperature on the growth of *Clostridium botulinum* from spores and vegetative cell inocula, *J. Appl. Bacteriol.* **30:**420–429 (1967).

10. BARKER, W. H., WEISSMAN, J. B., DOWELL, V. R., GUTMAN, L., AND KAUTTER, D. A., Type B botulism outbreak caused by a commercial food product, *J. Am. Med. Assoc.* **237:**456–459 (1977).

11. BENGSTON, U. A., Preliminary note on a toxin producing anaerobe isolated from the larvae of *Lucilla caesar*, *Public Health Rep.* **37:**164–170 (1922).

12. BLACK, R. E., AND ARNON, S. S., Botulism in the United States, 1976, *J. Infect. Dis.* **136:**829–832 (1977).

13. BLACK, R. E., AND GUNN, R. A., Hypersensitivity reactions associated with botulinal antitoxin, *Am. J. Med.* **69:**567–570 (1980).

14. BOROFF, D. A., AND SHU-CHEN, G., Radioimmunoassay for type A toxin of *Clostridium botulinum*, *Appl. Microbiol.* **25:**545–549 (1973).

15. BURKE, G. S., The occurrence of *Bacillus botulinus* in nature, *J. Bacteriol.* **4:**541–553 (1919).

16. BURKE, G. S., Notes on *Bacillus botulinus*, *J. Bacteriol.* **4:**555–565 (1919).

17. BURR, D. H., AND SUGIYAMA, H., Susceptibility to enteric botulinum colonization of antibiotic-treated adult mice, *Infect. Immun.* **36:**103–106 (1982).

18. California Department of Health Services, Type A botulism associated with commercial pot pie, *California Morbidity,* December 30, 1976 (51).

19. CARDELLA, M. A., Botulinum toxoids, in: *Botulism* (K. H. Lewis and K. Cassel, eds.), U.S. Public Health Service, Cincinnati, 1964.

20. CATO, E. P., GEORGE, W. L., AND FINEGOLD, S. M., Genus *Clostridium*, in: *Bergey's Manual of Systematic Bacteriology,* Volume 2 (P. H. A. SNEATH, N. S. MAIR, M. E. SHARPE, AND J. G. HOLD, eds.), pp. 1141–1200, Williams & Wilkins, Baltimore, 1986.

21. Centers for Disease Control, Botulism—Kentucky, *Morbid. Mortal. Weekly Rep.* **22:**417 (1973).

22. Centers for Disease Control, Follow-up: Botulism associated with commercial cherry peppers, *Morbid. Mortal. Weekly Rep.* **25:**148 (1976).

23. Centers for Disease Control, Botulism in the United States, 1899–1973: Handbook for Epidemiologists, Clinicians, and Laboratory Workers, p. 3 (1978).

24. Centers for Disease Control, Botulism from fresh foods—California, *Morbid. Mortal. Weekly Rep.* **34:**156–157 (1985).

25. CHERINGTON, M., Botulism: Ten-year experience, *Arch. Neurol.* **30:**432–437 (1974).

26. CHERINGTON, M., AND GINSBERG, S., Type B botulism: Neurophysiologic studies, *Neurology* **21:**43–46 (1971).

27. CHIA, J. K., CLARK, J. B., RYAN, C. A., AND POLLACK, M., Botulism in an adult associated with foodborne intestinal infection with *Clostridium botulinum*, *N. Engl. J. Med.* **315:**239–241 (1986).

28. CHIN, J., ARNON, S. S., AND MIDURA, T. F., Food and environmental aspects of infant botulism in California, *Rev. Infect. Dis.* **1:**693–696 (1979).

29. CLAY, S. A., RAMSEYER, J. D., FISHJMAN, L. S., AND SEDGWICK, R. P., Acute infantile motor unit disorder: Infant botulism, *Arch. Neurol.* **34:**236–243 (1977).

30. CORNBLATH, D. R., SLADSKY, J. T., AND SUMNER, A. J., Clinical electrophysiology of infantile botulism, *Muscle Nerve* **6:**448–452 (1983).

31. DAVIS, B. D., DULBECCO, R., EISEN, H. N., AND WOOD, W. B., *Microbiology,* pp. 672–674, Harper & Row, New York, 1967.

32. DAVIS, B. D., DULBECCO, R., EISEN, H. N., AND WOOD, W. B., *Microbiology,* pp. 828–831, Harper & Row, New York, 1967.

33. DAVIS, J. B., MATTMAN, L. H., AND WILEY, M., *Clostridium botulinum* in a fatal wound infection, *J. Am. Med. Assoc.* **146:**646–648 (1951).

34. DICKSON, E. C., Botulism: A clinical and experimental study, Rockefeller Inst. Med. Res. Monogr. No. 8, pp. 1–117 (1918).

35. DOLMAN, C. E., DARBY, G. E., AND LANE, R. F., Type E botulism due to salmon eggs, *Can. J. Public Health* **46:**135–141 (1955).

36. DOLMAN, C. E., TOMISCH, M., CAMPBELL, C. C. R., AND LAING, W. B., Fish eggs as a cause of human botulism: Two outbreaks in British Columbia due to type E and B botulinal toxins, *J. Infect. Dis.* **106:**5–19 (1960).

37. DONADIO, J. A., GANGAROSA, E. J., AND FAICH, G. A., Diagnosis and treatment of botulism, *J. Infect. Dis.* **124:**108–112 (1971).

38. DOWELL, V. R., AND HAWKINS, T. M., *Laboratory Methods in Anaerobic Bacteriology: CDC Laboratory Manual,* Centers for Disease Control, Atlanta, 1974.

39. DOWELL, V. R., MCCROSKEY, L. M., HATHEWAY, C. L., LOMBARD, G. L., HUGHES, J. M., AND MERSON, M. H., Coproexamination for botulinal toxin and *Clostridium botulinum*, *J. Am. Med. Assoc.* **238:**1829–1832 (1977).

40. EISEL, V., JARAUSCH, W., GORETSKY, K., HENSCHEN, A., ENGELS, J., WELLER, V., HABERMANN, E., AND NEIMANN, H., Tetanus toxin: Primary structure, expression in *E. coli*, and homology with botulinum toxins, *EMBO J.* **5:**2495–2502 (1986).

41. EISENBERG, M., AND BENDER, T. R., Botulism in Alaska, 1947 through 1974, *J. Am. Med. Assoc.* **235:**35–38 (1976).

42. EKLUND, M. W., POYSKY, F. T., AND BOATMAN, E. J., Bacteriophages of *Clostridium botulinum* types A, B, E, and F and nontoxigenic strains resembling type E, *J. Virol.* **3:**270–274 (1969).

43. EKLUND, M. W., POYSKY, F. T., REED, S. M., AND SMITH, C. A., Bacteriophage and the toxigenicity of *Clostridium botulinum* type C, *Science* **172:**480–482 (1971).

44. EL BISI, H. M., Radiation death kinetics of *C. botulinum* spores at cryogenic temperatures, in: *Botulism 1966* (M. Ingram and T. A. Roberts, eds.), pp. 89–107, Chapman & Hall, London, 1967.

45. ENGEL, W. K., Brief, small, abundant motor unit potentials, *Neurology* **25:**173–176 (1975).

46. *Federal Register,* Thermally processed low-acid foods packaged in hermetically sealed containers: Manufacture and processing, 38, No. 16, pp. 2398–2410, Jan. 24, 1973.

47. *Federal Register,* Thermally processed low-acid foods packaged in hermetically sealed containers: Records retention requirements, 39, No. 20, p. 3754, Jan. 24, 1974.

48. *Federal Register,* Thermally processed low-acid foods packaged in hermetically sealed containers: Miscellaneous amendments, 39, No. 63, p. 11,876, April 1, 1974.

49. FIOCK, M. A., DEVINE, L. F., GEARINGER, N. F., DUFF, J. T., WRIGHT, G. G., AND KADULL, P. J., Studies on immunity to toxins of *Clostridium botulinum*. VIII. Immunological response of man to purified bivalent AB botulinum toxoid, *J. Immunol.* **8:**277 (1962).

50. FIOCK, M. A., CARDELLA, M. A., AND GEARINGER, N. F., Studies on immunity to toxins of *Clostridium botulinum*. IX. Immunologic response of man to purified pentavalent A, B, C, D, E botulinum toxoid, *J. Immunol.* **90:**697–702 (1963).

51. GANGAROSA, E. J., DONADIO, J. A., ARMSTRONG, R. W., MEYER, K. F., BRACHMAN, P. S., AND DOWELL, V. R., Botulism in the United States, 1899–1969, *Am. J. Epidemiol.* **93:**93–100 (1971).

52. GIMENEZ, D. F., AND CICCARELLI, A. S., Another type of *Clostridium botulinum, Zentralbl. Bakteriol. Parasitenkd. Infektionskr. Hyg. Abt. 1* **215:**212–220 (1970).

53. GLASBY, C., AND HATHEWAY, C. L., Evaluation of fluorescent antibody tests as a means of confirming infant botulism, *J. Clin. Microbiol.* **20:**1209–1212 (1984).

54. GUNN, R. A., AND TERRANOVA, W. A., Botulism in the United States, 1977, *Rev. Infect. Dis.* **1:**722–725 (1979).

55. GUNNISON, J. B., CUMMINGS, J. R., AND MEYER, K. F., *Clostridium botulinum* type E, *Proc. Soc. Exp. Biol. Med.* **35:**278–280 (1936–1937).

56. GUTMAN, L., Pathophysiologic aspects of human botulism, *Arch. Neurol.* **33:**975–979 (1976).

57. GUYTON, A. C., AND MACDONALD, M. A., Physiology of botulinus toxin, *Arch. Neurol. Psychiatry* **57:**578–591 (1947).

58. HALL, J. D., MCCROSKEY, L. M., PINCOMB, B. J., AND HATHEWAY, C. L., Isolation of an organism resembling *Clostridium barati* which produces type F botulinal toxin from an infant with botulism, *J. Clin. Microbiol.* **21:**654–655 (1985).

59. HATHEWAY, C. L., Botulism, in: *Laboratory Diagnosis of Infectious Diseases: Principles and Practice,* Volume 1 (A. BALOWS, W. J. HAUSLER, JR., M. OHASHI, AND A. TURANO, eds.), pp. 111–133, Springer-Verlag, Berlin, 1988.

60. HATHEWAY, C. L., AND MCCROSKEY, L. M., Examination of feces and serum for diagnosis of infant botulism in 336 patients, *J. Clin. Microbiol.* **25:**2334–2338 (1987).

61. HATHEWAY, C. L., SNYDER, J. D., SEALS, J. D., SEALS, J. E., EDELL, T. A., AND LEWIS, G. E., Antitoxin levels in botulism patients treated with trivalent equine botulism antitoxin to toxin types A, B, and E, *J. Infect. Dis.* **150:**407–412 (1984).

62. HAUSCHILD, A. H. W., AND GAUVREAU, L., Food-borne botulism in Canada, 1971–84, *Can. Med. Assoc. J.* **133:**1141–1146 (1985).

63. Health and Welfare Canada, Restaurant-associated botulism from in-house bottled mushrooms—British Columbia, *Can. Dis. Weekly Rep.* **13:**35–36 (1987).

64. HOFFMAN, R. E., PINCOMB, B. J., SKEELS, M. R., AND BURKHART, M. J., Type F botulism, *Am. J. Dis. Child.* **136:**270–271 (1982).

65. HORWITZ, M. A., MARR, J. S., MERSON, M. H., DOWELL, V. R., AND ELLIS, J. M., A continuing common-source outbreak of botulism in a family, *Lancet* **1:**1–6 (1975).

66. HORWITZ, M. A., HUGHES, J. M., MERSON, M. H., AND GANGAROSA, E. J., Foodborne botulism in the United States, 1970–1975, *J. Infect. Dis.* **136:**153–159 (1977).

67. HUGHES, J. M., BLUMENTHAL, J. R., MERSON, M. H., LOMBARD, G. L., DOWELL, V. R., AND GANGAROSA, E. J., Clinical features of types A and B food-borne botulism, *Ann. Intern. Med.* **95:**442–445 (1981).

68. IIDA, H., Epidemiological and clinical observations of botulism outbreaks in Japan, In: *Proceedings of the First U.S.–Japan Conference on Toxic Microorganisms* (M. HERZBERG, ed.), pp. 357–359, U.S. Department of the Interior, Washington, D.C. 1970.

69. ISTRE, G. R., COMPTON, R., NOVOTNY, T., YOUNG, J. E., HATHEWAY, C. L., AND HOPKINS, R. S., Infant botulism: Three cases in a small town, *Am. J. Dis. Child.* **140:**1013–1014 (1986).

70. ITO, K. A., SESLAR, D. J., ERCERN, W. A., AND MEYER, K. F., The thermal and chlorine resistance of *Clostridium botulinum* types A, B, and E spores, in: *Botulism 1966* (M. Ingram and T. A. Roberts, eds.), pp. 108–122, Chapman & Hall, London, 1967.

71. JOHNSON, H. M., BRENNER, K., ANGELOTTI, R., AND HALL, H. E., Serological studies of types A, B, and E bot-

ulinal toxins by passive hemagglutination and bentonite floc-culation, *J. Bacteriol.* **91**:967–974 (1966).

72. JOHNSON, R. O., CLAY, S. A., AND ARNON, S. S., Diagnosis and management of infant botulism, *Am. J. Dis. Child.* **133**:586–593 (1979).

73. KAO, I., DRACHMAN, D. B., AND PRICE, D. L., Botulinum toxin: Mechanism of presynaptic blockade, *Science* **193**:1245–1258 (1976).

74. KAUTTER, D. A., LILLY, T., SOLOMON, H. M., AND LYNT, R. K., *Clostridium botulinum* spores in infant foods: A survey, *J. Food Protection* **45**:1028–1029 (1982).

75. KERNER, C. A. J., Neue Beobachtungen uber die in Wurttenbergso haufig vorfallenden todichen Vergiftungen durch in den Genuss geraucherter Wurste, Tübingen, 1829; cited in Dickson.[(34)]

76. KIMURA, J., *Electrodiagnosis in Diseases of Nerve and Muscle,* Davis, Philadelphia, 1983.

77. KOENIG, G. M., SPICKARD, A., CARDELLA, M. A., AND ROGERS, D. E., Clinical and laboratory observations on type B botulism in man, *Medicine* **43**:517–545 (1964).

78. KOENIG, G. M., DRUTZ, D. J., MUSHLIN, A. I., SCHAFFNER, W., AND ROGERS, D. E., Type B botulism in man, *Am. J. Med.* **42**:209–219 (1967).

79. LANDMAN, G., Ueber die Urasche der Darmstadter Bohnenvergiftung, *Hyg. Rundsch.* **10**:449–452 (1904).

80. LENCHS, J., Beitrage zur Kenntnis des Toxins und Antitoxins des *Bacillus botulinus, Z. Hyg. Infektionskr.* **65**:55–84 (1910).

81. L'HOMMEDIEU, C., STOUGH, R., AND BROWN, L., Potentiation of neuromuscular weakness in infant botulism by aminogylcosides, *J. Pediatr.* **95**:1065–1070 (1979).

82. LIU HONGDAO, Epidemiological and clinical analysis of 25 outbreaks of botulism, *Chin. J. Prev. Med.* **17**:195–197 (1983).

83. LONG, S. S., Epidemiologic study of infant botulism in Pennsylvania, *Pediatrics* **75**:928–934 (1985).

84. LONG, S. S., GAJEWSKI, J. L., BROWN, L. W., AND GILLIGAN, P. H., Clinical, laboratory, and environmental features of infant botulism in southeastern Pennsylvania, *Pediatrics* **75**:935–941 (1985).

85. LYNT, R. K., SOLOMAN, H. M., AND KAUTTER, D. A., Immunofluorescence among strains of *Clostridium botulinum* and other clostridia by direct and indirect methods, *J. Food Sci.* **36**:594–599 (1971).

86. MACDONALD, K. L., SPENGLER, R. F., HATHEWAY, C. L., HARGRETT, N. T., AND COHEN, M. L., Type A botulism from sauteed onions, *J. Am. Med. Assoc.* **253**:1275–1278 (1985).

87. MACDONALD, K. L., RUTHERFORD, G. W., FRIEDMAN, S. M., DIETZ, J. R., KAYE, B. R., MCKINLEY, G. F., TENNEY, J. H., AND COHEN, M. L., Botulism and botulism-like illness in chronic drug abusers, *Ann. Intern. Med.* **102**:616–618 (1985).

88. MACDONALD, K. L., COHEN, M. L., AND BLAKE, P. A., The changing epidemiology of adult botulism in the United States, *Am. J. Epidemiol.* **124**:794–799 (1986).

89. MACLENNAN, J. D., Anaerobic infection of war wounds in the Middle East, *Lancet* **2**:63–66 (1943).

90. MANN, J. M., MARTIN, S., HOFFMAN, R. E., AND MARRAZZO, S., Patient recovery from type A botulism: Morbidity assessment following a large outbreak, *Am. J. Public Health* **71**:266–269 (1981).

91. MANN, J. M., HATHEWAY, C. L., AND GARDINER, T. M., Laboratory diagnosis in a large outbreak of type A botulism. Confirmation of the value of coproexamination, *Am. J. Epidemiol.* **115**:598–605 (1982).

92. MANN, J. M., LATHROP, G. D., AND BANNERMAN, J. A., Economic impact of a botulism outbreak. Importance of the legal component in food-borne disease, *J. Am. Med. Assoc.* **249**:1299–1301 (1983).

93. MAYHEN, J. W., AND GORBACH, S. L., Rapid gas chromatographic technique for presumptive detection of *Clostridium botulinum* in contaminated food, *Appl. Microbiol.* **29**:297–299 (1975).

94. MCCROSKEY, L. M., AND HATHEWAY, C. L, Laboratory findings in adult botulism cases that suggest colonization of the intestinal tract, in: *Abstracts of the 86th Annual Meeting of the American Society for Microbiology,* p. 275, American Society for Microbiology, Washington, D.C., 1986.

95. MCCROSKEY, L. M., HATHEWAY, C. L., FENICIA, L., PASOLINI, B., AND AURELI, P., Characterization of an organism that produces type E botulinal toxin but which resembles *Clostridium butyricum* from the feces of an infant with type E botulism, *J. Clin. Microbiol.* **23**:201–202 (1986).

96. MERSON, M. H., AND DOWELL, V. R., Epidemiologic, clinical, and laboratory aspects of wound botulism, *N. Engl. J. Med.* **289**:1005–1010 (1973).

97. MESTRAMDEA, L. W., Rapid detection of *Clostridium botulinum* toxin by capillary tube diffusion, *Appl. Microbiol.* **27**:1017–1022 (1974).

98. MEYER, K. F., AND DUBOVSKY, B. J., The distribution of the spores of *B. botulinus* in California, *J. Infect. Dis.* **31**:541–555 (1922).

99. MEYER, K. F., AND GUNNISON, J. B., *Cl. botulinum* type D, sp. Nov., *Proc. Soc. Exp. Biol. Med.* **26**:88–89 (1928).

100. MIDURA, T. F., AND ARNON, S. S., Infant botulism: Identification of *Clostridium botulinum* and its toxin in faeces, *Lancet* **2**:934–936 (1976).

101. MIDURA, T. F., TACLINDO, C., NYGAARD, G. S., BODILY, H. L., AND WOOD, R. M., Use of immunofluorescence and animal tests to detect growth and toxin production by *Clostridium botulinum* in food, *Appl. Microbiol.* **16**:102–105 (1968).

102. MILLER, C. A., AND ANDERSON, A. W., Rapid detection and quantitative estimation of type A botulinum toxin by electroimmunodiffusion, *Infect. Immunol.* **4**:126–129 (1971).

103. MITSUI, N., KIRITANI, K., AND NISHIDA, S., A lysin(s) in lysates of *Clostridium botulinum* A190 induced by ultraviolet ray or mitomycin C, *Jpn. J. Microbiol.* **17**:353–360 (1973).

104. MOBERG, L. J., AND SUGIYAMA, H., Microbial ecological

basis of infant botulism as studied with germfree mice, *Infect. Immunol.* **25:**653–657 (1979).

105. MOLLER, V., AND SCHEIBEL, I., Preliminary report on the isolation of an apparently new type *Clostridium botulinum, Acta Pathol. Microbiol. Scand.* **48:**80 (1960).

106. MORRIS, J. G., JR., Current trends in therapy of botulism in the United States, in: *Biomedical Aspects of Botulism* (G. E. LEWIS, JR., ed.), pp. 317–326, Academic Press, New York, 1981.

107. MORRIS, J. G., SNYDER, J. D., WILSON, R., AND FELDMAN, R. A., Infant botulism in the United States: An epidemiologic study of the cases occurring outside California, *Am. J. Public Health* **73:**1385–1388 (1983).

108. ONO, T., KANASHIMADA, T., AND IIDA, H., Studies on the serum therapy of type E botulism (part III), *Jpn. J. Med. Sci. Biol.* **23:**177 (1970).

109. PICKETT, J., BERG, B., CHAPLIN, E., AND BRUNSTETTER-SHAFER, M., Syndrome of botulism in infancy, *N. Engl. J. Med.* **295:**770–772 (1976).

110. PIVNICK, H., JOHNSTON, M. A., THACKER, C., AND RUBIN, L. J., Effect of nitrite on destruction and germination of *Clostridium botulinum* and putrefactive anaerobes 3679 and 3679h in meat and in buffer, *Can. Inst. Food Technol. J.* **3:**103–109 (1970).

111. ROBERTS, T. A., AND HOBBS, G., Low temperature growth characteristics of clostridia, *J. Appl. Bacteriol.* **31:**75–88 (1968).

112. ROBERTS, T. A., AND INGRAM, M., Radiation resistance of spores of *Clostridium* species in aquaeous suspension, *Food Sci.* **30:**879–885 (1965).

113. ROBERTS, T. A., AND INGRAM, M., The resistance of spores of *Clostridium botulinum* type E to heat and radiation, *J. Appl. Bacteriol.* **28:**125–137 (1965).

114. RUSTIGIAN, R., AND CIPRIANI, A., The bacteriology of open wounds, *J. Am. Med. Assoc.* **133:**224–230 (1947).

115. SAKAGUCHI, G. S., SAKAGUCHI, S., KOZAKI, S., SUGII, S., AND OHISHI, I., Cross reaction in reversed passive hemagglutination between *Clostridium botulinum* type A and B toxins and its avoidance by the use of antitoxic component immunoglobin isolated by affinity chromatography, *Jpn. J. Med. Sci. Biol.* **27:**161–172 (1974).

116. SCHROEDER, K., AND TALLEFSRUD, A., Botulism from fermented trout, *Tidsskr. Nor. Laegeforen.* **82:**1084 (1962).

117. SEALS, J. E., SNYDER, J. D., EDELL, T. A., HATHEWAY, C. L., JOHNSON, C. J., SWANSON, R. C., AND HUGHES, J. M., Restaurant-associated type A botulism: Transmission by potato salad, *Am. J. Epidemiol.* **113:**436–444 (1981).

118. SEBALD, M., AND SAIMONT, G., Toxemie botulique. Interet de sa mise en evidence dans le diagnostic du botulisme humain de type B, *Ann. Microbiol. (Inst. Pasteur)* **124:**61–69 (1973).

119. SEGNER, W. P., AND SCHMIDT, C. F., Resistance of spores of marine and terrestrial strains of *Clostridium botulinum* type C, *Appl. Microbiol.* **22:**1030–1033 (1971).

120. SELLIN, L. C., THESLEFF, S., AND DASGUPTA, B. R., Different effects of types A and B botulinum toxin on transmitter release at the rat neuromuscular junction, *Acta Physiol. Scand.* **119:**127–133 (1983).

121. SHIELD, L. K., WILKINSON, R. G., AND RITCHIE, M., Infant botulism in Australia, *Med. J. Aust.* **1:**157 (1978).

122. SHIH, Y., AND CHAO, S., Botulism in China, *Rev. Infect. Dis.* **8:**984–990 (1986).

123. SHONE, C., WILTON-SMITH, P., APPLETON, N., HAMBLETON, P., MODI, N., GATLEY, S., AND MELLING, J., Monoclonal antibody-based immunoassay for type A *Clostridium botulinum* toxin is comparable to the mouse bioassay, *Appl. Environ. Microbiol.* **50:**63–67 (1985).

124. SMITH, L. D., *Botulism: The Organism, Its Toxins, the Disease,* pp. 15–33, Thomas, Springfield, Ill., 1977.

125. SMITH, L. D., The occurrence of *Clostridium botulinum* and *Clostridium tetani* in the soil of the United States, *Health Lab. Sci.* **15:**74–80 (1978).

126. ST. LOUIS, M. E., PECK, S. H., BOWERING, D., MORGAN, B., MILLING, M., KETTYLS, D., BLACK, W. A., TAUXE, R. V., AND BLAKE, P. A., Botulism from chopped garlic: Delayed recognition of a major outbreak, *Ann. Intern. Med.* **108:**363–368 (1988).

127. SUGIYAMA, H., *Clostridium botulinum* neurotoxin, *Microbiol. Rev.* **44:**419–448 (1980).

128. SUGIYAMA, H., AND MILLS, D. C., Intraintestinal toxin in infant mice challenged with *Clostridium botulinum* spores, *Infect. Immun.* **21:**59–63 (1978).

129. TACKETT, C. O., SHANDERA, W. X., MANN, J. M., HARGRETT, N. T., AND BLAKE, P. A., Equine antitoxin use and other factors that predict outcome in type A foodborne botulism, *Am. J. Med.* **76:**794–798 (1984).

130. TERRANOVA, W. A., BREMAN, J. G., LOCEY, R. P., AND SPECK, S., Botulism type B: Epidemiologic aspects of an extensive outbreak, *Am. J. Epidemiol.* **108:**150–156 (1978).

131. TERRANOVA, W. A., PALUMBO, J. N., AND BREMAN, J. G., Ocular findings in botulism type B, *J. Am. Med. Assoc.* **241:**475–477 (1979).

132. THOMPSON, J. A., GLASGOW, L. A., AND WARPINSKI, J. R., Infant botulism: Clinical spectrum and epidemiology, *Pediatrics* **66:**936–942 (1980).

133. TURNER, H. D., BRETT, E. M., GILBERT, R. J., CHOSH, A. C., AND LIEBSCHUETZ, H. J., Infant botulism in England, *Lancet* **1:**1277–1278 (1978).

134. United States Department of Agriculture, Home Canning of Fruits and Vegetables, Home and Garden Bulletin No. 8 (1975).

135. VAN ERMENGEM, E., Ueber einen neuen anaeroben Bacillus und seine Beziehungen zum Botulisms, *Z. Hyg. Infektionskr.* **26:**1–56 (1897).

136. VERMILYEA, B. L., WALKER, H. W., AND AYERS, J. C., Detection of botulinal toxins by immunodiffusion, *Appl. Microbiol.* **16:**21–24 (1968).

137. WAINWRIGHT, R. B., HEYWARD, W. L., MIDDAUGH, J. P.,

HATHEWAY, C. L., HARPSTER, A. P., AND BENDER, T. R., Food-borne botulism in Alaska, 1947–1985:Epidemiology and clinical findings, *J. Infect. Dis.* **157**:1158–1162 (1988).

138. WANG, Y., AND SUGIYAMA, H., Botulism in metronidazole-treated conventional adult mice challenged orogastrically with spores of *Clostridium botulinum* type A or B, *Infect. Immun.* **46**:715–719 (1984).

139. WELLS, C. L., SUGIYAMA, H., AND BLAND, S. E., Resistance of mice with limited intestinal flora to enteric colonization by *Clostridium botulinum*, *J. Infect. Dis.* **146**:791–796 (1982).

140. WILSON, R., MORRIS, J. G., SNYDER, J. D., AND FELDMAN, R. A., Clinical characteristics of infant botulism in the United States: A study of the non-California cases, *Pediatr. Infect. Dis.* **1**:148–150 (1982).

141. ZEZONES, H., AND HUTCHINGS, I. J., Thermal resistance of *Clostridium botulinum* (62A) spores as affected by fundamental food constituents, *Food Technol.* **19**:1003–1005 (1965).

12. Suggested Reading

ARNON, S. S., MIDURA, T. F., AND CLAY, S. A., Infant botulism: Epidemiological, clinical and laboratory aspects, *J. Am. Med. Assoc.* **237**:1946–1951 (1977).

Centers for Disease Control, Botulism in the United States, 1899–1977: Handbook for Epidemiologists, Clinicians, and Laboratory Workers (1978).

HATHEWAY, C. L., Botulism, in: *Laboratory Diagnosis of Infectious Diseases: Principles and Practice,* Volume 1 (A. BALOWS, W. J. HAUSLER, JR., M. OHASHI, AND A. TURANO, eds.), pp. 111–133, Springer-Verlag, Berlin, 1988).

MERSON, M. H., AND DOWELL, V. R., Epidemiologic, clinical, and laboratory aspects of wound botulism, *N. Engl. J. Med.* **289**:1005–1010 (1973).

SMITH, L. D., *Botulism: The Organism, Its Toxins, the Disease,* Thomas, Springfield, Ill., 1977.

CHAPTER 6

Brucellosis

Wendell H. Hall

1. Introduction

Brucellosis (undulant fever, Mediterranean fever, Malta fever, Bang's disease) is one of several zoonoses, a disease of animals transmissible to man.[94] The disease is caused by gram-negative bacilli of the genus *Brucella*. There are several species that cause human infections as well as animal brucellosis: *Brucella abortus* (cattle), *B. suis* (hogs), *B. melitensis* (goats, sheep), *B. canis* (dogs), and *B. rangiferi tarandi–B. suis*, biotype 4 (reindeer, caribou) (Table 1). *B. ovis* infects sheep and *B. neotomae* is found in desert wood rats, but neither species appears to cause human disease. Pregnant animals often have placentitis, and hence they may abort. The mammary gland is frequently involved in infected mammals, and the organism is usually present in their milk. Acute brucellosis in man is characterized by irregular fever, chills, sweats, and weakness. Chronic human brucellosis is often marked by fever, weakness, anxiety, and depression. There may be widespread granulomas in lymph nodes, bone marrow, liver, and spleen, as well as abscesses in bones, liver, spleen, kidneys, or brain. The public health importance of brucellosis in many countries is significant owing to economic losses from abortions in domestic animals and declining milk and meat production. The human disease is not contagious and causes few deaths. It does cause considerable debility, especially among people exposed either directly to infected animals or through ingestion of fresh milk or cheese.

Wendell H. Hall · Research Service, Veterans Administration Medical Center, Minneapolis, and Departments of Medicine and Microbiology, University of Minnesota Medical School, Minneapolis, Minnesota 55455.

2. Historical Background

In 1861 J. A. Marston wrote the first account of human brucellosis, describing his own symptoms while he served as a surgeon in the British Army Medical Service on the island of Malta.[80] The disease was then called Mediterranean gastric remittent fever. Surgeon David Bruce, also working on Malta, examined the spleen in five fatal cases, and in 1887 he briefly described methods for staining and cultivating the causative organisms on agar.[16] Because of their small size, Bruce called them micrococci. He also produced a fatal infection in an inoculated monkey and isolated the micrococci from its liver and spleen. The organism has since been named *Brucella* in his honor and the disease is called brucellosis. In 1897 surgeon M. L. Hughes in a book entitled *Mediterranean, Malta or Undulant Fever* wrote a description of the clinical course and pathology of human brucellosis in Malta.[61] Also in 1897 Professor A. E. Wright and D. Semple described the serum agglutination test using killed cultures of Bruce's "micrococci" as antigen to serologically separate brucellosis from typhoid fever.[129]

The British Army Medical Department soon thereafter established a Mediterranean Fever Commission. The members served on Malta from 1905 to 1907 and issued a series of seven reports. Dr. T. Zammit, a civilian employee of the Commission, discovered that nearly half the goats on Malta had agglutinins for *Brucella* in their serum. Horrocks, Zammit, and Kennedy found the typical "micrococci" in the blood, milk, and urine of Maltese goats. Zammit also fed *Brucella* to a healthy goat and reproduced the disease. In 1907 the link between the ingestion of fresh milk from Maltese goats and human brucellosis was convincingly demonstrated in a shipboard epidemic among the crew of the SS Joshua Nicholson.[87] Sixty-five goats were pur-

133

chased in Malta and shipped to New York via Antwerp. Nearly all the crew who drank fresh milk from the goats became ill with undulant fever. The serum agglutination test was positive in 32 goats and several had *Brucella* cultivated from their milk. The first proved human cases of brucellosis contracted in the United States were reported from Texas in 1911 by Gentry and Ferenbaugh.[40] They studied two patients who had been in contact with sick goats. *B. melitensis* was isolated from the patients' blood cultures.

In 1895 Professor B. Bang in Copenhagen first described *B. abortus* as the cause of contagious abortion in cattle.[7] Abortion was ascribed to placental infection with copious gelatinous exudate between the fetal membranes and uterine wall. Myriads of gram-negative bacilli were found within cells in the exudate. The bacilli grew on a serum gelatin agar if the atmospheric oxygen concentration was carefully adjusted. Using his cultures Bang reproduced the disease in pregnant heifers. In 1919 Theobold Smith discovered that the characteristic placentitis in the aborting cow was due to the presence of swarms of *B. abortus* within the cytoplasm of the fetal chorionic epithelium of the infected placenta.[112] Schroeder and Cotton in 1911 found *B. abortus* in the milk of apparently healthy cows in the United States (District of Columbia).[109] Morales-Otero had difficulty infecting healthy people fed *B. abortus* in pasteurized milk.[88] Normal adult subjects became infected when *B. abortus* was rubbed on abraded skin, but not when the skin was intact. In 1918 Alice Evans recognized the close resemblance of *B. abortus* to *B. melitensis* and suggested that human disease might result from drinking cows' milk containing *B. abortus*.[37]

The first isolation of *B. suis* was made from an aborted pig fetus by Jacob Traum in 1914.[86] The resemblance of the organism to *B. abortus* was noted. In 1931 Hardy *et al.*[52] reported on 300 patients with brucellosis in Iowa, including 35 cases caused by *B. suis*. They showed that human infections arose from contact with infected pigs. *B. suis* was more virulent than *B. abortus* in man.

The history of *B. canis* has been reviewed by the author in detail elsewhere.[47] The organism was discovered in 1964 by L. E. Carmichael as the cause of epidemics of abortion in beagle hounds raised in kennels for breeding, field trials, and research.[20,21] *B. canis* infections are widespread in household pets and stray dogs of various species in the United States, Mexico, Japan, and Europe. To date, there have been only 16 published cases of *B. canis* infections in man in the United States. In man the disease has been mild and not contagious.[48] Human cases arise chiefly from contact with infected dogs in laboratories.

3. Methodology

3.1. Sources of Data

In the United States, morbidity and mortality from brucellosis in man are accurately recorded. The diagnosis must be reported to the Department of Health of the state of origin. These data are accumulated annually and have been maintained by the Centers for Disease Control in Atlanta since 1933. Other relevant data have been reported, including age, sex, occupation, geographic incidence, and *Brucella* species.[5,18,39]

The world incidence of human brucellosis has been recorded by the World Health Organization and published in their annual WHO World Health Statistics Report. The reliability of these reports is variable. The occurrence of brucellosis in various animal species in the reporting countries is recorded in the FAO/WHO/OIE Animal Health Yearbook. The incidence, animal species, and *Brucella* species are reported for each country.[2]

3.2. Surveys

In the United States, surveys for human brucellosis have generally been made with the serum agglutination test among groups at high risk. The survey groups have included veterinary surgeons, abattoir workers, patients in institutions, and farm families. The reliability of the data is dependent on the antigens and serological procedures employed. Surveys have also reported using cultures of blood clots submitted to public health laboratories for serological tests.

Serological surveys for animal brucellosis have been widely done in the United States in dairy cattle and hogs. Infections in dairy herds have usually been traced through tests of pooled bulk milk by the ring test. The latter is very reliable in detecting infected herds. Individual infected cattle, pigs, and goats are usually found by the rapid plate serum agglutination test or slow tube agglutination test. Similar surveys of domestic animals have been done in Europe, particularly in the United Kingdom.

3.3. Laboratory Diagnosis

3.3.1. Isolation and Identification of the Organism.
In suspected cases of human brucellosis, cultures of blood, bone marrow, lymph nodes, granulomatous tissue, abscess pus, urine, or cerebrospinal fluid may be successful. Perhaps the most widely used culture method has been the double broth–agar medium of Castaneda.[22] The

preferred broth medium is trypticase soy or Albimi containing 1% sodium citrate. A square 120-ml bottle is employed, and on one side a layer of 2–3% agar is allowed to harden. Then 75 ml of sterile broth is added aseptically, and the bottle is closed with a sterile rubber stopper. Five to ten milliliters of blood is added aseptically, and if *B. abortus* is suspected, 10% carbon dioxide is added to the atmosphere. The bottle is incubated upright at 37°C and tilted every 2–3 days to allow the broth to spread over the agar. The agar should be examined before tilting for visible bacterial colonies, which, if *Brucella* are present, should appear in 1–2 weeks. Growth of *Brucella* on agar appears as smooth, translucent, blue-white to amber colonies. In the case of *B. canis* and *B. ovis* the colonies are rough and mucoid. Gram stains show small coccobacillary organisms without spores or capsules. *Brucella* in tissues are mildly acid-fast and may be demonstrated in the (animal) placenta and other infected animal tissues with either a modified Ziehl–Neelsen stain or fluorescent antibody stain.[26,125] *B. abortus* and *B. ovis* require 10% carbon dioxide for growth on primary cultures. The organisms are not motile. *Brucella* species pathogenic for man can be differentiated by means of biochemical and metabolic tests, immunological tests, and bacteriophage susceptibility (Table 1).[15,85] As can be seen from Table 1, there have been nine biotypes recognized for *B. abortus,* four biotypes for *B. suis,* three biotypes for *B. melitensis,* and one biotype each for *B. canis* and *B. rangiferi tarandi* (*B. suis,* biotype 4).

3.3.2. Serological and Immunological Tests. Serodiagnosis of brucellosis is most commonly made with the agglutination test. Commercial antigens are used for the slide agglutination test. This test is simple and quick, but it is not as accurate as the tube agglutination test. Unfortunately, there is no commercial antigen available for the tube test in the United States. A satisfactory antigen is the killed strain No. 1119 *B. abortus* antigen available from the Bureau of Animal Industry, U.S. Department of Agriculture, Ames, Iowa. The technique of the test is well described in the laboratory monograph written by Alton *et al.* (see Suggested Reading). In an active case of brucellosis, an agglutinin titer of 1 : 160 or higher is expected within 4–6 weeks of the onset. The titer will reach its peak in 2–3 months and then gradually declines. It may remain positive in low titers for as long as 1–5 years, especially in cases of chronic brucellosis with localized abscesses. In some subacute or chronic cases, a prozone of inhibition of agglutination may be present in low serum dilutions; hence, serum dilutions should be carried to 1 : 640 or higher. These prozones are associated with the so-called blocking anti-

bodies.[43] They may reach a titer of 1 : 40–1 : 80 and travel in electrophoresis with the IgG and IgA immunoglobulins.[132,133] The blocking test may be positive late in the course of brucellosis. The test has no proved diagnostic value except in suspected cases with a negative serum agglutination test. The Coombs antiglobulin agglutination test has been quite useful in patients with a negative or low titer agglutination test.[49] Coombs titers are generally higher than agglutinin titers and remain positive longer. The Coombs titer is also higher than that of the serum complement fixation test.[72,74,82] Fixation of complement requires the presence of antibody of the IgG class; neither IgA nor IgM antibody readily fixes complement.[74]

In 1965 Reddin *et al.*[102] showed that the first agglutinating antibodies to appear in acute brucellosis are sensitive to mercaptoethanol (ME). They are likely to fall in the 12–19 S class of IgM macroglobulins. Next to appear (2–3 weeks) were the ME-resistant agglutinins, belonging to the 7 S IgG immunoglobulin class. After clinical recovery, usually only ME-sensitive agglutinins were present. In patients with chronic suppurative brucellosis, only ME-resistant agglutinins were found. In persons with asymptomatic *Brucella* infections, the agglutinins were almost always entirely ME-sensitive macroglobulins. The usefulness of the ME agglutinin test in the diagnosis, staging, and prognosis of human brucellosis has been confirmed by many investigators.[24,38,73,74,77]

The various serological tests for brucellosis are not always specific, particularly when the titers of antibodies are low. Because of the presence of cross-reacting bacterial antibodies, one may observe low titers of *Brucella* antibodies in persons or animals infected with or immunized with *Francisella tularensis,*[96] *Yersinia enterocolitica* serotype 0 : 9,[25] or *Salmonella* serotypes group N.[25] Vaccination with cholera vaccine may also provoke *Brucella* agglutinins with titers as high as 1 : 160, and an even greater anamnestic response may occur in people previously exposed to *Brucella.*[35,36]

There are a number of relatively new serological methods available for diagnostic and epidemiological surveys for brucellosis in man and animals. These tests include precipitin (including immunodiffusion) tests,[41] the rose bengal plate agglutination test,[33] counterimmunoelectrophoresis,[32,33] passive hemagglutination,[103] enzyme-linked immunosorbent assay (ELISA) and radioimmunoassay (RIA),[6,54] and the card test.[106] The ELISA test appears to be the most useful. With a suitable antigen it is sensitive, specific, and economical.

A wide variety of extracts and fractions of *Brucella*

have been injected intradermally in man to elicit a local inflammatory response and detect hypersensitivity or allergy. Most of the skin test materials contain *Brucella* proteins as the active antigen. Brucellin and brucellergen are two widely used protein antigens. The skin test is quite sensitive but can be falsely negative in as many as 10% of cases of acute brucellosis.[104] Furthermore, many persons with positive tests lack any other sign of active brucellosis and often have no history of a previous attack. The skin test correlates poorly with serological tests.[104] The use of the skin test for diagnostic purposes may be confusing because it often provokes a significant serological response.[104] The skin test may be useful in epidemiological surveys to detect groups of exposed persons at greatest risk. Repeated testing might be necessary to detect skin test conversion rates and risks of continuing exposure. It is widely felt that *Brucella* skin tests are specific for brucellosis, but this has not been proved. It is not known whether repeated skin testing can sensitize the people tested.

The leukocyte migration inhibition test has been suggested as a simpler substitute for the skin test.[79] In a limited trial in five cases of human brucellosis compared to 12 other individuals, four of the five brucellosis cases had a lower migration index than did those without brucellosis. Two advantages were observed: collection of blood requires only one interview, and the immune status of the patient is not altered.

4. Biological Characteristics of the Organism

Table 1 shows the biochemical and antigenic differences in the four species and 17 biotypes of *Brucella* pathogenic for man. Cultures of *B. abortus, B. suis,* and *B. melitensis* on primary isolation on solid media grow in the form of antigenically active smooth (S) colonies. These cultures, when transferred in certain broth media, will dissociate to intermediate (I) and to antigenically inactive rough (R) and mucoid (M) forms.[56] The work of Braun established that the dissociation of *Brucella* was caused by inherent strain variations as well as environmental factors such as nutrients, metabolites, and serum.[12–14] There are several variants of *Brucella* which have been useful as live, avirulent but immunogenic vaccines. The most widely available stable variant is the strain 19 *B. abortus,* which has reduced virulence for guinea pigs, calves, and young heifers (2–6 months).[42] Strain 19 does not appear in the milk of vaccinated heifers and does not infect people exposed to the cattle. It can cause disease in veterinarians and

other persons inoculated with the vaccine.[116,119] Pickett and Nelson[99] reported finding smooth brown variants of *Brucella* from blood cultures of normal people by using citrated blood washed with distilled water. It was thought that washing removed *Brucella* antibody and also bacteriophage allowing growth of *Brucella* variants. The work has not been confirmed by others.

Brucella species lack capsules and exotoxins. Lipopolysaccharide (endotoxins) can be extracted from cell walls of smooth *B. abortus, B. suis,* and *B. melitensis* (but not rough *B. canis*). They are toxic for man and animals.[31] Differences in the toxicity of endotoxin from these species are associated with the presence or absence of the aminosugar, quinovosamine.[10] Both man and animals can be sensitized to endotoxins of smooth *Brucella* species.[30,117] In the sensitized animal, *Brucella* endotoxin induces fever, vascular injury, toxic hepatic changes, reduced adrenocortical function, leukopenia, low serum iron, and death.

One of the more striking manifestations of brucellosis in animals, particularly in cattle, pigs, and kennel-raised dogs, is the occurrence of epidemics of contagious abortions. Abortions may also occur in women, particularly with *B. melitensis* infection in the first trimester of pregnancy.[28,100,108,130] Pregnancy also appears to make females of many species of animals, including humans, more susceptible to brucellosis.[28] In pregnant ruminant ungulates (cows, sheep, goats) as well as pigs and dogs, *Brucella* can grow to enormous numbers in the placenta (fetal fluids and fetal placental chorions), leading to abortion in those species.[21,111] Extracts of their fetal fluids, fetal placenta, and chorion contain a substance promoting the growth of *B. abortus.*[71,76,111] It has been found to be a sugar-alcohol, erythritol.[71,76,111] Erythritol has not been found in the human placenta or in that of rats, guinea pigs, and rabbits.[76,111] Male genitalia of susceptible species (except dogs and man) contain erythritol.[71,111] Growth of *B. abortus* in newborn calves is stimulated by erythritol.[111] The growth of *B. suis* and *B. melitensis* in broth is also stimulated by erythritol, but growth of *B. canis* is not enhanced.[65,71,111] Virulent strains of *Brucella* are stimulated more by erythritol than are avirulent strains, and strain 19 *B. abortus* is not susceptible.[111]

5. Descriptive Epidemiology

5.1. Prevalence and Incidence

5.1.1. Mortality and Morbidity. The mortality rate of brucellosis in man was once about 3%. With effective

Table 1. Differentiation of *Brucella* Species Pathogenic for Man[a]

Species and biotypes	CO₂ requirement	H₂S production	Thionine a	b	c	Basic fuchsin b	c	A	M	Lysis by phage Tb at RTD[d]	Glutamic acid	Ornithine	Ribose	Lysine	Common host reservoir	Remarks
B. melitensis 1	−	−	−	+	+	+	+	−	+	−	+	−	−	−	Sheep, goats	Typical melitensis
2	−	−	−	+	+	+	+	+	+	−	+	−	−	−	Sheep, goats	
3	−	−	−	+	+	+	+	+	−	−	+	−	−	−	Sheep, goats	
B. abortus 1	+	+	−	−	−	+	+	+	−	+	+	−	+	−	Cattle	Typical abortus
2	+	+	−	−	−	−	−	+	−	+	+	−	+	−	Cattle	Rhodesian type
3	+	+	+	+	+	+	+	+	−	+	+	−	+	−	Cattle	
4	+	+	−	−	−	+	+	−	+	+	+	−	+	−	Cattle	British melitensis
5	−	−	−	+	+	+	+	−	+	+	+	−	+	−	Cattle	
6	−	+	−	+	+	+	+	+	−	+	+	−	+	−	Cattle	
7	−	−	−	+	+	+	+	+	+	+	+	−	+	−	Cattle	
8	+	+	−	+	+	+	+	+	+	+	+	−	+	−	Cattle	
9	+	+	+	+	+	+	+	+	−	+	+	−	+	−	Cattle	
B. suis 1	+	++	+	+	+	−	−	+	−	−	±	+	+	+	Pigs	American suis
2	−	−	+	+	+	−	−	+	−	−	+	+	+	−	Pigs, hares	Danish suis
3	−	−	+	+	+	+	+	+	−	−	+	+	+	+	Pigs	
4	−	−	+	+	+	+	+	−	+	−	+	+	+	+	Reindeer	*B. rangiferi tarandi*
B. canis 1	−	−	+	+	+	−	−	−	−	−	+	+	+	+	Dogs	Antigenically rough

[a] Modified from Brinley Morgan.[15]
[b] Growth on Albimi or trypticase agar with added dyes: a, 1:25,000; b, 1:50,000; c, 1:100,000.
[c] A, *B. abortus*; M, *B. melitensis*.
[d] Tbilisi (Tb) *Brucella* phage used at routine test dilution (RTD).

antibiotic therapy the mortality rate has dropped to about 1%. Mortality statistics therefore are not very useful. The annual number of deaths ascribed to human brucellosis in the United States in the period 1967–1976 varied from zero to six (average 2.2).[5] The number of reported cases of human brucellosis in the United States, 1968–1977, varied from 183 to 310 (average 232).[5] The annual incidence of human brucellosis per 100,000 population in the United States, 1968–1977, varied from 0.9 to 0.15 (average 0.11).[5] There was a steady decline in the annual number of cases from about 3500 in 1950 to about 200 in the early 1970s, with a moderate, temporary increase in 1974–1977 (average 269) (see Fig. 1). In the first half of 1986, only 32 cases were reported in the United States. This decline has been attributed to compulsory pasteurization of milk and milk products, as well as control of brucellosis in dairy cattle.

5.1.2. High-Risk Categories. Most cases of human brucellosis in the United States now occur in people directly exposed to infected animals (cattle, swine), their excreta, products of abortion, or carcasses.[18] The persons at greatest risk are abattoir workers engaged in killing and processing pigs infected with *B. suis,* probably as a result of exposure through skin contamination as well as exposure to aerosols.[53,70,128,133] *B. abortus* infections may also arise in abattoir workers handling infected bovine carcasses.[18,39] Farm families also have an increased risk through exposure to infected and aborting cattle or pigs.[114] The risk is also great in people who ingest unpasteurized or unsterilized milk or fresh cheese, especially if made from the milk of infected goats or sheep (*B. melitensis*).[34,122,131] Ingestion of unpasteurized milk from infected caribou and camels may also lead to brucellosis. Laboratory workers handling *Brucella* cultures have a high risk of acquiring brucellosis through accidents, aerosols, or inadequate sanitary precautions. A so-called "P3" laboratory is preferable.[127] Veterinarians have a high risk, especially if they work with aborting animals, remove retained placenta from infected animals or vaccinate animals with live *Brucella* vaccines (strain 19).[115,116] Nomads also have a high risk of brucellosis since they often depend upon fresh goat's milk for food, and live in close contact with the animals. If undernourished and iron-deficient, nomadic people may develop clinical brucellosis when given iron supplements.[92] Brucellosis is also a risk in persons (especially tourists) who take antacids or (Tagamet) cimetidine and ingest unpasteurized milk or fresh cheese.[121] People with achlorhydria may be at greater risk of brucellosis from ingestion because they lack the protection of the antibacterial action of gastric acidity. Patients with brucellosis often have gastric achlorhydria. Patients with peptic ulcer treated with a diet of unpasteurized milk are also at risk. Brucellosis may be a special risk for pregnant women, mostly in the second trimester of pregnancy, since brucellosis may lead to infection and abortion of the fetus. The risk is greatest in pregnant women exposed to goats or sheep or their fresh milk or cheese in countries where *B. melitensis* infections are common.[28,100,108,130]

5.2. Epidemic Behavior and Contagiousness

There have been several epidemics of human brucellosis in institutions traced to the ingestion of infected cows' milk. Most of these epidemics were caused by *B. suis* and arose from cattle exposed to infected pigs.[59,66] Since cattle are relatively resistant to *B. suis,* some of these outbreaks may have arisen from contamination of the cows' milk. Epidemics have also arisen from ingestion of fresh goats' or sheeps' cheese heavily infected with *B. melitensis.*[34,131] Brucellosis may also occur in epidemics in do-

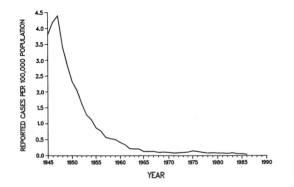

Figure 1. Number of reported cases of brucellosis per 100,000 population in the United States, 1945–1986. (Centers for Disease Control, Brucellosis Surveillance.)

mestic or wild animals. The widespread epidemics of abortions due to *B. canis* in kennel-raised dogs, especially in beagles, are an example.[20,47]

Brucellosis in man is not as contagious as it is in lower animals.[120] *Brucella* have been found in human milk, but babies have not been known to become infected by ingestion of human milk. *Brucella* may be found in the urine of some patients with brucellosis, but the disease apparently has not spread to their contacts. *Brucella* have been found in mosquitoes and hematophagous ticks feeding on bacteremic animals, but multiplication in the ticks and transmission to other animals or man through their bites have not been proved.[58] Ticks feeding on dogs bacteremic with *B. canis* were negative for *Brucella*.[91] There have been numerous laboratory-acquired acute *Brucella* infections.[84,93,127] One such outbreak may have been due to transmission via water contaminated by defective plumbing.[60] Experiments attempting to infect man artificially have suggested that transmission by ingestion often fails unless the dose is large and the strain virulent.[83,88,95] Infection is more readily produced by inoculation of abraded skin, injection through skin, or splashing on mucous membranes (conjunctiva).[88] Family studies have suggested that on farms, where unpasteurized cows' milk containing *B. abortus* is ingested, infection is most likely in people who ingest the most milk and have the closest contact with the infected cattle.[114]

5.3. Geographic Distribution

The number of reported cases of human brucellosis by state in the United States in 1984 is shown in Fig. 2. The largest number of cases occurred in Texas, California, and Florida.

The annual number of reported cases of human brucellosis by country was given in the World Health Statistics Report for 1973.[1] In order of occurrence, the countries reporting the largest numbers of cases in 1970–1971 were the USSR, Spain, Italy, Iran, Greece, Peru, Argentina, Mexico, France, Portugal, the United States, Poland, Australia, and New Zealand. The number of reported cases per year in Malta was only about 50, and in Spain there were more than 6000. The geographic distribution of various *Brucella* species in man varies with the incidence of brucellosis in various domestic animals.[81] *B. melitensis* infections occur in goats, sheep, and man in the Mediterranean countries, central Asia, Latin America, South America, Africa, and India.[2] *B. abortus* causes brucellosis in cattle and man in Europe, the USSR, the United States, Latin America, South America, Africa, and India.[2] Paradoxically, *B. abortus* infections appear to be increasing greatly in cattle

and in man in the oil-rich countries of the Near East, including Saudia Arabia, Kuwait, Iraq, and Iran.[2] The problem may be related to the importation and crowding of large numbers of cattle—both dairy and beef—with greater exposure of man through ingestion (unpasteurized milk, fresh cheese, ice cream) and direct contact with slaughtered animals and soil saturated with infected animal blood and products of abortion. Continued warfare and strife in the Near East probably increase the risk of contagion.

Brucellosis due to *B. suis* is found in pigs and man in the United States, the USSR, Europe, and southern Asia. *B. canis* infections have been found in man in the United States and in dogs in the United States, Mexico, Japan, and West Germany. *B. rangiferi tarandi* (*B. suis,* biotype 4) causes infections in caribou, reindeer, and man in Alaska, northern Canada, and Arctic USSR. *B. ovis* leads to epididymitis in rams in Australia and New Zealand but is not known to infect man. *B. neotomae* infects desert wood rats but not man in Utah (USA).

5.4. Temporal Distribution

In the United States, as in most of the Northern Hemisphere, the highest seasonal incidence of human brucellosis is in the spring and early summer with the onset in March to July.[5,78] The incidence declines in late summer, fall, and winter. The peak incidence in man falls a bit later in the spring than is the case for infected and aborting animals. In the latter, brucellosis reaches its peak in the late winter or early spring.[60] In the Southern Hemisphere, where the seasons are reversed, the peak incidence of human brucellosis occurs from October through December. This is the season when nomadic herdsmen bring their goats and sheep down from the mountain valleys to the coastal cities where they sell fresh cheese and milk.

5.5. Age

Human brucellosis can occur at any age, but the majority of cases in the United States are found in young men between the ages of 20 and 40.[17,78] This fact is related to the greater occupational hazards in young men. Doubt has been cast on the susceptibility of prepubertal children, because of the relative infrequency of clinical brucellosis in this age group. Nevertheless, children between the ages of 2 and 15 may become infected if they ingest fresh milk or fresh cheese containing *B. abortus* or *B. melitensis*.[78,122] The age distribution in females is often broader than in males. Females have less contact with infected animals.[78]

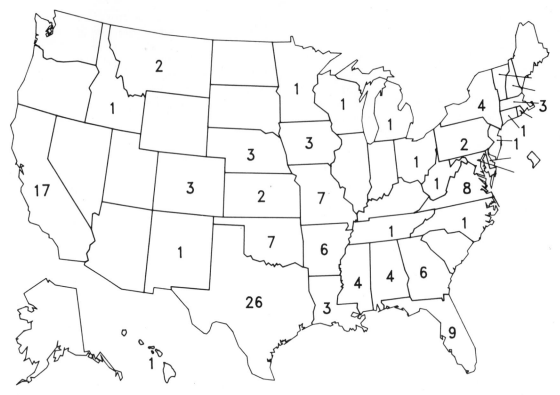

Figure 2. Reported cases of human brucellosis by state in the United States, 1984. Alaska none, Hawaii 1. From the CDC.

Infections in women more often arise at any age from ingestion of raw milk or fresh white goats' cheese.

5.6. Sex

In the United States, brucellosis is predominantly a disease of males; three-fourths of cases reported in Minnesota, 1945–1948, occurred in males.[79] This preponderance of males was true regardless of the species of *Brucella* found in blood cultures.[78] The male preponderance holds only between the ages of 13 and 55, because it is in that age group that men are more often exposed to infected animals. Female children and elderly women in Minnesota were infected as often as males of the same age. Females, therefore, are just as susceptible as males, but they are not more so, except perhaps during pregnancy.[78] In Minnesota there was no significant sex difference between urban and rural cases of brucellosis. Similar data for the United States in 1974 were collected by the CDC. Males represented 83% of the 235 cases of known sex. Epidemics of human brucellosis in the United States are now chiefly found in em-

ployees of packing houses. From 1965–1974, 94% of these employees with brucellosis were males.

5.7. Occupation

Human brucellosis in the United States has increasingly become a disease related to occupation. Infection by ingestion has been largely eliminated through control measures in dairy cattle and compulsory pasteurization of all dairy products. The disease is now seen chiefly in workers in abattoirs handling infected cattle or swine infected with *B. suis*.[18] In 1975, 55% of 309 human cases of brucellosis occurred in packing house employees, 4.2% in government abattoir inspectors, and 0.6% in rendering plant employees (total 60%). The livestock industry was the employer of 19.1% of the cases; these included livestock market employees 0.3%, livestock producers 17.5%, and veterinarians 1.3%. Other occupational categories included 1 laboratory worker, 5 homemakers, and 14 students or children.

The CDC studied the epidemiology of abattoir-associated human brucellosis, 1960–1972.[19] Their surveillance included 1644 cases. They also surveyed two abattoirs, 1960–1970, in Iowa and one in Illinois. Attack rates were higher for hog-kill employees having high frequencies of skin cuts, exposure to fresh animal blood and lymph, ingestion of potentially contaminated animal products, and conjunctival contact with animal tissue and infection. Although *B. suis*, type III, was recovered from the air in an abattoir during the time when infected swine were slaughtered, exposed guinea pigs and employees failed to become infected. In time, abattoir employees seemed to acquire immunity from infection. In the hog-kill department in abattoir C, the attack rate was only 3% in previously infected employees and 64% in previously noninfected employees.

In Florida, where in June 1976 only 36% of the counties had been certified as free of bovine brucellosis, human infections continued to occur mainly in persons working with livestock or milk production (84%). In 1974–1975 there was an increase in the number of cattle-associated human infections in both Florida and Montana.[9]

5.8. Other Factors

There are many possible sources of brucellosis. The chief source is direct contact with infected animals or their products (milk, cream, butter, fresh cheese, urine, blood, carcasses, abortion products). The animal sources include goats, sheep, cattle, water buffalo, horses, swine, caribou, reindeer, moose, elk, camel, llama, yak, zebu cattle, dogs. Infections in man have not been proved to arise from contaminated water, contaminated meat, or bites of infected insects. The disease has not been shown to be transmitted in man by sexual intercourse, though genital infections are known.

Genetic resistance to brucellosis has been demonstrated in rabbits by breeding a strain for resistance to challenge with *B. suis*.[64] There is no known racial or genetic difference in susceptibility to brucellosis in man. There must be several selective factors to account for the preference of the various species of *Brucella* for their natural animal hosts. One of the factors accounting for some of the selective pressure is the relative bactericidal capacity of the serum for the *Brucella* species.[45] Another important factor is the presence of progesterone and erythritol in the placenta and genitalia of the susceptible animals, and the consequent selective stimulation of growth of certain *Brucella* species.[4,71,111] Since the placenta is the site of the greatest multiplication of most *Brucella* species in cattle, swine, goats, and sheep, it seems likely that pregnancy increases susceptibility, especially in the first trimester.[28] The mechanism for this increase in susceptibility is not entirely clear though erythritol and progesterone play some part.[71,111] There are also important socioeconomic factors affecting susceptibility to brucellosis. Relapses of brucellosis among iron-deficient undernourished nomads given iron supplements and refeeding have already been mentioned.[92]

6. Mechanisms and Routes of Transmission

In the United States at this time, many cases of human brucellosis are probably acquired by way of cuts in the skin through direct contact with the carcasses of swine infected with *B. suis*.[19] In some states (Florida and Montana), the disease is usually acquired through direct contact with cattle infected with *B. abortus* or ingestion of dairy products from cattle.[9] There is indirect evidence that employees in hog-kill departments of abattoirs may also be infected by inhalation of aerosols and through splashing of blood and lymph into their conjunctival sac.[19,70] Veterinarians may acquire the disease by direct contact with aborting animals and their aborted fetus or placenta. Also, veterinary inspectors are directly exposed to the carcasses of infected animals. Veterinarians may also be infected by accidental inoculation percutaneously or into the conjunctival sac with live *B. abortus*, strain 19 vaccine.[116] Most human infections with *B. melitensis* are the result of ingestion of raw milk or fresh cheese from infected goats or sheep.[34,124,131]

7. Pathogenesis and Immunity

7.1. Pathogenesis

The incubation period in humans is 1–5 weeks. The pathogenesis of brucellosis in man and in lower animals varies with the *Brucella* species. *B. melitensis* is most invasive and produces the most severe illness and toxic effects.[11] *B. suis* is also quite invasive and produces more focal necrosis and suppuration in bones, liver, spleen, and lymph nodes. *B. abortus* is the least invasive. It usually produces a milder disease, and within involved organs there are granulomas usually without necrosis or suppuration. In man, *B. canis* causes bacteremia, lymphadenopathy, splenomegaly, and a mild illness.[89]

There have been few autopsy studies of human brucellosis and most of these have been after deaths resulting from unusual complications, such as infective endocarditis, suicide, ruptured mycotic aneurysm, encephalomeningitis, and pneumonia.[83] There have been a few illuminating pathological studies of tissue biopsies in man. In acute brucellosis caused by *B. abortus,* needle biopsy of the liver in 11 cases disclosed epithelioid cell granulomas with mononuclear cells but no necrosis or fibrosis.[118] Scattered necrotic liver cells were present in one case. No *Brucella* were seen or cultured from these liver biopsies. These findings were confirmed elsewhere in five liver biopsies and ten necropsies.[62] Similar granulomas have been found in biopsies of sternal bone marrow in patients with acute brucellosis caused by *B. abortus.*[123] Granulomas were made up of compact sheets of macrophages, variable numbers of lymphocytes, and occasional giant cells. Neutrophils and eosinophils were present in some cases. Bone marrow cultures were often positive for *B. abortus* in bacteremic cases.

The presence of *Brucella* in the cytoplasm of some cells has been noteworthy in a few cases of acute human brucellosis, as well as in many animals. Meyer[83] reported a case of a man dying of acute brucellosis 3 weeks after ingestion of a *B. suis* culture. *Brucella* cells were seen within alveolar septa of the lungs, in the cytoplasm of renal tubular cells, and in cells of Bowman's capsule. *Brucella* were thought to parasitize mesenchymal cells of various organs. In lower animals such as cattle, goats, swine, and dogs, in which brucellosis causes abortions, acute placentitis is common. Smith[112] first showed that the cytoplasm of the cells of the infected bovine fetal chorionic epithelium was crowded with *B. abortus.* Intracellular multiplication of bacteria destroyed the epithelium. Perivascular fibroblasts in the placenta were also seen to contain cytoplasmic *Brucella.*

Anderson *et al.* recently reported ultrastructural studies of placentitis in pregnant goats inoculated with *B. abortus.*[3,4] With transmission electron microscopy and sections of goat placentae stained with antibody-coated colloidal gold, they demonstrated *B. abortus* first in phagosomes of fetal trophoblasts and in the rough endoplasmic reticulum of chorioallantoic trophoblasts. Following necrosis of trophoblasts and chorioallantois, *B. abortus* was found within placental capillaries. Placental vasculitis followed. Placental trophoblasts became separated from the maternal syncytial epithelium and numerous *B. abortus* appeared in the connective tissue of chorionic villi. *B. abortus* cells were engulfed by trophoblasts through endocytosis and they multiplied in the rough endoplasmic reticulum. *B. abortus* was thought to utilize endoplasmic reticulum for synthesis and glycosylation of membrane proteins or else to catabolize trophoblastic secretory proteins.

In experimental animals, *B. abortus* have been observed in the cytoplasm of circulating neutrophilic leukocytes a few minutes after inoculation.[11] In the presence of human anti-*Brucella* serum, normal human neutrophils engulf *B. abortus* into phagocytic cytoplasmic vacuoles with subsequent loss of cytoplasmic granules.[90] The *Brucella* were not destroyed, apparently because the metabolic process necessary for leukocyte bactericidal effect was blocked by virulent *B. abortus.* In normal animals, within a few hours after inoculation of virulent *B. abortus,* the bacteria crowd the cytoplasm of phagocytic Kupffer cells in the liver where they are sequestered and inactivated in phagocytic vacuoles.[11,44] Phagocytic macrophages in the spleen are less able to kill *Brucella* than those in the liver.[44] Virulent *Brucella* have been observed *in vitro* to multiply rapidly in the cytoplasm of peritoneal monocytes from normal animals.[57] Transmission electron microscopy revealed that *B. abortus* grown in normal monocytes were localized in the cytoplasm within phagocytic vacuoles limited by a unit membrane.[69] *Brucella* lying within a phagocytic vacuole are protected there from the bactericidal effects of serum immunoglobulins and some antibiotics (tetracyclines and perhaps streptomycin[105,110]).

7.2. Immunity

There is evidence of some natural immunity to brucellosis in man. I have already commented upon the relative infrequency of the disease in children. This protection might be partly due to less occupational exposure, but young animals (calves, puppies) are also less susceptible than adults to brucellosis.[60] There is also a degree of acquired immunity to brucellosis in man following infection. Elderly veterinarians are relatively immune, as compared to young students.[126] The Mediterranean Fever Commission noted that attack rates of brucellosis were higher in young military recruits than in seasoned British personnel in Malta. I have mentioned the higher attack rates in new abattoir employees compared to older workers recovered from brucellosis.[19] The function of serum immunoglobulins and specific antibodies in immunity to brucellosis is uncertain.[45] Normal human serum containing "natural" antibody and complement kills *B. abortus* quickly. *B. suis* and *B. melitensis* are less susceptible, and *B. canis* is resistant.[45] Infants between 1½ and 4 months of age usually lack natural antibody; newborns appear to absorb it from ingested colostrum. In patients with acute brucellosis, serum bactericidal titers increase 1000-fold or more. Patients with chronic brucellosis lack serum killing of *Brucella* because it is blocked by a specific inhibitor, which can be found in either IgA or IgG serum fractions.[45,51]

Cellular immunity is probably more protective than

humoral immunity in brucellosis.[36] The cellular resistance of immune macrophages can be both specific and nonspecific. The specific circulating immunoglobulins are produced by B lymphocytes, but T lymphocytes are responsible for cell-mediated immunity. Activation of specific lymphocyte populations and consequent immunity can be demonstrated by lymphocyte transformation and macrophage migration inhibition.[67,68,107] The fate of *Brucella* within macrophages *in vivo* is not entirely certain. Immune serum enhances the *in vitro* uptake of *B. melitensis* by peritoneal macrophages of immune rabbits. Under aerobic conditions, *in vitro* growth of the bacteria is only briefly restricted, but under anaerobic conditions, the *Brucella* are killed by immune macrophages.[36] Recently, Krogstad and Schlesinger reviewed some functions of acids and acid hydrolases within cellular lysosomes against intracellular pathogens.[75] *Brucella* are considered to be facultative intracellular pathogens. It is likely that they are killed by acid hydrolases within the phagocytic vacuole after fusion of the phagosomes with lysosomes. The bacteria may survive if the phagosome ruptures (exocytosis) to allow the *Brucella* to escape intact from the cells. *Brucella* may also survive within phagosomes if weak bases enter the lysosomes or phagosomes and raise the pH.

8. Patterns of Host Response

The clinical host response in man is often an acute febrile illness beginning usually 1–5 weeks after exposure. Surveys of people exposed to brucellosis have shown that some with positive cultures of blood or urine are never febrile or ill. Furthermore, skin test and serological surveys disclose frequent subclinical infections among exposed groups. Infection is more common than clinical illness.[19,53,55,114]

8.1. Clinical Features

The onset is gradual. The most prevalent symptoms are weakness, malaise, chills, sweats, headache, backache, and arthralgia. Fever is common and may have an undulating course if untreated. Small, nontender cervical and axillary lymph nodes are often palpable. The spleen is enlarged in half the patients, and hepatomegaly is found in one-fourth. Both organs may be tender. Without treatment, patients with clinical brucellosis usually recover in 2–3 months. With effective chemotherapy, recovery is quicker, but relapses may be frequent.[46] Complications may occur in 10–35% of

patients with clinical brucellosis, especially if caused by *B. suis* or *B. melitensis*. Frequent complications include epididymitis, orchitis, abortions, hepatitis, calcifying abscesses of liver and spleen (with *B. suis*), and osteomyelitis of vertebrae. Rare complications are meningoencephalitis, chronic meningitis, infective endocarditis, pulmonary infections, pancytopenia with hypersplenism, interstitial nephritis, pyelonephritis, myocarditis, cholecystitis, ovarian abscess, bursitis, and septic arthritis. Death occurs in about 1% of treated patients and may be due to endocarditis, ruptured mycotic aneurysm, encephalitis, or suicide. About 10% of patients with clinical brucellosis may be ill for a year or more, with or without evidence of local infections. This syndrome has been called "chronic brucellosis." The concept of chronic brucellosis as an illness including vague anxiety and depression, in people having no previous acute febrile episode and only evidence of infection (positive skin test and serology) of unknown duration, has been discredited.[63,113,127] Nevertheless, there have been careful studies in some people with known exposure, chronic illness, and convincing serological and biopsy evidence of active brucellosis.[8] There is no known immunological deficit in patients with chronic brucellosis other than the presence of "blocking" antibodies. They may be anergic to *Brucella* antigens and to dinitrochlorobenzene, but their T lymphocytes may function normally as judged by erythrocyte-rosette formation and lymphocyte transformation.[23]

8.2. Diagnosis

The clinical diagnosis of acute brucellosis in man is based upon the presence of typical symptoms, the usual fever and other meager physical findings, supportive laboratory findings, and a history of exposure. Skin tests are not helpful and may stimulate misleading serological responses. The leukocyte count is normal or reduced, but there is often a relative lymphocytosis. The sedimentation rate is not useful. The serum agglutination titer is 1 : 160 or higher by the standard tube dilution method using *B. abortus* antigen prepared by the World Health Organization or the U.S. Department of Agriculture. With suitable methods (Albimi broth in Castaneda bottle plus 10% CO_2), *Brucella* species may be grown from venous blood or bone marrow in more than half of the acute cases. In chronic cases, blood cultures are usually negative, but with localized infections (abscesses) *Brucella* species may be grown by culture of pus.

The differential diagnosis may include infectious mononucleosis, viral hepatitis, lymphoma, tuberculosis, typhoid fever, typhus, tularemia, malaria, and influenza.

9. Control and Prevention

9.1. General Concepts

Brucellosis is primarily a disease of wild and domestic animals.[2,94] Man is only accidentally infected with a terminal infection which is not transmitted. Control of human brucellosis therefore depends upon elimination of the risk of infection spreading from animals to man. The risk of brucellosis from ingestion of contaminated milk, cheese, and other dairy products can be controlled by heating the milk (sterilization or pasteurization).[29] Prevention of human infections acquired through contact with infected animals is more difficult. In the United States, brucellosis caused by *B. abortus* in dairy cattle has been largely controlled, with the exception of a few states, by identifying infected herds through tests for *Brucella* antibodies in bulk milk and separating individual infected bovines by serum complement-fixation or agglutination tests.[94] The infected animals are then slaughtered. Infections of young (2–6 month) heifers can be prevented by vaccination with live strain 19 *B. abortus* vaccine.[27,94,101] Spread of *B. melitensis* infections in sheep and goats can be controlled with the use of live Rev-I *B. melitensis* vaccine.[36]

Control of *B. canis* infections in kennel-raised dogs has succeeded only when infected dogs have been identified by cultures of blood and urine or by periodic serological tests. The infected dogs must then be removed and destroyed.[20,47]

Control of brucellosis in swine remains an unsolved problem. Serological diagnosis is somewhat unreliable, and cultures are impractical for diagnosis and control.[67] Cell-mediated immune responses may be helpful.[67] There is no safe, effective vaccine approved for use in the United States in swine.[2] *B. suis* infections in employees of abattoirs might be prevented if protective clothing, goggles, masks, and gloves were required.[19]

9.2. Chemoprophylaxis

There are many antibiotics that inhibit or kill *Brucella* species.[50] Antibiotic therapy is effective in reducing mortality, preventing complications, and alleviating illness in man. Antibiotic-resistant strains of *Brucella* have not been a frequent problem, but posttreatment relapses often occur in man.[46] Antibiotic therapy in domestic animals with brucellosis is not cost-effective. Experimental *Brucella* infections in small laboratory animals can be suppressed or cured with antibiotics.[98] I am not aware of any success with chemoprophylaxis of brucellosis in animals or man.

9.3. Immunization

Vaccines have been used extensively in the USSR and China to immunize people exposed to *Brucella*.[2,36,58] Several reports have shown that large doses (150–200 million organisms) of live "avirulent" *B. abortus* BA/19 strain given s.c. 2–3 months prior to exposure reduce the risk of infection with *B. melitensis* by a factor of three to ten. Some local and systemic reactions occur. A safety trial of this vaccine was carried out in a prison in the United States.[119] The vaccine was given s.c. in a dose of 2.5×10^8 organisms to 16 volunteers. It produced local swelling in 13, systemic reactions in 4, and *Brucella* bacteremia in 1. The risk was judged to be substantial. This vaccine has not been approved for use in man in the United States.

The safety of the live streptomycin-dependent Rev-I strain of *B. melitensis* for use in man has also been tested.[119] Subcutaneous injection of 2.5×10^8 living organisms was followed by slight to moderate local soreness in 12 of 16 volunteers. Systemic reactions followed in 3 to 23 days in all but 2, and blood cultures showed *B. melitensis* on days 8 to 24 in all but 4 subjects. All 16 men were treated with tetracycline to abort their infection. The vaccine was found to be unsafe for use in man in the United States. Because the dose used was thought perhaps too large, another trial was made elsewhere.[97] Graded doses from 10^3 to 2.8×10^4 living Rev-I organisms were injected i.d. in ten young men. Local reactions were mild, but systemic reactions developed with the larger doses. Bacteremia was shown in three subjects. An immunological response was present even with small doses of Rev-I, but the safety margin was too narrow to recommend its use in man. Killed *Brucella* vaccines or antigenic *Brucella* fractions have been used in man, as well as in lower animals, but have not been proved to be protective in man.

10. Unresolved Problems

Prevention of human brucellosis in the United States will require continued efforts at detection and control of brucellosis in both domestic and wild animals. There remain unresolved problems with brucellosis in beef and dairy cattle in some states, such as California, Florida, and Texas. Improved testing of bulk milk supplies may identify foci in dairy herds, but simpler methods of serological testing are needed to detect infected herds of beef cattle. Human brucellosis in the United States often occurs in employees of abattoirs slaughtering heavily infected swine and cattle. Detection of infected swine by serological testing calls for better antigens and better methodology. Abattoir workers need protection from exposure to infective aerosols and infected animal blood and lymph, as well as from exposure through cuts and abrasions. Protective goggles, masks, gloves, and clothing might be an acceptable and effective precaution when slaughtering cattle and swine known to be infected. There is a need for a safe, effective vaccine for use in swine (reported to be available now in China).[2] A similar need for immunization of new abattoir workers is evident. *B. melitensis* infections can be largely eliminated in the United States if importation of fresh unpasteurized goats' cheese is prevented.

11. References

1. ABDUSSALAM, M., AND FEIN, D. A., Brucellosis as a world problem, *Dev. Biol. Stand.* **31**:9–23 (1976).
2. ALTON, G. G., AND PLOMMET, M., Brucellosis summit in Geneva, *WHO Chron.* **40**:19–21 (1986). See also 6th Report of Joint FAO/WHO Expert Committee on Brucellosis, *WHO Tech. Rep. Ser.* **740** (1986).
3. ANDERSON, T. D., MEADOR, V. P., AND CHEVILLE, N. F., Pathogenesis of placentitis in the goat inoculated with *Brucella abortus*. I. Gross and histologic lesions, *Vet. Pathol.* **23**:219–226 (1986).
4. ANDERSON, T. D., CHEVILLE, N. F., AND MEADOR, V. P., Pathogenesis of placentitis in the goat inoculated with *Brucella abortus*. II. Ultrastructural studies, *Vet. Pathol.* **23**:227–229 (1986).
5. Annual Summary—1977, *Morbid. Mortal. Weekly Rep.* **26**(53):1–80 (1978).
6. ARAJ, G. F., LULU, A. R., MUSTAFA, M. Y., AND KHATEEB, M. I., Evaluation of ELISA in the diagnosis of acute and chronic brucellosis in human beings, *J. Hyg.* **97**:457–469 (1986).
7. BANG, B., The etiology of epizootic abortion, *J. Comp. Pathol. Ther.* **10**:125 (1897).
8. BARRETT, G. M., AND RICKARDS, A. G., Chronic brucellosis, *Q. J. Med.* **22**:23–42 (1953).
9. BIGLER, W. J., HOFF, G. L., HEMMERT, W. H., TOMAS, J. A., AND JANOWSKI, H. T., Trends of brucellosis in Florida. An epidemiologic review, *Am. J. Epidemiol.* **105**:245–251 (1977).
10. BOWSER, D. V., WHEAT, R. W., FOSTER, J. W., AND LEONG, D., Occurrence of quinovosamine in lipopolysaccharide of Brucella species, *Infect. Immun.* **9**:772–774 (1974).
11. BRAUDE, A. I., Studies in the pathology and pathogenesis of experimental brucellosis. II. The formation of the hepatic granuloma and its evolution, *J. Infect. Dis.* **89**:87–94 (1951).
12. BRAUN, W., Dissociation in *Brucella abortus*: A demonstra-

tion of the role of inherent and environmental factors in bacterial variation, *J. Bacteriol.* **51**:327–349 (1946).
13. BRAUN, W., Studies on bacterial variation and selective environments. I. The nature of the selective serum factor affecting the variation of *Brucella abortus*, *J. Bacteriol.* **58**:291–297 (1949).
14. BRAUN, W., Studies on bacterial variation and selective environments. II. The effects of sera from Brucella-infected animals and from normal animals of different species upon the variation of *Brucella abortus*, *J. Bacteriol.* **58**:299–305 (1949).
15. BRINLEY, MORGAN, W. J., Brucellosis in Britain, *Ann. Sclavo* **19**:35–44 (1977).
16. BRUCE, D., Note on the discovery of a microorganism in Malta fever, *Practitioner* **39**:161–170 (1887).
17. *Brucellosis Surveillance*, Annual Summary—1974, pp. 1–11, CDC, (November 1975).
18. Brucellosis—United States, 1975, *Morbid. Mortal. Weekly Rep.* **25**:299–300 (1976).
19. BUCHANAN, T. M., HENDRICKS, S. L., PATTON, C. M., AND FELDMAN, R. A., Brucellosis in the United States, 1960–1972. An abattoir-associated disease. Part III. Epidemiology and evidence for acquired immunity, *Medicine* **53**:427–439 (1974).
20. CARMICHAEL, L. E., AND GEORGE, L. W., Canine brucellosis: Newer knowledge, *Dev. Biol. Stand.* **31**:237–250 (1976).
21. CARMICHAEL, L. E., AND KENNEY, R. M., Canine brucellosis: The clinical disease, pathogenesis and immune response, *J. Am. Vet. Med. Assoc.* **156**:1726–1734 (1970).
22. CASTANEDA, M. R., A practical method for routine blood cultures in brucellosis, *Proc. Soc. Exp. Biol. Med.* **64**:114–115 (1947).
23. CHUNG, S. C. S., Immunosuppression in chronic brucellosis, *Irish J. Med. Sci.* **147**:103–107 (1968).
24. COGHLAN, J. D., Antibodies in human brucellosis, *Br. Med. J.* **2**:269–271 (1967).
25. CORBEL, M. J., The serological relationship between *Brucella spp.*, *Yersinia enterocolitica* serotypes IX and *Salmonella* serotypes Kauffman–White group N, *J. Hyg.* **75**:151–171 (1975).
26. CORBEL, M. J., GILL, K. P. W., AND THOMAS, E. L., Methods for the identification of *Brucella*, Ministry of Agriculture, Fisheries and Food, Weybridge, England (pp. 48–50) (1978).
27. COTTON, W. E., BUCK, J. M., AND SMITH, H. E., Efficacy and safety of abortion vaccines prepared from *Brucella abortus* strains of different degrees of virulence, *J. Agr. Res.* **46**:291–314 (1933).
28. CRISCUOLO, E., AND DICARLO, F. C., El aborto y otras manifestaciones ginecobstetricas en el curso de la brucelosis humana, *Rev. Fac. Cien. Med. Univ. Nac. Cordoba* **12**:321 (1954).
29. DAVIES, G., AND CASEY, A., The survival of *Brucella abor-*

tus in milk and milk products, *Br. Vet. J.* **129**:345–353 (1973).

30. DIAZ, R., AND OYELEDUN, M. A., Studies of some biological activities of 'Brucella' exotoxin in normal and infected animals and the role of the hypersensitivity factor, *Ann. Sclavo* **19**:117–130 (1977).

31. DIAZ, R. L., JONES, L. M., AND WILSON, J. B., Antigenic relationship of the gram-negative organism causing canine abortion to smooth and rough brucellae, *J. Bacteriol.* **95**:618–624 (1968).

32. DIAZ, R., MARAVI-POMA, E., AND RIVERO, A., Comparison of counterimmunoelectrophoresis with other serological tests in the diagnosis of human brucellosis, *Bull. WHO* **53**:417–424 (1976).

33. DIAZ, R., MARAVI-POMA, E., DELGADO, G., AND RIVERO, A., Rose bengal plate agglutination and counterimmunoelectrophoresis tests on spinal fluid in the diagnosis of *Brucella* meningitis, *J. Clin. Microbiol.* **7**:236–237 (1978).

34. ECKMAN, M. R., Brucellosis linked to Mexican cheese, *J. Am. Med. Assoc.* **232**:636–637 (1975).

35. EISELE, C. W., MCCULLOGH, N. B., BEAL, G. A., AND ROTTSCHAEFER, W., Brucella agglutination tests and vaccination against cholera, *J. Am. Med. Assoc.* **135**:983–984 (1947).

36. ELBERG, S. S., Immunity to Brucella infection, *Medicine* **52**:339–356 (1973).

37. EVANS, A. C., Further studies on *Bacterium abortus* and related bacteria. II. A comparison of *Bacterium abortus* with *Bacterium bronchisepticus* and with the organism which causes Malta fever, *J. Infect. Dis.* **22**:580–593 (1918).

38. FARRELL, I. D., ROBERTSON, L., AND HINCHLIFFE, P. M., Serum antibody response in acute brucellosis, *J. Hyg.* **74**:23–28 (1975).

39. FOX, M. D., AND KAUFMANN, A. F., Brucellosis in the United States, 1965–1974, Center for Disease Control, *J. Infect. Dis.* **136**:312–316 (1977).

40. GENTRY, E. R., AND FERENBAUGH, T. L., Endemic Malta (Mediterranean) fever in Texas with isolation of the *Micrococcus melitensis* from two patients, *J. Am. Med. Assoc.* **57**:889 (1911).

41. GLENCHUR, H., SEAL, U. S., ZINNEMAN, H. H., AND HALL, W. H., Serum precipitins in human and experimental brucellosis, *J. Lab. Clin. Med.* **59**:220–230 (1962).

42. GRAVES, R. R., Story of John M. Buck's and Matilda's contribution to the cattle industry, *J. Am. Vet. Med. Assoc.* **102**:193–195 (1943).

43. GRIFFITTS, J. J., Agglutination and an agglutinin-"blocking" property in serums from known cases of brucellosis, *Public Health Rep.* **62**:865–875 (1947).

44. GUERRO, H., DETER, R. L., AND WILLIAMS, R. P., Infection at the subcellular level. II. Distribution and fate of intravenously injected brucellae within phagocytic cells of guinea pigs, *Infect. Immun.* **8**:694–699 (1973).

45. HALL, W. H., Studies of immunity to brucellosis and the bactericidal action of human blood against Brucella, Ph.D. thesis, University of Minnesota, Minneapolis (1950).

46. HALL, W. H., Brucellosis in man. A study of thirty-five cases due to Brucella abortus, *Minn. Med.* **36**:460–465 (1953).

47. HALL, W. H., Epidemic brucellosis in beagles, *J. Infect. Dis.* **124**:615–618 (1971).

48. HALL, W. H., History of brucella as a human pathogen, in: *Brucellosis: Clinical and Laboratory Aspects* (E. YOUNG AND M. CORBEL, eds.), p. 187, CRC Press, Boca Raton, (1989).

49. HALL, W. H., AND MANION, R. E., Comparison of the Coombs' test with other methods for Brucella agglutinins in human serum, *J. Clin. Invest.* **32**:96–106 (1953).

50. HALL, W. H., AND MANION, R. E., *In vitro* susceptibility of Brucella to various antibiotics, *Appl. Microbiol.* **20**:600–604 (1970).

51. HALL, W. H., MANION, R. E., AND ZINNEMAN, H. H., Blocking serum lysis of *Brucella abortus* by hyperimmune rabbit immunoglobulin A, *J. Immunol.* **107**:41–46 (1971).

52. HARDY, A. V., JORDON, C. F., BORTS, I. H., AND HARDY, G. C., Undulant fever with special reference to a study of Brucella infections in Iowa, *U.S. Natl. Inst. Health Bull.* **158**:1–89 (1931).

53. HEINMAN, H. S., AND DZIAMSKI, I. M., *Brucella suis* infection in Philadelphia. A survey of hog fever and asymptomatic brucellosis, *Am. J. Epidemiol.* **103**:88–100 (1976).

54. HEIZMANN, W., BOTZENHART, K., DOLLER, G., SCHANZ, D., HERMANN, G., AND FLEISCHMANN, K., Brucellosis: Serological methods compared, *J. Hyg.* **95**:639–653 (1985).

55. HENDERSON, R. J., AND HILL, D. M., Subclinical Brucella infection in man, *Br. Med. J.* **3**:154–156 (1972).

56. HENRY, B. S., Dissociation in the genus Brucella, *J. Infect. Dis.* **52**:374–402 (1933).

57. HOLLAND, J. J., AND PICKETT, M. J., A cellular basis of immunity in experimental Brucella infection, *J. Exp. Med.* **108**:343–360 (1958).

58. HOPTMAN, J., *Brucellosis in the USSR: A Review of the Literature*, National Institutes of Health, Bethesda, 1959.

59. HORNING, B. G., Outbreak of undulant fever due to *Brucella suis*, *J. Am. Med. Assoc.* **105**:1978–1979 (1935).

60. HUDDLESON, I. F., AND MUNGER, M., A study of an epidemic of brucellosis due to *Brucella melitensis*, *Am. J. Public Health* **30**:944–954 (1940).

61. HUGHES, M. L., *Mediterranean, Malta or Undulant Fever*, Macmillan & Co., London, 1897.

62. HUNT, A. C., AND BOTHWELL, P. W., Histological findings in human brucellosis, *J. Clin. Pathol.* **20**:267–272 (1967).

63. IMBODEN, J. B., CANTER, A., CLUFF, L. E., AND TREVER, R. W., Brucellosis. II. Psychologic aspects of delayed convalescence, *Arch. Intern. Med.* **103**:406–414 (1959).

64. IRWIN, M. R., AND BELL, F. N., On natural antibodies in the rabbit and hereditary resistance to infections of *Brucella suis*, *J. Infect. Dis.* **57**:74–77 (1935).

65. JONES, L. M., ZANARDI, M., LEONG, D., AND WILSON, J.

B., Taxonomic position in the genus *Brucella* of the causative agent of canine abortion, *J. Bacteriol.* 95:625–630 (1968).

66. JORDAN, C. F., BORTS, I. H., HARRIS, D. R., AND JENNINGS, J. R., Brucellosis. Consideration of its epidemiology, diagnosis and control, *Am. J. Public Health* 33:773–779 (1943).
67. KANEENE, J. M., ANDERSON, R. K., JOHNSON, D. W., ANGUS, R. D., MUSCOPLAT, C. C., PIETZ, D. E., VANDERWAGON, L. C., AND SLOANE, E. E., Cell-mediated immune responses in swine from a herd infected with Brucella suis, *Am. J. Vet. Res.* 39:1607–1611 (1978).
68. KANEENE, J. M., ANDERSON, R. K., JOHNSON, D. W., MUSCOPLAT, C. C., NICOLETTI, P., ANGUS, R. D., PIETZ, D. E., AND KLAUSNER, D. J., Whole-blood lymphocyte stimulation assay for measurement of cell-mediated immune responses in bovine brucellosis, *J. Clin. Microbiol.* 7:550–557 (1978).
69. KARLSBAD, G., KESSEL, R. W. I., dePETRIS, S., AND MONACO, L., Electron microscope observations of *Brucella abortus* grown within monocytes *in vitro*, *J. Gen. Microbiol.* 35:383–390 (1964).
70. KAUFMANN, A. F., FOX, M. D., BOYCE, J. M., ANDERSON, D. C., POTTER, M. E., MARTONE, W. J., AND PATTON, C. M., Airborne spread of brucellosis, *Ann. N.Y. Acad. Sci.* 353:105–114 (1980).
71. KEPPIE, J., Host and tissue specificity, *Symp. Soc. Gen. Microbiol.* 14:44–63 (1964).
72. KERR, W. R., COGHLAN, J. D., PAYNE, D. J. H., AND ROBERTSON, L., The laboratory diagnosis of chronic brucellosis, *Lancet* 2:1121–1183 (1966).
73. KERR, W. R., PAYNE, D. J. H., ROBERTSON, L., AND COOMBS, R. R. A., Immunoglobulin class of Brucella antibodies in human sera, *Immunology* 13:223–225 (1967).
74. KERR, W. R., McCAUGHEY, W. J., COGHLAN, J. D., PAYNE, D. J. H., QUAIFE, R. A., ROBERTSON, L., AND FARRELL, I. D., Techniques and interpretations in the serological diagnosis of brucellosis in man, *J. Med. Microbiol.* 1:181–193 (1968).
75. KROGSTAD, D. J., AND SCHLESINGER, P. H., Acid-vesicle function, intracellular pathogens, and the action of chloroquine against *Plasmodium falciparum*, *N. Engl. J. Med.* 317:542–549 (1987).
76. LOWRIE, D. B., AND KENNEDY, J. F., Erythritol and threitol in canine placenta. Possible implication in canine brucellosis, *FEBS Lett.* 23:69–72 (1972).
77. MACDONALD, A., AND ELMSLIE, W. H., Serological investigations in suspected brucellosis, *Lancet* 1:380–382 (1967).
78. MAGOFFIN, R. L., KABLER, P., SPINK, W. W., AND FLEMING, D., An epidemiologic study of brucellosis in Minnesota, *Public Health Rep.* 64:1021–1043 (1949).
79. MANN, P. G., AND RICHENS, E. R., Aspects of human brucellosis, *Postgrad. Med. J.* 49:523–525 (1973).
80. MARSTON, J. A., Report on fever (Malta), in: *Great Britain Army Medical Department Report for 1861*, pp. 486–521, London, 1863.
81. MATYAS, Z., AND FUJIKURA, T., Brucellosis as a world problem, *Dev. Biol. Stand.* 56:3–20 (1984).
82. McDEVITT, D. G., The relevance of the antihuman globulin (Coombs') test and the complement-fixation test in the diagnosis of brucellosis, *J. Hyg.* 68:173–187 (1970).
83. MEYER, K. F., Observations on the pathogenesis of undulant fever, in: *Essays in Biology in Honor of Herbert M. Evans*, pp. 439–459, University of California Press, Berkeley, 1943.
84. MEYER, K. F., AND EDDIE, B., Laboratory infections due to Brucella, *J. Infect. Dis.* 68:24–32 (1941).
85. MEYER, M. E., AND CAMERON, H. S., Metabolic characterization of the genus Brucella, *J. Bacteriol.* 82:387–410, 950–953 (1961).
86. MOHLER, J. R., Infectious abortion in cattle, in: *Annual Report, U.S. Bureau of Animal Industry*, 1913–1914, p. 30.
87. MOHLER, J. R., AND HART, G. H., Malta fever and the Maltese goat importance, in: *Annual Report, U.S. Bureau of Animal Industry*, 25:279 (1908).
88. MORALES-OTERO, P., Further attempts at experimental infections of man with a bovine strain of *Brucella abortus*, *J. Infect. Dis.* 52:54–59 (1933).
89. MORISSET, R., AND SPINK, W. W., Epidemic canine brucellosis due to a new species, *Brucella canis*, *Lancet* 2:1000–1002 (1969).
90. MORRIS, J. A., The interaction of *Brucella abortus* 544 and neutrophil polymorphonuclear leukocytes, *Ann. Sclavo* 19:143–150 (1977).
91. MUNFORD, R. S., WEAVER, R. E., PATTON, C., FEELEY, J. C., AND FELDMAN, R. A., Human disease caused by *Brucella canis*. A clinical and epidemiologic study of two cases, *J. Am. Med. Assoc.* 231:1267–1269 (1975).
92. MURRAY, M. J., MURRAY, A. B., MURRAY, M. B., AND MURRAY, C. J., The adverse effect of iron repletion on the course of certain infections, *Br. Med. J.* 2:1113–1114 (1978).
93. NELSON, K. E., RUBEN, F. L., AND ANDERSEN, B., An unusual outbreak of brucellosis, *Arch. Intern. Med.* 135:691–695 (1975).
94. NICOLETTI, P., The epidemiology of bovine brucellosis, *Advances Veterin. Sci. and Comp. Med.* 24:69–98, 1980.
95. NICOLLE, C., BURNET, E., AND CONSEIL, E., Le microbe de l'avortement épizootique se distingue de celui de la fièvre Méditerranéenne par l'absence de pouvoir pathogène pour l'homme, *C.R. Acad. Sci.* 176:1034–1036 (1923).
96. OHARA, S., SATO, T., AND HOMMA, M., Serological studies on *Francisella tularensis, Francisella novicida, Yersinia philomiragia*, and *Brucella abortus*, *Int. J. Syst. Bacteriol.* 24:191–196 (1947).
97. PAPPAGIANIS, D., ELBERG, S. S., AND CROUCH, D., Immunization against Brucella infections. Effects of graded doses of viable attenuated *Brucella melitensis* in humans, *Am. J. Epidemiol.* 84:21–31 (1966).
98. PHILLIPON, A. M., PLOMMET, M. G., KAZMIERCZAK, A., MARLY, J. L., AND NEVOT, P. A., Rifampin in the treatment

of experimental brucellosis in mice and guinea pigs, *J. Infect. Dis.* **136:**482–488 (1977).

99. PICKETT, M. J., AND NELSON, E. L., Observations on the problem of Brucella blood cultures, *J. Bacteriol.* **61:**229–237 (1951).

100. PORRECO, R. P., AND HAVERKAMP, A. D., Brucellosis in pregnancy, *Obstet. Gynecol.* **44:**597–602 (1974).

101. *Recommended Uniform Methods and Rules: Brucellosis Eradication,* U.S. Department of Agriculture, Animal and Plant Inspection Service, Hyattsville, Maryland, 1977.

102. REDDIN, J. L., ANDERSEN, R. K., KENNESS, R., AND SPINK, W. W., Significance of 7S and macroglobulin Brucella agglutinins in human brucellosis, *N. Engl. J. Med.* **272:**1263–1268 (1965).

103. RENOUX, M., PALAT, A., GUILLAUMIN, J. M., AND RENOUX, G., Hémagglutination passive, transformation lymphoblatique et migration des leucocytes appliquées au diagnostic des brucelloses, *Dev. Biol. Stand.* **31:**145–146 (1976).

104. ROBERTSON, L., WALLACE, J. G., BARROW, G. I., BRADSTREET, C. M. P., COGLAN, J. C., CUNLIFFE, A. C., FARRELL, I. D., HOWELLS, C. H. L., PAYNE, D. J. H., POLLACK, T. M., AND REID, D., Appraisal of the brucellin skin test. Report of a Working-Party to the Director of the Public Health Laboratory Service, *Lancet* **1:**676–678 (1972).

105. ROUX, J. RAMUZ, M., AND SERRE, J. C., Action de la chlortetracycline sur les Brucella intracellulaires, *Ann. Inst. Pasteur* **116:**49–62 (1969).

106. RUSSELL, A. O., PATTON, C. M., AND KAUFFMAN, A. F., Evaluation of the card test for diagnosis of human brucellosis, *J. Clin. Microbiol.* **7:**454–458 (1978).

107. SANDOK, P. L., HINSKILL, R. D., AND ALBRECHT, R. M., Migration inhibition of mouse macrophages by Brucella antigens, *Infect. Immun.* **4:**516–518 (1971).

108. SARRAM, M., FEIZ, J., FORUZANDEK, M., AND GAZANFARPOUR, P., Intrauterine fetal infection with *Brucella melitensis* as a possible cause of second-trimester abortion, *Am. J. Obstet. Gynecol.* **119:**657–660 (1974).

109. SCHROEDER, E. C., AND COTTON, W. E., Infectious abortion of cattle and the occurrence of its bacterium in milk. II. The bacillus of infectious abortion found in milk, in: *28th Annual Report, U.S. Bureau of Animal Industry* **28:**139 (1911).

110. SHAFFER, J. M., KUCERA, C. J., AND SPINK, W. W., The protection of intracellular Brucella against therapeutic agents and the bactericidal action of serum, *J. Exp. Med.* **97:**77–90 (1953).

111. SMITH, H., Biochemical challenge of microbial pathogenicity, *Bacteriol. Rev.* **32:**164–184 (1968).

112. SMITH, T., A characteristic localization of *Bacillus abortus* in the bovine fetal membranes, *J. Exp. Med.* **29:**451–456 (1919).

113. SPINK, W. W., What is chronic brucellosis? *Ann. Intern. Med.* **35:**358–374 (1951).

114. SPINK, W. W., Family studies on brucellosis, *Am. J. Med. Sci.* **227:**128–133 (1954).

115. SPINK, W. W., The significance of endotoxin in brucellosis.

Experimental and clinical studies, *Trans. Assoc. Am. Physicians* **67:**283–291 (1954).

116. SPINK, W. W., The significance of bacterial hypersensitivity in human brucellosis. Studies on infections due to strain 19, *Brucella abortus, Ann. Intern. Med.* **47:**861–874 (1957).

117. SPINK, W. W., AND ANDERSON, D., Experimental studies on the significance of endotoxin in the pathogenesis of brucellosis, *J. Clin. Invest.* **33:**540–548 (1954).

118. SPINK, W. W., HOFFBAUER, F. W., WALKER, W. W., AND GREEN, R. A., Histopathology of the liver in human brucellosis, *J. Lab. Clin. Med.* **34:**40–58 (1949).

119. SPINK, W. W., HALL, J. W., III, FINSTAD, J., AND MALLET, E., Immunization with viable Brucella organisms. Results of a safety test in humans, *Bull. WHO* **26:**409–419 (1962).

120. STANTIC-PAVLINIC, M., CEC, V., AND MEHLE, J., Brucellosis in spouses and the possibility of interhuman infection, *Infection* **11:**313–314 (1983).

121. STEFFEN, R. T., Antacids—A risk factor in travelers' brucellosis? *Scand. J. Infect. Dis.* **9:**311–312 (1977).

122. STREET, L., GRANT, W. W., AND ALVA, J. D., Brucellosis in childhood, *Pediatrics* **55:**416–421 (1975).

123. SUNDBERG, R. D., AND SPINK, W. W., The histopathology of lesions in the bone marrow of patients having brucellosis, *Blood* **1**(Suppl.):7–32 (1947).

124. THAPAR, M. K., AND YOUNG, E. J., Urban outbreak of goat cheese brucellosis, *Pediatr. Infect. Dis.* **5:**640–643 (1986).

125. THOMAS, K. W., AND MCCAUSLAND, I.P., The use of immunochemically purified anti-Brucella antibody in a direct fluorescent antibody test for *Brucella abortus, Vet. Immunol. Immunopathol.* **1:**343–352 (1980).

126. THOMSEN, A., Om kalvekastiningsfebrerens (svingefeberens) forekomst hos danske dyrlaeger, *Saertryk Maanedsskr. Dyrlaeger* **43:**46–57 (1931).

127. TREVER, R. W., CLUFF, L. E., PEELER, B. N., AND BENNETT, I. L., JR., Brucellosis. I. Laboratory-acquired acute infection. *Arch. Intern. Med.* **103:**381–397 (1959).

128. WHITE, P. C., JR., BAKER, E. F., JR., ROTH, A. J., WILLIAMS, W. J., AND STEPHENS, T. S., Brucellosis in a Virginia meat-packing plant, *Arch. Environ. Health* **28:**263–271 (1974).

129. WRIGHT, A. E., AND SEMPLE, D., On the employment of dead bacteria in the serum diagnosis of typhoid and Malta fever, *Br. Med. J.* **1:**1214–1216 (1897).

130. YOUNG, E. J., Human brucellosis. Review, *Rev. Infect. Dis.* **5:**821–845 (1983).

131. YOUNG, E. J., AND SUVANNOPARRAT, U., Brucellosis outbreak attributed to ingestion of unpasteurized goat cheese, *Arch. Intern. Med.* **135:**240–243 (1975).

132. ZINNEMAN, H. H., GLENCHUR, H., AND HALL, W. H., The nature of blocking antibodies in human brucellosis, *J. Immunol.* **83:**206–212 (1959).

133. ZINNEMAN, H. H., SEAL, U. S., AND HALL, W. H., Some molecular characteristics of blocking antibodies in human brucellosis. Soluble antigen–antibody complexes, *J. Immunol.* **93:**993–1000 (1964).

12. Suggested Reading

ALTON, G. G., JONES, L. M., AND PIETZ, D. E., *Laboratory Techniques in Brucellosis,* 2nd ed., WHO Monograph No. 55, Geneva, 1975.

HALL, W. H., AND KHAN, M. Y., Brucellosis, in: *Infectious Diseases,* 4th ed. (P. D. HOEPRICH, ed.), Harper & Row, New York, 1989.

HUDDLESON, I. F., *Brucellosis in Man and Animals,* The Commonwealth Fund, New York, 1943.

OLITZKI, A., *Immunological Methods in Brucellosis Research,* Parts I and II, Karger, Basel, 1970.

Reports of the Mediterranean Fever Commission, Parts 1–7, Harrison & Sons, London, 1905–1907.

SPINK, W. W., *The Nature of Brucellosis,* University of Minnesota Press, Minneapolis, 1956.

YOUNG, E. J., AND CORBEL, M. J., *Brucellosis: Clinical and Laboratory Aspects,* CRC Press, Boca Raton, 1989.

CHAPTER 7

Campylobacter Infections

David N. Taylor and Martin J. Blaser

1. Introduction

Campylobacters are slender, spiral or curved, micro-aerophilic gram-negative rods that cause diarrheal and systemic illness in humans and a number of diseases in wild and domestic animals. Because of morphological similarity with vibrios, these organisms were originally classified as *Vibrio fetus*.[103,204] *Campylobacter* (Greek for "curved rod") was proposed as a name of a new genus when it was found that these organisms differed in their biochemical characteristics from true members of the genus *Vibrio*. *C. jejuni* is now regarded as among the leading causes of diarrheal disease in humans. Other *Campylobacter* species that have been associated with diarrheal disease and are distinguished from *C. jejuni* by an inability to hydrolyze hippurate include *C. coli*, *C. fetus* subsp. *fetus*, *C. laridis*, *C. fennelliae*, *C. cinaedi*, *C. hyointestinalis*, and *C. upsaliensis* (Table 1). *C. fetus* also causes systemic infections in immunocompromised hosts.

The most recently discovered *Campylobacter* organism of significance is *C. pylori* (now *Helicobacter pylori*). This organism appears to be associated with gastritis and peptic ulcer disease in humans and unlike all other *Campylobacter* species does not now appear to have an animal host.

Although morphologically similar, taxonomic studies do not place *C. pylori* in the same group with the other campylobacters.[185] For this reason and because it is associated with a separate clinical entity,[10,67,132] *C. pylori* will not be discussed in this chapter. Other *Campylobacter* species that generally do not cause disease in humans include *C. sputorum* subsp. *sputorum* (a commensal organism isolated from the human oral cavity), *C. sputorum* subsp. *bubulus* from genital sites of cattle and sheep, *C. sputorum* subsp. *mucosalis* associated with intestinal disease in pigs, and *C. fetus* subsp. *venerealis* causing abortion and infertility in cattle.[103,203]

2. Historical Background

The first identification of *Campylobacter* was in 1909 during an investigation of infectious abortion, when Mac-Fadyean and Stockman,[128] two English veterinarians, isolated from placentas and aborted fetuses of cattle organisms that they called *Vibrio fetus*. Subsequently, similar organisms were found to cause infectious abortion in sheep.[128] *V. fetus* has become known as a major cause of enzootic and epizootic abortion in cattle and sheep.[203] Over the next 30 years, these organisms were isolated from calves[98] and swine with diarrhea[49] and from fowl with hepatitis and diarrhea.[203] Although *V. fetus* was at first believed to cause diarrheal illness in these hosts, this association has not been clearly documented.

David N. Taylor · Department of Bacterial Diseases, Walter Reed Army Institute of Research, Washington, D.C. 20307. **Martin J. Blaser** · Division of Infectious Diseases, Vanderbilt University School of Medicine, Nashville, Tennessee 37232.

Table 1. Characteristics of *Campylobacter* Species Isolated from Humans with Enteritis[a]

Campylobacter species	Growth 25°	Growth 42°	Hippurate hydrolysis	Susceptibility to (30 µg) Nalidixic acid	Susceptibility to (30 µg) Cephalothin	Catalase Production	0.1% TMAO[b]	Nitrate reduction	H₂S in TSI[c]	0.04% TTC[d]	Reservoir
C. jejuni	−	+[e]	+	S	R	+	−	+	−	+	Section 6
C. coli	−	+	−	S	R	+	−	+	d	+	Pigs
C. laridis[g]	−	+	−	R	R	+	+	+	−	−	Seagulls
C. hyointestinalis[h]	d	+	−	R	S	+	−	+	−	−	Pigs
C. fetus subsp. fetus	+	d	−	R	S	+	−	+	−	−	Cattle
C. cinaedi[i]	−	d	−	S	S[f]	+	−	+	−	+	Unknown
C. fennelliae[i]	−	d	−	S	S	+	−	−	−	+	Unknown
C. upsaliensis[j]	−	+	−	S	S	−/w	−	+	−	−	Dogs
C. cryoaerophilia	+	−	−	d	R	+	( )	( )	−	( )	Cattle, pigs

[a] +, positive; −, negative; d, variable; w, weak; S, susceptible; R, resistant.
[b] TMAO, anaerobic growth in trimethylamine N-oxide hydrochloride.
[c] TSI, triple sugar iron.
[d] TTC, triphenyltetrazolium chloride tolerance.
[e] Variants that grow poorly at 42°C may be cephalothin-sensitive, nitrate-negative,[209] or biochemically identical to *C. jejuni*.[225]
[f] Sensitive to cefazolin.
[g] Refs. 6, 31, 92, 125, 143, 200, 216.
[h] Refs. 53, 62.
[i] Refs. 56, 137, 170, 225, 230.
[j] Refs. 122, 136, 192, 209.

The first isolation of *V. fetus* from a human was in 1947 from the bloodstream of a pregnant woman who had an infectious abortion.[239] Over the next 30 years, there were occasional reports in the medical literature of isolation of these organisms from the bloodstream, cerebrospinal fluid, joint aspirates, endovascular tissue, and abscess cavities.[61] Most of the hosts were debilitated by alcoholism, neoplasm, diabetes mellitus, cardiovascular disease, or old age.[28,74] *V. fetus* was thought to be an unusual cause of systemic illness in debilitated hosts, and it was thus considered to be an opportunistic organism. However, in 1957, Elizabeth King[109] at the Centers for Disease Control (CDC) recognized that not all the *V. fetus* organisms were the same; she identified two groups with distinct serological and biochemical charcteristics. The majority of the isolates grew at 25 and 37°C, but the rest grew only at 37 and 42°C. She called this latter group "related vibrios" and noted that although they were isolated from the bloodstream, in each case the patient had had a diarrheal illness. She postulated that the "related vibrios" caused acute diarrheal illness, but because they were slow-growing and fastidious, they could not be isolated from fecal specimens.[109,110]

Based on King's and his own observations that the related vibrio was associated with diarrhea, Bokkenheuser concluded that this organism was probably present in feces, but could not be detected with the available laboratory techniques.[28] Cooper and Slee[42] in Australia isolated *V. fetus* (*C. jejuni*) from the stool of an immunocompromised patient with recurrent bacteremia and diarrhea by inoculating the patient's feces onto a horse blood agar plate containing cephalothin disks and incubating overnight in a carbon dioxide-enriched atmosphere. In 1972 Dekeyser *et al.* reported a positive stool culture for *Campylobacter* from a 22-year-old woman from whom *C. jejuni* had been isolated from the blood.[43] The stool isolate was obtained by filtering fecal specimens through a 0.65-µm Millipore filter with a syringe. Using this filtration procedure, Butzler *et al.* were able to isolate *Campylobacter* from 5.1% of 800 children in Brussels with diarrhea and only 1.3% of 1000 children without diarrhea.[36] Skirrow showed that an agar medium containing antibiotics could be used instead of filtration as a primary isolation technique and that *C. jejuni* was as important a cause of diarrheal disease in England as Butzler *et al.* had found it in Belgium.[201] The use of antibiotic-containing selective media combined with simple methods for obtaining a microaerobic atmosphere have made isolation of *Campylobacter* a routine procedure and have opened up the study of *Campylobacter* infections on a worldwide scale. By 1973, Veron and Chatlain[238] recognized that *V. fetus* and "related vibrios" had biochemical characteristics dissimilar to those of the Vibrionaceae, and a new genus, *Campylobacter*, was proposed. Under this scheme and later modification by Smibert,[203] King's "related vibrios" became *C. jejuni* and *C. coli*, and the opportunistic organisms became *C. fetus* subsp. *fetus*, respectively.[103,204,238]

In recent years it has been noted that some campylobacters, particularly the hippurate-negative group, are not thermotolerant and are susceptible to antibiotics, such as cephalothin and colistin, that are incorporated into selective isolation media. Steele *et al.*[209] have reported that *Campylobacter* can be isolated at 37°C on media without antibiotics by inoculating a stool suspension directly on a 0.45-μm Millipore filter that has been placed directly on a blood agar plate. This simplified version of Dekeyser's original isolation method has shown that there is a diversity of *Campylobacter* organisms that can be isolated from the stool.[69,122,136,137,226] At present, *C. jejuni* remains the most important cause of diarrheal disease in this group, and the importance of these "related" campylobacters as human pathogens has not yet been fully defined.

3. Methodology

3.1. Sources of Mortality Data

Limited information is available concerning the importance of *Campylobacter* in fatal diarrheal disease; however, judging from the frequency of *Campylobacter* infection in patients ill enough to seek medical attention, the bacterium may be a major cause of mortality due to diarrheal disease. In the developed countries in recent years, mortality due to diarrheal diseases has been low. Several deaths due to infection by *C. jejuni*[205] have been reported, and which have allowed for limited population-based estimates of mortality.[205] The uncommon human infections with *C. fetus* subsp. *fetus*, usually occurring in debilitated hosts, have sometimes been fatal.[28,61,200] Guillain–Barré syndrome and the hemolytic–uremic syndrome are uncommon complications of *C. jejuni* infections that are also potentially fatal (Section 8.1).

3.2. Sources of Morbidity Data

Since campylobacters produce diarrheal illnesses that are usually indistinguishable from those caused by other viral and bacterial enteric pathogens, it is not possible to obtain data on morbidity in the absence of laboratory identification of the organism. Most data on morbidity in Europe and the United States come from hospital-based or community-based studies of *Campylobacter* infections.[22,108,213] Surveys from hospitals and clinics have also been conducted in developing countries. At the International Center for Diarrheal Disease Research in Bangladesh, surveillance is based on culturing 4% of patients who come to the center with acute diarrheal disease.[212] In England and Wales, 200 public health and hospital laboratories report *Campylobacter* isolations to the Communicable Disease Surveillance Center.[202] In the United States, 42 states routinely report *Campylobacter* isolations to the Centers for Disease Control.[175]

3.3. Serological Surveys

Serological surveys using one or several antigens common to the majority of *Campylobacter* strains[172] have been performed among healthy populations in the United States, Bangladesh, and Thailand.[11,23,25] Surveys have been made to confirm the diagnosis in patients with diarrhea,[95,116,118] to investigate outbreaks,[96] to determine the etiology when multiple pathogens were isolated,[222] to investigate occupational exposure and other high-risk groups,[27,94,130] and to investigate the association of *Campylobacter* with postinfection complications such as reactive arthritis and Guillain–Barré syndrome.[99,116,117]

3.4. Laboratory Diagnosis

Stools or rectal swabs, the usual specimens submitted to the laboratory for examination,[101] must be inoculated to selective media to permit isolation of *Campylobacter*. The three most commonly used selective media are Skirrow's,[201] Butzler's,[35] and Campy-BAP,[13] all with rich basal media enriched with sheep or horse blood, and all containing antibiotics to inhibit the normal enteric flora. Both Campy-BAP and Butzler's media contain cephalosporins, which inhibit most strains of *C. fetus* subsp. *fetus* and many of the "atypical" organisms; for this reason, these organisms have rarely been associated with diarrheal illness.[9,112] Skirrow's medium is the least inhibitory to the enteric flora; however, in most patients with *Campylobacter* enteritis the titer of *Campylobacter* organisms per gram of stool ranges from 10^6 to 10^9,[15] a quantity easily detected with this medium. Butzler's media—Virion, which contains cefaperazone and is more inhibitory to competing flora, also appears to be very useful.[68,69,140] Blood-free media containing antibiotics have also been used successfully,[30,69,107] and several enrichment media have been found to support the growth of *Campylobacter*.[140,174] Enrichment methods are probably not necessary for detection of *Campylobacter* in diarrheal stools, but may be useful in detecting carriers.

Some campylobacters that cause diarrhea are inhibited by cephalothin or colistin that are present in the selective media, or by incubation at 42°C.[56,145,209,226] Steele demonstrated that a 0.45-μm cellulose acetate membrane filter placed directly on an antibiotic-free blood agar plate could be used to isolate *Campylobacter* at 37°C.[209] *Campylobacter* in saline solution are able to pass through the filter while other fecal flora do not. A 0.65-μm filter may offer better isolation rates than the 0.45 μm, although the number of contaminating bacteria is also increased.

Campylobacters require an atmosphere with an oxygen concentration of 5–10% for optimal growth. A microaerobic atmosphere may be produced by using *Campylobacter*-specific gas-generating kits[245] or by evacuating vacuum jars or bags and refilling with a mixture of 5% oxygen, 10% carbon dioxide, and 85% nitrogen. Campylobacters are capnophilic, although carbon dioxide is not essential for growth.[204] Incubation of plates in a candle jar may permit isolation from most positive specimens, but should best be used at 42°C.[245]

When using selective antibiotic media, optimal isolation of *C. jejuni* is obtained at an incubation temperature of 42°C; however, some *Campylobacter* species cannot be isolated at that temperature (Table 1). All organisms will grow at 37°C. Since *C. jejuni* is the most common, the use of the more selective media and the higher temperature for incubation is still recommended. If the membrane filter method is employed, the optimum incubation temperature is 37°C.

After incubation of cultures under these conditions for 24–48 h, colonies that are gray, mucoid, or wet-appearing, or discrete should be suspected of being *Campylobacter* and may be identified as such using standard biochemical tests[204] (Table 1). A rapid presumptive identification can be made by the following characteristics: (1) typical colonial morphology; (2) typical Gram stain showing gram-negative curved rods; (3) indication of oxidase and catalase positivity; and (4) motility. *Campylobacter* can be isolated from body fluids or tissues that do not have a normal flora using thioglycollate broth or biphasic media. Some commercial blood culture systems are superior to others for detection of bacteremia due to *Campylobacter* species.[244]

Direct examination of stools has been used as a rapid screening test for *Campylobacter* in developed countries.[82,83,154,156,169,193,195,228] These methods are usually specific, but are only about 50–75% sensitive. Staining with 1% aqueous basic fuchsin was reported to be the most sensitive method.[156,195] Sensitivity was increased in the presence of fecal leukocytes.[228]

Serological diagnosis is possible in which antibodies to the homologous strain or to a common acid-extracted antigen are detected.[11,116,214] DNA probes for the diagnosis of *Campylobacter* are still in the experimental stage.[229] Specific oligonucleotide probes have been produced and will eventually be useful when nonradioactive means of detection become available.[89]

A biotyping scheme for *C. jejuni*, *C. coli*, and *C. laridis* strains has been developed that is based on hippurate hydrolysis, rapid H_2S production, and DNA hydrolysis.[125] A phage typing system has also been developed for *C. jejuni* and *C. coli*.[72] The two most widely used serotyping systems for *C. jejuni* and *C. coli* are the Penner system, which identifies soluble, heat-stable (somatic, O) antigens by passive hemagglutination,[158] and the Lior system, which measures heat-labile (flagellar, H) antigens by slide agglutination.[126] There are over 90 reference serotypes defined by each of these systems. Both systems identify over 90% of *Campylobacter* isolated from humans and nonhuman sources.[97,157] The Lior system is easier to use and more rapid and consequently more applicable for use outside reference laboratories. Strains of a single serotype in one system may belong to multiple serotypes in another system. These two systems may eventually be combined to produce a system similar to *E. coli* serotyping based on both O and H antigen grouping.

4. Proof of Causation and Biological Characteristics of the Organism That Affect the Epidemiological Pattern

The evidence that *C. jejuni* is an etiological agent for human diarrheal disease can be summarized as follows: (1) In developed countries, *Campylobacter* has been isolated from the stools of 3–14% of patients presenting at hospitals with diarrhea, but only rarely from stool samples of controls (Table 2). (2) Outbreaks of gastrointestinal illness have occurred among previously healthy populations in which no other pathogen has been found, and *Campylobacter* has been isolated from the stools of patients but not from controls (Section 6). (3) In natural settings and in experimental models, *Campylobacter* has caused diarrheal illness in avian species[188] and in mammals such as puppies[168] and nonhuman primates.[231] (4) In several patients who had diarrheal illness, *Campylobacter* was simultaneously isolated from stool and blood.[42,43,109] (5) Rising titers of specific serum antibody to the infecting organisms have

Table 2. Isolation of *Campylobacter* from Fecal Cultures from Patients with Diarrhea and from Healthy Controls in the Developed Countries, 1973–1986

Reference	Location	Population	Patients with diarrhea				Healthy controls	
			No. studied	% with *C. jejuni*	% with *Salmonella*	% with *Shigella*	No. studied	% with *C. jejuni*
Butzler[36]	Belgium	Children	800	5.1			1000	1.3
Skirrow[201]	England	All ages	803	7.1			194	0
Brunton[33]	Scotland	All ages	196	8.7	2.5	6.7	50	0
Bruce[32]	England	All ages	280	13.9	4.3	3.9	156	0.6
Kendall[108]	England	All ages	3,250	14.9	2.1	1.1		
Severin[196]	Netherlands	All ages	584	10.8	10.0		120	0
Lopez-Brea[127]	Spain	All ages	446	4.5	12.1	1.3		
Delorme[44]	France	All ages	100	9.0	0	1.0	330	0
Graf[71]	Switzerland	All ages	665	5.7	12.6	0.9	800	0
Velasco[237]	Spain	All ages	6,970	7.3	10.2	5.4		
Figura[58]	Italy	Children	643	9.0	9.6	0		
Cevenini[38]	Italy	Children	561	8.0	7.3	0		
Svedhem[213]	Sweden	All ages	2,550	10.9	7.2	3.5		
Walder[242]	Sweden	All ages	5,771	6.9	4.1	1.7	2000	0.25
Pitkanen[162]	Finland	Adults	775	7.1	NR	NR		
Lassen[121]	Norway	All ages	7,700	3.0	4.7	2.9		
Steingrimsson[210]	Iceland	All ages	4,019	1.7	4.1	0.2		
Blaser[20]	USA	All ages	2,670	4.6	3.4	2.9	157	0
Blaser[22]	USA	All ages	8,097	4.6	2.3	1.0		
Pien[161]	Hawaii	All ages	471	8.7	4.2	3.8		
Pai[152]	Canada	Children	1,004	4.3	5.1	1.4	176	0
Thompson[227]	Canada	All ages	146,842	3.8	7.9	0.2		
Burke[34]	Australia	Children	975	7.4	5.7	1.3	975	0.6
Kirubakaran[111]	Australia	Children	386	4.4	12.2	3.4	332	0

been shown.[11,13,95,100,116,214] (6) Treatment of ill *Campylobacter*-infected patients with erythromycin, an agent to which most other recognized enteric pathogens do not respond, has been followed by rapid clearance of organisms and rapid remission of symptoms.[2,153,190] (7) Two volunteers ingested organisms in a glass of milk and developed a typical gastrointestinal illness after 3 days, and *Campylobacter* was isolated from their stools.[181,208] Finally, two strains of *C. jejuni* isolated from persons with diarrhea were fed to 110 American adult volunteers with sodium bicarbonate.[8,160] The minimum infective dose was 1000 organisms. With one strain (81–176) all became infected and 18 (46%) of 39 developed diarrhea with fecal leukocytes or fever after ingestion of 10^6 organisms. The findings thus fulfill the Henle–Koch postulates of causation [see Chapter 1 (Section 13)].

Campylobacters grow best at the body temperatures of warm-blooded hosts. *C. jejuni* has been identified as a part of the enteric flora in swine, dogs, cats, nonhuman primates, rodents, cattle, sheep, and other ruminants.[203] Optimal growth occurs at 42°C, the body temperature of fowl, and *C. jejuni* appears to be commensal in adult domestic fowl. *Campylobacter* appears to be an enteric pathogen for primates,[231] but its role as an enteric pathogen in other animal species is not well defined.

Viability of organisms under environmental conditions is temperature-dependent. *C. jejuni* will survive for weeks in water, feces, urine, and milk when kept at 4°C; however, at 25°C, viability persists for a few days or less.[15] *Campylobacter*, like *Salmonella*, is quite sensitive to low pH and will not survive longer than 5 min at a pH less than 2.3. At neutrality or alkaline pH, especially in bile, organisms may multiply and survive up to 3 months at 37°C.[15]

Of clinical isolates of *Campylobacter* in a Toronto

study, 15% were resistant to tetracycline and 15% to ampicillin.[105] Erythromycin resistance is generally reported to be less than 10%, but may be much greater and clinically significant in other areas.[223] *C. coli* isolated from animals or humans are more resistant to both erythromycin and tetracycline.[223,246] Ampicillin resistance was associated with chromosomally mediated β-lactamase production. Tetracycline resistance is carried on a 45-kb transmissible plasmid.[218,219] Kanamycin resistance in *C. coli* may be mediated on the same plasmid and may be due to synthesis of 3′-aminoglycoside phosphotransferase type III.[119,178] This type of aminoglycoside resistance was previously found only in gram-positive cocci and suggests that *Campylobacter* could acquire resistance plasmids from unrelated bacterial species.[120] Strains are generally susceptible to chloramphenicol, gentamicin, furazolidone, nalidixic acid, and the newer nalidixic acid analogues such as norfloxacin and ciprofloxacin.[40,198,234,235]

5. Descriptive Epidemiology

5.1. Prevalence and Incidence

It is now well established that *C. jejuni* is an important cause of diarrheal illness in the developed world in all age groups. Prevalence of *disease* caused by *Campylobacter* is based on the rate of isolation of the organism from patients with diarrheal illnesses. Inferences drawn from such studies must be tempered by knowledge of the surveillance artifacts implicit in laboratory-based culture surveys. Presence in a community of *infection* due to *Campylobacter* includes prevalence of isolation of the bacterium from the stools of healthy persons and the presence of antibodies to *Campylobacter* among a representative population sample. In the Denver area from 1982 to 1983 there were 24.4 reported cases of *C. jejuni* infections per 100,000 population.[205] Elsewhere in the United States, rates of reported cases ranged from 1.4 per 100,000 in Alabama to 33 per 100,000 in Washington.[60] In England and Wales, reported *Campylobacter* isolations now outnumber *Salmonella* isolations and are in the same range (20/100,000) as in the United States.[202] *Campylobacter* infections were estimated at nearly 100 per 100,000 population in hospital laboratory-based surveillance systems in Seattle, Washington and Haifa, Israel.[91,177] In England at the level of a community-based physician, the estimated annual rate of *Campylobacter* infection was 1100 per 100,000, approximately 50 times higher than estimates based on *Campylobacter*

isolations reported at the national level.[108] A similar incidence has been estimated for *Salmonella* infections in the United States.[37] Based on these prevalence data a case-fatality rate of 0.05 per 1000 has been estimated.[205] Rates of *Campylobacter* infections vary according to the age distribution and location of the study population.

Campylobacter infections have been evaluated as part of surveys on the etiology of diarrheal disease among persons coming to the hospital or clinic. In the developed world, *Campylobacter* ranks among the most commonly isolated bacterial pathogens from persons with diarrheal disease and is uncommonly isolated from populations of healthy controls (Table 2).

In developing countries, *Campylobacter* infection is hyperendemic and asymptomatic infection with *Campylobacter* is frequent (Table 3). The case-to-infection ratio is probably quite high. In developing countries, this ratio varies inversely according to age, suggesting that immunity is an important factor.[65] Furthermore, adults naturally and experimentally infected with *C. jejuni* were less susceptible to illness if they had preexisting antibody titers to *Campylobacter*.[27,160] Most *C. jejuni* infection in developed and developing countries is endemic.

5.2. Epidemic Behavior

In addition to endemic infection, outbreaks of disease associated with *Campylobacter* regularly occur in developed countries. Outbreaks do not occur where *Campylobacter* infections are hyperendemic such as in many areas of the developing world probably because of a high prevalence of postexposure immunity.[23,25] Outbreak investigations have provided much of the information about specific vehicles for transmission of infection (Section 6).

Investigations of outbreaks have shown that asymptomatic infection may occur in those exposed to an implicated vehicle[19,96] and that the spectrum of illness produced may be broad. In an outbreak at a summer camp, only 4 (10%) of 41 infected persons were sufficiently ill to seek medical attention.[19] Thus, surveillance based on culture reports from patients seeking medical attention will probably significantly undercount the number of cases and overestimate the severity of illness.

Secondary spread of infection does occur in close contact such as family members. In follow-up studies in Israel, 20 (10%) of 200 family contacts were found to excrete *Campylobacter*.[197] However, in most sporadic cases the source is not known and it is difficult to distinguish coprimary from secondary infections.

Table 3.   Isolation of *Campylobacter* from Fecal Cultures from Patients with Diarrhea and from Healthy Controls in the Developing Countries

Reference	Location	Year	Population	Patients with diarrhea		Healthy controls	
				No. studied	% with *Campylobacter*	No. studied	% with *Campylobacter*
	Asia						
Ringertz[176]	Indonesia	1980	0–9 yr	144	10	7	29
Blaser[14]	Bangladesh	1980	Children	204	12	141	18
Rajan[171]	India	1982	All ages	305	15	—	—
Glass[66]	Bangladesh	1983	All ages	3038	14	333	7
Nair[144]	India	1983	All ages	116	10	—	—
Lim[124]	Malaysia	1984	All ages	—	4	—	2
Ho[81]	Hong Kong	1985	0–2 yr	1957	2	1841	2
Young[249]	China	1986	0–15 yr	48	19	105	9
Taylor[a]	Thailand	1986	0–5 yr	1230	13	1230	11
	Africa						
Billingham[7]	Gambia	1981	All ages	287	14	383	4
De Mol[46]	Rwanda	1983	Children	271	14	203	3
Olusanya[150]	Nigeria	1983	5–39 yr	—	12	—	2
Georges[63]	Central African Republic	1984	0–15 yr	1197	11	748	7
Zaki[250]	Egypt	1986	All ages	3135	2	702	1
Megraud[a]	Algeria	1987	0–15 yr	868	16	376	15
Bokkenheuser[29]	S. Africa	1979	0–2 yr	78	35	63	16
Mauff[135]	S. Africa	1981	All ages	2323	4	—	—
	S. Africa	1981	0–2 white	—	5	—	—
	S. Africa	1981	0–2 black	—	13	—	—
Mackenjee[129]	S. Africa	1984	Hospital	126	21	128	5
	S. Africa	1984	Outpatient	352	7	—	—
Lastovica[123]	S. Africa	1986	Children	2951	10	—	—
	Latin America						
Hull[86]	Trinidad	1982	Children	60	12	—	2
Mata[134]	Costa Rica	1983	Children	233	8	—	—
Guerrant[75]	Brazil	1983	Children	40	8	—	—
Olarte[149]	Mexico	1983	Children	265	9	54	4
Figueroa[57]	Chile	1986	Children	35	6	—	—

[a]Presented at the IVth International Conference on *Campylobacter* infections (1987).

5.3. Geographic Distribution

Campylobacter infections are present in all parts of the world, as documented by studies of diarrheal disease on all inhabited continents (Tables 2 and 3). Isolations have been made from patients in tropical, temperate, and arctic climates. Travelers who have acquired *Campylobacter* infections in every region of the world represent a considerable proportion of the total cases in Scandinavian countries.[121,147,163,165] Similarly, persons from developed countries who are living in developing countries are also at risk for *Campylobacter* infection.[206,217,222] In northern climates such as Canada[227] and Iceland,[210] *Campylobacter* infections are reported more commonly among persons in rural areas. In Ontario, Canada the annual case rate was 80 per 100,000 in urban or nonfarm areas and 350 to 400 per 100,000 in farm areas where cases were often associated with raw milk ingestion.[227] High isolation rates in rural areas of Africa have been attributed to close association with domestic animals.[46]

The prevalence of *Campylobacter* infection is higher in developing than in developed areas (Table 3), and other enteric pathogens were frequently isolated with *Campylobacter*.[134,224] Studies of healthy children in rural South Africa,[29] rural Bangladesh,[14,66] Central African Republic,[65] and The Gambia[7] found that asymptomatic infection of young children was prevalent. In The Gambia, 7.6% of asymptomatic children 2–4 years old were infected, and in both South Africa and Bangladesh, 40% of children 9–24 months old were culture-positive on a single determination. In a longitudinal study, *Campylobacter* infections were found in 41% of 127 children who were cultured biweekly from birth until 6 months of age.[65] In developing countries, there is no difference in the isolation rate of *Campylobacter* from children with and without diarrhea. *Campylobacter* infections are uncommon in adults in developing countries; no difference in isolation rates was observed among adults with and without diarrhea in Bangladesh.[66] After infection, the duration of excretion of *Campylobacter* is shorter (about 7 days) than it is among persons in developed countries. The high *Campylobacter* isolation rate among persons with diarrhea is caused by frequent infection rather than prolonged convalescent excretion.[224]

5.4. Temporal Distribution

In industrialized countries in temperate climates there is a definite increase in isolation rate during the hot summer months and a definite decrease during the cold winter months.[20,225] In Scandinavian countries there is another peak after winter holiday seasons resulting from infections in travelers.[121,165] In tropical, developing countries there is usually no seasonal variation.[63,66]

5.5. Age and Sex

In industrialized countries there is a bimodal age distribution. The largest peak occurs in children less than 5 years old and a second peak occurs in young adults 20 to 29 years old (Fig. 1a). Among hospitalized patients, a third peak is observed among persons 60 to 80 years old.[163,225] In *Campylobacter* infections among children and young adults, males usually predominate[175] (Fig. 1a), and among older persons the ratio is equal or in favor of females. In Colorado, for example, males predominate in all age groups under 40 and the greatest difference between sexes was in infants, where the male-to-female ratio was over 2 : 1.[84] In keeping with the second peak of isolation in young adults,

Campylobacter is the predominant cause of diarrheal disease at American universities.[141,215] Eating undercooked chicken and close association with cats are recognized risk factors among university students.[45,215]

In developing countries, isolation rates are highest among children less than 1 year old and do not increase again in young adults (Fig. 1b). The highest isolation rate occurs in children 6 to 12 months old (Fig. 1b inset). In developing countries, one to two *Campylobacter* infections per year for children under 5 would be a conservative estimate. Serological surveys among healthy persons have shown a peak in *Campylobacter* IgG antibodies in children age 1 in Thailand and age 2 to 4 in Bangladesh.[23,25] Infection, even in infants, is frequently not associated with disease in areas of hyperendemicity.[65]

5.6. Occupation

There have been reports of infection immediately after occupational contact with cattle and sheep or with beef, swine, or chicken carcasses.[41,94,130] At present, there is no information to suggest that hospital personnel are at increased risk of infection.

5.7. Other Factors

Campylobacter infections may also be sexually transmitted in homosexual men.[170] Two new species, *C. cinaedi* and *C. fennelliae,* have been isolated from homosexual men[56,230] as well as have *C. fetus* subsp. *fetus*[47] and *C. hyointestinalis.*[53] Homosexuals who have been infected with multiple etiological agents appear to be at an increased risk of these *Campylobacter* species of low virulence. Prolonged or unusually severe *C. jejuni* infections have been recognized in patients with hypogammaglobulinemia[138,233] or AIDS.[51,91,247] Most patients infected with *C. fetus* subsp. *fetus* have been debilitated or compromised by chronic disease or were at the extremes of age.[9,26,48,207] Since most *C. fetus* subsp. *fetus* infections are detected by blood culture, it is possible that only the severe end of the spectrum of disease is recognized. When *C. fetus* subsp. *fetus* was isolated from stool in a milkborne outbreak, it caused a diarrheal disease indistinguishable from *C. jejuni.*[112]

6. Mechanisms and Routes of Transmission

Transmission of *Campylobacter* appears similar to that for other known enteric pathogens, i.e., transmission by

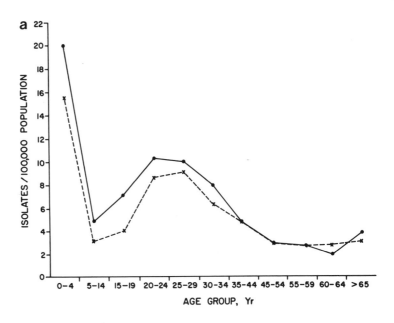

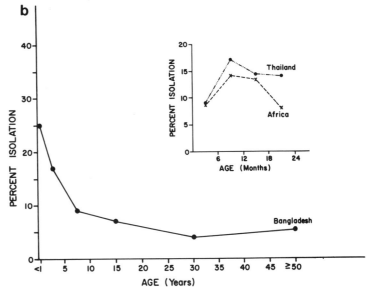

Figure 1. (a) Age-specific isolation rates of *Campylobacter* from persons with diarrhea in the United States in 1982. Solid line indicates males and dashed line indicates females.[60] (b) Age-specific isolation rates of *Campylobacter* from persons with diarrhea in Bangladesh in 1980.[66] Inset indicates the isolation rates from children less than 2 years old with diarrhea in the Central African Republic (Africa) in 1981–1982 and in Thailand in 1985.[63,224]

way of contaminated food and water or by oral contact with fecal material from infected animals or humans. This information comes from investigation of several large and small outbreaks and by inference from single cases. Increasing numbers of outbreaks are being reported in which contaminated water, or food, especially uncooked food, has been implicated as the vehicle. A history of travel to developing countries is common in some groups of *Campylobac-*

ter-positive patients[147,162]; consumption of contaminated food and water is considered the usual mode of transmission for travelers' diarrhea.

Since the animal species with which humans come into contact most frequently—including dogs, cats, cattle, sheep, goats, chickens, turkeys, swine, horses, and rodents[12,21]—have been shown to excrete *C. jejuni* in their feces, the potential reservoir for human infection is enormous. Serotypes of *Campylobacter* isolated from animals are essentially the same as those isolated from humans.

The best documented mode of transmission of *Campylobacter* infection is the ingestion of unpasteurized milk. Unpasteurized milk has been the source of numerous epidemics and appears to be an important cause of endemic disease in rural areas in the United Kingdom, the United States, and Australia.[112,114,115,167,182,183,220,241] Fecal excretion of *Campylobacter* in milk cows and cattle is common and probably the usual source of contamination. *Campylobacter* infection of the bovine udder (mastitis) also may be a source of milk contamination. *Campylobacter* remain viable in refrigerated milk for 3 weeks and when ingested in milk may be protected from the effect of gastric acid.[15] As few as 500 *Campylobacter* cells are infective when given with milk.[181] Persons who drink raw milk regularly have elevated levels of antibodies to *Campylobacter* compared to age-matched persons who do not drink raw milk.[27] *C. fetus* subsp. *fetus* has also been associated with diarrheal disease after the ingestion of raw milk.[112]

Waterborne outbreaks of *Campylobacter* infections have been reported in the United States, Europe, and Israel.[139,155,184,189,221,240] In the two largest outbreaks affecting 3000 persons in Vermont[240] and 2000 persons in central Sweden,[139] untreated surface water most likely contaminated drinking water systems. In smaller outbreaks at an English boarding school[155] and in a Florida town,[189] water in open-topped storage tanks became contaminated perhaps by feces from birds or rodents. In a national park in the Rocky Mountains of the western United States, ingestion of untreated surface water was the most important risk factor for *Campylobacter* infection, which was found to be a more common cause of diarrhea than giardiasis.[221] In Colorado ingestion of raw water is an important risk factor for sporadic cases.[85] *C. laridis* was the probable cause of a waterborne outbreak among 162 construction workers in Canada when lake water was cross-connected to the main drinking water supply.[31] This outbreak provided convincing evidence that *C. laridis* was a human diarrheal disease pathogen.

With *Campylobacter* excretion among domestic animals so common, it is not surprising that retail meats are frequently contaminated with *C. jejuni*. In surveys in the United States about 5% of beef or pork and 30% of poultry meats were found to be contaminated.[21,77,211] Outbreaks have been associated with undercooked chicken, and in England,[186] Sweden,[147] Washington,[78] and Colorado,[87] eating chicken, particularly undercooked chicken, appears to be a significant risk factor for sporadic *Campylobacter* infections.[45,147] It is possible that increasing reports of

Campylobacter infection in England may be partly due to the increased consumption of poultry in that country. An outbreak of *Campylobacter* infection occurred among new employees at a poultry abattoir and serological surveys indicate increased exposure among poultry workers.[41,94] Other outbreak reports have implicated cross-contamination of foods in kitchens[19,59,88] and contamination of shellfish with sewage.[73] Nonmeat products such as mushrooms may be contaminated in the soil.[50]

Human infection after contact with sick animals, especially puppies and kittens, was one of the first observed modes of transmission, but probably accounts for a relatively small proportion of the total cases.[16,54,191,201]

As with other enteric infections, infected humans may be a reservoir for further transmission of infection, but *Campylobacter* is microaerophilic and sensitive to desiccation. Person-to-person transmission has been reported[18,151]; however, the index case has usually been a young child not yet toilet-trained. There have been several reports of vertical transmission of *Campylobacter* infection from symptomatic or asymptomatic mothers to their neonates.[1,80,104,106] Among 19 reported cases of premature labor, abortion, and perinatal sepsis due to *Campylobacter* species, *C. fetus* subsp. *fetus* was isolated in 9 and *C. jejuni/coli* in 10.[200] Considering that *C. jejuni* infection is many more times (ca. 500) more common than *C. fetus* subsp. *fetus* infection, *C. fetus* must be considered to have a propensity for these complications.[9,175] Neonatal infections may be severe. A nosocomial outbreak of meningitis occurred in a neonatal nursery in France.[70] Transmission has not been demonstrated from asymptomatic food handlers or hospital personnel, nor has chronic or convalescent fecal carriage of *Campylobacter* been a source of transmission. There has been a report of laboratory-acquired infection,[148] but transmission to hospital personnel from patients or specimens in the hospital appears to be uncommon.

7. Pathogenesis and Immunity

The minimal dose of *Campylobacter* producing human infections is not known. A volunteer who ingested 10^6 organisms in milk became ill within 3 days.[200] In a large milkborne outbreak, for most patients the onset of illness was 2–7 days after drinking the contaminated milk.[166] For most pathogens, the length of the incubation period is inversely related to the dose ingested. The marked sensitivity of *Campylobacter* to gastric pH[15] suggests that it would take a high dose to infect 50–100% of subjects. The ID_{50} when given with sodium bicarbonate was 10^8.[8]

Infection leads to multiplication of organisms in the intestine; patients shed 10^6–10^9 *Campylobacter*/g stool,[15] concentrations similar to those in *Salmonella* and *Shigella* infections. The sites of tissue injury include the jejunum, ileum, and colon,[15,110] although whether the small or large intestine is more commonly affected is not known. In both organs, acute exudative and hemorrhagic inflammation may occur, and the appendix, mesenteric lymph nodes, and gallbladder may also be affected by the inflammatory process.[4,201] Patients with severe clinical manifestations frequently have colonic involvement. The pathological lesion may include infiltration of the lamina propria with acute and chronic inflammatory cells and destruction of epithelial glands with crypt abscess formation.[17] This nonspecific colitis may mimic that seen in other types of infectious colitis, acute ulcerative colitis, or Crohn's disease. A pseudomembranous colitis has also been described.

The mechanism(s) by which *C. jejuni* causes disease is not known. There is evidence for cytotoxins, enterotoxins, invasive and adherence properties.[55,93,113,243] *C. jejuni* enterotoxin appears to be immunologically related to the heat-labile (LT) toxin of *Escherichia coli,* but is not produced by genes that are homologous with LT gene probes.[3] Although strains have different pathogenic properties,[113] as yet there is no well-defined association between the clinical illness and any virulence property. In developed countries over 50% of patients with enteritis caused by *C. jejuni* have bloody diarrhea,[22] while in developing countries the proportion varies from 10 to 30%.[66,224] *Campylobacter* serotypes show little geographic variation and there is no other strain difference that can account for the difference in the severity of the illness. Immunity to *Campylobacter* infection, which is higher among persons in developing countries, may prevent illness or modify the illness to a less severe form.[160] Hippurate-negative *Campylobacter* strains may be less virulent than *C. jejuni,* which is hippurate-positive. In most surveys from developed countries, hippurate-negative strains account for a small proportion of the total number of *Campylobacter* isolates; however, *C. coli* accounts for 30 to 40% of strains isolated in Hong Kong[81] and the Central African Republic,[64] a sufficient number to make an impact on the observed spectrum of illness.

Most intestinal isolates of *C. jejuni* are killed by normal human serum (serum-sensitive) while extraintestinal isolates may be either serum-sensitive or serum-resistant.[24] Extraintestinal isolates from normal hosts are usually serum-resistant, and extraintestinal isolates from impaired hosts are serum-sensitive as are the intestinal isolates.[9] Serum-resistance in *C. jejuni* strains has been associated with the total amount of LPS produced.[9,159] The LPS may serve as a type of capsule that protects the organism from the killing activity of serum.

Studies in Canada,[102] the United States,[16] the United Kingdom,[166] and Sweden[213] have shown the median duration of excretion to be 2–3 weeks from onset of symptoms. Almost all patients were culture-negative by 2 months. In developing countries the duration of excretion is 7 to 10 days.[66,224] A longer excretion period was observed in Thailand among children less than 1 year old (14 days) compared to older children (8 days), suggesting that previous immunity may shorten the convalescent excretion period.[224]

Patients infected with *Campylobacter* develop specific serum antibodies.[11,96,116,214] The IgM antibodies rise and fall earlier than the IgG and do not reach the height of the IgG titer rise. Titers of both classes of antibodies appear to decline within several months of infection.[11] Serum antibodies developed in response to infection with one *Campylobacter* strain are cross-reactive with heterologous strains.[142] In developing countries, IgG antibody titers to *Campylobacter* antigens peak in the first few years of life and then decline while IgA antibody titers continue to increase throughout life[23,25]; repeated infections may stimulate specific IgA production, but have little effect on systemic IgG production. After acute infection, IgA appears in the serum more rapidly than IgG and is predominantly in polymeric form.[133] Intestinal antibodies have also been detected.[160,248] Uninfected individuals have low-titer antibody to specific organisms. Volunteers with elevated serum and intestinal antibody levels to *Campylobacter* proteins become infected, but are protected from illness.[160] Similarly, habitual raw milk drinkers were protected from illness when exposed to contaminated raw milk that led to illness in other persons.[27]

8. Patterns of Host Response

8.1. Clinical Features

The consequences of infection with *C. jejuni* vary from asymptomatic excretion to death. The infection-to-case ratio is not known, but in one large outbreak, 25% of those infected were found to be asymptomatic.[166] In Sweden, 11% of persons with *Campylobacter* enteritis required hospitalization.[242]

In general, the symptoms and signs of *Campylobacter* infection are not so distinctive that the physician would be able to distinguish it from illness caused by other enteric pathogens. At the mild end of the spectrum, symptoms may last for 24 h and be indistinguishable from those seen with a viral gastroenteritis. Such patients usually do not seek medical attention; the occurrence of those cases has been detected only in outbreaks.[19,220] In industrialized nations, bloody diarrhea or the presence of fecal leukocytes is often a helpful clinical indication of *Campylobacter* infection.

Most information on the clinical features of *Campylobacter* infection is based on hospital- or laboratory-based studies and is thus biased toward those who are the most severely ill and who have diarrheal illnesses. In a multicenter study[22] in the United States where diarrhea was the criterion for stool culture, *Campylobacter* infection was associated with abdominal pain (79%), fever ≥ 37.8°C (74%), and a history of bloody diarrhea (46%). Among those 10 to 29 years old, 31% of persons with a history of fever and ten or more fecal leukocytes had *Campylobacter* enteritis. The abdominal pain has been so severe on occasion as to mimic acute appendicitis.[164,201] Fever has been noted in up to 80% of these patients, although children have been febrile less frequently; convulsions have been reported.[79] A prodrome of constitutional complaints, chiefly fever, may be more prominent than the enteric symptoms.[1,102,152]

Illness usually lasts less than 10 days, but up to 20% of the patients studied in the hospital-based series had a more prolonged and severe illness, with persistently high fever and frequently grossly bloody stools.[20] With bloody diarrhea and abdominal pain being common manifestations, many were thought to have an acute bout of inflammatory bowel disease or a surgical abdomen before *Campylobacter* infection was diagnosed.[17,164] *Campylobacter* colitis may mimic the early presentation of ulcerative colitis. *Campylobacter* infection may be a cause of exacerbation of inflammatory colitis, but there is no evidence that it plays a role in the etiology of these diseases. Endoscopic examination is often helpful in differentiating infectious from idiopathic types of colitis.[236] Cultures obtained by endoscopy at the site of mucosal ulceration may be positive when stool cultures are negative.[4] *Campylobacter* colitis also may present as a surgical abdomen because of severe abdominal pain or bleeding.

Rarely, *Campylobacter* may infect the biliary tract, giving rise to cholecystitis, pancreatitis, or obstructive hepatitis.[162,163,173] It may cause peritonitis in patients receiving peritoneal dialysis, and has occasionally been isolated from the urinary tract in women.

A reactive arthritis is the most common postinfectious complication of *Campylobacter* infection. Similar to *Shigella*, *Salmonella*, and *Yersinia* infection, this complication is associated with HLA-B27 in about 60% of the cases.[5,76,90,117,194,232] In Scandinavia 1 to 2% of patients with *Campylobacter* enteritis develop arthritis beginning 4 days to 4 weeks after the onset of diarrhea.[52] In Australia, 38% of patients with Guillain–Barré syndrome had serological evidence of a recent *Campylobacter* infection.[99] *Campylobacter* infection was the most frequently identified risk factor for this syndrome. Cases of Guillain–Barré syndrome that were serologically associated with *Campylobacter* infections were more severe than cases not associated with *Campylobacter* infection (B. Dwyer, personal communication). Although a history of diarrheal disease was found in many with positive serology, *Campylobacter* species were rarely isolated from stool specimens. Cases of Guillain–Barré syndrome were found to occur 9 months after the peak months of *Campylobacter* isolations from stool specimens. Erythema nodosum and migrating urticaria also have been associated with *Campylobacter* infections.[162,163] Hemolytic-uremic syndrome has been reported following *Campylobacter* infection, but other organisms such as *E. coli* 0157 : H7 that have been associated with this syndrome were not sought.[39]

Illness is frequently self-limited and usually ends within 10 days; however, one or more relapses can occur. Those with more severe symptoms may have presistence of illness for 1 month or longer. Campylobacters are susceptible *in vitro* to a wide variety of antimicrobial agents.[105,234,235,246] Because erythromycin is safe, easy to administer, and has less of an inhibitory effect on fecal flora than other antibiotics, it is the recommended therapy. However, most clinical trials performed in adults or children have not found that erythromycin significantly alters the clinical course of *Campylobacter* infection.[2,131,146,153,179,180] Only one study in Peru demonstrated that children with bloody diarrhea benefited from erythromycin therapy if treatment was begun early in the course of illness.[190] Treatment of susceptible organisms shortens the duration of convalescent excretion, which in areas of poor sanitation may be useful. *Campylobacter* strains are highly susceptible to the new analogues of nalidixic acid such as norfloxacin and ciprofloxacin and limited clinical studies have shown a good response in adults.[187]

8.2. Diagnosis

The diagnosis of *Campylobacter* infection is based on a positive stool culture or a positive blood culture. The frequency of bacteremia was low (about 1%) in one series of patients hospitalized for acute *Campylobacter* enteritis.[225] Not all commercial blood culture methods support the growth of *Campylobacter*.[244]

Serological diagnosis may be useful in industrialized countries where background asymptomatic infection rates are low. Serodiagnostic techniques may also be useful in determining the role of *Campylobacter* in abortion, postinfectious syndromes, inflammatory bowel disease, and other late manifestations of *Campylobacter* infection.

Serotyping and biotyping of *C. jejuni* and *C. coli* have been useful in epidemiological investigations to determine associated cases and the source of infection. Typing has so far not identified strains of different virulence potential.

9. Control and Prevention

Since poultry, livestock, pets, and wild animals are the major reservoir for these organisms, control is based on interruption of transmission to humans from animals, animal products, or environmental sources contaminated by animals. Awareness of the necessity for hand-washing after contact with animals or animal products and the importance of proper cooking and storage of foods of animal origin are as important for preventing *Campylobacter* infections as they are for *Salmonella* infections. Similarly, consuming only pasteurized milk and treated water is an important sanitary measure for the prevention of illness by individuals.

Control of nosocomial transmission from patients hospitalized with *Campylobacter* infection is another important consideration. As such, "excretion precautions" are recommended for infected infants, children, and adults with fecal incontinence. In general, the bases for control of enteric infection in the hospital are sanitary disposal of excretions and contaminated linens, and hand-washing by the patient and by staff members after contact with the patient, especially following contact with excreta. For *Campylobacter* infection, precautions should be maintained for the duration of the illness.

To date, there have been no reports of transmission of *Campylobacter* infection by asymptomatic excretors. Asymptomatically infected food handlers or hospital employees need not be excluded from work, but the need for hand-washing after defecation should be stressed to these individuals. Erythromycin treatment rapidly eliminates *Campylobacter* from the stool and would be useful for persons working as food handlers or in hospitals.

Recommendations are different when persons are infected with *Campylobacter* and continue to have diarrhea. Because of the known risk of transmission of other enteric pathogens from individuals with diarrhea, food handlers

and symptomatic hospital employees with patient-care responsibilities should not be permitted to work until the diarrheal episode has ended.

Because of the diversity of serotypes of *C. jejuni*, the possibility of vaccination for prevention of infection is limited. However, identification of group antigens could make immunization feasible.

10. Unresolved Problems

Epidemiological and clinical research during the last 10 years has done much to define the disease and the sources of infection. The priorities should be directed at public health prevention. First, we must learn how to produce poultry and livestock that are not infected with *Campylobacter*. This strategy would not eliminate *Campylobacter* because of the vast reservoir in wild animals and birds, but it should decrease the number of human infections considerably. Efforts also should be directed at determining how to process meat so that it is not contaminated with animal feces containing campylobacters.

Cheaper and simpler diagnostic methods should be available so that a greater number of patients can be cultured for *Campylobacter*, which in turn might lead to better surveillance and more opportunities to investigate outbreaks to find additional modes of transmission. Efforts should be made to introduce simple and inexpensive isolation methods into all diagnostic microbiology laboratories. This should be combined with training in isolation techniques for technicians. Research on new diagnostic methods such as simple antigen detection kits and nonradioactive DNA probes should be pursued and a simple, standardized serotyping scheme should be widely available and routinely used.

The pathogenesis of *Campylobacter* infection, the host mechanisms that allow most infections to be self-limited, and the occurrence and mediators of immunity are still not well understood. Research in the area of pathogenesis and immunity should continue and may help provide the basis for effective prophylaxis or intervention.

11. References

1. ANDERS, B. J., LAUER, B. A., AND PAISLEY, J. W., *Campylobacter* gastroenteritis in neonates, *Am. J. Dis. Child.* **135**:900–902 (1981).
2. ANDERS, B. J., LAUER, B. A., PAISLEY, J. W., AND RELLER, L. B., Double-blind placebo controlled trial of erythromycin

for treatment of *Campylobacter* enteritis, *Lancet* **1**:131–132 (1982).

3. BAIG, B. H., WACHSMUTH, I. K., MORRIS, G. K., AND HILL, W. E., Probing of *Campylobacter jejuni* with DNA coding for *Escherichia coli* heat-labile enterotoxin [letter], *J. Infect. Dis.* **154**:542 (1986).

4. BAYERDORFFER, E., HOCHTER, W., SCHWARZKOPF-STEIN-HAUSER, G., BLUMEL, P., SCHMIEDEL, A., AND OTTEN-JANN, R., Bioptic microbiology in the differential diagnosis of enterocolitis, *Endoscopy* **18**:177–181 (1986).

5. BENGTSSON, A., AHLSTRANS, C., LINDSTROM, F. D., AND KIHLSTROM, E., Bacteriological findings in 25 patients with Reiter's syndrome (reactive arthritis), *Scand. J. Rheumatol.* **12**:157–160 (1983).

6. BENJAMIN, J. S., LEAPER, S., OWEN, R. J., AND SKIRROW, M. B., Description of *Campylobacter laridis*, a new species comprising the nalidixic acid resistant thermophilic *Campylobacter* (NARTC) group, *Curr. Microbiol.* **8**:231–238 (1983).

7. BILLINGHAM, J. D., *Campylobacter* enteritis in The Gambia, *Trans. R. Soc. Trop. Med. Hyg.* **75**:641–644 (1981).

8. BLACK, R. E., LEVINE, M. M., CLEMENTS, M. L., HUGHES, T. P., AND BLASER, M. J., Experimental *Campylobacter jejuni* infections in humans, *J. Infect. Dis.* **157**:472–479 (1988).

9. BLASER, M. J., Extraintestinal *Campylobacter* infections, *West. J. Med.* **144**:353–354 (1986).

10. BLASER, M. J., Gastric *Campylobacter*-like organisms, gastritis, and peptic ulcer disease, *Gastroenterology* **93**:371–383 (1987).

11. BLASER, M. J., AND DUNCAN, D. J., Human serum antibody response to *Campylobacter jejuni* infection as measured in an enzyme-linked immunosorbent assay, *Infect. Immun.* **44**:292–298 (1984).

12. BLASER, M. J., AND RELLER, L. B., *Campylobacter* enteritis, *N. Engl. J. Med.* **305**:1444–1452 (1981).

13. BLASER, M. J., BERKOWITZ, I. D., LaFORCE, F. M., CRAVENS, J., RELLER, L. B., AND WANG, W.-L. L., *Campylobacter* enteritis: Clinical and epidemiologic features, *Ann. Intern. Med.* **91**:179–185 (1979).

14. BLASER, M. J., GLASS, R. I., IMDADUL HUQ, M., STOLL, B., KIBRIYA, G. M., AND ALIM, A. R. M. A., Isolation of *Campylobacter fetus* subsp. *jejuni* from Bangladeshi children, *J. Clin. Microbiol.* **12**:744–747 (1980).

15. BLASER, M. J., HARDESTY, H. L., POWERS, B., AND WANG, W.-L. L., Survival of *Campylobacter fetus* subsp. *jejuni* in biological milieus, *J. Clin. Microbiol.* **11**:309–313 (1980).

16. BLASER, M. J., LaFORCE, F. M., WILSON, N. A., AND WANG, W.-L. L., Reservoirs for human campylobacteriosis, *J. Infect. Dis.* **141**:665–669 (1980).

17. BLASER, M. J., PARSONS, R. B., AND WANG, W.-L. L., Acute colitis caused by *Campylobacter fetus* ssp. *jejuni*, *Gastroenterology* **78**:448 (1980).

18. BLASER, M. J., WALDMAN, R. J., BARRETT, T., AND ERLANDSON, A. L., Outbreaks of *Campylobacter* enteritis in two extended families: Evidence for person-to-person transmission, *J. Pediatr.* **98**:254–257 (1981).

19. BLASER, M. J., CHECKO, P., BOPP, C., BRUCE, A., AND HUGHES, J. M., *Campylobacter* enteritis associated with foodborne transmission, *Am. J. Epidemiol.* **116**:886–894 (1982).

20. BLASER, M. J., RELLER, L. B., LEUCHTEFELD, N. W., AND WANG, W.-L. L., *Campylobacter* enteritis in Denver, *West. J. Med.* **136**:287–290 (1982).

21. BLASER, M. J., TAYLOR, D. N., AND FELDMAN, R. A., Epidemiology of *Campylobacter jejuni* infections, *Epidemiol. Rev.* **5**:157–176 (1983).

22. BLASER, M. J., WELLS, J. G., FELDMAN, R. A., POLLARD, R. A., ALLEN, J. R., AND the Collaborative Diarrheal Disease Study Group, *Campylobacter* enteritis in the United States: A multicenter study, *Ann. Intern. Med.* **98**:360–365 (1983).

23. BLASER, M. J., BLACK, R. E., DUNCAN, D. J., AND AMER, J., *Campylobacter jejuni*-specific serum antibodies are elevated in healthy Bangladeshi children, *J. Clin. Microbiol.* **21**:164–167 (1985).

24. BLASER, M. J., SMITH, P. F., AND KOHLER, P. F., Susceptibility of *Campylobacter* isolates to the bactericidal activity of human serum, *J. Infect. Dis.* **151**:227–235 (1985).

25. BLASER, M. J., TAYLOR, D. N., AND ECHEVERRIA, P., Immune response to *Campylobacter jejuni* in a rural community in Thailand, *J. Infect. Dis.* **153**:249–254 (1986).

26. BLASER, M. J., PEREZ, G. P., SMITH, P. F., PATTON, C., TENOVER, F. C., LASTOVICA, A. J., AND WANG, W.-L. L., Extraintestinal *Campylobacter jejuni* and *Campylobacter coli* infections: Host factors and strain characteristics, *J. Infect. Dis.* **153**:552–559 (1986).

27. BLASER, M. J., SAZIE, E., AND WILLIAMS, L. P., The influence of immunity on raw milk-associated *Campylobacter* infection, *J. Am. Med. Assoc.* **257**:43–46 (1987).

28. BOKKENHEUSER, V., *Vibrio fetus* infection in man. I. Ten new cases and some epidemiologic observations, *Am. J. Epidemiol.* **91**:400–409 (1970).

29. BOKKENHEUSER, V. D., RICHARDSON, N. J., BRYNER, J. H., ROUX, D. J., SCHUTTE, A. B., KOORNHOF, H. J., FREIMAN, I., AND HARTMAN, E., Detection of enteric campylobacteriosis in children, *J. Clin. Microbiol.* **9**:227–232 (1979).

30. BOLTON, F. J., HUTCHINSON, D. N., AND COATES, D., Blood-free selective medium for isolation of *Campylobacter jejuni* from feces, *J. Clin. Microbiol.* **19**:169–171 (1984).

31. BROCZYK, A., THOMPSON, S., SMITH, D., AND LIOR, H., Water-borne outbreak of *Campylobacter laridis*-associated gastroenteritis [letter], *Lancet* **1**:164–165 (1987).

32. BRUCE, D., ZOCHOWSKI, W., AND FERGUSON, I. R., *Campylobacter* enteritis, *Br. Med. J.* **2**:1219 (1977).

33. BRUNTON, W. A. T., AND HEGGIE, D., *Campylobacter* associated diarrhea in Edinburgh, *Br. Med. J.* **2**:956 (1977).

34. BURKE, V., GRACEY, M., ROBINSON, J., PECK, D., BEAMAN, J., AND BUNDELL, C., The microbiology of child-

hood gastroenteritis: *Aeromonas* species and other infective agents, *J. Infect. Dis.* **148:**68–74 (1983).

35. BUTZLER, J.-P., AND SKIRROW, M. B., *Campylobacter* enteritis, *Clin. Gastroenterol.* **8:**737–765 (1979).

36. BUTZLER, J.-P., DEKEYSER, P., DETRAIN, M., AND DEHAEN, F., Related vibrio in stools, *J. Pediatr.* **82:**493–495 (1973).

37. CHALKER, R., AND BLASER, M. J., A review of human salmonellosis. III. Magnitude of infection in the United States, *Rev. Infect. Dis.* **10:**111–123 (1988).

38. CEVENINI, R., VAROLI, O., RUMPIANESI, F., MAZZARACCHIO, R., NANETTI, A., AND LA PLACA, M., A two-year longitudinal study on the etiology of acute diarrhea in young children in northern Italy, *Microbiologica* **8:**51–58 (1985).

39. CHANOVITZ, B. N., HARTSTEIN, A. I., ALEXANDER, S. R., TERRY, A. B., SHORT, P., AND KATON, R., *Campylobacter jejuni*-associated hemolytic–uremic syndrome in a mother and daughter, *Pediatrics* **71:**253–256 (1983).

40. CHAU, P. Y., LEUNG, Y. K., AND NG, W. W., Comparative in vitro antibacterial activity of ofloxacin and ciprofloxacin against some selected gram-positive and gram-negative isolates, *Infection* **14:**S237–S239 (1986).

41. CHRISTENSON, B., RINGER, A., BLUCHER, C., BILLAUDELLE, H., GUNDTOFT, K. N., ERIKSSON, G., AND BOTTIGER, M., An outbreak of *Campylobacter* enteritis among the staff of a poultry abattoir in Sweden, *Scand. J. Infect. Dis.* **15:**167–172 (1983).

42. COOPER, I. A., AND SLEE, K. J., Human infection by *Vibrio fetus, Med. J. Aust.* **1:**1263–1267 (1971).

43. DEKEYSER, P., GOSSVIN-DETRAIN, M., BUTZLER, J.-P., AND STERNON, J., Acute enteritis due to related vibrio: First positive stool cultures, *J. Infect. Dis.* **125:**390–392 (1972).

44. DELORME, L., LAMBERT, T., BRANGER, C., AND ACAR, J. F., Enteritis due to *Campylobacter jejuni* in the Paris area, *Med. Malad. Infect.* **9:**675–681 (1979).

45. DEMING, M. S., TAUXE, R. V., BLAKE, P. A., DIXON, S. E., FOWLER, B. S., JONES, T. S., LOCKAMY, E. A., PATTON, C. M., AND SIKES, R. O., *Campylobacter* enteritis at a university: Transmission from eating chicken and from cats, *Am. J. Epidemiol.* **126:**526–534 (1987).

46. DE MOL, P., BRASSEUR, D., HEMELHOF, W., KALALA, T., BUTZLER, J.-P., AND VIS, H. L., Enteropathogenic agents in children with diarrhoea in rural Zaire, *Lancet* **1:**516–518 (1983).

47. DEVLIN, H. R., AND MCINTYRE, L., *Campylobacter fetus* subsp. *fetus* in homosexual males, *J. Clin. Microbiol.* **18:**999–1000 (1983).

48. DHAWAN, V. K., ULMER, D. D., NACHUM, R., RAO, B., AND SEE, R. B., *Campylobacter jejuni* septicemia: Epidemiology, clinical features and outcome, *West. J. Med.* **144:**324–328 (1986).

49. DOYLE, L. P., A vibrio associated with swine dysentery, *Am. J. Vet. Res.* **5:**3–5 (1944).

50. DOYLE, M. P., AND SCHOENI, J. L., Isolation of *Campylobacter jejuni* from retail mushrooms, *Appl. Environ. Microbiol.* **51:**449–450 (1986).

51. DWORKIN, B., WORMSER, G. P., ABDOO, R. A., CABELLO, F., AGUERO, M. E., AND SIVAK, S. L., Persistence of multiply antibiotic-resistant *Campylobacter jejuni* in a patient with the acquired immune deficiency syndrome, *Am. J. Med.* **80:**965–970 (1986).

52. EASTMOND, C. J., RENNIE, J. A., AND REID, T. M., An outbreak of *Campylobacter* enteritis: A rheumatological follow-up survey, *J. Rheumatol.* **10:**107–108 (1983).

53. EDMONDS, P., PATTON, C. M., GRIFFIN, P. M., BARRETT, T. J., SCHMID, G. P., BAKER C. N., LAMBERT, M. A., AND BRENNER, D. J., *Campylobacter hyointestinalis* associated with human gastrointestinal disease in the United States, *J. Clin. Microbiol.* **25:**685–691 (1987).

54. ELLIOT, D. L., TOLLE, S. W., GOLDBERG, L., AND MILLER, J. B., Pet-associated illness, *N. Engl. J. Med.* **313:**985–995 (1985).

55. FAUCHERE, J. L., ROSENAU, A., VERON, M., MOYEN, E. N., RICHARD, S., AND PFISTER, A., Association with HeLa cells of *Campylobacter jejuni* and *Campylobacter coli* isolated from human feces, *Infect. Immun.* **54:**283–287 (1986).

56. FENNELL, C. L., TOTTEN, P. A., QUINN, T. C., PATTON, D. L., HOLMES, K. K., AND STAMM, W. E., Characterization of *Campylobacter*-like organisms isolated from homosexual men, *J. Infect. Dis.* **149:**58–66 (1984).

57. FIGUEROA, G., ARAYA, M., IBANEZ, S., CLERC, N., AND BRUNSER, O., Enteropathogens associated with acute diarrhea in hospitalized infants, *J. Pediatr. Gastroenterol. Nutr.* **5:**226–231 (1986).

58. FIGURA, N., AND ROSSOLINI, A., A prospective etiological and clinical study on gastroenteritis in Italian children, *Boll. Ist. Sieroter. Milan.* **64:**302–310 (1985).

59. FINCH, M. J., AND BLAKE, P. A., Foodborne outbreaks of campylobacteriosis: The United States experience, 1980–1982, *Am. J. Epidemiol.* **122:**262–268 (1985).

60. FINCH, M. J., AND RILEY, L. W., *Campylobacter* infections in the United States: Results of an 11-state surveillance, *Arch. Intern. Med.* **144:**1610–1612 (1984).

61. FRANKLIN, B., AND ULMER, D. D., Human infection with *Vibrio fetus, West. J. Med.* **120:**200–204 (1974).

62. GEBHART, C. J., EDMONDS, P., WARD, G. E., KURTZ, H. J., AND BRENNER, D. J., "*Campylobacter hyointestinalis*" sp. nov.: A new species of *Campylobacter* found in the intestines of pigs and other animals, *J. Clin. Microbiol.* **21:**715–720 (1985).

63. GEORGES, M. C., WACHSMUTH, I. K., MEUNIER, D. M., NEBOUT, N., DIDIER, F., SIOPATHIS, M. R., AND GEORGES, A. J., Parasitic, bacterial, and viral enteric pathogens associated with diarrhea in the Central African Republic, *J. Clin. Microbiol.* **19:**571–575 (1984).

64. GEORGES-COURBOT, M. C., BAYA, C., BERAUD, A. M., MEUNIER, D. M. Y., AND GEORGES, A. J., Distribution and serotypes of *Campylobacter jejuni* and *Campylobacter coli* in

enteric *Campylobacter* strains isolated from children in the Central African Republic, *J. Clin. Microbiol.* **23**:592–594 (1986).

65. GEORGES-COURBOT, M. C., BERAUD-CASSEL, A. M., GOUANDJIK, I., AND GEORGES, A. J., Prospective study of enteric *Campylobacter* infections in children from birth to 6 months in the Central African Republic, *J. Clin. Microbiol.* **25**:836–839 (1987).

66. GLASS, R. I., STOLL, B. J., HUQ, M. I., STRUELENS, M. J., BLASER, M., AND KIBRIYA, A. K., Epidemiology and clinical features of endemic *Campylobacter jejuni* infection in Bangladesh, *J. Infect. Dis.* **148**:292–296 (1983).

67. GOODWIN, C. S., ARMSTRONG, J. A., AND MARSHALL, B. J., *Campylobacter pyloridis*, gastritis, and peptic ulceration, *J. Clin. Pathol.* **39**:353–365 (1986).

68. GOOSSENS, H., DE BOECK, M., AND BUTZLER, J.-P., A new selective medium for the isolation of *Campylobacter jejuni* from human faeces, *Eur. J. Clin. Microbiol.* **2**:389–393 (1983).

69. GOOSSENS, H., DE BOECK, M., COIGNAU, H., VLAES, L., VAN DEN BORRE, C., AND BUTZLER, J.-P., Modified selective medium for isolation of *Campylobacter* spp. from feces: Comparison with Preston medium, a blood-free medium, and a filtration system, *J. Clin. Microbiol.* **24**:840–843 (1986).

70. GOOSSENS, H., HENOCQUE, G., KREMP, L., ROCQUE, J., BOURY, R., ALANIO, G., VLAES, L., HEMELHOF, W., VAN DEN BORRE, C., MACART, M., AND BUTZLER, J.-P., Nosocomial outbreak of *Campylobacter jejuni* meningitis in newborn infants, *Lancet* **2**:146–149 (1986).

71. GRAF, J., SCHAR, G., AND HEINZER, I., *Campylobacter-jejuni*-enteritis in der Schweiz, *Schweiz. Med. Wochenschr.* **110**:590–595 (1980).

72. GRAJEWSKI, B. A., KUSEK, J. W., AND GELFAND, H. M., Development of a bacteriophage typing system for *Campylobacter jejuni* and *Campylobacter coli*, *J. Clin. Microbiol.* **22**:13–18 (1985).

73. GRIFFIN, M. R., DALLEY, E., FITZPATRICK, M., AND AUSTIN, S. H., *Campylobacter* gastroenteritis associated with raw clams, *J. Med. Soc. N.J.* **80**:607–609 (1983).

74. GUERRANT, R. L., LAHITA, R. G., WINN, W. C., AND ROBERTS, R. B., Campylobacteriosis in man: Pathogenic mechanisms and review of 91 bloodstream infections, *Am. J. Med.* **65**:584–592 (1978).

75. GUERRANT, R. L., KIRCHHOFF, L. V., SHIELDS, D. S., NATIONS, M. K., LESLIE, J., DE SOUSA, M. A., ARAUJO, J. G., CORREIA, L. L., SAUER, K. T., MCCLELLAND, K. E., TROWBRIDGE, F. L., AND HUGHES, J. M., Prospective study of diarrheal illnesses in northeastern Brazil: Patterns of disease, nutritional impact, etiologies, and risk factors, *J. Infect. Dis.* **148**:986–997 (1983).

76. GUMPEL, J. M., MARTIN, C., AND SANDERSON, P. J., Reactive arthritis associated with *Campylobacter* enteritis, *Ann. Rheum. Dis.* **40**:64–65 (1981).

77. HARRIS, N. V., THOMSON, D., MARTIN, D. C., AND NOLAN, C. M., A survey of *Campylobacter* and other bacterial contaminants of pre-market chicken and retail poultry and meats,

King County, Washington, *Am. J. Public Health* **76**:401–406 (1986).

78. HARRIS, N. V., WEISS, N. S., AND NOLAN, C. M., The role of poultry and meats in the etiology of *Campylobacter jejuni/coli* enteritis, *Am. J. Public Health* **76**:407–410 (1986).

79. HAVALAD, S., CHAPPLE, M. J., KAHAKACHCHI, M., AND HARGRAVES, D. B., Convulsions associated with *Campylobacter* enteritis, *Br. Med. J.* **280**:984–985 (1980).

80. HERSHKOWICI, S., BARAK, M., COHEN, A., AND MONTAG, J., An outbreak of *Campylobacter jejuni* infection in a neonatal intensive care unit, *J. Hosp. Infect.* **9**:54–59 (1987).

81. HO, B. S. W., AND WONG, W. T., A one-year survey of *Campylobacter* enteritis and other forms of bacterial diarrhoea in Hong Kong, *J. Hyg.* **94**:55–60 (1985).

82. HO, D. D., AULT, M. J., AULT, M. A., AND MURATA, G. H., *Campylobacter* enteritis: Early diagnosis with Gram's stain, *Arch. Intern. Med.* **142**:1858–1860 (1982).

83. HODGE, D. S., PRESCOTT, J. F., AND SHEWEN, P. E., Direct immunofluorescence microscopy for rapid screening of *Campylobacter* enteritis, *J. Clin. Microbiol.* **24**:863–865 (1986).

84. HOPKINS, R. S., AND OLMSTED, R. N., *Campylobacter jejuni* infection in Colorado: Unexplained excess of cases in males, *Public Health Rep.* **100**:333–336 (1985).

85. HOPKINS, R. S., OLMSTED, R., AND ISTRE, G. R., Endemic *Campylobacter jejuni* infection in Colorado: Identified risk factors, *Am. J. Public Health* **74**:249–250 (1984).

86. HULL, B. P., SPENCE, L., BASSETT, D., SWANSTON, W. H., AND TIKASINGH, E. S., The relative importance of rotavirus and other pathogens in the etiology of gastroenteritis in Trinidadian children, *Am. J. Trop. Med. Hyg.* **31**:142–148 (1982).

87. ISTRE, G. R., BLASER, M. J., SHILLAM, P., AND HOPKINS, R. S., *Campylobacter* enteritis associated with undercooked barbecued chicken, *Am. J. Public Health* **74**:1265–1267 (1984).

88. ITOH, T., SAITO, K., MARUYAMA, T., SAKAI, S., OHASHI, M., AND OKA, A., An outbreak of acute enteritis due to *Campylobacter fetus* ssp. *jejuni* at a nursery school in Tokyo, *Microbiol. Immunol.* **24**:371–379 (1980).

89. JABLONSKI, E., MOOMAW, E. W., TULLIS, R. H., AND RUTH, J. L., Preparation of oligodeoxynucleotide–alkaline phosphatase conjugates and their use as hybridization probes, *Nucleic Acids Res.* **14**:6115–6128 (1986).

90. JOHNSEN, K., OSTENSEN, M., MELBYE, A. C., AND MELBY, K., HLA-B27-negative arthritis related to *Campylobacter jejuni* enteritis in three children and two adults, *Acta Med. Scand.* **214**:165–168 (1983).

91. JOHNSON, K. E., AND NOLAN, C. M., Community-wide surveillance of *Campylobacter jejuni* infection: Evaluation of a laboratory-based method, *Diagn. Microbiol. Infect. Dis.* **3**:389–396 (1985).

92. JOHNSON, R. J., NOLAN, C., WANG, S. P., SHELTON, W. R., AND BLASER, M. J., Persistent *Campylobacter jejuni* infection in an immunocompromised patient, *Ann. Intern. Med.* **100**:832–834 (1984).

93. JOHNSON, W. M., AND LIOR, H., Cytotoxic and cytotonic

factors produced by *Campylobacter jejuni, Campylobacter coli,* and *Campylobacter laridis, J. Clin. Microbiol.* **24:**275–281 (1986).

94. JONES, D. M., AND ROBINSON, D. A., Occupational exposure to *Campylobacter jejuni* infection [letter], *Lancet* **1:**440–441 (1981).

95. JONES, D. M., ELDRIDGE, J., AND DALE, B., Serological response to *Campylobacter jejuni/coli* infection, *J. Clin. Pathol.* **33:**767–769 (1980).

96. JONES, D. M., ROBINSON, D. A., AND ELDRIDGE, J., Serological studies in two outbreaks of *Campylobacter jejuni* infection, *J. Hyg.* **87:**163–170 (1981).

97. JONES, D. M., SUTCLIFFE, E. M., AND ABBOTT, J. D., Serotyping of *Campylobacter* species by combined use of two methods, *Eur. J. Clin. Microbiol.* **4:**562–565 (1985).

98. JONES, F. S., AND LITTLE, R. B., Etiology of infectious diarrhea (winter scours) in cattle, *J. Exp. Med.* **53:**835–843 (1931).

99. KALDOR, J., AND SPEED, B. R., Guillain–Barre syndrome and *Campylobacter jejuni:* A serological study, *Br. Med. J. (Clin. Res.)* **288:**1867–1870 (1984).

100. KALDOR, J., PRITCHARD, H., SERPELL, A., AND METCALF, W., Serum antibodies in *Campylobacter* enteritis, *J. Clin. Microbiol.* **18:**1–4 (1983).

101. KAPLAN, R. L., GOODMAN, L. J., BARRETT, J. E., TRENHOLME, G. M., AND LANDAU, W., Comparison of rectal swabs and stool cultures in detecting *Campylobacter fetus* subsp. *jejuni, J. Clin. Microbiol.* **15:**959–960 (1982).

102. KARMALI, M. A., AND FLEMING, P. C., *Campylobacter* enteritis in children, *J. Pediatr.* **94:**527–533 (1979).

103. KARMALI, M. A., AND SKIRROW, M. B., Taxonomy of the genus *Campylobacter,* in: *Campylobacter Infection in Man and Animals* (J.-P. BUTZLER, ed.), pp. 1–20, CRC Press, Boca Raton, 1985.

104. KARMALI, M. A., AND TAN, Y. C., Neonatal *Campylobacter* enteritis, *Can. Med. Assoc, J.* **122:**192–193 (1980).

105. KARMALI, M. A., DE GRANDIS, S., AND FLEMING, P. C., Antimicrobial susceptibility of *Campylobacter jejuni* with special reference to resistance patterns of Canadian isolates, *Antimicrob. Agents Chemother.* **19:**593–597 (1981).

106. KARMALI, M. A., NORRISH, B., LIOR, H., HEYES, B., MONTEATH, A., AND MONTGOMERY, H., *Campylobacter* enterocolitis in a neonatal nursery, *J. Infect. Dis.* **149:**874–877 (1984).

107. KARMALI, M. A., SIMOR, A. E., ROSCOE, M., FLEMING, P. C., SMITH, S. S., AND LANE, J., Evaluation of a blood-free, charcoal-based selective medium for the isolation of *Campylobacter* organisms from feces, *J. Clin. Microbiol.* **23:**456–459 (1986).

108. KENDALL, E. J., AND TANNER, E. I., *Campylobacter* enteritis in general practice, *J. Hyg.* **88:**155–163 1982).

109. KING, E. O., Human infections with *Vibrio fetus* and a closely related vibrio, *J. Infect. Dis.* **101:**119–129 (1957).

110. KING, E. O., The laboratory recognition of *Vibrio fetus* and a closely related vibrio isolated from cases of human vibriosis, *Ann. N.Y. Acad. Sci.* **98:**700–711 (1962).

111. KIRUBAKARAN, C., DAVIDSON, G. P., DARBY, H., HANSMAN, D., MCKAY, G., MOORE, B., AND LEE, P., *Campylobacter* as a cause of acute enteritis in children in South Australia. I. A 12-month study with controls, *Med. J. Aust.* **2:**333–335 (1981).

112. KLEIN, B. S., VERGERONT, J. M., BLASER, M. J., EDMONDS, P., BRENNER, D. J., JANSSEN, D., AND DAVIS, J. P., *Campylobacter* infection associated with raw milk: An outbreak of gastroenteritis due to *Campylobacter jejuni* and thermotolerant *Campylobacter fetus* subsp. *fetus, J. Am. Med. Assoc.,* **255:**361–364 (1986).

113. KLIPSTEIN, F. A., ENGERT, R. F., SHORT, H., AND SCHENK, E. A., Pathogenic properties of *Campylobacter jejuni:* Assay and correlation with clinical manifestations, *Infect. Immun.* **50:**43–49 (1985).

114. KORLATH, J. A., OSTERHOLM, M. T., JUDY, L. A., FORFANG, J. C., AND ROBINSON, D. A., A point-source outbreak of campylobacteriosis associated with consumption of raw milk, *J. Infect. Dis.* **152:**592–596 (1985).

115. KORNBLATT, A. N., BARRETT, T., MORRIS, G. K., AND TOSH, F. E., Epidemiologic and laboratory investigation of an outbreak of *Campylobacter* enteritis associated with raw milk, *Am. J. Epidemiol.* **122:**884–889 (1985).

116. KOSUNEN, T. U., PITKANEN, T., PETTERSSON, T., AND PONKA, A., Clinical and serological studies in patients with *Campylobacter fetus* spp. *jejuni* infection: II. serological findings, *Infection* **9:**279–282 (1981).

117. KOSUNEN, T. U., PONKA, A., KAURANEN, O., MARTIO, J., PITKANEN, T., HORTLING, L., AITTONIEMI, S., PENTTILA, O., AND KOSKIMIES, S., Arthritis associated with *Campylobacter jejuni* enteritis, *Scand. J. Rheumatol.* **10:**77–80 (1981).

118. KOSUNEN, T. U., RAUTELIN, H., PITKANEN, T., PONKA, A., AND PETTERSSON, T., Antibodies against an acid extract from a single *Campylobacter* strain in hospitalized *Campylobacter* patients, *Infection* **11:**189–191 (1983).

119. KOTARSKI, S. F., MERRIWETHER, T. L., TKALCEVIC, G. T., AND GEMSKI, P., Genetic studies of kanamycin resistance in *Campylobacter jejuni, Antimicrob. Agents Chemother.* **30:**225–230 (1986).

120. LAMBERT, T., GERBAUD, G., TRIEU-CUOT, P., AND COURVALIN, P., Structural relationship between the genes encoding 3′-aminoglycoside phosphotransferases in *Campylobacter* and in gram-positive cocci, *Ann. Inst. Pasteur Microbiol.* **136B:**135–150 (1985).

121. LASSEN, J., AND KAPPERUD, G., Epidemiological aspects of enteritis due to *Campylobacter* spp. in Norway, *J. Clin. Microbiol.* **19:**153–156 (1984).

122. LASTOVICA, A. J., AND AMBROSIO, R. E., Plasmid profiles of clinical isolates of *Campylobacter* with no or weak catalase activity, *S. Afr. Med. J.* **70:**337–338 (1986).

123. LASTOVICA, A. J., LE ROUX, E., CONGI, R. V., AND PENNER, J. L., Distribution of sero-biotypes of *Campylobacter jejuni* and *C. coli* isolated from paediatric patients, *J. Med. Microbiol.* **21:**1–5 (1986).

124. LIM, Y. S., JEGATHESAN, M., AND WONG, Y. H., *Campylo-*

bacter jejuni as a cause of diarrhoea in Kuala Lumpur, Malaysia, *Med. J. Malaysia* **39**:285–288 (1984).

125. LIOR, H., New, extended biotyping scheme for *Campylobacter jejuni, Campylobacter coli,* and "Campylobacter laridis," *J. Clin. Microbiol.* **20**:636–640 (1984).

126. LIOR, H., WOODWARD, D. L., EDGAR, J. A., LAROCHE, L. J., AND GILL, P., Serotyping of *Campylobacter jejuni* by slide agglutination based on heat-labile antigenic factors, *J. Clin. Microbiol.* **15**:761–768 (1982).

127. LOPEZ-BREA, M., MOLINA, D., AND BAQUERO, M., *Campylobacter* enteritis in Spain, *Trans. R. Soc. Trop. Med. Hyg.* **73**:474 (1979).

128. MacFADYEAN, F., AND STOCKMAN, S., Report of the Department Committee Appointed by the Board of Agriculture and Fisheries to Inquire into Epizootic Abortion, Volume 3, His Majesty's Stationery Office, London (1909).

129. MACKENJEE, M. K., COOVADIA, Y. M., COOVADIA, H. M., HEWITT, J., AND ROBINS-BROWNE, R. M., Aetiology of diarrhoea in adequately nourished young African children in Durban, South Africa, *Ann. Trop. Paediatr.* **4**:183–187 (1984).

130. MANCINELLI, S., PALOMBI, L., RICCARDI, F., AND MARAZZI, M. C., Serological study of *Campylobacter jejuni* infection in slaughterhouse workers, *J. Infect. Dis.* **156**:856 (1987).

131. MANDAL, B. K., ELLIS, M. E., DUNBAR, E. M., AND WHALE, K., Double-blind placebo-controlled trial of erythromycin in the treatment of clinical *Campylobacter* infection, *J. Antimicrob. Chemother.* **13**:619–623 (1984).

132. MARSHALL, B. J., Perspective: *Campylobacter pyloridis* and gastritis, *J. Infect. Dis.* **153**:650–657 (1986).

133. MASCART-LEMONE, F. O., DUCHATEAU, J. R., OOSTEROM, J., BUTZLER, J.-P., AND DELACROIX, D. L., Kinetics of anti-*Campylobacter jejuni* monomeric and polymeric immunoglobulin A1 and A2 responses in serum during acute enteritis, *J. Clin. Microbiol.* **25**:1253–1257 (1987).

134. MATA, L., SIMHON, A., PADILLA, R., DEL MAR GAMBOA, M., VARGAS, G., HERNANDEZ, F., MOHS, E., AND LIZANO, C., Diarrhea associated with rotaviruses, enterotoxigenic *Escherichia coli, Campylobacter,* and other agents in Costa Rican children, 1976–1981, *Am. J. Trop. Med. Hyg.* **32**:146–153 (1983).

135. MAUFF, A. C., AND CHAPMAN, S. R., *Campylobacter* enteritis in Johannesburg, *S. Afr. Med. J.* **59**:217–218 (1981)..

136. MEGRAUD, F., AND BONNET, F., Unusual campylobacters in human faeces, *J. Infect.* **12**:275–276 (1986).

137. MEGRAUD, F., AND ELHARRIF, Z., Isolation of *Campylobacter* species by filtration, *Eur. J. Clin. Microbiol.* **4**:437–438 (1985).

138. MELAMED, I., BUJANOVER, Y., IGRA, Y. S., SCHWARTZ, D., ZAKUTH, V., AND SPIRER, Z., *Campylobacter* enteritis in normal and immunodeficient children, *Am. J. Dis. Child.* **137**:752–753 (1983).

139. MENTZING, L. O., Waterborne outbreaks of *Campylobacter* enteritis in central Sweden, *Lancet* **2**:352–354 (1981).

140. MERINO, F. J., AGULLA, A., VILLASANTE, P. A., DIAZ, A.,

SAZ, J. V., AND VELASCO, A. C., Comparative efficacy of seven selective media for isolating *Campylobacter jejuni, J. Clin. Microbiol.* **24**:451–452 (1986).

141. MURRAY, B. J., *Campylobacter* enteritis: A college campus average incidence and a prospective study of the risk factors for exposure, *West. J. Med.* **145**:341–342 (1986).

142. NACHAMKIN, I., AND HART, A. M., Western blot analysis of the human antibody response to *Campylobacter jejuni* cellular antigens during gastrointestinal infection, *J. Clin. Microbiol.* **21**:33–38 (1985).

143. NACHAMKIN, I., STOWELL, C., SKALINA, D., JONES, A. M., HOOP, R. M., II, AND SMIBERT, R. M., *Campylobacter laridis* causing bacteremia in an immunosuppressed patient, *Ann. Intern. Med.* **101**:55–57 (1984).

144. NAIR, G. B., BHATTACHARY, S. K., AND PAL, S. C., Isolation and characterization of *Campylobacter jejuni* from acute diarrhoeal cases in Calcutta, *Trans. R. Soc. Trop. Med. Hyg.* **77**:474–476 (1983).

145. NG, L. K., STILES, M. E., AND TAYLOR, D. E., Comparison of basal media for culturing *Campylobacter jejuni* and *Campylobacter coli, J. Clin. Microbiol.* **21**:226–230 (1985).

146. NOLAN, C. M., JOHNSON, K. E., COYLE, M. B., AND FALER, K., *Campylobacter jejuni* enteritis: Efficacy of antimicrobial and antimotility drugs, *Am. J. Gastroenterol.* **78**:621–626 (1983).

147. NORKRANS, G., AND SVEDHEM, A., Epidemiological aspects of *Campylobacter jejuni* enteritis, *J. Hyg.* **89**:163–170 (1982).

148. OATES, J. D., AND HODGIN, U. G., Laboratory-acquired *Campylobacter* enteritis, *South. Med. J.* **74**:83 (1981).

149. OLARTE, J., AND PEREZ, G. I., *Campylobacter jejuni* in children with diarrhea in Mexico City, *Pediatr. Infect. Dis.* **2**:18–20 (1983).

150. OLUSANYA, O., ADEBAYO, J. O., AND WILLIAMS, B., *Campylobacter jejuni* as a bacterial cause of diarrhoea in Ile-Ife, *J. Hyg.* **91**:77–80 (1983).

151. OOSTEROM, J., DEN UYL, C. H., BANFFER, J. R., AND HUISMAN, J., Epidemiological investigations on *Campylobacter jejuni* in households with a primary infection, *J. Hyg.* **93**:325–332 (1984).

152. PAI, C. H., SORGER, S., LACKMAN, L., SINAI, R. E., AND MARKS, M. I., *Campylobacter* gastroenteritis in children, *J. Pediatr.* **94**:589–591 (1979).

153. PAI, C. H., GILLIS, F., TUOMANEN, E., AND MARKS, M. I., Erythromycin in treatment of *Campylobacter* enteritis in children, *Am. J. Dis. Child.* **137**:286–288 (1983).

154. PAISLEY, J. W., MIRRETT, S., LAUER, B. A., ROE, M., AND RELLER, L. B., Dark-field microscopy of human feces for presumptive diagnosis of *Campylobacter fetus* subsp. *jejuni* enteritis, *J. Clin. Microbiol.* **15**:61–63 (1982).

155. PALMER, S. R., GULLY, P. R., WHITE, J. M., PEARSON, A. D., SUCKLING, W. G., JONES, D. M., RAWES, J. C., AND PENNER, J. L., Water-borne outbreak of *Campylobacter* gastroenteritis, *Lancet* **1**:287–290 (1983).

156. PARK, C. H., HIXON, D. L., POLHEMUS, A. S., FERGUSON,

C. B., AND HALL, S. L., A rapid diagnosis of *Campylobacter* enteritis by direct smear examination, *Am. J. Clin. Pathol.* **80:**388–390 (1983).

157. PATTON, C. M., BARRETT, T. J., AND MORRIS, G. K., Comparison of the Penner and Lior methods for serotyping *Campylobacter* spp., *J. Clin. Microbiol.* **22:**558–565 (1985).

158. PENNER, J. L., AND HENNESSEY, J. N., Serotyping *Campylobacter fetus* subsp. *jejuni* on the basis of somatic (O) antigens, *J. Clin. Microbiol.* **12:**732–737 (1980).

159. PEREZ, G. I., AND BLASER, M. J., Lipopolysaccharide characteristics of pathogenic campylobacters, *Infect. Immun.* **47:**353–359 (1985).

160. PERLMAN, D. M., BLACK, R. E., LEVINE, M. M., AND BLASER, M. J., Immunity to *Campylobacter jejuni* following challenge in volunteers, Presented at the IVth International Workshop on *Campylobacter* Infections, Goteborg, Sweden, pp. 16–18 (1987).

161. PIEN, F. D., HSU, A. K., PADUA, S. A., ISAACSON, S., AND NAKA, S., *Campylobacter jejuni* enteritis in Honolulu, Hawaii, *Trans. Soc. Trop. Med. Hyg.* **4:**492–494 (1983).

162. PITKANEN, T., PETTERSSON, T., PONKA, A., AND KOSUNEN, T. U., Clinical and serological studies in patients with *Campylobacter fetus* spp. *jejuni* infection. I. Clinical findings, *Infection* **9:**274–278 (1981).

163. PITKANEN, T., PONKA, A., PETTERSSON, T., AND KOSUNEN, T. U., *Campylobacter* enteritis in 188 hospitalized patients, *Arch. Intern. Med.* **143:**215–219 (1983).

164. PONKA, A., PITKANEN, T., AND KOSUNEN, T. U., *Campylobacter* enteritis mimicking acute abdominal emergency, *Acta Chir. Scand.* **147:**663–666 (1981).

165. PONKA, A., PITKANEN, T., SARNA, S., AND KOSUNEN, T. U., Infection due to *Campylobacter jejuni:* A report of 524 outpatients, *Infection* **12:**175–178 (1984).

166. PORTER, I. A., AND REID, T. M. S., A milk-borne outbreak of *Campylobacter* infection, *J. Hyg.* **84:**415–419 (1980).

167. POTTER, M. E., BLASER, M. J., SIKES, R. K., KAUFMANN, A. F., AND WELLS, J. G., Human *Campylobacter* infection associated with certified raw milk, *Am. J. Epidemiol.* **117:**475–483 (1983).

168. PRESCOTT, J. F., AND BARKER, I. K., *Campylobacter* colitis in gnotobiotic dogs, *Vet. Rec.* **107:**314–315 (1980).

169. PRICE, A. B., DOLBY, J. M., DUNSCOMBE, P. R., AND STIRLING, J., Detection of *Campylobacter* by immunofluorescence in stools and rectal biopsies of patients with diarrhoea, *J. Clin. Pathol.* **37:**1007–1013 (1984).

170. QUINN, T. C., GOODELL, S. E., FENNELL, C., WANG, S.-P., SCHUFFLER, M. D., HOLMES, K. K., AND STAMM, W. E., Infections with *Campylobacter jejuni* and *Campylobacter*-like organisms in homosexual men, *Ann. Intern. Med.* **101:**187–192 (1984).

171. RAJAN, D. P., AND MATHAN, V. I., Prevalence of *Campylobacter fetus* subsp. *jejuni* in healthy populations in southern India, *J. Clin. Microbiol.* **15:**749–751 (1982).

172. RAUTELIN, H., AND KOSUNEN, T. U., An acid extract as a common antigen in *Campylobacter coli* and *Campylobacter jejuni* strains, *J. Clin. Microbiol.* **17:**700–701 (1983).

173. REDDY, K. R., FARNUM, J. B., AND THOMAS, E., Acute hepatitis associated with *Campylobacter* colitis, *J. Clin. Gastroenterol.* **5:**259–262 (1983).

174. RIBEIRO, C. D., AND PRICE, T. H., The use of Preston enrichment broth for the isolation of 'thermophilic' campylobacters from water, *J. Hyg.* **92:**45–51 (1984).

175. RILEY, L. W., AND FINCH, M. J., Results of the first year of national surveillance of *Campylobacter* infections in the United States, *J. Infect. Dis.* **151:**956–959 (1985).

176. RINGERTZ, S., ROCKHILL, R. C., RINGERTZ, O., AND SUTOMO, A., *Campylobacter fetus* subsp. *jejuni* as a cause of gastroenteritis in Jakarta, Indonesia, *J. Clin. Microbiol.* **12:**538–540 (1980).

177. RISHPON, S., EPSTEIN, L. M., SHMILOVITZ, M., KRETZER, B., TAMIR, A., AND EGOZ, N., *Campylobacter jejuni* infections in Haifa subdistrict, Israel, summer 1981, *Int. J. Epidemiol.* **13:**216–220 (1984).

178. RIVERA, M. J., CASTILLO, J., MARTIN, C., NAVVARRO, M., AND GOMEZ-LUS, R., Aminoglycoside-phosphotransferases APH (3')-IV and APH (3″) synthesized by a strain of *Campylobacter coli, J. Antimicrob. Chemother.* **18:**153–158 (1986).

179. ROBINS-BROWNE, R. M., COOVADIA, H. M., BODASING, M. N., AND MACKENJEE, M. K., Treatment of acute nonspecific gastroenteritis of infants and young children with erythromycin, *Am. J. Trop. Med. Hyg.* **32:**886–890 (1983).

180. ROBINS-BROWNE, R. M., MACKENJEE, M. K., BODASING, M. N., AND COOVADIA, H. M., Treatment of *Campylobacter*-associated enteritis with erythromycin, *Am. J. Dis. Child.* **137:**282–285 (1983).

181. ROBINSON, D. A., Infective dose of *Campylobacter jejuni* in milk, *Br. Med. J.* **282:**1584 (1981).

182. ROBINSON, D. A., AND JONES, D. M., Milk-borne *Campylobacter* infection, *Br. Med. J. Clin. Res.* **282:**1374–1376 (1981).

183. ROBINSON, D. A., EDGAR, W. J., GIBSON, G. L., MATCHEFF, A. A., AND ROBERTSON, L., *Campylobacter* enteritis associated with consumption of unpasteurized milk, *Br. Med. J.* **1:**1171–1173 (1979).

184. ROGOL, M., SECHTER, I., FALK, H., SHTARK, Y., ALFI, S., GREENBERG, Z., AND MIZRACHI, R., Waterborne outbreak of *Campylobacter* enteritis, *Eur. J. Clin. Microbiol.* **2:**588–590 (1983).

185. ROMANIUK, P. J., ZOLTOWSKA, B., TRUST, T. J., LANE, D. J., OLSEN, G. J., PACE, N. R., AND STAHL, D. A., *Campylobacter pylori,* the spiral bacterium associated with human gastritis, is not a true *Campylobacter* sp., *J. Bacteriol.* **169:**2137–2141 (1987).

186. ROSENFIELD, J. A., ARNOLD, G. J., DAVEY, G. R., ARCHER, R. S., AND WOODS, W. H., Serotyping of *Campylobacter jejuni* from an outbreak of enteritis implicating chicken, *J. Infect.* **2:**159–165 (1985).

187. RUIZ-PALACIOS, G. M., Norfloxacin in the treatment of bac-

terial enteric infections, *Scand. J. Infect. Dis.* **48**:S55–S63 (1986).

188. RUIZ-PALACIOS, G. M., ESCAMILLA, E., AND TORRES, N., Experimental *Campylobacter* diarrhea in chickens, *Infect. Immun.* **34**:250–255 (1981).

189. SACKS, J. J., LIEB, S., BALDY, L. M., BERTA, S., PATTON, C. M., WHITE, M. C., BIGLER, W. J., AND WITTE, J. J., Epidemic campylobacteriosis associated with a community water supply, *Am. J. Public Health* **76**:424–428 (1986).

190. SALAZAR-LINDO, E., SACK, R. B., CHEA-WOO, E., KAY, B. A., PISCOYA, Z. A., LEON-BARUA, R., AND YI, A., Early treatment with erythromycin of *Campylobacter jejuni*-associated dysentery in children, *J. Pediatr.* **109**:355–360 (1986).

191. SALFIEDL, N. J., AND PUGEH, E. J., *Campylobacter* enteritis in young children living in households with puppies, *Br. Med. J.* **294**:21–22 (1987).

192. SANDSTEDT, K., URSING, J., AND WALDER, M., Thermotolerant *Campylobacter* with no or weak catalase activity isolated from dogs, *Curr. Microbiol.* **8**:209–213 (1983).

193. SAZIE, E. S., AND TITUS, A. E., Rapid diagnosis of *Campylobacter* enteritis, *Ann. Intern. Med.* **96**:62–63 (1982).

194. SCHAAD, U. B., Reactive arthritis associated with *Campylobacter* enteritis, *Pediatr. Infect. Dis.* **1**:328–332 (1982).

195. SCHWARTZ, R. H., BRYAN, C., RODRIGUEZ, W. J., PARK, C., AND McCOY, P., Experience with the microbiologic diagnosis of *Campylobacter* enteritis in an office laboratory, *Pediatr. Infect. Dis.* **2**:298–301 (1983).

196. SEVERIN, W. P. J., *Campylobacter* en enteritis, *Ned. Tijdschr. Geneeskd.* **122**:499–504 (1978).

197. SHMILOVITZ, M., KRETZER, B., AND ROTMAN, N., *Campylobacter jejuni* as an etiological agent of diarrheal diseases in Israel, *Isr. J. Med. Sci.* **18**:935–940 (1982).

198. SHUNGU, D. L., WEINBERG, E., AND GADEBUSCH, H. H., In vitro antibacterial activity of norfloxacin (MK-0366, AM-715) and other agents against gastrointestinal tract pathogens, *Antimicrob. Agents Chemother.* **23**:86–90 (1983).

199. SIMOR, A. E., AND WILCOX, L., Enteritis associated with *Campylobacter laridis*, *J. Clin. Microbiol.* **25**:10–12 (1987).

200. SIMOR, A. E., KARMALI, M. A., JADAVJI, T., AND ROSCOE, M., Abortion and perinatal sepsis associated with *Campylobacter* infection, *Rev. Infect. Dis.* **8**:397–402 (1986).

201. SKIRROW, M. B., *Campylobacter* enteritis: A "new" disease, *Br. Med. J.* **2**:9–11 (1977).

202. SKIRROW, M. B., *Campylobacter* enteritis: The first five years, *J. Hyg.* **89**:175–184 (1982).

203. SMIBERT, R. M., The genus *Campylobacter*, *Ann. Rev. Microbiol.* **32**:700–773 (1978).

204. SMIBERT, R. M., Genus *Campylobacter* Sebald and Veron 1963, 907^AL, in: *Bergey's Manual of Systematic Bacteriology* (N. R. KRIEG AND J. G. HOLT, eds.), pp. 111–118, Williams & Wilkins, Baltimore, 1984.

205. SMITH, G. S., AND BLASER, M. J., Fatalities associated with *Campylobacter jejuni* infections, *J. Am. Med. Assoc.* **253**:2873–2875 (1985).

206. SPEELMAN, P., STRUELENS, M. J., SANYAL, S. C., AND GLASS, R. I., Detection of *Campylobacter jejuni* and other potential pathogens in travelers' diarrhoea in Bangladesh, *Scand. J. Gastroenterol.* **18**(Suppl. 84):19–23 (1983).

207. SPELMAN, D. W., DAVIDSON, N., BUCKMASTER, N. D., SPICER, W. J., AND RYAN, P., *Campylobacter* bacteraemia: A report of 10 cases, *Med. J. Aust.* **145**:503–505 (1986).

208. STEELE, T. W., AND McDERMOTT, S., *Campylobacter* enteritis in South Australia, *Med. J. Aust.* **2**:404–406 (1978).

209. STEELE, T. W., SANGSTER, N., AND LANSER, J. A., DNA relatedness and biochemical features of *Campylobacter* spp. isolated in Central and South Australia, *J. Clin. Microbiol.* **22**:71–74 (1985).

210. STEINGRIMSSON, O., THORSTEINSSON, S. B., HJALMARSDOTTIR, M., JONASDOTTIR, E., AND KOLBEINSSON, A., *Campylobacter* ssp. infections in Iceland during a 24-month period in 1980–1982, *Scand. J. Infect. Dis.* **17**:285–290 (1985).

211. STERN, N. J., HERNANDEZ, M. P., BLANKENSHIP, L., DEIBEL, K. E., DOORES, S., DOYLE, M. P., NG, H., PIERSON, M. D., SOFOS, J. N., SVEUM, W. H., AND WESTHOFF, D. C., Prevalence and distribution of *Campylobacter jejuni* and *Campylobacter coli* in retail meats, *J. Food Prot.* **47**:595–599 (1985).

212. STOLL, B. J., GLASS, R. I., BANU, H., HUQ, M. I., KHAN, M. U., AND HOLT, J. E., Surveillance of patients attending a diarrhoeal disease hospital in Bangladesh, *Br. Med. J.* **285**:1185–1188 (1982).

213. SVEDHEM, A., AND KAIJSER, B., *Campylobacter fetus* subspecies *jejuni:* A common cause of diarrhea in Sweden, *J. Infect. Dis.* **142**:353–359 (1980).

214. SVEDHEM, A., GUNNARSSON, H., AND KAIJSER, B., Diffusion-in-gel enzyme-linked immunosorbent assay for routine detection of IgG and IgM antibodies to *Campylobacter jejuni*, *J. Infect. Dis.* **148**:82–92 (1983).

215. TAUXE, R. V., DEMING, M. S., AND BLAKE, P. A., *Campylobacter jejuni* infections on college campuses: A national survey, *Am. J. Public Health* **75**:659–660 (1985).

216. TAUXE, R. V., PATTON, C. M., EDMONDS, P., BARRETT, T. J., BRENNER, D. J., AND BLAKE, P. A., Illness associated with *Campylobacter laridis*, a newly recognized *Campylobacter* species, *J. Clin. Microbiol.* **21**:222–225 (1985).

217. TAYLOR, D. N., AND ECHEVERRIA, P., Etiology and epidemiology of travelers' diarrhea in Asia, *Rev. Infect. Dis.* **8** (Suppl. 2):S136–S141 (1986).

218. TAYLOR, D. E., DE GRANDIS, S. A., KARMALI, M. A., AND FLEMING, P. C., Transmissible tetracycline resistance in *Campylobacter jejuni*, *Lancet* **2**:797 (1980).

219. TAYLOR, D. E., DE GRANDIS, S. A., KARMALI, M. A., AND FLEMING, P. C., Transmissible plasmids from *Campylobacter jejuni*, *Antimicrob. Agents Chemother.* **19**:831–835 (1981).

220. TAYLOR, D. N., PORTER, B. W., WILLIAMS, C. A., MILLER, H. G., BOPP, C. A., AND BLAKE, P. A., *Campylobacter* enteritis: A large outbreak traced to commercial raw milk, *West. J. Med.* **137**:365–369 (1982).

221. TAYLOR, D. N., MCDERMOTT, K. T., LITTLE, J. R., WELLS, J. G., AND BLASER, M. J., *Campylobacter* enteritis from untreated water in the Rocky Mountains, *Ann. Intern. Med.* **99:**38–40 (1983).

222. TAYLOR, D. N., ECHEVERRIA, P., BLASER, M. J., PITARANGSI, C., BLACKLOW, N., CROSS, J., AND WENIGER, B. G., Polymicrobial aetiology of travellers' diarrhoea, *Lancet* **1:**381–383 (1985).

223. TAYLOR, D. N., BLASER, M. J., ECHEVERRIA, P., PITARANGSI, C., BODHIDATTA, L., AND WANG, W. L., Erythromycin-resistant *Campylobacter* infections in Thailand, *Antimicrob. Agents Chemother.* **31:**438–442 (1987).

224. TAYLOR, D. N., ECHEVERRIA, P., PITARANGSI, C., SERIWATANA, J., BODHIDATTA, L., AND BLASER, M. J., The influence of strain characteristics and immunity on the epidemiology of *Campylobacter* infections in Thailand, *J. Clin. Microbiol.* **26:**863–868 (1988).

225. TEE, W., KALDOR, J., AND DWYER, B., Epidemiology of *Campylobacter* diarrhoea, *Med. J. Aust.* **145:**499–503 (1986).

226. TEE, W., ANDERSON, B. N., ROSS, B. C., AND DWYER, B., Atypical campylobacters associated with gastroenteritis, *J. Clin. Microbiol.* **25:**1248–1252 (1987).

227. THOMPSON, J. S., CAHOON, F. E., AND HODGE, D. S., Rate of *Campylobacter* spp. isolation in three regions of Ontario, Canada, from 1978 to 1985, *J. Clin. Microbiol.* **24:**876–878 (1986).

228. THORSON, S. M., LOHR, J. A., DUDLEY, S., AND GUERRANT, R. L., Value of methylene blue examination, dark-field microscopy, and carbol-fuchsin Gram stain in the detection of *Campylobacter* enteritis, *J. Pediatr.* **106:**941–943 (1985).

229. TOMPKINS, L. S., AND KRAJDEN, M., Approaches to the detection of enteric pathogens, including *Campylobacter,* using nucleic acid hybridization, *Diagn. Microbiol. Infect. Dis.* **4:**71S–78S (1986).

230. TOTTEN, P. A., FENNELL, C. L., TENOVER, F. C., WEZENBERG, J. M., PERINE, P. L., STAMM, W. E., AND HOLMES, K. K., *Campylobacter cinaedi* (sp. nov.) and *Campylobacter fennelliae* (sp. nov.): Two new *Campylobacter* species associated with enteric disease in homosexual men, *J. Infect. Dis.* **151:**131–139 (1985).

231. TRIBE, G. W., AND FRANK, A., Campylobacter in monkeys, *Vet. Rec.* **106:**365–366 (1980).

232. VAN DE PUTTE, L. B., BERDEN, J. H., BOERBOOMS, M. T., MULLER, W. H., RASKER, J. J., REYNVAAN-GROENDIJK, A., AND VAN DER LINDEN, S. M., Reactive arthritis after *Campylobacter jejuni* enteritis, *J. Rheumatol.* **7:**531–535 (1980).

233. VAN DER MEER, J. W. M., MOUTON, R. P., DAHA, M. R., AND SCHUURMAN, R. K. B., *Campylobacter jejuni* bacteraemia as a cause of recurrent fever in a patient with hypogammaglobulinaemia, *J. Infect.* **12:**235–239 (1986).

234. VANHOOF, R., VANDERLIDEN, M. P., DIERICKX, R., LAUWERS, S., YOURASSOWSKI, E., AND BUTZLER, J. P.,

235. VANHOOF, R., HUBRECHTS, J. M., ROEBBEN, E., NYSSEN, H. J., NULENS, E., LEGER, J., AND SCHEPPER, N., The comparative activity of pefloxacin, enoxacin, ciprofloxacin and 13 other antimicrobial agents against enteropathogenic microorganisms, *Infection* **14:**294–298 (1986).

236. VAN SPREEUWEL, J. P., DUURSMA, G. C., MEIJER, C. J., BAX, R., ROSEKRANS, P. C., AND LINDEMAN, J., *Campylobacter* colitis: Histological, immunohistochemical and ultrastructural findings, *Gut* **26:**945–951 (1985).

237. VELASCO, A. C., MATEOS, M. L., MAS, G., PEDRAZA, A., DIEZ, M., AND GUTIERREZ, A., Three-year prospective study of intestinal pathogens in Madrid, Spain, *J. Clin. Microbiol.* **20:**290–292 (1984).

238. VERNON, M., AND CHATLAIN, R., Taxonomic study of the genus *Campylobacter* (Sebald and Veron) and designation of the neotype strain for the type species, *Campylobacter fetus* (Smith and Taylor) Sebald and Veron, *Int. J. Syst. Bacteriol.* **23:**122–134 (1973).

239. VINZENT, R., DUMAS, J., AND PICARD, N., Septicemie grave au cours de la grossesse due a un vibrion: avortment consecutif, *Bull. Acad. Natl. Med.* **131:**90–93 (1947).

240. VOGT, R. L., SOURS, H. E., BARRETT, T., FELDMAN, R. A., DICKINSON, R. J., AND WITHERELL, L., *Campylobacter* enteritis associated with contaminated water, *Ann. Intern. Med.* **96:**292–296 (1982).

241. VOGT, R. L., LITTLE, A. A., PATTON, C. M., BARRETT, T. J., AND ORCIARI, L. A., Serotyping and serology studies of campylobacteriosis associated with consumption of raw milk, *J. Clin. Microbiol.* **20:**998–1000 (1984).

242. WALDER, M., Epidemiology of *Campylobacter* enteritis, *Scand. J. Infect. Dis.* **14:**27–33 (1982).

243. WALKER, R. I., CALDWELL, M. B., LEE, E. C., GUERRY, P., TRUST, T. J., AND RUIZ-PALACIOS, G. M., Pathophysiology of *Campylobacter* enteritis, *Microbiol. Rev.* **50:**81–94 (1986).

244. WANG, W. L., AND BLASER, M. J., Detection of pathogenic *Campylobacter* species in blood culture systems, *J. Clin. Microbiol.* **23:**709–714 (1986).

245. WANG, W. L., LUECHTEFELD, N. W., BLASER, M. J., AND RELLER, L. B., Effect of incubation atmosphere and temperature on isolation of *Campylobacter jejuni* from human stools, *Can. J. Microbiol.* **29:**468–470 (1983).

246. WANG, W. L., RELLER, L. B., AND BLASER, M. J., Comparison of antimicrobial susceptibility patterns of *Campylobacter jejuni* and *Campylobacter coli*, *Antimicrob. Agents Chemother.* **26:**351–353 (1984).

247. WHEELER, A. P., AND GREGG, C. R., *Campylobacter* bacteremia, cholecystitis, and the acquired immunodeficiency syndrome, *Ann. Intern. Med.* **105:**804 (1986).

248. WINSOR, D. K., JR., MATHEWSON, J. J., AND DUPONT, H. L., Western blot analysis of intestinal secretory immunoglobulin A response to *Campylobacter jejuni* antigens in

Susceptibility of *Campylobacter fetus* subsp. *jejuni* to twenty-nine antimicrobial agents, *Antimicrob. Agents Chemother.* **14:**553–556 (1978).

patients with naturally acquired *Campylobacter* enteritis, *Gastroenterology* **90**:1217–1222 (1986).

249. YOUNG, D. M., BIAO, J., ZHENG, Z., HADLER, J., AND EDBERG, S. C., Isolation of *Campylobacter jejuni* in Hunan, the People's Republic of China: Epidemiology and comparison of Chinese and American methodology, *Diagn. Microbiol. Infect. Dis.* **5**:143–149 (1986).

250. ZAKI, A. M., DUPONT, H. L., ALAMY, M., ARAFAT, R., AMIN, K., AWAD, M. M., BASSIOUNI, L., IMAN, I. Z., EL MALIH, G. S., EL MARSAFIE, A., MOHIELDIN, M. S., NAGUIB, T., RAKHA, M. A., SIDAROS, M., WASEF, N., WRIGHT, C. E., AND WYATT, R. G., The detection of enteropathogens in acute diarrhea in a family cohort population in rural Egypt, *Am. J. Trop. Med. Hyg.* **35**:1013–1022 (1986).

12. Suggested Reading

BLASER, M. J., AND RELLER, L. B., *Campylobacter* enteritis, *N. Engl. J. Med.* **305**:1444–1452 (1981).

BLASER, M. J., TAYLOR, D. N., AND FELDMAN, R. A., Epidemiology of *Campylobacter jejuni* infections, *Epidemiol. Rev.* **5**:157–176 (1983).

BLASER, M. J., WELLS, J. G., FELDMAN, R. A., POLLARD, R. A., ALLEN, J. R., AND the Collaborative Diarrheal Disease Study Group, *Campylobacter* enteritis in the United States: A multicenter study, *Ann. Intern. Med.* **98**:360–365 (1983).

BUTZLER, J.-P. (ed.), *Campylobacter Infection in Man and Animals*, CRC Press, Boca Raton, 1985.

PEARSON, A. D., SKIRROW, M. B., LIOR, H., AND ROWE, B. (ed.), *Campylobacter III: Proceedings of the Third International Workshop on Campylobacter Infections*, Public Health Laboratory Service, London, 1985.

WALKER, R. I., CALDWELL, M. B., LEE, E. C., GUERRY, P., TRUST, T. J., AND RUIZ-PALACIOS, G. M., Pathophysiology of *Campylobacter* enteritis, *Microbiol. Rev.* **50**:81–94 (1986).

CHAPTER 8

Chancroid

George P. Schmid

1. Introduction

Chancroid is a sexually transmitted disease characterized by one or more genital ulcers, often accompanied by painful inguinal lymphadenopathy. The etiologic agent is *Haemophilus ducreyi,* a fastidious, small gram-negative rod.

2. Historical Background

Although chancroid is an ancient disease, it was not clinically differentiated from syphilis until 1852. *H. ducreyi* was identified in 1889 by Ducrey, who found a single organism, compatible with *H. ducreyi,* in smears of exudate from serially passaged ulcers[2]; other workers later isolated the organism. Subsequently, chancroid became recognized as a disease associated with poverty and prostitution, occurring in the wake of traveling carnivals and commonly among troops in World War I.

3. Methodology

3.1. Sources of Mortality Data

H. ducreyi does not spread beyond the genital area and fatalities do not occur.

George P. Schmid · Division of STD/HIV Prevention, Center for Prevention Services, Centers for Disease Control, Atlanta, Georgia 30333.

3.2. Sources of Morbidity Data

In the United States, chancroid is a reportable disease and state health departments and the Centers for Disease Control, to whom the state health departments report their cases, compile statistics on the number of cases reported by physicians. Outside the United States, reporting requirements vary by country.

Unfortunately, chancroid is a difficult disease to confirm by laboratory methods. Culture of *H. ducreyi* is notoriously difficult and direct detection and serologic methods have not been well developed. Thus, the large majority of cases reported worldwide are based on clinical diagnosis, and chancroid can be confused with other diseases. Because of this diagnostic confusion, chancroid is overreported in some areas and underreported in others.

3.3. Surveys

The absence of a widely available serologic test, combined with the fact that the large majority of symptomatic individuals seek medical treatment, preclude surveys for previous or subclinical disease. The best incidence figures for chancroid come from surveys done in sexually transmitted disease or medical clinics.

3.4. Laboratory Diagnosis

3.4.1. Isolation and Identification of Organism. Culture is the only definitive means of diagnosis, but the sensitivity of culture depends on the presence of personnel who are experienced in working with *H. ducreyi,* the type and number of media used, and the conditions under which plates are incubated. The sensitivity of culture from patients

173

suspected of having chancroid ranges from 0 to as high as 80%, depending largely on the above factors.[3]

Although many methods have been used to culture *H. ducreyi,* blood and chocolate agars, both containing vancomycin (3 μg/ml) to suppress contaminating organisms, are the media currently used. Rabbit blood is used for the blood agar and 1% hemoglobin is used for the chocolate agar, although some workers prefer 5% chocolated horse blood instead of hemoglobin. The addition of 3–5% fetal calf serum to either medium appears to enhance the growth of at least some strains.[13]

Material is obtained from the base of the ulcer with either a cotton swab or a wire loop, inoculated onto plates, and the plates are then well streaked to allow the best chance of observing colonies of *H. ducreyi.* Plates should be incubated at 33°C in a candle jar, in the bottom of which should be a moist (but not soaked) paper towel to provide humidity. Although it is sometimes recommended that plates be incubated up to 7 days, the highest yield of *H. ducreyi* will be at 48 or 72 h. Colonies of *H. ducreyi* are small (1–2 mm), gray, and can be differentiated from colonies of other bacteria because they can be pushed intact across the top of the agar. Colonies meeting these criteria, which are oxidase-positive when tested using tetramethyl-*p*-phenylenediamine (the dimethyl reagent will produce a negative result), and which contain small, gram-negative bacilli or coccobacilli, can be presumptively identified as *H. ducreyi.* Further biochemical testing will definitively identify *H. ducreyi.*[1]

3.4.2. Serologic and Immunologic Diagnostic Methods. Although a complement fixation serologic test and the Ito-Reenstierna skin test (using a suspension of killed *H. ducreyi*) have been used for the confirmation of chancroid, they are, because of cross-reactivity with other bacteria, unreliable and no longer available. Recently developed serologic tests using modern techniques, including dot blotting[10] and Western blotting,[15] appear more promising. These tests, however, need further development and testing, and are currently only research tools. No reliable, commercially available, serologic test is available.

Direct detection of *H. ducreyi* in ulcer exudate by immunofluorescence using monoclonal antibodies directed against epitopes on *H. ducreyi* offers a promising diagnostic alternative.[10]

4. Biological Characteristics of the Organism

H. ducreyi is a short, nonmotile, non-spore-forming, gram-negative rod. On agar, colonies are almost invariably

smaller than colonies of other bacteria isolated from the genital tract, gray, and translucent. However, small and scattered large colonies of *H. ducreyi* may occur on the same plate. An important diagnostic feature is that colonies can be pushed intact along the surface of the agar. On primary isolation plates, it is common for only a few colonies to be present and be outnumbered by colonies of commensal bacteria; a dissecting microscope is helpful in identifying colonies of *H. ducreyi.*

The virulence factors of *H. ducreyi* have not been described. Lesions can be produced in rabbits and, with serial passage on agar, some strains lose their ability to produce lesions, suggesting the loss of one or more unidentified virulence factors.

H. ducreyi has acquired resistance to penicillins, sulfonamides, and tetracyclines by acquiring plasmids encoding resistance to these drugs; resistance to tetracyclines in some cases is chromosomally mediated. Six plasmids, most of which are known to encode for antimicrobial resistance, have been described in *H. ducreyi* and, as with other bacteria, offer epidemiologic tools for distinguishing similarities among strains isolated in varying geographic areas.[6]

5. Descriptive Epidemiology

5.1. Prevalence and Incidence

Determining the prevalence and incidence of chancroid is difficult because of the problem of accurate diagnosis.

In the United States, a mean of 878 cases were reported annually between 1971 and 1980, an incidence of 0.4/100,000. Since 1980, however, numerous outbreaks of chancroid have occurred and the number of cases reported annually has risen dramatically. In 1987, 5047 cases were reported, an increase of 48% over 1986 and the largest number of cases since 1949.[12]

Outside the United States, chancroid is very common in developing countries in Central and South America, Africa, and Asia, while in Europe chancroid occurs sporadically. In many developing countries, chancroid is the most common cause of genital ulcers, while in the United States this is the case only in exceptional outbreak situations.[4]

5.2. Epidemic Behavior and Contagiousness

Unlike many other sexually transmitted diseases, chancroid occurs in only selected communities in the United States.[12] In communities where it has become established, disease occurs at a level commensurate with sexual activity by infected individuals. In communities where chancroid is first appearing, successful control depends upon prompt recognition of the disease by clinicians and immediate identification and treatment of sexual partners. If the individual introducing chancroid has intercourse with a limited number of partners and these partners are not highly sexually active, control efforts may be successful in eliminating disease from the community. Sudden, large outbreaks have occurred among men, however, when female prostitutes have been the source of infection. These outbreaks have proven to be very difficult to control because the illegality and anonymity of prostitution makes locating infected individuals difficult. In addition, in the United States, several outbreaks have occurred among illegal entrants, further hampering control efforts.

The likelihood of chancroid being transmitted during a single act of unprotected intercourse is unclear, but a figure of 63% for male-to-female transmission was derived in a small study.[7]

5.3. Geographic Distribution

In the United States, the largest number of cases has occurred in New York City, but numerous Florida cities, Boston, Dallas, Los Angeles/Long Beach, and Orange County (California) have also had significant numbers of cases. Several other cities continually have small numbers of cases, and small outbreaks have been successfully terminated in several other cities.[12]

Specific geographic distribution is generally lacking outside the United States. Upon reviewing national statistics from countries scattered throughout the world, it appears that chancroid occurs frequently in the large majority of developing countries. Scattered cities in Europe have reported cases.

5.4. Temporal Distribution

Chancroid occurs throughout the year.

5.5. Age

Since national age distribution data are not collected, age-specific data come from information gathered during outbreaks. Cases in males are generally most common in the 20–24-year age group, but the mean and median age are higher, indicating that a significant number of men older than 20–24 acquire disease. Age distribution data in women are less well defined because of the relative paucity of cases

in women, but the onset of disease in females is generally at a younger age than in men.

5.6. Sex

In nine outbreaks in the United States between 1981 and 1987, the male : female ratio was 3 : 1–25 : 1, and was highest in outbreaks involving prostitutes.[12] The preponderance of cases in males is due largely to the role prostitution plays in selected outbreaks and, less so, to the fact that disease in men is almost always symptomatic and easily visible, while ulcers in women may occasionally occur in the vagina and be less symptomatic and thus not reported.

5.7. Race

Reported cases of chancroid have occurred preponderantly in blacks and, less so, in Hispanics, than in other racial groups. It is unlikely, however, that this distribution of cases reflects racial predisposition. Instead, it likely reflects socioeconomic status and reporting sources (most cases are reported from public clinics), types of outbreaks (outbreaks involving illegal entrants involve principally Hispanics), frequency of prostitute visitation, and attitudes toward such factors as condom usage and rates of circumcision (which may predispose to chancroid).

5.8. Occupation

Occupation *per se* does not predispose to acquiring chancroid, although individuals involved in certain jobs, e.g., seamen or military personnel on leave, may be more likely to have contact with infected individuals.

5.9. Occurrence in Different Settings

During times of war, chancroid becomes relatively common in military personnel because of the high prevalence of prostitute visitation.

5.10. Socioeconomic Factors

Chancroid is said to increase during times of poverty and war and, to some degree, this is true. This increase undoubtedly does not reflect poor nutrition or crowded living conditions, but rather a matrix of availability of medical care, knowledge of and attitudes toward STDs, sexual habits, reporting sources, and prevalence of prostitution (for alcohol, money, or drugs). The latter factor may be related to living standards in that during times of austerity, prostitution becomes more common.

6. Mechanisms and Routes of Transmission

Chancroid is sexually transmitted and lesions outside the genital tract are rare, but may occur from oral or anal intercourse, or autoinoculation.

7. Pathogenesis and Immunity

Lesions arise in the areas of the male genital tract that are most easily traumatized: the prepuce of uncircumcised men and the coronal sulcus area of circumcised men. In women, most lesions are found on the external genitalia and only occasionally on the vaginal walls or cervix; perianal lesions may occur and do not appear to necessarily result from anal sex.[7,8,14] The usual incubation period is about 3–7 days, but longer incubation periods are common. Whether some degree of immunity occurs is unknown, but second infections may occur.

8. Patterns of Host Response

8.1. Clinical Features

At the site of inoculation, an inflamed macule or papule appears and rapidly erodes into an ulcer; many patients simply recall a "sore" developing without a distinct macule or papule stage. About one-half of patients have more than one ulcer, but it is unusual to have more than four.[8,14] Typically, an ulcer caused by *H. ducreyi* is deep, has a ragged, nonindurated margin with an erythematous edge, and a beefy, necrotic base. Superficial ulcers, however, may occur. A diagnostic feature of chancroidal ulcers is that they are exquisitely painful, making examination difficult—retraction of the prepuce due to phimosis may be impossible. Ulcers may coalesce and form large, serpiginous ulcerations that partly encircle the penis.

As the disease progresses, as many as one-half of men develop unilateral or bilateral inguinal adenopathy, which is characteristically painful even though nodes may be small. Large, fluctuant lymph nodes (buboes) may occur, a finding not seen in genital herpes or syphilis. In the absence of effective antimicrobial therapy and, occasionally, needle drainage, buboes frequently rupture. Lymphadenopathy in women is unusual, presumably because of differences in lymphatic drainage.

Asymptomatic colonization of *H. ducreyi* of the penis, cervix, and mouth has been described but appears to be rare.[5,7] Ulcers of the cervix or vagina may occur with little or no symptomatology.

Without treatment, tissue destruction may be significant but *H. ducreyi* does not spread outside the genital tract. Patients eventually heal their infection after several (unpleasant) months, but often with scarring.

8.2. Diagnosis

Because few laboratories have media for culture of *H. ducreyi*, Gram stain diagnosis of chancroid is not specific, and there is no standardized serologic test, diagnosis of chancroid is often made on clinical grounds. In cases where ulcers are of "typical appearance" and painful, and accompanied by painful, large inguinal lymph nodes, clinical diagnosis is reasonably accurate. Unfortunately, many cases are not so characteristic and other causes of genital ulceration (syphilis and genital herpes) and painful, large inguinal lymph nodes (lymphogranuloma venereum) must be differentiated from chancroid.[9] All patients with a genital ulcer should have a darkfield examination and serologic test for syphilis performed to exclude, as best as possible, syphilis; *Treponema pallidum* coinfects about 10% of chancroid cases. Genital herpes may be accompanied by painful, inguinal lymphadenopathy but rarely causes buboes, and is typically accompanied by multiple, shallow ulcerations preceded by vesicles. Lymphogranuloma venereum is often confused with chancroid, but in lymphogranuloma venereum it is unusual for the ulcer to be present at the time inguinal lymphadenopathy is prominent.

Gram-stained smears of ulcer material are sometimes used to diagnose chancroid, but the diagnostic utility of the Gram stain has not been well studied. Ulcers often contain many species of bacteria, some of which may appear like *H. ducreyi* on smear. Diagnostic specificity is probably enhanced by identifying as presumptive *H. ducreyi* only smears showing strands of bacteria, sometimes appearing like "railroad tracks," along mucous strands. Finding organisms compatible with *H. ducreyi* in a bubo aspirate is more specific, but is uncommon. Monoclonal antibodies have been developed to *H. ducreyi* and may offer a specific immunofluorescence means of visualizing *H. ducreyi* in ulcer or bubo exudate.[10]

9. Control and Prevention

9.1. General Concepts

In the United States, cases of chancroid must be reported to local health authorities. Cases should be treated with an appropriate antimicrobial and interviewed to elicit the names of all sexual partners. These partners should be examined and treated, whether lesions are present or not, because they may be in the incubation stage or asymptomatic carriers of *H. ducreyi*.

Outbreaks of disease occurring in an area where chancroid is first appearing must be aggressively managed if there is to be any hope of eliminating chancroid from the area. Identifying and locating prostitutes is crucial in these efforts, but often difficult because of the anonymity of prostitution and evidence that exchange of illegal drugs for sex has been the form of payment in some outbreaks. If initial control efforts fail and chancroid becomes established, elimination becomes very difficult.

9.2. Antibiotic and Chemotherapeutic Approaches to Prophylaxis

H. ducreyi has, primarily via plasmids, developed resistance to several antimicrobials. Currently, treatment with either erythromycin, 500 mg, orally, four times a day for 7 days, or ceftriaxone, 250 mg, intramuscularly, once, are effective therapies for cases or sex partners.[11]

9.3. Immunization

No vaccine is available.

10. Unresolved Problems

The largest scientific impediment in controlling chancroid is the lack of simple, accurate diagnostic tests. The development of rapid diagnostic techniques would greatly enhance the ability to differentiate causes of genital ulcers and lead to immediate efforts to locate sexual partners; currently such efforts are diluted by the uncertainty over whether the patient really has chancroid. Improved culture techniques and an accurate serologic test would enhance the ability to determine whether asymptomatic carriage is more common than thought, as well as aid in accurately determining the prevalence of chancroid.

11. References

1. ALBRITTON, W. L., PLUMMER, F. A., SOTTNEK, F. O., AND KRAUS, S. J., *Haemophilus ducreyi* and *Calymmatobacterium granulomatis,* in: *Manual of Clinical Microbiology,* 4th ed. (E. H. LENNETTE, A. BALOWS, W. J. HAUSLER, JR., AND J. J. SHADOMY, eds.), pp. 869–873, American Society for Microbiology, Washington, D.C., 1985.
2. DUCREY, A., Experimentelle untersuchungen uber den Ansteckungsstoff des weichen Schankers und uber die Bubonen, *Monatsh. Prakt. Dermatol.* **9:**387 (1889).
3. DYLEWSKI, J., NSANZE, H., MAITHA, G., AND RONALD, A. Laboratory diagnosis of *Haemophilus ducreyi:* Sensitivity of culture media, *Diagn. Microbiol. Infect. Dis.* **4:**241–245 (1986).
4. Editorial, Chancroid, *Lancet* **2:**747–748 (1982).
5. KINGHORN, G. R., HAFIZ, S., AND McENTEGART, M. G., Genital colonisation with *Haemophilus ducreyi* in the absence of ulceration, *Eur. J. Sex. Transm. Dis.* **1:**89–90 (1983).
6. McNICOL, P. J., AND RONALD, A. R., The plasmids of *Haemophilus ducreyi, J. Antimicrob. Chemother.* **14:**561–564 (1984).
7. PLUMMER, F. A., D'COSTA, L. J., NSANZE, H., DYLEWSKI, J., KARASIRA, P., AND RONALD, A. R., Epidemiology of chancroid and *Haemophilus ducreyi* in Nairobi, Kenya, *Lancet* **2:**1293–1295 (1983).
8. PLUMMER, F. A., D'COSTA, L. J., NSANZE, H., KARASIRA, P., MacLEAN, I. W., PIOT, P., AND RONALD, A. R., Clinical and microbiologic studies of genital ulcers in Kenyan women, *Sex. Transm. Dis.* **12:**193–197 (1985).
9. SALZMAN, R. S., KRAUS, S. J., MILLER, R. G., SOTTNEK, F. O., AND KLERIS, G. S., Chancroidal ulcers that are not chancroid: Cause and epidemiology, *Arch. Dermatol.* **120:**636–639 (1984).
10. SCHALLA, W. O., SANDERS, L. L., SCHMID, G. P., TAM, M. R., AND MORSE, S. A., Use of dot-immunobinding and immunofluorescence assays to investigate clinically suspected cases of chancroid, *J. Infect. Dis.* **153:**879–887 (1986).
11. SCHMID, G. P., The treatment of chancroid, *Rev. Infect. Dis.* 1990 (in press).
12. SCHMID, G. P., SANDERS, L. L., BLOUNT, J. H., AND ALEXANDER, E. R., Chancroid in the United States: Reestablishment of an old disease, *J. Am. Med. Assoc.* **258:**3265–3268 (1987).
13. SOTTNEK, F. O., BIDDLE, J. W., KRAUS, S. J., WEAVER, R. E., AND STEWART, J. A., Isolation and identification of *Haemophilus ducreyi* in a clinical study, *J. Clin. Microbiol.* **12:**170–174 (1980).
14. TAYLOR, D. N., DUANGMANI, C., SUVONGSE, C., O'CONNOR, R., PITARANGSI, C., PANIKABUTRA, K., AND ECHEVERRIA, P., The role of *Haemophilus ducreyi* in penile ulcers in Bangkok, Thailand, *Sex. Transm. Dis.* **11:**148–151 (1984).
15. VAN DYCK, E., KAVUKA, M., VERVOORT, T., AND PIOT, P., Detection of serum IgG antibodies to *Haemophilus ducreyi* in an enzyme immune assay, presented at the International Society for STD Research, August 3, 1987, Atlanta.

12. Suggested Reading

KROCKTA, W. P., AND BARNES, R. C., Genital ulceration with regional adenopathy, *Infect. Dis. Clin. North Am.* **1**(1):217–233 (1987).

RONALD, A. R., AND ALBRITTON, W. L., Chancroid and *Haemophilus ducreyi,* in: *Sexually Transmitted Diseases* (K. K. HOLMES, P. A. MÅRDH, P. F. SPARLING, P. J. WIESNER, W. CATES JR., S. M. LEMON, AND W. E. STAMM, eds.), pp. 263–272, McGraw–Hill, New York, 1990.

CHAPTER 9

Chlamydial Infections

E. Russell Alexander and H. Robert Harrison

1. Introduction

There are five quite different disease patterns that result from human infection with chlamydial organisms. Infection with *Chlamydia trachomatis,* by far the most important as a human pathogen, may result in trachoma, a variety of other syndromes that accompany ocular or genital infection, or lymphogranuloma venereum (LGV). *C. psittacii* has one human disease manifestation—psittacosis. The fifth pattern is respiratory disease caused by *C. pneumoniae*. This species of *Chlamydia* was previously unclassified and was referred to as TWAR strains[26] (after Taiwan and Acute Respiratory studies, from which they were first recovered).

Trachoma causes a cicatrizing keratoconjunctivitis, and its sequelae of keratitis, pannus, entropion, and trichiasis occur in severe form in certain endemic areas, primarily the hot, arid parts of the world. Trachoma is the leading infectious cause of blindness.

From a genital reservoir, *C. trachomatis* is transmitted sexually to cause a variety of diseases (Table 1). In the adult female, other disease manifestations include cervicitis, salpingitis, urethral syndrome, and possibly postpartum endometritis. In the male, they include urethritis, epididymitis, and proctitis. (Both sexes may contract inclusion conjunctivitis.) Infant chlamydial diseases include inclusion conjunctivitis of the newborn, pneumonia, and possibly bronchiolitis and otitis media. In the United States, and in other Western countries where it has been studied, *C. tra-*

chomatis is the most prevalent sexually transmitted organism. In infancy, it is the leading single cause of pneumonia in the first 6 months of life.

LGV is a systemic sexually transmitted disease with worldwide distribution, particularly prevalent in warmer climates. The bubonic form is of declining importance in the United States, although proctitis due to the agent is more often recognized.

Psittacosis is an interstitial pneumonia or generalized toxic disease of children and adults that is transmitted from infected avian species. It has become an infrequent disease, except from occupational exposure or exposure to infected psittacine house pets.

C. pneumoniae causes a range of respiratory disease from pharyngitis and otitis media to bronchitis and interstitial pneumonia.[25] Clinically and, to a great extent, epidemiologically, the manifestations are very similar to those caused by *Mycoplasma pneumoniae*. From present knowledge it is exclusively a human disease.

2. Historical Background

The description of trachoma is ancient, trachoma being one of the earliest of human diseases to be recognized as a distinct clinical entity.[70] It was described in the Ebers papyrus (1500 B.C.). The name *trachoma* was first used by Dioscorides in 60 A.D., and the stages of the disease were described by Galen a century later. From the Middle Eastern reservoir, it spread throughout Europe in many waves from the time of the Crusades to Napoleon, being known as both "Egyptian and military ophthalmia."[70] In the last century, the disease has decreased in incidence in many of the temperate climates of the world. It has disappeared from Eu-

E. Russell Alexander and H. Robert Harrison · Division of Sexually Transmitted Diseases, Center for Prevention Services, Centers for Disease Control, Atlanta, Georgia 30333. *Present address of E. R. A.:* Seattle–King County Department of Public Health, Seattle, Washington 98104.

Table 1.   Disease Manifestations of *Chlamydia*

Chlamydia trachomatis
 Trachoma
 Oculogenital diseases

Adult	Female	Male	Infant
a. Conjunctivitis	b. Cervicitis	f. Urethritis	i. Conjunctivitis
	c. Salpingitis	g. Epididymitis	j. Pneumonia
	d. Urethral syndrome	h. Arthritis (Reiter's	k. Bronchiolitis
	e. Postpartum endometritis	syndrome)	

 Lymphogranuloma venereum
Chlamydia psittacii
 Psittacosis
Chlamydia pneumoniae

rope, for example, and is essentially gone from foci that existed in the central United States. Although sulfonamide treatment was introduced in 1938, and tetracyclines and macrolides in the following decade, they cannot be credited with this change. Rather, it has appeared to follow improvements in the standard of living and of hygiene practices. Trachoma has persisted in hot, dry climates and is still a major cause of blindness in those developing countries.

In 1907, Halberstaedter and von Prowazek[27] described cytoplasmic inclusion bodies in epithelial scrapings from trachoma cases. They named them "chlamydozoa" or "mantle bodies" because reddish elementary particles appeared to be embedded in a blue matrix or mantle. Two years later, the same investigators reported inclusions in infants with nongonococcal ophthalmia neonatorum. Lindner[44] named this disease "inclusion blenorrhea" and reproduced ocular disease in nonhuman primates from a mother's genital secretion. Inclusions were demonstrated in female genital epithelium and in nongonococcal urethritis (NGU) scrapings. Material from each of these sources and from infant conjunctivitis was used to produce follicular conjunctivitis in monkeys. Thus, it was believed as early as 1910 that trachoma and ocular genital diseases were caused by similar agents, and the vertical transmission of these agents was postulated.

In 1911, Nicolle *et al.*[53] in Tunis passed trachoma secretions through Berkefeld V filters and succeeded in producing a conjunctivitis in an ape and a chimpanzee, established to be trachoma by transmission to human conjunctiva. In the 1930s, Julianelle[40] for trachoma and Thygeson[70] for inclusion conjunctivitis expanded these studies with the use of smaller filters. After Bedson had described the unique developmental cycle of the psittacosis

agent. Thygeson recognized that the same cycle held true for the agent of inclusion conjunctivitis. Thus, Bedson[5] in 1953, noting the morphological similarity of the developmental cycles of the agents, termed them members of the psittacosis–LGV group of atypical viruses. This concept was strengthened by the finding by Rake that they all shared a common complement-fixing antigen.[57]

In the period 1930–1950, the clinical and epidemiological features of trachoma and inclusion conjunctivitis were described[40,71]—all on the basis of cytological morphological identification. In 1938, the first effective therapy of trachoma occurred with the introduction of sulfanilimides, although it was recognized early that these drugs did not kill the agents. In the search for *in vitro* isolation techniques for Chlamydiae, the chorioallantois of the embryonated hen's egg and a wide variety of tissue-culture systems were explored. These attempts failed, and Chlamydiae were believed to be a virus with propensity for epithelial growth. Machiavello in 1944 and Stewart in 1950 claimed organism growth in the yolk sac of embryonated eggs, but their findings could not be confirmed. It remained for Tang *et al.*[68] in China in 1957 to clearly isolate the agent of trachoma in yolk sac treated with streptomycin to retard bacterial contamination and to demonstrate that this material caused inclusion-positive conjunctivitis in the monkey model. Collier and Sowa[15] confirmed this finding in African studies in The Gambia and, in addition, showed serological response to the agent in human sera. They also showed that the antigen responsible for seroconversion was common to the psittacosis and LGV groups of agents. An explosion of trachoma research followed, including studies in Saudi Arabia, Egypt, Taiwan, and San Francisco. As the trachoma agent was studied, it became clear that it was not a virus but a small bacterium that shared with viruses the property of obligate intracellular parasitism. The agent of inclusion conjunctivitis and NGU was identified by Jones *et al.*[38] in 1959, using yolk-sac techniques. In the period 1960–1980, the development of cell cultures for isolation[22] and microimmunofluorescence methods for antigen identification, immunotyping, and measurement of host response[76,77] has permitted clinical and epidemiological characteristics of *C. trachomatis* diseases to be expanded.

Psittacosis and LGV were first described clinically much later than trachoma (1874[39] and 1786,[35] respectively), but in both cases their real definition took place in the first half of this century. The understanding of the biology of the organisms developed more rapidly than with the trachoma and inclusion-conjunctivitis agents, primarily because of their greater virulence and host range. In particular, their pathogenicity for mice and for the embryonated yolk sac permitted the development of isolation methods and of serological methods (a complement-fixation test was developed as early as 1930).[4] With the advent of tissue-culture methods, the exploration of the molecular biology of chlamydiae has expanded considerably.[3]

C. pneumoniae disease was first described by Grayston in 1986.[25] The agent had been recovered from the eye of a primary school child in 1965 in a prospective study of trachoma in Taiwan. Two decades later, it was noted that this antigen recognized antibody in the serum of children and adults with respiratory disease.[25]

3. Methodology

3.1. Sources of Mortality Data

For none of the diseases caused by *Chlamydia* is there significant mortality, and the rare deaths associated with infant chlamydial pneumonitis or psittacosis are usually in persons with serious accompanying underlying disease. Fatal outcome has no importance in the epidemiology of these conditions.

3.2. Sources of Morbidity Data

Trachoma is not a reportable disease in the United States. For the last 30 years, the World Health Organization (WHO) and many national health agencies have accumulated data on trachoma occurrence by clinical surveys, for planning control efforts, but no continuing statistics on incidence are available. In the United States the oculogenital chlamydial diseases are not uniformly reportable, but there

is some degree of reporting in approximately half of the states. So far, all are underreported. Other estimates have been made from sexually transmitted disease clinics where the ratio of nongonococcal to gonococcal disease has been used, along with other prevalence data, to estimate annual incidence.[81] LGV is a reportable disease, but because of its rarity, data are usually available only in annual summaries published by the U.S. Public Health Service. Psittacosis is reportable, and data on incidence are published weekly in the *Morbidity and Mortality Weekly Report* and are summarized in *Surveillance Reports* by the Centers for Disease Control. In addition, the same centers accumulate data on the occurrence of psittacosis in pet birds or in fowl flocks when these animals are submitted to state laboratories for inspection. There are no data on the incidence of *C. pneumoniae* infections and all of the information so far has come from two laboratories in Seattle and London. Seroepidemiological studies show that the infection is a common one in many countries.

3.3. Surveys

Trachoma-control programs, often supported by the WHO, have depended on clinical surveys of trachoma prevalence and of trachoma sequelae, including blindness. The WHO has helped to standardize survey methods.[86] Most recently, these have been combined with more general surveys of visual acuity and blindness. Traditionally, such surveys do not utilize laboratory confirmation by chlamydial cytology, isolation, or serological methods, other than in research studies. This is not necessary for trachoma, since the disease is well defined clinically.

Oculogenital chlamydial diseases are not regularly the subject of surveys, but data on incidence and prevention are available from research studies. These have included studies in STD clinics, prospective studies in pregnant women, rare studies of chlamydial genital carriage in normal populations, and surveys in infants. These studies have utilized isolation of *Chlamydia* from the genital tract. Seroepidemiological studies have been rare, due to the relative difficulty of the methods available (see Section 3.4,3).

There are no significant survey data for LGV, psittacosis, or *C. pneumoniae* infections in the United States.

3.4. Laboratory Diagnosis

3.4.1. Cytological Identification. For *C. trachomatis,* the organism can be identified in cytological scrapings or in tissue specimens by recognition of characteristic intracytoplasmic inclusions.[87] Such identification in con-

Table 2.   Choice of Diagnostic Tests[a]

| Diagnostic tests[b] | Trachoma | Oculogenital disease | | | | LGV | Psittacosis | C. pneumoniae disease |
| | | Conjunctivitis | | Urethra | Cervix | | | |
		Adult	Infant					
Cytology								
Iodine	±	−	±	−	−	−	−	−
FA	+	+	+	±	±	−	−	−
Giemsa	+	±	+	−	±	−	−	−
Serology								
CF	−	−	−	−	−	+	+	±
MIF	+	±	±	±	±	+	+	+
Isolation								
Yolk sac	±	±	±	±	±	+	+	±
Mice	−	−	−	−	−	±	+	±
Tissue culture	+	+	+	+	+	+	+	±
Antigen detection								
Direct FA	+	+	+	+	+	−	−	±
EIA	+	+	+	+	+	−	−	±

[a]Modified from Schachter and Dawson.[61] +, method of choice; ±, possible, but not optimal; −, not recommended.
[b]CF, complement fixation; EIA, enzyme immunoassay; MIF, microimmunofluorescence.

junctival epithelial cells, and less frequently in cervical epithelial cells, constituted the only identification possible from the time when trachoma and oculogenital diseases were first recognized, at the turn of the century, until the organism was isolated in embryonated eggs in 1957.

With regard to cytological smears, an essential component is the quality of the smear itself. If discharge is present, this should be gently removed, since inclusions are not recognizable in dead or dying cells. Fresh epithelial cells are necessary and are best obtained by a spatula or curette. They should be collected from the upper fornix for trachoma, the lower conjunctiva for inclusion conjunctivitis, from the transitional epithelium for the cervix, and from the anterior male urethra. They can be stained with Giemsa stain (the time-honored method, and probably still the first choice in most laboratories), by fluorescent-antibody (FA) methods, and by iodine staining (to demonstrate glycogen in the inclusions). The sensitivity and specificity of these methods differ among laboratories, but in experienced hands the Giemsa stain and FA test are roughly equivalent for ocular specimens (see Table 2). Iodine stains are more suitable for identification of inclusions in cell cultures, and are not useful for genital specimens, since other glycogen may also be seen in uninfected cells from those sites.[60] Giemsa stain of cytological scrapings has the advantage of permitting examination of the inflammatory response. For trachoma in particular, this has proved to be useful, since

the cellular response is often characteristic (the presence of lymphoid and plasma cells and giant macrophages known as Leber cells). For inclusion conjunctivitis and genital disease, this is less true, but it does permit the opportunity to assess the presence or absence of other bacteria. On the other hand, the FA method has the advantage of specific identification of *C. trachomatis*. Potentially, it can permit separate identification of immunotypes, but in practice, the broadly reacting antiserum to LGV is used for clinical specimens.

Cytological examination of ocular scrapings is still widely used and, as indicated in Table 2, is quite sensitive. Cytological identification of scrapings of the cervix or urethra is very insensitive, and is described only to indicate that it has been attempted. The most sensitive method for identification of *C. trachomatis* of the genital tract is isolation. Antigen detection by direct fluorescent antibody (DFA) staining or by enzyme immunoassay are somewhat less sensitive and specific, but are widely used.[31] *C. trachomatis* can be recognized in tissue sections by Giemsa stain, by IF methods, and by electron microscopy. All these methods have been used in human disease and in experimental models.

C. trachomatis cannot be recognized cytologically with any consistency in bubo aspirates in LGV using any of the staining methods. Inclusions have been seen in biopsy material, but this is a poor method of identification. Similarly, *C. psittacii* is rarely recognized in cytological preparations and rarely in tissue secretions. FA methods and Giemsa stains have been used effectively in tissue secretions of experimental animal models of *C. psittacii* infection, but are not useful in human diagnosis. *C. pneumoniae* strains are difficult to isolate and have been recovered both from the embryonated egg and from tissue culture.[25] They can also be recognized by DFA antigen detection methods if genus-specific conjugate is used.

3.4.2. Isolation

a. C. trachomatis. The method of choice for recovery of *C. trachomatis* is by cell culture. Cells used are McCoy cells, the HeLa-229 cell line, BHK-21 cells, or L-929 cells. A necessary step in cell cultivation of *C. trachomatis* strains other than LGV is centrifugation of the inoculum into the cells. In addition, the cells are treated in some manner to enhance infection; Gordon *et al.*,[22] who developed the modern cell-culture technique, used irradiation of McCoy cells. Hobson *et al.*[32] and others have shown that irradiation is not necessary, but does enhance growth of the organism, probably by enlarging cells and permitting greater intracytoplasmic growth. IUdR,[84] cytochalasin B,[63] and cycloheximide[58] have been used as substitutes for irradiation. In most hands, the best result are obtained with cycloheximide-treated McCoy cells, and it is the most widely used method at present. Specimen material is inoculated into individual vials with cell sheets on coverslips within them or into wells of microtiter plates that have been implanted with cells. They can be examined at 48–96 h after inoculation. Intracytoplasmic inclusions are recognized by iodine stain, by Giemsa stain, or by FA techniques. The most commonly used stain is iodine, which permits rapid identification. When either iodine stains or FA methods are used, *C. trachomatis* will be identified. Giemsa staining will permit identification of *C. psittacii* strains in cell cultures, but since this is usually not necessary, iodine stains are most widely used. The sensitivity of the culture methods is enhanced by one additional passage through cells. Whether or not this step is necessary depends on the degree of sensitivity required for the isolate. LGV strains may be readily isolated in the same system as for the trachoma and oculogenital strains, although they grow more readily in cell culture and do not require cell pretreatment or centrifugation.

Isolation of *C. trachomatis* from yolk sac was historically the first method of agent recovery. However, it is far less sensitive than tissue culture, and more often there is contamination with other bacteria in clinical specimens. For those reasons, it is no longer used diagnostically. For LGV, yolk sac is as sensitive as cell culture.[62] The method consists of inoculation of specimen material into the yolk sac of 7-day-old embryonated chicken eggs. They are examined daily (candled) from days 3 to 13. Impression smears of yolk sac are examined microscopically for elementary bodies. Yolk-sac material is ground and reinoculated and is considered negative after two blind passages. The method is slow and cumbersome and has more opportunity for bacterial superinfection or cross-contamination than the cell-culture method, particularly when multiple passages are required. However, in cultivation of LGV, the organisms are usually recognized in the initial or second passage. In most laboratories, yolk-sac isolation is the method of choice for LGV. Mouse inoculation is another possible method for LGV isolation. Intracranial inoculation is more effective than intranasal instillation, but both are inferior to yolk-sac inoculation. Trachoma and inclusion-conjunctivitis strains will not grow in mice.

b. C. psittacii. These agents will grow in cell culture, in yolk sac, and in mice, by a variety of routes of inoculation. Cultivation in yolk sac or embryonated chick egg is most commonly used in laboratories that are accustomed to this method, as is true of mouse inoculation. This may be accomplished by intraperitoneal, intracerebral, or intranasal inoculation. Since cell-culture methods are now more widely available because of greater interest in *C. trachomatis* infection, they will probably be more widely used. In experienced laboratories, the methods have equal sensitivities. Care must be taken with any of these methods when attempting to recover *C. psittacci* strains, since they are more likely to result in accidental laboratory infections and in cross-contamination.

c. C. pneumoniae Strains. These strains have been isolated from the yolk sac of embryonated eggs, and from HeLa cell tissue culture. There is no consistent preference in method and often the strains are difficult to passage. Antigen has been recognized in tissue culture cells where no strain could be recovered. There is a need for a more reliable method of isolation.[25] A presumptive identification of *C. pneumoniae* antigen in respiratory tract specimens can be accomplished by demonstration of antigen with genus-specific, but not with *C. trachomatis* species-specific antibody, both of which are commercially available in DFA kits for *C. trachomatis* identification.

3.4.3. Antigen and Nucleic Acid Probes.
In recent years, two other diagnostic methods have been evaluated and widely used, and a third is currently undergoing evaluation. They are direct fluorescent antibody smear (DFA), enzyme immunoassay (EIA), and genetic probe methods.

There are a number of DFA kits commercially available. Although they differ primarily in their specificity and in their ease of laboratory measurement, the general principle is the same. A cytological smear is fixed (at which stage it can be stored), stained with a fluorescein monoclonal antibody, and examined under a fluorescence microscope. Elementary bodies are recognized as small apple-green dots and with practice can be recognized with as few as four per slide. The specificity of the diagnosis will relate to the specificity of the monoclonal antibody. When the test is performed by experienced persons, the sensitivity can be as high as 90% but is more often 70–80%. The specificity is usually 98% or greater. Thus, it is an excellent screening test for high-risk populations, but less useful in low-prevalence populations.[56,65]

The EIA class of tests are designed for immunochemical detection of solubilized antigenic components. They have been designed with use of plastic beads to absorb *Chlamydia* lipopolysaccharide from chemical material[31] or that of antigen capture in a sandwich format.[49] All of them use enzyme-conjugated antibody and a recognition system. They share the same sensitivity and specificity with DFA methods.

Both DFA and EIA are less expensive, technologically easier, and less difficult to transport than cell culture.[31] However, they have decreased sensitivity and some loss of specificity. The DFA has the advantage of a verifiable sample quality, a rapid test (as little as one half hour), and no restriction as to specimen site. EIA requires less training and experience as its indicator is more objective; it is more suitable for batch processing; and can be automated.

Nucleic acid probes are in the process of development and a number will soon be commercially available. So far, they are less sensitive than culture, although they are highly specific. They have the potential of ease of transport, automated batch processing, and the potential of differentiation of chlamydial or gonococcal disease on the same specimen. As with antigen identification methods, there is the drawback that no organism is available for further identification (e.g., serological markers, or testing for antibiotic sensitivity). Also, they may be more expensive than culture.

3.4.4. Serological and Immunological Diagnostic Methods

C. trachomatis. Although a variety of serological methods have been used in the past, the FA method, first developed by Bernkopf and then by McComb and Nichols, has been simplified and standardized in an indirect micro-immunofluorescence (MIF) test by Wang and Grayston.[75] At present, this is the most commonly used test for evaluation of host response to trachoma or to oculogenital *C. trachomatis* agents. For LGV, the complement-fixation (CF) test can be used, although the MIF test remains more sensitive and specific.

The MIF test employs yolk-sac- or cell-culture-grown *C. trachomatis* of all known immunotypes as antigen. Antigen dots are placed on a slide in a specific pattern. They are attached to the slide in a diluted yolk-sac suspension. Serial dilutions of serum, tears, or local secretions are applied followed by fluorescein-conjugated anti-human globulin. An obvious advantage of the test is that the conjugate may be prepared against any immunoglobulin class, thus permitting titration of IgG-, IgM-, or IgA-specific antibody. A counterstain is added to the conjugate to permit clearer identification of specific fluorescence in the dots to which antibody-containing serum has been applied. If differentiation among antibodies to specific immunotypes is sought, the antigens can be evaluated separately. For many purposes, antigen pools can be used.

A CF test is available to measure host response to any chlamydial infection.[48] It is still the most commonly used test for psittacosis and LGV, but it is too insensitive for trachoma or oculogenital infections. Usually, the antigen for the CF is obtained from a yolk-sac-grown LGV strain and is prepared by boiling and treatment with phenol. For *C. pneumoniae* strains, the CF test is intermediate in sensitivity. A CF response can be recognized in approximately two thirds of cases showing response by MIF.[80]

Other serological tests that have been evaluated and rejected for lack of sensitivity or specificity are microagglutination, hemagglutination (direct and indirect), and immunodiffusion. A radioisotope immune precipitation test has been studied and appears to be sensitive, but lacks specificity (and is relatively expensive). Several enzyme immunoassay serological tests have been developed utilizing broadly reactive antigens, usually of LGV serotypes. They are capable of genus antibody detection.[21] Although sensitive, these tests will measure antibody to any chlamydiae. The cross-reaction with *C. pneumoniae* antibody makes them difficult to use for *C. trachomatis*. Because of their high sensitivity, they may have utility as screening tests in low-risk populations. One of these tests, adapted to detect infant IgM, has particular utility in the diagnosis of infant pneumonia, and, for this purpose, may be as sensitive as MIF.[45]

For many years, skin-test hypersensitivity to an LGV antigen (prepared from bubo pus) was used for diagnosis of LGV (Frei test).[62] Before more sensitive and specific antibody measurements were available, it was a useful diagnostic aid. However, because cases of LGV are usually not seen early, conversion from negative to positive is rarely observed. In addition, the possibility that positive skin tests merely reflect earlier infections due to other chlamydiae, along with the relative insensitivity of the test and the difficulty in standardizing antigen, have rendered the test obsolete.

Another immunological method of importance to epidemiological studies is the immunotyping of *C. trachomatis* organisms. Earlier, using a method that employed the protection from type-specific toxic death resulting from massive intravenous inoculation in mice (a method adopted from analogous methods in rickettsial research), it was learned that there were specific immunotypes of *C. trachomatis*. Type-specific immunity could be demonstrated, and it appeared that there was some relationship of immunotype to broad disease categories.[2] Wang *et al.*[76] subsequently showed that a far simpler method of immunotyping could be developed using an MIF method. By this method, 12 immunotypes that cause trachoma and oculogenital disease have been identified, and another 3 associated with LGV. No such immunotyping method has been applied to *C. psittacii* or *C. pneumoniae*, although specific immunotypes may well exist. Immunotyping of *C. trachomatis* strains has no broad diagnostic significance other than the differentiation of LGV and oculogenital strains, but immunotyping can be used as a marker of strains in epidemiological investigations.

4. Biological Characteristics of the Organism

Chlamydiae are unusual in that they are obligate intracellular parasites (characteristic of viruses), but they have other characteristics of bacteria. In fact, they were thought to be viruses for many years and were termed *Bedsonia* or *Miyagawanella*. However, it became clear that they had a complex cell wall (similar to gram-negative bacteria in composition), both DNA and RNA, prokaryotic ribosomes, and metabolic enzymes that would permit independent existence, except that they lack energy-production mechanisms.[3] Moulder[51] has thus termed the chlamydiae "energy parasites" and credited their obligate intracellular parasitism to this trait.

The other unusual characteristic of the chlamydiae is their reproductive cycle (Fig. 1). The extracellular form of the organism is the elementary body, and it alone is infectious. Following attachment, the elementary body enters the host cell by a phagocytic process, which is induced by the chlamydial particle. If the particles are live, or do not have antibody attached, they prevent lysosomal fusion and permit replication in the phagosome. Within 6–8 h of ingestion, the elementary body is reorganized into a reticulate body (sometimes called an initial body). This larger, thin-walled body diverts the host cell's synthetic functions for its own metabolic purpose and proceeds to divide by binary fission. In this stage, the reticulate bodies are not infectious. After 18–24 h, the reticulate bodies become reorganized again into elementary bodies (and thus become infectious again). Subsequently, elementary bodies may disrupt and exit the host cell to infect new cells. The full cycle takes about 40 h. These intracytoplasmic collections of elementary bodies constitute the inclusions that may be seen in cytological smears stained by Giemsa or immunofluorescence methods.

Although all chlamydiae share a genus-specific antigen, there is little DNA homology between *C. trachomatis*, *C. psittacii*, and *C. pneumoniae* strains.[10] The three species of chlamydiae are distinguished by several features. The inclusions of *C. trachomatis* accumulate glycogen and

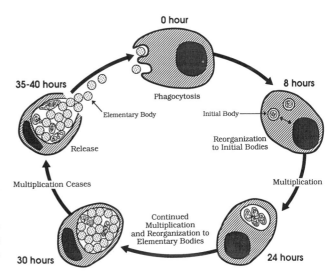

Figure 1. Life cycle of chlamydial organisms. The cycle begins when small elementary bodies infect the host cell by inducing active phagocytosis. During the next 8 h, they reorganize into the larger reticulated initial bodies, which then divert the cell's synthetic functions to their own metabolic needs, and begin to multiply by binary fission. About 24 h after infection, the daughter organisms begin reorganizing into infectious elementary bodies. At about 30 h, multiplication ceases, and by 35–40 h, the disrupted host cell dies, releasing new elementary bodies that can infect other host cells and thus continue the cycle. From Alexander.[1]

0 hour
Phagocytosis
35-40 hours
Elementary Body
8 hours
Initial Body
Reorganization to Initial Bodies
Release
Multiplication
Multiplication Ceases
Continued Multiplication and Reorganization to Elementary Bodies
30 hours
24 hours

thus stain with iodine, whereas the inclusions of *C. psittacii* and *C. pneumoniae* do not. The inclusions of *C. trachomatis* are more compact than those of *C. psittacii* and *C. pneumoniae*. A third difference is their response to sulfonamides: *C. trachomatis* is sensitive and *C. psittacii* and *C. pneumoniae* are not.

C. trachomatis can be further subdivided into strains that cause LGV and strains that cause oculogenital infections. They differ significantly in their biological activity. LGV strains (3 serotypes) are more invasive and can invade many tissues in addition to epithelial cells (e.g., lymphnode invasion, forming the characteristic bubo). This property permits more active cell-to-cell transmission in cell culture and the use of animal inoculation (e.g., mouse) for diagnostic purposes. The oculogenital strains consist of 12 serotypes. They are not readily invasive in tissue culture and *in vivo* grow only in columnar epithelial cells (conjunctivae, respiratory tract, urethra, cervix, rectal mucosa).

C. psittacii will survive for long periods (years) in tissues frozen at − 20°C and can persist in dry bird feces for months. Protein (e.g., serum albumin) will aid stability of *Chlamydia*. *C. trachomatis* strains will lose infectivity within 48 h at room temperature. They are heat-labile, being inactivated in minutes at 56°C. They are inactivated by common disinfectants (e.g., formalin, phenol).

5. Descriptive Epidemiology

5.1. Trachoma

5.1.1. Prevalence and Incidence. Prevalence surveys of trachoma in endemic countries are repeated frequently for control purposes. In hyperendemic areas, the prevalence of trachoma is essentially 100% by the 2nd or 3rd year of life.[37] Active disease, however, is most common in children, who constitute the reservoir of the disease. By adult life, active infection becomes infrequent, although the sequelae of the disease continue to produce the damaging effects that result in visual defect and blindness. In such areas, trachoma constitutes the major cause of blindness.

In areas of moderate endemicity, infection and disease occur later, often beginning at school entry and going through young adult life.[23] The disease is milder in such settings and sequelae are mild, rarely leading to blindness. Often, within such areas, microfoci of severe disease will persist in certain family groups, where a full range of severity will be found.

The United States represents a nonendemic area where trachoma persists only in isolated population segments. As

in the hyperendemic areas, this disease status is constantly changing as betterment of living standards results in decreasing prevalence. Thus, in southwestern American Indian populations 22 years ago, 10% of Indian schoolchildren were found to have active trachoma at school entrance.[19] Today (1988), active trachoma is absent. However, in such areas, sequelae of trachoma can still be seen in the majority of the older population segment.

5.1.2. Epidemic Behavior and Contagiousness. Trachoma is never seen in epidemic form, although perhaps it could return to susceptible populations under disaster conditions if disruption were to result in marked disturbance of hygienic practices. In hyperendemic areas, it persists and is transmitted by a variety of practices that permit eye-to-eye transmission. This may include use of common washing utensils or use of eye drops. The availability of water for washing will greatly affect its transmission. The transmission is potentiated by a variety of ecological factors. In particular, the presence of flies amplifies the transmission of disease. The occurrence of bacterial eye infections (also transmitted by flies) and the effect of dust on eye irritation also facilitate active infection. When trachoma is reintroduced in nonendemic areas, it is not contagious as long as the conditions do not facilitate the transmission.

5.1.3. Geographic Distribution. The trachoma-hyperendemic areas of the world are North Africa and sub-Saharan Africa, the Middle East, drier regions of the Indian subcontinent, and Southeast Asia. Foci of trachoma persist in Australia, the South Pacific, and Latin America.

Within the United States, there are no remaining areas of endemicity. At the turn of the century, there was an endemic focus in the south central United States (extending to Texas). A hospital in Missouri devoted to the treatment of trachoma was closed only at midcentury. Similar disappearance of endemic trachoma occurred in Europe, Russia, and the Mediterranean in the same period.

5.1.4. Temporal Distribution. Throughout the world, trachoma vanishes as changes occur in standards of living, particularly the availability of water and the control of flies. Thus, the trends are usually ones of decrease. Within many endemic areas, there are seasonal changes that closely follow the seasonal increase in fly prevalence and the accompanying bacterial conjunctivitis. In some sites (e.g., northern India), two such peaks may occur each year. Such changes will not affect the prevalence of chronic trachoma or the blinding sequelae.

5.1.5. Age. The relationship to age is discussed in Section 5.1.1.

5.1.6. Sex. In hyperendemic areas, there is no sex differential in young children—the reservoir of active trachoma. In adults, reinfection disease occurs more frequently in women taking care of children, although there is no evidence that this alters the relative prevalence of blinding sequelae, which are equally prevalent in both sexes.

5.1.7. Race. There is no evidence for racial differences.

5.1.8. Occupation. There are no occupational factors that cannot be related to socioeconomic factors.

5.1.9. Socioeconomic Factors. These are predominant epidemiological factors. The important aspects appear to be water availability, fly occurrence, health and hygienic practices, and crowding.[38] Studies in Saudi Arabia by Nichols *et al.*[52] depicted the decrease of trachoma occurring with the creation of small towns replacing rural foci where trachoma had been hyperendemic. Striking differences could be shown among cities, small towns, and oasis villages. In the United States, as in many other countries, trachoma has vanished with improvement in the standard of living.

5.1.10. Other Factors. Although nutritional factors have been questioned as a possible contributing factor, there is no clear evidence that such is the case, and the factors of water shortage, exposure to bacterial conjunctivitis, fly transmission, and the amplifying factor of dust irritation appear to be most important. Jones[37] summarizes these conditions as those that contribute to "ocular promiscuity" (in contrast to the amplifying factors of "sexual promiscuity" for genital *C. trachomatis* infections) (also see Section 6.1).

5.2. Oculogenital Diseases

5.2.1. Prevalence and Incidence

a. Adult Inclusion Conjunctivitis. No incidence or prevalence data in either males or females are available for this illness.

b. Cervicitis. Overall population estimates for chlamydial infection are difficult to obtain. However, figures have been obtained for different subgroups. Among pregnant women enrolling for prenatal care, 3–25% have been found to be infected, depending on the group examined. In venereal disease clinics,[14] up to 30% of symptomatic women have cervical chlamydiae. The prevalence in asymptomatic partners of males with urethritis may be as high as 50%.[67] In asymptomatic nonpregnant college students, chlamydiae were found in the cervixes of 5%.

Etiology in symptomatic cervicitis is more difficult to define, since multiple organisms may be involved. However, chlamydiae have been isolated from 34 to 63% of women with clinical cervicitis.[8]

c. Salpingitis. In the United States, over 200,000 women per year are hospitalized for active pelvic inflammatory disease, and it is estimated that another million are treated as outpatients. If tubal cultures taken at laparoscopy are regarded as identifying the etiological organism, then *C. trachomatis* causes approximately 20–40% of salpingitis in this country and almost 60% in Sweden.[46] Serological data have also implicated *C. trachomatis* as a causal agent in peritonitis or perihepatitis or both (Fitz-Hugh–Curtis syndrome).[78]

d. Female Urethral Syndrome. The prevalence of acute urethral syndrome is unknown. An estimated 5 million women per year in the United States are seen for symptoms suggestive of urinary-tract infection. As many as 30% of these *may* have acute urethral syndrome (acute dysuria, frequent urination, "sterile" urine). Studies suggest that approximately 30% of the cases of acute urethral syndrome are due to *C. trachomatis.*[64,82]

e. Postpartum Endometritis. In one study, 7 (22%) of 32 women with *C. trachomatis* cervical infection during pregnancy developed late postpartum endometritis (48 h–6 weeks postdelivery).[74] In other studies the association has been less or not found.[7,83]

f. Male Urethritis. In the United States, more than half the estimated 2 million cases of acute urethritis are of nongonococcal etiology. *C. trachomatis* causes 30–50% of these cases.[33] In some populations, e.g., student health clinics, *C. trachomatis* is far more common than gonococcus as a cause of urethritis.

g. Epididymitis. This severe complication of acute urethritis occurs in approximately 500,000 men per year in the United States. Roughly half these cases are caused by *C. trachomatis.*[34]

h. Arthritis (Reiter's Syndrome). In studies in the United Kingdom, it has been estimated that Reiter's syndrome occurs in about 1% of NGU.[41] An estimate from Finland is 2%.[36] Sexually acquired reactive arthritis (see Section 8.2.1h) as a complication of NGU without the classic triad of Reiter's syndrome occurs four times more frequently.[41]

i. Infant Inclusion Conjunctivitis and Pneumonia. Approximately 25% of infants exposed to *C. trachomatis* in the birth canal will develop conjunctivitis and 10%, pneumonia.[1] If a conservative figure of 10% maternal carriage rate is used, 3.0 million babies born each year in the United States would yield 75,000 cases of inclusion conjunctivitis and 30,000 cases of chlamydial pneumonia. *C. trachomatis* has been estimated to cause 20–30% of all pneumonia in infants under 6 months of age ill enough to require hospitalization.

5.2.2. Epidemic Behavior and Contagiousness. The chlamydial oculogenital diseases behave like other STDs. The increasing incidence and prevalence of chlamydial infection paralleled that of gonorrhea and may reasonably be termed epidemic at this time.

In the United Kingdom and Sweden, where both gonococcal urethritis and NGU are reportable, the incidence of both diseases rose rapidly from the early 1960s. In fact, the start of the epidemic increase in Sweden preceded the start in the United States by about 4 years. The rest of the curve is very much the same as the United States for gonorrhea. In the mid-1970s, Sweden saw a plateau for the incidence of gonorrhea (the United States experienced the same phenomenon in 1978). In Sweden, the incidence of chlamydial infections is decreasing. Chlamydial infections are probably as contagious as gonorrheal infections, but studies to evaluate this have not been done.

Chlamydia and gonorrhea occur together frequently. *C. trachomatis* is recovered from 20–30% of men with gonorrhea, for example; postgonococcal urethritis is now recognized as a chlamydial infection following a gonococcal infection as a result of simultaneous exposure (with *C. trachomatis* having a longer incubation period). Chlamydial and gonococcal infection may occur together in the cervix and presumably may occur in salpingitis.

Chlamydial conjunctivitis may be transmitted through infected persons by contact. There is no evidence that chlamydial pneumonia can be transmitted in any other way than at birth.

5.2.3. Geographic Distribution. The agent and its various clinical pictures have a worldwide prevalence; it has been identified in all populations in which STDs have been examined.

5.2.4. Temporal Distribution. No seasonal variation is recognized.

5.2.5. Age, Sex, Race, Occupation, Occurrence in Different Settings, Socioeconomic Factors, and Other Factors. *C. trachomatis,* like other genital pathogens, has been found with increased frequency among individuals who are younger, more often nonwhite, unmarried, and of lower socioeconomic status. Both males and females with infection tend to have had more sexual experience in terms of the number of recent sexual partners. Pregnant women with *C. trachomatis* also tend to be of lower gravidity. These factors also characterize the infants who contract conjunctivitis or pneumonia. No distinctive characteristics of diseased versus nondiseased infected infants have been found. Infant conjunctivitis develops at 5–14 days of life (rarely later to 6 weeks, which may be recurrences). Infant pneumonia develops from 2 weeks to 4 months of age. The occurrence of *C. trachomatis* pneumonia in older children and adults is rarely seen.

5.3. Lymphogranuloma Venereum

5.3.1. Prevalence and Incidence. Reported cases of LGV have been decreasing in the last few years from 394 in 1974 to 300 in 1987[13] (the rates have changed from 0.2 to 0.1/100,000 population).

5.3.2. Epidemic Behavior and Contagiousness. LGV is transmitted by sexual contact, but the degree of contagiousness has not been measured. Likewise, the epidemic behavior of the disease has not been well documented. The disease was more prevalent in the United States in the first half of this century than it is at present, and except for some increase among the most sexually active homosexual population, it remains a disease of decreasing incidence in the United States today.

5.3.3. Geographic Distribution. In the early part of this century, LGV was more common in the southeastern United States. The present geographic distribution shows a higher prevalence in some of these states (e.g., Virginia, Georgia, and Louisiana). When examined by city, the highest prevalences are in Washington, D.C., Atlanta, Houston, and New York. Although some of this concentration can be attributed to better diagnosis in certain centers, it is clear that this also reflects imported disease, particularly in merchant seamen and military personnel. Regarding the source of infection overseas, the disease is more often seen in tropical climates, notably in Africa, Central America, and tropical areas of Asia.

5.3.4. Temporal Distribution. There are no data on temporal distribution.

5.3.5. Age and Sex. This disease is recognized more often in midadult life and more often in males than in females.

5.3.6. Race. Although a greater susceptibility of blacks was postulated in years past, such a hypothesis cannot be substantiated, and no difference in racial susceptibility is believed to exist.

5.3.7. Other Factors. The only other population group that appears to be at higher risk are sexually active homosexuals. In recent studies in large cities such as New York, San Francisco, and Seattle, isolates have been found among homosexuals, particularly in men with proctitis.

5.4. Psittacosis

5.4.1. Prevalence and Incidence. Psittacosis is a relatively rare disease in the United States. In 1987, 98 cases were reported (0.4/1,000,000 population).[11] Most of these cases are associated with exposure to psittacine birds of domestic or foreign origin. Cases associated with poultry processing decreased in the 1970s and then stabilized. An exception was 1984 when a particular outbreak reversed that trend.[12]

All birds entering the United States (except from Canada) are required by the U.S. Department of Agriculture to undergo a 30-day quarantine, during which time they are treated with chlortetracycline. So far, strains remain susceptible to tetracycline. It has recently been proposed that the quarantine period be extended to 45 days, particularly for larger psittacine birds. The current importation is about 700,000 birds per year.

5.4.2. Epidemic Behavior and Contagiousness. In 1929, epidemic disease from infected psittacine birds spread from Argentina to England, Germany, and the United States as infected psittacine birds were transported to those countries. Discovery of the cause of this disease and its treatment resulted in control of epidemic disease by the 1950s and cessation of such outbreaks. From 1979 to 1984, there were no significant outbreaks in the United States. In 1984 an outbreak occurred in turkey slaughtering plants.

Human-to-human transmission can occur from a heavily infected pneumonia case, but such occurrence is extremely rare and is of no significance in the epidemiology of the disease. The important epidemiological source remains either psittacine birds or poultry flocks.

5.4.3. Geographic Distribution. Cases are broadly distributed in the United States, but in recent years there have been more cases reported from mountain and Pacific coast states (57% in 1987). Few cases are reported from the northwest central and southeastern states. Although this reflects, in part, the distribution of psittacine birds, it also reflects increased disease awareness and better diagnostic facilities in these states.

5.4.4. Temporal Distribution. The distribution of cases has no distinct seasonal pattern.

5.4.5. Age, Sex, Race, and Occupation. Cases occur more often in midadult life and more often in males than in females, reflecting the increased exposure in these groups. There is no evidence of racial predilections. Regarding occupation, most cases of psittacosis in recent years have occurred in owners of pet birds, employees of the commercial pet-bird trade, bird fanciers, pigeon fanciers, and a variety of miscellaneous avian exposures. Since 1974, few cases have occurred in poultry producers and processors, although the potential for such occurrence still exists. Only about 10% of cases occur in persons without clear-cut exposure. Thus, the majority (93% from 1975 to

1984) of cases occur in persons exposed through vocational or avocational activities.[12]

5.4.6. Socioeconomic Factors. Socioeconomic status is not of epidemiological significance.

5.5. *C. pneumoniae* Infections

5.5.1. Prevalence and Incidence. There are no population-based studies of prevalence or incidence of these infections. Serological studies of Finnish military recruits, of pneumonia sera submitted to the state serum institute in Denmark, of hospitalized patients in Halifax, Nova Scotia, and of both college students and pneumonia patients in Seattle are remarkably similar in showing that 20–60% of adults have specific *C. pneumoniae* antibody.[80] Too little time has elapsed to be able to comment on the incidence. What is becoming clear is that the agent is not constantly present in a given community, but whether seasonality or cyclicity is present is not known.

5.5.2. Epidemic Behavior and Contagiousness. Four different epidemics of pneumonia were studied by Kleemola and colleagues and were shown to be caused by *C. pneumoniae*.[43] These were in garrisons of military recruits in Finland and occurred between 1977 and 1985. In three instances they occurred in spring, and in one instance in summer and fall. The epidemics lasted 5–7 months. In one of the epidemics the disease was also widespread in an adjacent civilian community. Attack rates varied from 60 to 80 per 1000 men. Human-to-human transmission was suggested but not proven.

5.5.3. Geographic Distribution. Seroepidemiological studies in Denmark, Finland, Canada, Taiwan, Japan, Panama, and Seattle have shown antibody to be widely prevalent (20–60% of adults).[80] Serological studies of what appears to be a similar strain from Iran have shown widespread antibody in the United Kingdom. Population-based seroepidemiological studies have not been done to date.

5.5.4. Temporal Distribution. It is known that the disease can occur in any season, and it is also apparent that there can be long gaps of time (at least 2–3 years) when there is no evidence of transmission in a community. On the other hand, age prevalence curves have been remarkably similar in the different settings where they have been studied, suggesting that the periods of absent transmission are not too long.

5.5.5. Age and Sex. In reported seroepidemiological studies,[80] the most rapid rise in age-specific prevalence occurs in the age group 5–20 years. This is similar to the age characteristics for *M. pneumoniae* pneumonia, which has peak attack rates in the adolescent and young adult. The age-specific prevalence slowly increases during adult years from about 30 to 60% prevalence.

Consistent for all large-sample studies is a significant excess of women over men. That excess is not as large as the excess in *C. trachomatis* antibody. This fact, along with the absence of any neonatal peak, suggests that sexual transmission is not a major transmission route.

5.5.6. Race, Occupation, Occurrence in Different Settings, and Socioeconomic Factors. There are no data on these factors. Most of the samples studied to date have been white, but antibody has been noted in black and native American subjects. There are no clear-cut occupational associations, but there is surprising uniformity in seroepidemiology from quite divergent samples. Again, this is very similar to the epidemiological findings for *M. pneumoniae* infection.

6. Mechanisms and Routes of Transmission

6.1. Trachoma

The conjunctival epithelium of humans constitutes the reservoir of infection for trachoma. It is passed from eye to eye by direct contact. In some instances, this is aided by local practices. For example, in India, it is usual for dye to be applied around the eye, with a small stick or with the finger. This is applied to adult women first and then down to children of both sexes—from the oldest to the youngest. In many Southeast Asian countries, washcloths are applied to the face—again from eldest to youngest, and in crowded areas of poverty, usually the same cloth without a change of water. Both are ideal methods for transmission.

Transmission is also potentiated by flies. They will differ as to species, but in each case they are capable of carrying infected secretions from face to face, where they may be self-inoculated into the eye. Jones[37] showed by use of fluorescein dyes that ocular discharges could be transferred from person to person in the usual family setting in a matter of minutes. He referred to the sum of these various methods of transfer of infected secretions as "ocular promiscuity" and suggested that this characterizes the epidemiological pattern of endemic trachoma in much the same manner as genital promiscuity characterizes the method of transmission for oculogenital diseases.

Two other factors play some part in the transmission of endemic trachoma in certain areas of the world—perhaps in preparing the eye for more severe infection. One is the occurrence of bacterial conjunctivitis—often also fly-transmitted. In certain settings, seasonal epidemics of bacterial conjunctivitis precede the peak of trachoma infectivity by a few weeks. A variety of bacterial pathogens have been implicated, particularly certain *Haemophilus* and *Neisseria* species. It is surmised that the bacterial infections increase both conjunctival and corneal inflammation, and thus amplify their subsequent response to trachomatous infection. Anyone who has been in such areas at the height of the fly season can attest to the intensity of fly infestation. Flies cover the faces of children, particularly around the eyes, where there is conjunctival discharge.

A second set of factors less well understood are the environmental factors that characterize many of the foci of greatest prevalence. These are dust and sunlight—both irritants to conjunctiva and to cornea and both hypothesized to aid *C. trachomatis* in its damaging effects. It is difficult to measure these influences, but trachoma remains most prevalent and most damaging in those locations where these factors predominate.[37]

6.2. Oculogenital Diseases

The columnar cells of the adult male urethra and female endocervix are felt to be the reservoirs of infection. Asymptomatic infection seems to be the rule: more than 50% of infected men and women with positive urethral or cervical cultures have no complaints or discharge. The organism is transmitted via sexual contact. Recent evidence suggests that *C. trachomatis* also infects the female urethra.

In women, *C. trachomatis* is responsible for a proportion of acute and chronic cervicitis on examination, but how much is difficult to say, since it is often accompanied by other pathogens (e.g., *Mycoplasma hominis*, *Ureaplasma urealyticum*, *Trichomonas vaginalis*, herpes, cytomegalovirus). Urethral syndrome or acute urethritis may be a result of simultaneous infection, spread from infected cervical secretions, or trauma during intercourse. The exact mode is not clear. The organism is responsible for 20–40% of cases of salpingitis, presumably via direct extension. Postpartum endometritis, thought to be at least partly due to *C. trachomatis*, also occurs via direct extension.[83]

In males, the major illnesses (urethritis and epididymitis) are due to direct extension of infection from the primary urethral focus. Hematogenous dissemination has never been documented in either sex. Adult inclusion conjunctivitis is felt to be transmitted via hand-to-eye contact from infected genital foci.

The only documented mode of transmission of infection to infants is vertically by passage through an infected cervix. No hard evidence for transplacental or postnatal infection exists.

6.3. Lymphogranuloma Venereum

The reservoir of infection is the cervix of the asymptomatic female and, to a lesser extent, for the male homosexual, the rectal mucosa of the asymptomatic male. It is spread exclusively by sexual contact. In the male, primary lesions appear on the penis, usually on the glans (occasionally in the urethra), or the wall of the rectum, and in the female on the labia or on the wall of the vagina. Such lesions are usually painless and may be hidden, adding to the risk of transmission. Extragenital sites for primary lesions include hands (especially fingers) and tongue. Although secondary and tertiary lesions are the ones most easily diagnosed and are the stages of disease that result in damaging sequelae, it is the painless primary lesions that are the source for sexual transmission.

6.4. Psittacosis

The predominant source for human disease are infected avian species, all of which are potential reservoirs. Meyer[47] listed 130 species known to be such sources in 1967, and the list could no doubt be lengthened. The risk of exposure is greatly increased in those occupations in which handling birds or their carcasses is common. The most common avian sources are parrots and parakeets, usually resulting in sporadic cases from pet birds. In recent years, about two thirds were from psittacine species. Pigeons are another source, as are poultry, particularly turkeys. Wild birds have infrequently been documented as a source. Domestic and other lower mammals are infected with *C. psittacii* strains, but they rarely cause human disease. Those infections that have been documented are from laboratory animals. In the overwhelming majority of cases, psittacosis occurs in persons in whom bird processing or handling is a vocation or avocation. Casual exposure is extremely rare.

Transmission between humans can take place, and on rare occasions such transmission has been documented. It has resulted from close exposure to extremely sick or fatal cases. In only one instance has psittacosis been spread between humans through mildly ill or asymptomatic cases.

The route of infection is airborne, and the primary site of infection is the lower respiratory tract. The involvement is in the alveoli, with very little evidence of bronchial or upper-respiratory-tract infection.

6.5. *C. pneumoniae* Infections

There is no evidence for other than human-to-human transmission of *C. pneumoniae* infection. Clearly human epidemics occur, as described in the pneumonia epidemics in military trainees in Finland.[43] Because TWAR was originally thought to be a member of the psittacine species and because it can infect experimental animals, an extensive search for antibody in serum of domestic pets was made and has yielded no evidence for an animal reservoir. In addition, there is no epidemiological evidence to suggest an unusual frequency of animal contact in cases.[25]

7. Pathogenesis and Immunity

7.1. Trachoma

In the early stages of disease, trachoma appears as a follicular conjunctivitis with hyperemia, edema, and distortion of the vascular pattern of the conjunctiva. This is accompanied by papillary hypertrophy of the conjunctiva. The follicles are, in fact, lymphoid germinal centers. In these initial stages, there is involvement of both palpebral and bulbar conjunctivae. Such conjunctival follicles can occur as a response to a number of stimuli, both infectious and toxic. The infant conjunctiva cannot so respond for a number of weeks, and thus chlamydial ocular infection of the newborn (inclusion conjunctivitis) is afollicular, even though the strains are very similar (e.g., as shown by the disease produced in the experimental monkey eye). The chronic follicular conjunctivitis of trachoma heals by scarring. These scars lead to distortion of the lids. This, in turn, results in inability of the lids to close completely, allowing dust particles to damage the cornea. Similarly, the lid distortion results in trichiasis, or inversion of lashes, which adds to the trauma to the cornea. Both these sequelae of trachoma contribute to blindness.[37] The incubation period is not known. In human volunteer studies and experimental studies in the nonhuman primate it is 5–12 days. It is important to note that in both experimental situations, infection will not occur with simple corneal exposure, but only after vigorous application of concentrated inoculum. Therefore, it might be surmised that the natural incubation period is somewhat longer.

Acute corneal involvement includes follicles, which often ring the limbus and, after rupture, lead to corneal defects termed Herbert's pits. Punctate erosions of the cornea occur (epithelial keratitis). Inflammatory infiltrates of the cornea may be seen. A characteristic feature of trachoma is the vascularization of the cornea, with swelling of the corneal–scleral border, which constitutes pannus. This is an important component of trachoma diagnosis.

Collectively, these features of trachoma constitute the acute and chronic conjunctivitis and their blinding sequelae. The occurrence of these features in all populations increases with age, although the age at which they occur will depend on the intensity of disease in each sample.

All these changes have been reproduced experimentally in the monkey, but never with the initial infection, which produces only acute follicular conjunctivitis leading to minimal scarring. Pannus is only a result of reinfection (exogenous reinfection or endogenous relapse).[24] Whether this is true for human disease has never been substantiated. If it is, then the disease that is characterized as trachoma (with pannus) is never a primary infection. Nevertheless, it is clear in human disease that the serious sequelae that lead to blindness occur only as a result of many reinfections, abetted by the many other causes of corneal diseases in hyperendemic trachomatous populations including bacterial infections and various environmental factors (e.g., dust, sunlight). It has been speculated that nutritional factors may also play a role.

If reinfection is a necessary factor for severe trachoma, what is the role of immunity? In the experimental animal, after infection, for a short period, there is immunity to reinfection with homologous strains (but no immunity to heterologous rechallenge). In the few studies that were made with what are now recognized as relatively crude and antigenically weak vaccines, there was transient immunity to rechallenge. When this immunity waned, not only were the experimental animals susceptible to reinfection, but also the severity of disease produced by such rechallenge was enhanced (a phenomenon similar to that seen in other experimental vaccines, such as those for *M. pneumoniae* and respiratory syncytial virus). Whether such a period of hyperreactivity exists in natural human infection has not been determined, but immunity in nature is fleeting. Infection in man and in experimental animals produces both local and circulatory immune responses, but these antibodies do not appear to be protective. One epidemiological fact continues to kindle interest in the prospect of producing an effective vaccine for trachoma—the observation that in all endemic situations studied, active trachoma decreases with age. Although the age at which this occurs will vary with the intensity of disease in the population, eventually the older segment of the population no longer has active disease, suggesting that immunity eventually prevails. This occurs at an early enough age in some populations that one cannot attribute it to decrease in ocular promiscuity alone. It is the aim of proponents of vaccine development to create a vaccine that would mimic the natural occurrence. To date, our knowledge of the immunology of trachoma is relatively primitive (particularly cellular immunity), as is our knowledge of the antigens of *C. trachomatis*.

7.2. Oculogenital Diseases

There are several useful unifying principles in regard to the oculogenital infections caused by *C. trachomatis*: (1) The organism infects superficial columnar epithelial cells in various sites (endocervix, urethra, epididymis, endometrium, salpinx, conjunctiva, nasopharynx, lower respiratory tract) and appears to have little propensity for invasion of or destruction of deeper tissue. (2) The clinical features of chlamydial infection seem to be produced by the host inflammatory response, rather than by the inherent destructiveness of the organism. (3) *C. trachomatis* infections may be present and asymptomatic ("latent" or "silent" infection) for prolonged periods of time. For example, infants have been documented to shed organisms from conjunctivae for up to 2 years postdelivery. Similarly, women with cervical infection have been culture-positive for over 15 months. (4) The stimuli that convert latent infection to chronic disease, or that determine symptomatic versus asymptomatic primary infection, are unknown. (5) At least in some cases (pregnant women), infection can occur, recur, and persist even in the presence of serum antibody. Cell-mediated immune responses (as measured by lymphocyte blastogenic response) appear to be associated with clearing infection, although the evidence is far from clear.

The incubation periods for oculogenital syndromes vary with the syndrome. Urethritis appears to have an incubation period of 5–14 days. This is longer than the incubation period for gonococcal urethritis, which is 2–7 days. When they occur as a result of concurrent exposure, the chlamydial urethritis usually occurs later, which accounted for the entity known as postgonococcal urethritis that occurred in some cases of gonococcal urethritis treated with penicillin only. The incubation period for cervicitis is probably the same as urethritis, but because of the slow and infrequent development of symptoms, is harder to define. The incubation period for chlamydial salpingitis is longer usually following cervical infection by 2–3 weeks. The incubation period for conjunctivitis of infants, children, or adults is 5–12 days. In the case of ophthalmia neonatorum, chlamydial ophthalmia most often has onset in the second week of life as opposed to gonococcal conjunctivitis which occurs characteristically in the first week. Chlamydial pneumonia of infancy has onset between 3 and 12 weeks of age. From prospective studies it appears to follow the earliest recognition of posterior nasopharyngeal infection by a week or so. Rectal infection is rarely discovered before the second month of life.

In all illnesses so far studied, the surface chlamydial infection appears to produce an early polymorphonuclear inflammatory response at the surface and a later subepithelial infiltration of lymphocytes, plasma cells, monocytes, and eosinophils. Inclusions have been seen in cervix, conjunctiva, salpinx, and infant airways. Although the antigen load, in terms of inclusions seen, does not appear great, the immune response appears to be profound. In infants with chlamydial pneumonitis, for example, large interstitial and peribronchiolar lymphoid infiltrates and organizing nodules with germinal centers can be seen; these are the "infiltrates" seen on chest radiography.

The preliminary evidence available indicates that chlamydial infections may produce chronic sequelae. The observations are not unexpected, since the intense inflammatory response produced by chlamydial infection can lead to tissue destruction, fibrosis, and scarring. Data from Sweden suggest that chlamydial salpingitis has a higher postinfectious incidence of involuntary infertility and ectopic pregnancy than does gonorrheal disease. Distal tubal obstruction has been reproduced in the nonhuman primate by repeated salpingeal infection.[55] Furthermore, obliterative bronchiolitis has been observed in the lung-biopsy specimen taken from an infant recovering from chlamydial pneumonitis.

At this point, the investigation of the immunopathogenesis of oculogenital *C. trachomatis* infections is in its infancy. Many interesting and significant observations are still to come. For example, in the case of oculogenital diseases, it appears that such immunotypes may cause adult pneumonias in immunocompromised hosts.[66] The pathogenesis of such reactivation disease is not understood.

7.3. Lymphogranuloma Venereum

The primary lesion of LGV is usually painless and may often be missed. The incubation period is variable and has been described as 3–30 days. The primary lesion may be a papule, an ulcer or erosion, a vesicle, or a urethritis. Rarely, the site may be extragenital. Pathologically, there is nothing specific about these lesions. Proctitis commonly accompanies primary anorectal infection.

In most instances, it is the secondary lesions that bring the disease to medical attention. These are involvement of lymph nodes, producing the characteristic bubo. The

bubonic form occurs in males more often than females (9 : 1), in part due to differences in lymphatic drainage patterns. Both inguinal and femoral node chains can be involved (when both are involved, the characteristic groove sign results—a groove between the two chains). Systemic signs (fever, myalgia) may occur at this time, but leukocytosis is rare. Large mononuclear cells proliferate within the nodes, and foci become necrotic. These foci may proceed to suppuration and rupture of the nodes, developing draining fistulas. Alternatively, the nodes may spontaneously harden and then heal. In approximately 5% of cases, a chronic lymphadenopathy may occur, which may persist for many years.

What are sometimes referred to as tertiary lesions of LGV are analogous to the sequelae of trachoma in that they are the result of scarring. They include strictures of the rectum and vagina and fistulas that may be rectovaginal or may involve the urethra. These lesions are characterized by destruction of mucosal epithelium with scarring and plasma-cell infiltration. Extragenital involvement may rarely involve the conjunctivae, the skin (e.g., fingers), the oral mucosa—each with respective lymph-node involvement. Even less frequent are syndromes of meningitis, salpingitis, arthritis, and pneumonitis.

LGV elicits a marked host response. Nonspecifically, this is reflected in a hypergammaglobulinemia that may result in a reversal of albumin/globulin ratio. Specifically, broad and intense response can be measured with chlamydial antigens. For that reason, CF antibodies are uniformly elevated, and this generally insensitive test is useful in this disease, utilizing *C. psittacii* antigen. Using specific MIF antigens, a brisk response is noted, which is characteristically broad (responding to many *C. trachomatis* antigens). Although the immunological response can be readily measured, less is known concerning immunity in this disease. Reinfection has not been reported, but chronic disease can occur. Cellular immunity is poorly studied in this infection, but skin-test reactivity and the prominent tissue damage in lymph nodes suggest that such immunity is operative.

7.4. Psittacosis

The respiratory tract is the organ of entry and initial multiplication. The incubation period is between 6 and 15 days (rarely longer). In the experimental monkey, initial respiratory infection is followed by regional lymphadenopathy (tracheobronchial lymph nodes). Bacteremia occurs, followed by involvement of the reticuloendothelial system with early hepatic infection and persistent splenic infection.

Monocytic and polymorphonuclear infiltration of the tracheal wall marks the initial respiratory lesions, but in human specimens from fatal cases, bronchiolar involvement is not found. The characteristic lesion of psittacosis is a serofibrinous alveolar exudate that results in focal or lobar consolidation. The alveoli contain both fibrinous red cells and polymorphonuclear cells. In later stages, alveolar septal-cell hyperplasia with phagocytic infiltration occurs.

The splenomegaly results from lymphoid infiltration with an increase in mononuclear phagocytic cells. Focal necrosis and granulomata may occur in the liver. CNS involvement occurs infrequently and is characterized by congestion and edema of the brain or spinal cord.

Host response to *C. psittacii* infection can be measured in a number of ways, and it is clear that both circulating and cellular immune responses occur. On the other hand, there is no evidence for lasting immunity in either animal or man following this infection. Reinfection is well documented, as is persistent infection under some circumstances.

7.5. *C. pneumoniae* Infections

The pathogenesis of *C. pneumoniae* infections is not understood. There have been no lung biopsies, deaths, and there is no experimental model. Our knowledge is limited to clinical observation and the analogy to *M. pneumoniae* pneumonia. The incubation period for *C. pneumoniae* infection is not known, although limited observations on case-to-case interval suggest it may be as long as 3–4 weeks. Reinfection has been documented, even in the same epidemic.[43]

8. Patterns of Host Response

8.1. Trachoma

8.1.1. Clinical Features. The initial response to infection with *C. trachomatis* is a conjunctivitis. This involves both palpebral and bulbar conjunctivae, and in both areas, congestion and edema are the first responses, with papillary hypertrophy prominent in the palpebral conjunctiva. This is followed by follicle formation (except for infants less than 6 weeks of age, in whom follicle formation is not possible). Follicles can also be found on the bulbar conjunctiva. Those that form on the limbal border are most characteristic. After rupture, they leave shallow scars, which are termed Herbert's pits. In hyperendemic trachoma, severe disease is more characteristic of the upper tarsus. The conjunctivitis produces an ocular discharge that

is initially serous, but with congestion can become serosanguinous. Since trachomatous conjunctivitis is usually a subacute process, necrosis is minimal, and therefore pure trachomatous disease is not particularly purulent (with the exception of infant conjunctivitis, which has either purulent or mucopurulent discharge). Unfortunately, in hyperendemic areas, bacterial infection often accompanies the initial disease, and thus the discharge is often very purulent. In trachoma, corneal involvement is usually present, producing punctate erosions of the epithelium with cellular infiltrates of the central corneal epithelium and anterior stroma (keratitis). Particularly characteristic of hyperendemic trachoma is a neovascularization (pannus) at the superior limbus. This sign is an important component in the diagnosis of trachoma.

In either classic trachoma or adult inclusion conjunctivitis, the most damaging aspects of the disease are the sequelae of reinfection. Follicles of the palpebral conjunctiva scar, which results in distortion of the lids. This may result in trichiasis (inturning of the lashes to scrape the cornea) and entropion (distortion of the lid margins secondary to scarring, resulting in failure of the lids to close, in turn resulting in disturbance of the protective cleansing action of the lids and therefore further corneal scarring, particularly in dusty environments). These changes, along with the recurrent keratitis, in company with multiple reinfections and bacterial superinfections result in loss of visual acuity and may result in blindness.

All these change are seen, but to a lesser degree, in adult inclusion conjunctivitis. The difference in sequelae between trachoma and inclusion conjunctivitis is probably related more to the greater number of reinfections in hyperendemic trachoma and the adverse physical environment (including the effect of fly-borne bacterial conjunctivitides) than it is to the biological difference between trachomatous and oculogenital chlamydial strains. When reinfection has been studied in nontrachomatous environments (e.g., the studies of Mordhorst[50] in Denmark), each of the sequelae of trachoma has been recognized, but in lesser severity. Also, the potentiation of chlamydial conjunctivitis by bacterial superinfection has been reproduced in a cat model, utilizing a psittacine strain.[16]

8.1.2. Diagnosis. Epidemiologically, trachoma is recognized in restricted areas of the world (see Section 5.1.3) and within those areas can most often be found in populations with poor hygiene and under conditions that favor "ocular promiscuity" (often also favoring fly-borne bacterial conjunctivitis). Other isolated population segments in nonendemic countries may have endemic trachoma.

According to WHO definitions,[85] the clinical diagnosis of trachoma can be made if two of the following signs are present: (1) lymphoid follicles on the upper tarsal conjunctiva; (2) typical conjunctival scarring; (3) vascular pannus; (4) limbal follicles or their sequelae—Herbert's pits. Scales of severity and activity have been used to classify trachoma. The most commonly used staging is called the MacCallan classification, which progresses from immature follicles (I) to mature follicular disease (II), active follicles with scarring (III), and scars and other sequelae without activity (IV).

For epidemiological survey purposes, Dawson *et al.*[20] have more recently devised a scale of intensity based on three gradations of follicle activity and papillary hypertrophy. For the potentially disabling irreversible lesions, simple three-grade scores for congenital and corneal scarring and for trichiasis or enteropion or both have also been devised. This method leads to more reproducible and epidemiologically valid results in surveys.

Other syndromes can cause follicular conjunctivitis, including viral and bacterial infections, toxic follicular conjunctivitis, vernal catarrh and atopic conjunctivitis (allergic in origin), and a variety of rarer forms of chronic follicular conjunctivitis of unknown etiology.

The laboratory diagnosis of trachoma depends on the recovery of *C. trachomatis* from conjunctival scrapings or the demonstration of characteristic inclusions in the cytoplasm of conjunctival epithelial cells obtained from such scrapings. These may most easily be recognized with Giemsa stain, but if MIF methodology is available, the sensitivity of this cytological method is greater.

An advantage of the Giemsa stain in cytological diagnosis is the recognition of the characteristic inflammatory response. Whereas viral conjunctivitis usually elicits a lymphocytic response, and vernal catarrh and atopic conjunctivitis can be recognized by the presence of eosinophils or granules, the characteristic picture in trachoma or inclusion conjunctivitis is a mixture of polymorphonuclear leukocytes, immature lymphoid cells, and plasma cells. Also, Leber cells (giant macrophages containing ingested material) are often seen. This inflammatory response, while not in itself diagnostic, may aid in the cytological diagnosis of trachoma.

Although antibodies to *C. trachomatis* may invariably be recognized in the sera of trachomatous patients by MIF methods, it is unusual to detect an antibody rise, since the disease is most often recognized in its chronic state and therefore reflects only past infection with a *C. trachomatis* strain.

8.2. Oculogenital Diseases

8.2.1. Clinical Features (see Table 1)

a. Adult Inclusion Conjunctivitis. Adult inclusion conjunctivitis in both the male and the female is an acute follicular conjunctivitis with edema, mucopurulent exudate, and erythema. Inclusions can be found on scrapings of either the tarsal plate or the lower palpebral conjunctiva, and chlamydiae can be cultured from either site. Infection is thought to occur from infected genital-tract secretions via hand-to-eye contact. The illness is self-limited, although treatment will shorten the clinical course. Progression to trachoma has not been documented, but pannus and conjunctival scarring may result from reinfection.

b. Cervicitis. Chlamydial infection of the endocervix is often associated with a purulent endocervical discharge, congestion, and inflammation. The essential finding is the presence of mucopus (discoloration) on a cervical swab. Initially the criterion of ten or more polymorphonuclear leukocytes per microscopic field was also used,[8] but the difficulties of standardizing the smears made this unreproducible. A more reliable criterion, in addition to mucopurulent exudate, was bleeding induced by swabbing the endocervical mucosa (friability of the mucosa).[29] Approximately 50% of women with chlamydial cervicitis are asymptomatic, but almost 80% will have an abnormal cervical appearance. The difficulty in diagnosing chlamydial cervicitis is that the findings present are often the same as those found with cervicitis of other etiologies.[8] Furthermore, the cervix is often infected with several other organisms simultaneously (e.g., *T. vaginalis, M. hominis, U. urealyticum,* herpes simplex, *Neisseria gonorrhoeae*).

Under the proper stimulus (as yet undefined), chlamydial cervicitis may progress to salpingitis, or to postpartum endometritis in pregnant women, and it may be associated with urethral syndrome. Endometrial infection has been shown to follow cervical infection in more than one third of cases.[29] An inflammation of Bartholin's gland may also be caused by *C. trachomatis.* Hand-to-eye contact may lead to adult inclusion conjunctivitis. Without progression to other sites, chlamydial cervical infection may remain active but silent, or it may be cleared by the host either spontaneously or with treatment. Another potential diagnostic problem is differentiation from lymphocytic interstitial pneumonia (LIP) associated with human immunodeficiency virus (HIV) and Epstein–Barr virus (EBV) infections. Usually they do not occur at the same age. *C. trachomatis* pneumonia is rare after 4 months of age and LIP is rare before 6 months of age, characteristically occurring in the second year of life. Tachypnea, rather than repetitive cough, is characteristic of LIP and the radiographic pattern is more diffuse in LIP. Although both may have hyperglobulinemia, eosinophilia is not characteristic of LIP.

c. Salpingitis. Chlamydial pelvic inflammatory disease is similar in presentation to that caused by other organisms, with the exception that it tends to be of more gradual than acute onset and to exhibit low-grade fever, and often has elevation of the erythrocyte sedimentation rate ($>$ 30 mm/h). Like gonorrheal illness, it tends to occur in younger, more sexually active women, and as a first rather than recurrent episode. Major signs and symptoms include fever, lower abdominal pain, and adnexal and uterine tenderness on pelvic examination. The diagnosis of chlamydial infection has proven difficult, however, since the organism may reside solely in the salpinx. Thus, cervical or cul-de-sac cultures may yield gonorrhea or anaerobes, yielding a false diagnosis. The clearest results have been obtained in Sweden using laparoscopy with tubal biopsy, but this is neither a universally available nor an accepted technique for mild illness. If results from an animal model of salpingitis utilizing a psittacine strain are valid, it would seem that endometrial cultures most clearly reflect tubal infection.[55] The contribution of chlamydial salpingitis to involuntary infertility and to ectopic pregnancy in the United States is not known, although both have increased in parallel with increase in the incidence of salpingitis. Assuming 1 million cases of salpingitis per year in the United States and 15–20% resulting in bilateral tubal occlusion, it has been estimated that 150,000–200,000 women per year become infertile as a result of salpingitis—at least one quarter of which can be attributed to chlamydial infection.

An uncommon complication of salpingitis is perihepatitis (Fitz-Hugh–Curtis syndrome), assumed to be caused by peritoneal spread of the infection. Studies have implicated *C. trachomatis* as etiological agent in a proportion of these cases. It would appear that the complications have an important immunological component, and it is hypothesized that they occur as a result of reinfection with heterologous immunotypes.[78]

d. Female Urethral Syndrome. This syndrome is the equivalent in women of NGU in men. It is predominantly manifest as frequency dysuria, with sterile pyuria on microscopic and cultural examination, in young, sexually active women. In this specifically defined group, one study revealed a 62% (10 of 16) prevalence of *C. trachomatis* as the etiological agent.[64] Other studies show a lesser contribution.[82] Often, there is a history of a new sexual partner in the month prior to symptoms. Untreated, the urethral syndrome will resolve with time. Long-term sequelae are as yet undetermined.

e. Postpartum Endometritis. *C. trachomatis* cervical infection in pregnant women has been associated with the development of postpartum endometritis, with onset more than 48 h after delivery in approximately one third of cases.[74] The disease is not different clinically from that due to other organisms.[83]

f. Male Urethritis. Chlamydial infection of the adult male urethra is the most common single cause (60–70%) of "nongonococcal urethritis" (NGU) or "postgonococcal urethritis." This is a syndrome of dysuria with or without discharge, with pus cells on Gram smear of an endourethral swab, in which *N. gonorrhoeae* can be neither seen nor cultured. The disease occurs in young, sexually active males and is at least equal in prevalence to gonococcal urethritis in the United States. Untreated, it may lead to epididymitis or resolve spontaneously. Treatment shortens the clinical course.[33]

g. Epididymitis. *C. trachomatis* is the most common cause of "idiopathic" acute epididymitis in sexually active man under 35 years of age with no underlying genitourinary pathology.[34] The prevalence of the organism in the urethra, semen, and epididymis of these men far exceeds that of *N. gonorrhoeae*, coliforms, or *Pseudomonas* species. Patients with chlamydial epididymitis tend to have a more chronic course, with more induration of the epididymis, than those with other etiological diagnoses.

The illness will resolve spontaneously, although treatment hastens recovery. The incidence of infertility following chlamydial epididymitis is unknown. However, chlamydial epididymitis is often associated with oligozoospermia.

h. Arthritis (Reiter's Syndrome). One of the most serious complications of NGU is Reiter's syndrome. Symptoms appear 1–4 weeks after onset of urethritis. The arthritis is usually asymmetric, involving large joints of the lower extremities or sacroiliac joints. In most patients, arthritis may be the only manifestation. Achilles tendon and plantar fasciae may also be affected. This condition has been termed sexually acquired reactive arthritis (SARA). The full expression (termed Reiter's syndrome) may additionally involve eyes, skin, and mucous membranes. Ocular involvement ranges from a transient mild conjunctivitis to severe uveitis. Skin lesions may involve the penis (balanitis) and a keratoderma of the palms and soles. The mucous-membrane lesions are small ulcers of the palate, tongue, and oral mucosa. Symptoms eventually will cease, even without treatment, but recurrences are common.[41] Other infections (not sexually transmitted), such as shigella and salmonella, can also cause Reiter's syndrome.

C. trachomatis has been recovered from at least one third of cases of SARA, but serological evidence suggests that one half to two thirds are a result of this infection. Antibody responses are much higher than are usually seen in NGU, suggesting that a brisk immunological response is a part of the condition. A genetic predisposition to the development of SARA is marked by the presence of histocompatibility determinant HLA-B27 in two thirds of cases. Additional evidence for *Chlamydia* etiology comes from examining synovium or synovial fluid cells with fluorescein-labeled monoclonal antibody to *C. trachomatis*. Two thirds of patients examined with SARA showed such antigen along with high titers of serum antibody, suggesting that SARA results directly from the presence of *Chlamydia* elementary bodies in the joint.[42,69]

i. Infant Inclusion Conjunctivitis. Inclusion conjunctivitis of the newborn is by far the most common cause of neonatal conjunctivitis in the United States and is estimated to be ten times as prevalent as gonococcal ophthalmia neonatorum. Approximately 25% of infants born to cervix-positive mothers will develop some degree of chlamydial conjunctivitis, involving one or both eyes. The illness most commonly has an incubation period of 1–3 weeks. Infants then present with varying degrees of conjunctival erythema, edema, and mucopurulent discharge. Physical examination shows a *nonfollicular* conjunctivitis (as distinct from the conjunctival disease of older children and adults) with diffuse erythema of the conjunctivae. Fever and systemic findings are absent. Untreated, the disease course is quite variable. Generally, the conjunctivitis remits within 3–4 weeks, although asymptomatic shedding may persist indefinitely. Occasionally, reexacerbations may occur for unknown reasons. Chronic sequelae do occur; in one study, micropannus was observed in a small percentage of infants 1 year following infection.

j. Infant Pneumonia. *C. trachomatis* pulmonary infection has been estimated to cause 20–30% of all hospitalized pneumonia in infants less than 6 months old.[36] Approximately 10% of infants born to cervix-positive mothers will develop pulmonary disease. These infants typically present between 3 and 12 weeks of age, although younger patients have been seen. They have a history of chronic congestion and of a chronic staccato, machine-gun-like cough.[6] They are usually afebrile, with minimal malaise, but may have a history of poor growth and weight gain. On examination, they tend to be congested and tachypneic and to have diffuse rales on physical examination. Conjunctivitis is sometimes present. Laboratory examination characteristically reveals eosinophilia ($> 300–400/mm^3$), hyperglobulinemia (especially IgM), and elevated anti-chlamydial antibody titers. Chest radiographs show hyperexpanded lungs with variable degrees and patterns of infiltrates. The organism itself may be cultured from nasopharynx, tracheal aspirate material, or lung biopsy, if obtained. Although pneumonia is best studied, other forms of lower-respiratory-tract disease can occur (e.g., bronchiolitis).

Untreated, the illness tends to be chronic, with multiple exacerbations and remissions, but with gradual recovery over weeks to months. Although placebo-controlled therapy trials have not been performed, appropriate antibiotic therapy does eliminate shedding of the organism and probably shortens the course of the illness.

8.2.2. Diagnosis. The major epidemiological features of chlamydial genital diseases are that they occur in predominantly younger, more sexually active adults who are more often single, of lower socioeconomic status, and more often nonwhite. This is the pattern expected in a sexually transmitted disease. Infant disease may be expected in a proportion of those born to infected women.

In all of the syndromes listed below, antigen detection by DFA or EIA may be substituted for culture as long as one is not dealing with a low-risk group, when predictive power of the test becomes a problem.

a. Adult Inclusion Conjunctivitis. The diagnosis is suspect if a follicular conjunctivitis is present. Wright- or Giemsa-stained conjunctival scrapings will reveal inclusion-containing epithelial cells if done carefully and examined in an experienced laboratory. Chlamydial culture is the diagnostic procedure of choice. Similar diseases are caused by bacteria (including *Neisseria meningitidis* and *N. gonorrhoeae*) and viruses (especially adenovirus). Bacterial conjunctivitis is usually purulent, without follicles.

b. Cervicitis. Clinical features include mucopurulent discharge, ectopy (redness), with edema, friability, and congestion. Laboratory diagnosis is difficult, at best, since a positive chlamydial endocervical swab or paired serological fourfold titer change is required. Wright- or Giemsa-stained cervical scrapings examined for inclusions are not generally helpful. Other organisms associated with a similar picture include *N. gonorrhoeae*, *M. hominis*, herpes simplex, and possibly *T. vaginalis* and *U. urealyticum*. The presence of mucopurulent exudate is most frequently associated with chlamydial or gonococcal infection.

c. Salpingitis. Epidemiological and clinical features are discussed in Section 8.2.1c. Laboratory diagnosis is most definitively made with tubal culture of biopsy under laparoscopy. Endometrial culture has the best correlation with tubal infection. Other sites in which chlamydiae may be cultured with less reliability include cervix and pelvic cul-de-sac. Serologically, a fourfold or greater rise in anti-chlamydial antibody is usually demonstrable.

Other agents associated with salpingitis include *N. gonorrhoeae*, gram-negative enteric organisms such as *Escherichia coli*, and anaerobic flora.

d. Female Urethral Syndrome. Diagnosis of chlamydial etiology is, first, by exclusion of other bacterial etiology on urine and urethral culture and, second, by the culturing of *C. trachomatis* from the urethra or cervix. Other etiological agents include coliforms, staphylococci, and possibly ureaplasmas.

e. Postpartum Endometritis. Information on this syndrome is still limited. However, diagnosis may be established by obtaining *C. trachomatis* from endometrial curetting, aspirates, or swabs. The diagnosis is suspect if *C. trachomatis* is obtained on cervical culture. A serological change also occurs in this infection. Endometritis is also caused by *N. gonorrhoeae*, coliforms, and anaerobes.

f. Male Urethritis. Diagnosis is similar to that of urethral syndrome, except that in this case gonococcal infection must be ruled out. The other known cause of NGU is *U. urealyticum.* In 20–30% of cases, no agent is isolated or serological conversion demonstrated.

g. Epididymitis. Diagnosis is made by exclusion of bacterial agents in urine, urethra, or epididymis (coliforms, *Pseudomonas, N. gonorrhoeae*) and by culture of *C. trachomatis* from urethra or epididymal aspirate, or both, or demonstration of seroconversion.

h. Arthritis (Reiter's Syndrome). In either SARA or Reiter's syndrome, the diagnosis is made by recovery of *C. trachomatis* from the urethra of a clinically compatible case or the demonstration of a fourfold rise in specific antibody, or both. Alternatively, the presence of IgM *C. trachomatis* antibody, or the presence of high titers of IgG antibody, is presumptive evidence of chlamydial involvement. Antigen detection in synovial biopsy or synovial fluid is a recently developed method.[69]

i. Infant Inclusion Conjunctivitis. Conjunctival scraping (stained by Giemsa or FA methods) or culture for *C. trachomatis* are the procedures of choice. Gonococcal ophthalmia neonatorum and other bacterial agents may be excluded by culture and Gram smear. Chemical conjunctivitis (silver nitrate) rarely presents as late as chlamydial disease.

j. Infant Pneumonia. Diagnosis of chlamydial disease is made with a compatible clinical history and physical examination, eosinophilia, hyperinflation, and hyperglobulinemia, coupled with a positive tracheal aspirate, nasopharyngeal, or lung biopsy culture. Serological diagnosis using paired sera may be accomplished retrospectively in patients on antibiotics who are culture-negative.

Since this disease occurs early in infancy, active infection may be suspected with a high titer of specific IgG antibody (particularly if it is simultaneously compared with maternal titer) or by a high titer of specific IgM antibody (> 1:32 by MIF).

Agents that cause similar pictures are *Bordetella pertussis* and *B. parapertussis*, cytomegalovirus, respiratory syncytial virus, and adenovirus. Recent evidence has also suggested *Pneumocystis carinii* as an etiological agent.

8.3. Lymphogranuloma Venereum

8.3.1. Clinical Features. The primary lesion of LGV may develop on the penis, labia, vagina, or cervix, or within the urethra, anus, or rectum, often resulting in proctitis. Rarely, it may be extragenital (e.g., fingers or tongue). Since it is usually painless and may be papular, ulcerative, or bullous, it rarely will cause the patient to seek medical attention, and is usually not recognized historically. The secondary lesion of LGV consists of lymphadenopathy, which may follow the primary lesion in 1–6 weeks. With genital involvement, either inguinal or femoral lymph-node chains may be involved, starting with a single node, but progressing to involve the whole chain. Abscesses form within the nodes, which expand to necrotic foci that may become fluctuant, spontaneously rupture, and leave chronic draining fistulas. These necrotic abscessed nodes are the buboes that characterize this disease—and are most commonly the initial recognition of it. The fact that a far greater number of males than females are recognized to have buboes (up to tenfold in some reports) probably reflects the anatomical differences in lymphatic drainage from the various sites. The vaginal and cervical infections often drain to retroperitoneal chains, as do the anorectal primaries, which may produce manifestations more often confused with appendicitis or inguinal hernia. In the bubo stage, fever, myalgia, and headache may reflect systemic response to the lymphatic infection, and leukocytosis may result. Buboes may spontaneously subside and should not be surgically incised or drained, but may be aspirated. Rarely, chronic lymphadenopathy may result from this disease. The tertiary stage of disease consists of chronic inflammation and scarring, which may result in stricture and fistulas. These changes may follow acute LGV by 5–10 years. Urethral strictures may occur, as may penile fistulas. Anal strictures and rectovaginal fistulas are more often the sequelae in females (perhaps because of the more silent involvement of retroperitoneal lymph nodes). The current increase in the incidence of anorectal LGV in male homosexuals in the United States may be expected to result in increased recognition of resultant anal strictures due to tertiary LGV in the future.

Much rarer clinical manifestations reflect unusual extragenital sites of primary infection, such as axillary buboes with finger sites or submaxillary buboes for oral lesions. Other rare reported manifestations of LGV include meningitis, arthritis, pneumonitis, and conjunctivitis.

8.3.2. Diagnosis. Epidemiologically, LGV is found in sexually active persons, particularly those with past histories of other STDs. At one time, it was prevalent in blacks in the southern United States, but this is probably no longer true. Since the disease is more prevalent in African and Southeast Asian countries, another epidemiological feature of the occurrence in the United States has been overseas contact, such as is found in port cities or in returning military personnel who have served in these areas. In recent years, however, the disease has been found more frequently in the more sexually active male homosexual population in the United States. This segment probably represents the most frequent source of infection in the United States today.

Clinically, the primary lesion rarely comes to medical attention, and the most commonly recognized stage is that of the bubo. They are most often recognized in males, and then by inguinal or femoral node-chain involvement. If both chains are involved, the "groove sign" is seen, the groove being formed between enlarged nodes of both chains. Although highly characteristic of this disease, it is seen in only 15–20% of cases.

The differential diagnosis of LGV includes syphilis (although characteristically the nodes are hard and separate in that disease), granuloma inguinale, and chancroid. Other causes of lymphadenopathy such as various viral infections or cat-scratch disease can often be differentiated by the discrete and often tender adenopathy they produce and more usually involvement of other chains of nodes. Herpes genitalis may present with lymphadenopathy. Bacterial lymphadenitis may mimic LGV, but sites of invasion should be recognized, and, of course, in these instances, bacteria will be recognized in node aspirates. Lymphoma and leukemia are also a part of the differential diagnosis.

The laboratory diagnosis is most definitively made by tissue culture of bubo aspirate. However, if the node is necrotic enough to rupture spontaneously, it may be too late to recover active organisms. (In the past, yolk-sac culture or mouse inoculation was used for diagnosis, but tissue-culture methods are more sensitive.)

The Frei antigen—a skin test made of a partially purified elementary body suspension of yolk-sac-grown LGV—was used widely for diagnosis and is still available in the United States today. However, cell-culture isolation and serological methods have supplanted the Frei test. The poor sensitivity and specificity and the delay in development of the latter test have made it obsolete.

As with other chlamydial infections, the definitive serological method is the MIF method. However, in the case of LGV, as with psittacosis, CF antibodies usually result from infection within a few weeks of the initial infection and characteristically result in high titers ($> 1:64$). The CF test is group-specific and may be performed with either LGV or psittacosis yolk-sac- or cell-culture-prepared antigens. Although cross-reactions with the oculogenital trachoma strains would be expected, the general insensitivity of the CF test results in few patients with the oculogenital syndromes who have detectable CF antibody, and then usually at low titer.

8.4. Psittacosis

8.4.1. Clinical Features. The most common human manifestation of infection is an atypical pneumonia. It may be a relatively mild systemic disease (like mycoplasmal pneumonia) or a more severe one (like influenza). An alternative presentation is an acute septic-like illness with fever and chills and little pneumonitis. Liver and spleen enlargement may occur (particularly in the latter toxic form). Without treatment, fever may extend into the 2nd week, and before chemotherapy, the case-fatality rate averaged 20%, being higher in those 50 years of age and older. With apparent recovery, relapse may later occur—sometimes a matter of years following the original infection. In the 1136 cases reported in the United States in 1975–1984, pneumonia occurred in 54%.[12] Other common symptoms are headache, weakness, and myalgia. Rarely, manifestations such as arthralgia, meningiomas, abdominal pain, photophobia, pleuritis, or pericarditis may result.

8.4.2. Diagnosis. Serological diagnosis is most often employed. The CF test (insensitive for trachoma or oculogenital disease) is sensitive enough for this disease. The usual criterion is a fourfold increase in titer from acute to convalescent sera, but single titers above 1:64 are highly suggestive. *C. psittacii* can be isolated in yolk sac in embryonated eggs, in mice, or in tissue-culture systems. The best source for isolation is sputum or bronchial aspirate. Whole blood (heparinized or citrated), serum, or plasma may occasionally yield the agent. Isolation is more common in the 2nd week of disease.

8.5. *C. pneumoniae* Infections

8.5.1. Clinical Features. The limited observations to date suggest that *C. pneumoniae* organisms cause a range of respiratory disease from pharyngitis and otitis media through bronchitis to pneumonia.[25] Illness is more frequent in school-aged children and young adults. It is also apparent that the majority of infections are of low-grade manifestation or are asymptomatic. There appears to be some tendency for more severe manifestations to be seen in the adolescent or young adult. In general, the disease is mild and no fatalities have been recorded. Onset of illness is gradual and symptoms are often extended over a number of weeks. In all these characteristics, *C. pneumoniae* disease is very similar to *M. pneumoniae* disease.

These initial observations came from prospective observational studies in college students and in a health cooperative in Seattle,[25] and from a series of epidemics described in Finland.[43] Pharyngitis (often with laryngitis) appears to precede lower-respiratory-tract disease in most cases, often by a week or more. Pneumonia and bronchitis are often prolonged in course and relapses are common, even when treated with an antibiotic. Lung lesions are more often unilobular and are often circumscribed lesions, although bilateral interstitial infiltrates may occur. Rarely, pleural effusions and atelectasis have occurred.

The antibiotics of choice are tetracycline or erythromycin. Tetracycline is contraindicated in children (under age 10) and pregnant women. The response to antibiotic is not dramatic and no controlled clinical trials have been reported.

8.5.2. Diagnosis. The organisms may be recovered from respiratory secretions but recovery by culture is poor.[25] Often, when inclusions are seen in tissue culture, they grow poorly in serial passage. Some isolates have grown only in the yolk sac of embryonated eggs. A second method of identification has been by antigen recognition in respiratory secretions. Elementary bodies can be seen in cytological smears of respiratory secretions when stained by fluorescein-conjugated monoclonal antibodies to TWAR species. Specific conjugates are not commercially available but the range of DFA kits for chlamydia that are available contain both genus-specific and *C. trachomatis* specific kits. By demonstration of antigen with genus-specific and its absence in *C. trachomatis*-specific, one can infer the presence of TWAR antigen. Specific diagnostic reagents should be available soon.

Circulating antibodies in serum can be found in all cases of *C. pneumoniae* disease. Two patterns of response have been described using MIF as the measure.[80] The first is one of slow development of IgG and IgM antibody over 1–2 months, with subsequent loss of IgM antibody. This would appear to be a primary type of response. The second response is one of rapid IgG response in the absence of any IgM response and is more often noted in older individuals. This is more characteristic of a secondary or reinfection response.

When CF antibodies are measured on the same serum sets, a CF response is noted in two thirds of patients in whom an MIF response can be measured for the first pattern ("primary response"). No CF antibody is measured in sera for the second pattern (reinfection pattern). Thus, CF antibodies may be useful in screening for primary infection but will not be useful for reinfection disease or for seroepidemiological studies. Serological studies show *C. pneumoniae* antibody prevalence rising steeply between ages 5 and 20 and then reaching a plateau of about 40% in adult years, reflecting a rather prevalent infection.

9. Control and Prevention

9.1. Trachoma

9.1.1. General Concepts. Eradication of trachoma has occurred in large segments of the world, not as a result of specific control programs, but following the changes in life-style that accompany a raised standard of living. However, in those areas of the world where trachoma remains hyperendemic, such changes are not likely to occur, and in fact, impairment of visual acuity due to trachoma may further delay such development. Therefore, much national and international effort has been expended (with significant contributions from the WHO) on trachoma control programs. In the last few decades, trachoma control programs have been based almost entirely on the mass application of locally applied antibiotics. The results have been far from encouraging. After initial response, trachoma returns to become endemic again. Dawson *et al.*[20] have reviewed this subject and suggested that efforts be modified and that programs should be expanded to include the following elements:

1. Assessment of the problem and of the effect of intervention
2. Allocation of resources
3. Chemotherapeutic intervention
4. Surgical intervention to correct lid deformation
5. Training and utilization of local health aides and other nonspecialized health workers
6. Health education and community participation

With regard to treatment, satisfactory practical methods have still not been developed.[17] Topical tetracyclines are effective, but too often, following intensive large-scale chemotherapy, there is failure to follow this by intermittent family-based topical treatment, which depends on easy local availability of inexpensive topical preparations and on vigorous health education by local health workers. Such workers should not only ensure adequate family antibiotic treatment but also actively educate the family regarding the importance of water for hand-washing, reduction of crowding, identification and control of breeding sites of eye-seeking flies, and improvement of personal hygiene.

9.1.2. Antibiotic and Chemotherapeutic Approaches. Community-based antibiotic treatment programs are in a sense, prophylaxis of reinfection, which is the damaging aspect of trachoma. As stated above, the change in emphasis on use of antibiotics is not one of change of treatment modality, but the community application. As is being learned in many public-health programs, lasting effects cannot be produced by large, centrally directed mass programs. Success has been achieved in those countries where trachoma control becomes an ongoing part of the broad community-based public-health program.[72]

Choice of antibiotic depends on availability, price, and ease of administration. With the exception of rifampin, no significant antibiotic resistance has developed to *C. trachomatis*. Thus, the choices lie with sulfonamides, tetracyclines, erythromycin, and certain other macrolides. Strategies of treatment and control of trachoma have been studied with regard to cost-effectiveness.[59] In areas of high endemicity, mass therapy with ocular antibiotics must be the first resort. When oral antibiotics (tetracycline or doxycycline) are administered as a supplement, the healing rates improve. The use of oral antibiotics can be shown to be a cost-effective strategy, particularly in communities where fewer than 20% of children have active trachoma.[72] Oral administration is theoretically preferable, but topical eye ointments or suspensions have been more practical.

9.1.3. Immunization. Soon after *C. trachomatis* was first recovered in eggs, laboratories in London, Boston, and Taipei (later Seattle) began developing vaccines for trachoma.[22] Even though reinfection can readily occur in humans following prior trachoma, it was found in monkey models that hyperimmunization with vaccine could prevent reinfection, at least under the somewhat artificial environment of an animal trial. In one instance, a similar result was obtained in blind volunteers. However, each of the candidate vaccines was made with relatively crude whole-organism preparations, and all of them gave only fleeting protection. Even more discouraging was the finding that both in

animal experiments and in human trials, subsequent rechallenge might result in more severe disease than occurred in rechallenge after natural infection (a phenomenon that has also been seen in other experimental vaccines of low antigenic potency). At that point, all vaccine trials were abandoned, pending further study of the molecular biology of the organism, with the hope of discovering antigenic subunits that might result in a more permanent immunity. Such efforts are about to move from the laboratory bench to animal testing.

9.2. Oculogenital Diseases

9.2.1. General Concepts. Since these are STDs, control measures are similar to those for gonorrhea and syphilis. *C. trachomatis* should be sought by culture or antigen detection methods in persons with STD complaints or history. Current recommendations include treatment of all persons with urethritis (gonococcal or nongonococcal), mucopurulent cervicitis, pelvic inflammatory disease, and epididymitis in men under age 35 as if they had both gonococcal and chlamydial infection.[14] They should be treated with a penicillin-like antibiotic (or alternative where penicillin-resistant strains exceed 3%) and a tetracycline antibiotic (or erythromycin in pregnant women). Other individuals recommended for *C. trachomatis* treatment are asymptomatic contacts to patients with the four syndromes mentioned above and others with established gonococcal or chlamydial infections. Similarly, sexual partners of persons with gonococcal infection should be treated. All of these could be treated without a positive laboratory test if diagnostic laboratory sources are limited. Then diagnostic screening can be saved for highest risk groups. These would be central city women who are sexually active and who are below age 25, particularly adolescents. Of particular concern are those with a history of prior STD. When possible, contact tracing should be pursued. Both cases and contacts should be treated concurrently and should avoid intercourse (or use condoms) during treatment. In pregnant women, culture and treatment is indicated to protect against postpartum maternal and neonatal consequences.

9.2.2. Prophylaxis. In infected males and nonpregnant females, treatment with tetracyclines, erythromycin, or sulfonamides eliminates infection and therefore provides prophylaxis against the complications of that infection.[14]

Treatment of women during pregnancy or immediately postdelivery will eliminate infection and may protect against postpartum fever and endometritis. Furthermore, for the treatment to be effective during pregnancy, the sexual partner must be treated simultaneously to prevent reinfection. Tetracyclines and sulfonamides are contraindicated during pregnancy; erythromycin remains the only safe and effective drug. If further study elucidates prenatal fetal or maternal complications of infection, or both, routine first-trimester cervical culture and treatment of positive women and partners may be a theoretically useful prophylactic procedure.

For infants, effective prevention of chlamydial disease occurs by treating mothers and partners prior to delivery. Since silver nitrate prophylaxis is ineffective against chlamydiae, topical erythromycin or tetracycline eye prophylaxis at birth for the prevention of inclusion conjunctivitis should be considered. Preliminary results suggest that prenatal treatment prevents inclusion conjunctivitis and infant pneumonia and that neonatal eye prophylaxis with erythromycin or tetracycline prevents inclusion conjunctivitis to some extent but not pneumonia.[28]

Antibiotic resistance of *C. trachomatis* has not been and is not currently a clinical problem.

9.2.3. Immunization. No immunization for oculogenital diseases is available.

9.3. Lymphogranuloma Venereum

9.3.1. General Concepts. Prevention of LGV depends on the recognition and treatment of infected persons. Problems exist in both these aims. Although classic cases of LGV are easily recognized, relapse of old disease may occur, particularly in debilitated persons. Furthermore, the occurrence of relatively silent disease in anogenital carriers, particularly in sexually active homosexuals, and the difficulty in availability of simple diagnostic tests result in rather persistent endemic foci. For LGV, unique among other chlamydial diseases, a specific highly effective method of chemotherapy is also lacking. Sulfonamides were classically used, but more commonly today, tetracycline therapy is preferred. The major difficulty is in assessing the effect of therapy, particularly in treatment of the embryonic or tertiary stage.

9.3.2. Prophylaxis and Immunization. No prophylaxis or immunization for LGV is available.

9.4. Psittacosis

9.4.1. General Concepts. Control of psittacosis depends on control of avian sources of infection. Control of the 1929 pandemic of psittacosis was accomplished by bans on the importation of psittacine birds. This was followed by a method of certification of clean flocks, but many of these

efforts were damaged by poor supervision, smuggling, and contamination of susceptible birds from clean flocks during shipment. An effective method for controlling psittacosis in parakeets has been developed—a chlortetracycline-impregnated seed. Current requirements for quarantine of imported birds are for 30 days of treatment. This is probably not enough, and it has been proposed that this be extended to 45 days. It is probable that some birds have suppressed infections that reactivate during shipment following quarantine. The remaining problems are ones of assuring more adequate response to control regulations.

The control of occupational disease in the poultry-processing industry appears to have been successful in recent years, although there is no developed public-health program. The epidemics in 1974 served to alert the industry to the problem, and the infection in poultry flocks tends to be rapidly recognized and treated. It is also probable that human disease continues to occur, but is quickly recognized, treated, and not reported in these workers.

9.4.2. Prophylaxis and Immunization. There is no prophylaxis in humans, and although experimental psittacosis vaccines have been developed in birds, they are not cheap enough to replace antibiotic treatment of birds. There is no need to develop human vaccine for such an infrequent disease.

10. Unresolved Problems

10.1. Trachoma

For trachoma, there is no problem of diagnosis, since clinical recognition is relatively simple. The formidable problem is the development of a simple, safe, and easily applied (once daily) chemotherapeutic agent and a public-health structure that will assure its application. A vaccine would be far more useful, but development of one depends on a greatly expanded understanding of the immunology and molecular biology of this agent.

10.2. Oculogenital Diseases

10.2.1. Epidemiology and Disease Spectrum. There have been no significant additions to our knowledge of the disease spectrum in the last 5 years. Syndromes such as otitis media, prostatitis, diarrhea, or pharyngitis have not been shown to be caused by *C. trachomatis*. Reports that claimed to find a significant contribution of chlamydia to pharyngitis were based on serological evidence. It is now clear[59] that this phenomenon and the unexplained increment of antibody in early childhood were both a function of cross-reacting antibody to TWAR organisms.

10.2.2. Diagnostic Tests. Chlamydial culture and serological techniques are time-consuming and expensive; they are not easily usable as screening techniques. Large-scale diagnosis and treatment of *C. trachomatis* infections as a public-health risk of the magnitude of gonorrhea will require either huge amounts of monetary investment or development of cheaper and more rapid diagnostic techniques.

10.2.3. Host Response. Data from individuals with asymptomatic infection have shown that infection may persist in the presence of both serum and local antibody. The contribution of other arms of the immune response to clearance of infection is very largely unknown.

10.2.4. Control. Control of oculogenital infections due to *C. trachomatis* constitutes a large-scale public-health problem. As has been discussed in other sections, true control of these infections will require definition of all the illnesses caused by *C. trachomatis,* and all modes of transmission of infection, coupled with the development of rapid and easily applicable diagnostic techniques.

10.3. Lymphogranuloma Venereum

The outstanding problem in this case, as with the oculogenital syndromes, is the development of a rapid, inexpensive diagnostic method. In this instance, further study of optimal chemotherapy is also needed.

10.4. Psittacosis

In this instance, it would seem that the basic tools are at hand. A vaccine for birds or a more effective antibiotic feed method that would assure eradication of avian infection in less than 30 days would assure better cooperation by the industry.

10.5. *C. pneumoniae* Infections

There are many research needs for this newly discovered agent. Culture and serological methods need to be further adapted for this organism. Basic epidemiological and natural history studies are needed. Although serological studies indicate a ubiquitous agent, there appear to be periods of occurrence and absence in given locations. The transmission of the organism, its infectivity and incubation period need to be defined. Methods of treatment, control, and prevention require extensive research.

11. References

1. ALEXANDER, E. R., Chlamydia: The organism and neonatal infection, *Hosp. Pract.* **14:**63–69 (1979).
2. ALEXANDER, E. R., WANG, S.-P., AND GRAYSTON, J. T., Further classification of TRIC agents from ocular trachoma and other sources by the mouse toxicity prevention tests, *Am. J. Ophthmal.* **63:**1469–1478 (1967).
3. BECKER, Y., The Chlamydia: Molecular biology of procaryotic obligate parasites of eucaryocytes, *Microbiol. Rev.* **42:**274–306 (1978).
4. BEDSON, S. P., The use of the complement-fixation reaction in the diagnosis of human psittacosis, *Lancet* **2:**1277–1280 (1935).
5. BEDSON, S. P., The psittacosis–lymphogranuloma group of viruses, *Br. Med. Bull.* **9:**226–227 (1953).
6. BEEM, M. O., AND SAXON, E. M., Respiratory-tract colonization and a distinctive pneumonia syndrome in infants infected with *Chlamydia trachomatis. N. Engl. J. Med.* **296:**306–310 (1977).
7. BERMAN, S., HARRISON, H. R., BOYCE, W. T., HAFFNER, J. J., LEWIS, M., AND ARTHUR, J. B., Low birth weight, prematurity and post partum endometritis: Association with prenatal cervical *Mycoplasma hominis* and *Chlamydia trachomatis* infections, *J. Am. Med. Assoc.* **257:**1189–1194 (1987).
8. BRUNHAM, R. C., PAAVONEN, J., STEVENS, C. E., KIVIAT, N., KUO, C. C., CRITCHLOW, C. W., AND HOLMES, K. K., Mucopurulent cervicitis: The ignored counterpart in women of urethritis in men, *N. Engl. J. Med.* **311:**1–6 (1984).
9. CALDWELL, H. D., AND KUO, C. C., Serologic diagnosis of lymphogranuloma venereum by counterimmunoelectrophoresis with a *Chlamydia trachomatis* protein antigen, *J. Immunol.* **118:**442–446 (1977).
10. CAMPBELL, L. A., KUO, C. C., AND GRAYSTON, J. T., Characterization of the new chlamydia agent TWAR as a unique organism by restriction endonuclease analysis and by DNA–DNA hybridization, *J. Clin. Microbiol.* **25:**1911–1916 (1987).
11. Centers for Disease Control, *Morbidity and Mortality Weekly Report Summary of Notifiable Disease: United States 1985,* **34:**3–4 (1987).
12. Centers for Disease Control, *Psittacosis Surveillance, Summary (1975–84),* 1987.
13. Centers for Disease Control, *Sexually Transmitted Disease Statistics 1987,* Issue No. 136, 1988.
14. Centers for Disease Control, *Chlamydia trachomatis* infections. Policy guidelines for prevention and control, *Morbid. Mortal. Weekly Rep.* (Suppl.) **34:**53S–74S (1988).
15. COLLIER, L. H., AND SOWA, JR., Isolation of trachoma virus in embryonated eggs, *Lancet* **1:**993–994 (1958).
16. DAROUGAR, S., MANNICKENDAM, M. A., EL-SHIEKH, H., TREHARNE, J. D., WOODLAND, R. M., AND JONES, B. R., Animal models for the study of chlamydial infections of the

eye and genital tract, in: *Nongonococcal Urethritis and Related Infections* (D. HOBSON AND K. K. HOLMES, eds.), pp. 186–198, American Society for Microbiology, Washington, D.C., 1977.

17. DAWSON, C., Therapy of diseases caused by Chlamydia organisms: *Int. Ophthalmol. Clin.* **13:**93–101 (1972).

18. DAWSON, C. R., AND SCHACHTER, J., Strategies for treatment and control of blinding trachoma: Cost effectiveness of topical systemic antibiotic, *Rev. Infect. Dis.* **7:**768–773 (1985).

19. DAWSON, C. R., HANNA, L., AND JAWETZ, E., Controlled treatment trials of trachoma in American Indian children, *Lancet* **2:**961–963 (1967).

20. DAWSON, C. R., JONES, B. R., AND TARIZZO, M. L., Trachoma control: Programmes for the prevention of blindness, Presented at the National Society for Prevention of Blindness, Committee on Ophthalmia Neonatorum, San Francisco, 1980.

21. FINN, M. P., OHLIN, A., AND SCHACTER, J., Enzyme-linked immunosorbent assay for immunoglobulin G and M antibodies to *Chlamydia trachomatis* in human sera, *J. Clin. Microbiol.* **17:**848–852 (1983).

22. GORDON, F. B., HARPER, I. A., GUAN, A. L., TREHARNE, J. D., DWYER, R. SR. C., AND GARLAND, J. A., Detection of Chlamydia (Bedsonia) in certain infections of man. I. Laboratory procedures: Comparison of yolk sac and cell culture for detection and isolation, *J. Infect. Dis.* **120:**451–462 (1969).

23. GRAYSTON, J. T., AND WANG, S.-P., New knowledge of chlamydiae and the diseases they cause, *J. Infect. Dis.* **132:**87–105 (1975).

24. GRAYSTON, J. T., AND WANG, S.-P., The potential for vaccine against infection of the genital tract with *Chlamydia trachomatis, J. Am. Vener. Dis. Assoc.* **5:**78–79 (1978).

25. GRAYSTON, J. T., KUO, C. C., WANG, S. P., AND ALTMAN, J., A new *Chlamydia psittacii* strain called TWAR from acute respiratory tract infections, *N. Engl. J. Med.* **315:**161–168 (1986).

26. GRAYSTON, J. T., KUO, C. C., CAMPBELL, L. A., AND WANG, S. P., *Chlamydia pneumoniae* sp nov for chlamydia strain TWAR, *Int. J. Syst. Bacteriol.* (Jan. 1989).

27. HALBERSTAEDTER, L., AND VON PROWAZEK, S., Uber Zelleinschliesse parasitarer Natur beim Trachom, *Arb. Kais. Gesund.* **26:**44–47 (1907).

28. HAMMERSCHLAG, M. R., CHANDLER, J. W., ALEXANDER, E. R., ENGLISH, M., CHIANG, W.-T., KOUTSKY, L., ESCHENBACH, D. A., AND SMITH, J. R., Erythromycin ointment for ocular prophylaxis of neonatal chlamydial infection, *J. Am. Med. Assoc.* **244:**2291–2293 (1980).

29. HANDSFIELD, H. H., JASMAN, L. L., ROBERTS, P. L., HANSON, V. W., KOTHENBENTEL, R. C., AND STAMM, W. E., Criteria for selective screening for *Chlamydia trachomatis* infection in women attending family planning clinics, *J. Am. Med. Assoc.* **255:**1730–1734 (1986).

30. HARRISON, H. R., ENGLISH, M. G., LEE, C. K., AND ALEXANDER, E. R., *Chlamydia trachomatis* infant pneumonitis. Comparison with matched controls and other infant pneumonitis, *N. Engl. J. Med.* **298:**702–708 (1978).

31. HIPP, S. S., YANGSOOK, H., AND MURPHY, D., Assessment of enzyme immunoassay and immunofluorescence test for detection of *Chlamydia trachomatis, J. Clin. Microbiol.* **25:**1938–1943 (1987).

32. HOBSON, D., JOHNSON, F. W. A., REES, E., AND TAIT, A., Simplified method for diagnosis of genital and ocular infections with Chlamydia, *Lancet* **2:**555–557 (1974).

33. HOLMES, K. K., HANDSFIELD, H. H., WANG, S.-P., WENTWORTH, P. B., TURCK, M., ANDERSON, J. B., AND ALEXANDER, E. R., Etiology of nongonococcal urethritis, *N. Engl. J. Med.* **292:**1199–1206 (1975).

34. HOLMES, K. K., BERGER, R. E., AND ALEXANDER, E. R., Acute epididymitis: Etiology and therapy, *Arch. Androl.* **3:**309–316 (1979).

35. HUNTER, J. S., *A Treatise on the Venereal Disease*, London, 1786.

36. KOUSA, M., SAIKKU, P., RICHMOND, S., AND LASSUS, A., Frequent association of chlamydial infection with Reiter's syndrome, *Sex. Transmit. Dis.* **5:**57–61 (1978).

37. JONES, B. R., Prevention of blindness from trachoma, *Trans. Ophthalmol. Soc. U.K.* **95:**16–33 (1974).

38. JONES, B. R., COLLIER, L. H., AND SMITH, C. H., Isolation of a virus from inclusion blennorrhea, *Lancet* **1:**902–905 (1959).

39. JUERGENSEN, T., *Handbuch der Speziellen Pathologie und Therapie*, Apparate 2:3, *Handbuch der Krankheiten des Respirations*, Vogel, Leipzig, 1874.

40. JULIANELLE, L. A., *The Etiology of Trachoma*, The Commonwealth Fund, New York, 1938.

41. KEAT, A. C., THOMAS, B. J., TAYLOR-ROBINSON, D., PEGRUM, G. D., MAINI, R. N., AND SCOTT, J. T., Evidence of *Chlamydia trachomatis* infection in sexually acquired reactive arthritis, *Ann. Rheum. Dis.* **39:**431–437 (1980).

42. KEAT, A., DIXEY, J., SONNEX, C., THOMAS, B., OSBORN, M., AND TAYLOR-ROBINSON, D., *Chlamydia trachomatis* and reactive arthritis: The missing link, *Lancet* **1:**72–74 (1987).

43. KLEEMOLA, M., SAIKKU, P., VISAKORPI, R., WANG, S.-P., AND GRAYSTON, J. T., Epidemics of pneumonia caused by TWAR, a new chlamydia organism, in military trainees in Finland, *J. Infect. Dis.* **157:**230–236 (1988).

44. LINDNER, K., Zur Trachomforschung, *Z. Augenheilkd.* **22:**547–549 (1909).

45. MAHONEY, J. B., CHERNESKY, M. A., BROMBERG, K., AND SCHACTER, J., Accuracy of immunoglobulin M immunoassay for diagnosis of chlamydia infections in infants and adults, *J. Clin. Microbiol.* **24:**731–735 (1986).

46. MÅRDH, P.-A., An overview of infectious agents of salpingitis, their biology and recent advances in methods of detection, *Am. J. Obstet. Gynecol.* **138:**933–951 (1980).

47. MEYER, K. F., The host spectrum of psittacosis–lymphogranuloma venereum (PL) agents, *Am. J. Ophthalmol.* **63:**1225–1246 (1967).

48. MEYER, K. F., EDDIE, B., AND SCHACHTER, J., Psittacosis–lymphogranuloma venereum agents, in: *Diagnostic Procedures for Viral and Rickettsial Infections*, 4th ed. (E. H.

LENNETTE AND N. J. SCHMIDT, eds.), pp. 869–903, American Public Health Association, New York, 1969.

49. MOHANTY, K. C., O'NEILL, J. J., AND HAINBLING, M. H., Comparison of enzyme immunoassays and cell culture for detecting *Chlamydia trachomatis, Genitourin. Med.* **62:**175–176 (1986).

50. MORDHORST, C. H., WANG, S.-P., AND GRAYSTON, J. T., Childhood trachoma in a nonendemic area, *J. Am. Med. Assoc.* **239:**1765–1771 (1978).

51. MOULDER, J. W., The relation of the psittacosis group (chlamydiae) to bacteria and viruses, *Annu. Rev. Microbiol.* **20:**107–130 (1966).

52. NICHOLS, R. I., BOBB, A. A., HADDAD, A., AND McCOMB, D. E., Immunofluorescent studies of the microbiologic epidemiology of trachoma in Saudi Arabia, *Am. J. Ophthalmol.* **63:**1372–1408 (1967).

53. NICOLLE, C., CUENOD, A., AND BLAISOT, L., Étude experimentalle du trachome, *Arch. Inst. Pasteur Tunis* **3:**185–188 (1911).

54. PAAVONEN, J., KIVIAT, N., BRUNHAM, R. C., STEVENS, C. E., KUO, C. C., STAMM, W. E., MIETTINEN, A., SOULES, M., ESCHENBACH, D. A., AND HOLMES, K. K., Prevalence and manifestations of endometritis among women with cervicitis, *Am. J. Obstet. Gynecol.* **152:**280–286 (1985).

55. PATTON, D., KUO, C. C., WANG, S.-P., AND HALBERT, S. A., Distal tubal obstruction induced by repeated *Chlamydia trachomatis* salpingeal infection in pig-tailed macaques, *J. Infect. Dis.* **155:**1292–1299 (1987).

56. PHILLIPS, R. S., HAUFF, P. A., KAUFMANN, R. S., AND ARONSON, M. D., Use of a direct fluorescent antibody test for detecting *Chlamydia trachomatis* cervical infection in women seeking routine gynecologic care, *J. Infect. Dis.* **156:**575–581 (1987).

57. RAKE, G., SHAFFER, M. F., AND THYGESON, P., Relationship of agents of trachoma and inclusion conjunctivitis to those of lymphogranuloma–psittacosis group, *Proc. Soc. Exp. Biol. Med.* **99:**545–547 (1942).

58. RIPA, K. T., AND MARDH, P.-A., Cultivation of *Chlamydia trachomatis* in cyclohexamide-treated McCoy cells, *J. Clin. Microbiol.* **6:**328–330 (1977).

59. SCHACHTER, J. S., Human *Chlamydia psittacii* infection, in: *Chlamydia Infections* (D. ORIEL, G. RIDGWAY, J. S. SCHACHTER, D. TAYLOR-ROBINSON, AND M. WARD, eds.), pp. 311–320, Cambridge University Press, London, 1986.

60. SCHACHTER, J., AND DAWSON, C. R., Comparative efficacy of various diagnostic methods for chlamydial infection, in: *Nongonococcal Urethritis and Related Infections* (D. HOBSON AND K. K. HOLMES, eds.), pp. 337–341, American Society for Microbiology, Washington, D.C., 1977.

61. SCHACHTER, J., AND DAWSON, C. R., *Human Chlamydial Infections,* p. 218, PSG, Littleton, Mass., 1978.

62. SCHACHTER, J., SMITH, D. E., DAWSON, C. R., ANDERSON, W. R., DELLER, J. J., JR., HOKE, A. W., SMARTT, W. H., AND MEYER, K. F., Lymphogranuloma venereum. I. Comparison of Frei test, complement fixation test, and isolation of the agent, *J. Infect. Dis.* **120:**372–375 (1969).

63. SOMPOLINSKY, D., AND RICHMOND, S., Growth of *Chlamydia trachomatis* in McCoy cells treated with cytochalasin B, *Appl. Microbiol.* **28:**912–914 (1974).

64. STAMM, W. E., WAGER, K. F., AMSEL, R., ALEXANDER, E. R., TURCK, M., COUNTS, G. W., AND HOLMES, K. K., Causes of the acute urethral syndrome in women, *N. Engl. J. Med.* **303:**409–415 (1980).

65. STAMM, W. E., HANSEN, H. R., ALEXANDER, E. R., CLES, L. D., SPENCE, M. R., AND GUINN, T. C., Diagnosis of *Chlamydia trachomatis* infections by direct immunofluorescence staining of genital secretions: A multicenter trial, *Ann. Intern. Med.* **101:**638–641 (1984).

66. TACK, K. J., RASP, F. L., HANTO, D., PETERSON, P. K., O'LEARY, M., SIMMONS, R. L., AND SABATH, L. D., Isolation of *Chlamydia trachomatis* from the lower respiratory tract of adults, *Lancet* **2:**116 (1980).

67. TAIT, I. A., REES, E., HOBSON, D., BYNG, R. E., AND TWEEDIE, C. K., Chlamydial infection of the cervix in contacts of men with nongonococcal urethritis, *Br. J. Vener. Dis.* **56:**37–41 (1980).

68. T'ANG, F. F., CHANG, H. L., HUANG, Y. T., AND WANG, K. C., Trachoma virus in chick embryo, *Natl. Med. J. China* **43:**81–86 (1957).

69. TAYLOR-ROBINSON, D., THOMAS, B. J., DIXEY, J., OSBORNE, M. F., FURR, P. M., AND KEAT, A. C., Evidence that *Chlamydia trachomatis* causes seronegative arthritis in women, *Ann. Rheum. Dis.* **47:**295–299 (1988).

70. THYGESON, P., Trachoma virus: Historical background and review of isolates, *Ann. N.Y. Acad. Sci.* **98:**6–13 (1962).

71. THYGESON, P., AND STONE, W., JR., The epidemiology of inclusion conjunctivitis, *Arch. Ophthalmol.* **27:**91–122 (1942).

72. THYLEFORS, B., Development of trachoma control programs and the involvement of natural resources, *Rev. Infect. Dis.* **7:**774–776 (1985).

73. TREHARNE, J. D., The community epidemiology of trachoma, *Rev. Infect. Dis.* **7:**760–764 (1985).

74. WAGER, G. P., MARTIN, D. H., KOUTSKY, L., ESCHENBACH, D. A., DALING, J. R., CHIANG, W. T., ALEXANDER, E. R., AND HOLMES, K. K., Puerperal infectious morbidity: Relationship to route of delivery and to antepartum *Chlamydia trachomatis* infections, *Am. J. Obstet. Gynecol.* **138:**1028–1033 (1980).

75. WANG, S.-P., AND GRAYSTON, J. T., Immunologic relationship between genital TRIC, lymphogranuloma venereum, and related organisms in a new microtiter indirect immunofluorescence test, *Am. J. Ophthalmol.* **70:**367–374 (1970).

76. WANG, S.-P., KUO, C. C., AND GRAYSTON, J. T., A simplified method for immunological typing of trachoma–inclusion conjunctivitis–lymphogranuloma venereum organisms, *Infect. Immun.* **7:**356–360 (1973).

77. WANG, S.-P., GRAYSTON, J. T., ALEXANDER, E. R., AND HOLMES, K. K., A simplified microimmunofluorescence test with trachoma lymphogranuloma venereum (*Chlamydia tra-*

chomatis) antigens for use as a screening test for antibody, *J. Clin. Microbiol.* **1**:250–255 (1975).

78. WANG, S.-P., ESCHENBACH, D. A., HOLMES, K. K., WAGER, G., AND GRAYSTON, J. T., *Chlamydia trachomatis* infection in Fitz-Hugh–Curtis syndrome, *Am. J. Obstet. Gynecol.* **138**: 1034–1035 (1980).

79. WANG, S.-P., KUO, C. C., BARNES, R. C., STEPHENS, R. S., AND GRAYSTON, J. T., Immunotyping of *Chlamydia trachomatis* with monoclonal antibodies, *J. Infect. Dis.* **152**:791–800 (1985).

80. WANG, S.-P., AND GRAYSTON, J. T., Microimmunofluorescence serological studies with the TWAR organisms, in: *Chlamydia Infections* (D. Oriel, G. Ridgway, J. S. Schachter, D. Taylor-Robinson, and M. Ward, eds.), pp. 329–332, Cambridge University Press, London, 1986.

81. WASHINGTON, A. E., JOHNSON, R. E., SANDERS, L. L., BARNES, R. C., AND ALEXANDER, E. R., Incidence of *Chlamydia trachomatis* infections in the United States using reported *Neisseria gonorrhoeae* as a surrogate, in: *Chlamydia Infections* (D. ORIEL, G. RIDGWAY, J. S. SCHACHTER, D. TAYLOR-ROBINSON, AND M. WARD, eds.), pp. 987–990, Cambridge University Press, London, 1986.

82. WATHNE, B., HOVELIUS, B., AND MARDH, P. A., Causes of frequency and dysuria in women, *Scand. J. Infect. Dis.* **19**:223–229 (1987).

83. WATTS, D. H., AND ESCHENBACH, D. A., The role of *Chlamydia trachomatis* in post-partum endometritis, in: *Chlamydia Infections* (D. ORIEL, G. RIDGWAY, J. S. SCHACHTER, D. TAYLOR-ROBINSON, AND M. WARD, eds.), pp. 245–250, Cambridge University Press, London, 1986.

84. WENTWORTH, B. B., AND ALEXANDER, E. R., Isolation of *Chlamydia trachomatis* by use of 5-iodo-2-deoxyuridine-treated cells, *Appl. Microbiol.* **27**:912–916 (1974).

85. World Health Organization Report, Fourth W.H.O. Scientific Group on Trachoma Research, No. 330, Geneva, 1966.

86. World Health Organization, *World Health Organization Guide to Trachoma Control*, WHO, Geneva, 1981.

87. YONEDA, C., DAWSON, C. R., DAGHFOUS, T., HOSHIWARA, I., JONES, P., MESSADI, M., AND SCHACHTER, J., Cytology as a guide to the presence of chlamydial inclusions in Giemsa-stained conjunctival smears in severe endemic trachoma, *Br. J. Ophthalmol.* **59**:116–124 (1975).

12. Suggested Reading

BATTEIGER, B. E., AND JONES, R. B., Chlamydia infections, *Infect. Dis. Clin. North Am.* **1**:55–81 (1987).

HOLMES, K. K., MARDH, P. A., SPARLING, P. F., WEISNER, P. J., CATES, W., LEMON, S. M., AND STAMM, W. E., (eds.), *Sexually Transmitted Diseases*, Chapters 15–17, McGraw–Hill, New York, 1990.

SCHACHTER, J., AND CALDWELL, H. D., Chlamydiae, *Annu. Rev. Microbiol.* **34**:285–309 (1980).

SCHACHTER, J., AND DAWSON, C. R., *Human Chlamydial Infections*, PSG, Littleton, Mass., 1978.

TAYLOR-ROBINSON, D., AND THOMAS, B. J., The role of *Chlamydia trachomatis* in genital-tract and associated diseases, *J. Clin. Pathol.* **33**:205–233 (1980).

THOMPSON, S. E., AND WASHINGTON, A. E., Epidemiology of sexually transmitted *Chlamydia trachomatis* infections, *Epidemiol. Rev.* **5**:96–123 (1983).

CHAPTER 10

Cholera

Abram S. Benenson

1. Introduction

Cholera is an acute epidemic dehydrating diarrhea, usually sudden in onset and, if not properly treated, fatal in as many as half those affected. While a similar clinical entity can be caused by other agents, the term is usually reserved for all diarrheal illnesses caused by *Vibrio cholerae,* and expanded to include those with only a few loose bowel movements.

Cholera is the most dramatic of diseases. Periodically, it has spread out of its homeland in Asia as devastating pandemics with high fatality rates. A healthy individual could be dead within a few hours, so that to wish cholera on a person was a most serious curse in eastern Europe. The illness is equally dramatic in its response to treatment; literally within minutes after treatment with fluid and electrolytes is initiated, a moribund individual can become essentially well, other than a continuing diarrhea.

Governments have fallen and the political map of Europe has been shaped by outbreaks of cholera. More than any other disease, it forced the intrusion of society (government) into the privacy of one's castle to eliminate conditions presumed to cause the disease, leading ultimately to the establishment of boards of health with legal authority to limit a citizen's activities. The desire to prevent country-to-country spread led to the establishment of the International Quarantine Commission. The study of its spread laid an early foundation for development of modern methods of infectious-disease epidemiology.

Abram S. Benenson · Graduate School of Public Health, San Diego State University, San Diego, California 92182.

2. Historical Background

There is every reason to believe that cholera had existed on the Indian subcontinent for many centuries before the Europeans first arrived. At the beginning of the 16th century, the Portugese clearly described the picture of classic cholera. As India became better known to the Europeans, catastrophic outbreaks were reported, especially related to military movements and the aggregation of large numbers of pilgrims attending religious fairs. There is no evidence in any available language that the disease had spread to adjacent countries such as Burma, Ceylon, and Java.

However, on seven occasions since 1817, the classical disease poured out of Bengal, extending far beyond its normal habitat, and attacked large populations in many countries. The First Pandemic lasted from 1817 to 1823, reaching China and Japan to the east; to the west, it spread to the shores of the Mediterranean and Zanzibar on the east coast of Africa. The pandemic ended when the disease completely disappeared from any region outside India.

The Second Pandemic began in 1829. The disease spread to Persia, into Russia, Poland, Austria, Prussia, England, Ireland, and France. It came to the New World in 1832 on ships traveling to Quebec. It reached New York on June 23, 1832, Philadelphia on July 5, and spread through the rest of the country until 1835. Outbreaks of cholera occurred in Mexico, Cuba, Nicaragua, and Guatemala until 1837. The impact of the disease in Europe is evidenced by several historical episodes. In Newburn, England, on January 15, 1832, 50 people, almost one tenth of the entire population, were attacked between nightfall and noon the next day; by the end of the epidemic, which lasted 1 month, half of the population had had the disease and one in eight had died.[75,100]

In 1840, cholera was reintroduced into China by British troops transferred from India; the disease was carried westward in 1842 from China, reentering western Asia and Europe. It reentered the United States in 1848 through both New York and New Orleans, and during 1849 and 1850 rampaged through the country as what was called "America's greatest scourge."[28] In 1849, it was carried from New Orleans to Panama and then to San Francisco. By 1852, the disease had generally disappeared, but still smoldered in the region of Russia and Poland. It was in this pandemic that John Snow appreciated the relationship between water and cholera and was motivated to write his classic report, *On the Mode of Communication of Cholera*,[100] in 1849.

The Third Pandemic is stated by Pollitzer[92] to have begun in 1852, extending to Persia and Mesopotamia and to Europe. It covered northern Europe as a whole, but especially affected England, permitting Snow to complete his studies of the relationship of the disease to the water supply and describe the "most terrible outbreak of cholera which ever occurred in this kingdom," which was centered on the now-famous Broad Street pump.[100] In 1854, cholera entered the United States, and again the disease spread eastward to China and Japan. By 1859, Europe was free of the disease.

The Fourth Pandemic began in 1863 and lasted until 1873 or 1875. The disease reached southern France and Italy, coming through Arabia and Egypt. From 1865 to 1867, cholera was again prevalent in the United States, complicated by the movement of military personnel in the aftermath of the Civil War. However, the mortality rate did not reach 5% in any community in 1866; in 1833, the death of 5–15% of the population of a locality had not been unusual; in 1849, the mortality rate had seldom reached 10%; and in 1856, the rate was low compared to the earlier experiences, but 50,000 are estimated to have died in the United States.[28] Disease continued in Europe, and in 1873, New Orleans and the Mississippi Basin were once again seriously invaded. Outbreaks continued until about 1877–1879.

The Fifth Pandemic, which started in 1881, provided Robert Koch the opportunity to study the disease in Egypt and Calcutta and to identify in 1883 the pathogen that produces the disease. A steamer with infected patients arrived in New York in October 1887; the application of newly learned laboratory methods was credited with the control of the secondary cases. In 1892, ships again arrived with cholera patients with no spread. However, South America was afflicted, as were Africa and eastern Asia.

The Sixth Pandemic began in 1899; disease persisted in eastern Europe until 1923.

The Seventh Pandemic, which is at present extant, originated in 1958 with endemic disease in Sulawesi (Celebes) in Indonesia. This disease was caused by a variant of *V. cholerae* that had been isolated in 1903 in the El Tor Quarantine Station, on the Sinai peninsula, from an individual not considered to have cholera, and the organism was originally considered to be nonpathogenic (for discussion, see Section 4). In early July 1961, an international regatta of dragon boats was held in Kuching, Sarawak, with representatives from Sulawesi. Cholera broke out with 270 cases and 61 deaths.[40] The disease spread to Macao, Hong Kong, and the Philippines, and by 1965 cholera had spread westward into eastern Europe and Africa with incursions into Italy, Spain, and Portugal. The disease still persists throughout most of Africa. Occasional imported cases occur in other European countries and in the United States.

3. Methodology

3.1. Sources of Mortality Data

Cholera being one of the diseases dreaded by man, reporting of its occurrence has been required since records have been kept. Unfortunately, the accuracy of the reporting has reflected the competence of the health-care delivery system and its practitioners, often modified by political and economic motivations. The carefully collected statistical data contributed by the dedicated physicians of the Indian Medical Service are most valuable. However, the reporting was based on the cases seen in the treatment facilities; deaths in rural areas could well have been overlooked, and overreporting occurred, unless bacteriology was carried out on all cases, by inclusion of cases of acute dehydrating diarrhea from causes other than *V. cholerae*, such as the entity of "nonvibrio cholera."[73]

Cholera is reportable to the local health authority by the most rapid means, with rapid transmission to the World Health Organization (WHO). The information coming from infected areas is then disseminated to all health administrations. Unfortunately, this has often resulted in the imposition of restrictive measures, such as requirement of vaccination for all travelers coming from the infected area, use of prophylactic antibiotics, prohibition of movement of food and even metal ore from the infected areas, restriction of the mail, and other irrelevant activities, often with economic implications. This, too, has led to concealment rather than reporting of the disease.

Complicating this, the appearance of cholera within a country is considered by some to indicate failure on the part of public-health officials. A misguided "scientific" approach may obscure the data. As one example, the health authorities of East Pakistan directed in 1958 that cholera and cholera deaths could be reported only if bacteriologically confirmed; because laboratory facilities were essentially not available, subsequent statistical data indicated a marked increase in mortality from "diarrhea" and "dysentery," but no cholera. A diagnostic complication was observed in reviewing a "Cholera Register" covering the period 1937–1964 in an East Bengal rural health center. This record carefully preserved the identity, age, and outcome of every case reported as cholera to the district sanitary inspector. The entries on almost all children were lined out with the notation "Worms," deleting them from the final official report of cholera cases. In the experience of the Pakistan–SEATO Cholera Research Laboratory (CRL), the passage of a few ascarids either in the stools or in the vomitus of cholera patients was usual.

3.2. Sources of Morbidity Data

The problems associated with mortality data pertain even more to morbidity data. Added to this is the fact that the vast majority of illnesses caused by *V. cholerae* are manifested by a diarrheal bout no different from that frequently experienced in all parts of the world. Without bacteriological investigation of diarrheal attacks in endemic areas, it is impossible to assess accurately the morbidity caused by *V. cholerae*.

3.3. Surveys

Many surveys have been carried out, using bacteriological and serological methods, usually as components of research projects such as those carried out in East Pakistan–Bangladesh. They have included surveillance of the total population of a community,[78] serological surveys of a random sample of a large population sample,[85] and an organized surveillance system of large populations for diarrheal symptoms with bacteriological and/or serological identification of the etiological organisms.[15]

3.4. Laboratory Diagnosis

3.4.1. Isolation and Identification of the Organism.
The cholera vibrio is one of the easiest bacteria to culture.[41] It grows readily on simple nutrient media at temperatures ranging from 22 to 40°C; maximal growth occurs at 37.5°C. The organisms are sensitive to acid and killed at a pH below 3; their tolerance to alkalinity is the basis of most selective media, which are needed only when

the vibrios are relatively few in number, as in the stools of asymptomatic carriers. In the rice-water stool of the classic cholera patient, the vibrios are the predominant organisms and are easily isolated on simple nutrient agar, often as a pure culture. On gelatin agar (GA) (3% gelatin, 1% trypticase, and 1% NaCl in 1.7% agar), colonies of *V. cholerae* are surrounded by a halo formed by the gelatinase produced by the vibrio[98]; this becomes more obvious if the plates are refrigerated for 15 min before examination. Unfortunately, vibrios do not grow on the usual "enteric" media, such as eosin–methylene blue agar (EMB) or *Salmonella–Shigella* (SS) agar; they may grow on MacConkey's agar and on some lots of deoxycholate agar.

In carriers and antibiotic-treated and convalescent patients, the use of selective media or enrichment before plating is necessary. Selective media, such as alkaline taurocholate–tellurite–gelatin agar (TTGA)[83] or thiosulfate–citrate–bile salt–sucrose agar (TCBS),[79] permit use of heavy inocula. Incubation of the specimen overnight in alkaline (pH 8.5–8.6) peptone water or in other vibrio enrichment media before plating suppresses the growth of other organisms without inhibiting the growth of the vibrios. Vibrios survive well in transport media.[37] In some, such as the Cary–Blair modification of Stuart's medium, the organisms remain viable without significant multiplication; in others, such as alkaline taurocholate–tellurite–peptone media, multiplication of vibrios occurs. Unfortunately, when the specimen contains "noncholera" vibrios, these tend to overgrow and may obscure the presence of cholera vibrios after incubation for more than 24 h.[84]

Barua and Gomez[7] have shown the feasibility of submitting a fecal specimen to the laboratory by wetting blotting paper (but not filter paper) with the liquid stool and placing this in a moisture-tight plastic bag.

Rapid diagnosis is made possible by the heavy bacterial load in the cholera stool; 82% of cases in Dacca had vibrio counts greater than 10^5/ml[84]; Huber[65] found counts greater than 10^7/ml in 12 of the 23 cases he studied in Manila. Direct examination of a wet mount of fecal material (a rectal swab immersed in 0.3–0.5 ml broth) by dark-field or phase-contrast microscopy reveals the rapid, darting motility characteristic of vibrios. Wet mounts can then be treated with preservative-free sera directed against the two serotypes, Ogawa and Inaba (see Section 4); the homologous vibrios are immediately immobilized, providing a specific diagnosis within 3–5 min in 50–70% of cases positive by standard culture. On reexamination of the broth after 6–18 h at 37°C, 85–96% of positive cases were detected.[13,57] Sack and Barua[95] showed the effectiveness of the direct and the indirect immunofluorescent techniques in detecting infection when the cholera stool contained more than 10^6 and 10^7 vibrios/ml, respectively; the positive diagnosis was available in 1½ h. Barua[6] found enough growth on nutrient agar plates after incubation for 4–5 h at 37°C to recognize the typical vibrio colonies in the stereomicroscope and permit specific group-O1 serotype agglutination.

A series of 263 consecutive diarrhea cases at the Pakistan–SEATO CRL were followed in 1964 by daily rectal swabs plated directly, and, after enrichment, on TTGA and GA plates, and by antibody titrations on paired sera taken on admission and more than 6 days later. Vibrios were isolated on the day of admission from 93% of the 178 whose stools were positive at some time; a rise in bacterial agglutinins was found in 5 who were consistently negative on culture. In this series, positive cultures were found in 97% of the 183 with cholera; in 90% of these cases, vibrios were isolated from the admission specimen.[10]

3.4.2. Serological Diagnostic Methods. Infection with *V. cholerae* elicits antibody responses directed against the antigens of the vibrios themselves and against the soluble exotoxin (enterotoxin) they elaborate. Antibodies to the specific vibrio antigens can result from natural infection or immunization; however, infection with organisms sharing common antigens with vibrios[93] may elicit antibodies, and the heat-labile enterotoxin (LT) of the geographically more widely distributed *Escherichia coli* is antigenically similar to the enterotoxin of *V. cholerae*.

Bacterial agglutinins directed against live vibrios are present in the convalescent patient, but shortly fall to low or undetectable levels.[55] A microtiter technique for bacterial-agglutinin testing was developed; of 364 bacteriologically positive cases with a second serum on the 6th or later day, a diagnostic rise in titer was seen in 90%. However, of those in the 0- to 4-year age group, only 78% showed a titer rise.[16]

The vibriocidal technique described by McIntyre and Feeley[80] was also modified to the microtiter system. This was more sensitive than agglutinin testing and no less specific. In a series of 370 bacteriologically positive cases, fourfold or greater rises were observed in over 96%.[17] Among bacteriologically negative cases, a significant rise in titer was observed in 9 individuals; 6 of these were close relatives of a patient with bacteriologically confirmed cholera; 3 had also received cholera vaccine. Only in 3 others (0.8%) was a significant titer rise observed, but since exposure could not be documented, these could represent false-positive reactions. The vibriocidal test was positive in 7.3% of cases that did not exhibit a rise in agglutinins; in only 0.5% did the reverse obtain.

The microtiter techniques made possible the use of fingertip blood. This provides an ideal technique for field surveys; in a population that is needle-shy, samples were obtained from every individual present in the community who had been preselected for bleeding.[85]

The antibody directed against the enterotoxin can be quantified by a variety of techniques: neutralization,[18] passive hemagglutination,[42] or ELISA.[60] Since licensed cholera vaccines have not contained cholera toxoid, any antitoxin detected in the serum is a consequence of natural infection and not from vaccine. However, as noted above, the enterotoxin of *V. cholerae* and the LT of *E. coli* are antigenically similar, so that an antitoxin rise alone cannot be taken as proof of cholera.

4. Biological Characteristics of the Organism

V. cholerae is a gram-negative, slightly curved rod about 1.5 μm long and 0.4 μm wide. A single polar flagellum imparts to the organism a rapid darting motion that caused Robert Koch to compare the appearance of the organism in a hanging drop to the swarming of gnats on a summer evening. The range of temperature over which the vibrio grows is wide and includes the ambient temperature of tropical areas. The organisms grow well in alkaline media, but they are very sensitive to acidity. They are differentiated from related organisms by being oxidase-, gelatin-, indol-, and mannitol-positive; inositol-negative; lysine- and ornithine-decarboxylase-positive; and arginine-dihydrolase-negative. They form no gas from glucose and have a guanosine–cytosine base ratio of 42–47%.

Gardner and Venkatraman[48] divided vibrios serologically; those that were agglutinated by O-subgroup 1 (often shortened to O1) antiserum included the organisms isolated from patients with typical Asiatic cholera. These organisms were further differentiated into the Inaba and Ogawa serotypes by the use of sera absorbed to remove the common group 1 antigen. There is suppressed formation of the Inaba antigen in the Ogawa organisms; this becomes manifest when the organisms are grown at 20°C,[68] so that the organisms now are agglutinated by both specific antisera, the characteristic of the Hikojima serotype.

In 1906, Gotschlich[56] reported at the El Tor Quarantine Station on the Sinai peninsula the recovery of vibrios from patients without cholera symptoms that were agglutinated by anticholera sera they differed from the classic organisms by elaborating a soluble hemolysin. They were isolated from the intestinal contents of persons dying of illnesses that were not considered to be cholera clinically or anatomically, and therefore the organisms were considered to constitute a separate El Tor biotype that did not cause cholera. They were later accepted to be the etiological agent of outbreaks of localized choleralike disease that occurred in Sulawesi (Celebes), called "El Tor disease" or "paracholera." As noted in Section 2, the present pandemic of cholera began with the spread of this disease out of Sulawesi into Hong Kong and the Philippines in 1961, but not until 1962 was the disease caused by the El Tor vibrio considered to be cholera from the point of view of the application of international sanitary regulations.[36] Paradoxically, the El Tor vibrios involved in the current pandemic have lost their hemolytic potency, but do differ from the classic strains in that fresh isolates from agar plates agglutinate chicken erythrocytes in a direct slide test (classic strains do not), give a positive Voges–Proskauer test, are sensitive to polymyxin B, and are resistant to Mukerjee's group IV cholera phage.[47]

The different biological properties of the two biotypes do influence their epidemic behavior. The classic vibrios persist in water for only short periods of time,[14] and isolations from sewage have been rare. The El Tor vibrio, on the other hand, survives and in some circumstances actually persists in natural water supplies. The growth rate of the El Tor strains is more rapid, and they overgrow classic organisms in mixed cultures.[9] In culturing night soil, Bart *et al.*[5] recovered classic Inaba vibrios very rarely while disease was occurring in the community; when both classic and El Tor biotypes were concurrently causing disease, El Tor strains were isolated ten times more frequently from the night soil. This may be related to the observations of Colwell and her group, who have found that, under conditions replicating those that occur in the environment, cholera vibrios that were considered viable by their reaction with fluorescent antibody failed to grow on laboratory culture media.[22] When these organisms were injected into ligated rabbit ileal loops, the loops filled with fluid, as did those injected with culturable vibrios, and from these loops vibrios grew on artificial media as a pure culture.[31] A nonpathogenic strain derived from classical vibrios was subjected to the conditions leading to nonculturability; when the organisms failed to grow on selective and nonselective media and in broth, they were fed to two volunteers and within a few days vibrios were recovered from the stools of both on usual culture media.[32] These findings complicate the interpretation of the results of environmental surveillance; viable *V. cholerae* were detected in river and pond waters from the Matlab study area in concentrations of 100 to 1000 organisms/ml from water samples from which vibrios could not be isolated by standard techniques. Using microcosms of Matlab village water, Colwell found that the

different biotypes and serotypes of *V. cholerae* O1 showed a similar pattern of entry into a nonculturable stage after more than 3 days of incubation at 25°C.[32] These dormant vibrios in water sources were attached to the copepods in the zooplankton; while nonculturable, they retain their infectivity and under certain conditions they can revert to a culturable form. While these studies do not clarify why El Tor strains are more frequently isolated from the environment, they indicate the need for new studies. In any case, it is evident that these dormant forms constitute a reservoir for this disease.

The clinical disease produced by the classic and El Tor biotypes do not differ.[105] However, comparing the incidence of infection and disease among family contacts of patients in the latter community, an infection/case/ratio of 36 : 1 was found among El Tor Ogawa contacts, compared to 4 : 1 among contacts of cases with classic Inaba disease.[4] These differences in infection/case ratios have been taken to indicate that the El Tor strains are less virulent. That this is not necessarily so is suggested by the findings in the Dacca area in 1973.[70] Secondary infections occurred in 31% of the family contacts of cases hospitalized at the Cholera Research Laboratory for cholera caused by El Tor organisms; 78.6% of these were symptomatic, and 20% of the infected individuals required hospitalization. In this series, the infection/symptomatic case ratio was 1.3 : 1; the infection/ hospitalized case ratio was 4.7 : 1.

These data can be interpreted to indicate that the greater ability of the El Tor biotype to survive in the environment results in a greater likelihood of dissemination. This can result in more frequent ingestion of the organisms, but at lower doses, resulting in a greater likelihood of asymptomatic or mild infections. Given comparable exposures, the susceptible individuals might develop comparable disease. The answer can be obtained only by volunteer studies.

Vibrios that do not agglutinate in O group-1 sera have been called "NCV" (noncholera) or "NAG" (nonagglutinable) vibrios. Because of similarity in numerical taxonomy, DNA base composition, isozymic analysis, and DNA–DNA hybridization analyses, these organisms have been combined with the classic cholera strains into the taxospecies and genospecies of *V. cholerae*, but constituting differing serotypes. This results in confusion and apprehension in the public mind when the recovery of ubiquitous "NCVs" from local waters is reported as contamination with cholera vibrios.[67] These organisms are now usually designated as non-O1 *V. cholerae* strains. While these are most frequently nonpathogenic environmental contaminants, some strains have been shown to produce an enterotoxin neutralized by cholera antitoxin[41] and have been incriminated as the causal agent of acute choleralike diarrhea.[81] In 1968, an outbreak of gastroenteritis caused by these organisms occurred in the Sudan, producing 544 cases with at least 31 deaths.[66]

The enterotoxin (choleragen) elaborated by cholera vibrios has a molecular weight of approximately 84,000. It is composed of two subunits, A and B, joined by sulfhydryl bonds. The B subunit (choleragenoid) is nontoxic but antigenic and has a total molecular weight of approximately 56,000; the A subunit has a molecular weight of 28,000. Strains of *V. cholerae* vary in their production of enterotoxin, which is controlled by a chromosomal gene. Enterotoxin production by *E. coli*, on the other hand, is mediated by a plasmid; the toxins are immunologically cross-reactive.[104]

Heating destroys the A subunit, and only the nontoxic B subunit remains. The B subunit is a potent antigen, and antitoxin in the convalescent cholera patient is specifically directed against this portion of the toxin.

In addition to enterotoxin, cholera vibrios also elaborate mucinase and neuraminidase, which contribute to the pathogenesis of the organism, as well as a host of other enzymes.

5. Descriptive Epidemiology

5.1. Prevalence and Incidence

The incidence of cholera disease is determined by a multiplicity of environmental and host factors. These include the degree of crowding, the level of sanitation of the community, and the presence in the population of this organism as well as other less well defined host factors. The high frequency of subclinical infections further increases the inaccuracy of any data. Studies in Dacca have shown that wide variations of rates occur within a geographic area; for example, over a 2-year period in Dacca Municipality, the rates were 55/100,000 and 33/100,000; within individual political units of Dacca City, however, the rates varied from 0 to 220.[76] In the Philippines in 1961, the incidence rate was 123/100,000[38]; in Taiwan in 1962, the rate was 3.4/100,000.[116] These data are based on those who came for medical treatment. Close surveillance of the vaccinees in the Matlab vaccine trials of 1963 and 1964 disclosed diarrheal rates of 470/100,000 and 560/100,000, respectively. The incidence of infection by *V. cholerae* can be monitored by serological follow-up and regular stool cultures. In an endemic area, an infection rate of 2740/100,000 was found in a community over a 10-week period with not a single case of diarrheal disease suggestive

of cholera; 5 mild diarrheas were seen from which *V. cholerae* were isolated.[78] Hospitalization rates in the Matlab study area of cholera cases caused by the classical biotype during the period 1966–1972 averaged 1.3/1000 per year; during 1973–1980, when the disease was caused by the El Tor biotype, the rate was 2.9/1000 (2900/100,000).[51]

5.2. Epidemic Behavior and Contagiousness

There have been seven major pandemics of cholera, of which the Seventh, still prevailing, began in 1961 (see Section 2). The spread of cholera vibrios through unsanitary areas is easily understood on a strictly fecal–oral basis. What is not clear is why each of the pandemics has been followed by an interval during which there is no evidence that *V. cholerae* persisted in any areas outside the Indian subcontinent. Cholera had existed in the Philippines until 1937; from that time until its reintroduction in 1961, despite the practice of good bacteriology, not a single isolation of *V. cholerae* was made.

The persistence of cholera in the Indian subcontinent suggests some special characteristics; the contagiousness of cholera varies with the physical state of the subject and the dose of organisms ingested. There may be a very much greater susceptibility among those who live on the Indian subcontinent than in other parts of the world, or there may be environmental or cultural practices that increase the probability of exposure to large doses of vibrios. There is no evidence that a racial factor is involved.

As a general hypothesis, an epidemic of cholera can be considered to be a group of common-source outbreaks,[76] usually from foods or from contaminated water. When the level of contamination of water is low, water still constitutes an important hazard if it is used for food preparation without being boiled. This was observed in the preparation of the Bengali dish of *panta bhat,* in which leftover rice is covered with water, held at ambient temperatures, and ingested on the following day. When this rice-handling was duplicated in the laboratory using water with minimal vibrio contamination, the vibrio count increased by several orders of magnitude when a small amount of sodium chloride was present.[14] The water source of many households is easily contaminated once the organism is introduced into a household, especially if there are small children and the water is obtained from dug wells within the household area that are exposed to surface contamination.

The importance of dose was clearly demonstrated by Hornick *et al.,*[64] who found that 10^3 vibrios, ingested by volunteers after 2 g sodium bicarbonate had been taken, produced asymptomatic excretion of vibrios; a dose of 10^4–

10^6 produced simple diarrhea in about 60% of the volunteers. Clinical cholera requiring intravenous treatment occurred in 1 of 8 who received 10^5 organisms, 6 of 23 (26%) of those who received 10^6, and 1 of 2 who received 10^8 vibrios.

5.3. Geographic Distribution

The homeland of epidemic cholera is in the Indian subcontinent, where each year cases of cholera have been recorded and out of which the pandemics have spread. The El Tor vibrio had been recognized as the cause of localized outbreaks of "paracholera" in Indonesia since 1937.[36] Since 1961, however, this biotype has spread out of Indonesia, first through eastern Asia and the Philippines, then westward to involve all of Asia, much of Europe, and most of Africa. Figure 1 covers the period until 1986. In 1987, there was a large outbreak of disease in Angola, which continued in 1988; a smaller outbreak occurred in Tanzania. In 1988, a large outbreak attributed to the consumption of contaminated drinking water was reported to have occurred in rural areas of China. Intrusions into Europe have been

temporary, while those in Africa have continued unabated. In 1977, cholera extended into Oceania with outbreaks in the Gilbert Islands[107] and in 1978 in Nauru.[109] During March to May 1978, a severe epidemic hit the Republic of Maldives, where no cholera had been known for the previous 50 years. There was a total of 11,303 clinical cases for an overall attack rate of 7700/100,000 with 252 deaths and a case-fatality rate of 2.2%. On some islands, 30% of the population were sick within a span of 2–3 months. Deaths occurred within a few hours of onset, and as many as 4 cases came from one house. The outbreak was attributed to contamination of the water in the many superficial wells.[108] The interrelationships of health programs became apparent: chlorination of the wells to kill the vibrios also killed the larviparous fish that were effective in controlling breeding of the culicine vectors of dengue. Thus, cholera control increased the danger of dengue hemorrhagic fever.[30]

From 1873 to 1972, the United States had been free of naturally acquired cholera. In August 1973, a case of typical cholera occurred in a 51-year-old man from the Gulf Coast town of Port Lavaca, Texas. He had not been out of

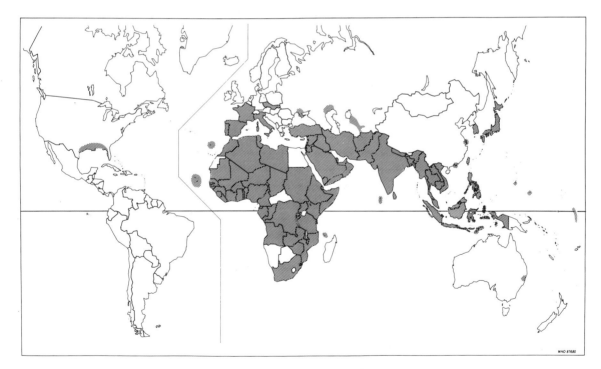

Figure 1. Countries, or areas within countries, that reported cholera during the present pandemic—1961–1986. Courtesy of the World Health Organization.

the country since military service in the 1950s; no source case or secondary cases were found.[106] In August 1978, *V. cholerae* was isolated in southwest Louisiana along the Gulf Coast from a 44-year-old man with dehydrating diarrhea. An additional three individuals positive for vibrios had diarrhea, but were not hospitalized. Four more hospitalized cases of vibrio-positive diarrhea were found, and the organisms were recovered from three patient contacts, for a total of 11 infected persons. All had recently eaten boiled or steamed crabs, and vibrios were recovered from infected crabs boiled less than 8 min or steamed less than 25 min. Vibrios were also recovered from the sewage of six towns, three with no known infection. The isolates were hemolytic, in contrast to the nonhemolytic pandemic strains, and had bacteriophage sensitivities different from those of the pandemic strains; their characteristics were identical to those of the Port Lavaca strain. The geographic association of this area with that of the Lavaca case and the similar characteristics of the isolates suggest that there has been an ongoing focus of cholera in this portion of the United States since at least 1973.[21] In 1986, 12 cases of cholera were diagnosed in Louisiana, 10 with severe diarrhea, and 7 were hospitalized. Eleven had eaten crabs or shrimp within 5 days.[27] An additional case occurred in Atlanta, Georgia, in a woman who had eaten oysters from an approved oyster bed in Texas.[88]

Cholera was present in Spain from July to November 1977, with 267 cases reported, including 141 cases in Malaga province, a popular resort area.[112] In November 1979, a small outbreak occurred on the island of Sardinia with 10 cases, 6 of which were hospitalized, and the water and clams from a lagoon receiving raw sewage were infected.[113]

Cholera was reported in 1988 by 30 countries, with endemic disease in 12 African countries, 11 Asian, 1 American state (8 cases in Louisiana), and in Australia.[114] Other countries probably have had disease without reporting their cases; e.g., Bangladesh is not listed, and there are suspicious gaps in the map of Africa (Fig. 1). Four countries in Europe (Federal Republic of Germany, Netherlands, Switzerland, and the United Kingdom), and Canada reported only imported cases. Japan, Hong Kong, and the United States reported imported as well as indigenous cases (Table 1). The Australian case was that of a 2½-year-old boy with diarrhea and dehydration in a town on the Albert/Logan river system of Queensland; toxigenic cholera vibrios have been intermittently isolated from this river system since 1977, when they were recovered from a patient. Thus, it becomes evident that environmental persistence of *V. cholerae* O1 occurs; however, these organisms may be

Table 1.   Cases of Cholera Notified to WHO, 1988[a]

Area	No. of countries	No. of reported cases[b]
Africa	12	23,186
America	2	10 (2)
Asia	11	20,872 (34)
Europe	4	14 (14)
Oceania	1	1
World total	30	44,083 (50)

[a]From *WHO Weekly Epidemiol. Rec.* **64**:141 (1989).
[b]Numbers in parentheses are imported cases.

nontoxigenic and their presence in a diarrhea patient may be coincidental rather than causal.

During 1978, cholera occurred in Japan among those who ate lobsters imported from Southeast Asia; no secondary cases occurred. While there have been many importations of cholera into European countries, Australia, and Canada, secondary cases have rarely occurred. During 1980, nine imported cases occurred in the United States, most of them from Indochinese refugees, with no secondary spread. This did happen in Italy, in Spain, and in Portugal, but the outbreaks were of short duration. The 1973 outbreak in Naples lasted from August through October.[2] The 1974 outbreak in Portugal affected all but one district of the country; the first case occurred on April 24, and the country was declared free of disease on November 29.[19] The persistence of cholera is a reflection of the level of sanitation in the population group into which the organism is introduced; while the organisms may be endemic in some areas, such as Louisiana and Queensland, persisting in an environmental reservoir, disease is extremely sporadic when sanitary standards are high.

5.4. Temporal Distribution

In endemic areas, cholera appears with a quite constant seasonal distribution, which varies from community to community. Thus, in Dacca, the annual peak occurs in November and December; in Matlab Bazaar, 25 miles away, in January and February. With the shift to the El Tor biotype, the seasonal peak advanced, peaking in October and November.[51] In Calcutta, 125 miles away, the outbreak usually peaks in May and June. A relationship in this area to the monsoon would be expected; at the beginning of the monsoon in Dacca in April or May, there are often outbreaks as the early rains wash contamination into water sources, but after this, cholera essentially disappears until the end of the monsoon season. In Calcutta, the peak occurs at the height of the monsoon; however, one must take into account the very different environmental conditions that pertain in the crowded bustee areas (native quarters) of Calcutta and the more open areas in East Bengal.

5.5. Age

The age distribution is a reflection of the endemicity of the disease. In the Dacca area, hospitalization rates were highest among those less than 10 years of age.[76] In the Matlab vaccine study area in 1963 and 1964, disease rates among those 0–4 years of age were 11.7 and 16.3 per thousand; among those over 15, the rate were 1.8 and 1.5 per thousand.[15] This is consistent with the observation that about 50% of the children in the 5–9 age group with no history of vaccination or disease have detectable vibriocidal antibody.[85] On the other hand, when cholera strikes a native population, the highest incidence of serious disease is usually found in the older age group. In Taiwan, those over 55 were particularly susceptible, with an incidence two to three times as great as that of those younger than 35.[116] In the Philippines, the incidence among those over 20 was twice as great as that of those under 20.[38] In later years, the incidence was greatest among the children.

5.6. Sex

The distribution of cases by sex reflects the degree of exposure to the prevailing mechanisms of transmission. In Dacca, when males predominated in the population, there were more male than female cases. When the source of infection was from "charitable feeding centers," the incidence rates were higher for females over the age of 15.[71] In the Philippines, in the first year of the epidemic, of those over 40 the incidence among men was twice that among women.[38] In Taiwan, there was an excess of females in the age groups 20–29 and 40–49, which is consistent with the practice of the women in the household nursing the sick. In Dacca, when the index case was a male over 15, the secondary infection rate among family members was 6.3%; when the index case was a woman or a child under 15, the secondary infection rates were 44.4 and 31.9%, respectively.[69]

5.7. Race

No specific racial predisposition has been evident that cannot be explained by socioeconomic factors. A racial or genetic characteristic is often proposed to explain the country-to-country variation in severity of disease. In 1964, cholera in Saigon was caused by El Tor vibrios; the duration of purging was so short that antibiotic efficacy was not demonstrable. When the El Tor strain spread into India and East Pakistan, the pattern of full-blown disease was no less severe than that produced by the classic organism.[105] While this could be associated with genetic factors, one cannot exclude the differences in behavioral patterns. As an example, in Bengal, the traditional food item of *panta bhat*, as noted in Section 5.2, may ensure that the Bengali is exposed to a very large inoculum and therefore experiences more severe infections.[14] This may well be complicated by host factors produced by malnutrition, which may adversely affect gastric acidity and which has been shown to inhibit the mucosal immune response to intraluminal toxoid or toxin in rats.[3]

5.8. Occupation

Yen[116] was impressed by the numbers of patients who were farmers, fishermen, or laborers who had been exposed to considerable heat and sun with consequent severe thirst and consumption of large amounts of water; he attributed the higher incidence of disease in these groups to loss of salts through excessive sweating. It must be noted that the greater the amount of water one drinks in unsanitary areas, the greater is the likelihood of ingesting an infectious dose of vibrios.

5.9. Occurrence in Family and Other Settings

In Taiwan, Yen[116] reported a prevalence rate of bacteriological positivity of 9500/100,000 among those living in the household of a cholera patient. This contrasts with a rate of 340/100,000 among neighbors living within 500 m of the house of the index patient and 302/100,000 among residents of the rest of the village.

When an intensive study was made to uncover cases with milder diarrhea among family contacts of patients admitted to the Cholera Research Laboratory Hospital in Dacca City, a secondary attack rate of 11.1%, or 11,100/100,000, was found.[87] In the rural Matlab vaccine-trial population, infection with *V. cholerae* had occurred in 10.7% of family contacts, or 10,700/100,000[15]; 3.5% of the contacts (3500/100,000) had diarrhea. In the Philippines, 18.2% of family contacts were infected, but only 1.7% required hospitalization.[103]

Cholera had been a traditional affliction of those situations in which large numbers of people aggregate, especially if sanitary facilities are rudimentary. Most usually, this has been associated with religious festivals and fairs, but it is also a concomitant of refugee settlements in areas where the organisms are endemic, such as occurred among the East Pakistani refugees in India in 1971.

5.10. Socioeconomic Factors

Cholera is traditionally the disease of the poor. The failure of Pettenkofer to acquire cholera when he drank the culture fluid in his famous dispute with Robert Koch, and the illnesses of his students when they repeated the gesture,[39] have been taken to be indicative of the miserable salaries paid to laboratory technicians in those days; in fact, he was probably immune because of earlier exposures to cholera. The high prevalence of cholera in the poor segments of the community leads to the debate whether poverty, and the consequent nutritional deficiencies, evokes a greater host susceptibility to the disease, or whether the high incidence is due to the poor sanitary conditions under which the poor are forced to live, or a combination of the two.

5.11. Other Factors

A host factor of greatest importance is the gastric acidity. In the outbreak in Jerusalem in 1970, the disease afflicted many persons in the upper social classes. These patients were predominantly achlorhydric or had had a subtotal gastrectomy.[50] Studies carried out among volunteers showed that even among those who are not achlorhydric, there are a group whom Hornick et al.[64] designated "nonsecretors" because their gastric contents were still alkaline 30 min after ingestion of 2 g sodium bicarbonate. It was in this group that the greatest susceptibility to experimental infection was found; after a challenge of 10^6 vibrios given orally with bicarbonate, 7 of 11 "secretors" versus 21 of 23 "nonsecretors" were infected.[64] The possibility that malnutrition is associated with impaired gastric acidity provides a logical relationship between socioeconomic class and susceptibility to cholera.

Glass et al.[52] have reported the association between susceptibility to cholera and the O blood group. While there was no difference in the proportion of contacts who became infected, severe cases were much more likely to be in the O blood group and less likely to have AB blood—68% of severely ill patients were in the O group in contrast to 36% of the asymptomatic infections. None of the severely ill

patients were in the AB blood group. In the population, 32% were O and 8% AB, suggesting that the pressure of cholera accounts for the very low prevalence of O group members in this population.

6. Mechanisms and Routes of Transmission

Cholera is transmitted by the fecal–oral route. While the vomitus in the acute case may be heavily contaminated, this is essentially a reflux of intestinal contents. The nonoffensive odor-free cholera stool with a volume as great as 20 liters/day, containing approximately 10^7 vibrios/ml, is the primary source of potentially massive environmental pollution.

Infection occurs when these organisms enter the body in food or drink. In the classic study of John Snow, the water supplied by the Southwark and Vauxhall Company to several of the south districts of London was in essence diluted sewage; the identity of the water supplier could be recognized by adding silver nitrate and observing the heavy precipitate of silver chloride, probably contributed by urinary contamination. The water of the Broad Street pump had its own special flavor, favored by some. In general, the usual vibrio burden of waters is not great. In the Matlab study area, the incidence of diarrhea associated with V. cholerae was not lower in those families that used tubewell water (generally bacteria-free) than in those that used surface waters for drinking.[34] However, that water can play an important part in the transmission of cholera was demonstrated by the 1974 outbreak in Portugal, when a widely distributed bottled water was shown to have spread the disease.[20]

Foods can be contaminated by the classic transmitters of the enteric disease, e.g., fecal-feeding flies, foul fingers, or by adding water containing V. cholerae to foods that are not subsequently reheated. Given an infective dose and the absence or neutralization of gastric acidity, infection of the nonimmune individual will occur.

The reservoir of V. cholerae has been considered to be man since no other animal species has been found consistently infected, even though some studies have succeeded in recovering O1 vibrios from animal sources.[96] V. cholerae organisms have been recovered from Chesapeake Bay,[31] from Bangladeshi waters,[23] from surface waters in Kent, England,[8] and from sewage in Brazil.[110] These isolations may be very significant. As noted in Section 5.3, there is very strong evidence for persistence of organisms infective for man along the Gulf Coast in Louisiana and Texas, and Queensland.

7. Pathogenesis and Immunity

7.1. Pathogenesis

The incubation period of cholera is stated to be from a few hours to 5 days, usually 2–3 days, after ingesting the infecting dose. In one outbreak, the incubation periods were considered to range from 4 to 203 h, but other exposures were not ruled out.[54] For disease to occur, the ingested vibrios must first survive the transit through the stomach, which can be achieved because of achlorhydria, by neutralization of the acidity by food, or by very rapid transit through the stomach in water. On reaching the alkaline small intestine, the vibrios multiply. The epithelial lining of the small intestine is protected by a mucous layer; the mucinase elaborated by the organisms provides a method for breaching this barrier.[97] Reaching the intestinal mucosa, the organisms lie in apposition to the brush-border surface of the cell by an adherence factor. The enterotoxin they produce attaches by its B subunit to the GM_1 ganglioside present in the brush border. Neuraminidase (or sialidase) is also elaborated by the vibrio, and this actually may convert other gangliosides to GM_1, providing more receptors for the toxin.[61] After a lag period of about 45 min, there begins an outpouring of fluid and salts into the lumen of the bowel. During the interval (which does not occur if the cell membrane is broken so that the toxin can enter directly toward its site of activity),[49] the sulfhydryl bonds between the A and B subunit are broken, and the A subunit penetrates through the cell wall into the interior of the cell to the locus of adenylate cyclase activity. This is now activated, resulting in an accumulation of cyclic AMP, which is associated with the increase in fluid transudate. This fluid has the same osmotic pressure as the serum and contains 45 meq bicarbonate and 16 meq potassium per liter of fluid.

These physiological changes occur with no morphological changes in the gut mucosa, other than some congestion, goblet-cell hyperplasia, and a mononuclear-cell inflammatory exudate.[46]

This outpouring of fluid produces dehydration, the loss of bicarbonate produces metabolic acidosis, and potassium loss results in hypokalemia. The severely dehydrated cholera patient presents with sunken eyes, wrinkled skin, rapid breathing, bizarre P waves and flat T waves on the electrocardiogram, and absent peripheral pulses and blood pressure. While cholera patients may be semicomatose, they can be roused and sometimes, despite absence of any detectable peripheral pulse, will stand and walk. Basal rales indicative of heart failure are often present. Studies by Harvey et al.[58] demonstrated that with acidosis, there is a shutdown of the peripheral circulation with central overload, so that in essence the patients go into cardiac failure. When Harvey and her group administered intravenous bicarbonate solution, raising the blood pH to 7.4, the circulatory abnormalities were corrected dramatically.

The loss of potassium is manifested by flat T waves on the electrocardiogram, but evidence of hypokalemia was rarely evident clinically. However, many anecdotal episodes were recounted in which convalescent cholera patients would suddenly drop dead on resuming normal activity; these were in cases that had been managed without potassium replacement. No such episodes were uncovered in the thousands of cholera cases treated by the Pakistan–SEATO Cholera Research Laboratory, now the International Centre for Diarrhoeal Disease Research, Bangladesh.

7.2. Immunity

The difference in age-specific disease incidence in endemic areas is ample evidence that immunity to cholera is real and important. However, second attacks have been documented 11–60 months after the initial illness[115]; the infection rates were significantly higher with the heterologous than with the homologous serotype.

In a study of the Matlab experience over the period 1968–1977, it was estimated that 29 individuals should have experienced a second hospitalization for cholera if there were no resulting immunity. In fact, there were only three instances, all among children (ages 5, 5, and 2 years at the initial hospitalization), with a second hospitalization within 2 years. Two were infected with the original biotype and serotype (both with the Inaba serotype, one with the classical and the other the El Tor biotype); the third case had an initial infection with an El Tor Ogawa organism followed by an El Tor Inaba 2 years later.[51] In volunteer studies, Cash et al.[25] rechallenged 27 men who had had diarrhea following their first challenge 4–12 months previously. None of 20 developed diarrhea after homologous challenge; 1 became stool-positive for vibrios but remained asymptomatic. Of 6 given a heterologous oral challenge, 4 developed diarrhea and 1 had an asymptomatic infection. Protection here was evidently antibacterial rather than antitoxic, since there is no difference in the enterotoxin elaborated by the different serotypes. Studies of disease among contacts of cholera cases indicated that the presence of vibriocidal antibodies protected against colonization by the vibrios and prevented disease in those who were colonized. The presence of IgG to cholera toxin or to lipopolysaccharide, however, had no protective effect on either event.[53]

8. Patterns of Host Response

8.1. Clinical Features

The spectrum of disease elicited by infection by *V. cholerae* ranges from a completely asymptomatic infection, through an ordinary diarrhea, to a violent dehydrating diarrhea with an acute onset and death within as short a time as 4 h if untreated. Volunteer studies suggest that the severity of the disease is related to the severity of the challenge, the interval between ingestion of the challenge dose and onset of symptoms being 36–53 h, with extreme ranges from 14 to 143 h; the severe cases had the shorter incubation periods.[24]

Classic cholera presents typically as a painless diarrhea; the stool initially is brown, but very shortly becomes rice-water in character, completely inoffensive, and essentially odorless, containing flecks of mucus. Vomiting occurs not infrequently, but appears several hours *after* the onset of purging and is apparently the consequence of acidosis or dehydration or both, since it ceases completely after proper treatment has been started. As body fluid is lost, the eyes become sunken, tissue turgor is lost, the blood pressure falls, the pulse becomes inapparent, and the patient becomes semicomatose and goes into shock. Replacement of the lost fluid and electrolytes[91] corrects the extraintestinal chemical imbalances, but purging persists for as long as 7 days. The diarrhea usually stops at the time that antibody (coproantibody) appears in the stool.[44] When an antibiotic such as tetracycline is given, purging stops within 48 h, and the bacteria disappear from the stool; in the untreated individual, the vibrios are shed for at least a week.

Cases of cholera with "ordinary" diarrhea cannot be differentiated by any clinical criteria from cases of diarrhea from any other cause; laboratory studies are required.

Women in the third trimester of pregnancy are severely affected by cholera. Dehydration is more severe than among nonpregnant women or those in the second trimester of pregnancy; 50% of the fetuses are stillborn. Fetal death is usual when the mother had an absent or thready radial pulse. With modern replacement therapy, maternal deaths no longer occur, but fetal death has usually occurred before the woman presents for treatment.[59] Cholera among children is in general similar to that in adults, but dehydration was less severe in those under 2 years of age; coma on admission was most frequent among those 2–10 years of age. Children tended to have prolonged drowsiness or semi-stupor lasting as much as 15 h to 8 days after initial rehydration had been accomplished; sometimes this was related to hypokalemia. In Dacca, coma and convulsions due to hypo-

glycemia were observed in 1.4% of children aged 2–10. While closer observation of intake and output was needed to keep the children from going into shock, the prognosis with modern therapy is excellent, with a case-fatality rate below 1%, even in a rural treatment center.[74]

8.2. Diagnosis

Cholera must be suspected when there is a sharp outbreak of severe dehydrating diarrhea appearing in a small geographic area or in a group of individuals associated with a common source of infection. Isolated cases are unusual, but a severe dehydrating diarrhea, with vomiting beginning several hours after the diarrhea, suggests cholera. The severe cholera case usually cannot be differentiated clinically on admission from cases of severe "nonvibrio cholera"; however, the purging in the latter rarely continues for more than 24–48 h.[73] Many of these cases are due to enterotoxigenic *E. coli* or other pathogens. In children, a "white diarrhea" can be produced by rotavirus. Laboratory support is necessary to identify the etiological agent, with isolation of the organism or the demonstration of an antibody rise directed against *V. cholerae* confirming the case as one of cholera (see Section 3.4).

9. Control and Prevention

9.1. General Concepts

The ultimate control of cholera is based on high levels of sanitation and personal hygiene to assure that fecally shed organisms are not ingested in sufficient numbers to cause disease. This involves the availability of adequate facilities for sanitary disposal of feces, effective hand-washing after defecation, the availability of water supplies free of vibrios, and a level of culinary standards in the home and in the commercial food establishment sufficient to prevent fecal contamination of foods that may be held at room temperature (which should in any case be brief, as stressed in Chapter 4). Until this ideal is realized, control of cholera will depend on pragmatic measures.[11]

The cholera patient who excretes large quantities of fecal fluid containing 10^{7-8} vibrios/ml is capable of seriously contaminating the home environment, resulting in secondary infections within the household. This is particularly true of children, especially those who are not yet toilet-trained. Removal of cases to a treatment facility permits safe handling of the stool, as well as assures survival from this onetime dramatically fatal disease by proper intravenous or oral treatment, or both, with electrolytes and fluid. This allays the panic and hysteria that so often are associated with an outbreak of cholera. The chronic carrier sheds a relatively low number of organisms, and while carriers have been implicated in the introduction of vibrios into a new area,[116] they are not important within the epidemic itself. While shedding of vibrios for as long as 11 years has been documented in "Cholera Dolores,"[1] no secondary cases have been found that could be attributed to her over the years of close surveillance. Other studies have indicated the unimportance of the known long-term carrier in spreading disease.[45,69]

The frequency of asymptomatic infections in which organisms are shed for several days invalidates any possibility that strict isolation of cases would be beneficial in epidemic control. Even though it was cholera that induced the establishment of the International Quarantine Commission, quarantine has had a negative value. Quarantine posts were established along major routes of travel, which are avoided by migrants and the poor among whom the disease predominates. Worse yet, quarantine has too often been associated with restrictive measures; in the current pandemic, boatloads of food were dumped, shipments of commercial items like iron ore delayed, and mail service interrupted when they came from a country that had reported the presence of cholera. The predictable result was deliberate concealment of the presence of cholera in a country.

Reporting the presence of the disease in an area is of the utmost importance. Because cholera is so often similar to "ordinary" diarrhea, routine bacteriological monitoring of diarrhea cases is important, using culture media that will detect the presence of *V. cholerae,* so that the earliest cases will be detected and reported and a possible epidemic anticipated. This will then permit health authorities to prepare necessary supplies and to alert the medical profession with regard to the proper management of the cholera case. This was well demonstrated when cholera entered the Philippines in 1961; as the disease appeared in individual communities, case-fatality rates as high as 50% were often seen, but only during the first few days of the attack.

9.2. Antibiotic and Chemotherapeutic Approaches to Prophylaxis

Tetracycline (and other broad-spectrum antibiotics as well as furazolidone) is an effective vibriocidal compound and rids the patient of the organisms within a very short period. These agents are valuable for the prophylaxis of members of the patients' hearth-group, those with whom he eats, among whom secondary cases are so frequent.[77]

However, the use of such agents for mass prophylaxis results in the predictable emergence of organisms resistant to the antimicrobial agent used. In Tanzania, vibrio isolates in 1977 were sensitive to tetracycline; after 5 months of use of the drug therapeutically and in mass prophylaxis, 76% of isolates were resistant.[82] This resistance was attributed to one of two plasmids that were transferable among *V. cholerae* strains and also to other members of the enteric group of bacteria such as *E. coli.*[111] Tetracycline was an effective antibiotic in the East Pakistan–Bangladesh study area from 1963 to 1980 when some cholera patients failed to respond as expected to treatment and the isolated organisms were found to be resistant *in vitro* to tetracycline, ampicillin, kanamycin, streptomycin, and trimethoprim–sulfamethoxazole.[26] After about 6 months, isolates were again antibiotic-sensitive.[51]

9.3. Immunization

Cholera vaccines over the years have consisted of a mixture of the Inaba and Ogawa serotypes, usually heat-killed and phenol-preserved. Carefully controlled studies carried out in East Pakistan and in the Philippines have shown beyond any doubt that these vaccines do indeed induce immunity against natural infection[12] and that lipopolysaccharide (LPS) itself was effective, that a monovalent Ogawa vaccine afforded protection against both Inaba and Ogawa infections, and that protection against infection with El Tor organisms was comparable whether the vaccine was prepared with El Tor or with classic organisms.

Vaccine was much more effective among adults than among children in the Matlab field studies; e.g., the Ogawa LPS was effective only among adults in protecting against Inaba disease. These studies have been carried out in endemic populations; the superior protection afforded to adults was clearly a secondary response. With some vaccines, two doses were necessary to produce a significant level of protection to children.[86]

While the protection afforded by bacterial cholera vaccine is real and significant, this protection is unfortunately transient. With all trials, except for the first, in which an unusually potent vaccine was used, protection was no longer present after 3–6 months. This means that an immunization program must be scheduled annually to be carried out not earlier than 6 months before the appearance of cholera is expected; such precise timing cannot be assured.

The mechanism of action of the antibacterial vaccine is not entirely clear. An inverse association between cholera attack rates and the level of vibriocidal antibodies in a population has been shown.[12] The administration of vaccine to children raises the mean antibody level to that of unim-munized adults; they then experience the attack rate found in the older group. That the effectiveness of a vaccine might differ significantly between indigenous and foreign popula-tions is suggested by the report that a whole-cell cholera vaccine induced a marked rise in IgA against *V. cholera* LPS in the breast milk of Pakistani women, but not in Swedish women.[102] Freter[43] has shown that parenteral cholera vaccine produced detectable levels of coproan-tibodies, and that antibacterial antibody in intestinal loops of an experimental animal does not inhibit bacterial growth, but the vibrios are now found free in the lumen rather than attached to the mucosal surface. With individuals, however, volunteer studies have shown that infection occurred after oral challenge with 10^6 organisms as frequently among those with as those without vibriocidal antibody.[25]

There would seem to be a greater hope for protection from an antitoxin directed against the enterotoxin. In the dog, Curlin and Carpenter,[33] using crossed circulations, have clearly shown that the presence of antitoxin in the blood supplying an isolated loop protected the loop against vibrio challenge. Pierce *et al.*[90] have demonstrated in the dog that a solid immunity followed the instillation of toxoid into the lumen of the bowel; to be effective, the oral antigen required a preliminary parenteral injection of toxoid.[3] Pro-tection could be solid in the absence of demonstrable cir-culating antitoxin. This immunity depends on the local pro-duction of secretory IgA in mucosal plasma cells[89]; Barry and Pierce[3] have shown that protein deficiency impairs this response.

Field trials have been carried out in Bangladesh with a toxoid preparation free of LPS; overall protection of only 26% was seen against Inaba disease only in the 5–14 age group, and it was present only during the first 90 days.[35] Results of studies with toxoid in volunteers have been disap-pointing, with no protection despite good levels of induced circulating antitoxin following oral ingestion of purified toxoid. Under the same test conditions, excellent homolo-gous and heterologous protection was shown among those with earlier cholera diarrhea.[72]

A field trial has been carried out using a killed whole-cell vaccine (WC) and the same vaccine containing the B subunit of cholera toxin (BS-WC). These were given orally in three doses to children and women and elicited signifi-cant protection, greater with BS-WC than WC alone. Again, protection began to fall after a few months.[29]

The greatest hope for induced immunity might be by establishing stable mutants of *V. cholerae* that elaborate only B subunit (choleragenoid) and cannot revert to toxin production. A candidate strain has been described by Honda

and Finkelstein[63]; since it retains the ability to adhere to the mucosal surface, it should provide effective antibacterial immunity after oral administration without producing dis-ease. The duration of that immunity, and proof that the strain cannot produce disease in any people, need to be demonstrated.

As indicated above, no vaccines now available are ef-fective for more than a very short period of time,[101] and immunization programs generally tend to miss those who are most likely to be exposed to cholera. More important, immunization has had a negative effect on cholera control because health authorities squander scarce resources carry-ing out immunizations rather than improving sanitary condi-tions. Emphasis has been placed on whether or not there was the proper entry on the yellow immunization certifi-cate, on the assumption that this assured freedom from in-fection; unfortunately, vaccination, even when effective in preventing disease, did not prevent asymptomatic infec-tion.[15] The elimination of vaccination as a requirement for international travel has been an advance in the control of cholera.

9.4. Prevention of Death

The single most important advance in the control and prevention of cholera, of course, has been the improvement in treating the disease, which has changed cholera from a rapidly lethal disease to one of short-term incapacity. The moribund, pulseless patient is restored to general health—with the exception of the small intestine—literally within minutes by the intravenous infusion of an alkaline isotonic solution containing potassium; the ability of the intestinal mucosal cells to be stimulated by glucose and amino acids to absorb sodium ions has made it possible to effectively maintain the rehydrated state and to completely treat the moderately severely dehydrated cases with an oral solution. This extends the treatment capability to the village level rather than the sophisticated medical center. For intravenous treatment, the WHO Diarrhea Treatment Solution [contain-ing 13 meq K^+, 48 meq HCO_3^- equivalence, prepared with 4 g NaCl, 6.5 g sodium acetate (or 5.4 g sodium lactate), 1 g KCl, and 8 g glucose/liter], Ringer's lactate, or a homemade 5:4:1 solution of 5 g NaCl, 4 g $NaHCO_3$ (or equivalent), and 1 g KCl/liter is effective. The oral solution, containing 3.5 g NaCl, 1.5 g KCl, 2.5 g $NaHCO_3$, and 20.0 g glucose (or 40 g sucrose)/liter, can be prepared locally, or the dry salts can be obtained in packets for mixing with a liter of water, under national or UNICEF programs. Cereals can be used in place of glucose, adding some protein in addition and permitting the use of a household item. Starch from rice, corn, wheat, potato, sorghum, millet, and plantain are under study; they are more effective than glucose in decreasing vomiting and total stool volume.

Effective antibiotics play only a secondary role, serving only to shorten the period over which replacement fluids must be administered; the latter are the keys to survival. Oral rehydration therapy has not only saved the lives of innumerable cholera patients, but its expanding use for the management of diarrhea regardless of cause has been a major factor in improving child survival globally.

10. Unresolved Problems

There would be value in having a vaccine that was generally acceptable and had a long duration of effectiveness and in which the cold chain was not a critical element. An attenuated organism[63] must be shown to be stable in transportation under adverse conditions and to be innocuous when administered to immunodeficient recipients. Perhaps a subunit vaccine[62] or an oral toxoid preparation[90] will provide the long-lasting protection not now available.

The worldwide dissemination of cholera still needs definition. Are there other foci like the Gulf Coast of the United States in which vibrios persist and which become the source of isolated rare cases? Since *V. cholerae* strains are found in various waters in widely different geographic areas,[8,110] this becomes a more probable explanation than fecal droppings from airplanes.[94]

The therapy of cholera has been well developed; the problem has been that of achieving its implementation, particularly in underdeveloped countries in which the disease predominates. Still unresolved is the definition' of the factors in host resistance that make this a disease of the poor; if a replaceable deficit in diet could be defined, appropriate food supplementation could be considered, such as the addition of iodine to table salt.

Cholera is acquired by fecal–oral transmission; it occurs rarely in well-sanitated areas. Can we hope for sanitary improvements in the Third World to assure safe disposal of feces, and provision of water safe for drinking and in sufficient quantity to permit appropriate hand-washing?

Progress in the understanding of cholera and its etiology, pathogenesis, epidemiology, and treatment has advanced by orders of magnitude in the past 25 years. Those who have been involved are proud of the accomplishments and look forward to the day when cholera is no longer considered a problem—a day that is well within sight.

11. References

1. AZURIN, J. C., BASACA-SEVILLA, V., ALVERO, M., SULLESTA, E., KOBARI, K., AND KOTERA, K., A long-term carrier of cholera: Cholera Dolores, in: *Proceedings of the 14th Joint Conference,* US–Japan Cooperative Medical Science Program Cholera Panel, Symposium on Cholera, Karatsu, pp. 24–29, National Institute of Health, Tokyo, 1978.
2. BAINE, W. B., ZAMPIERI, A., MAZZOTTI, M., ANGIONI, G., GRECO, D., DI AIOIA, M., IZZO, E., GANGAROSA, E. J., AND POCCHIARI, F., Epidemiology of cholera in Italy in 1973, *Lancet* **2:**1370–1374 (1974).
3. BARRY, W. S., AND PIERCE, N. F., Impaired mucosal immune response to cholera toxin/toxoid in protein-deprived rats, in: *Proceedings of the 14th Joint Conference,* US–Japan Cooperative Medical Science Program Cholera Panel, Symposium on Cholera, Karatsu, pp. 115–123, National Institute of Health, Tokyo, 1978.
4. BART, K. J., HUQ, Z., KHAN, M., AND MOSLEY, W. H., Seroepidemiologic studies during a simultaneous epidemic of infection with El Tor Ogawa and classical Inaba *Vibrio cholerae, J. Infect. Dis.* **121:**S17–S24 (1970).
5. BART, K. J., KHAN, M. V., AND MOSLEY, W. H., Isolation of *Vibrio cholera* from nightsoil during epidemics of classical and El Tor cholera in East Pakistan, *Bull. WHO* **43:**421–429 (1970).
6. BARUA, D., Laboratory diagnosis of cholera cases and carriers, in: *Principles and Practice of Cholera Control,* Public Health Papers No. 40, pp. 47–52, WHO Geneva, 1970.
7. BARUA, D., AND GOMEZ, C. Z., Blotting-paper strips for transportation of cholera stools, *Bull. WHO* **37:**798 (1967).
8. BASHFORD, D. J., DONOVAN, T. J., FURNISS, A. L., AND LEE, J. F., *Vibrio cholera* in Kent, *Lancet* **1:**436–437 (1979).
9. BASU, S., BHATTACHARYA, P., AND MUKERJEE, S., Interaction of *Vibrio cholerae* and *Vibrio El Tor, Bull. WHO* **34:**371–378 (1966).
10. BENENSON, A. S., Laboratory diagnosis of cholera, in: *Annual Progress Report, Oct. 1963–Oct. 1964,* Pakistan-SEATO Cholera Research Laboratory, Dacca, 1964.
11. BENENSON, A. S., The control of cholera, *Bull. N.Y. Acad. Med.* **47:**1204–1210 (1971).
12. BENENSON, A. S., Review of experience with whole-cell and somatic antigen vaccines, in: *Proceedings of the 12th Joint Conference,* US–Japan Cooperative Medical Science Program Cholera Panel, Symposium on Cholera, Sapporo, pp. 228–244, National Institute of Health, Tokyo, 1976.
13. BENENSON, A. S., ISLAM, M. R., AND GREENOUGH, W. B., III, Rapid identification of *Vibrio cholerae* by dark-field microscopy, *Bull. WHO* **30:**827–831 (1964).
14. BENENSON, A. S., ZAFAR AHMAD, S., AND OSEASOHN, R. O., Person-to-person transmission of cholera, in: *Proceedings of the Cholera Research Symposium,* Honolulu, PHS Publ. 1328, pp. 332–336, U.S. Government Printing Office, Washington, D.C., 1965.

15. BENENSON, A.S., MOSLEY, W. H., FAHIMUDDIN, M., AND OSEASOHN, R. O., Cholera vaccine field trials in East Pakistan. 2. Effectiveness in the field, *Bull. WHO* **38:**359–372 (1968).

16. BENENSON, A. S., SAAD, A., AND PAUL, M., Serological studies in cholera. 1. Vibrio agglutinin response of cholera patients determined by a microtechnique, *Bull. WHO* **38:**267–276 (1968).

17. BENENSON, A. S., SAAD, A., AND MOSLEY, W. H., Serological studies in cholera. 2. The vibriocidal antibody response of cholera patients determined by a microtechnique, *Bull. WHO* **38:**277–285 (1968).

18. BENENSON, A. S., SAAD, A., MOSLEY, W. H., AND AHMED, A., Serological studies in cholera. 3. Serum toxin neutralization—Rise in titre in response to infection with *Vibrio cholerae*, and the level in the "normal" population of East Pakistan, *Bull. WHO* **38:**287–295 (1968).

19. BLAKE, P. A., ROSENBERG, M. L., BANDEIRA COSTA, J., SOARES FERREIRA, P., LEVY GUIMARAES, C., AND GANGAROSA, E. J., Cholera in Portugal, 1974. I. Modes of transmission, *Am. J. Epidemiol.* **105:**337–343 (1977).

20. BLAKE, P. A., ROSENBERG, M. L., FLORENCIA, J., BANDEIRA COSTA, J., DO PRADO QUINTINO, L., AND GANGAROSA, E. J., Cholera in Portugal, 1974. II. Transmission by bottled mineral water, *Am. J. Epidemiol.* **105:**344–348 (1977).

21. BLAKE, P. A., ALLEGRA, D. T., SNYDER, J. D., BARRETT, T. J., MCFARLAND, L., CARAWAY, C. T., FEELEY, J. C., CRAIG, J. P., LEE, J. V., PUHR, N. D., AND FELDMAN, R. A., Cholera—A possible endemic focus in the United States, *N. Engl. J. Med.* **302:**305–309 (1980).

22. BRAYTON, P. R., AND COLWELL, R. R., Fluorescent antibody staining method for enumeration of viable environmental *Vibrio cholerae* O1, *J. Microbiol. Methods* **6:**309–314 (1987).

23. BRAYTON, P. R., TAMPLIN, M. L., HUQ, A., AND COLWELL, R. R., Enumeration of *Vibrio cholerae* O1 in Bangladesh waters by fluorescent-antibody direct viable counts, *Appl. Environ. Microbiol.* **53:**2862–2865 (1987).

24. CASH, R. A., MUSIC, S. I., LIBONATI, J. P., SNYDER, M. J., WENZEL, R. P., AND HORNICK, R. B., Response of man to infection with *Vibrio cholerae*. I. Clinical, serologic and bacteriologic responses to a known inoculum, *J. Infect. Dis.* **129:**45–52 (1974).

25. CASH, R. A., MUSIC, S. I., LIBONATI, J. P., CRAIG, J. P., PIERCE, N. F., AND HORNICK, R. B., Response of man to infection with *Vibrio cholerae*. II. Protection from illness afforded by previous disease and vaccine, *J. Infect. Dis.* **130:**325–333 (1974).

26. Centers for Disease Control, Multiply antibiotic-resistant O-group 1 *Vibrio cholerae*—Bangladesh, *Morbid. Mortal. Weekly Rep.* **29:**109–110 (1981).

27. Centers for Disease Control, Cholera in Louisiana—Update, *Morbid. Mortal. Weekly Rep.* **35:**687–688 (1986).

28. CHAMBERS, J. S., *The Conquest of Cholera, America's Greatest Scourge,* Macmillan Co., New York, 1938.

29. CLEMENS, J. D., HARRIS, J. R., KHAN, M. R., KAY, B. A., YUNUS, M., SVENNERHOLM, A.-M., SACK, D. A., CHAKRABORTY, J., STANTON, B. F., KHAN, M. U., ATKINSON, W., AND HOLMGREN, J., Field trial of oral cholera vaccines in Bangladesh, *Lancet* **2:**124–127 (1986).

30. CLYDE, D. F., Personal communication (1980).

31. COLWELL, R. R., BRAYTON, P. R., GRIMES, D. J., ROSZAK, D. B., HUQ, S. A., AND PALMER, L. M., Viable but non-culturable *Vibrio cholerae* and related pathogens in the environment: Implications for release of genetically engineered microorganisms, *Biotechnology* **3:**817–820 (1985).

32. COLWELL, R. R., TAMPLIN, M. L., BRAYTON, P. R., GAUZENS, A. L., TALL, B. D., HERRINGTON, D., LEVINE, M. M., HALL, S., HUQ, A., AND SACK, D. A., Environmental aspects of *Vibrio cholerae* in transmission of cholera, Abstracts, Twenty Third Joint Conference on Cholera, pp. 33–34, National Institutes of Health, Washington, D.C., 1987.

33. CURLIN, G. T., AND CARPENTER, C. C. J., JR., Antitoxic immunity to cholera in isolated perfused canine ileal segments, *J. Infect. Dis.* **121:**S132–S136 (1970).

34. CURLIN, G. T., AZIZ, K. M. A., AND KHAN, M. R., The influence of drinking tubewell water on diarrhea rates in Matlab Thana, Bangladesh, in: *Proceedings of the 12th Joint Conference,* US–Japan Cooperative Medical Science Program Cholera Panel, Symposium on Cholera, Sapporo, pp. 48–54, National Institute of Health, Tokyo, 1976.

35. CURLIN, G. T., LEVINE, R. L., AZIZ, K. M. A., MIZANUR RAHMAN, A. S. M., AND VERWEY, W. F., Serological aspects of a cholera toxoid field trial in Bangladesh, in: *Proceedings of the 12th Joint Conference,* US–Japan Cooperative Medical Science Program Cholera Panel, Symposium on Cholera, Sapporo, pp. 276–285, National Institute of Health, Tokyo, 1976.

36. DE MOOR, C. E., A non-haemolytic El Tor vibrio as the cause of an outbreak of paracholera in West New Guinea—The El Tor problem and pandemic paracholera in the West Pacific, *Trop. Geogr. Med.* **15:**97–107 (1963).

37. DEWITT, W. E., GANGAROSA, E. J., HUQ, I., AND ZARIFI, A., Holding media for the transport of *Vibrio cholerae* from field to laboratory, *Am. J. Trop. Med. Hyg.* **20:**685–688 (1971).

38. DIZON, J. J., ALVERO, M. G., JOSEPH, P. R., TAMAYO, J. F., MOSLEY, W. H., AND HENDERSON, D. A., Studies of cholera El Tor in the Philippines. 1. Characteristics of cholera El Tor in Negros Occidental province, November 1961 to September 1962, *Bull. WHO* **33:**627–636 (1965).

39. EVANS, A. S., Pettenkofer revisited: The life and contributions of Max von Pettenkofer (1818–1902), *Yale J. Biol. Med.* **46:**161–176 (1973).

40. EVANS, A. S., Personal communication.

41. FINKELSTEIN, R. A., Cholera, *CRC Crit. Rev. Microbiol.* **2:**553–623 (1973).

42. FINKELSTEIN, R. A., AND PETERSON, J. W., *In vitro* detection of antibody to cholera enterotoxin in cholera patients and laboratory animals, *Infect. Immun.* **1:**21–29 (1970).

43. FRETER, R., Studies of the mechanism of action of intestinal antibody in experimental cholera, *Tex. Rep. Biol. Med.* **27**:299–316 (1969).

44. FRETER, R., DE, S. P., MONDAL, A., SHRIVASTAVA, L., AND SUNDERMAN, F. W., JR., Coproantibody and serum antibody in cholera patients, *J. Infect. Dis.* **115**:83–87 (1965).

45. FUKUMI, H., Detection of cholera vibrio at quarantine stations and its significance for quarantine against cholera, in: *Proceedings of the 12th Joint Conference,* US–Japan Cooperative Medical Science Program Cholera Panel, Symposium on Cholera, Sapporo, pp. 55–62, National Institute of Health, Tokyo, 1976.

46. GANGAROSA, E. J., BEISEL, W. R., BENYAJATI, C., SPRINZ, H., AND PIYARATIN, P., The nature of the gastrointestinal lesion in Asiatic cholera and its relation to pathogenesis: A biopsy study, *Am. J. Trop. Med. Hyg.* **9**:125–135 (1960).

47. GANGAROSA, E. J., BENNETT, J. V., AND BORING, J. R., III, Differentiation between *Vibrio cholerae* and *Vibrio cholerae* biotype El Tor by the polymyxin B disc test: Comparative results with TCBS, Monsur's, Mueller–Hinton and nutrient agar media, *Bull. WHO* **35**:987–990 (1967).

48. GARDNER, A. O., AND VENKATRAMAN, K. V., The antigens of the cholera group of vibrios, *J. Hyg.* **35**:262–282 (1935).

49. GILL, D. M., AND KING, C. A., The mechanism of action of cholera toxin in pigeon erythrocyte lysates, *J. Biol. Chem.* **250**:6424–6432 (1975).

50. GITELSON, S., Gastrectomy, achlorhydria and cholera, *Isr. J. Med. Sci.* **7**:663–667 (1971).

51. GLASS, R. I., BECKER, S., HUQ, M. I., STOLL, B. J., KHAN, M. U., MERSON, M. H., LEE, J. V., AND BLACK, R. E., Endemic cholera in rural Bangladesh, 1966–1980, *Am. J. Epidemiol.* **116**:959–970 (1982).

52. GLASS, R. I., HOLMGREN, J., HALEY, C. E., KHAN, M. R., SVENNERHOLM, A.-M., STOLL, B. J., ELAYET HOSSAIN, K. M., BLACK, R. E., YUNUS, M., AND BARUA, D., Predisposition for cholera of individuals with O blood group, *Am. J. Epidemiol.* **121**:791–796 (1985).

53. GLASS, R. I., SVENNERHOLM, A.-M., KHAN, M. R., HUDA, S., HUQ, M. I., AND HOLMGREN, J., Seroepidemiological studies of El Tor cholera in Bangladesh: Association of serum antibody levels with protection, *J. Infect. Dis.* **51**:236–242 (1985).

54. GOH, K. T., LAM, S., KUMARAPATHY, S., AND TAN, J. L., A common source foodborne outbreak of cholera in Singapore, *Int. J. Epidemiol.* **13**:210–215 (1984).

55. GOODNER, K., SMITH, H. L., JR., AND STEMPEN, H., Serologic diagnosis of cholera, *J. Albert Einstein Med. Cent.* **8**:143–147 (1960).

56. GOTSCHLICH, F., Uber Cholera und Cholera-ähnliche Vibrionen unter den aus Mekka zurückkehrenden Pilgern, *Z. Hyg. Infektionskr.* **53**:281 (1906).

57. GREENOUGH, W. B., III, BENENSON, A. S., AND ISLAM, M. R., Experience in darkfield examination of stools from diarrheal patients, in: *Proceedings of the Cholera Research Symposium,* PHS Publ. 1328, pp. 56–58, U.S. Government Printing Office, Washington, D.C., 1965.

58. HARVEY, R. M., ENSON, Y., LEWIS, M. L., GREENOUGH, W. B., III, ALLY, K. M., AND PANNO, R. A., Hemodynamic studies on cholera: Effects of hypovolemia and acidosis, *Circulation* **37**:709–729 (1968).

59. HIRSCHHORN, N., ALLAUDDIN CHOWDHURY, A. K. M., AND LINDENBAUM, J., Cholera in pregnant women, *Lancet* **1**:1230–1232 (1969).

60. HOLMGREN, J., AND SVENNERHOLM, A.-M., Enzyme-linked immunoabsorbent assays for cholera serology, *Infect. Immun.* **7**:759–763 (1973).

61. HOLMGREN, J., LONNROTH, I., AND SVENNERHOLM, A., Tissue receptor for cholera exotoxin: Postulated structure from studies with G_{M1} ganglioside and related glycolipids, *Infect. Immun.* **8**:208–214 (1973).

62. HOLMGREN, J., SVENNERHOLM, A., LONNROTH, I., FALL-PERSSON, M., MARKMAN, B., AND LUNDBECK, H., Development of improved cholera vaccine based on subunit toxoid, *Nature* **269**:602–604 (1977).

63. HONDA, T., AND FINKELSTEIN, R. A., Selection and characteristics of a *Vibrio cholerae* mutant lacking the A (ADP-ribosylating) portion of the cholera enterotoxin, *Proc. Natl. Acad. Sci. USA* **76**:2052–2056 (1979).

64. HORNICK, R. B., MUSIC, S. I., WENZEL, R., CASH, R., LIBONATI, J. P., SNYDER, M. J., AND WOODWARD, T. E., The Broad Street pump revisited: Response of volunteers to ingested cholera vibrios, *Bull. N.Y. Acad. Med.* **47**:1181–1191 (1971).

65. HUBER, G. S., The significance of the number of vibrios seen in rice-water stools, in: *Proceedings of the Cholera Research Symposium,* Honolulu, PHS Publ. 1328, pp. 41–45, U.S. Government Printing Office, Washington, D.C., 1965.

66. KAMAL, A. M., Outbreak of gastro-enteritis by nonagglutinable (NAG) vibrios in the Republic of Sudan, Oct.–Nov. 1968, *J. Egypt. Public Health Assoc.* **46**:125–159 (1971).

67. KAPER, J., LOCKMAN, H., COLWELL, R. R., AND JOSEPH, S. W., Ecology, serology, and enterotoxin production of *Vibrio cholerae* in Chesapeake Bay, *Appl. Environ. Microbiol.* **37**:91–103 (1979).

68. KAUFFMANN, F., On the serology of the *Vibrio cholerae, Acta Pathol. Microbiol. Scand.* **27**:283–299 (1950).

69. KHAN, A. Q., Role of carriers in the intrafamilial spread of cholera, *Lancet* **1**:245–246 (1967).

70. KHAN, M. U., AND SHAHIDULLAH, M., Pattern of intrafamilial spread of cholera, in: *Proceedings of the 14th Joint Conference,* US–Japan Cooperative Medical Science Program Cholera Panel, Symposium on Cholera, Karatsu, pp. 30–34, National Institute of Health, Tokyo, 1978.

71. KHAN, M. U., SHAHIDULLAH, M., AHMED, W. U., PURIFICATION, D., AND KHAN, M. A., The eltor cholera epidemic in Dhaka in 1974 and 1975, *Bull. WHO* **61**:653–659 (1983).

72. LEVINE, M. M., NALIN, D. R., CRAIG, J. P., HOOVER, D., BERGQUIST, E. J., WATERMAN, D., HOLLEY, P., LIBONATI, J. P., HORNICK, R. B., AND PIERCE, N. F., Immunity to

cholera, in: *Proceedings of the 13th Joint Conference, US–Japan Cooperative Medical Science Program Cholera Panel, Symposium on Cholera, 1977, Atlanta, pp. 308–334, DHEW Publ. (NIH) 78-1590, 1978.

73. LINDENBAUM, J., GREENOUGH, W. B., III, BENENSON, A. S., OSEASOHN, R., RIZVI, S., AND SAAD, A., Non-vibrio cholera, *Lancet* **1**:1081–1083 (1965).

74. LINDENBAUM, J., AKBAR, R., GORDON, R. S., JR., GREENOUGH, W. B., III, HIRSCHHORN, N., AND ISLAM, M. R., Cholera in children, *Lancet* **1**:1066–1068 (1966).

75. LONGMATE, N., *King Cholera: The Biography of a Disease*, p. 49, Hamish Hamilton, London, 1966.

76. MARTIN, A. R., MOSLEY, W. H., BISWAS SAU, B., AHMED, A., AND HUQ, I., Epidemiologic analysis of endemic cholera in urban East Pakistan, 1964–1966, *Am. J. Epidemiol.* **89**:572–582 (1969).

77. MCCORMACK, W. M., CHOWDHURY, A. M., JAHANGIR, N., FARIDUDDIN AHMED, A. B., AND MOSLEY, W. H., Tetracycline prophylaxis in families of cholera patients, *Bull. WHO* **38**:787–792 (1968).

78. MCCORMACK, W. M., SHAFIQUL ISLAM, M., FAHIMUDDIN, M., AND MOSLEY, W. H., A community study of inapparent cholera infections. *Am. J. Epidemiol.* **89**:658–664 (1969).

79. MCCORMACK, W. M., DEWITT, W. E., BAILEY, P. E., MORRIS, G. K., SOEHARJONO, P., AND GANGAROSA, E. J., Evaluation of thiosulfate–citrate–bile salts—sucrose agar, a selective medium for the isolation of *Vibrio cholerae* and other pathogenic vibrios, *J. Infect. Dis.* **129**:497–500 (1974).

80. MCINTYRE, O. R., AND FEELEY, J. C., Passive serum protection of the infant rabbit against experimental cholera, *J. Infect. Dis.* **114**:468–465 (1964).

81. MCINTYRE, O. R., FEELEY, J. C., GREENOUGH, W. B., III, BENENSON, A. S., HASSAN, S. I., AND SAAD, A., Diarrhea caused by non-cholera vibrios, *Am. J. Trop. Med. Hyg.* **14**:412–418 (1969).

82. MHALU, F. S., MMARI, P. W., AND IJUMBA, J., Rapid emergence of El Tor *Vibrio cholerae* resistant to antimicrobial agents during first six months of fourth cholera epidemic in Tanzania, *Lancet* **1**:345–347 (1979).

83. MONSUR, K. A., Bacteriological diagnosis of cholera under field conditions, *Bull. WHO* **28**:387–389 (1963).

84. MONSUR, K. A., RIZVI, S., AND AHMED, S. Z., Limitations of current methods of laboratory diagnosis of cholera, in: *Proceedings of the Cholera Research Symposium*, Honolulu, pp. 38–40, PHS Publ. 1328, U.S. Government Printing Office, Washington, D.C., 1965.

85. MOSLEY, W. H., BENENSON, A. S., AND BARUI, R., A serological survey for cholera antibodies in rural East Pakistan. 1. The distribution of antibody in the control population of a cholera-vaccine field-trial area and the relation of antibody titre to the pattern of endemic cholera, *Bull. WHO* **38**:327–334 (1968).

86. MOSLEY, W. H., AZIZ, K. M. A., MIZANUR RAHMAN, A. S. M., ALAUDDIN CHOWDHURY, A. K. M., AND AHMED, A., Field trials of monovalent Ogawa and Inaba cholera vaccines

in rural Bangladesh—Three years of observation, *Bull, WHO* **49**:381–387 (1973).

87. Pakistan–SEATO Cholera Research Laboratory, Cholera in East Pakistan families, 1962–1963, *Bull. WHO* **32**:205–209 (1965).

88. PAVIA, A. T., CAMPBELL, J. F., BLAKE, P. A., SMITH, J. D., MCKINLEY, T. W., AND MARTIN, D. L., Cholera from raw oysters shipped interstate, *J. Am. Med. Assoc.* **258**:2374 (1987).

89. PIERCE, N. F., The role of antigen form and function in the primary and secondary intestinal immune responses to cholera toxin and toxoid in rats, *J. Exp. Med.* **148**:195–206 (1978).

90. PIERCE, N. F., KANIECKI, E. A., AND NORTHRUP, R. S., Protection against experimental cholera by antitoxin, *J. Infect. Dis.* **126**:606–616 (1972).

91. PIERCE, N. F., CASH, R. A., HIRSCHHORN, N., MAHALANABIS, D., NALIN, D. L., RAHMAN, M. M., AND SACK, R. B., Management of cholera and other acute diarrheas in adults and children, in: *Principles and Practice of Cholera*, Public Health Papers No. 40 (revised), pp. 61–75, WHO, Geneva, 1978.

92. POLLITZER, R., Cholera, *WHO Monogr. Ser.* **43**:11–49 (1959).

93. POLLITZER, R., Cholera, *WHO Monogr. Ser.* **43**:267–270 (1959).

94. RONDLE, C. J. M., RAMESH, B., KRAHN, J. B., AND SHERRIFF, R., Cholera: Possible infection from aircraft effluent, *J. Hyg.* **81**:361–371 (1978).

95. SACK, R. B., AND BARUA, D., The fluorescent antibody technique in the direct examination of cholera stool, in: *Proceedings of the Cholera Research Symposium*, Honolulu, pp. 50–56, PHS Publ. 1328, U.S. Government Printing Office, Washington, D.C., 1965.

96. SANYAL, S. C., SINGH, S. J., TIWARI, I. C., SEN, P. C., MARWAH, S. M., HAZARIKA, U. R., SINGH, H., SHIMADA, T., AND SAKAZAKI, R., Role of household animals in maintenance of cholera infection in a community, *J. Infect. Dis.* **130**:575–579 (1974).

97. SCHRANK, G. D., AND VERWEY, W. F., Distribution of cholera organisms in experimental *Vibrio cholerae* infections: Proposed mechanisms of pathogenesis and antibacterial immunity, *Infect. Immun.* **13**:195–203 (1976).

98. SMITH, H. L., AND GOODNER, K., Detection of bacterial gelatinases by gelatin–agar plate methods, *J. Bacteriol.* **76**:662–665 (1958).

99. SNOW, J., *On the Mode of Communication of Cholera*, John Churchill, London, 1849.

100. SNOW, J., *On the Mode of Communication of Cholera*, 2nd ed., "much enlarged," John Churchill, London, 1855; reprinted in: *Snow on Cholera* (being a reprint of two papers by John Snow, M.D.) (W. H. FROST, ed.), pp. 1–139, Commonwealth Fund, New York, 1936.

101. SOMMER, A., AND MOSLEY, W. H., Ineffectiveness of cholera vaccination as an epidemic control measure, *Lancet* **1**:1232–1235 (1973).

102. SVENNERHOLM, A. M., HANSON, L. A., HOLMGREN, J., LINDBLAD, B. S., NILSSON, B., AND QUERESHI, F., Different secretory immunoglobulin A antibody responses to cholera vaccination in Swedish and Pakistani women, *Infect. Immun.* **30:**427–430 (1980).

103. TAMAYO, J. F., MOSLEY, W. H., ALVERO, M. G., JOSEPH, P. R., GOMEZ, C. Z., MONTAGUE, T., DIZON, J. J., AND HENDERSON, D. A., Studies of cholera El Tor in the Philippines. 3. Transmission of infection among household contacts of cholera patients, *Bull. WHO* **33:**645–649 (1965).

104. VASIL, M. L., HOLMES, R. K., AND FINKELSTEIN, R. A., Conjugal transfer of a chromosomal gene determining production of enterotoxin in *Vibrio cholerae, Science* **187:**849–850 (1975).

105. WALLACE, C. K., CARPENTER, C. C. J., MITRA, P. P., SACK, R. B., KHANDRA, S. R., WERNER, A. S., DUFFY, T. P., OLEINICK, A., AND LEWIS, G. W., Classical and El Tor cholera: A clinical comparison, *Br. Med. J.* **2:**447–449 (1966).

106. WEISSMAN, J. B., DEWITT, W. E., THOMPSON, J., MUCHNICK, C. N., PORTNOY, B. L., FEELEY, J. C., AND GANGAROSA, E. J., A case of cholera in Texas, 1973, *Am. J. Epidemiol.* **100:**487–498 (1974).

107. World Health Organization, Cholera in 1977, *Weekly Epidemiol. Rec.* **53:**117–118 (1978).

108. World Health Organization, Prompt control of a cholera epidemic in Maldives, *WHO Chron.* **33:**187–188 (1979).

109. World Health Organization, Cholera in 1978, *Weekly Epidemiol. Rec.* **54:**129–131 (1979).

110. World Health Organization, Cholera surveillance—Brazil, *Weekly Epidemiol. Rec.* **54:**257 (1979).

111. World Health Organization, Cholera surveillance—Rapid emergence of resistant *Vibrio cholerae* strains, *Weekly Epidemiol. Rec.* **54:**333–334 (1979).

112. World Health Organization, Cholera surveillance, *Weekly Epidemiol. Rec.* **55:**93–94 (1980).

113. World Health Organization, Cholera surveillance—Italy, *Weekly Epidemiol. Rec.* **55:**15 (1980).

114. World Health Organization, Cholera in 1988, *Weekly Epidemiol. Rec.* **64:**141–148 (1989).

115. WOODWARD, W. E., Cholera reinfection in man, *J. Infect. Dis.* **123:**61–66 (1971).

116. YEN, C. H., A recent study of cholera with reference to an outbreak in Taiwan in 1962, *Bull. WHO* **30:**811–825 (1964).

12. Suggested Reading

CRAIG, J. P., Cholera toxins, in: *Microbiol Toxins,* Volume 2A, pp. 189–254, Academic Press, New York, 1971.

FINKELSTEIN, R. A., Cholera, *CRC Crit. Rev. Microbiol.* **2:**553–623 (1973).

POLLITZER, R., Cholera, *WHO Monogr. Ser.* **43:**11–49 (1959).

SNOW, J., *On the Mode of Communication of Cholera,* 2nd ed., "much enlarged," John Churchill, London, 1855, in: *Snow on Cholera* (being a reprint of two papers by John Snow, M.D.) (W. H. FROST, ed.), pp. 1–139, Commonwealth Fund, New York, 1936.

VAN HEYNINGEN, W. E., AND SEAL, J. R., *Cholera: The American Scientific Experience, 1947–1980,* Westview Press, Boulder, Colo., 1983.

World Health Organization, *Principles and Practice of Cholera Control,* WHO Public Health Papers No. 40, WHO, Geneva, 1978.

CHAPTER 11

Diphtheria

Paul F. Wehrle

1. Introduction

Diphtheria is an acute infectious and communicable disease involving primarily the tonsils, pharynx, larynx, or nose, and occasionally other mucous membranes or skin. A false membrane is formed in one or more of these locations. This is the site of production of the diphtheria toxin, which is responsible for the general symptomatology and subsequent damage of many organs, including cardiac and central nervous system tissue. Although the incidence of the disease has declined substantially with improved immunization, the continuing occurrence of cases in most countries and the relatively high case-fatality ratios of 5–10% emphasize its importance.

2. Historical Background

Although presumably recognized as a clinical entity by Hippocrates (4th century B.C.), it is mentioned by another name in the Babylonian Talmud (A.D. 352–427). Aretaeus (2nd or 3rd century A.D.) clearly described it as "ulcera Syriaca." Aetius (6th century A.D.) provided the first clear description of epidemic diphtheria and mentioned palatal paralysis as a sequel. The chronicles of early monks contained descriptions of the epidemics of A.D. 856, 1004, and 1039. The characteristic membrane was noted by Baillou in

his description of an epidemic in Paris in 1576. He suggested tracheotomy, but did not use the procedure. Additionally, clinical descriptions were left by Tulp (1640), Fothergill (1748), and Huxham (1757). Samuel Bard of New York (1771) provided a classic description of diphtheria, entitled *Angina Suffocativa*. Bretonneau, in an important monograph, gave the disease its present name (1826). He described the typical clinical characteristics more completely and differentiated it from scarlatinal angina and spasmodic croup. Klebs (1883) first saw the diphtheria bacillus and associated it with the disease, and Loeffler (1884) first cultivated the organism on artificial media, established the causal relationship of the diphtheria bacillus, differentiating it from pseudodiphtheritic organisms, and identified asymptomatic infections (carriers) among healthy children. Roux and Yersin (1888) demonstrated that tissue damage was produced by an extracellular heat-labile toxin produced by the bacteria and transported to various sites through the circulation. Later, von Behring (1890–1893) showed that serum obtained from animals immunized against diphtheria toxin could be used for the prevention and treatment of the disease. Park contributed to the information on the bacteriology and serology of diphtheria (1892–1906) and with Beebe (1893) clearly documented the asymptomatic carrier state suggested earlier by Loeffler. The Schick test for susceptibility was introduced in 1913. In 1951, Freeman described the role of bacteriophage in toxigenicity. Pappenheimer, Gill, and associates (1952–1973) have clarified the molecular mechanisms involved in the pathogenesis of the disease. The comparatively early development of the information concerning the epidemiology, etiology, and pathogenesis of this disease has been helpful in guiding research in other infectious-disease models.[16]

Paul F. Wehrle · Department of Pediatrics, University of Southern California and Los Angeles County–University of Southern California Medical Center, Los Angeles, California 90033.

3. Methodology

The control of diphtheria is dependent on prompt and accurate recognition of individual cases and deaths, identification and treatment of carriers of virulent organisms, and complete and timely reporting to appropriate health authorities. In the United States, diphtheria is considered a Class 2 disease with case reports regularly required by all health jurisdictions wherever the disease occurs. Specifically, a case report must be sent to local health authorities by telephone, telegraph, or other rapid means. These are then forwarded to the next superior health jurisdiction weekly by mail, except that the first recognized case in an area or the first case outside the limits of a known affected local area is to be reported by telegraph.

3.1. Sources of Mortality Data

The diphtheria case-fatality ratios with pharyngeal and respiratory-system involvement have approximated 10% for many years. Since deaths are customarily reported more completely than are cases, this provides substantial confidence that case reporting is reasonably complete. Reporting has been remarkably consistent for many years for both cases and deaths due to diphtheria.[8,10]

3.2. Sources of Morbidity Data

Cases of diphtheria reported under the Class 2 requirements are tabulated weekly in the *Morbidity and Mortality Weekly Report* published by the Centers for Disease Control (CDC), Atlanta, Georgia.[9] This report, with a circulation in excess of 78,000, is mailed regularly to those physicians and health jurisdictions requesting this service. Additionally, an annual summary including all cases and deaths reported during each calendar year is compiled in September of the following year and is similarly forwarded to all individuals requesting such information.[11]

3.3. Surveys

Detailed analyses of the prevalence of diphtheria in particular population groups or geographic locations, or unusual trends in the type of organisms involved or the site of disease, are analyzed by the staff of the CDC. These data are published periodically in *Diphtheria Surveillance* as important developments occur. The most recent report, No. 12, provides a summary of the 1971–1975 experience and was published in July 1978.[10]

Few surveys, by either Schick test or serology, have been conducted during recent years. Earlier data from Africa and India suggested that conversion to Schick-negative status occurred earlier in tropical climates and was often associated with increased prevalence of the cutaneous form of the disease. Surveys of military-recruit populations within the United States by Worchester and Cheever,[38] confirmed a decade later by Liao in 1954, indicate that Schick negativity without prior immunization was seen more frequently in the southern United States. Widespread immunization, as is now practiced in virtually all countries, has greatly diminished the value of such surveys.

3.4. Laboratory Diagnosis

Corynebacterium diphtheriae is an obligate aerobe that grows rapidly on the surface of many types of artificial media. The organisms are club-shaped gram-positive nonspore-bearing rods, and are without flagellae or capsules. The bacteria are somewhat tapered and vary from 2 to 6 μm in length and from 0.5 to 1.0 μm in diameter. On stained smears from the pharynx or after being cultured, the organisms may form characteristic "Chinese letter" figures. Considerable experience is required for interpretation of direct examination of pharyngeal smears, and even in the best of hands, direct examination is not a substitute for culture and additional tests as noted. After cultivation on blood agar or Loeffler's medium, metachromatic granules are seen after methylene blue or toluidine blue staining.

3.4.1. Isolation and Identification of *C. diphtheriae*. For primary isolation, blood agar, Loeffler's coagulated serum medium, or blood or chocolate agar plates with potassium tellurite may be used. The use of tellurite provides a selective medium, since the growth of normal flora is inhibited. The characteristic rough, dry, yellow or gray colonies (blood agar) or black colonies (tellurite) of *C. diphtheriae* appear within 12–24 h, although occasionally additional incubation is required. Some other organisms from the respiratory tract also form black colonies with tellurite, so appropriately stained smears from individual colonies are required for presumptive identification. Fluorescent-antibody techniques have proven more accurate for immediate diagnosis than direct examination of properly stained preparations,[37] although specially prepared reagents are required.[1]

Diphtheria bacilli ferment glucose and maltose, producing acid but not gas. A rapid-fermentation technique originally developed for *Neisseria* may be used. Thus, it is possible to readily distinguish *C. diphtheriae* from other corynebacteria that may be present in suspected diphtheritic lesions. The addition of catalase (+) and urease (−) tests will provide additional assurance of identity. On the basis of colony growth and other characteristics, the organisms have been classified as gravis, mitis, intermedius, and minimus. The relative pathogenicity of these types, and that of smooth or rough strains, may not be as important as believed earlier in toxin production, epidemiological behavior, or specific clinical forms of the disease following infection in man, although biotype gravis is associated more frequently with fatal illness.[27]

Since only those strains of *C. diphtheriae* that are infected (lysogenic) with beta-prophage or a related phage carrying the *tox* gene produce diphtheria toxin, the presence of an organism morphologically consistent with *C. diphtheriae* is not necessarily an indication that it is the cause of the clinical syndrome observed. Under certain nutritional conditions and for certain strains (PW8) of the organism, toxin may represent more than 5% of the total bacterial protein synthesized and more than 75% of the total protein secreted by the organisms. This provides an index of the pathogenicity of the specific strain of *C. diphtheriae* identified, although clinical disease and death have been associated with nontoxigenic strains.[11,31]

After organisms with the colony and individual morphology consistent with *C. diphtheriae* have been identified and the typical fermentation characteristics evaluated, the presence of toxin may be determined by animal inoculation or gel-diffusion tests. In the former, 0.1 ml of a heavy suspension of the bacilli washed from the Loeffler slant is inoculated intradermally into the shaved side of a guinea pig. After 4 h, the animal is given 500 U diphtheria antitoxin intraperiotoneally, and 30 min later a second sample of the test suspension is injected intradermally at a separate site. If toxigenic *C. diphtheriae* are present, the characteristic necrotic lesions should appear within 48–72 h. A modification of this test has been used, employing 1.0 ml of the bacterial suspension in each of two animals, one protected in advance with antitoxin, and, as end point, death of the unprotected animal in 48–72 h. In some laboratories, rabbits are preferred for the intradermal test.

An alternate technique for toxin demonstration is a modification of the agar gel-diffusion test, utilizing a petri plate of peptone–maltose–lactate agar with 20% horse serum. A strip of filter paper moistened with antitoxin is placed on the agar surface, and test and control inocula are streaked perpendicular to and crossing the filter-paper strip. The presence of toxin production can be readily identified by thin lines of precipitate as in other precipitin-in-gel test techniques. The antitoxin utilized must be highly purified and free from nonspecific cross-reactive substances; false-negative reactions have been a problem in some laboratories.

A significant proportion of reported cases are associated with infection by nontoxigenic organisms, regardless of laboratory techniques utilized. A greater proportion of cutaneous (145 of 431) than of fatal respiratory (2 of 27) cases were presumably caused by this biotype.[11]

3.4.2. Serological and Immunological Diagnostic Methods. The Schick test was employed frequently in the past for determining susceptibility of the individual to the toxin. The test was accomplished by injecting intradermally $\frac{1}{50}$ guinea pig minimum lethal dose into the volar surface of the forearm; suitable heat-inactivated toxin control material was inoculated into the opposite forearm. Erythema, and sometimes severe local reactions reaching a peak at 48–72 h, indicated susceptibility. Since this test could not be quantitated, and since it represented an uncomfortable and at times inaccurate estimate, the determination of susceptibility is now accomplished by serological techniques. These include indirect hemagglutination-inhibition and radioimmunoassay techniques.[25,29] Of these, the latter have been used most frequently and are remarkably accurate.[29]

Serological tests are not necessary for the confirmation of diphtheria in the individual patient, but are useful to evaluate host response after various immunization routines and to answer specific epidemiological questions.

4. Biological Characteristics of the Organism

C. diphtheriae organisms are susceptible to drying, heat, and sunlight and do not remain viable in the environment for more than a few hours or days at most. Although several species of animals are susceptible to the toxin, and experimental infections can be induced, the occurrence of naturally acquired disease appears to be restricted to man. This biological characteristic is of particular interest, since the *tox* gene stimulates the production of an enzyme specific for cells of higher forms of life, while produced and maintained in a bacterial host.[31] The specific mode of action of the toxin has been described in mammalian cell cultures and tissue extracts.[17,30]

Actually, both clinical and epidemiological data suggest that the production of toxin may be an important survival mechanism for *C. diphtheriae*.[14] Local tissue destruction at the site of pseudomembrane formation appears to favor bacterial multiplication. The abundance of organisms would logically lead to greater ease of transmission on contact, particularly among children and those living in close quarters. Greater spread has been observed from clinical cases than from those with inapparent or silent carrier states.

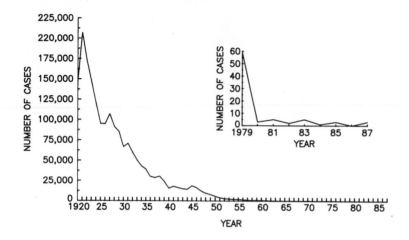

Figure 1. Diphtheria: reported cases, United States, 1920–1987.

In addition to the greater ease of transmission from clinical cases, it has become apparent that carriage of virulent organisms is less prevalent among well-immunized populations, thus providing additional evidence that local tissue damage may favor transmission of this infection. It should be noted that both cases and carriers may be found in comparatively well-immunized populations.

5. Descriptive Epidemiology

In the United States during the last several decades, the trend of diphtheria cases and deaths has been progressively downward. When deviations from this trend have occurred, they have usually reflected unusual concentrations of cases in selected and poorly immunized groups within the total populations.

5.1. Prevalence and Incidence

In 1920, the annual incidence of clinical cases of diphtheria approached 200/100,000 population, and the case-fatality ratio was between 15 and 20/100,000 (see Fig. 1). This ratio of cases to deaths has continued with decreasing numbers of cases.[12,13,27] In 1972, the incidence had declined to 0.07/100,000 population and the case-fatality ratio to 0.01/100,000. Since 1972, the incidence has continued downward, although the case-fatality ratio has declined even more rapidly. The earlier ratios approximating 10% have fallen to as low as 1.6% in 1975.

This change in the case-fatality ratio reflects a marked increase in the proportion of cases of cutaneous diphtheria with comparatively low mortality rates. For example, in

1975, 101 cases of noncutaneous diphtheria (predominantly respiratory-tract) with 5 deaths were reported, a case-fatality ratio of 4.9%. Additionally, 203 cases of cutaneous diphtheria were also reported with no deaths. Since two thirds of the total cases reported were cutaneous in type, the 5 deaths among the 304 total patients provided the lowest case-fatality ratio, 1.6%, reported to date in the United States.[10]

In the 7-year interval 1980 through 1986, only 19 cases were reported. This represents an average of fewer than 3 cases per year. In 1986 no cases were reported (see Fig. 2).

5.2. Epidemic Behavior and Contagiousness

Since effective immunization has been available, the occurrence of epidemic disease has been limited almost entirely to countries with localized populations with inadequate or no prior immunization. Because individuals with clinical disease may transmit organisms to others with comparative ease, carrier rates of 5 or 10% are frequently seen among close contacts. In contrast, among well-immunized populations, carriage of virulent diphtheria bacilli is uncommon, although both carriers and cases may be found.

5.3. Geographic Distribution

During the period 1971–1975, 30 states and Puerto Rico reported one or more cases of diphtheria. The average annual incidence in the United States was 0.11 case/100,000 population per year. An example of a localized outbreak occurred in the state of Washington, which reported 51% of the cases reported from the entire nation. This state also reported the greatest average annual inci-

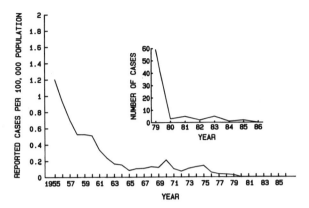

Figure 2. Diphtheria: by year, United States, 1955–1986.

dence (3.55 cases/100,000 population). This sharp localization reflected an unusually great incidence of diphtheria among American Indian populations in the state, and the cases reported among Indians were almost entirely cutaneous diphtheria with extremely low case-fatality ratios.[10]

5.4. Temporal Distribution

In temperate climates, diphtheria is predominantly a disease of the colder months. In the United States, the month of lowest incidence is July, while the most frequent occurrence of both cutaneous and respiratory forms of the disease is from October through April.[8,10]

5.5. Age

Traditionally, diphtheria has been a disease primarily of young children. From 1971 through 1975, 189 of the 751 cases of respiratory and other noncutaneous diphtheria reported in the United States were among children between 5 and 9 years of age. Thus, approximately 25% of all cases occurred within this age group, a pattern in sharp contrast to that reported for the cutaneous form of the disease. In the latter, all but 16 of 428 cases in whom age was reported were 20 years of age or older, and it is of considerable interest to note that 10 of the 16 children with cutaneous diphtheria were American Indians.[10] Reported cases of diphtheria by age for 1978 are indicated in Fig. 3.

5.6. Sex

As is usual with most communicable diseases, there is a tendency toward a predominance among males in both cases

and deaths. For diphtheria between 1971 and 1975 in the United States, 424 of the 751 cases (56.4%) of respiratory diphtheria occurred among males, with the differences between the sex distribution of the cases remaining relatively constant throughout all age groups. This is in sharp contrast to the cutaneous form of the disease, of which 382 of the 428 cases (89.2%) occurred among males. This is of particular interest in that 239 of the 382 males (62.6%) were 40 or more years of age.[10] The relative importance of differences in exposure or immunization in affecting these ratios is unknown.

5.7. Race

There is no known specific racial susceptibility factor. During the last several years, it is apparent that the cases and deaths per 100,000 per year reported among white and black have been remarkably similar. In contrast, the rates for all other races combined are substantially higher. It is of particular interest that this higher rate represented cases among the American Indian populations, a group that represented only 30% of all "other races" in the 1970 census. The rate among these Indians varied from 10 to 100 times the rate observed in other populations. These differences were even more striking when the cutaneous form of the disease was considered.[31]

5.8. Occupation

There are no occupational factors of importance, although substantial numbers of cases of cutaneous diphtheria occurred among unimmunized American soldiers subjected to field conditions in the tropics during World War II.[4]

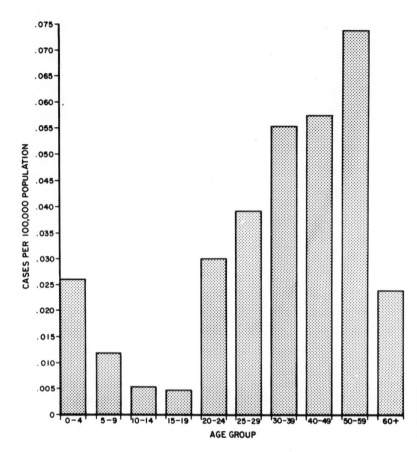

Figure 3. Diphtheria: reported case rates by age group, United States, 1978. Cases of unknown ages are excluded. From the CDC, personal communication.

There were 5700 cases (rate of 0.22/1000) and 67 deaths in the U.S. Army between 1942 and 1945.[24]

5.9. Occurrence in Different Settings

Although diphtheria has been a problem for children and young adults subjected to crowding or unfavorable living conditions, such as the soldiers noted above, improved immunization levels have greatly reduced the impact of crowding and poor personal hygiene. Increased prevalence of carriers of toxigenic strains has been reported in custodial hospitals[19] and in other selected populations.[20] The recent increase in cutaneous diphtheria among crowded and impoverished Indian populations emphasizes the need for greater attention to appropriate immunization as well as to socioeconomic factors.

5.10. Socioeconomic Factors

These are important primarily as they govern the availability of immunization against diphtheria and as they influ-

ence human behavior toward its acceptance.[23,36] Facilities that favor improved personal hygiene may be important in reducing the incidence of cutaneous diphtheria.

5.11. Other Factors

Although nutritional and genetic factors are important in some diseases, they do not appear to have an important influence on diphtheria incidence. The overriding behavioral pattern worthy of note is the willingness to accept appropriate primary and booster immunization at appropriate intervals.

6. Mechanisms and Routes of Transmission

C. diphtheriae organisms are carried normally in the upper respiratory tract, particularly tonsillar tissue, of otherwise healthy carriers. By droplet infection or hand-to-mouth contact, these organisms may be transferred to susceptible individuals. With pseudomembrane formation, the number of organisms appears to increase with greater probability of transfer. The nasal form of the disease may favor spread, due to the mild symptomatology and presence of the organisms in the nose as well as the pharynx.

The route of transmission for cutaneous diphtheria appears to be by droplets and direct physical contact. Patients with cutaneous forms of the disease have been shown to frequently harbor *C. diphtheriae* in the respiratory tract and to have greater spread of infection to other household contacts than among household contacts of patients with respiratory forms of the infection.[2,3] Factors associated with crowding, e.g., shared towels and linens, may also be important in favoring spread of infection, since the organism may survive for several hours or even days.

7. Pathogenesis and Immunity

C. diphtheriae is not an invasive microorganism, and consequently it is dependent on elaboration of toxin to induce local and systemic signs of disease in persons who lack antibody to the toxin. The relative importance of IgG and IgA is unknown. Local trauma, surgical procedures, and abrasions or injuries of the mucous membrane or skin appear to favor replication of these organisms in susceptible individuals, but quantitative data are lacking.[28] The elaboration of toxin at these sites induces local necrosis, leukocyte response, and exudate with the formation of the typical pseudomembrane, which may be easily recognized clinically. This necrotic reaction may progress visibly within hours and often extends beyond the original point of involvement, as in the extension of the pseudomembrane from the tonsil to include the palate and uvula or downward to include the larynx and trachea. *C. diphtheriae* bacteremia does not occur in diphtheria, and involvement of kidney, heart, and neural tissue is dependent on systemic toxemia or circulating toxin in the bloodstream.

8. Patterns of Host Response

Spread of *C. diphtheriae* is dependent on transfer of the infection from healthy carriers to those who then develop subclinical or recognized disease and then to susceptible individuals. A broad spectrum of involvement is seen, ranging from the healthy carrier to virulent organisms through mild and frequently unrecognized disease to typical clinical involvement and fulminant, rapidly fatal illnesses. Fortunately, the majority of infections are either asymptomatic or very mild, and among those clinically recognized, ap-

proximately 10% terminate with fatal consequences. Perhaps due to earlier recognition and consequently less extensive toxin absorption, cutaneous diphtheria is seldom fatal.

Prior to the development of the present effective vaccines, a substantial portion of the population developed immunity to the toxin following pharyngeal carriage of virulent organisms. Cutaneous infections may also be important in providing naturally acquired antibody to the toxin.[5] Small amounts of toxin, insufficient to cause recognizable disease, appear to be absorbed and provide an immunological stimulus without apparent clinical illness. Historically, the Schick test has been used to evaluate the immune status of various populations. Although this test has been supplanted by serological techniques, the waning of passively acquired immunity in the young infant during the early months of life and the increasing proportion of children and adults indicating an immune response to this test provided an index of the relative prevalence of virulent toxin-producing *C. diphtheriae* in various localities.

Similar to the development of immunity following carriage of virulent organisms, clinical disease generally leads to lasting immunity. Since second attacks have been reported, the patient should be immunized during convalescence.

8.1. Clinical Features

Following an incubation period of between 1 and 10 days, averaging 2–5 days, the illness begins gradually with moderate fever, malaise, and sore throat. The temperature rarely exceeds 102°F.

Several clinical types of disease have been recognized. The most frequent is the tonsillar or pharyngeal type, in which the pseudomembrane formation is limited to the tonsil or the tonsil area and adjacent pharynx. More extensive involvement of the upper respiratory region is termed nasopharyngeal diphtheria; here, the membrane extends to involve nasal, tonsillar, and adjacent tissue. In this form, edema involving the cervical lymph glands and adjacent tissues may be extensive, a condition termed bullneck diphtheria. In this form, the toxemia is prominent and the prognosis more guarded.

A hemorrhagic form of the disease with prominent petechiae in the mucous membranes may be seen. The accompanying thrombocytopenia has been correlated with severe myocarditis; in this form of the disease, the outlook is grave.

The laryngeal involvement may be seen as a primary disease (diphtheritic croup) or in combination with tonsillar and tracheobronchial involvement. With involvement of the larynx and lower airways, potential obstruction of these passages poses an additional clinical problem. While tracheotomy is lifesaving with laryngeal involvement, it may be difficult or impossible to assure an adequate airway when extensive involvement of the trachea and bronchi is present.[21,28]

Additionally, a nasal form of the disease has been recognized. Since these patients have milder systemic symptoms, the nasal discharge is infectious, and recognition and proper treatment may be delayed, this form may be more hazardous to household and other contacts.

Finally, cutaneous or wound diphtheria has been recognized in tropical climates, but was an infrequent problem until recently in the United States. In 1971–1975 inclusive, 30% of all cases of diphtheria reported were of the cutaneous variety. In this form, the necrotic pseudomembrane formation occurs on the skin, often at the site of prior trauma or infection by other microorganisms, and may involve any area of the skin, including the genital region, ears, and lower extremities.

8.2. Diagnosis

The diagnosis is suspected clinically by the appearance of the necrotic pseudomembrane in the respiratory tract or on the skin surface. A history of diphtheria among contacts, lack of prior immunization, and poor hygienic conditions (as in "skid-row" populations) should increase the need to consider this disease.

Confirmation is by recovery of *C. diphtheriae* in culture, including fermentation and catalase tests followed by appropriate tests for toxin formation. The presence of a local lesion and the recovery of toxigenic organisms provides confirmation. Although historically the diagnosis was confirmed by direct examination of smears from the lesions after appropriate staining with methylene blue or toluidine blue, the technique is not sufficiently accurate, even when performed by experienced personnel, except possibly to confirm a presumptive clinical diagnosis. If diphtheria is seriously suspected, appropriate antitoxin and antibiotic therapy must be given promptly, since there is evidence that delay of therapy substantially increases the chance of death.[28] The Schick test during acute and convalescent stages is no longer used, and serological confirmation of the disease is cumbersome and unnecessary.

8.3. Differential Diagnosis

Conditions included in the differential diagnosis of diphtheria include streptoccoal pharyngitis and tonsillitis, infectious mononucleosis, adenovirus infections, and peritonsillar abscess. In each, the acute inflammatory response in the tonsillar area, together with substantial exudate, may prove confusing. A foreign body in the nose, a frequent problem in young children, can closely simulate nasal diphtheria. The cutaneous form of diphtheria may resemble impetigo, tinea, or other fungal infections or cutaneous infections with atypical acid-fast bacilli. Laryngeal and tracheal diphtheria clinically resembles croup or tracheobronchitis due to other causes. Inspection of the larynx is helpful in evaluating this syndrome.

Although other characteristics of the aforenamed conditions are often helpful to the clinician in reaching the correct diagnosis, frequently even experienced clinicians must rely on appropriate cultures to exclude diphtheria. If diphtheria is a serious possibility, particularly if the patient appears toxic and has not been immunized previously, and particularly if cases of diphtheria are known in the vicinity, antitoxin should be given and antibiotic therapy instituted promptly.

It should be noted that use of equine antitoxin introduces another variable in the differential diagnosis, since in addition to the initial risk of anaphylaxis, serum sickness can be expected in at least 10% of recipients during the 2 weeks following antitoxin administration. The resulting fever, urticaria, adenopathy, and positive heterophil reaction may prove confusing to the inexperienced clinician.

9. Therapy

Treatment includes the prompt administration of antitoxin in doses of 30,000 to a maximum of 80,000 U. A useful guide for antitoxin dosage calculation is 10,000 U per infected organ per day of illness prior to treatment. The calculated quantity of antitoxin should be given as a single dose. The weight or age of the patient is disregarded in determining the dose to be given. The intravenous route is preferred, and a 10% solution of antitoxin in isotonic saline is infused over 1 h after appropriate skin tests for hypersensitivity have been completed.

Although antibiotics have no effect on toxin already elaborated or absorbed, either erythromycin or parenteral penicillin therapy should be administered, to eradicate the organism as rapidly as possible and reduce the hazard to those attending the patient. General supportive therapy must be provided, with particular attention to the airway in those patients with laryngeal or tracheal involvement.[21] Strict isolation is required until respiratory secretions or skin lesions are no longer infectious. Masks and gowns are required for hospital personnel, and hand-washing is mandatory after attending patients.

Major complications of clinical importance include thrombocytopenia, myocarditis, and cranial- or peripheral-nerve involvement.[22,26,28,32] The thrombocytopenia reflects significant systemic toxin absorption and appears to represent platelet destruction. It is most frequently seen with bullneck disease and in patients with delayed treatment. Petechiae and significant bleeding occur, and replacement therapy with blood or platelets may be required.

Myocarditis frequently follows thrombocytopenia. All patients with diphtheria should have platelet counts and electrocardiograms at daily or more frequent intervals to anticipate coagulation and myocardial conduction defects. Although pacemakers have been used successfully for defects in myocardial conduction, severe direct myocardial involvement is not amenable to such measures. Glucocorticoids have been recommended for myocarditis, but convincing proof of efficacy is not available.

Involvement of cranial or peripheral nerves is customarily seen during convalescence. Generally, pharyngeal paralysis appears earlier, while an illness resembling Guillain–Barré syndrome appears late in convalescence, and its appearance may occasionally be delayed for several weeks. Although function customarily returns ultimately, paralysis may be permanent.

10. Control and Prevention

With present knowledge of the etiology and pathogenesis of this disease, the effectiveness of the currently available vaccines, and present surveillance of diphtheria, excellent control and even virtual eradication has been achieved.

10.1. General Concepts

Diphtheria should be suspected in any patient presenting with a necrotic lesion of the upper respiratory tract or skin surface. This is particularly true in those who have not been immunized or reside in areas where diphtheria has been recognized previously. Nasal and pharyngeal swabs must be obtained and special efforts should be made to secure material from the area adjacent to and beneath the edge of the lesion itself. If *C. diphtheriae* is identified, the case should be promptly reported to health authorities, and nasal and pharyngeal swabs should be obtained from each contact. A search for contacts should proceed promptly prior to the final determination of the toxigenicity of the original isolate. Booster or primary immunization against diphtheria should be provided for all contacts and appropriate

erythromycin or penicillin therapy for those found to be positive. Each contact harboring *C. diphtheriae* should be examined at least daily and the temperature recorded twice daily for 1 week. Although administration of antitoxin in doses of 2000–10,000 U was recommended for all unimmunized persons exposed to diphtheria, and particularly for those harboring virulent organisms, there is little evidence that this reduced the incidence of disease.[15] Daily surveillance to detect the first symptoms and signs of disease with appropriate active immunization and treatment of those found infected is at least equally useful for household contacts of cases and does not result in unnecessary sensitization to horse serum or serum sickness. Should signs and symptoms consistent with diphtheria appear, prompt treatment with antitoxin and appropriate antibiotics should be provided.

Should asymptomatic persons be found on incidental culture, or cultures obtained for another purpose, to harbor a toxigenic strain of *C. diphtheriae*, they should be isolated and treated with appropriate antibiotic therapy for at least 10 days. Prior to release from isolation, both cases and carriers must have two successive negative nose and throat cultures obtained at 24-h intervals after antibiotic therapy has been terminated for at least 48 h.

10.2. Antibiotic and Chemotherapeutic Approaches to Prophylaxis

Since both erythromycin and penicillin have been shown to be effective in the eradication of *C. diphtheriae* from both carriers and cases, all persons harboring toxigenic strains of this organism should receive treatment. The course of therapy recommended is from 7 to 10 days. Antimicrobial resistance has not been recognized, and failure to eradicate the organism suggests noncompliance with treatment recommendations. If the organism has not been eradicated after therapy, another course of treatment is indicated. Tonsillectomy to interrupt the carrier state is no longer warranted.

10.3. Immunization

The control and perhaps virtual eradication of diphtheria from a population is dependent on universal immunization against this disease. Several schedules for vaccine administration have been evaluated, and all have provided adequate response.[6] The physical state of the vaccine and the route of administration influence the type and magnitude of antibody response.[7]

Present recommendations include the routine immunization of infants beginning at 4–6 weeks of age with diphtheria–pertussis–tetanus (DPT) vaccine, utilizing three doses at 2-month intervals. An additional dose is administered at 15 months of age, and a final dose of DPT vaccine is recommended at age 6 years. For older children and adults, the adult-type diphtheria–tetanus (Td) antigen should be used.[33–35] This contains substantially less (only 10%) diphtheria toxoid than DPT, thus reducing reactions and the need for prior tests for toxoid reactivity among older children and adults. When given at 10-year intervals, this is adequate to maintain immunity against both tetanus and diphtheria and is the preparation to be used for primary immunization of those older than 6 years of age who have not been previously immunized. Prompt responses to booster doses given 10–33 years after primary immunization have been reported.[18] Present vaccine formulations have been well tolerated with minimal reactions, except for DPT. Here, the reactivity has been almost exclusively attributed to the pertussis component.

11. Unresolved Problems

Since the causative organism has been thoroughly studied by many investigators, the mechanism of toxin production has been elucidated, and the molecular mechanisms involved in the pathogenesis of the disease itself have been described and confirmed, the disease stands as a model for many other health problems.[14] Despite this information and the availability of effective vaccines, diphtheria continues to occur with considerable frequency. In the United States during recent years, the incidence has ranged from 435 clinical cases reported in 1970 to a progressive decline since that time.

Continued surveillance for evidence of clinical disease and for identification of particular populations of high susceptibility such as American Indians is indicated. The major unresolved problem for diphtheria, and for some other diseases against which effective vaccines have been available for years, is how to best motivate the individual to seek and accept immunization and how to motivate the health worker to think immunization. This is particularly true for diseases currently of low or waning incidence.

With improved surveillance and better immunization coverage, even with no improvement in present vaccines, the goal of zero cases of diphtheria per year in the United States was reached in 1986, although it is probable that occasional cases will be reported during the next few years.

ACKNOWLEDGMENTS

Figures 1–3 were kindly provided by Michael B. Gregg, M.D., Centers for Disease Control, Atlanta.

12. References

1. ALLEN, J. C., AND CLUFF, L. E., Identification of toxinogenic *C. diphtheriae* with fluorescent antitoxin: Demonstration of its nonspecificity, *Proc. Soc. Exp. Biol. Med.* **112**:194–199 (1963).

2. BELSEY, M. A., AND LeBLANC, D. R., Skin infections and the epidemiology of diphtheria: Acquisition and persistence of *C. diphtheriae* infections, *Am. J. Epidemiol.* **102**:179–184 (1975).

3. BELSEY, M. A., SINCLAIR, T. M. M., RODER, M. R., AND LeBLANC, D. R., *Corynebacterium diphtheriae* skin infections in Alabama and Louisiana, *N. Engl. J. Med.* **280**:135–141 (1969).

4. BLATTNER, R. J., Epidemiology of diphtheria: Role of cutaneous infection [editorial], *J. Pediatr.* **74**:991–993 (1969).

5. BRAY, J. P., BURT, E. G., POTTER, E. V., POON-KING, T., AND EARLE, D. P., Epidemic diphtheria and skin infections in Trinidad, *J. Infect. Dis.* **126**:34–40 (1972).

6. BROWN, G. C., VOLK, V. K., GOTTSHALL, R. Y., KENDRICK, P. L., AND ANDERSON, H. D., Responses of infants to DTP-P vaccine used in nine injection schedules, *Public Health Rep.* **79**:585–601 (1964).

7. BUTLER, W. T., ROSSEN, R. D., AND WENDE, R. D., Effect of physical state and route of inoculation of diphtheria toxoid on the formation of nasal secretory and serum antibodies in man, *J. Immunol.* **104**:1396–1400 (1970).

8. Centers for Disease Control, *Diphtheria Surveillance*, HEW Publ. (HSM) 72-8087, Report No. 11, 1969–1970 Summary, December 31, 1971.

9. Centers for Disease Control, *Morbidity and Mortality Weekly Report*, HEW Publ. (CDC) 78-8017, Volume 26, No. 49, December 9, 1977.

10. Centers for Disease Control, *Diphtheria Surveillance*, HEW Publ. (CDC) 78-8087, Report No. 12, 1971–1975 Summary, July 1978.

11. Centers for Disease Control, *Morbidity and Mortality Weekly Report, Annual Summary 1977*, HEW Publ. (CDC) 78-8241, Volume 26, No. 53, September 1978.

12. Centers for Disease Control, Leads from the MMWR, diphtheria, tetanus and pertussis: Guidelines for vaccine prophylaxis and other preventive measures, *J. Am. Med. Assoc.* **254**:885–900 (1985).

13. DOEGE, T. C., HEATH, C. W., JR., AND SHERMAN, I. L., Diphtheria in the United States, 1959–1960, *Pediatrics* **30**:194–205 (1962).

14. DOULL, J. A., STOKES, W. R., AND McGINNES, G. F., The

incidence of clinical diphtheria among family contacts subsequent to the discovery of carriers, *J. Prev. Med.* **11**:191–204 (1928).

15. DOWLING, H. F., Diphtheria as a model, *J. Am. Med. Assoc.* **226**:550–553 (1973).
16. ENGLISH, P. C., Diphtheria and theories of infectious disease: Centennial appreciation of the critical role of diphtheria in the history of medicine, *Pediatrics* **76**:1–9 (1985).
17. GILL, D. M., PAPPENHEIMER, A. M., JR., BROWN, R., AND KURNICK, J. T., Studies on the mode of action of diphtheria toxin. VII. Toxin-stimulated hydrolysis of nicotinamide adenine dinucleotide in mammalian cell extracts, *J. Exp. Med.* **129**:1–21 (1969).
18. GOTTLIEB, S., MARTIN, M., MCLAUGHLIN, F. X., PANARO, R. J., LEVINE, L., AND EDSALL, G., Long-term immunity to diphtheria and tetanus: A mathematical model, *Am. J. Epidemiol.* **85**:207–218 (1967).
19. GRAY, R. D., AND JAMES, S. M., Occult diphtheria infection in a hospital for the mentally subnormal, *Lancet* **1**:1105–1106 (1973).
20. HEATH, C. W., JR., AND ZUSMAN, J., An outbreak of diphtheria among skid-row men, *N. Engl. J. Med.* **267**:809–812 (1962).
21. LANG, W. S., Diphtheria at the present time, *Laryngoscope* **75**:1092–1102 (1965).
22. LEDBETTER, M. K., CANNON, A. B., II, AND COSTA, A. F., The electrocardiogram in diphtheritic myocarditis, *Am. Heart J.* **68**:559–611 (1964).
23. MARCUSE, E. K., AND GRAND, M. G., Epidemiology of diphtheria in San Antonio, Texas, 1970, *J. Am. Med. Assoc.* **224**:305–310 (1973).
24. MCGUINNESS, A. C., Diphtheria in preventive medicine in World War II, Volume IV (J. B. COATES, JR., ed.), Office of the Surgeon General, Department of the Army, Washington, D.C., 1958.
25. MILLIAN, S. J., CHERUBIN, C. E., SHERWIN, R., AND FUERST, H. T., A serologic survey of tetanus and diphtheria immunity in New York City, *Arch. Environ. Health* **15**:776–781 (1967).
26. MORALES, A. R., VICHITBANDHA, P., CHANDRUANG, P., EVANS, H., AND BOURGEOIS, C. H., Pathological features of cardiac condition disturbance in diphtheric myocarditis, *Arch. Pathol.* **91**:1–7 (1971).
27. MUNFORD, R. S., ORY, H. W., BROOKS, G. F., AND FELDMAN, R. A., Diphtheria deaths in the United States, 1959–1970, *J. Am. Med. Assoc.* **229**:1890–1893 (1974).
28. NAIDITCH, M. J., AND BOWER, A. G., Diphtheria, *Am. J. Med.* **17**:229–245 (1954).

29. NELSON, L. A., PERI, B. A., RIEGER, C. H. L., NEWCOMB, R. W., AND ROTHBERG, R. M., Immunity to diphtheria in an urban population, *Pediatrics* **61**:703–710 (1978).
30. PAPPENHEIMER, A. M., JR., AND BROWN, R., Studies of the mode of action of diphtheria toxin. VI. Site of the action of toxin in living cells, *J. Exp. Med.* **127**:1073–1986 (1969).
31. PAPPENHEIMER, A. M., JR., AND GILL, D. M., Diphtheria, *Science* **182**:353–358 (1973).
32. POWARS, D., MATHIES, A., AND WEHRLE, P., Diphtheria: Thrombocytopenia, myocarditis and peripheral polyneuritis, *Clin. Res.* **20**:272 (1972) (abstract).
33. RUBEN, F. L., NAGEL, J., AND FIREMAN, P., Antitoxin responses in the elderly to tetanus-diphtheria (Td) immunization, *Am. J. Epidemiol.* **108**:145–149 (1948).
34. SHEFFIELD, F. W., IRONSIDE, A. G., AND ABBOTT, J. D., Immunization of adults against diphtheria, *Br. Med. J.* **2**:249–250 (1978).
35. SISK, C. W., AND LEWIS, C. E., Reactions to tetanus–diphtheria toxoid (adult), *Arch. Environ. Health* **11**:34–36 (1965).
36. STEWART, J. C., JR., Analysis of the diphtheria outbreak in Austin, Texas, 1967–69, *Public Health Rep.* **85**:949–954 (1970).
37. WHITAKER, J. A., NELSON, J. D., AND FINK, C. W., The fluorescent antitoxin test for the immediate diagnosis of diphtheria, *Pediatrics* **27**:214–218 (1961).
38. WORCHESTER, J., AND CHEEVER, F. S., The Schick status of 18,000 young adult males, *N. Engl. J. Med.* **240**:954 (1949).

13. Suggested Reading

BENENSON, A. S., *Control of Communicable Diseases in Man,* 14th ed., American Public Health Association, New York, 1985.

BURNET, M., AND WHITE, D. O., *Natural History of Infectious Disease,* 4th ed., Cambridge University Press, London, 1972.

DAVIS, B. D., DULBECCO, R., EISEN, H. N., GINSBERG, H. S., AND WOOD, W. B., JR., *Microbiology,* 3rd ed., Harper & Row, New York, 1980.

HARPER, P. A., *Preventive Pediatrics,* Appleton–Century–Crofts, New York, 1962.

Report of the Committee on Infectious Diseases, 20th ed., American Academy of Pediatrics, Evanston, Ill., 1986.

WEHRLE, P. F., AND TOP, F. H., SR., *Communicable and Infectious Diseases,* 9th ed., Mosby, St. Louis, 1981.

CHAPTER 12

Escherichia coli Diarrhea

Herbert L. DuPont and John J. Mathewson

1. Introduction

During the 1940s and 1950s, a series of outbreaks of diarrhea in hospital newborn nurseries were reported in which the etiological agent appeared to be *Escherichia coli* identified by serotype. These strains became known as enteropathogenic *E. coli* (EPEC). Although it is generally recognized that these strains are responsible for diarrhea among children under 2 years of age, only now are we beginning to understand how they produce disease.

In 1969, a strain of *E. coli* was shown to be responsible for diarrhea in a group of British soldiers stationed in the Middle East. The strain was later shown to produce an exotoxin that caused fluid accumulation in a ligated rabbit loop preparation. Such enterotoxigenic *E. coli* (ETEC) strains have proven to be causes of diarrhea with a worldwide distribution. The strains are responsible for approximately 40% of the diarrhea among United States travelers to developing countries.

Certain nonenterotoxigenic *E. coli* strains are pathogenic by virtue of possessing the ability to penetrate intact epithelial cells. These enteroinvasive *E. coli* (EIEC) strains produce bacillary dysentery clinically indistinguishable from that produced by *Shigella* strains. This form of diarrhea is not common.

Herbert L. DuPont and John J. Mathewson · Program in Infectious Diseases and Clinical Microbiology, The University of Texas Medical School at Houston, Houston, Texas 77225.

Enterohemorrhagic *E. coli* (EHEC) strains have recently been shown to cause hemorrhagic colitis, which is a distinctive clinical syndrome characterized by bloody diarrhea with little or no fever. EHEC belong primarily to serotypes O157:H7 and O26:H11. These strains have also been strongly incriminated in the development of hemolytic uremic syndrome as a sequela.

In this chapter, we will review information available about EPEC, ETEC, EIEC, and EHEC. Since the organisms are biochemically similar (each represents an *E. coli*), they will be discussed in the same sections even though their clinical features and epidemiology are distinctly different.

2. Historical Background

In 1945, Bray[7] identified an organism with similar antigenic properties in stools obtained from 42 of 44 infants who acquired a diarrheal illness during a hospital-nursery outbreak. A few years later, Giles *et al.*[26] and Taylor *et al.*[87] described similar outbreaks of diarrhea due to serotype-identified *E. coli*. During the 1950s, serological procedures were outlined that allowed the fingerprinting of *E. coli* strains according to their somatic (O) and flagellar (H) antigens.[19,42,43] It was reported soon thereafter that EPEC strains had a worldwide distribution. Recently, much has been learned about the pathogenic mechanisms of these strains, although much remains to be resolved.

Taylor *et al.*[88] reported in 1961 that *E. coli* isolated from stools of a number of children with a diarrheal syndrome give a positive rabbit-loop reaction (dilatation from transudation of fluid and electrolytes), while strains recovered from healthy infants, from well water, or from the urine of patients with urinary-tract infections produced a negative reaction. In 1970, an O148 strain of *E. coli* was reported to have produced diarrhea in British soldiers stationed in the Middle East.[73] This strain was later shown to be enterotoxigenic. In 1970, two different enterotoxins were shown to be produced by *E. coli* pathogenic for swine.[84] The toxins could be differentiated by a variation in heat susceptibility. In 1971, it was shown that for disease to be produced, ETEC had to colonize the upper gut of the infected host,[14,28,78] and later, colonization fimbriae were identified with this adherence property.[20] ETEC strains have been shown to be the most important cause of diarrhea among United States travelers to Mexico (see Section 5.1).

EIEC strains were first demonstrated as causative agents of diarrhea in Japan[63] and Brazil.[92] The similarity of these strains to shigellae in causing bacillary dysentery was demonstrated in volunteer studies.[14] Except for two widespread outbreaks in the United States associated with contaminated food,[50,93] these strains have been shown to be rare causes of diarrhea in nearly all parts of the world.

In 1982, two large outbreaks of diarrhea caused by EHEC strains were recognized in the United States.[69] Both outbreaks were associated with the consumption of undercooked hamburger. In 1984, it became clear that O157:H7 was also a cause of sporadic diarrheal illness.[68] It was also recognized at that time that hemolytic uremic syndrome could be a sequela of infection by EHEC strains.

3. Methodology

3.1. Sources of Mortality Data

Since *E. coli* diarrhea is not a reportable disease, little is known about the actual incidence and mortality of illness. It is necessary to rely on outbreak data or information obtained from prevalence surveys. The mortality of EPEC diarrhea has varied widely from 0 to as high as 70%. The average mortality rate is 5–6%,[6,44] with an age-specific mortality rate in the neonatal period of 16%.[44] Risk factors that relate directly to increased mortality are age, in that the neonatal period and prematurity are associated with higher death rates, and strain variation, in that EPEC strains appear to differ in virulence. *E. coli* O111 is generally associated

with a more striking clinical illness and higher mortality rate.[12] There is a prevailing attitude that mortality of EPEC illness has lessened in recent years.

ETEC strains produce mild disease in healthy persons from the United States traveling in Latin America, but severe choleralike illness has been reported in patients studied in cholera-endemic areas.[28,78] Mortality is unusual with ETEC, but it undoubtedly occurs in areas of the world where health standards are low and where fluid and electrolyte replacement is not established in those with dehydrating illness.

EIEC is thought to be a rare cause of bacillary dysentery. There are no accurate data on mortality rates, but reported studies suggest that deaths would be unusual.[50,92] These reports describe the disease primarily in healthy Western adults and children in developing countries. There is good reason to consider the mortality to approximate that seen in shigellosis.

Since EHEC infections are newly recognized, almost nothing is known about mortality, although infection by *E. coli* O157:H7 has been associated with the development of hemolytic uremic syndrome, which has a mortality rate of about 10% if untreated.

3.2. Sources of Morbidity Data

Since *E. coli* diarrhea is not a reportable disease, data on morbidity must come from survey information.

3.3. Surveys

Sporadic cases and hospital-nursery outbreaks of EPEC diarrhea have been documented in nearly every country where appropriate studies have been carried out. Three types of studies have been done to determine the importance of EPEC illness: surveys of the relative frequency of recovering EPEC strains in populations with diarrhea, study of newborn-nursery outbreaks of EPEC disease, and surveillance of the strains during short periods in communities under study. While it is impossible to state the prevalence and incidence of diarrhea with accuracy, in approximately 10% of diarrhea episodes in infants and young children, an EPEC strain can be recovered from stools. Surveillance studies during community epidemics have verified the epidemic potential for EPEC.

Surveys of ETEC, EIEC, and EHEC diarrhea have been restricted to short-term studies of diarrhea cases and outbreaks in several regions around the world.

3.4. Laboratory Diagnosis

3.4.1. Isolation and Identification of Organisms.

The methodology for *E. coli* isolation is readily available in microbiology texts, and any diagnostic laboratory that performs bacteriological isolation can isolate *E. coli* with proficiency. Biochemically, diarrheagenic *E. coli* are not distinct from the nonpathogenic *E. coli* always present in the intestine. *E. coli* strains that cause illness can only be differentiated from normal flora strains by the demonstration of a virulence property. This has always presented a problem for the routine clinical bacteriology laboratory because demonstration of *E. coli* virulence properties requires sophisticated methodology generally available only in research and reference laboratories. This diagnostic problem has limited what we know about the epidemiology of *E. coli* diarrhea.

E. coli strains can be differentiated by the serological typing system originally developed by Kauffmann.[42] Two different antigens are important in this scheme. Somatic (O) antigens consist mainly of the lipopolysaccharide portion of the cell wall and are heat-stable. Flagellar antigens, also called H antigens, are destroyed by heating to 100°C. Capsular or K antigens also exist but are now rarely used in serotyping. Complete serotyping, a requirement to definitively classify an *E. coli* strain to be EPEC, includes a determination of both the O and H antigen types. There are approximately 164 O groups and 57 H groups. Table 1 lists the 12 O serogroups considered to be EPEC.

In serotyping, it is necessary to do more than O-group typing because avirulent strains may show similar O groups but lack similarity when O–H groups are compared. To perform serotyping, at least three steps are required.[19,22]

1. Screening of suspected EPEC strains is done using polyvalent pools consisting of the O antisera of groups recognized as EPEC. Strains that do not agglutinate in these pools are not EPEC.
2. Strains that are positive in these pools are then tested for agglutination as heated and unheated antigens in the appropriate O and H typing antisera.
3. Strains that react in an individual O or H typing serum are then titrated against that antiserum to confirm it is an EPEC.

ETEC are diagnosed by the demonstration of the production of one or both of the enterotoxins that they produce. Generally, five to ten *E. coli* strains per patient need to be tested for both toxins. The reference assay for the detection of heat-labile enterotoxin (LT) and heat-stable toxin (ST) is the ligated rabbit ileal-loop assay. Bacteria-free supernatant is injected into ileal loops prepared surgically in a rabbit.

Table 1. Important *E. coli* Serotypes[a]

EPEC	ETEC	EIEC	EHEC
O44	O6:H16 or H⁻	O28:H⁻	O26:H11
O55	O8:H9 or H⁻	O112:H⁻	O157:H7
O86	O15:H11 or H⁻	O115:H⁻	
O111	O20:H⁻	O124:H⁻	
O114	O25:H42 or H⁻	O136:H⁻	
O119	O27:H7 or H20	O143:H⁻	
O125	O63:H12 or H⁻	O144:H⁻	
O126	O78:H11, H12, or H20	O147:H⁻	
O127	O85:H7	O152:H⁻	
O128	O115:H11 or H40	O164:H⁻	
O142	O128:H7 or H21	O167:H⁻	
O158	O148:H28		
	O159:H20		
	O167:H5		

[a]EPEC, enteropathogenic; ETEC, enterotoxigenic; EIEC, enteroinvasive; EHEC, enterohemorrhagic.

Swelling of the loop caused by transudation of fluid and electrolytes within 5–6 h is indicative of ST and swelling within 12–18 h is indicative of LT. This assay has been replaced with several other more practical assays which we will discuss.

LT is often detected using tissue culture techniques. Cell-free supernatants containing LT cause morphological changes and steroidogenesis in Y-1 adrenal cells which can be neutralized by specific anti-LT sera. ST can be detected in the suckling-mouse assay. Cell-free culture supernatants containing ST cause fluid accumulation in the intestines of 2- to 3-day-old mice, which is measured by the gut-to-body-weight ratio. Recently, immunological methods for detection of LT and ST have become available.[34,89] Most of these methods are enzyme-linked immunosorbent assays (ELISA). Also, DNA probes that hybridize with the genes that encode LT and ST have been developed.[57] These probes have proven extremely useful for large-scale field studies because of the ease of testing many hundreds of strains. In the past, ETEC testing had been a limiting factor for the size of many field trials.

Pathogenicity of a *Shigella* or EIEC strain can be verified by testing in the guinea pig eye (Sereny) model.[83] A heavy suspension of bacteria is dropped into the conjunctival sac of a guinea pig, and 1–7 days later purulent keratoconjunctivitis is seen if the strain possesses the ability to invade epithelial cells. DNA probes are now available to test directly for the presence of genes encoding for invasiveness.[5]

One can screen for the presence of EHEC strains by looking for the ability to ferment sorbitol, which is unusual among *E. coli* strains, along with the inhibition of motility in media containing H7 antiserum.[23] Also, strains can be checked for the production of Shiga toxin in a tissue culture assay.[61]

3.4.2. Serological and Immunological Diagnostic Methods.

Although each of the *E. coli* types that produce diarrhea commonly elicits an immunological response, serology has not been employed routinely as a diagnostic tool. Also, the importance of serum antibody response has been questioned because the intestinal secretory IgA (sIgA) response is more relevant in intestinal infections. Study of the sIgA response has been limited due to technical difficulties, which are just now beginning to be solved and applied to the study of enteric diseases.[95]

During infection with an EPEC strain, seroconversion has been documented,[24,38] but the diverse number of serogroups makes this a poor diagnostic tool. Perhaps serological surveys in populations may play a role in determining the extent of exposure to prevalent strains of EPEC.

In ETEC diarrhea, seroconversion to anti-LT antibody is common,[11,21,79] but not invariable. An ELISA was developed for the detection of IgG and IgM antibody to LT that has allowed the characterization of specific immunoglobulin.[74] Measurement of anti-LT antibody may be useful in determining previous exposure to LT-ETEC and hence in determining resistance to naturally occurring infection.[21] Also, ELISAs have recently been developed to detect serum antibody to colonization factor antigens.[10] Perhaps these assays will allow the characterization of specific antibody response to these antigens.

During infection with EIEC, a serological response can be documented.[14] In view of the similarity to bacillary dysentery, most probably the frequency of seroconversion will correlate with the presence of dysentery (bloody mucous stools), which indicates the extent of mucosal invasion.[13]

No serological methods are available to study the immune response to EHEC strains, because the organism is newly recognized.

4. Biological Characteristics of the Organisms

Volunteer experiments have been conducted to establish the virulence of EPEC strains. In 1950, Neter and Shumway[60] produced illness in an infant by feeding an O111 strain of *E. coli*. This strain as well as an O55 strain were fed to additional adult volunteers and the severity of illness was shown to be directly related to dose.[24,38] Adults were found to be relatively resistant to infection. Additional volunteer studies have confirmed the earlier experiments demonstrating the pathogenicity of EPEC strains for adults.[47]

Recently, EPEC strains have been defined as specific serogroups of *E. coli* that have been epidemiologically incriminated as causes of diarrhea but do not produce conventional enterotoxins and are not invasive.[18] The serogroups recognized as EPEC are listed in Table 1. Biopsies from children infected with O119 have shown a characteristic lesion consisting of localized adherence of microcolonies, cupping of the enterocyte, and destruction of the microvilli.[72] There is no evidence of invasion. Cravioto *et al.*[9] developed a tissue culture model of this adherence property using HEp-2 cells. Later, it was discovered that there were at least two patterns of adherence to the HEp-2 cells: localized and diffuse.[82] Localized adherence, which is encoded by genes carried on a plasmid, is most clearly related to pathogenicity among strains of EPEC.[3] A DNA probe has been isolated and should be useful in studying the epidemiology of these strains.[58] *E. coli* strains exhibiting HEp-2 cell adherence but not belonging to traditional EPEC serogroups have also been associated with diarrhea in U.S. travelers to Mexico and Mexican children.[52,53] Pathogenicity of these isolates has been shown in adult volunteers.[54]

ETEC strains possess a number of virulence properties that relate to their persistence and pathogenicity for men and animals. Both enterotoxins (LT and ST) have been shown to be encoded for by genes carried on plasmids. Plasmids encoding for enterotoxin production tend to be associated with certain *E. coli* serotypes (Table 1) and are easily lost on subculture. Many ETEC strains that occur in nature produce ST alone, LT alone, or both.

LT is a complex protein that resembles cholera toxin in antigenicity and biological activity.[48] There is a single A subunit associated with five identical B subunits. The B subunits appear to be involved in binding to the membrane of the enterocyte. The A subunit enters the cell, causing the production of cyclic AMP, which in turn results in the net secretion of fluids and electrolytes from the cell.

ST is a very small molecule that is poorly antigenic. Two types of ST are recognized: human and porcine ST. Both are important in human disease. The mechanism of action of ST is not as well understood. It is known that this toxin causes fluid accumulation by increasing the intercellular concentrations of cyclic GMP.

ETEC strains show a high degree of host specificity that probably relates to the organism's ability to proliferate in the

Table 2. Adherence Fimbriae of Enterotoxigenic *E. coli*

Surface antigen	Natural host
K88	Piglet
K99	Calf, lamb
987-type	Piglet
CFA/I	Human
CFA/II	Human
E8775	Human

small bowel of the infected animal and not to differences in any enterotoxin produced. The colonization potential of an ETEC strain generally relates to the presence of fimbrial antigens that serve as ligands in an intestinal binding process. Table 2 lists the known surface antigens that are probably important to intestinal colonization by ETEC strains. K88, K99, and 987-type fimbrial antigens serve as adherence factors for strains of ETEC pathogenic for animals. There is little evidence that strains pathogenic for animals are commonly transmitted to man. This probably relates to the prerequisite of human-adapted colonization factor antigens (CFAs). A K88-positive ETEC strain highly pathogenic for swine was fed to a group of adult volunteers in a dose of 10^{10} viable cells and disease failed to occur, apparently because the strain did not replicate in the upper gut of the men.[14] Human ETEC strains isolated from patients with diarrhea often have one of three colonization fimbriae designated CFA/I, CFA/II, and E8775. The antigens often show a relationship to serotype (Table 3). These adherence properties can be demonstrated by showing colonization in the upper gut of infant rabbits, which can be confirmed by immunofluorescence. There is an unexplained ubiquity of ETEC in the developing but not the industrialized portions of the world. Environmental factors characteristic of these areas must be important prerequisites for persistence of ETEC strains.

Table 3. Relationship of Colonization Factor Antigen and Serotype in Human Enterotoxigenic *E. coli* Strains

CFA	Serotypes
CFA/I	O15:H11, O15:H−, O25:H42, O25:H−, O63:H12, O63:H−, O73:H11, O78:H12
CFA/II	O6:H16, O6:H−, O8:H9, O8:H−
E8775	O25:H42, O23:H−, O115:H40, O167:H5

EIEC strains possess *Shigella*-like invasive properties that probably represent the important biological activity favoring persistence in nature. This ability to invade epithelial cells is also encoded for by genes carried on a plasmid and are the same as those found in shigellae.[5] The resemblance of these strains to shigellae is further seen in their possession of common antigens.[19] There is a relationship between EIEC and *E. coli* serotype. Table 1 lists the recognized EIEC serotypes. It is unknown why these strains are not more important causes of illness.

EHEC strains are thought to cause disease by production of high levels of Shiga-like toxin.[61] Recently, a fimbrial antigen was described that might enhance the persistence of the organisms in the intestine.[40] There is some evidence that cattle may be an environmental reservoir of EHEC.

5. Descriptive Epidemiology

5.1. Prevalence and Incidence

Studies of diarrhea cases based on hospital data indicate that EPEC strains are responsible for between 10 and 40% of illness presenting to such facilities.[4,33] The frequency of EPEC in stools of diarrhea cases is higher when hospital cases are compared to outpatients.[4] In the reports with the highest frequency of EPEC disease, a single strain usually could be identified in many of the cases, indicating a communitywide epidemic. Three geographically distinct areas were involved in one outbreak. In the three epidemic census tracts, attack rates were 73, 118, and 55/1000 among nonwhite infants less than 1 year of age. Of index households, 50% had one or more asymptomatic pharyngeal carriers of the epidemic strain, while next-door neighbors and distant community household members harbored the strain in the pharynx in 33 and 0%, respectively. Intestinal carriage in the three household groups was 18, 3, and 0%, respectively. Kessner *et al.*[44] carried out a prospective examination of EPEC in a defined geographic area in Illinois and Indiana. An extensive community epidemic of diarrhea due to *E. coli* O111 during the summer, autumn, and winter of 1960 and 1961 was documented. Age-specific attack rates for the 0- to 6-month age group ranged from 1800 to 3700/100,000. Carrier rates of asymptomatic contacts of index cases ranged from 5 to 10%. Pal *et al.*[64] described a community outbreak that occurred in India. The morbidity for the population under study was 0.16%, with age-specific attack rates for the 0- to 2-year-old group of 0.98% and for the 6- to 11-month age group, 2.4%. During another community outbreak in Atlanta, EPEC strains were isolated from 12.7/1000 persons at risk and from 125/1000 infants less than 1 year of age.[6] EPEC strains are responsible for epidemic or sporadic diarrhea as well as community epidemics.[33]

ETEC has variably been reported to cause between 0 and 86% of diarrhea cases in North America.[17,29,32,39,66] The more comprehensive 2-year surveys have indicated that these strains are unusual causes of endemic diarrhea in North America.[32,66] ETEC strains may, however, produce epidemics of diarrhea. Such epidemics have been associated with the consumption of food or water contaminated with ETEC.[14,49,71,96] Also, outbreaks have been documented in hospital nurseries.[31,76] ETEC infection is more common in developing countries. These organisms were the most frequently isolated pathogen among Mexican children with diarrhea.[54] During the first 3 years of life, Mexican children showed a progressive rise in IgG anti-LT antibody that was statistically greater than that seen for Houston children.[74] Latin Americans possess high serum antibody titers to LT, while North Americans possess relatively low titers.[21] The titer of LT antibody most probably reflects prior exposure to LT-producing *E. coli* and directly relates to resistance to infection.[21] ETEC strains are the most important cause of diarrhea among U.S. travelers in Latin America,[15,29,55] being responsible for 40–60% of disease. Persons from the United States develop resistance to infection as they remain at risk to develop disease.

EIEC strains are unusual causes of endemic or epidemic diarrhea. Two outbreaks associated with contaminated food have been documented in the United States.[50,93] EIEC has also been shown to be a cause of endemic diarrhea in Brazil.[92]

EHEC has been incriminated in both endemic and epidemic diarrhea in the United States, Canada, and Europe.[68,69] Outbreaks have occurred in nursing homes, day-care centers, schools, and the community. Investigations have demonstrated that sporadic cases of hemorrhagic colitis occur widely.[68]

5.2. Epidemic Behavior and Contagiousness

EPEC strains have a predilection for spread within the hospital, particularly in nursery populations. Although the organism is spread within the community, the hospital probably plays a role in transmission to community members.[4,44] In a community outbreak of EPEC disease, 37% of the cases had been hospitalized within the preceding 30 days, while an additional 17% had direct contact with hospitals.[44] Factors related to contagiousness of EPEC other than exposure to hospitals are age, sex, race, and degree of crowding.

ETEC diarrhea shows epidemic spread to susceptible persons under unusual exposure, which may result from a hospital confinement or travel to a part of the world where ETEC strains are endemic.

Epidemic behavior and contagiousness of EIEC and EHEC strains are unknown.

5.3. Geographic Distribution

EPEC diarrhea occurs with a worldwide distribution. The first large outbreaks were recognized in industrialized urban parts of the world. This may have been due to greater reporting and the availability of more sophisticated identification techniques. Recently, EPEC diarrhea has been reported more often in studies of endemic diarrhea in developing countries.[54,58,82]

ETEC diarrhea has been shown to be common only in developing parts of the world. Only two reports suggest that ETEC strains might be common causes of endemic diarrhea in the United States.[27,80] The infection has been reported to occur with frequency in Asia,[28] Brazil,[30] Mexico,[15,54] and Africa.[77] Outbreaks of illness among adults due to ST-only strains have been reported in Japan.[45]

EIEC strains have a worldwide distribution, but have been reported to be a frequent cause of diarrhea only in Brazil.[92]

E. coli O157:H7 has only been identified in developed nations. There are no reports of illness due to this organism in developing countries.

5.4. Temporal Distribution

EPEC diarrhea occurs year-round, and although some investigators have found a peak summertime incidence,[6,32,33] others have shown the disease to have a fall–winter peak.[44] The time of year probably does not greatly influence disease rates.

ETEC diarrhea also occurs year-round. Many of the published studies were conducted during the summer months, and therefore there is a predominance of ETEC isolation during the warmer months. Since most of the areas of the world where ETEC is commonly found to be associated with diarrhea are tropical, it may be that a strong seasonal pattern will not be found.

There is no information about the temporal distribution of EIEC or EHEC infections.

5.5. Age

Perhaps the best study of the relationship of age to EPEC is that of Kessner *et al.*[44] The median age at the time of hospitalization was 8 months and 2 weeks. The distribution by age groups was: 0–18 months, < 86%; 1 year, 65%; neonatal, 9%. In the community survey, the age distribution of those with positive stool culture, regardless of symptoms, mirrored the age group hospitalized for diarrhea. Most published studies have confirmed that nearly all episodes of culturally confirmed EPEC diarrhea are seen in infants under 2 years of age, with more than half being in the group less than 6 months of age. In Houston, EPEC disease was documented to occur 20 times more frequently in infants below 6 months of age compared to children 1–2 years of age.[97] One study indicated that approximately 25% of infants were infected with an EPEC strain during the first year of life, and the prevalence of EPEC intestinal excretion by a group of infants less than 1 year of age was 1%.[90]

In ETEC diarrhea, most cases of infection occur in children in areas where disease is endemic, as determined by the natural history of antibody to LT during the first 3 years of life plus the observation that adults living in these areas are immune to infection. Little information is available concerning age-specific attack rates.

No information is available about the relationship of age to EIEC or EHEC disease.

5.6. Sex

As with many other infections, males show a higher infection rate due to EPEC strains. An overall male/female ratio of 1.4 has been reported.[44] Others have documented male predominance.[6,35]

Insufficient information is available to determine whether a sex relationship exists for the other diarrheal diseases due to *E. coli.*

5.7. Race

The published studies show a correlation of infection with exposure to hospitals and crowded living conditions, which probably explains the greater occurrence of EPEC in nonwhite children in the United States.[6,44] In rural Guatemala, among a primitive culture wherein hospital exposure was nonexistent and breast-feeding was prevalent, EPEC diarrhea was not encountered during the neonatal period despite shedding of potentially infectious strains by the mothers.[51] EPEC disease occurred later during weaning from breast-feeding in this population. It may be that race is only important in enhancing the probability of exposure and in decreasing the tendency toward breast-feeding.

Insufficient data are available to determine whether

there are racial influences on ETEC, EIEC, and EHEC diarrhea.

5.8. Occupation

EPEC is a disease of infants. Those persons taken into tropical climates by their employment might be expected to be at risk for ETEC disease. Occupational factors relating to exposures to EIEC and EHEC are unknown.

5.9. Occurrence in Different Settings

EPEC strains produce diarrhea primarily in hospital populations, particularly in nurseries housing newborn infants. Hospitalized infants and children attending day-care centers represent the major reservoirs for community spread.

ETEC diarrhea is a particular problem among groups traveling from low-risk (United States, northwestern Europe, Canada, and Japan) to high-risk areas (Latin America, Asia, and Africa). It is also a problem among infants and children in these high-risk areas. Hospital outbreaks of ETEC diarrhea have been reported.[31,76] EIEC organisms have been reported as a rare cause of foodborne outbreaks in the United States.[50,93] These organisms have been found rarely in most parts of the world. An exception appears to be Brazil, where there is an unexplained prevalence of EIEC-associated diarrhea.[92] Hemorrhagic colitis has been shown to occur only in developed nations.[68,69]

5.10. Socioeconomic Factors

Socioeconomic factors are important in EPEC diarrhea primarily as they influence crowding, sanitation, breast-feeding, and exposure to hospitals. There is no known relationship between socioeconomic factors and other diarrheal diseases due to *E. coli,* although it can be assumed that the same factors that influence EPEC illness are also important.

6. Mechanisms and Routes of Transmission

Within hospital environments, EPEC organisms are transmitted by direct contact, spread by dust, and from fomites. During one outbreak of diarrhea due to an EPEC strain, nursing personnel and family members were shown to be asymptomatic excretors of the epidemic strain,[8] suggesting a possible role in the transmission of the agent. In the same study, recovery of an EPEC from stools of mothers just before delivery was documented in 13% (361 mothers), with subsequent isolation of the same serotype of *E. coli* from 40% of the newborn infants of the culture-positive mothers. Asymptomatic adult carriers of EPEC strains undoubtedly play a role in disease transmission to infants and young children.[35,44,62] During one community epidemic, the infecting strain was commonly isolated from pharyngeal cultures, and respiratory symptoms were noted.[8] Others have noted the association of respiratory symptoms and EPEC diarrhea.[35,44] It is possible that a respiratory route of transmission may play a role in disease transmission. As with other enteric diseases, fecal–oral transmission is the most likely mode for spread. Person-to-person contact spread has been suggested by the epidemiological patterns of infection.[44] In a longitudinal study of 40 households, EPEC infection correlated with crowded sleeping arrangements, pork and chicken consumption, and intimate contact with household pets.[86] In one family outbreak, a pet dog was shown to be the index case.

From the available studies, it appears that ETEC strains are spread through ingestion of contaminated food.[81,91] In our studies in Mexico, when students ate at public eating establishments, they were more likely to develop ETEC diarrhea than if they consumed meals prepared by themselves in their own apartments.[91] Food sampled from public eating facilities was commonly found to be contaminated with coliforms. Sack *et al.*[81] found a small percentage of foods in the United States to be contaminated with ETEC. Due to the large inoculum necessary to produce diarrhea in healthy adults ($> 10^8$ viable cells),[14] it is likely that food or water are the most important vehicles of disease transmission.

The important transmission kinetics of EIEC are unknown, largely because of the rarity of infection by these strains. All the major documented outbreaks have been associated with consumption of food contaminated with these organisms.[50,93]

Little is known about the transmission of EHEC strains, except that several of the reported outbreaks were correlated with eating hamburgers usually at fast food outlets.[69]

7. Pathogenesis and Immunity

Several histopathological studies have shown that there is a characteristic lesion associated with EPEC infection.[18,72] The EPEC are seen by electron microscopy as microcolonies that adhere to epithelial cells with destruction of the brush border, but with no evidence of invasion. Pedestal formation has also been noted. This lesion can be duplicated in an animal model[56] and there is a tissue culture

model (HEp-2 cell assay) available.[9] This adherence property is encoded for by genes carried on a plasmid[3] and has been named the enteroadherence factor (EAF). The product of the EAF gene is unknown and most probably is not fimbrial in nature.[48] Although toxins are suggested by the nature of the lesion in EPEC infection and a few toxins have been reported,[48] it now appears that if enterotoxins are present, they are unrecognized. Although EPEC strains appear to produce illness in adults, the disease is primarily a disease of newborns and young infants. The age distribution suggests that protective immunity develops. The nature and extent of immunity are unknown.

Prior to the development of illness, ETEC strains must colonize the toxin-sensitive upper intestine before elaborating secretory enterotoxins. Specific fimbrial antigens on the surface of ETEC strains have been shown to mediate adherence of the *E. coli* to the mucosa of the small bowel. Table 2 lists the recognized colonization factor antigens of ETEC according to natural hosts. In the small intestine of piglets, the K88 antigen appears to bind to a receptor on the villous epithelial cell.[1,37,85] Attachments of ETEC to the upper gut depend not only on the fimbriae of the bacteria but also on the presence of specific receptors for the fimbriae.[75] Some strains of pigs genetically lack the receptor for K88, making them immune to disease due to K88-bearing organisms. Antigenically different fimbriae, K88, K99, 987-type, and type 1 (common) pili, adhere equally to porcine intestinal epithelium.[36] These ligands probably bind to different receptors in view of a lack of competitive inhibition of bacterial adherence.[36] ETEC strains infecting humans usually possess one of three recognized colonization factor antigens (CFAs) known as CFA/I, CFA/II, and E8775. Once an ETEC has adhered to the upper gut of the infected host, enterotoxins produce changes in ion flux across the mucosa of the small intestine. The two classical *E. coli* enterotoxins affect intestinal secretion through two different pathways. ST shows more rapid onset of action, and the effect is of shorter duration than LT.

Natural immunity to ETEC infection occurs when persons remain at high risk for infection. In a study of students attending school in Mexico, the attack rate was inversely related to the length of time the student had lived in the endemic area.[15] Newly arrived students from the United States suffered from diarrhea at a rate of 40% per month, compared to a rate of 20% for the same time period for those students from the United States who had been in Mexico for approximately a year or longer. Newly arrived students from Venezuela did not show an increase in illness, indicating immunity from prior exposure in Venezuela to agents prevalent in Mexico. A decreased frequency and lowered severity of illness among Latin American students correlated with an apparent resistance to ETEC infection. An inverse relationship was found between the geometric mean antibody titer (GMT) to LT and the occurrence of diarrhea associated with LT-producing *E. coli*.[21] Ruiz-Palacios *et al.*[74] examined the titer of IgG and IgM antitoxin antibodies from birth to 3 years of age among children from the United States and Mexico by an ELISA. IgG antitoxin antibodies fell to low levels from birth to 3 months (presumably from natural decay of maternally acquired immunoglobulin) and rose thereafter. The titers were significantly higher among Mexican children than those from the United States. We have found the GMTs of 3-year-old children from Houston to be essentially the same as those found for adults from various parts of the United States. The lack of exposure to ETEC in the United States appears to explain the remarkable susceptibility to infection among persons from the United States traveling in developing countries. Immunity to ETEC infection does not appear to be strictly antitoxic in origin, since Latin American students exposed to ETEC strains rarely excrete the organism in stools asymptomatically, in contrast to the common finding of asymptomatic fecal shedding of strains in United States students.[15,65] These data suggest that antibacterial immunity is operative because virulent strains are excluded from gut colonization. This could represent intestinal antibody to adhesion fimbriae and/or somatic antigens or other factors.

The pathogenic mechanisms of EIEC are the same as those of shigellae. These organisms invade the colonic mucosa and spread laterally in the epithelium, causing ulcer formation and clinical dysentery. It can be assumed that immunity to EIEC is similar to that seen in shigellosis. Experiments using monkeys have shown that immunity to *Shigella* develops after infection, but the immunity is serotype specific.[25] EHEC apparently causes disease by adherence to the mucosa of the transverse colon mediated by a newly described fimbrial antigen.[40] *E. coli* O157:H7 strains have been shown to elaborate large quantities of Shiga-like toxin that is thought to be responsible for the tissue damage seen in this infection. Since hemorrhagic colitis is a newly recognized disease, little information is available concerning immunity to infection.

8. Patterns of Host Response

In EPEC infection, unapparent infection and transient colonization are common, especially among older children

and adults. In one study, 15–20/1000 normal children between birth and 5 years of age harbored an EPEC strain in their stools.[67] Another study found prevalence of EPEC excretion to be 1% for infants less than 1 year of age.[35] In a 1-year longitudinal study of 40 households, transient excretion, infection defined as excretion longer than 4 weeks, and clinical illness were most common in young children.[86] The rate of excretion of EPEC in this study was approximately 11% in children under 1 year of age, while the rate in adults was 5%. Overt illness was seen in 25% of children under 1 year of age who had an EPEC detected in their stools. Illness is uncommon in older children and adults, even though they often carry the organism.

ETEC excretion commonly occurs asymptomatically in persons exposed to these strains.[15,65] It appears that highly susceptible individuals most commonly develop overt disease when exposed to ETEC strains, in contrast to those partially immune, in whom excretion without illness characteristically occurs, and to those with natural immunity through prior exposure, in whom neither disease nor excretion can be documented.

In EIEC infection, as experimentally induced in volunteers, asymptomatic excretion was common and seroconversion occurred without overt illness.[14]

No data are available to describe the host response to infection with EHEC strains.

8.1. Clinical Features

While there is marked variation in the duration and severity of EPEC illness, the most common findings are: fever (60%), diarrhea (> 90%), respiratory symptoms (50%), abdominal distension suggesting paralytic ileus (10%), and convulsions (< 1%).[44] Dehydration may be seen in one third of cases, especially in infants under 1 year of age, and hypernatremia and metabolic acidosis commonly occur.[35] Illness usually lasts about 1 week, yet protracted illness occurs, as well as fatalities.[4,12] In fatal cases and in certain outbreaks of more virulent disease, a picture of septicemia and widespread intestinal inflammation and necrosis is found. A more severe disease with a higher percentage of fatalities has been seen in infection with the O111 serogroup of *E. coli*.[12,86] Mortality is higher for ill infants who are less than 1 month of age.[44]

In ETEC diarrhea, the disease resembles mild cholera in most cases, where the most common finding is watery diarrhea. In contradistinction to cholera, abdominal pain and cramps (which may be severe) are common in *E. coli* diarrhea, and low-grade fever may be seen. In our experience in Mexico, the average illness in adults consists of passage of 8–12 unformed stools over a 4- to 5-day period. In volunteers with experimentally induced illness, the clinical syndrome in the most severe cases consisted of passage of 5–10 watery stools per day lasting as long as 19 days. We have recently seen a patient in Houston with ETEC infection present with a choleralike illness requiring more than 30 liters of intravenous fluids to maintain hydration. Of significance was that this person had had a previous gastric resection for peptic-ulcer disease. Fatalities are unusual with ETEC disease and probably occur only in the very young, the elderly, and those with marginal cardiovascular reserves. The illness associated with ST-only (strains that produce only ST) *E. coli* appears to be quite similar to that produced by ST/LT strains.[45,76]

EIEC strains produce an illness indistinguishable from shigellosis (bacillary dysentery). Fever, abdominal pain, and bloody mucous stools are frequently seen.[14,93] As in shigellosis, the disease is usually self-limiting, and fatalities are probably unusual.

Hemorrhagic colitis is a distinctive clinical syndrome.[69] It normally starts as watery diarrhea and abdominal cramps and progresses to grossly bloody diarrhea with little or no fever. The average duration of symptoms is around 8 days. There does, however, appear to be a spectrum of clinical disease with some patients having only watery diarrhea with no blood in the stool or fever.[68] EHEC has also been associated with hemolytic uremic syndrome as a common sequela to infection with these organisms.[68,69]

8.2. Diagnosis

The features of *E. coli* infections relevant to diagnosis are summarized in Table 4.

EPEC diarrhea should be considered in any outbreak that develops in a hospital nursery or on a pediatric hospital ward. In this setting, serotyping is the only way to identify these strains because of the epidemic potential of these strains. Because of the variable clinical syndrome depending on strain variation and host response, any diarrheal illness in a hospitalized pediatric population should be considered EPEC in origin. Serotyping of *E. coli* from children with sporadic community-acquired diarrhea is of questionable importance and probably does not justify the cost. More studies need to be conducted to determine the importance of the HEp-2 cell adherence assay and the EAF probe in detecting diarrheagenic strains of *E. coli* related to EPEC in endemic diarrhea.

ETEC intestinal infection should be considered in any traveler from the United States, Canada, or northwestern Europe who develops diarrhea without high fever while traveling in Latin America, Asia, or Africa. Unfortunately, the routine diagnostic laboratory is presently unable to assay for LT and ST, which are available only in research and

Table 4.   Features of *E. coli* Infections

	EPEC	ETEC	EIEC	EHEC
Laboratory diagnosis	Serotyping, DNA probe	ST and LT detection	Sereny test, DNA probe	Serotyping
Prevalence	10–40% of hospitalized diarrhea	Rare in USA Travelers' diarrhea 40–60%	Rare	Developed countries
Outbreaks	Nurseries	Travelers, infants	Foodborne	Foodborne
Geographic	Worldwide	Developing nations	Worldwide	Developed countries
Temporal	Summer peak	Year-round, summer peak	Unknown	Unknown
Age	< 2 yr	Travelers, infants	Unknown	Unknown

reference laboratories. ELISAs and DNA probes are now being developed for use in the routine diagnostic laboratory.

EIEC infection should be suspected in a patient with bacillary dysentery (bloody mucous stools with prevalent fecal leukocytes on microscopic examination) in whom stool cultures are negative for shigellae. The routine diagnostic laboratory can make a presumptive identification of EIEC by the biochemical reactions of these organisms. EIEC strains, unlike most *E. coli* strains, are lysine decarboxylate negative and are nonmotile. Presumptively identified strains must then be confirmed in a reference laboratory by DNA probe or the Sereny (guinea pig eye) test.[83]

EHEC diarrhea should be suspected in patients with bloody stools and little or no fever. These strains can be definitively identified only by serotyping them as O157:H7 or possibly O26:H11. The clinical laboratory can screen for these strains by looking for *E. coli* that ferment sorbitol and whose motility can be blocked by antisera to H7 or H11.[23]

9. Control and Prevention

9.1. General Concepts

Since *E. coli* diarrhea is not a reportable condition, we do not have adequate information about the epidemiology and optimal control and intervention procedures. It is clear that during EPEC outbreaks, standard public-health and infection-control procedures are important in terminating transmission. Isolation of cases, cohorting by area and nursing personnel, institution of strict hand-washing, and prevention of common exposure to equipment, bedding, or solutions are all indicated.

In ETEC diarrhea of travelers, careful selection of food by individuals and institutions and enforcement of food hygiene in public eating establishments by departments of public health are the major areas for disease control. For an individual, the selection of a restaurant where a history free of acquisition of diarrheal disease can be elicited from those who frequent the establishment is probably the most important single consideration. Beyond this, ingestion of hot and steaming foods and beverages, carbonated bottled drinks, and citrus fruits, and avoidance of leafy green vegetables, cold meats, desserts, fresh cheese, and milk, are advisable when traveling in parts of the world where food sanitation is substandard. Consumption of tapwater in rural parts of the developing world is never advisable.

In EIEC diarrhea, it is not known whether person-to-person spread occurs or whether, due to a large inoculum

responsible for disease, food and water represent the important vehicles of transmission. No specific information on the control of EIEC or EHEC are available.

9.2. Antibiotic and Chemotherapeutic Approaches to Prophylaxis

The most important factor in treatment of any diarrheal disease is the maintenance of fluid and electrolyte balance by rehydration. The value of antimicrobial agents in the control of hospital outbreaks of EPEC diarrhea has not been established. The strains identified in these outbreaks were generally susceptible to the aminoglycosides and polymyxins.[2,6,24,41,59,70,94] Several of these studies demonstrated an apparent effect when neomycin, gentamicin, or colymycin was administered to infants and children during hospital outbreaks. Problems in other reports have related to development of antibiotic resistance by the infecting strain during therapy or failure to affect the spread of the epidemic.[35,59] EPEC strains recently isolated have been very resistant to antimicrobial agents and these R factors are apparently carried on the same plasmid as the EAF genes.[46]

In studies of ETEC diarrhea, a variety of antimicrobial agents have been used with success in preventing illness among travelers from low-risk to high-risk areas. The drugs include doxycycline, trimethoprim, trimethoprim/sulfamethoxazole, furazolidone, and norfloxacin. A chemical compound, bismuth subsalicylate, has also been found to prevent diarrhea in a group of students from the United States traveling in Mexico.[16] While prophylaxis is not recommended for routine use by travelers, these means of intervention may have value in certain high-risk groups during brief exposures. Groups for which chemoprophylaxis may be useful include businessmen, politicians, the aged, the medically disabled, and those who have had severe diarrhea in the past. Problems to anticipate as groups begin using chemoprophylaxis include adverse reaction to the drugs, selection of more resistant bacterial enteropathogens, and increase in prevalence of resistant pathogens.

Drug prevention of EIEC and EHEC diarrhea is not feasible in view of the facts that populations at high risk are unknown and antibiotic administration is of unknown benefit.

9.3. Immunization

No immunizing agents are available for EPEC, ETEC, EIEC, or EHEC infections. Efforts are currently underway to develop a vaccine against ETEC infection using genetic engineering techniques.

10. Unresolved Problems

In EPEC disease, the most important issues to be resolved are the mechanisms of intestinal adherence, the importance of the different adherence patterns, and the pathogenicity and relationship of HEp-2-cell-adherent *E. coli* that do not belong to traditional EPEC serotypes. Further studies using the EAF probe should allow the elucidation of the importance of EPEC strains in endemic diarrhea in developing nations.

In ETEC diarrhea, the most pressing problems still center around assays to identify ST and LT in the routine diagnostic laboratory. Progress is being made in this area and practical serological procedures should be available in the near future. Also, since ETEC disease represents an important childhood illness and immunity occurs naturally, there is great interest in the development of immunoprophylactic agents.

The prevalence and epidemiology of EIEC diarrhea need to be clarified further. This should now be accomplished by using the newly developed DNA probes in field-based studies to determine the prevalence and epidemiology of these organisms.

Hemorrhagic colitis is the most recently recognized of the *E. coli* diarrheas. Much needs to be learned concerning the prevalence, epidemiology, pathogenic mechanisms, detection, and immune response to this O157:H7 strain. An especially important problem is to determine the exact relationship of EHEC infection to the development of hemolytic uremic syndrome.

As we continue work with virulent *E. coli* strains, it is essential that we reserve the term enteropathogenic *E. coli* (EPEC) as a designation for those strains that include the specific serotypes that have been epidemiologically incriminated as pathogens. All *E. coli* that cause diarrhea should be referred to as a group as diarrheagenic *E. coli*. Diarrheagenic *E. coli* compose a diverse group of strains that should be classified by the pathogenic mechanisms they possess.

11. References

1. ARBUCKLE, J. B. R., The location of *Escherichia coli* in the pig intestine, *J. Med. Microbiol.* **3:**333–340 (1970).
2. BAKER, C. J., BARRET, F. F., AND CLARK, D. J., Antibiotic

susceptibility patterns of enteropathogenic *Escherichi coli* isolates, *South. Med. J.* **67:**412–414 (1974).
3. BALDINI, M. M., KAPER, J. B., LEVINE, M. M., CANDY, D. C. A., and MOOM, H. W., Plasmid-mediated adhesion in enteropathogenic *Escherichia coli*, *J. Pediatr. Gastroenterol. Nutr.* **2:**534–538 (1983).
4. BELNAP, W. D., AND O'DONNELL, J. J., Epidemic gastroenteritis due to *Escherichia coli* O-111: A review of the literature, with epidemiology, bacteriology, and clinical findings of a large outbreak, *J. Pediatr.* **47:**178–193 (1955).
5. BOILEAU, C. R., D'HAUTEVILLE, H. M., AND SANSONETTI, P. J., DNA hybridization technique to detect *Shigella* species and enteroinvasive *Escherichia coli*, *J. Clin. Microbiol.* **20:**959–961 (1984).
6. BORIS, M., THOMASON, B. M., HINES, V. D., MONTAGUE, T. S., AND SELLERS, T. F., A community epidemic of enteropathogenic *Escherichia coli* O126:B16:NM gastroenteritis associated with asymptomatic respiratory infection, *Pediatrics* **33:**18–29 (1964).
7. BRAY, J., Isolation of antigenically homogeneous strains of *Bact. coli neapolitanum* from summer diarrhoea of infants, *J. Pathol. Bacteriol.* **57:**239–247 (1945).
8. COOPER, M. L., KELLER, H. M., WALTERS, E. W., PARTIN, J. C., AND BOYE, D. E., Isolation of enteropathogenic *Escherichia coli* from mothers and newborn infants, *Am. J. Dis. Child.* **97:**255–266. (1959).
9. CRAVIOTO, A., GROSS, R. J., SCOTLAND, S. M., AND ROWE, B., An adhesive factor found in strains of *Escherichia coli* belonging to traditional enteropathogenic serotypes, *Curr. Microbiol.* **3:**95–99 (1979).
10. DEETZ, T. R., EVANS, D. J., JR., EVANS, D. G., AND DU-PONT, H. L., Serologic responses to somatic O and colonization-factor antigens of enterotoxigenic *Escherichia coli* in travelers, *J. Infect. Dis.* **140:**114–118 (1979).
11. DONTA, S. T., SACK, D. A., WALLACER, B., DUPONT, H. L., AND SACK, R. B., Tissue-culture assay of antibodies to heat-labile *Escherichia coli* enterotoxins, *N. Engl. J. Med.* **291:**117–121 (1974).
12. DRUCKER, M. M., POLIACK, A., YEVIEN, R., AND SACKS, T. G., Immunofluorescent demonstration of enteropathogenic *Escherichia coli* in tissue of infants dying with enteritis, *Pediatrics* **46:**855–864 (1970).
13. DUPONT, H. L., HORNICK, R. B., DAWKINS, A. T., SNYDER, M. J., AND FORMAL, S. B., The response of man to virulent *Shigella flexneri* 2a, *J. Infect. Dis.* **119:**296–299 (1969).
14. DUPONT, H. L., FORMAL, S. B., HORNICK, R. B., SNYDER, M. J., LIBONATI, J. P., SHEAHAN, D. G., LABREC, E. H., AND KALAS, J. P., Pathogenesis of *Escherichia coli* diarrhea, *N. Engl. J. Med.* **285:**1–9 (1971).
15. DUPONT, H. L., OLARTE, J., EVANS, D. G., PICKERING, L. K., AND EVANS, D. J., JR., Comparative susceptibility of Latin American and United States students to enteric pathogens, *N. Engl. J. Med.* **295:**1520–1521 (1976).
16. DUPONT, H. L., ERICSSON, C. D., JOHNSON, P. C., BITSURA, J. M., DUPONT, M. W., AND DE LA CABADA, F. J., Prevention

of travelers' diarrhea by the tablet formulation of bismuth subsalicylate, *J. Am. Med. Assoc.* **257**:1347–1350 (1987).

17. ECHEVERRIA, P., BLACKLOW, N. R., AND SMITH, D. H., Role of heat-labile toxigenic *Escherichia coli* and reovirus-like agent in diarrhoea in Boston children, *Lancet* **2**:1113–1116 (1975).

18. EDELMAN, R., AND LEVINE, M. M., Summary of a workshop on enteropathogenic *Escherichia coli*, *J. Infect. Dis.* **147**:1108–1118 (1983).

19. EDWARDS, P. R., AND EWING, W. H., The genus *Escherichia*, in: *Identification of Enterobacteriaceae*, 3rd ed., Burgess Publishing, Minneapolis, 1972.

20. EVANS, D. J., JR., EVANS, D. G., AND DUPONT, H. L., Virulence factors of enterotoxigenic *Escherichia coli*, *J. Infect. Dis.* **136**:S118–S123 (1977).

21. EVANS, D. J., JR., RUIZ-PALACIOS, G., EVANS, D. G., DUPONT, H. L., PICKERING, L. K., AND OLARTE, J., Humoral immune response to heat-labile enterotoxin of *Escherichia coli* in naturally acquired diarrhea and antitoxin determination by passive immune hemolysis, *Infect. Immun.* **16**:781–788 (1977).

22. FARMER, J. J., JR., DAVIS, B. R., CHERRY, W. B., BRENNER, D. J., DOWELL, V. R., JR., AND BOLOWS, A., "Enteropathogenic serotypes" of *Escherichia coli* which really are not, *J. Pediatr.* **90**:1047–1049 (1977).

23. FARMER, J. J., JR., AND DAVIS, B. R., H7 antiserum–sorbitol fermentation medium: A single tube screening method for detecting *Escherichia coli* O157:H7 associated with hemorrhagic colitis, *J. Clin. Microbiol.* **22**:620–625 (1985).

24. FERGUSON, W. W., AND JUNE, R. C., Experiments on feeding adult volunteers with *Escherichia coli* 111, B4, a coliform organism associated with infant diarrhea, *Am. J. Hyg.* **55**:155–169 (1952).

25. FORMAL, S. B., HALE, T. L., KAPFER, C., COGAN, J. P., SNOY, P. J., CUNG, R., WINGFIELD, M. E., ELISBERG, B. L., AND BARON, L. S., Oral vaccination of monkeys with an invasive *Escherichia coli* K-12 hybrid expressing *Shigella flexneri* 2a somatic antigen, *Infect. Immun.* **46**:465–469 (1984).

26. GILES, C., SANGSTER, G., AND SMITH, J., Epidemic gastroenteritis of infants in Aberdeen during 1947, *Arch. Dis. Child.* **24**:45–53 (1949).

27. GORBACH, S. L., AND KHURANA, C. M., Toxigenic *Escherichia coli*: A cause of infantile diarrhea in Chicago, *N. Engl. J. Med.* **287**:933–936 (1972).

28. GORBACH, S. L., BANWELL, J. G., CHATTERJEE, B. D., JACOBS, B., AND SACK, R. B., Acute undifferentiated human diarrhea in the tropics. I. Alterations in intestinal microflora, *J. Clin. Invest.* **50**:881–889 (1971).

29. GORBACH, S. L., KEAN, B. H., EVANS, D. G., EVANS, D. J., JR., AND BESSUDO, D., Travelers' diarrhea and toxigenic *Escherichia coli*, *N. Engl. J. Med.* **292**:933–936 (1975).

30. GUERRANT, R. L., MOORE, R. A., KIRCHENFIELD, P. M., AND SANDE, M. A., Role of toxigenic and invasive bacteria in acute diarrhea of childhood, *N. Engl. J. Med.* **293**:567–573 (1975).

31. GUERRANT, R. L., DICKENS, M. D., WENZEL, R. P., AND KAPIKIAN, A. Z., Toxigenic bacterial diarrhea: Outbreak involving multiple strains, *J. Pediatr.* **89**:885–891 (1976).

32. GURWITH, M. J., AND WILLIAMS, T. W., Gastroenteritis in children: A two-year review in Manitoba. I. Etiology, *J. Infect. Dis.* **136**:239–247 (1977).

33. GURWITH, M. HINDE, D., GROSS, R., AND ROWE, B., A prospective study of enteropathogenic *Escherichia coli* in endemic diarrheal disease, *J. Infect. Dis.* **137**:292–297 (1978).

34. GUSTAFSSON, B., AND MOLLBY, R., GM1 ganglioside enzyme-linked immunosorbent assay for detection of heat-labile enterotoxin produced by human and porcine *Escherichia coli* strains, *J. Clin. Microbiol.* **15**:298–301 (1982).

35. IRONSIDE, A. G., TUXFORD, A. F., AND HEYWORTH, B., A survey of infantile gastroenteritis, *Br. Med. J.* **3**:20–24 (1970).

36. ISAACSON, R. E., FUSCO, P. C., BRINTON, C. C., AND MOON, H. W., *In vitro* adhesion of *Escherichia coli* to porcine small intestinal epithelial cells: Pili as adhesive factors, *Infect. Immun.* **21**:392–397 (1978).

37. JONES, G. W., AND RUTTER, J. M., Role of K88 antigen in the pathogenesis of neonatal diarrhea caused by *Escherichia coli* in piglets, *Infect. Immun.* **6**:918–927 (1972).

38. JUNE, R. C., FERGUSON, W. W., AND WORFEL, M. T., Experiments in feeding adult volunteers with *Escherichia coli* 55, B5 a coliform organism associated with infant diarrhea, *Am. J. Hyg.* **57**:222–236 (1953).

39. KAPIKIAN, A. Z., KIM, H. W., AND WYATT, R. G., Human reoviruslike agent as the major pathogen associated with "winter" gastroenteritis in hospitalized infants and young children, *N. Engl. J. Med.* **294**:965–972 (1976).

40. KARCH, H., HEESEMAN, J., LAUFS, R., O'BRIEN, A. D., TACKET, C. O., AND LEVINE, M. M., A plasmid of enterohemorrhagic *Escherichia coli* O157:H7 is required for expression of a new fimbrial antigen and adhesion to epithelial cells, *Infect. Immun.* **55**:455–461 (1987).

41. KASLOW, R. A., TAYLOR, A., JR., DWECK, H. S., BOBO, R. A., STEELE, C. D., AND CASSADY, G., JR., Enteropathogenic *Escherichia coli* infection in a newborn nursery, *Am. J. Dis. Child.* **128**:797–801 (1974).

42. KAUFFMANN, F., The serology of the *coli* group, *J. Immunol.* **57**:71–100 (1947).

43. KAUFFMANN, F., AND DUPONT, A. J., *Escherichia* strains from infantile epidemic gastroenteritis, *Acta Pathol. Microbiol. Scand.* **27**:552–564 (1950).

44. KESSNER, D. M., SHAUGHNESSY, H. J., GOOGINS, J., RASMUSSEN, C. M., ROSE, M. J., MARSHALL, A. L., JR., ANDELMAN, S. L., HALL, J. B., AND ROSENBLOM, P. J., An extensive community outbreak of diarrhea due to enteropathogenic *Escherichia coli* O111:B4. I. Epidemiologic studies, *Am. J. Hyg.* **76**:27–43 (1962).

45. KUDOH, Y., ZEN-YOJI, H., MATSUSHITA, S., SAKAI, S., AND MARUYAMA, T., Outbreaks of acute enteritis due to heat-stable enterotoxin producing strains of *Escherichia coli*, *Microbiol. Immun.* **21**:175–178 (1977).

46. LAPORTA, M. Z., SILVA, M. L. M., SCALETSKY, C. A., AND TRABULSI, L. R., Plasmids coding for drug resistance and localized adherence to HeLa cells in enteropathogenic *Escherichia coli* O55:H⁻ and O55:H6, *Infect. Immun.* **51**:715–717 (1986).

47. LEVINE, M. M., BERGQUIST, E. J., NALIN, D. R., WATERMAN, D. H., HORNICK, R. B., YOUNG, C. R., SCOTMAN, S., AND ROWE, R., *Escherichia coli* strains that cause diarrhoea but do not produce heat-labile or heat-stable enterotoxins and are non-invasive, *Lancet* **1**:1119–1122 (1978).

48. LEVINE, M. M., KAPER, J. B., BLACK, R. E., AND CLEMENTS, M. L., New knowledge of pathogenesis of bacterial enteric infections as applied to vaccine development, *Microbiol. Rev.* **47**:510–550 (1983).

49. MACDONALD, K. L., EIDSON, M., STROHMEYER, C., LEVY, M. E., WELLS, J. G., PUHR, N. D., WACHSMUTH, K., HARGRETT, N. T., AND COHEN, M. L., A multistate outbreak of gastrointestinal illness caused by enterotoxigenic *Escherichia coli* in imported semisoft cheese, *J. Infect. Dis.* **151**:716–720 (1985).

50. MARIER, R., WELLS, J. G., SWANSON, R. C., CALLAHAN, W., AND MEHLMAN, I. J., An outbreak of enteropathogenic *Escherichia coli* foodborne disease traced to imported French cheese, *Lancet* **2**:1376–1378 (1973).

51. MATA, L. J., AND URRUTIA, J. J., Intestinal colonization of breast-fed children in a rural area of low socioeconomic level, *Ann. N.Y. Acad. Sci.* **176**:93–109 (1971).

52. MATHEWSON, J. J., JOHNSON, P. C., DUPONT, H. L., MORGAN, D. R., THORNTON, S. A., WOOD, L. V., AND ERICSSON, C. D., A newly recognized cause of travelers' diarrhea: Enteroadherent *Escherichia coli*, *J. Infect. Dis.* **151**:471–475 (1985).

53. MATHEWSON, J. J., JOHNSON, P. C., DUPONT, H. L., SATTERWHITE, T. K., AND WINSOR, D. K., Pathogenicity of enteroadherent *Escherichia coli* studied in adult volunteers, *J. Infect. Dis.* **154**:524–527 (1986).

54. MATHEWSON, J. J., OBERHELMAN, R. A., DUPONT, H. L., DE LA CABADA, F. J., AND GARIBAY, E. V., Enteroadherent *Escherichia coli* as a cause of diarrhea among children in Mexico, *J. Clin. Microbiol.* **25**:1917–1919 (1987).

55. MERSON, M. H., WELLS, J. G., FEELEY, J. C., SACK, R. B., CHEECH, W. B., KAPIKAN, A. Z., GANGAROSA, E. J., MORRIS, G. K., AND SACK, D. A., Travelers' diarrhea in Mexico: A prospective study of physicians and family members attending a congress, *N. Engl. J. Med.* **294**:1299–1305 (1976).

56. MOON, H. W., WHIP, S. L., ARGENZIO, R. A., LEVINE, M. M., AND GIANELLA, R. A., Attaching and effacing activities of rabbit and human enteropathogenic *Escherichia coli* in pig and rabbit intestines, *Infect. Immun.* **41**:1341–1351 (1983).

57. MOSELY, S. L., ECHEVERRIA, P., SERIWATANA, J., TIRAPAT, C., CHAICUMPA, W., AND FALKOW, S., Identification of enterotoxigenic *Escherichia coli* by colony hybridization using three gene probes, *J. Infect. Dis.* **145**:863–869 (1982).

58. NATARO, J. P., BALDINI, M. M., KAPER, J. B., BLACK, R. E., BRAVO, N., AND LEVINE, M. M., Detection of an adherence factor of enteropathogenic *Escherichia coli* with a DNA probe, *J. Infect. Dis.* **152**:560–565 (1985).

59. NETER, E. Enteritis due to enteropathogenic *Escherichia coli*, *J. Pediatr.* **55**:223–239 (1959).

60. NETER, E., AND SHUMWAY, C. N., *E. coli* serotype D433: Occurrence in intestinal and respiratory tracts, cultural characteristics, sensitivity to antibiotics, *Proc. Soc. Exp. Biol. Med.* **75**:504–507 (1950).

61. O'BRIEN, A. D., LIVELY, T. A., AND CHEN, M. S., *Escherichia coli* O157:H7 strains associated with hemorrhagic colitis in the United State produce a *Shigella dysenteriae* 1 (Shiga)-like cytotoxin, *Lancet* **1**:702 (1983).

62. OCKLITZ, H. W., AND SCHMIDT, E. F., Enteropathogenic *Escherichia coli* serotypes: Infection of the newborn through mother, *Br. Med. J.* **2**:1036–1038 (1957).

63. OGAWA, H., NAKAMURA, A., AND SAKAZAKI, R., Pathogenic properties of "enteropathogenic" *Escherichia coli* from diarrheal children and adults, *Jpn. J. Med. Sci. Biol.* **21**:333–349 (1968).

64. PAL, S., RAO, C. K., KERESELIDZE, T., KRISHNASWAMI, A. K., MURTY, D. K., PANDIT, C. G., AND SHRIVASTAV, J. B., An extensive community outbreak of enteropathogenic *Escherichia coli* O86:B7 gastroenteritis, *Bull. WHO* **41**:851–858 (1969).

65. PICKERING, L. K., DUPONT, H. L., EVANS, D. G., EVANS, D. J., JR., AND OLARTE, J., Isolation of enteric pathogens from asymptomatic students from the United States and Latin America, *J. Infect. Dis.* **135**:1003–1005 (1977).

66. PICKERING, L. K., EVANS, D. J., JR., MUNOZ, O., DUPONT, H. L., COELLA-RAMIREZ, P., VOLLET, J. J., CONKLIN, R. H., OLARTE, J., AND KOHL, S., Prospective study of enteropathogens in children with diarrhea in Houston and Mexico, *J. Pediatr.* **93**:383–388 (1978).

67. RAMSAY, A. M., Acute infectious diarrhoea, *Br. Med. J.* **2**:347–350 (1968).

68. REMIS, R. S., MACDONALD, K. L., RILEY, L. W., PUHR, B. S., WELLS, J. G., DAVIS, B. R., BLAKE, P. A., AND COHEN, M. L., Sporadic cases of hemorrhagic colitis associated with *Escherichia coli* O157:H7, *Ann. Intern. Med.* **101**:624–626 (1984).

69. RILEY, L. W., REMIS, R. S., HELGERSON, S. D., McGEE, H. B., WELLS, J. G., DAVIS, B. R., HERBERT, R. J., OLCOTT, E. S., JOHNSON, L. M., HARGRETT, N. T., BLAKE, P. A., AND COHEN, M. L., Hemorrhagic colitis associated with a rare *Escherichia coli* serotype, *N. Engl. J. Med.* **308**:681–685 (1983).

70. ROGERS, K. B., BENSON, P. R., FOSTER, W. P., JONES, L. F., BUTLER, E. B., AND WILLIAMS, T. C., Phthalylsulphacetamide and neomycin in the treatment of infantile gastroenteritis, *Lancet* **2**:599–604 (1956).

71. ROSENBERG, M. I., KOPLAN, J. P., WACHSMUTH, I. K., WELLS, J. G., GANGAROSA, I. J., GUERRANT, R. L., AND SACK, D. A., Epidemic diarrhea at Crater Lake from enterotoxigenic *Escherichia coli*: A large waterborne outbreak, *Ann. Intern. Med.* **86**:714–718 (1977).

72. ROTHBAUM, R., MCADAMS, A. J., GIANELLA, R., AND PARTIN, J. C., A clinicopathologic study of enterocyte-adherent *Escherichia coli:* A cause of protracted diarrhea in infants, *Gastroenterology* **83**:441–454 (1982).

73. ROWE, B., TAYLOR, J., AND BETTELHEIM, K. A., An investigation of travellers' diarrhoea, *Lancet* **1**:1–5 (1970).

74. RUIZ-PALACIOS, G. M., EVANS, D. G., EVANS, D. J., JR., AND DUPONT, H. L., Enzyme-linked immunosorbent assay (ELISA) for detection of antibody to heat-labile enterotoxin of *Escherichia coli, Abstr. Annu. Meet. Am. Soc. Microbiol.* p. 60 (1978).

75. RUTTER, J. M., BURROWS, M. R., SELLWOOD, R., AND GIBBONS, R. A., A genetic basis for resistance to enteric disease caused by *E. coli, Nature* **257**:135–136 (1975).

76. RYDER, R. W., WACHSMUTH, I. K., BUXTON, A. E., EVANS, D. G., DUPONT, H. L., MASON, E., AND BARRET, F. F., Infantile diarrhea produced by heat-stable enterotoxigenic *Escherichia coli, N. Engl. J. Med.* **295**:849–853 (1976).

77. SACK, D. A., KAMINSKY, D. C., SACK, R. B., WAMOLA, I. A., ORSKOV, F., ORSKOV, I., SLACK, R. C. B., ARTHUR, R. R., AND KAPIKIAN, A. Z., Enterotoxigenic *Escherichia coli* diarrhea of travelers: A prospective study of American Peace Corps volunteers, *Johns Hopkins Med. J.* **141**:64–70 (1977).

78. SACK, R. B., GORBACH, S. L., BANWELL, J. G., JACOBS, B., CHATTERJEE, B. D., AND MITRA, R., Enterotoxigenic *Escherichia coli* isolated from patients with severe cholera-like disease, *J. Infect. Dis.* **123**:378–385 (1971).

79. SACK, R. B., JACOBS, B., AND MITRA, R., Antitoxin responses to infections with enterotoxigenic *Escherichia coli, J. Infect. Dis.* **129**:330–335 (1974).

80. SACK, R. B., HIRSCHHORN, N., BROWNLEE, I., CASH, R. A., WOODWARD, W. E., AND SACK, D. A., Enterotoxigenic *Escherichia coli*-associated diarrheal disease in Apache children, *N. Engl. J. Med.* **292**:1041–1045 (1975).

81. SACK, R. B., SACK, D. A., MEHLMAN, I. J., ORSKOV, F., AND ORSKOV, I., Enterotoxigenic *Escherichia coli* isolated from food, *J. Infect. Dis.* **235**:313–317 (1977).

82. SCALETSKY, I. C. A., SILVA, M. L. M., AND TRABULSI, L. R., Distinctive patterns of adherence of enteropathogenic *Escherichia coli* to HeLa cells, *Infect. Immun.* **45**:534–536 (1984).

83. SERENY, B., Experimental shigella keratoconjunctivitis: A preliminary report, *Acta Microbiol. Acad. Sci. Hung.* **2**:293–296 (1955).

84. SMITH, H. W., AND GYLES, C. L., The relationship between two apparently different enterotoxins produced by enteropathogenic strains of *Escherichia coli* of porcine origin, *J. Med. Microbiol.* **3**:387–401 (1970).

85. SMITH, H. W., AND LINGGOOD, M. A., Observation on the pathogenic properties of the K88 Hly, and Ent plasmids of *Escherichia coli* with particular reference to porcine diarrhoea, *J. Med. Microbiol.* **4**:467–485 (1971).

86. SMITH, M. H. D., NEWELL, K. W., AND SULIANTI, J., Epidemiology of enteropathogenic *Escherichia coli* infection in nonhospitalized children, *Antimicrob. Agents Chemother.* **5**:77–83 (1965).

87. TAYLOR, J., POWELL, B. W., AND WRIGHT, J., Infantile diarrhea and vomitting: A clinical and bacteriological investigation, *Br. Med. J.* **2**:117–125 (1949).

88. TAYLOR, J., WILKINS, M. P., AND PAYNE, J. M., Relations of rabbit gut reaction to enteropathogenic *Escherichia coli, Br. J. Exp. Pathol.* **42**:43–52 (1961).

89. THOMPSON, M. R., BRANDWEIN, H., LABINE-RACKE, AND GIANNELA, R. A., Simple and reliable enzyme-linked immunosorbent assay with monoclonal antibodies for the detection of *Escherichia coli* heat-stable enterotoxins, *J. Clin. Microbiol.* **20**:59–64 (1984).

90. THOMSON, S., WATKINS, A. G., AND GRAY, O. P., *Escherichia coli* gastroenteritis, *Arch. Dis. Child.* **31**:340–345 (1956).

91. TJOA, W., DUPONT, H. L., SULLIVAN, P., PICKERING, L. K., HOLGUIN, A. H., OLARTE, J., EVANS, D. G., AND EVANS, D. J., JR., Location of food consumption and travelers' diarrhea, *Am. J. Epidemiol.* **106**:61–66 (1977).

92. TRABULSI, L. R., AND DE TOLEDO, M. R. F., *Escherichia coli* serogroup O115 isolated from patients with enteritis: Biochemical characteristics and experimental pathogenicity, *Rev. Inst. Med. Trop. San Palo* **11**:358–362 (1969).

93. TULLOCH, E. F., JR., RYAN, K. J., FORMAL, S. B., AND FRANKLIN, F. A., Invasive enteropathogenic *Escherichia coli* dysentery: An outbreak in 28 adults, *Ann. Intern. Med.* **79**:13–17 (1973).

94. WHEELER, W. E., Spread and control of *Escherichia coli* diarrheal disease, *Ann. N.Y. Acad. Sci.* **66**:112–117 (1969).

95. WINSOR, D. K., JR., Mathewson, J. J., AND DUPONT, H. L., Western blot analysis of intestinal secretory IgA response to *Campylobacter jejuni* antigens in patients with naturally acquired Campylobacter enteritis, *Gastroenterology* **90**:1217–1222 (1986).

96. WOOD, L. V., WOLFE, W. H., RUIZ-PALACIOS, G., FOSHEE, W. S., CORMAN, L. I., MCCLESKEY, F., WRIGHT, J. A., AND DUPONT, H. L., An outbreak of gastroenteritis due to heat-labile enterotoxin-producing strain of *Escherichia coli, Infect. Immun.* **41**:931–934 (1983).

97. YOW, M. D., MELNICK, J. L., BLATTNER, R. J., STEPHENSON, W. B., ROBISON, N. W., AND BURKHARDT, M. A., The association of viruses and bacteria with infantile diarrhea, *Am. J. Epidemiol.* **92**:33–39 (1970).

12. Suggested Reading

DUPONT, H. L., FORMAL, S. B., HORNICK, R. B., SNYDER, M. J., LIBONATI, J. P., SHEAHAN, D. G., LABREC, E. H., AND KALAS, J. P., Pathogenesis of *Escherichia coli* diarrhea, *N. Engl. J. Med.* **285**:1–9 (1971).

DUPONT, H. L., AND PICKERING, L. K., *Infections of the Gastrointestinal Tract: Microbiology, Pathophysiology, and Clinical Features,* Plenum Medical, New York, 1980.

EDELMAN, R., AND LEVINE, M. M., Summary of a workshop on enteropathogenic *Escherichia coli, J. Infect. Dis.* **147:**1108–1118 (1983).

LEVINE, M. M., KAPER, J. B., BLACK, R. E., AND CLEMENTS, M. L., New knowledge of the pathogenesis of bacterial enteric infections as applied to vaccine development, *Microbiol. Rev.* **47:**510–550 (1983).

RILEY, L. W., REMIS, R. S., HELGERSON, S. D., MCGEE, H. B., WELLS, J. G., DAVIS, B. R., HEBERT, R. J., OLCOTT, E. S., JOHNSON, L. M., HARGRETT, N. T., BLAKE, P. A., AND COHEN, M. L., Hemorrhagic colitis associated with a rare *Escherichia coli* serotype, *N. Engl. J. Med.* **308:**681–685 (1983).

CHAPTER 13

Gonococcal Infections

Jonathan Zenilman and Paul J. Wiesner

1. Introduction

Gonococcal infections have plagued the human race for centuries. A complex interaction of human sexual behavior, social and health-related factors, and biological characteristics of *Neisseria gonorrhoeae* determines the epidemiology of gonorrhea. The term *gonorrhea,* which means "a flow of seed," is inadequate to encompass the vast array of clinical manifestations of gonococcal infection. After the gonococcus initially infects columnar and transitional epithelium (eye, oropharynx, respiratory tract, anal canal, uterine cervix, urethra), serious complications can arise through tubal strictures or bacteremia.

In 1988, about 2 million cases of uncomplicated gonococcal infections are estimated to have occurred in the United States. Acute and chronic gonococcal salpingitis cases contribute significantly to the estimated 850,000 cases of pelvic inflammatory disease that can lead to ectopic pregnancy and infertility, often in young women of minority race who are economically disadvantaged. The direct and indirect costs of women with pelvic inflammatory disease, last estimated in 1984, exceed $2.6 billion.[103]

Prevention and control of gonococcal infection depend upon individual and community education, high standards of diagnosis and treatment, appropriately targeted screen-ing, counseling, and contact tracing. Prerequisites to effective prevention programs are community recognition of the devastating effects of gonococcal complications, commitment to the primacy of primary prevention, and epidemiological focusing of efforts on populations that account for the transmission of most of the infections in a community.

2. Historical Background

Allusions to gonococcal infection may have been made in early Chinese writings, the Book of Leviticus, and by Hippocrates and Galen. In 1879, Neisser identified the gonococcus, and by 1885 Bumm cultivated the bacteria *in vitro.* In the early 1880s, Karl Credé experimented with the topical application of silver nitrate in preventing gonococcal ophthalmia neonatorum. In 1956, Stuart[94] described a transport medium for gonococci, and by 1964, Thayer and Martin[96] had developed a medium that selectively cultivated gonococci from genital, anal, and oral swabs, excluding most normal flora.

In the early 1960s, the incidence of gonorrhea in the United States began a precipitous 12-year rise[6] while the relative resistance of the gonococcus to most antimicrobial agents gradually increased. In 1972, state efforts to control gonorrhea were financed by federal grants. In 1976, for the first time in almost 20 years, the reported cases of uncomplicated gonococcal infection decreased in the United States. However, in 1976, the gonococcus joined the list of bacterial species that produce plasmid-mediated β-lactamase.

By 1985, a multiplicity of plasmid-mediated and chromosomally mediated antimicrobial resistances added addi-

Jonathan Zenilman · Division of Sexually Transmitted Diseases, Center for Prevention Services, Centers for Disease Control, Atlanta, Georgia 30333. *Present address:* Division of Infectious Diseases, Johns Hopkins Hospital, Baltimore, Maryland 21205. **Paul J. Wiesner** · Training and Laboratory Program Office, Centers for Disease Control, Atlanta, Georgia 30333. *Present address:* Dekalb County Board of Health, Decatur, Georgia 30030.

tional threats to effective treatment of *N. gonorrhoeae*. Nearing the close of the 20th century, biogenetic techniques have greatly expanded our understanding of the basic microbiology of the gonococcus, but only modest inroads have been made against the infection itself.

3. Methodology

3.1. Sources of Mortality Data

Fatalities from acute gonococcal infection are rare events, usually resulting from endocarditis or meningitis[74] complicating disseminated gonococcal infection (DGI). Data on mortality from sequelae of gonococcal infection, such as pelvic inflammatory disease (PID) and ectopic pregnancy, are unreliable because the conditions listed on death certificates are rarely specifically linked to the infection. For example, a recent study estimated the mortality from PID (all causes) to be 0.29 death per 100,000 women age 15–44.[36] However, because the underlying microbial etiology is not listed, determining how many of these were related to gonococcal PID is impossible.

3.2. Sources of Morbidity Data

Gonorrhea is a reportable disease in all 50 states. Many areas now also report antibiotic-resistant strains that are identified. Physicians, laboratories, and institutions have been required to report either positive culture results or the diagnosis, name, address, demographic data, and identity of the reporter to local or state health departments, depending on the jurisdiction. Data on all reportable infectious diseases, including sexually transmitted diseases (STDs), are reported from the states to the federal Centers for Disease Control (CDC). Weekly incidence of gonorrhea is reported in the CDC publication *Morbidity and Mortality Weekly Report*. Additionally, national statistical summaries of STD data are published periodically by CDC.[16]

In the United States military, gonorrhea and other STD reporting is a function of the Preventive Medicine Units (PMU) for each of the armed services. Military bases located in the United States usually coordinate reporting and disease intervention activities with the local county or state health department. Bases located overseas report STD morbidity to the appropriate Preventive Medicine Command through the PMUs.

Outside the United States, reporting requirements vary. Most countries do not have national-based surveillance for gonorrhea. The areas with the most complete reporting of gonococcal disease are Great Britain and the Scandinavian countries.

For a case to be included in the national morbidity statistics, it must be first diagnosed, then reported, and finally correctly tabulated. Misdiagnosis, underdiagnosis, and underreporting probably occur frequently. The extent of these errors, or reporting bias, is partially determined and corrected by special surveys.

Interpretation of disease incidence data must be carefully performed, taking into account possible confounding factors, such as reporting bias, demographic trends, and sexual behavior.

3.3. Surveys

Screening programs and surveys have served a multitude of purposes in guiding emphasis of the national and state control programs. For example, the Gonorrhea Screening Program, which provides free cultures for women, has been instrumental in identifying large numbers of asymptomatically infected women. Studies of reporting habits among private physicians are prone to reporting bias. For example, in one Seattle study, the underreporting of private-sector gonorrhea was estimated to be over 90%.[32] These results must be tempered by another study from Alaska, demonstrating that although private physicians may underreport, in surveys, they may actually overestimate the incidence of gonorrhea in their practice.[26] Demographic surveys have indicated that persons infected with gonorrhea are geographically concentrated, and that targeting intervention efforts in these areas may be productive.[84] Microbiological surveys, such as the Gonococcal Isolate Surveillance Project,[19] have been useful in determining the prevalence of gonococcal strains with antimicrobial resistance. These data, in turn, may be useful in developing recommendations for therapy.

3.4. Microbiological Diagnosis[67]

In most clinical situations, selective culture media, such as Modified Thayer–Martin or Martin–Lewis media, are used. These media contain antibiotics (e.g., vancomycin, colistin, and nystatin) that suppress overgrowth of common contaminants, such as fungi, gram-negative rods, and *Staphylococcus aureus*. A small proportion of gonococci are hypersusceptible to vancomycin and may result in false-negative cultures on selective medium.[48] However, these situations are unusual.

In uncomplicated gonococcal infection, presumptive

identification of the organism is made on the basis of growth on selective media, characteristic microbial and colony morphology, and a positive oxidase test. Laboratory diagnosis of *N. gonorrhoeae* is confirmed by either sugar fermentation reactions or serological techniques. Typically, the gonococcus will ferment glucose, but not maltose, sucrose, or lactose. Recently, highly specific monoclonal antibody reagents have been developed for direct immunofluorescent staining (DFA) and coagglutination methods of culture confirmation.

Specificity of culture without confirmation varies by anatomical site, correlated with the presence of commensal organisms which could produce false-positive results. Specificity of presumptive laboratory diagnosis of urethral cultures (i.e., identification without confirmation by sugar fermentation or monoclonal antibodies) in men is over 95%. For cervical specimens in women, specificity is estimated to be 85%. In pharyngeal, rectal, and ocular infections, this proportion is lower and all isolates from these and other unusual sites should be confirmed. *All* isolates from children and others in whom sexual abuse or assault is a consideration should be confirmed and saved.

In practice, cultures should be obtained from the anatomical sites corresponding to the patient's sexual exposures by history. Pharyngeal and rectal cultures should be performed if indicated. Additionally, up to 30% of women have rectal coinfection with cervical gonorrhea (irrespective of history of rectal intercourse), and routine rectal culture is recommended for all women because cervical cultures are relatively insensitive.

Estimates of culture sensitivity are approximately 80% for a single endocervical culture and greater than 98% for urethral culture in men.[35] Rectal cultures probably have a sensitivity similar to cervical cultures. Either site may, therefore, be the sole site where infection can be detected. Pharyngeal culture sensitivity is probably somewhat less.[44] In all cases, specificity should approach 100% if confirmatory procedures are used.

If possible, Gram stains of urethral and cervical exudates should be performed when specimens for culture are obtained.[35] In men, demonstration of typical gram-negative diplococci within polymorphonuclear leukocytes in a urethral smear is 96% sensitive and almost 100% specific for the diagnosis of gonococcal infection when the examination is conducted by well-trained technicians. In women, whereas specificity remains high when similarly trained technicians perform the examinations, sensitivity falls to the range of 50%. Gram stain diagnosis is useful in establishing the diagnosis and in facilitating treatment at the initial patient encounter. However, Gram stains of specimens from the rec-

tum and pharynx are not recommended. Culture should still be performed in all cases when the diagnosis must be confirmed and, more importantly, to allow for antimicrobial susceptibility and β-lactamase testing (see below).

Laboratory diagnosis of gonococcal infection from normally sterile sites, such as blood, synovial fluid, cerebrospinal fluid (CSF), and conjunctivae, is often challenging. In these cases, the selective media used for genital cultures *should not* be used. Blood and synovial fluid should be cultured on enriched broth medium. Most commercially available blood culture sets now contain a medium for culturing fastidious organisms, such as the *Neisseriaceae* and *Hemophilus* species. Synovial fluid, conjunctival discharge, and CSF should also be cultured directly onto supplemented chocolate agar and placed in a CO_2 incubator as soon as possible. Gram stains of conjunctival discharge, joint fluid, and CSF may be a useful adjunct.

In gonococcal septicemia (DGI), sensitivity of blood culture, under the best conditions, is often less than 50%. However, the presence of positive blood cultures often correlates with the type of DGI syndrome. For example, in cases of dermatitis–synovitis (without frank arthritis), half have documented septicemia.

Use of immunological techniques to detect gonococcal infection is problematic at best. Antibody detection systems (e.g., complement fixation, immunofluorescence, radioimmunoassays, agglutination) were the first immunological techniques developed; however, all suffer from poor sensitivity. Serological tests are both poorly sensitive and relatively nonspecific. The more recent antigen detection systems, especially the solid-phase enzyme-linked immunosorbent assays (ELISA), are a marked improvement. However, they still suffer from two important limitations. First, use of these tests in screening situations (prevalence generally in the range of 1–3%) results in a high proportion of false-positive results.[63] Second, without culture, testing of antimicrobial susceptibility is impossible.

3.4.1. Testing for Antimicrobial Susceptibility. With the recent upsurge in incidence of gonococcal infections resistant to antibiotics, susceptibility testing has become increasingly important. β-Lactamase testing is relatively simple, and is performed by reacting a colorimetric reagent directly with a colony from the primary culture. Direct antimicrobial susceptibility testing can be done either by disk diffusion on supplemented agar, or by the technically more complex agar-dilution method.

CDC has recommended that all isolates be tested for β-lactamase production.[17] Direct susceptibility testing should be performed on *all* isolates from cases where initial treatment failure can result in severe sequelae (e.g., DGI, endocarditis, ophthalmia, and invasive soft-tissue infections). In other cases, susceptibility testing should be performed as resources permit.

3.4.2. Posttreatment Cultures. Posttreatment cultures have been a cornerstone of gonorrhea control programs. However, less than 30% of patients routinely return for posttreatment cultures. Aggressive follow-up of nonreturnees is dependent on a number of factors, especially the available resources and the response rate.[88]

4. Biological Characteristics of the Organism

N. gonorrhoeae is a fastidious aerobic gram-negative diplococcus that grows best at 35–36°C on a rich medium (such as chocolate agar) containing hemoglobin and a variety of other nutrients, in a moist atmosphere containing at least 3% CO_2. Characteristic colonies are small, rounded, and glistening gray after 24 h of incubation, and are nonhemolytic on blood agar.

In the early 1960s, a relationship between gonococcal colony morphology and virulence was established. Sharply bordered colonies, which contain organisms with pili, were associated with infection in humans, whereas diffuse colonies, consisting of organisms without pili, were associated with lessened virulence. Pili are thin, proteinaceous extensions of cytoplasm that appear to be important for gonococcal adherence to mucosal surfaces and inhibition of phagocytosis.

Besides pilin, the gonococcal cell membrane contains lipopolysaccharide (LPS) and three integral major outer membrane proteins (OMP). Gonococcal LPS has endotoxin activity similar to LPS found in the walls of other gram-negative bacteria. Gonococcal LPS has also been found to have a cytotoxic effect on human Fallopian tube mucosa.[66] Antibodies against gonococcal LPS have recently been found to stimulate chemotaxis.[24] Protein I, the major gonococcal OMP, is a genetically stable marker that has been used to develop a monoclonal antibody-based serological typing system.[55] Protein I serves as a porin, forming a voltage-dependent aqueous channel for the selective passage of aqueous phase solutes through the hydrophobic outer membrane.[111] Protein II has functionally many similarities to pilin. It is a group of proteins that are involved in gonococcal adhesion to epithelial cells and neutrophils. Protein II also demonstrates antigenic diversity and rapid antigenic variation. Protein III is common to all gonococci, and is closely associated with protein I. Although the function of protein III is incompletely understood, it appears to play

an important role in the pathogenesis of DGI. Gonococci from patients with DGI are resistant to killing by human serum. Blocking IgG, which binds to protein III, inhibits complement-mediated phagocytosis and killing of these serum-resistant gonococci.[65] The target site for blocking IgG appears to be protein III.[50] Other more recently described proteins are H8 antigen, which may play a role in the pathogenesis of DGI, and an iron-transport protein, which may play a role in the pathogenesis of mucosal infection.

Over the past 10 years, antibiotic resistance has become an important clinical problem. This topic will be discussed in Section 5.8.

5. Descriptive Epidemiology

Useful data on the trends of reported cases of gonococcal infection are available in countries where most cases are seen in public, specialized clinics (United Kingdom), where most laboratory tests are performed in a single central laboratory (Denmark), or where few changes in reporting habits have occurred (United States). In these countries, the epidemic nature of the disease is undisputed; similar circumstances are also likely in the rest of the world.

5.1. Prevalence and Incidence

The reported cases of uncomplicated gonococcal infection in the United States are depicted in Fig. 1. Total number of reported cases peaked in 1978, with 1,013,436, and has since decreased to 780,905 in 1987. Changes in cases reported among women reflect not only cases presenting for treatment, but also additional case-finding by screening. Trends in acute gonococcal urethritis in men are less influenced by efforts of health workers to find cases.

Since 1978, reported cases have decreased. The reasons for this decrease are probably multifactorial including institution of the control program and greater public awareness. Behavioral changes among high-risk groups have had an impact. For example, among homosexual men, gonorrhea incidence has decreased 80–90% since 1980.[13,37] Probably equally important in explaining this decrease are demographic factors. Since gonorrhea is a disease primarily of young adults, as the postwar "baby-boom" generation gets older, the number of individuals at risk for gonorrhea actually decreases. When adjustment is made for population changes, gonorrhea rates have not decreased as much as the reported cases.[80]

Reported cases help define trends, but they need to be

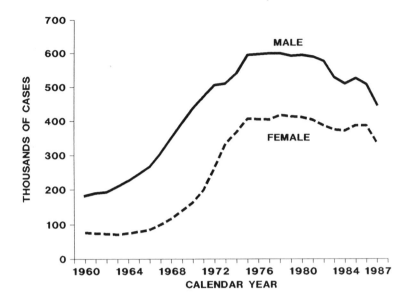

Figure 1. Gonorrhea by sex, United States, calendar years 1960–1987.

supplemented by special surveys that count cases in other systems and assess reporting patterns. Published surveys of reporting habits have been challenged because of physicians' low response rates and their tendency to overestimate the number of cases they actually see.[26] Methods to assess magnitude include surveys of randomly selected physicians who prospectively record all clinical encounters for a specified time, and surveys of randomly selected individuals diagnosed by culture. By these approaches, we estimate that the actual incidence is approximately twice the reported incidence of disease.

Serious forms of gonococcal infection, such as ophthalmia, acute and recurrent salpingitis, epididymitis, and DGI, have not been systematically recorded even in those countries, such as the United Kingdom and Denmark, that have more complete data on uncomplicated infections. Special studies provide us with estimates of incidence of these complications, and are summarized in the clinical sections.

5.2. Epidemic Behavior and Contagiousness

The spread of gonorrhea in a community is related not only to sexual behavior and the risk of transmission of the disease on exposure, but also to the natural course of the disease, the health behavior of infected individuals, and behavior of the medical practitioner.

Figure 2 shows the relationship of incubation period,

symptoms, and transmission rates to the spread of gonorrhea; it should be useful in correcting several myths about the spread of this disease. It is incorrect to assume that all men with urethral gonorrhea develop typical acute urethritis,[38] that the vast majority of women with gonorrhea have no symptoms, or that the cycle of transmission goes from asymptomatic women to symptomatic men and back again. Tracing the course of gonorrhea in Fig. 2 will illustrate these points. Begin with uninfected women being exposed to infected men: the majority of men who infect women have no or atypical urethral symptoms, and the disease is quite effectively transmitted (50–70%). Once infected, many of these women will develop either acute salpingitis (20–40%) or a constellation of less specific symptoms (20–30%) (e.g., perineal syndrome, vaginal discharge, abnormal uterine bleeding) within 3–45 days of infection. The remaining 30–60% of infected women will have minimal or no symptoms, yet carry the gonococcus endocervically for 3–12 months.

Next, consider the uninfected men shown in the lower right corner of Fig. 2 who will be exposed mainly to women who are unaware of symptoms; transmission of gonorrhea probably occurs 20–30% of the time.[40] Although the majority of men with urethral infection develop frank urethritis (80%), some have atypical signs and symptoms (15–18%). The tendency to seek treatment for either typical or atypical presentations of gonorrhea will vary among different social and psychological groups, so that the perceived incubation

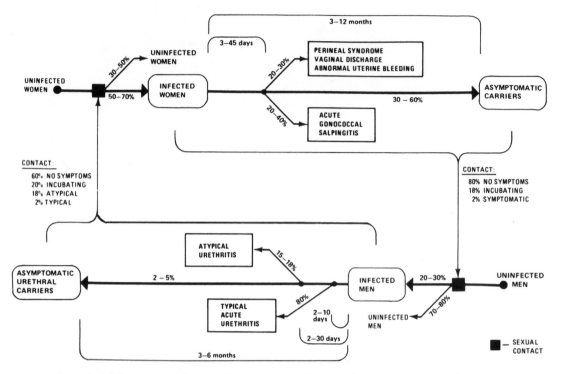

Figure 2. Relationship of incubation period, symptoms, and transmission rates to the spread of gonorrhea.

period may well vary from 2 to 30 days if the patient seeks medical advice at all. Some asymptomatic urethral carriers may be of long duration (2–5%) and are very important vectors of gonorrhea; thus, the cycle repeats itself.

Most gonococcal infections are transmitted from asymptomatic individuals or from those who do not recognize atypical signs and symptoms of the disease.[70] This is true for *both* sexes. Thus, both men and women who seek care for acute symptomatic urethritis or symptomatic pelvic infection will in all but rare cases have acquired their infection from *infected sexual partners* who have no symptoms. Last, infected women frequently have symptoms, and many men have no symptoms. These asymptomatic men accumulate in high-risk populations and may be major contributors to the spread of disease in the community.

Lesbians rarely transmit the disease to their partners,[83] but the principles of heterosexual transmission of disease in general hold true for homosexual men; the major sources of spread are from asymptomatic urethral and anorectal infections.[73] Homosexual men can develop symptomatic proctitis with anorectal infection, but the majority are asymptomatic. The course of urethral infection in gay men is similar to that in heterosexual men. Pharyngeal gonococcal infection is usually asymptomatic in both sexes and, although quite common among gay men, is an unlikely, but possible, source of disease transmission.

5.3. Geographic Distribution

Reported case rates of gonorrhea vary widely among the states. These variations may reflect population factors, such as socioeconomic status, and disease attack rates. The rates may also reflect differences in local control programs, such as case-finding activity, reporting practices, and the availability of public clinics. More recently, the influence of behavioral factors such as drug abuse (especially "crack" cocaine) and the effect of AIDS-risk reduction activities have become appreciated.

In 1987, the highest gonorrhea rates in the United States occurred in the Southeast (Fig. 3). The range of disease rates was from 573/100,000 (Florida) to 33/100,000 (Vermont). The highest gonorrhea rates occur in large cities. In 1987, 16 cities had rates above 1000/100,000, with the highest rates in Atlanta (2932), Washington, D.C. (2288), and Detroit (1776). These are rates (per 100,000) for the overall population. If the groups at highest risk are consid-

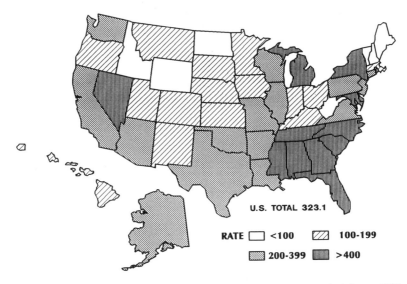

Figure 3. Reported cases of gonorrhea per 100,000 population by state, United States, 1987.

ered, for example, sexually active persons between the ages of 15 and 34, the rates within these subgroups would be much higher. Additionally, because of the "core theory" phenomenon,[84] smaller defined areas within these cities such as zip codes or census tracts may have local disease rates as much as three or four times these rates. Typically, most severely affected are inner-city areas with lower socioeconomic status. Racial minorities, especially blacks and Hispanics, have the highest disease rates (Section 5.6). This predilection holds true even when corrected for socioeconomic status and when underreporting bias in other groups is accounted for. Disease rates are generally lower in areas of lower population density, with the lowest rates seen in rural areas.

5.4. Temporal Distribution

A marked seasonality of reported cases has been found ever since data began to be collected in the United States. Consistently, the incidence of reported disease is at least 20% higher in August through October than in February through May. The seasonality of reported gonorrhea cases may reflect combinations of greater mobility, leisure time, and sexual activities in the summer, and increased antibiotic use in the winter.[47] The large, rapid changes over a 3- to 6-month period suggest that the spread of gonorrhea may be related to rather modest changes in human behavior.

5.5. Age and Sex

Young adults (20–24 years of age) are at greatest risk of acquiring gonorrhea; the second-highest risk group is teenagers (15–19 years of age). Teenage females are at higher risk than teenage males (Fig. 4).

5.6. Race

Although race distribution for cases is not calculated, on a national basis early studies found the reported incidence for black men to be higher than for white men in the same age groups. The higher rates among blacks undoubtedly result in part from the geographic distribution of disease in socioeconomically deprived areas and higher rates of reporting from black patients, who are more often seen in public clinics. However, in one study,[75] even after correcting for census tract on the basis of socioeconomic status, the prevalence of gonococcal infection among black women was higher than among white women who received endocervical culture. The higher rates of gonorrhea among blacks as compared to whites may also reflect the quality of preventive and therapeutic health services available to the two groups. In addition, some have suggested that persons with blood type B (of ABO group) may be more susceptible to gonorrhea, and black populations are more at risk because their gene pool is more likely type B.[30]

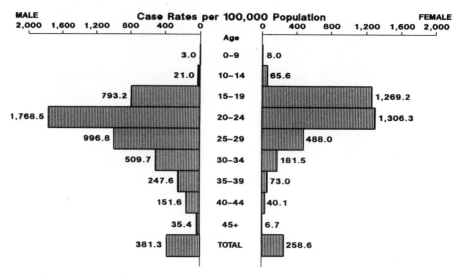

Figure 4. Age-specific case rates of gonorrhea by sex, United States, calendar year 1987.

5.7. Occupational and Socioeconomic Factors

No reliable data are available on occupation-specific risks for gonorrhea. In general, prostitutes are at higher risk than the general population.

Many factors could potentially have contributed to the current epidemic of gonorrhea including: gonococcal antibiotic resistance; differential infectiousness or transmissibility of the organism, the capacity of the gonococcus to cause symptoms or perception of symptoms in various groups; sexual behavior; methods and rates of contraception; homosexuality; illness behavior; other associated high-risk behaviors such as drug abuse; and the quality of clinical and preventive care services available to different groups likely to be infected.

The contributions of most of these factors are not easy to document because of insufficient trend data and means of measuring the variable under study. For example, sexual behavior, especially among adolescents, is a very complex issue. Although premarital intercourse among men rose steadily from the end of World War II to the early 1980s, among women the increase was dramatic only after 1967.[23] Even the relationship between the number of sexual partners per unit time and the risk of acquiring gonorrhea is somewhat ambiguous.[4] Similarly, the emergence of anonymous sex within gay bathhouses in the mid-1970s set the stage for increases in STDs in gay men during this period.[110] "Crack" cocaine abuse, and the phenomenon of "sex for drugs" prostitution that accompanies crack use,

has led to substantial increases in resistant gonorrhea and syphilis within areas where crack abuse is a problem, typically inner-city areas. "Crack" cocaine has no known biological effect on susceptibility to gonococcal infection. Increased disease rates among these groups appear to be related to behavioral changes brought on by the introduction of this drug, e.g., an increased number of anonymous sexual contacts.

Quantitative evaluation of the contribution of these behaviors to STD morbidity is difficult to perform. Additionally, the dynamic nature of the population at risk, and the rapid behavioral changes that may occur make assessment even more difficult. For example, "crack" abuse has been recognized as an important contributory factor only since 1986.

5.8. Antimicrobial Resistance

At the end of World War II, when penicillin became widely available, the recommended dose for gonorrhea treatment was 200,000 U of aqueous procaine penicillin G (APPG). Over the next 20 years, the minimum inhibitory concentration of penicillin gradually increased. By 1979, the recommended dose had increased 200-fold, to 4.8×10^6 U.[42] Still, antibiotic resistance was not perceived to be an important clinical problem. Since 1976, however, the picture has dramatically changed, with the introduction of multiple types of drug resistance (Table 1), and necessitat-

**Table 1.   Antimicrobial Resistance
in *N. gonorrhoeae***

Plasmid-mediated
   Penicillin (PPNG)
   Tetracycline (TRNG)
Chromosomally mediated
   Penicillin
   Tetracycline
   Cephalosporins
   Spectinomycin

ing revision of treatment and control recommendations. Diagnosis of resistant organisms can only be made in the laboratory.

5.8.1. Penicillinase-Producing *N. gonorrhoeae*. In 1976, the first cases of plasmid-mediated PPNG were discovered in the United States, with source contacts from Southeast Asia and west Africa. Although a number of different size plasmids have been described, the two most commonly identified are 3.2 MDa and 4.4 MDa.

Although initially concentrated in small epidemics in coastal cities,[49] by 1987 PPNG had become firmly entrenched in the United States, with cases being reported from every state and most large metropolitan areas. Over 20% of gonococcal disease in Miami and Detroit is now PPNG, and other cities such as New York, Philadelphia, Los Angeles, Seattle, and Denver have experienced large outbreaks of PPNG.[14,15,20] In 1987, CDC surveillance data estimated that almost 3% of all gonorrhea in the United States was PPNG (Fig. 5). PPNG accounts for 40–60% of all gonorrhea in parts of Africa and Asia.

Inappropriate use of oral antibiotics, as either self-treatment or prophylaxis, has been implicated in contributing to the high prevalence of PPNG in the Philippines and in south Florida.[113] However, using risk-factor profiles to identify PPNG patients may be useful only during the period when the strain is introduced into a community. When PPNG and other resistant infections become endemic (usually at > 3% of total gonorrhea), the epidemiological characteristics of PPNG patients are almost identical to those of ordinary gonorrhea patients.[17]

At least half of patients with PPNG who are treated with either APPG or amoxicillin will not respond to therapy. Additionally, strains with the 4.4 MDa plasmid often contain chromosomally mediated resistance determinants to tetracycline, and have decreased susceptibility to second- and third-generation cephalosporins.[100]

5.8.2. Chromosomally Mediated Resistance. CMRNG was first identified in 1983 in a large outbreak in North Carolina.[27] CMRNG results as a cumulative effect of multiple genetic mutations, resulting in altered outer-membrane permeability to antibiotics and changes in the periplasmic penicillin-binding proteins.[12,25] Mechanistically, CMRNG therefore really represents a number of different types of antibiotic resistance.

Clinically important CMRNG organisms are usually resistant to penicillin and tetracycline, and also meet CDC definition of cefoxitin resistance. Organisms with multiple-drug resistance are common. The minimum inhibitory con-

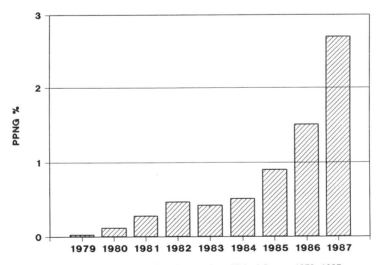

Figure 5. PPNG percent of total gonorrhea, United States, 1979–1987.

centration (MIC) to ceftriaxone may be increased tenfold compared to that of susceptible organisms, although still well within the therapeutic margin.

Testing for CMRNG requires direct susceptibility testing and, therefore, accurate prevalence data are not available. CMRNG is thought to be widely prevalent in Asia and Africa, again corresponding to areas in which there is widespread prophylactic use of antibiotics. In the United States, data from the Gonococcal Isolate Surveillance Project (GISP) in 1987 indicate that 9% of all isolates have chromosomally mediated resistance to penicillin, tetracycline, and cefoxitin. A geographical distribution of disease was evident, with the highest proportions of CMRNG being found in the southeast and the lowest in the Pacific Northwest. All isolates were susceptible to ceftriaxone and spectinomycin.

5.8.3. Plasmid-Mediated Tetracycline Resistance (TRNG). TRNG is characterized by high-level tetracycline resistance (MIC > 8 μg/ml).[57] Diagnosis can be made only by susceptibility determination. Usually, the organisms are susceptible to other antibiotics, although a number of small outbreaks of combined PPNG–TRNG were reported in 1985 and 1986. However, cases of TRNG that are treated with tetracycline as sole therapy have a greater than 90% risk of treatment failure.

The tetracycline resistance determinant is the *tetM* gene located on a 25.2-MDa plasmid. This plasmid is thought to have evolved through a recombinant event, in which a *tetM* transposon inserted into another plasmid normally found in some gonococci, the 24.5-MDa conjugative plasmid.[68] TRNG has spread rapidly. The first cases were identified in New Hampshire in 1982, and by 1986 had been identified in 17 states. Data from GISP surveillance indicate that TRNG prevalence may be as high as 3% nationwide, and as high as 15% in some localities, in particular Baltimore and Philadelphia.

Discovery of TRNG was a major factor in recommending against use of tetracycline as sole therapy for gonococcal infection. With current treatment recommendations, TRNG should not present much of a clinical problem. However, from a public health standpoint, this organism is of concern because of its ability to readily transfer plasmids with resistant determinants to other gonococci and closely related species. For example, the 25.2-MDa plasmid has been found in meningococci and may mediate conjugal transfer of β-lactamase plasmids to meningococci *in vitro*.[82] Transfer of the resistance determinant to *Chlamydia trachomatis* has not occurred, and is not thought to be a potential problem.

5.8.4. Spectinomycin   Resistance. Spectinomycin resistance was first described in 1981 in patients from Southeast Asia. Outside that area, spectinomycin-resistant organisms are isolated only sporadically. For example, during 1985–1986, only ten spectinomycin-resistant isolates were identified in the United States, six of which were linked to an overseas source contact.[112] In Southeast Asia, emergence and maintenance of spectinomycin-resistant gonococcal subpopulations has been linked to high background levels of its use.[9]

Microbiologically, clinically important spectinomycin resistance is a single-step, high-level mutation resulting in MIG > 2000 μg/ml, suggesting a ribosomal mechanism. It is easily diagnosed by the commonly used antimicrobial susceptibility techniques. Spectinomycin resistance may coexist with other plasmid- or chromosomally mediated types of resistance. All reported cases to date have been susceptible to ceftriaxone.

6. Mechanisms and Routes of Transmission

The major mode of transmission of gonococcal infection in adults is through sexual intercourse (see Section 5.2).

Nonsexual transmission of gonorrhea is extremely rare among adults. Although survival of gonococci can be demonstrated on inanimate objects, such as toilet seats,[33] epidemiological data implicating fomites in transmission are lacking. Although nonsexual transmission in children is possible in rare situations, sexual transmission must always be considered in the management of childhood infections. Infants born to infected mothers can acquire conjunctival infection and orogastric colonization before delivery (with premature rupture of fetal membranes) or during delivery. Children up to the age of 5 years rarely acquire the disease from fomites or inoculation with infected adult secretions. However, in all children, family situations must be examined because sexual abuse, frequently involving a close member of the household, may be the mode of transmission. Most cases of gonorrhea in adolescent children are acquired through sexual intercourse.

7. Pathogenesis and Immunity

7.1. Pathogenesis

The incubation period for gonococcal infection of all types is 1–7 days. The majority of patients with urethritis will exhibit symptoms within 72 h of infection. In women, since cervical infection is often asymptomatic, the incubation period is harder to define.

Gonococcal infection is initiated by intimate contact of

the gonococcus with either epithelial or mucus-secreting cells, usually a nonciliated columnar epithelial surface. Gonococci taken directly from exudate are infectious when inoculated into another human, but serial passage in the laboratory results in reduced virulence. Artificial conditions select against virulence factors, such as the presence of pili and protein II (see Section 4).

Employing an *in vitro* Fallopian tube organ-culture system, investigators have observed the entire process of mucosal infection, and have delineated four phases[66]:

1. Mucosal attachment to nociliated cells, mediated by gonococcal pili
2. Endocytosis of gonococci by epithelial cells
3. Movement of endocytic vacuole within the ingesting cell; intracellular replication
4. Egestion of gonococci by either exocytosis or rupture of epithelial host (usually by third day)

In most cases, natural infection is usually accompanied by an intense local polymorphonuclear inflammatory response. Systemic symptoms, however, are unusual.

In about 1% of cases, mucosal infection, often asymptomatic, will progress to septicemia. As discussed in Section 4, serum-resistant organisms may be involved. Patients with defects in the terminal components of complement are also at higher risk for DGI.[76]

7.2. Immunity

When purified antigens, such as pilin, outer membrane protein I, and LPS, are employed in sensitive assays, most patients with gonococcal infection can be shown to produce humoral antibody. However, these responses are generally short-lived. Transient antibodies have also been found in genital secretions.[98]

Secretory IgA is produced in both men and women in response to mucosal gonococcal infection.[53] The gonococcus neutralizes the activity of secretory IgA by two routes. Gonococci produce IgA proteases, which destroy the host's secretory immunoglobulin. Second, gonococci are capable of a process called phase variation in which the pili, against which the immunoglobulin is directed, can shift antigenic determinants, producing new pilin protein against which the immunoglobulin is ineffective.

Since gonococci are antigenically heterogeneous for many of these cell constituents, immunity may be highly strain-specific.[58] Because of the large antigenic variety involved, the transient nature of the immunological response, and the ability of many pathogenic gonococci to produce an IgA protease that neutralizes any type-specific secretory antibody, previous infection has little effect on susceptibility to future infection with *N. gonorrhoeae*.

In addition, serum from individuals who presumably have never had a gonococcal infection contains "natural antibody" that is bactericidal for all gonococci except those causing disseminated infection.[87] This class of antibody is thought to arise from previous infection or from colonization with nonpathogenic *Neisseriae,* such as meningococci. As noted in Section 4, "serum-resistant" gonococci, which cause the majority of DGI cases, preferentially bind (to the receptor site, protein III) a blocking antibody found in normal serum that successfully competes with bactericidal antibody, thereby protecting the pathogen from complement-mediated destruction.

8. Patterns of Host Response

Gonorrhea has been one of the most intensively studied infectious diseases. However, much still remains to be learned. For example, we know that asymptomatic infections among both men and women are common and are important in disease transmission. However, the term *asymptomatic* may be used too loosely. Since neither patient nor physician may perceive mild symptoms as indicative of an STD, many cases are missed, go untreated, and remain infectious despite a definite host response of a variety of humoral antibodies, local IgA, and cellular hypersensitivity.

8.1. Clinical Features

8.1.1. Urethritis in Men.[43] Purulent discharge followed by dysuria are the most common symptoms. Although most men have one or both symptoms within 1 week of infection, perhaps 5% of cases never develop signs or symptoms.

The major differential diagnosis is gonococcal urethritis (GCU) and nongonococcal urethritis (NGU). Although GCU is more frequently associated with purulent discharge and dysuria, the diagnosis cannot be confirmed or excluded by history and physical examination alone.[45] Gonorrhea is diagnosed by urethral smear and Gram stain, and confirmed by culture (Section 3.4). Coinfection with *C. trachomatis* is common.

Untreated gonococcal urethritis will usually resolve within 6 months. Since the vast majority of symptomatic men seek early treatment, there are few epidemiological data on the sequelae of untreated gonococcal urethritis. In developing countries, where chronic untreated infections still occur, paraurethral and preputial abscesses, fistula formation, and urethral strictures occur frequently.

Prostatitis and epididymitis are other sequelae. However, recent data suggest that in younger patients, these complications may, in most cases, be due to infection with *C. trachomatis*.[7]

8.1.2. Endocervicitis. In most women with gonococcal cervicitis, purulent exudate and cervical friability can be detected by a careful visual speculum examination. Infected women may have nonspecific complaints such as increased vaginal discharge, abnormal menses (increased flow or dysmenorrhea), dyspareunia, or dysuria. Patients often do not associate these symptoms with STD. Labial tenderness and Bartholin's and Skene's gland abscesses are less frequent signs of infection. Fifty percent of women are asymptomatic at presentation. Bimanual examination of the pelvis is mandatory in evaluating women with gonococcal infection. As many as half of women with endocervical gonorrhea may have upper-tract signs, such as adnexal tenderness, at initial evaluation.[77]

Coinfection with other genitourinary pathogens is common. *C. trachomatis* cervicitis, *Trichomonas vaginalis* vaginitis, and nonspecific vaginosis may be present in 30–50% of patients with gonococcal cervicitis.[42] Diagnosis of gonococcal cervicitis is made by culture. Gram stain of cervical secretions may be useful but has poor sensitivity (see Section 3.4). Because of the high proportion of coinfection by *C. trachomatis*, treatment regimens currently in use (e.g., ceftriaxone plus tetracycline) are effective against both pathogens.

8.1.3. Upper-Genital-Tract Infection and Pelvic Inflammatory Disease (PID). PID is the most important complication of gonorrhea. Ascending infection from the endocervix through the uterine cavity to the Fallopian tubes usually occurs within one to two menstrual cycles in 10–20% of women with untreated or undertreated gonococcal infection.[106] PID is actually a spectrum of soft-tissue infections, including endometritis and salpingitis. Leakage of infected material can result in tubo-ovarian abscess and/or pelvic peritonitis. Tubal damage results in impairment of host defense mechanisms, such as ciliary action, setting the stage for superinfection and possible abscess formation. Tubal scarring, the major long-term sequela of PID, leads to increased susceptibility for repeated episodes of PID, increased incidence of tubal infertility, and higher risk to develop ectopic pregnancy.

Patients at highest risk for developing PID are under 25 years old, have had previous episodes of PID, have multiple sexual partners, and have an intrauterine device. Use of oral contraceptives as a risk factor for PID is still a subject of considerable debate.[103]

In over 50% of cases, *N. gonorrhoeae* or *C. trachomatis* is isolated.[95,97] Combined infection is common. Other microorganisms implicated in PID are gram-negative rod enterics, anaerobes, Group B streptococci, and the genital tract mycoplasmas.

Clinical diagnosis of PID has been traditionally made by documenting the combination of lower abdominal pain, abnormal cervical or vaginal discharge, and tenderness on bimanual exam.[105] Fever occurs in only half the cases. Women with PID may have crampy, dull lower abdominal pain occurring with menses, or irregular menses over several cycles before the disease becomes overt. On bimanual examination, the signs in PID are uterine traction tenderness, adnexal tenderness, or adnexal enlargement. Although adnexal abscesses are unusual in gonococcal PID, clinical suspicion should lead to further evaluation, such as by sonography. The wide spectrum of disease, including mild cases, and the relative nonspecificity of clinical signs, make accurate clinical diagnosis often difficult. Laparoscopic studies have demonstrated clinicopathological correlation in only two thirds of cases.[46] Therefore, careful clinical observation of the patient is extremely important.

Distinguishing between PID caused by *N. gonorrhoeae*, *C. trachomatis*, and other microorganisms is important but often difficult. Laparoscopic evaluation, although invasive, gives the best diagnostic yield, and is being used more widely. Without laparoscopy, properly performed endocervical Gram stains and culture are the only way to make a microbiological diagnosis. However, diagnostic sensitivity and specificity are both substantially compromised. Culdocentesis without frank pus may not be entirely reliable because specimens may be contaminated with vaginal flora.

Because of the diagnostic problems, treatment regimens for PID are designed to include adequate antimicrobial coverage for *N. gonorrhoeae*, *C. trachomatis*, gram-negative organisms, and anaerobes. Hospitalization may be necessary in severe cases. In addition, if foreign bodies such as IUDs are present, they should be removed.

8.1.4. Anorectal Infections. Anorectal gonorrhea occurs predominantly in homosexual men with a history of receptive rectal intercourse, and in women with endocervical gonorrhea, in which 30–50% of patients have coexistent rectal infection.[54,61] In women, infection is not related to rectal intercourse; infected perineal secretions are thought to cause a secondary anorectal mucosal infection.

Most anorectal infections in women are asymptomatic. In homosexual men, symptoms such as tenesmus, mucoid discharge, hematochezia, perianal irritation, and constipation are seen more frequently. Anoscopy in symptomatic cases may show erythema, exudate, and friable mucosa in the anal canal and terminal rectum.[79] In asymptomatic cases, however, anoscopy is often normal.[61]

The differential diagnosis of anorectal gonorrhea, especially in homosexual men, includes rectal herpes and *C. trachomatis.*[70] Because of the large number of asymptomatic cases, and poor performance specificity of rectal Gram stain, diagnosis of anorectal gonorrhea is more accurately made by culture.

8.1.5. Pharyngeal Infection. Pharyngeal infection usually results from oral sexual exposure to an infected partner.[72,109] Among patients with anogenital gonorrhea, pharyngeal infection has been demonstrated in some studies in 3–7% of heterosexual men, 5–20% of women, and 10–25% of homosexual men.[44] Among pregnant women, the proportion may be higher. Exudative pharyngitis and sore throat are seen in symptomatic cases; however, pharyngeal gonorrhea in most cases is asymptomatic, and sore throat in some patients may be more related to a postfellatio syndrome rather than an infectious process.[86] Asymptomatic pharyngeal infection resulting in DGI has been well described.

Diagnosis of pharyngeal gonorrhea is made only by culture. Because of the presence of a large number of commensal *Neisseriaceae*, careful attention must be paid to confirmation of the diagnosis. Although there are reports of pharyngeal isolation of *C. trachomatis,*[51] the clinical significance of this remains open to question. Pharyngeal gonorrhea is more difficult to cure than gonorrhea at other mucosal sites. Spectinomycin fails to cure about 50% of the cases.[52] Therefore, when antibiotic-resistant infection is suspected, ceftriaxone should be used. Paradoxically, in studies where patients were followed without antibiotic treatment, spontaneous loss of gonococci from the throat, without evidence of disease, often occurred.[44,101]

8.1.6. Gonococcal Perihepatitis. This syndrome is probably caused by direct spread of the gonococcus to the capsule of the liver from a pelvic focus, via either the peritoneal cavity or lymphatics. Again, chlamydia is in the differential diagnosis. Patients, usually women with mucopurulent cervicitis or PID, have right-upper-quadrant pain, and mild elevation of liver enzymes. Jaundice is unusual and sonographic studies of the gallbladder and biliary tree are within normal limits. Perihepatitis usually resolves with antibiotic therapy of the underlying infectious process.

8.1.7. Disseminated Gonococcal Infection. Asymptomatic transient gonococcemia probably occurs frequently. Approximately 0.5–1.0% of patients with gonorrhea develop DGI. Patients with the DGI syndrome have a local infection, either rectal, urogenital, or pharyngeal, that is commonly asymptomatic. Host and organism factors are both important. As described earlier, organisms from patients with DGI are more likely to have properties such as serum resistance. Organisms that cause DGI are generally more sensitive to antibiotics than those found in routine

anogenital infection.[108] However, DGI due to PPNG or CMRNG does occur, and must be considered in areas where antibiotic resistance is a problem. DGI occurs more commonly in women than men; pregnant women are at highest risk, probably because of suppressed cell-mediated immunity. Persons with complement defects are at higher risk. Increasingly, DGI is being caused by organisms with antibiotic resistance. DGI caused by PPNG[18,81] and CMRNG organisms have been described, and are probably in proportion to their prevalence in the general community.

DGI syndromes can be separated clinically into two groups.[59,64,71] The first includes patients with chills, fever, or polyarthralgias and tenosynovitis (which are not usually migratory, but additive), who have 3–20 petechial, papular, pustular, hemorrhagic, or necrotic skin lesions (usually a combination of more than one type) on the distal extremities. Fingers, toes, hands, wrists, and ankles are most likely to be involved in an asymmetrical fashion. Painful skin lesions may bring the patient to the physician. Blood cultures are positive for *N. gonorrhoeae* in about half these cases. These clinical findings, together with cultures from mucosal sites, allow a definite or probable diagnosis of DGI in about 85% of cases. Aspiration of small joints is usually not productive. Gram stain or culture of skin lesions is usually negative; however, gonococci can usually be demonstrated by fluorescent antibody techniques.

The second common syndrome is a septic arthritis, usually monarticular, affecting large joints. The knee is involved most commonly. The signs and symptoms are those of any acute joint-space infection where purulent material is rapidly accumulating. Although the septic arthritis is secondary to a bacteremic process, blood cultures at this stage are rarely positive. Gram stain and culture of synovial fluid are mandatory diagnostic tests in any suspected septic arthritis, and are positive in about half the cases of gonococcal arthritis. The culture-negative cases are thought to result from either immune-complex deposition, or intraarticular killing of the organisms prior to arthrocentesis. DGI generally responds rapidly to appropriate antibiotic therapy.

In a small proportion of patients with DGI, severe complications such as meningitis, endocarditis, toxic hepatitis, and septic seeding of other organs can develop.[41] Fortunately, these complications are rare.

8.1.8. Gonococcal Ophthalmia. Gonococcal ophthalmia occurs in two groups: neonates born to women with endocervical gonorrhea, and adults who are exposed to infected secretions.[99,102]

Neonatal gonococcal ophthalmia is now rare in the United States, because of prenatal screening and universal prophylaxis; chlamydial ophthalmia is more common.[1] In developing countries, however, this disease is still a major cause of blindness, and is more common than chlamydial disease.[31] Infants with gonococcal ophthalmia may also have infection at other sites, such as the throat, anal canal, and respiratory tract. Incubation periods longer than 3 days are not unusual. Clinically, diffuse redness and conjunctival swelling are first seen, followed by a profuse, purulent discharge, from which the organism can be easily identified by Gram stain and culture. Corneal scarring and blindness can occur if left untreated.

Adult gonococcal ophthalmia has been increasingly reported. The patients are typically young adults with anogenital gonorrhea or recent exposure. In one study, infected urine had been used as a folk remedy for acute hemorrhagic viral conjunctivitis.[2] Purulent keratoconjunctivitis is seen clinically. Compared to the neonatal cases, corneal involvement was reported more often.

Diagnosis of gonococcal eye disease is made by Gram stain and culture. Care must be exercised in confirming the culture result. Cases of "pseudogonococcal ophthalmia" due to *Branhamella,* other *Neisseria,* and *Acinetobacter* have been reported.[90] Antibiotic-resistant infections such as PPNG should be considered where these organisms are prevalent. Because of the grave sequelae of this disease, all isolates should be tested for antimicrobial susceptibility.

Neonatal gonococcal ophthalmia can be prevented by maternal screening and treatment, where indicated. Additionally, neonatal ocular prophylaxis, first instituted by Credé, is one of the triumphs of preventive medicine.[29] In the United States, all but one require routine prophylaxis at birth with either erythromycin, silver nitrate, or tetracycline. The latter two have recently been shown to be equally effective in a large study done in Kenya.[60]

8.1.9. Pediatric Gonorrhea.[28,78] Gonococcal infections in prepubertal children are probably underreported. Clinically, in young girls, either symptomatic or asymptomatic vulvovaginitis may be seen.[3] Urethritis has been described in boys, and anorectal, rectal, and pharyngeal infection may be seen in both sexes.

Since nonsexual transmission of gonorrhea in children is extremely rare,[10,69] sexual exposure and child sexual abuse must be seriously considered when the diagnosis is made.[89] Because of the forensic implications, specific diagnosis is imperative.[107] The chain of custody must be maintained, cultures from all sites should be confirmed by experienced laboratories, and positive specimens should be archived.

9. Control and Prevention

9.1. Principles of Control

For control through public health intervention, we emphasize the importance of establishing priorities among gonorrhea cases for the implementation of measures such as intensive case-finding activities and epidemiological treatment. In other words, public-health authorities attempt to identify gonorrhea cases where intervention will have the highest yield in potential cases that will be prevented by the intervention (see Sections 9.1.2, 9.1.3). The mistaken assumption that every case of gonorrhea is equally important for the further spread of disease must be dispelled. Failure to treat gonorrhea cases and to promote primary prevention among groups with a high rate of disease transmission significantly limits the chances of success. Different degrees of control are possible in different environments. Control programs in many developed countries are currently focused on efforts to decrease the prevalence of the disease. In other areas, attempts may be made to prevent only serious sequelae, i.e., gonococcal ophthalmia neonatorum and gonococcal PID.

9.1.1. Clinical Services. Provision of easily accessible clinical services and proficient laboratory support services are essential to control programs. Clearly, it is futile to engage in widespread screening and elaborate efforts to locate sexual partners while waiting periods in clinics are long, patients with symptoms are being turned away, and the misdiagnosis and mismanagement of known cases are common. The establishment of practical clinical services should precede attempts at more sophisticated intervention and may in itself have a significant effect on the control of gonorrhea in some communities. To increase accessibility, all services related to the control of gonorrhea should be rendered free of charge or at least not denied because of an inability to pay.

The prevention of gonococcal ophthalmia neonatorum is, perhaps, the only substantial intervention that is not rooted in STD clinical services. Even ophthalmia prophylaxis requires trained clinical personnel. Community education and promotion of primary prevention (e.g., abstinence, partner selection, personal prophylaxis) should be informed and focused by epidemiological information derived from clinical facilities.

9.1.2. Epidemiological Process. Because of the large reservoir of asymptomatic and minimally symptomatic cases, especially in women, gonorrhea cannot be controlled solely by the application of diagnosis and treatment to cases with apparent symptoms. Public-health intervention is targeted both at identifying potentially infected individuals and in preventing the further transmission of disease.

Direct disease control activities are usually a function of local health departments. Ideally, the epidemiological process should focus on five groups: new patients, sexual partners of patients, patients with repeated infections, health-care providers, and community sources of health information. The basic information to be obtained from patients is directed toward identifying potentially infected partners and should include age, race, sex, place of residence, mobility, and special sociobehavioral features (e.g., prostitution, employment). Health-care providers for the population at highest risk must be determined. Simple measures for doing so include: (1) finding out from patients and their sexual partners where they are seeking health care; (2) making a survey of health-care providers located near the places of residence of high-risk groups; and (3) seeking "hidden" health-care providers (e.g., pharmacists, hotel physicians). In addition, a sample of physicians should be visited to find out the extent of their services to gonorrhea patients, if there is reason to suspect that a significant proportion of cases are not being reported. Health-care providers serving high-risk groups must be assisted in the correct diagnosis and treatment of gonorrhea and encouraged to use appropriate intervention techniques.

Each community may have unique sources of health information. The quality and influence of these sources (peers, media, social groups, churches, opinion leaders) will vary for subgroups within the community. Liaison with these information sources should be sought by local health authorities.

9.1.3. Transmitters or Nontransmitters. Special emphasis must be placed on finding those infected. Patients who are most likely to be efficient transmitters of the disease[85] deserve special emphasis in case-finding activities. Generally, efficient transmitters are those who are either asymptomatic or tend to ignore symptoms, who have a large number of different sexual partners, and who have limited access to medical care. A good indicator of a group with a high proportion of transmitters is the rate of repeated infection in the group.

9.1.4. Culture Screening. Because of cost considerations, culture screening for case detection in gonorrhea control must be targeted to high-risk groups. The cost-effectiveness of screening will depend on the prevalence of the disease in the population and can be increased by concentrating on the high-risk groups. However, although this measure will find cases at a lower cost per case, control-effectiveness will depend on the proportion of existing cases

missed by the screening procedure and other control strategies.

Populations screened should be carefully selected. For example, women presenting with signs or symptoms of other STDs, women distinguished by behavioral or demographic factors characteristic of high-risk groups (e.g., prostitutes), and women from groups in which the prevalence of the disease is high should be those selected for initial screening. The concept of repeated screening may be applied in a retrospective or prospective fashion. Retrospectively, women and men with a history of gonococcal infection should be screened whenever they visit a health facility; prospectively, patients treated for gonorrhea should be reexamined in 1 week, and for high-risk groups again in 5 weeks, after completion of treatment. Available resources will determine the number of screenings and the combinations of initial and repeat screenings that are possible within each locality. In most circumstances, only women should be screened for gonorrhea; nevertheless, the most intensive screenings should be done in the populations most likely to transmit infection. In high-prevalence areas, screening in different clinical settings should also be considered (e.g., in antenatal, gynecological, or family-planning clinics). Endocervical culture is the preferred screening method.

9.1.5. Epidemiological Treatment. Epidemiological treatment consists of providing full therapeutic doses of antibiotics to persons recently exposed to gonorrhea while awaiting the results of laboratory tests to confirm a diagnosis. This practice is recommended because of the significant chance that the patient has been infected, the serious consequences of the disease, the relative safety and efficacy of treatment, the frequency with which people in high-risk groups default on appointments, and the risk of the spread of the disease in the community.

a. Counseling to Obtain the Simultaneous Treatment of Sexual Partners. Since the treatment of patients in isolation would have insufficient effect on disease transmission, every gonorrhea patient should receive counseling with the aim of ensuring that: (1) the patient will return for reexamination; (2) the patient will advise his or her sexual partners to seek examination and treatment; (3) the patient will abstain from sexual contact until the sexual partners have been examined and treated; and (4) should the patient be reinfected in the future, he or she will bring recent sexual partners along to the health-care facility.

b. More Intensive Case Management. These techniques range from brief motivational educational sessions with individual patients to systems utilizing referral cards and to actual personal interviews with patients that will enable public-health workers to visit the patients' sexual partners in the community and offer treatment. Individual personal interviews to learn the names and whereabouts of sexual contacts and, in particular, community visits by health workers to locate these contacts may be possible in some areas. Whatever methods for providing epidemiological treatment to patients' sexual partners are used, they need not be used uniformly for all patients.

   c. Priorities for Epidemiological Services. The aim of contact tracing is to provide epidemiological treatment for those most likely to have transmitted the disease recently and most likely to continue transmitting it in the future. Contact tracing also requires the accessibility of the index case to the counselor or public-health worker. Granting this, priority for epidemiological services should be given to these groups of patients, symptomatic men, and members of high-risk groups (Table 2). When the sexual partners of these groups of patients are examined, the rate of asymptomatic infection is high. If the control organization is still weak, it may initially be most practical for epidemiological services to concentrate on men with symptomatic gonococcal urethritis.

   9.1.6. Health Education. Health education has been widely accepted as an important tool in the control of STDs because of increased recognition of the behavioral and sociocultural factors involved in their prevention, transmission, diagnosis, and treatment. Medical and organizational measures by themselves have proven to be unsatisfactory. In some countries, sex and health education is neglected, particularly among the young. The consequent ignorance about the STDs may hinder their control, because infected patients may be slow to take advice.

   Decisions and action to adopt control and preventive measures in relation to the STDs depend on several factors, such as information and misconceptions about these diseases, changes in beliefs about them and in attitudes toward

Table 2. Examples of Priority Criteria for Disease Intervention[a]

Prostitutes
Women with pelvic inflammatory disease
Symptomatic men
Cases of treatment failure (possibility of resistance)
Residence within a defined "core" area
Antimicrobial-resistant infection
Use of "crack" cocaine
Large number of sexual contacts

[a]These are examples of criteria used by different communities. Not all may be applicable to any one community.

them, prevailing cultural views and social norms, and the way patients are received by the STD health providers.

   Health-education activities may be aimed at making the public aware of the STD problem in the community, at seeking the active cooperation of groups and individuals in control activities, at informing groups at risk about control and preventive measures and motivating them to adopt these measures, at educating young people to consider the health-related aspects of their sexuality, at preparing personnel for their educational functions in the control program, and at orienting services at the relevant clinics toward the needs of their clients.

9.2. Personal Prophylaxis

   The overall value of physical and chemical means of personal prophylaxis is limited by factors of motivation, acceptance, and use. The effectiveness of condoms and diaphragms plus spermicide is poor in some populations, both for contraception and for disease prevention, because of poor compliance by users. The effectiveness of the condom must be emphasized to the public to encourage its use by those concerned about disease prevention.

   Condoms, when used appropriately, are highly effective in preventing transmission of gonorrhea and other STDs.[21] Latex condoms are recommended, since natural membrane condoms contain pores, which may not offer a complete transmission barrier to small viral particles, such as HIV. These pores are not present in latex condoms.

   Some intravaginal capsules, jellies, and creams contain gonocidal compounds in addition to spermicides. Some have been shown to possess a significant *in vitro* effect against the gonococcus after a 1-min exposure, and a recent study has shown that prophylactic use of nonoxynol-9-containing jelly may reduce the incidence of gonococcal and chlamydial infection.[62] Coordinating the use of these preparations with family-planning programs needs further emphasis.

9.3. Control of Antibiotic-Resistant *N. gonorrhoeae*

   As described in Section 5.8, there are multiple types of clinically important antimicrobial resistance. The rapidity with which these organisms can spread is impressive. For example, in PPNG epidemics in Miami and Detroit, the proportion of gonococci identified as PPNG rose from less than 5% to over 20% in less than a year. TRNG, first identified in 1985, was diagnosed in 17 states by 1986, and in 1987, accounted for 3% of gonococcal infections in the national antimicrobial surveillance system.

The cornerstone of controlling antibiotic resistance is early diagnosis, facilitating effective early treatment. Besides β-lactamase testing, antimicrobial susceptibility testing should be performed on as many specimens as possible to detect CMRNG and TRNG organisms. In the absence of universal testing, subsets should be periodically evaluated to gauge the background levels of resistance.

Eradication of these organisms from the United States is no longer practical. Contact tracing is labor-intensive, expensive, and generally succeeds with antibiotic-resistant gonorrhea only during the period when the organism is introduced into a community (introductory phase). The short incubation period, presence of asymptomatic infection, and relatively high transmission efficiency all conspire against effective eradication of an established focus of disease. Additionally, many outbreaks of PPNG have recently been linked to cocaine-abusing ("crack") populations, groups in which disease-intervention effort is difficult. In other words, once a resistant strain becomes endemic, it has the same epidemiological characteristics as endemic, antibiotic-sensitive gonorrhea.

CDC currently recommends that all gonococcal infections be treated with drugs effective against resistant organisms (such as ceftriaxone). (Table 3). Although this policy results in higher drug costs, it eliminates the need for follow-up of patients initially treated with PPNG-ineffective drugs, such as penicillin. Educational programs should be instituted to persuade private-sector physicians, emergency rooms, and other health-care providers to adopt a presumptive treatment policy. Patients diagnosed with PPNG, TRNG, or CMRNG should have posttreatment cultures documenting their cure.

Table 3. Current Regimens for Therapy of Gonorrhea

1. Ceftriaxone, 250 mg intramuscularly, one dose
2. Spectinomycin, 2 g intramuscularly, one dose[a]
3. Ciprofloxacin, 500 mg, orally, one dose[b]

In addition, all patients treated for gonorrhea should also be cotreated[c] (for chlamydial infection) with oral: tetracycline, 500 qid, or doxycycline, 100 mg bid, or erythromycin, 500 mg qid

[a]Spectinomycin is not effective for pharyngeal gonorrhea.
[b]Should not be given to adolescents or pregnant women.
[c]Because of widespread resistance, these drugs should not be used as single-drug therapy for gonorrhea.

9.4. Possibilities of Immunization

Three potential vaccine candidates exist: two constituents of the cell envelope—outer membrane protein and certain LPS complexes—and the filamentous proteinaceous pili. Most recent work has been directed toward developing a vaccine against the outer membrane protein or pilin moieties. It is unlikely and unknown whether these antigens would make the most successful vaccine, since there are advantages and disadvantages to each.

Outer membrane proteins: Over 70 serotypes have been identified,[56] and there are undoubtedly more. They are of special interest because they induce bactericidal antibody. However, they have not been the sole constituents of any currently used vaccine, and absolute purity may be very difficult to achieve.

Pili are antigenically diverse. Initial approaches to a gonococcal vaccine targeted pili antigens. However, not only was there too much antigenic diversity to produce an effective vaccine, but the gonococcal colonies are also capable of producing structurally similar but antigenically distinct pili,[11,22,91] thereby making this vaccine approach unworkable.

A vaccine will have to undergo extensive testing before it can be considered ready for clinical evaluation. In its most acceptable form, the vaccine should be composed of highly purified and well-characterized subcellular material. The mechanism by which this component causes pathogenicity and induces immunity should be understood. Any hope for the eventuality of vaccine trials in humans is tempered with difficulties in design and definition of relevant clinical and ethical endpoints.

9.5. Antibiotic Prophylaxis against Gonococcal Infection

There are few data about the efficacy of systemically administered prophylactic antibiotics for gonorrhea, although the idea is certainly not new. Patients have self-medicated almost as long as antibiotics have been available, especially where prescriptions are not required. In two recent studies, 60% of Singaporean prostitutes admitted to self-administered prophylaxis.[34] On the other hand, in England, where antibiotics are more strictly regulated, urinalysis of STD clinic patients found antibiotics in only 4% of the cases.[8] Clinical studies with penicillin[5] and minocycline[39] as postexposure prophylaxis found both to be effective in preventing infection with sensitive strains. However, these studies were conducted over 20 years ago.

With the increased levels of antibiotic resistance, antibiotic prophylaxis becomes less attractive. First, presumptively, it is difficult to know what the susceptibilities of the infecting strains will be. Second, and more important, prophylactic antibiotic use has been implicated in the development of antibiotic resistance, not only in *N. gonorrhoeae*, but in many other organisms, such as *Salmonella* from beef animals treated with antimicrobials[92] and multiple organisms from nosocomial infections.

10. Unresolved Problems

In a very real sense, the global problem of gonococcal infections is a scientific, social, and political one with interesting and serious medical consequences. The pathophysiology and relationship between *N. gonorrhoeae* and other possible coinfecting organisms, such as *C. trachomatis*, and the possible effect of gonococcal infection on transmission of other STD, such as that caused by HIV, need to be elucidated. Development of a gonococcal vaccine has proven to be an enormous challenge, not in the least due to unusual biological characteristics of the organism, such as antigenic phase variation, that allow it to successfully evade host defense mechanisms. The increased incidence and expanding spectrum of antimicrobial resistance are indicative of the remarkable ability of the gonococcus to adapt to adverse environments, and therefore, resistance monitoring should become an integral part of control programs.

Besides the aforementioned biological factors, there are behavioral issues that require further research. For example, patients with gonorrhea are at high risk to develop reinfection via new sexual exposure(s). The personal suffering of individuals, often the poorest in society, and the direct and indirect economic burden caused by gonococcal infections are not recognized by decision makers in communities. The stigma of having an STD contributes substantially to this apathy. Application of existing knowledge and technology could prevent enormous suffering and save the productivity of many citizens.

Similar social factors have until recently slowed the full development of a comprehensive research program into the control and prevention of this infection. Clinically, the current pandemic of HIV infection is driving advances in basic social, immunological, epidemiological, and behavioral research that is also required to address the gonococcal problem. Methods of primary prevention for all STDs should have definite positive spin-offs for gonorrhea control.

11. References

1. ALEXANDER, E. R., AND HARRISON, H. R., Role of *Chlamydia trachomatis* in perinatal infection, *Rev. Infect. Dis.* **5:**713–719 (1983).
2. ALFONSO, E., FRIEDLAND, B., HUPP, S., OLSEN, K., SENIKOWICH, K., SKLAR, V. E. F., AND FORSTER, R. K., *Neisseria gonorrhoeae* conjunctivitis. An outbreak during an epidemic of acute hemorrhagic conjunctivitis, *J. Am. Med. Assoc.* **250:**794–795 (1983).
3. ALTCHEK, A., Pediatric vulvovaginitis, *Pediatr. Clin. North Am.* **19:**559–580 (1972).
4. ARAL, S. O., SCHAFFER, J. E., MOSHER, W. D., AND GATES, W., JR., Gonorrhea rates: What denominator is most appropriate? *Am. J. Public Health* **78:**702–703 (1988).
5. BABIONE, R. W., HEDGECOCK, L. G., AND RAY, J. P., Naval experience with oral use of penicillin as a prophylaxis, *U.S. Armed Forces Med. J.* **3:**973–990 (1952).
6. BARNES, R. C., AND HOLMES, K. K., Epidemiology of gonorrhea, *Epidemiol. Rev.* **6:**1–30 (1984).
7. BERGER, R. E., ALEXANDER, E. R., MONDA, G. D., ANSELL, J., McCORMICK, G., AND HOLMES, K. K., *Chlamydia trachomatis* as a cause of acute idiopathic epididymitis, *N. Engl. J. Med.* **298:**301–304 (1978).
8. BIGNELL, C. J., FLANNIGAN, K., AND MILLAR, M. R., Antimicrobial substances in urine of patients attending department of genitourinary medicine, *Genitourin. Med.* **62:**264–266 (1986).
9. BOSLEGO, J. W., TRAMONT, E. C., TAKAFUJI, E. T., DINIEGA, B. M., MITCHELL, B. S., SMALL, J. W., KHAN, W. N., AND STEIN, D. C., Effect of spectinomycin use on the prevalence of spectinomycin-resistant and of penicillinase-producing *Neisseria gonorrhoeae*, *N. Engl. J. Med.* **317:**272–278 (1987).
10. BRANCH, G., AND PAXTON, R., A study of gonococcal infections among infants and children, *Public Health Rep.* **80:**347–352 (1965).
11. BRITIGAN, B. E., COHEN, M. S., AND SPARLING, P. F., Gonococcal infection: A model of molecular pathogenesis, *N. Engl. J. Med.* **312:**1683–1694 (1985).
12. CANNON, J. G., AND SPARLING, P. F., The genetics of the gonococcus, *Annu. Rev. Microbiol.* **38:**111–113 (1984).
13. Centers for Disease Control, Declining rates of rectal and pharyngeal gonorrhea among males—New York City, *Morbid. Mortal. Weekly Rep.* **33:**295–297 (1984).
14. Centers for Disease Control, Penicillinase-producing *Neisseria gonorrhoeae*—United States, Florida, *Morbid. Mortal. Weekly Rep.* **35:**12–14 (1986).
15. Centers for Disease Control, Multiple strain outbreak of penicillinase-producing Neisseria gonorrhoeae—Denver, Colorado, *Morbid. Mortal. Weekly Rep.* **35:**534–543 (1986).
16. Centers for Disease Control, Sexually transmitted disease statistics—1988, U.S. Public Health Service, Atlanta, 1989.
17. Centers for Disease Control, Antibiotic-resistant strains of

Neisseria gonorrhoeae: Policy guidelines for detection, management, and control, *Morbid. Mortal. Weekly Rep.* **36**(Suppl. 5S):1S–18S (1987).

18. Centers for Disease Control, Disseminated gonorrhea caused by penicillinase-producing *Neisseria gonorrhoeae, Morbid. Mortal. Weekly Rep.* **36**:161–167 (1987).

19. Centers for Disease Control, Sentinel surveillance system for antimicrobial resistance in clinical isolates of *Neisseria gonorrhoeae, Morbid. Mortal. Weekly Rep.* **36**:585–593 (1987).

20. Centers for Disease Control, Outbreak of a distinct strain of penicillinase-producing *Neisseria gonorrhoeae*—King County, Washington, *Morbid. Mortal. Weekly Rep.* **36**:757–759 (1987).

21. Centers for Disease Control, Condoms for Prevention of Sexually Transmitted Diseases, *Morbid. Mortal. Weekly Rep.* **37**:133–137 (1988).

22. DALLABETTA, G., AND HOOK, E. W., III, Gonococcal infections, *Infect. Dis. Clin. North Am.* **1**:25–54 (1987).

23. DARROW, W. W., Sexual behavior in America: Implications for the control of sexually transmitted diseases, in: *Sexually Transmitted Diseases* (Y. FELMAN, ed.), pp. 261–280, Churchill–Livingstone, Edinburgh, 1986.

24. DENSEN, P., GULATI, S., AND RICE, P. A., Specificity of antibodies against *Neisseria gonorrhoeae* that stimulate neutrophil chemotaxis, *J. Clin. Invest.* **80**:78–87 (1987).

25. EASMON, C. S. F., Gonococcal resistance to antibiotics, *J. Antimicrob. Chemother.* **16**:409–417 (1985).

26. EISENBERG, M. S., AND WIESNER, P. J., Reporting and treating gonorrhea: Results of a statewide survey in Alaska, *J. Am. Vener. Dis. Assoc.* **3**:79–83 (1976).

27. FARUKI, H., KOHMESCHER, R. N., MCKINNEY, W. P., AND SPARLING, P. F., A community-based outbreak of infection with penicillin-resistant *Neisseria gonorrhoeae* not producing penicillinase (chromosomally-mediated resistance), *N. Engl. J. Med.* **313**:607–611 (1985).

28. FOLLAND, D. S., BURKE, R. E., HINMAN, A. R., AND SCHAFFNER, W., Gonorrhea in preadolescent children: An inquiry into source of infection, *Pediatrics* **60**:153–156 (1977).

29. FORBES, G. B., AND FORBES, G. M., Silver nitrate and the eyes of the newborn: Crede's contribution to preventive medicine, *Am. J. Dis. Child.* **121**:1–5 (1971).

30. FOSTER, M. T., AND LABRUM, A. L. T., Relation of infection with *Neisseria gonorrhoeae* to ABO blood groups, *J. Infect. Dis.* **133**:329–330 (1976).

31. FRANSEN, L., NSANZE, H., KLAUSS, V., VAN DER STUYFT, P., D'COSTA, L., BRUNHAM, R. C., AND PIOT, P., Ophthalmia neonatorum in Nairobi, Kenya: The roles of *Neisseria gonorrhoeae* and *Chlamydia trachomatis, J. Infect. Dis.* **153**:862–869 (1986).

32. GALE, J. L., AND HINDS, M. W., Male urethritis in King County, Washington 1974–75: 1. Incidence, *Am. J. Public Health* **68**:20–25 (1978).

33. GILBAUGH, J. H., AND FUCHS, P. C., The gonococcus and the toilet seat, *N. Engl. J. Med.* **301**:91–93 (1979).

34. GOH, C. L., MEIJA, P., SNG, E. H., RAJAN, V. S., AND THIRUMOORHTY, T., Chemoprophylaxis and gonococcal infections in prostitutes, *Int. J. Epidemiol.* **13**:344–346 (1984).

35. GOODHART, G. E., OGDEN, J., ZAIDI, A. A., AND KRAUS, S. K., Factors affecting the performance of smear and culture for the detection of *Neisseria gonorrhoeae, Sex. Transm. Dis.* **9**:63–68 (1982).

36. GRIMES, D. A., Deaths due to sexually transmitted diseases, *Am. Med. Assoc.* **255**:1727–1729 (1986).

37. HANDSFIELD, H. H., Declining incidence of gonorrhea among homosexually active men—Minimal effect on risk of AIDS, *West. J. Med.* **143**:469–470 (1985).

38. HANDSFIELD, H. H., LIPMAN, T. O., HARNISCH, J. B., TRONCA, E., AND HOLMES, K. K., Asymptomatic gonorrhea in men: Diagnosis, natural course, prevalence, and significance, *N. Engl. J. Med.* **290**:117–123 (1970).

39. HARRISON, W. O., HOOPER, R. R., WIESNER, P. J., CAMPBELL, A. F., KARNEY, W. W., REYNOLDS, G. H., JONES, O. G., AND HOLMES, K. K., A trial of minocycline given after exposure to prevent gonorrhea, *N. Engl. J. Med.* **300**:1074–1078 (1979).

40. HOLMES, K. K., JOHNSON, D. W., AND TROSTLE, H. J., An estimate of the risk of men acquiring gonorrhea by sexual contact with infected females, *Am. J. Epidemiol.* **91**:17–24 (1970).

41. HOLMES, K. K., COUNTS, G. W., AND BEATY, H. N., Disseminated gonococcal infection, *Ann. Intern. Med.* **74**:979–993 (1971).

42. HOOK, E. W., AND HOLMES, K. K., Gonococcal infections, *Ann. Intern. Med.* **102**:229–243 (1985).

43. HOOTEN, T. M., AND BARNES, R. C., Urethritis in men, *Infect. Dis. Clin. North Am.* **1**:165–178 (1987).

44. HUTT, D. M., AND JUDSON, F. N., Epidemiology and treatment of oropharyngeal gonorrhea, *Ann. Intern. Med.* **104**:655–658 (1986).

45. JACOBS, N. F., AND KRAUS, S. K., Gonococcal and nongonococcal urethritis in men. Clinical and laboratory differentiation, *Ann. Intern. Med.* **82**:7–12 (1975).

46. JACOBSON, L., AND WESTROM, L., Objectivized diagnosis of pelvic inflammatory disease, *Am. J. Obstet. Gynecol.* **18**:35 (1975).

47. JAFFE, H. W., ZAIDI, A. A., THORNSBERRY, C., REYNOLDS, G. H., AND WIESNER, P. J., Trends and seasonality of antibiotic resistance of *Neisseria gonorrhoeae, J. Infect. Dis.* **136**:684–688 (1977).

48. JAFFE, H. W., LEWIS, J. S., AND WIESNER, P. J., Vancomycin-sensitive *Neisseria gonorrhoeae, J. Infect. Dis.* **144**:198 (1981).

49. JAFFE, H. W., BIDDLE, J. W., JOHNSON, S. R., AND WIESNER, P. J., Infections due to penicillinase-producing *Neisseria gonorrhoeae* in the United States: 1976–80, *J. Infect. Dis.* **144**:191–197 (1981).

50. JOINER, K. A., SCALES, R., WARREN, K. A., FRANK, M. M., AND RICE, P A., Mechanism of action of blocking im-

munoglobulin G for *Neisseria gonorrhoeae*, *J. Clin. Invest.* **76:**1765–1772 (1985).

51. JONES, R. B., RABINOVITCH, R. A., KATZ, B. P., BATLEIGER, B. E., WUINN, T. S., TERHO, P., AND LAPWORTH, M. A., *Chlamydia trachomatis* from the rectum and pharynx of heterosexual patients at risk for genital infection, *Ann. Intern. Med.* **102:**757–762 (1985).

52. JUDSON, F. N., EHRET, J. M., AND HANDSFIELD, H. H., Comparative study of ceftriaxone and spectinomycin for treatment of pharyngeal and anorectal gonorrhea, *J. Am. Med. Assoc.* **253:**1417–1419 (1985).

53. KEARNS, D. H., O'REILLY, R. J., LEE, L., AND WELCH, B. G., Secretory IgA antibodies in the urethral exudate of men with uncomplicated urethritis due to *Neisseria gonorrhoeae*, *J. Infect. Dis.* **127:**99–101 (1973).

54. KLEIN, E. J., FISHER, L. S., CHOW, A. W., AND GUZE, L. B., Anorectal gonococcal infection, *Ann. Intern. Med.* **86:**340–346 (1977).

55. KNAPP, J. S., TAM, M. R., NOWINSKI, R. C., HOLMES, K. K., AND SANDSTROM, E. G., Serological classification of *Neisseria gonorrhoeae* with use of monoclonal antibodies to gonococcal outer membrane protein I, *J. Infect. Dis.* **150:**44–48 (1984).

56. KNAPP, J. S., SANDSTROM, E. G., AND HOLMES, K. K., Overview of epidemiological and clinical applications of auxotype/serovar classification of *Neisseria gonorrhoeae*, in: *The Pathogenic Neisseriae* (G. K. Schoolnik, ed.), pp. 6–12, American Society for Microbiology, Washington, D.C., 1985.

57. KNAPP, J. S., ZENILMAN, J. M., BIDDLE, J. W., PERKINS, G. H., DEWITT, W. E., THOMAS, M. L., JOHNSON, S. R., AND MORSE, S. A., Frequency and distribution in the United States of *Neisseria gonorrhoeae* with plasmid-mediated, high-level resistance to tetracycline, *J. Infect. Dis.* **155:**819–822 (1987).

58. KOHL, P. K., AND BUCHANAN, T. M., Serotype-specific bactericidal activity of monoclonal antibodies to protein I of *Neisseria gonorrhoeae*, in: *The Pathogenic Neisseria* (G. K. Schoolnik, ed.), pp. 442–444, American Society for Microbiology, Washington, D.C., 1985.

59. KOSS, P. G., Disseminated gonococcal infection—The tenosynovitis–dermatitis and suppurative arthritis syndromes, *Cleveland Clin. Q.* **52:**161–173 (1985).

60. LAGA, M., PLUMMER, F. A., AND PIOT, P., Prophylaxis of gonococcal and chlamydial ophthalmia neonatorum, *N. Engl. J. Med.* **318:**653–657 (1988).

61. LEBEDOFF, D. A., AND HOCHMAN, E. B., Rectal gonorrhea in men: Diagnosis and treatment, *Ann. Intern. Med.* **92:**463–466 (1980).

62. LOUV, W. C., AUSTIN, H., ALEXANDER, W. J., STAGNO, S., AND CHEEKS, J., A clinical trial of nonoxynol-9 for preventing gonococcal and chlamydial infections, *J. Infect. Dis.* **158:**518–523 (1988).

63. MARTIN, R., COOPES, S., NEAGLE, P., ENGLAND, E. H., AND WENTWORTH, B. B., Comparison of Thayer–Martin,

Transgrow, and Gonozyme for detection of *Neisseria gonorrhoeae* in a low-risk population, *Sex. Transm. Dis.* **13:**108–110 (1986).

64. MASI, A. T., AND EISENSTEIN, B. I., Disseminated gonococcal infection and gonococcal arthritis: II. Clinical manifestations, diagnosis, complications, treatment, prevention, *Semin. Arthritis Rheum.* **10:**173–197 (1981).

65. MCCUTCHAN, J. A., KATZENSTEIN, D., NORQUIST, D., CHIKAMI, G., WUNDERLICH, A., AND BRAUDE, A. I., Role of blocking antibody in disseminated gonococcal infection, *J. Immunol.* **121:**1884–1888 (1978).

66. MCGEE, Z. A., JOHNSON, A. P., AND TAYLOR-ROBINSON, D., Pathogenic mechanisms of *Neisseria gonorrhoeae*: Observations on damage to human fallopian tubes in organ culture by gonococci of colony type 1 or type 4, *J. Infect. Dis.* **143:**413–422 (1981).

67. MORELLO, J. A., JANDA, W. M., AND BOHNHOFF, M. *Neisseria* and *Branhamella*, in: *Manual of Clinical Microbiology* (E. H. Lennette, A. Balows, W. J. Hausler, and H. J. Shadomy, eds.), pp. 179–192, American Society for Microbiology, Washington, D. C., 1985.

68. MORSE, S. A., JOHNSON, S. R., BIDDLE, J. W., AND ROBERTS, M. C., High-level tetracycline resistance in *Neisseria gonorrhoeae* is result of acquisition of streptococcal *tetM* determinant, *Antimicrob. Agents Chemother.* **30:**664–670 (1987).

69. NEINSTEIN, L., GOLDDENRING, J., AND CARPENTER, S., Nonsexual transmission of sexually transmitted diseases: An infrequent occurrence, *Pediatrics* **74:**67–76 (1984).

70. *Neisseria gonorrhoeae* and gonococcal infections, Report of a WHO Scientific Group, Technical Report Series, No. 616, WHO, Geneva, 1978.

71. O'BRIEN, J. P., GOLDENBERG, D. L., AND RICE, P. A., Disseminated gonococcal infection: A prospective analysis of 49 patients and a review of pathophysiology and immune mechanisms, *Medicine* **62:**395–406 (1983).

72. OSBORNE, N. G., AND GRUBIN, L., Colonization of the pharynx with *Neisseria gonorrhoeae*: Experience in a clinic for sexually transmitted disease, *Sex. Transm. Dis.* **6:**253–256 (1979).

73. OSTROW, D. G., AND ALTMAN, N. L., Sexually transmitted diseases and homosexuality, *Sex. Transm. Dis.* **10:**208–215 (1983).

74. PASQUIERELLO, C. A., PLOTKIN, S. A., RICE, R. J., AND HACKNEY, J. R., Fatal gonococcal septicemia, *Pediatr. Infect. Dis.* **4:**204–206 (1984).

75. PEDERSON, A. H. B., AND BONIN, P., Screening females for asymptomatic gonococcal infection, *Northwest. Med.* **70:**225–261 (1971).

76. PETERSON, B. H., LEE, T. J., SNYDERMAN, R., AND BROOKS, G. F., *Neisseria meningitidis* and *Neisseria gonorrhoeae* bacteremia associated with C6, C7, or C8 deficiency, *Ann. Intern. Med.* **90:**917–920 (1979).

77. PLATT, R., RICE, P. A., AND MCCORMACK, W. M., Risk of acquiring gonorrhea and prevalence of abnormal adnexal

findings among women recently exposed to gonorrhea, *J. Am. Med. Assoc.* **250:**3205–3209 (1983).

78. POTTERAT, J. J., MARKEWICH, G. S., AND ROTHENBERG, R., Prepubertal infections with *Neisseria gonorrhoeae:* Clinical and epidemiologic significance, *Sex. Transm. Dis.* **5:**1–3 (1978).

79. QUINN, T. C., STAMM, W. E., GOODELL, S. E., MKRTICHIAN, E., BENEDETTI, J., COREY, L., SCHUFFLER, M. D., AND HOLMES, K. K., The polymicrobial origin of intestinal infection in homosexual men, *N. Engl. J. Med.* **309:**576 (1983).

80. RICE, R. J., ARAL, S. O., BLOUNT, J. H., AND ZAIDI, A. A., Gonorrhea in the United States 1975–1984: Is the giant only sleeping? *Sex. Transm. Dis.* **14:**83–87 (1987).

81. RINALDI, R. Z., HARRISON, W. O., AND FAN, P. T., Penicillin-resistant gonococcal arthritis: A report of four cases, *Ann. Intern. Med.* **97:**43–45 (1982).

82. ROBERTS, M. C., AND KNAPP, J. S., Transfer of β-lactamase plasmids from *Neisseria gonorrhoeae* to *Neisseria meningitidis* and commensal *Neisseria* by the 25.2 megadalton conjugative plasmid, *Antimicrob. Agents Chemother.* **32:**1430–1432 (1988).

83. ROBERTSON, P., AND, SCHACHTER, J., Failure to identify venereal disease in a lesbian population, *Sex. Transm. Dis.* **8:**75–76 (1981).

84. ROTHENBERG, R. B., The geography of gonorrhea, *Am. J. Epidemiol.* **117:**688–694 (1983).

85. ROTHENBERG, R. B., AND POTTERAT, J. J., Temporal and social aspects of gonorrhea transmission: The force of infectivity, *Sex. Transm. Dis.* **15:**88–92 (1988).

86. SACKEL, S. G., ALPERT, S., FIUMARA, N. J., DONNER, A., LAUGHLIN, C. A., AND MCCORMACK, W. M., Orogenital contact and the isolation of *Neisseria gonorrhoeae, Mycoplasma hominis,* and *Ureaplasma urealyticum* from the pharynx, *Sex. Transm. Dis.* **6:**64–68 (1979).

87. SARAFIAN, S. K., TAM, M. R., AND MORSE, S. A., Gonococcal protein-I-specific opsonic IgG in normal human serum, *J. Infect. Dis.* **148:**1025–1032 (1983).

88. SCHMID, G. P., JOHNSON, R. E., BRENNER, E. R., AND The Cooperative Study Group, Symptomatic response to therapy of men with gonococcal urethritis: Do all need post-treatment cultures? *Sex. Transm. Dis.* **14:**37–40 (1987).

89. SGROI, S., Pediatric gonorrhea and child sexual abuse: The venereal disease connection, *Sex. Transm. Dis.* **9:**154–156 (1982).

90. SPARK, R. P., DAHLBERG, P. W., AND LaBELLE, J. W., Pseudogonococcal ophthalmia neonatorum, *Am. J. Clin. Pathol.* **72:**471–473 (1979).

91. SPARLING, P. F., CANNON, J. G., AND So, M., Phase and antigenic variation of pili and outer membrane protein II of *Neisseria gonorrhoeae, J. Infect. Dis.* **153:**196–201 (1986).

92. HOLMBERG, S. E., OSTERHOLM, M. T., SENGER, K. A., AND COHEN, M. L., Drug-resistant salmonella from animals fed antimicrobials, *N. Engl. J. Med.* **311:**617–622 (1984).

93. STRADER, K. W., WISE, C. M., WASILAUKAS, B. L., AND

94. STUART, R. D., Transport problems in public health bacteriology: Use of transport media and other devices to maintain viability of bacteria in specimens, *Can. J. Public Health* **49:**114–122 (1956).

95. SWEET, R. L., Pelvic inflammatory disease and infertility in women, *Infect. Dis. Clin. North Am.* **1:**199–215 (1987).

96. THAYER, J. D., AND MARTIN, J. E., JR., A selective medium for the cultivation of *Neisseria gonorrhoeae* and *Neisseria meningitidis, Public Health Rep.* **79:**49 (1964).

97. THOMPSON, S. E., AND HAGER, W. D., Acute pelvic inflammatory disease, *Sex. Transm. Dis.* **4:**105–113 (1977).

98. TRAMONT, E. C., Inhibition of adherence of *Neisseria gonorrhoeae* by human genital secretions, *J. Clin. Invest.* **59:**117–124 (1977).

99. ULLMAN, S., ROUSSEL, T. J., CULBERTSON, W. W., FORSTER, R. K., ALFONSO, E., MENDELSOHN, A. D., HEIDEMANN, D. G., AND HOLLAND, S. P., *Neisseria gonorrhoeae* keratoconjunctivitis, *Ophthalmology* **94:**525–531 (1987).

100. VAN KLINGEREN, B., ANSINK-SHIPPER, M. C., DESSENS-KROON, M., HUIKESHOVEN, M. H., AND WOUDSTRA, R. K., Relationship between auxotype, plasmid pattern, and susceptibility to antibiotics in penicillinase-producing *Neisseria gonorrhoeae, J. Antimicrob. Chemother.* **16:**143–147 (1985).

101. WALLIN, J. E., AND SIEGEL, M. S., Pharyngeal *Neisseria gonorrhoeae:* Coloniser or pathogen, *Br. Med. J.* **1:**1462–1463 (1979).

102. WAN, W. L., FARKAS, G. C., MAY, W. N., AND ROBIN, J. B., The clinical characteristics and course of adult gonococcal conjunctivitis, *Am. J. Ophthalmol.* **102:**575–583 (1986).

103. WASHINGTON, A. E.,, GOVE, S., SCHACHTER, J., AND SWEET, R. L., Oral contraceptives, *Chlamydia trachomatis* infection, and pelvic inflammatory disease, *J. Am. Med. Assoc.* **253:**2246–2250 (1985).

104. WASHINGTON, A. E., ARNO, B. S., AND BROOKS, M. A., The economic cost of pelvic inflammatory disease, *J. Am. Med. Assoc.* **255:**1735–1738 (1986).

105. WASSERHEIT, J. N. Pelvic inflammatory disease and inferitility, *Md. Med. J.* **36:**58–63 (1987).

106. WESTROM, L., Incidence, prevalence, and trends of acute pelvic inflammatory disease and its consequences in industrialized countries, *Am. J. Obstet. Gynecol.* **138:**880–892 (1980).

107. WHITTINGTON, W. L., RICE, R. J., BIDDLE, J. W., AND KNAPP, J. S., Incorrect identification of *Neisseria gonorrhoeae* from infants and children, *Pediatr. Infect. Dis. J.* **7:**3–10 (1988).

108. WIESNER, P. J., HANDSFIELD, H. H., AND HOLMES, K. K., Low antibiotic resistance of gonococci causing disseminated infection, *N. Engl. J. Med.* **288:**1221–1222 (1973).

109. WIESNER, P. J., TRONCA, E., BONIN, P., PEDERSON, A. H. B., AND HOLMES, K. K., Clinical spectrum of pharyngeal gonococcal infection, *N. Engl. J. Med.* **284:**181–185 (1973).

SALZER, W. L., Disseminated gonococcal infection caused by chromosomally mediated penicillin-resistant organisms, *Ann. Intern. Med.* **104:**365–366 (1986).

110. WILLIAM, D. C., Sexually transmitted diseases in gay men: An insider's view, *Sex. Transm. Dis.* **6:**278–280 (1979).

111. YOUNG, J. D. E., BLAKE, M., MAURO, A., AND COHN, Z. A., Properties of the major outer membrane protein from *Neisseria gonorrhoeae* incorporated into model lipid membranes, *Proc. Natl. Acad. Sci. USA* **80:**3831–3835 (1983).

112. ZENILMAN, J. M., NIMS, L. J., MENEGUS, M. A., NOLTE, F., AND KNAPP, J. S., Spectinomycin-resistant gonococcal infections in the United States, 1985–1986, *J. Infect. Dis.* **156:**1002–1004 (1987).

113. ZENILMAN, J. M., BONNER, M., SHARP, K. L., RABB, J., ALEXANDER, E. R., AND The Dade County Public Health Unit, Penicillinase-producing *Neisseria gonorrhoeae* in Dade County, Florida: Evidence of core-group transmitters and the impact of illicit antibiotics, *Sex. Transm. Dis.* **15:**45–50 (1988).

12. Suggested Reading

BARNES, R. C., AND HOLMES, K. K., Epidemiology of gonorrhea: Current perspectives, *Epidemiol. Rev.* **6:**1–30 (1984).

Discusses long-term epidemiological trends of gonorrhea, programmatic aspects of gonorrhea control programs, and differentiation of disease transmitters into "efficient" and "nonefficient" categories.

Centers for Disease Control, Policy Guidelines for the Detection, Management, and Control of Antibiotic-Resistant *Neisseria gonorrhoeae. Morbidity and Mortality Weekly Report* 1987 (Suppl. 5S).

Clinical aspects of antibiotic-resistant gonococcal infection are discussed, including laboratory diagnosis, treatment. Staged intervention programs are presented, based on the relative prevalence of resistant strains.

Centers for Disease Control, 1989 Sexually Transmitted Disease Treatment Guidelines. *Morbidity and Mortality Weekly Report* 1989 (Suppl. s-8). (Available free from CPS-DSTD Technical Information Service, Mailstop E-06, Centers for Disease Control, Atlanta, GA 30333.)

EASMON, C. S. F., AND ISON, C. A., *Neisseria gonorrhoeae:* A versatile pathogen, *J. Clin. Pathol.* **40:**1088–1097 (1987).

Article by the foremost British authorities on gonococcal disease in which the laboratory techniques of diagnosis and pathophysiology are discussed. Extensively discusses the various mechanisms of gonococcal antibiotic resistance.

HOLMES, K. K., MARDH, P.-A., SPARLING, P. F., AND WIESNER, P. J., (ed.), *Sexually Transmitted Diseases,* McGraw–Hill, New York, 1989.

This encyclopedic volume covers historical, clinical, behavioral, and epidemiological aspects of all sexually transmitted diseases. There are especially good sections on organizing effective STD services.

HOOK, E. W., III, AND HOLMES, K. K., Gonococcal infections, *Ann. Inter. Med.* **102:**229–243 (1985).

Comprehensive review of the pathophysiology, pathogenesis, and clinical syndromes associated with gonococcal infection, oriented to a broad audience.

ROTHENBERG, R. B., The geography of gonorrhea: Empirical demonstration of core group transmission, *Am. J. Epidemiol.* **117:**688–694 (1983).

In this article, the "core theory" (Section 5.3), which states that gonorrhea incidence rates have a specific geographic distribution, is developed. The core theory is now becoming the basis for focused intervention programs.

CHAPTER 14

Haemophilus influenzae Type b

Stephen L. Cochi and Joel I. Ward

1. Introduction

Invasive disease caused by *Haemophilus influenzae* type b (Hib) is recognized as a leading infectious disease health problem, primarily for young children (Table 1). An estimated 20,000 persons develop invasive Hib disease each year in the United States, and it has also been estimated that during the first 5 years of life the cumulative incidence of disease is one episode in every 200 children.[84] Hib is the most important cause of bacterial meningitis in the United States; in addition, it causes a wide variety of other severe infections characterized by invasion of the bloodstream with involvement of organ systems other than the CNS. Despite the availability of effective antimicrobials, Hib remains a substantial cause of mortality and morbidity.

The current annual number of cases and deaths due to Hib disease in the United States are similar to those of paralytic poliomyelitis during the peak epidemic years from 1951 to 1955 (Table 2). This comparison is an additional indication of the importance of Hib disease and the need to develop means to prevent the disease.

Within the last two decades, there has been a considerable accumulation of knowledge regarding the epidemiology, pathogenesis, and immunology of Hib disease that has

Stephen L. Cochi · Division of Immunization, Center for Prevention Services, Centers for Disease Control, Atlanta, Georgia 30333. Joel I. Ward · Harbor–UCLA Medical Center, UCLA School of Medicine, Torrance, California 90509.

proven useful in efforts to prevent the disease. These advances have led to the development of effective vaccines, which in turn has ushered us into an era where control of Hib disease is now becoming a reality. For purposes of this review, invasive Hib disease is distinguished from mucosal infections (such as otitis media, bronchitis, and sinusitis); the latter are generally caused by nonencapsulated *H. influenzae* and occur by extension from colonized respiratory passages to contiguous body sites (see Section 8). Mucosal infections generally do not result in bacteremia and hence are rarely life-threatening. The vaccines developed to date for *H. influenzae* disease are intended to prevent only type b invasive disease and will have little or no impact on the incidence of mucosal infections and other infections due to non-type b strains. Thus, the preventive measures reviewed in this chapter are directed toward invasive Hib disease and do not include strategies for preventing non-type b mucosal infections.

2. Historical Background

H. influenzae was first described in 1892 by Robert Pfeiffer,[314] who noted the presence of the organism in the purulent sputum of patients with influenza during the major 1889–1892 outbreak of influenza in Europe. He proposed that the organism was the cause of influenza,[315] and it became known as the "Pfeiffer influenza bacillus." Although there remained some doubt about the etiological role

277

Table 1. Public Health Importance of Invasive
Haemophilus influenzae **Type b (Hib) Disease in the**
United States

Characteristic	Annual morbidity/mortality/cost
Incidence	10,000 Hib meningitis cases
	8–10,000 cases of other invasive
	Hib disease
Deaths	1000 children
Neurologic sequelae	3000 children
Total medical costs[a]	$425 million

[a]Estimate of the Institute of Medicine, National Academy of Sciences, 1985.

of Pfeiffer's organism as a cause of influenza, it was not until the influenza pandemic of 1918 that its etiological role was seriously questioned. In 1920, the Society of American Bacteriologists changed the name of the organism to *H. influenzae* to acknowledge the historic association with influenza and to emphasize its requirement of blood factors for growth (*Haemophilus:* "blood-loving").[457] In 1933 Smith *et al.*[392] established that influenza was caused by a virus and finally refuted any remaining confusion about an association between *H. influenzae* and the influenza syndrome.

During the 1930s, classic work by Margaret Pittman demonstrated that *H. influenzae* existed in encapsulated and unencapsulated forms, and she identified six capsular types (types a–f).[323] She also observed that virtually all *H. influenzae* isolates from CSF and blood were capsular type b, and demonstrated that type b horse antiserum conferred protection against lethal systemic infection in rabbits.[324] At about the same time, studies by Fothergill and Wright showed a strong relationship between the age-specific risk for Hib meningitis and the absence of bactericidal antibodies, leading these investigators to propose that the bactericidal activity of serum conferred immunity against Hib

Table 2. Relative Morbidity and Mortality of
Invasive *Haemophilus influenzae* **Type b (Hib) Disease**
and Poliomyelitis in the United States

Measure	Hib diease (1980s)	Poliomyelitis (1951–1955)
Annual cases	20,000	(total) 28,000–57,000 (paralytic) 10,000–21,000
Annual deaths	1,000	1,000–3,100

meningitis.[133] This hypothesis provided an explanation for the observed protective effects of maternally acquired antibody in very young infants and the protection in older children afforded by antibody acquired by natural exposure to the organism.

Prior to the availability of antimicrobial therapy, Hib meningitis and most other forms of invasive Hib disease were virtually always fatal.[429] The first effective therapy for Hib disease was developed during the 1930s using antiserum produced from the immunization of horses with whole formalinized strains of Hib.[136,429] A mixture of antiserum and complement was usually given intrathecally twice daily. Despite this therapy, the reported case-fatality ratio was more than 80%.[136] During the late 1930s, methods were devised to prepare hyperimmune rabbit sera for immunotherapy of Hib meningitis.[2,5,8] Using a mouse protection assay, it was shown that absorption of the whole-cell hyperimmune Hib antisera with purified type b capsular polysaccharide removed most of its protective activity.[7] The clinical use of rabbit type b antiserum, in conjunction with sulfonamides, in children with Hib meningitis reduced the case-fatality ratio to 24%,[4] as compared to case-fatality ratios of 72–88% with sulfonamides alone[3,6] and 54–82% with sulfonamides combined with horse antiserum therapy.[4] Rabbit antiserum combined with sulfonamides was also used successfully for children with other invasive Hib disease, such as epiglottitis and empyema.[4,6]

The advent of more effective antimicrobial agents focused attention on the treatment rather than prevention of Hib disease. While progress continued to occur in our understanding of the pathogenesis and immunology of the disease, there was a hiatus in research directed toward developing means to prevent Hib disease. This hiatus ended during the early 1970s, when two groups of investigators purified and characterized the type b polysaccharide [polyribosyl-ribitol phosphate (PRP)]. In adults it was shown that serum antibodies to PRP were bactericidal and opsonophagocytic, and protected against invasive infection in mouse, rat, and monkey protection models.[25,214,345,360] Thus, evidence accumulated that antibody to the type b polysaccharide was a potential vaccine immunogen. The protective efficacy of a PRP vaccine against invasive Hib disease in children 18–71 months of age was established in a prospective, randomized field trial in Finland initiated in 1974. The results of 4-year follow-up of children in this trial were published in 1984.[3] These studies culminated in the licensure of PRP vaccine in the United States in April 1985, the first vaccine available for the prevention of Hib disease (see Section 9.2.1). The first Hib conjugate vaccine, one of a group of second-generation vaccines that alter the PRP antigen so as to enhance its immunogenicity, was licensed in December 1987, for routine use in children at 18 months of age (see Section 9.2.3). The prospect of actively immunizing young infants, the age group at highest risk for Hib disease, awaits the results of additional studies with newer Hib conjugate vaccines.[443]

3. Methodology

3.1. Sources of Mortality Data

The only national data available on deaths caused by invasive *H. influenzae* disease are compiled by the National Center for Health Statistics (NCHS). The NCHS receives copies of death certificates from each county and codes and tabulates the recorded diagnosis using the International Classification of Diseases (ICD-9) codes. The questions that arise with death-certificate data concern the accuracy of the recorded diagnosis, the completeness of reporting, and the lack of a comprehensive set of ICD codes encompassing all forms of invasive Hib disease. To assess the completeness and validity of these data, death-certificate data from 1962 to 1968 were compared with population-based retrospective studies of Hib meningitis from four separate areas of the United States.[127] Only 58% of the confirmed cases of fatal *H. influenzae* meningitis in the four study areas were listed as *H. influenzae* meningitis on the NCHS registry. More recent evaluations of the completeness and validity of the NCHS death data have not been published.

Surveillance of invasive *H. influenzae* disease based on datasets that compile ICD-9 hospital discharge diagnoses has been shown to be more sensitive for meningitis than for bacteremic disease without meningitis.[450]

The most reliable mortality data are derived from hospital-based and population-based studies of invasive Hib disease.[84] Passive surveillance from the National Bacterial Meningitis Surveillance Study, a passive surveillance system with variable participation from 27 states that represent 52% of the U.S. population, has provided estimates of age-specific case-fatality ratios of Hib meningitis.[357]

3.2. Sources of Morbidity Data

In the United States, invasive *H. influenzae* disease is not a nationally reportable disease. Consequently, national data on the incidence and morbidity of invasive Hib disease are not readily available from a single source. National estimates are derived by extrapolation from community-based or hospital-based studies[84] (see Section 5.1). Population-based studies with active surveillance efforts provide the most accurate estimates on the incidence of Hib disease, and are particularly useful for evaluating risk factors for Hib disease (see Section 5). Passive surveillance from the National Bacterial Meningitis Surveillance Study provides another source of epidemiological data on Hib meningitis, but these data are affected by substantial underreporting of disease.[357] Hospital-based studies, although not providing accurate incidence data, have improved our understanding of the clinical spectrum, complications, and long-term sequelae of Hib disease (see Section 8.1).

Studies that are laboratory-based are useful for determining the incidence of Hib meningitis, because virtually all patients with the disease are hospitalized and the organism can usually be isolated by routine culture of blood and CSF, or the diagnosis can be confirmed by antigen detection assays. However, the diagnosis of invasive Hib disease other than meningitis depends upon clinical criteria and recognition of the need to obtain blood cultures or cultures of other normally sterile body fluids, such as joint fluid or pleural fluid. Case definitions dependent upon blood cultures are likely to underestimate the true incidence of Hib disease, because of nonuniform use of blood and other cultures by different physicians. Also, negative cultures may occur in children who have received antimicrobials prior to obtaining cultures.

3.3. Surveys

Several well-conducted surveys of Hib pharyngeal carriage have been done in different populations (see Section 5.1.2). However, few studies with systematically obtained serological data are available, except data collected in the context of vaccine immunogenicity studies or studies of high-risk populations. Historical difficulties in performing assays of antibody to the capsular polysaccharide of Hib, and the lack of standardized methodology resulting in variability in quantitation of antibody,[451] have been impediments to comparing serological results among different surveys.

3.4. Laboratory Diagnosis

H. influenzae is a small gram-negative coccobacillus that on Gram stain of clinical specimens can be pleomorphic, especially in specimens from patients who have received β-lactam antimicrobials. Its variable morphology can lead to misinterpretation of stained smears.

The laboratory identification of *H. influenzae* is dependent upon the organism's nutritional requirements for X and V factors for growth. The X factor is a heat-stable, iron-containing protoporphyrin essential for activity of the electron-transport chain and for aerobic growth. The V factor, a coenzyme, is a heat-labile factor supplied by NAD. Both of these factors are present within erythrocytes, and are released in chocolate agar by heat or enzyme lysis of the red cells. The growth requirements for X and V factors remain the primary basis for the laboratory differentiation of *H. influenzae* from other *Haemophilus* species.

Fermentation and other metabolic activities of the organism are variable among strains and therefore are not particularly useful for identification. However, a biotyping scheme, based on the metabolism of indole, urea, and ornithine decarboxylase activity, has been used to subtype strains. Although not essential for growth, some strains grow better in 5 to 10% CO_2. *H. influenzae* grows in almost any enriched liquid or solid medium that contains X and V factors. After overnight incubation on an enriched medium, colonies appear that are 0.5 to 1.5 mm in diameter and rough or granular in appearance. Encapsulated strains usually produce slightly larger, mucoid or glistening colonies. The encapsulated strains (serotypes a–f) can be typed serologically with specific antiserum by agglutination or Quellung reaction.

Media that can selectively detect Hib have been developed. Enriched agar medium containing bacitracin (to inhibit growth of other organisms) and anticapsular antiserum has been used.[269] On this medium Hib organisms grow selectively and produce a halo as a result of the interaction between the organism's capsule and antiserum in the medium. Other organisms with capsules that cross-react may also produce halos, but usually are distinguished from Hib by colony morphology and biochemical reactions. Antiserum agar medium is useful for pharyngeal carriage studies because of its rapidity of identifying Hib, sensitivity, and specificity when working with cultures of oropharyngeal secretions containing many species of bacteria including nontypable *H. influenzae*.

4. Biological Characteristics of the Organism

Several surface structures of *H. influenzae* appear to be important in the pathogenicity of the organism. Like many bacterial pathogens, its outermost structure is its polysaccharide capsule. Six antigenically and biochemically distinct capsular polysaccharide serotypes have been described and designated types a through f. The type b capsule is of primary importance inasmuch as type b organisms account for 95% of all strains that cause invasive disease.[100,170,258, 309,412]

The type b capsular polysaccharide consists of a repeating polymer of ribosyl and ribitol phosphate having a 1–1 linkage (Fig. 1). This capsular antigen, released both *in vitro* and *in vivo*, can be detected with specific immunological techniques now used for rapid diagnosis.[98,105,176,204,216,256,311,354,375,410,421,432,442,446] Commercially obtained reagent kits using latex agglutination methods are most widely used to detect the type b capsular antigen in body fluids. Although the capsule of Hib and some other encapsulated bacteria may share similar antigenic determinants, cross-reactions causing false-positive antigen

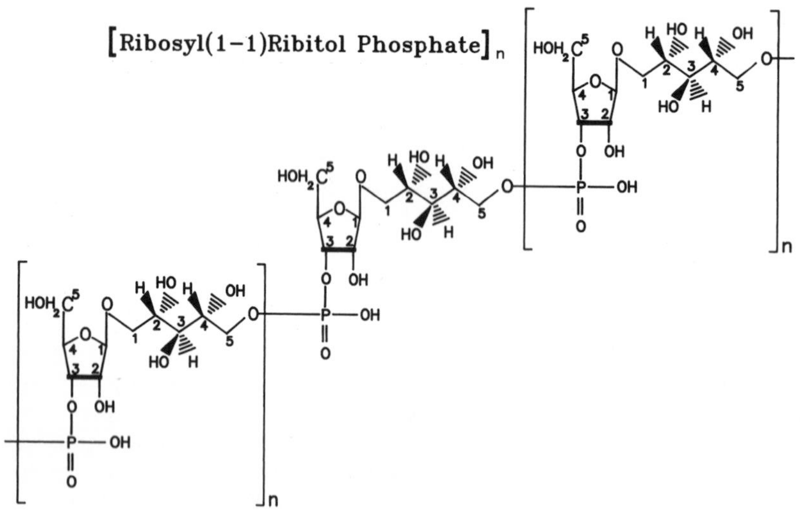

Figure 1. Repeating-unit chemical structure of *Haemophilus influenzae* type b capsular polysaccharide (Hib), shown in its protonated form: $(\rightarrow 3)$-β-D-Rib$_f$-$(1\rightarrow 1)$-D-Ribol-5-$(PO_2H)\rightarrow$. Adapted from Zon and Robbins.[471]

tests for Hib rarely occur in clinical practice. Strains without capsules also cause disease, but they rarely cause bacteremia, except in neonates, immunocompromised adults, or compromised children in developing countries (see Section 8).

Other important elements of the *H. influenzae* cell envelope include lipopolysaccharide (LPS; endotoxin) and a number of outer-membrane proteins (OMPs), many with yet undefined functions. Methods have been developed for differentiating isolates of Hib by differences in electrophoretic mobility patterns of the major OMPs, and this has been useful for epidemiological studies.[46,162,247] To date, specific OMP patterns have not clearly been associated with virulence. However, the possibility has been suggested that strains of different OMP subtypes may cause a differing clinical spectrum of illness.[402] LPS or endotoxin of Hib is important in the pathogenicity of the organism, and appears to have little antigenic diversity,[187] although there is variability in LPS electrophoretic patterns after passage *in vivo* or *in vitro*.[413] Therefore, electrophoretic characterization of endotoxin has not been useful as an epidemiological tool.

Multilocus enzyme electrophoresis is a method used to characterize isoenzymes of the organism. This method has been used to distinguish different genotypes of Hib for epidemiological purposes.[286,325,326] This procedure appears to have the greatest genetic discriminating power when sufficient numbers of enzymes are analyzed.

Pili or fimbriae are protein filaments extending from the outer membrane of the organism and appear to mediate attachment of the organism to host epithelial cells.[90,185,321] The expression of pili appears to be reversible. The role of these structures in the pathogenesis of disease is unknown.

Another important biological feature of *H. influenzae* has been the development of resistance to various antimicrobials, in particular ampicillin and chloramphenicol. Ampicillin was the primary antimicrobial for therapy of disease until the mid-1970s, when resistance to it was first noted.[74,75,82,87,212,228,356,411,414,418,455] Since then, ampicillin resistance has become widespread, now ranging between 5 and 50% of all isolates in various parts of the world.[39,50,68,76,115,188,200,209,212,215,265,289,316,328,353,366,400,433] The mechanism of resistance usually involves plasmid-mediated β-lactamase enzyme production,[386] and resistant strains are often characterized by their plasmid or β-lactamase enzyme content. While most isolates have been associated with the production of a distinctive β-lactamase enzyme termed TEM-1, since 1979 a new β-lactamase enzyme called Rob β-lactamase has been identified[107] and non-β-lactamase-mediated resistance has been described.

Of particular recent concern has been the finding of resistance to chloramphenicol, which is usually mediated by an enzyme, chloramphenicol acetyltransferase.[264,344] Although chloramphenicol-resistant strains are rare in the United States, in some areas of the world they are increasing in prevalence.[69] Unfortunately, strains resistant to both ampicillin and chloramphenicol have been reported from the United States,[76,227,264,301,422] Thailand,[383] Mexico,[186] Australia,[134] the United Kingdom,[328] Denmark,[39] and Spain.[69] More than 50% of recently reported clinical isolates in Barcelona, Spain, were multiply resistant.[69] In some areas, the development of these multiply resistant strains has necessitated therapy with alternative antimicrobials, such as newer and more expensive third-generation cephalosporins.[107] This situation further underscores the need to maintain antimicrobial surveillance and to find effective means to prevent Hib disease.

5. Descriptive Epidemiology

5.1. Incidence and Prevalence

5.1.1. Incidence of Endemic (Primary) Disease. Although a nationwide system for reporting of invasive Hib disease does not exist, several population-based studies have been conducted within the past 30 years, making it possible to estimate the incidence, magnitude, and spectrum of endemic invasive Hib disease in the United States. *H. influenzae* causes about 20,000 cases of invasive (bacteremic) disease annually. More than 95% of all invasive *H. influenzae* clinical isolates are serotype b; virtually all isolates from infants and young children are serotype b.[100,170,258,309,412] Invasive Hib disease occurs endemically, as true communitywide epidemics have not been observed. Hib disease is very uncommon above 5 years of age (less than 15% of all disease), due presumably to the age-related acquisition of natural immunity. Thus, epidemiological studies of invasive Hib disease tend to focus on defining disease patterns in the principal risk group, children less than 5 years of age.

In the United States prior to 1976, incidence studies were restricted to Hib meningitis. In these earlier studies, the annual incidence varied from 19 to 63 cases per 100,000 children younger than 5 years of age per year in different population groups (Table 3).[45,132,137,139–141,266,268,291,306,351,390,403] Differences in the methodologies and rigor of case-finding efforts may explain, in part, the variability in incidence. Differences in exposure or host susceptibility factors also might affect the magnitude of risk in a given population. Several studies suggested an increasing inci-

Table 3.   Comparison of Rates of *Haemophilus influenzae* Meningitis and Other Invasive Disease among Children Younger Than 5 Years of Age

Geographic area	Study period	Annual incidence of *H. influenzae*		Ref.
		Meningitis	All invasive disease[a]	
United States				
Olmsted Co., MN	1959–1970	40		141
Franklin Co., OH	1960–1968	35		390
Allegheny Co., PA	1961–1970	32		266, 268
Charleston Co., SC	1961–1971	38		140
Tennessee	1963–1971	23		132
Bernalillo Co., NM	1964–1971	38		139
Baltimore, MD	1965–1975	19		351
Mecklenburg Co., NC	1966–1970	63		306
Vermont	1967–1970	35		141
Rhode Island	1970–1974	27		403
Los Angeles, CA	1975	31		45
Fresno Co., CA	1976–1978	60	90	170
Alaska (non-Natives)	1980–1982	69	129	438
Colorado (6 months)	1981–1982	68	112	210
Jefferson Co., AL	1981–1983	62	NA[b]	9
Monroe Co., NY	1982–1983	55	86	336
Dallas Co., TX	1982–1984	67	109	284
Minnesota	1982–1984	45	67	284
Atlanta, GA	1983–1984	57	82	85
Europe				
Sweden	1971–1980	27	NA	79
	1981–1983	31	NA	416
Finland	1976–1981	NA	41	310
	1978	27	NA	423
The Netherlands		22	NA	393
High-risk populations				
Australia Aboriginals	1985–1986	NA	1100	193
U.S. Navajos	1968–1973	173	NA	92
	1974–1980	153	214	94
U.S. Alaskan Eskimos	1971–1980	440	572	436
Natives[c]	1980–1982	282	601	438
U.S. Apaches	1973–1982	254	NA	249

[a]Cases per 100,000 persons younger than 5 years of age.
[b]NA, not available.
[c]Natives include: Eskimo, Indian, mixed Eskimo, mixed Indian, Aleut.

dence since 1960[141,268,291,306,390] while others have not.[351] However, only two studies examined population-based data for a defined population over time.[141,390] In Franklin County, Ohio, a two- to threefold increase in Hib meningitis incidence in children was noted between 1942 and 1968, although there was little change in the incidences of pneumococcal or meningococcal meningitis. Fraser *et al.*

observed a three- to fourfold increase in incidence if Hib meningitis in Olmsted County, Minnesota, between 1935 and 1970 and inconclusively explored a variety of possible explanations for this finding, including improvements in bacteriological techniques, increases in the availability of diagnostic facilities, increases in the proportion of persons in the population who belonged to known high-risk groups, and changes in the age distribution of the study population. These observations were later extended in a study of the same study population during the period 1950–1981; a stepwise increase in the incidence of Hib meningitis was demonstrated with each decade since 1950.[291]

In contrast to earlier studies, those conducted during the past 15 years (Table 3) have evaluated all invasive forms of Hib disease. These studies have demonstrated a consistently higher attack rate of meningitis, ranging from 45 to 69 cases per 100,000 children less than 5 years of age per year and little change over time.[9,85,170,210,284,336,438] It is not known whether these higher rates of disease are due to improvements in diagnosis and surveillance or to changes in risk factors, such as increased use of day-care facilities, which may have contributed to a true increase in disease incidence. In addition, recent studies have provided estimates of the incidence of other forms of invasive Hib disease, ranging from 22 to 60 cases per 100,000 children less than 5 years of age. Therefore, the combined incidence of all invasive Hib disease ranges from 67 to 129 cases per 100,000 children per year.[9,85,170,210,284,336,438] Based on these estimates, invasive Hib disease affects approximately 1 in 200 children in the United States during the first 5 years of life.[84]

With the exception of North America and parts of Europe, the epidemiology of invasive Hib disease has not been studied in depth. In Sweden,[79,350,416] Finland,[310,423] and The Netherlands,[393] *H. influenzae* is the most common cause of bacterial meningitis. In these countries the incidence of Hib meningitis varies from 22 to 31 per 100,000 children younger than 5 years of age per year, about one third to one half that in the United States (Table 3). Hib also ranks as the leading cause of bacterial meningitis in Canada, with an incidence similar to that in the United States.[424] In other parts of Europe, including the United Kingdom[62,108,460] and Norway,[308] and in most developing countries, meningococcal disease is reported to be more common than Hib meningitis. Since 1980 in the United Kingdom, however, reported invasive Hib disease has exceeded reported meningococcal disease, perhaps because of the increasing recognition of the importance of this pathogen.[460] The only data outside the United States that examine whether Hib disease incidence may have increased over time are from a retrospective study of Scandinavian countries over a 25-year period. The authors noted an increase in Hib meningitis incidence beginning during the 1970s, but could only speculate as to its origin.[350]

Population-based incidence figures for most developing countries are not available; however, *H. influenzae* appears to rank first as a cause of bacterial meningitis in some studies of hospitalized patients, and second or third behind meningococcal and pneumococcal disease in others.[65,180,462] These studies do not specifically address the comparative incidence in young children.

Investigators in Australia have reported an exceptionally high rate of invasive Hib disease among Aboriginal children in central Australia, with an attack rate of 1100 cases per 100,000 children younger than 5 years of age per year[193] (Table 3). Other high-risk populations include Native American Navajo, Apache, Yakima, and Athabascan, Native Alaskans and Native North Americans.[92,94,145,249,299,435,436,438,461,462]

5.1.2. Prevalence and Other Characteristics of the Carrier State.

Human beings are the only natural hosts for *H. influenzae,* which is carried in the upper respiratory tract. Although Hib is transmitted by respiratory droplets or contact with respiratory secretions, the patterns of transmission can be complex because carriage is usually asymptomatic. Both encapsulated and unencapsulated strains of *H. influenzae* are considered part of the normal bacterial flora of the upper airway. Since Hib may pass from a patient with disease to a series of several other persons, who remain asymptomatic carriers, before the organism again causes illness, the incubation period cannot be accurately assessed. Despite a low point prevalence of pharyngeal carriage (1–5%), most young children become colonized during the first 2 to 5 years of life.[3,111,243,259,269,270,275,368,417] In some settings the point prevalence of pharyngeal carriage may be higher. Stephenson *et al.*[398] reported a 15% prevalence of Hib colonization among healthy children attending daycare. The cumulative rate of pharyngeal acquisition of encapsulated type b strains is such that by 5 years of age most children will have acquired Hib and thereby develop specific immunity.[10,43,133,164,179,189,360,368,372,373,398] Colonization rates are highest in closed populations exposed to a case, such as household or day-care center classroom contacts of a patient with disease.[43,164,267] Type b strains may persist in the nasopharynx for months[243,267] and often are not eliminated by antimicrobials that do not enter respiratory secretions.[10,372,373] Culture of throat swabs with antiserum agar appears to be the most sensitive method for detecting Hib carriage.[270] However, a recent study suggested that latex agglutination assays to detect Hib capsular polysaccharide antigen in nasopharyngeal swabs may be more sensitive, easier to perform, rapid, and less expensive than culture methods, but specificity has not yet been fully evaluated.[198]

To prevent the possible nosocomial transmission of Hib, respiratory isolation of hospitalized patients with invasive Hib disease for 24 h after initiating effective antimicrobial therapy is recommended, based on the assumption that transmission of the organism is eliminated or suppressed within 24 h.[143] However, studies have shown that children with invasive Hib disease may remain colonized with Hib following the discontinuation of their antimicrobial therapy.[10,267,372,373] Four studies have evaluated the duration and intensity of Hib colonization of children receiving systemic antimicrobial therapy.[10,146,282,294] Alpert et al.[10] cultured 35 children with Hib meningitis and found 6 (17%) patients colonized on day 6 of therapy, and one of these patients on day 10. However, all patients were only lightly colonized. Murphy et al.[282] recovered Hib from 2 of 24 patients with Hib meningitis after the first 24 h of therapy (1 of 11 patients treated with ceftriaxone and 1 of 13 patients treated with ampicillin). The positive cultures were obtained on days 2 and 6 of therapy, respectively, in broth culture only, suggesting that the bacteria were present in the pharynx in low concentrations. Gilsdorf[146] obtained multiple culture specimens on 26 patients more than 25 h after beginning therapy; none of 83 specimens were positive for Hib. Ogle et al.[294] studied 38 children and did not recover Hib from the pharynx of any child beyond 14 h of effective antimicrobial therapy. These data suggest that recovery of the Hib organism from the pharynx is suppressed after 24 h of effective therapy and the current standard of respiratory isolation for the initial 24 h of hospitalization is appropriate.

5.2. Contagiousness of the Organism

Although the contagious potential of invasive Hib disease has generally been considered to be limited, certain circumstances can lead to outbreaks or direct secondary transmission of disease. Instances of direct secondary Hib disease transmission have been reported since 1909,[110,157] but only since 1978 has the risk of secondary Hib disease for contacts of a case been more accurately characterized. The data on transmission of disease among household contacts, day-care center contacts, and other institutional settings have led to a general recognition of the potential for invasive Hib disease to spread to contacts, particularly those less than 2 years of age.[1,166,330] It is important to distinguish "secondary" disease, that occurring following direct contact with a child with invasive Hib disease, from "primary" or endemic disease, which occurs following contact with an asymptomatic Hib carrier (Fig. 2). With secondary transmission, the child transmitting the organism is ill; thus, the exposed children at risk because of close contact can be identified. Secondary disease is usually defined as illness occurring within 1–60 days following con-

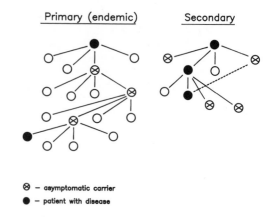

Figure 2. Primary and secondary *Haemophilus influenzae* type b disease.

tact with another child who has Hib disease, although some of the earlier studies of household contacts examined only the 30-day period following disease onset in the index patient. The issue of secondary disease has received considerable attention because chemoprophylaxis with rifampin is an available control measure (see Section 9.1.1). Nonetheless, secondary disease represents only a small proportion of all Hib disease (< 5%).

5.2.1. Risk of Secondary Disease in Household Settings. Six studies have estimated the risk of secondary disease in household contacts of a case in the month (30 days) following onset of disease in an index case[43,66,130,150,166,170,434] (Table 4). Few data exist to determine the risk beyond 30 days.[170] One of the six studies has been excluded from the summary in Table 4, because not all of the secondary cases were proven by culture. Two of the studies were limited to contacts of patients with meningitis.[150,434] Overall, the attack rate for contacts of all ages was 0.3%, representing a risk about 600-fold higher than the age-adjusted risk in the general population.[434] However, attack rates varied significantly by age of the contacts; the attack rate was more than 6% in contacts less than 1 year old, 3.3% in children less than 2 years old, 1.6% in children 24–47 months old, 0.06% in children 4–5 years old, and 0% in children 6 years or older. Among the household contacts, 64% of secondary cases occurred within the first week of disease onset in the index patient, 20% during the second week, and 16% during the third and fourth weeks.[1] Thus, the risk of secondary disease in the household setting is confined almost exclusively to children less than 4 years old (especially those less than 2 years old), and is concentrated in the first 2 weeks after onset of disease in the index case.

Table 4. Risk of Secondary *Haemophilus influenzae* Type b Disease in Household Contacts within 30 Days after Onset in the Index Case

Geographic area	Study period	Reference	Percent risk (secondary cases/total household contacts)				
			0–11 mo	12–23 mo	24–47 mo	48–71 mo	All ages
Multistate	1977–1978	Ward[434]	6.0 (3/50)	1.4 (1/69)	1.5 (4/259)	0.1 (1/1309)	0.2 (9/4311)
Pittsburgh, PA	1972–1979	Campbell[66]	6.8 (2/29)	0 (0/29)	0 (0/106)	0 (0/130)	not reported
Fresno Co., CA	1977–1978	Granoff[170]	4.2 (1/224)[a]		0 (0/38)	0 (0/39)	0.3 (1/396)
Boston, MA	1974–1976	Glode[150]	5.7 (2/35)[a]		3.5 (2/57)	0 (0/79)	0.7 (4/555)
Multistate	1979–1981	Band[43]	0 (0/35)[a]		3.3 (3/92)	0 (0/73)	0.5 (3/604)
Total			3.3 (9/269)[a]		1.6 (9/552)	0.06 (1/1630)	0.3 (17/5866)

[a]These figures are for ages 0–23 mo combined.

Also, the risk of secondary Hib disease appears to be no different following exposure to a patient with meningitis or other invasive Hib disease. In contrast, secondary transmission of meningococcal disease occurs in all age groups, although the risk is also higher in younger persons and most secondary cases also occur within 2 weeks of the index case. For endemic meningococcal disease in the absence of chemoprophylaxis, the risk among household contacts is about 0.4%, an overall risk comparable to that observed for Hib disease.[409]

For household contacts there appears to be a relationship between disease risk and the prevalence of Hib pharyngeal carriage among household contacts of a case.[43,104,158, 267,419] Michaels *et al.* observed that 52 of 67 families of a child with Hib meningitis or epiglottitis, studied soon after the child was hospitalized, had at least one other family member colonized with Hib. This was usually a sibling; the carriage rate among siblings of meningitis cases was 56%.[267] Similar to the age-related risk for secondary Hib disease, a stepwise decrease in carrier rates was found with increasing age; the rate was 71% (39/55) in those 0–4 years old, 44% (30/68) in those 5–10 years old, 23% (3/13) in those 11–20 years old, and 9% (11/119) for parents. Furthermore, Hib colonization persisted for at least 6 months in 39 of the 67 families, with 40% of culture-negative siblings and mothers of index children subsequently becoming colonized. This might explain the occasional occurrence of late secondary cases. Few fathers were colonized at any time. In a similar, but smaller study, Turk[419] detected Hib carriers in 13 of 28 families, and in 9 of the 13 families with three or more children. Persistence of the organism within families for up to 6 months was also demonstrated. Band *et al.*[43] cultured 976 household contacts soon after children with invasive Hib disease were hospitalized and found a pattern of pharyngeal colonization similar to that of Michaels *et al.* Colonization rates were highest in contacts younger than 6 years of age (34%), and declined with increasing age, to a rate of 12% for parents. Siblings had higher carriage rates (30%) than unrelated household contacts (22%). Interestingly, carriage rates were highest for contacts exposed to case-patients with nonmeningitic invasive disease.

5.2.2. Risk of Secondary Disease in Day-Care Settings. In recent years, out-of-home day-care for young children has become commonplace. It is currently estimated that about 40% of children under 5 years of age attend some type of day-care facility either full-time or part-time. Thus, an increasing number of young children are exposed to infectious diseases in these facilities, and outbreaks of several infectious agents have been documented, including outbreaks of Hib disease.[159,166,408] Of particular importance as the number of children attending day-care in the United States has increased, is whether the day-care environment enhances the transmission of invasive Hib disease. Controversy exists about the degree of risk of secondary Hib disease among day-care contacts exposed to a child with invasive Hib disease. Four studies have estimated this risk for day-care classroom contacts of a case during the 60-day period following onset of disease in the index case[130,254,283,296] (Table 5). An additional report[43] studied only secondary cases occurring within 30 days of an index case. Three of the studies listed in Table 5 demonstrated a substantial risk, 1.7–3.2%, for contacts younger than 24 months of age,[43,130,254] a risk comparable to that of household contacts of a similar age (see Tables 4 and 5). One of these studies also showed that the risk was similar for different clinical syndromes (2.8% for meningitis versus 2.6% for other invasive disease) and for different geograph-

Table 5.   Risk of Secondary *Haemophilus influenzae* Type b Disease in Day-Care Classroom Contacts[a] 0–23 Months of Age Who Did Not Receive Rifampin[b]

Geographic area	Study period	Case finding[c]	Secondary cases/total day-care contacts	Attack rate (%)	95% Confidence interval	Ref.
Multistate[a]	1979–1981	P	1/31	3.2	0.1–17	43
Multistate[d]	1983–1984	R	10/376	2.7	1.1–4.3	130
Dallas County	1982–1984	P	0/361	0	0–1.0	283
Minnesota	1982–1984	P	0/370	0	0–1.0	296
Oklahoma	1984–1986	P	5/292	1.7	0.6–4.3	254

[a] Within 60 days after onset of diease in the index case child (with the exception of a 30-day study period for Ref. 143).
[b] Adapted from Broome *et al.*[61]
[c] P, prospective; R, retrospective.
[d] The attack rates were: Seattle=3.3%, Oklahoma=2.7%, Atlanta=2.2%. None of the secondary cases in Seattle were identified before the study.

ic regions in a study of three areas.[130] However, two other studies failed to demonstrate any increased risk for secondary disease in day-care contacts.[283,296] There is no obvious explanation for the disparate findings, although there can be considerable variation in secondary Hib disease risk over time, in different day-care settings, and perhaps by geographic region.[1,61,101,257] Increased risk, when observed, has been largely confined to day-care classroom contacts less than 24 months of age. This is in contrast to the household setting, where substantial risk (an attack rate = 1.6%) exists in children 24–47 months of age (Table 4). The secondary attack rates among children 24–47 months of age attending day-care and who did not receive rifampin chemoprophylaxis were low: 0.5% (1/194) in Oklahoma, 0.4% (1/226) in Dallas County, 0.0% (0/716) in Minnesota, and 0.0% (0/379) in the multistate study by Fleming *et al.* Recommendations for use of rifampin chemoprophylaxis differ as a result of the controversy over differences in assessed disease risk in different studies of secondary spread in day-care settings (see Section 9.1.1).

Among the studies that showed an elevated risk among day-care classroom contacts, several additional findings supported the view that the day-care environment may enhance the transmission of Hib disease. Fleming *et al.*[130] showed that the risk of secondary disease for children in other classrooms at a day-care center where a case had occurred was not significantly greater than the expected endemic disease risk in a population of equivalent age, suggesting that nonclassroom contacts need not be considered at increased risk. Furthermore, controlling for age by multivariate regression analysis, they found that children attending day-care more hours per week were more likely to transmit and acquire secondary disease. Specifically, no

child with primary disease who attended a day-care facility less than 18 h/week was associated with secondary disease, and no child who attended a day-care facility less than 25 h/week acquired secondary disease. Specific day-care characteristics such as classroom size and age range, acceptance of drop-ins, and so forth did not appear to be associated with secondary disease, although these analyses were not definitive. The authors of the study concluded that, although the overall risk for most day-care contacts of a case was small, the risk for young classroom contacts approached that of household contacts. Finally, Band *et al.*[43] obtained pharyngeal cultures on 429 day-care classroom contacts of a child with primary invasive Hib disease, and found relatively high colonization rates (teachers, 8%; children, 23%), presumably because of sufficiently close contact with the index patients to lead to transmission of the organism.

Another study in Pittsburgh[245] confirmed the observation that increased Hib carriage rates occurred among household and day-care classroom contacts of a child with invasive Hib disease. They prospectively studied Hib colonization in six day-care facilities where children had developed invasive Hib disease, and evaluated the carriage rates in household contacts of colonized children from the day-care facilities. Carriage rates in households of carriers were then compared with carriage rates in 14 households of children who had invasive Hib disease. The colonization rate in day-care classroom contacts of an index case was 23% (28/124), ranging from 8% to 100% in the six facilities. The colonization rate in the household contacts of an index case was 26% (11/43); siblings had a higher carriage rate (53%, 9/17) than parents (8%, 2/26; $p = 0.002$). In addition, within families of the asymptomatically colonized day-care children, 25% of household members were colonized despite lack of direct contact with the index patients. This colonization rate was comparable to that of household contacts of index patients (26%). The authors concluded that household contacts of colonized day-care children are also a reservoir of Hib, and the findings suggested that the day-care environment may enhance the transmission of Hib.

5.2.3. Risk of Secondary Disease in Other Institutional Settings. Secondary Hib disease transmission in chronic-care institutions for children has been reported.[42,155,373,464] One outbreak affected 5 of 30 young children with chronic illness within a 6-month period, while another affected 4 of 11 young children within 16 days. Nosocomial transmission of invasive Hib disease among elderly adults in a nursing home setting has been reported.[391] Only one instance of secondary transmission in children in an acute-care hospital has been reported.[49] Presumed transmission occurred from a 4-month-old child with Hib septic arthritis to another 4-month-old child sharing the same room who developed Hib meningitis, while hospitalized, 38 days after the initial exposure. The OMP profile of the two isolates was identical and previously had been observed infrequently from patients with Hib disease in that geographic area. Considering the large number of Hib cases yearly, the lack of similar such reports suggests that the risk of nosocomial transmission in acute-care hospitals is very low. A recent as yet unpublished outbreak in South Africa of multiply resistant Hib suggests that there is potential for nosocomial Hib disease transmission when large numbers of susceptible children are kept in close quarters and resistant strains are prevalent.

5.3. Geographic Distribution

Whether there are true differences in the incidence of invasive Hib disease internationally is not known with certainty because, outside of North America and Europe, there have been few population-based studies with active surveillance (see Section 5.1). In the United States, there has been some variability in the reported incidence of Hib disease in different populations, but no obvious geographic clustering is evident from these studies. Some of the variability in incidence, but certainly not all, can be explained by differences in methods of case finding. However, one prospective, laboratory-based incidence study that used similar methodology in two different geographic areas (Dallas County and Minnesota) during the same time period (1982–1984) found substantially different incidences of invasive Hib disease in children under 5 years of age (109 versus 67 cases per 100,000).[284] A second explanation is

differences in the prevalence of risk factors in the population that result in differing incidences by area. For example, three differences noted in the Dallas and Minnesota populations were the higher proportion of patients in Dallas who were enrolled in day-care centers (see Section 5.9), the longer total hours per week in day-care in Dallas, and the higher proportion of black children in Dallas (see Section 5.7). Other possible explanations that have been proposed are that there may be true differences in attack rates by geographic area due to differing environmental or host susceptibility factors, or as yet undefined differences in the invasive potential of different strains of Hib.

5.4. Seasonal Distribution

A characteristic bimodal seasonal pattern has been observed in several studies, with one peak between September and December, a decrease in cases in January and February, and a second peak between March and May.[60,142,209,357,438] This has been shown in the United States generally, and also in Alaska. In contrast, the peak incidence of both pneumococcal and meningococcal meningitis is between January and March.[357] The reason for these differences is not known. In one multistate study,[357] the biphasic seasonal pattern observed for Hib meningitis existed for northern states only, with the early spring peak essentially absent in the southern states, although the number of cases studied from the southern states was small. It has been suggested that the seasonality of births may contribute to this pattern[142]; however, the biphasic pattern of Hib disease appears to be more accentuated than could be explained by seasonal factors in birth cohorts. Furthermore, the same pattern of seasonal peaks in Hib disease has been found among children 1 year of age and older.[60]

5.5. Age

The most important epidemiological feature of invasive Hib disease is its age-related incidence, a feature that has been appreciated for more than half a century.[135] Young age is associated with the highest incidence of disease; risk is highest between the ages of 6 and 12 months. The age-related incidence of Hib disease has been evaluated with similar methods in several recent population-based surveillance studies in Alaska, Atlanta, Fresno, Minnesota, and Dallas, which are summarized in Table 6 and Fig. 3.[85,170,284,438] Although not as well studied, approximately 15% of invasive *H. influenzae* disease occurs in persons 5 or more years of age, most of whom are older adults, often with underlying disease that has increased dis-

Table 6.   Age-Specific Incidence of Invasive *H. influenzae* Disease, U.S. Population-Based Studies, 1976–1984

Age (months)	Meningitis only		All invasive disease		Cumulative[b] percentage of disease (%)
	Median	Range	Median	Range	
0–5	101	59–141	148	98–197	10–15
6–11	179	143–279	275	218–452	37–43
12–17	146	88–184	223	123–248	60–61
18–23	62	20–64	92	57–107	64–68
24–35	31	18–39	50	37–70	75–78
36–47	17	5–26	31	7–39	80–83
48–59	4	2–16	11	7–41	84–86
(0–59)	(60)	(45–69)	(90)	(68–129)	—
≥60	0.2	0.1–0.2	1.3	1.2–2.4	100

[a]Cases per 100,000 population per year. Range of point estimates from five studies, including Alaska 1980–82 (excluding Eskimos, Indians), Atlanta 1983–84, Fresno Co. 1976–78, Dallas 1982–84, Minnesota 1982–84.
[b]Cumulative percentage and incidence data for ages ≥ 60 months are based on studies from Alaska, Atlanta, and Fresno Co. where active surveillance for all age groups was conducted.

ease susceptibility. Furthermore, a substantial proportion of the invasive disease in older individuals may be due to non-type b strains (see Section 8.1).

Approximately 85% of all invasive *H. influenzae* dis-

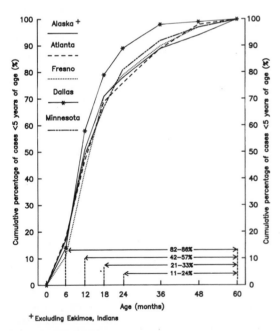

Figure 3. Age distribution of invasive *Haemophilus influenzae* disease in children under 5 years of age, U.S. population-based studies, 1976–1984.

ease occurs in children under 5 years of age, and in this age group disease is due almost exclusively to type b strains. Invasive disease is relatively uncommon in infants less than 6 months old (< 15% of cases), presumably because of less exposure, transplacental acquisition of maternal antibody, and protection conferred by breast-feeding. Figure 3 shows the cumulative proportion of disease by age during the first 5 years of life, which is important when considering strategies for prevention. For example, assuming the availability of a perfect vaccine that could be given universally (i.e., 100% vaccine efficacy and 100% immunization rates), vaccinating all children at 24 months of age might be expected to reduce the incidence of Hib disease in the first 5 years of life by only 11–24%, whereas vaccinating children by 6 months of age could prevent 85% of all childhood Hib disease.

Each type of invasive disease has a characteristic age occurrence, but as a group the clinical syndromes, other than meningitis and cellulitis, tend to occur at older ages[100,438] (Fig. 4). In most U.S. populations studied, the peak incidence of meningitis occurs in children 6 to 9 months of age and declines markedly after 2 years of age.[137,139–141] Hib cellulitis tends to occur during the first year of life, and epiglottitis generally occurs in children over 2 years of age. Interestingly, meningitis accounts for a relatively small proportion of episodes of invasive disease in adults (Fig. 4), while pneumonia is more common.

In populations with especially high disease incidence, such as Native Americans, the age-specific incidence is shifted toward younger children (Table 3).[92,94,249,435,

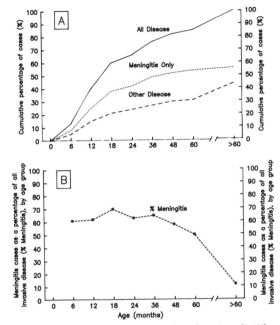

* Data from studies in Alaska (N=144), Atlanta (N=135) and Fresno (N=102)

Figure 4. Cumulative percentage of invasive *Haemophilus influenzae* disease by age and disease type. Data from studies in Alaska ($N = 144$), Atlanta ($N = 135$), and Fresno ($N = 102$).

436,438) Native American groups at increased risk include Apache,[249] Navajo,[92,94] Yakima,[229] Canadian[461] and Athabascan Indians,[438] and Alaskan Eskimos,[145, 435,436,438] but not Pima Indians.[468] Among Native Americans in southwestern Alaska, the incidence of Hib disease peaks in children 4–7 months of age, with similar peak attack rates of meningitis observed in Navajo (4–5 months) and Apache (4–6 months) children.[94,249] Antibody studies in the Alaskan children showed that antibody titers to Hib were significantly higher in newborns (reflecting high levels of maternal antibody) and at 48–60 months of age than were titers in a composite U.S. reference population.[435,436] The risk of invasive Hib disease in Alaskan Natives is concentrated in the first year of life, with 59% of all invasive disease occurring in children under 12 months of age, and 85% occurring in children under 18 months of age.[438] Similarly, 81% of Hib meningitis in Navajos occurs in children under 12 months of age.[94] This age distribution contrasts with other U.S. populations in which 42–57% of invasive disease occurs in children under 12 months of age (Fig. 3). The social structure of Native American groups, usually with large families in small dwellings and with con-

fined living conditions for much of the year, suggests that early or intense exposure to Hib at home or in the community may explain the early age of disease onset and the development of immunity at an earlier age than in other groups.

The age-specific incidence may be shifted toward older preschool children in populations with low incidences of Hib disease.[79,310,350,393,416,423] In Finland, the peak incidence of Hib meningitis is reported in children at about 12 months of age.[309] Beyond this age, the incidence of invasive Hib disease declines less precipitously than in most U.S. populations studied, with approximately 60% of childhood invasive Hib disease occurring in children older than 18 months of age.[310] In contrast, in the United States the figure is only about 30% (Fig. 3). Such a shift suggests less intense exposure to Hib than in U.S. and high-risk populations, although other factors cannot be ruled out.

The relative frequency of meningitis caused by *H. influenzae* in U.S. school-age children 6 to 15 years old was retrospectively examined in a hospital-based study at four tertiary care hospitals in three states during 1974–1978.[459] Hib ranked second behind *Neisseria meningitidis* as a cause of bacterial meningitis in this age group. However, the incidence rate was not compared to that in children under 6 years of age.

5.6. Sex

Although most studies show approximately equal rates of disease in boys and girls, several population-based studies[85,351,438] and national surveillance data from passively reported cases of meningitis[357] found attack rates to be 1.2- to 1.5-fold higher in boys than in girls.

5.7. Race and Ethnicity

Population-based active surveillance studies have identified blacks as having increased risk for invasive Hib disease. The incidence of Hib meningitis has consistently been shown to be two to four times higher for black as compared to white children less than 5 years of age.[45, 132,139,140,306,351, 403] Also, the incidence of all invasive Hib disease was 1.6- to 4-fold higher in blacks compared with whites.[85,170] High incidences of invasive Hib disease have also been observed in Hispanics[45,170] and Native Americans[92,94,145,229,248,435,436,438,461,468] (see Section 5.1). A study in Dallas, however, found no difference in the incidence of Hib disease between white and Hispanic children.[284]

Although some investigators have suggested that racial and ethnic differences in incidence of Hib disease may be due to genetically determined differences in host suscepti- bility[173] (see Section 5.13), this hypothesis is unproven because of confounding socioeconomic variables that are associated both with race/ethnicity and with disease (see Section 5.10). Factors that may increase exposure by chil- dren to carriers of the Hib organism, such as household crowding, number of siblings, and day-care, are exceed- ingly difficult to separate from host susceptibility factors, such as an increased predisposition to Hib disease. So- cioeconomic factors affect family size and structure, and therefore could influence the likelihood of exposure to Hib bacteria. Studies are needed that analyze both host suscepti- bility factors and exposure risk factors, including so- cioeconomic factors, using multivariate analysis to assess the independent effects of potential risk factors that may be highly correlated with each other, such as black race and household crowding. In one study in Atlanta, there was no increased risk in blacks compared with whites once the independent effects of household crowding, day-care, and family income on risk were accounted for by multivariate analysis.[85]

5.8. Occupation

There are no data to suggest any relationship of oc- cupation, including adults who work in hospital or day-care settings, to risk of Hib disease in the small number of adults reported with invasive Hib disease.

5.9. Occurrence in Day-Care Settings

Three population-based studies have evaluated whether day-care attendance is associated with increased risk of pri- mary (endemic) invasive Hib disease.[85,210,336] All found that children attending day-care were at significantly higher risk for invasive Hib disease than children not in day-care (Fig. 5). One study estimated that up to 50% of all invasive Hib disease may be attributable to day-care attendance.[85] Each study used different methodology.

The first published report suggesting that day-care at- tendance was a risk factor for primary Hib disease was a cohort study conducted in Monroe County, New York.[336] This study defined day-care as any licensed child-care facil-

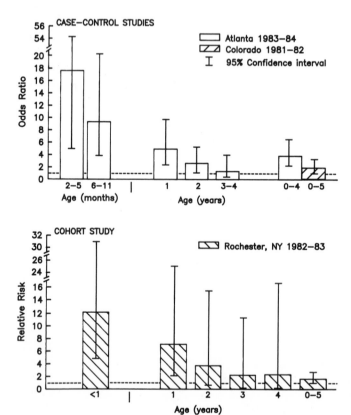

Figure 5. Relative risks (odds ratios) for attendance at day-care, by age group, primary invasive *Haemophilus influenzae* type b disease.

ity where three or more unrelated children are supervised by a nonparent for 3 or more hours each day, and only examined risk in licensed day-care facilities. No cases were reported in unlicensed day-care facilities. Overall, the relative risk for Hib disease among children under 6 years of age attending licensed day-care was 1.7 (95% confidence interval: 1.1–2.8) (Fig. 5). However, the relative risk varied by age; children under 1 year of age were at highest risk, and risk declined with increasing age. Attack rates for Hib disease were significantly higher only among children under 36 months of age in licensed day-care as compared to children of a similar age who did not attend licensed day-care. Several limitations of this study have been reviewed.[59] Because data were not available from unlicensed facilities, there may have been substantial underestimation of the total number of children attending day-care facilities and an overestimation of the relative risk of Hib disease due to day-care attendance (in both licensed and unlicensed facilities). A second consideration was that the Monroe County study did not separate primary and secondary Hib cases in the analysis. The study also did not examine the interaction of day-care attendance with other potential risk factors and confounding factors, the effects of which might wholly or partially account for the apparent association of day-care attendance with risk for Hib disease. Despite these limitations, the study was a landmark.

Two subsequent studies evaluated day-care attendance and other potential risk factors for Hib disease using multivariate analysis, so that the independent effect of day-care attendance as a risk factor could be examined. A case–control study conducted in Atlanta during 1983–1984 showed an overall relative risk, by univariate analysis, for children under 5 years of age of 3.9 (95% confidence interval: 2.3–6.6) (Fig. 5). In the multivariate model, day-care attendance was an independent risk factor; risk was highest in children under 1 year of age, and declined with increasing age similar to that of the Monroe County study. There was suggestive but inconclusive evidence that an increasing number of hours per week of attendance at day-care was associated with an increasing relative risk of disease.

The other study using multivariate analysis to evaluate day-care attendance as a risk factor for Hib disease was a case–control study conducted in Colorado during 1981–1982.[210] By univariate analysis, the overall relative risk for children under 6 years of age was 1.9 (95% confidence interval: 1.2–3.2). However, in contrast to the other two studies, the relative risk was significantly increased only for children $\geq$ 12 months of age (odds ratio = 3.7, 95% confidence interval 1.6–8.5). Risk increased with the size of the day-care facility, providing the first clear evidence that spe-

cific characteristics of the day-care setting may be associated with risk of Hib disease.

5.10. Socioeconomic Factors

The interplay of multiple factors affecting exposure to the Hib organism and host susceptibility appears to determine the risk of invasive Hib disease. Socioeconomic factors that may increase the likelihood of exposure to Hib among children, and thereby increase the risk of Hib disease, include large household size,[170,268,300] crowding,[268] and greater population density.[132] Other socioeconomic factors that could be considered surrogates for increased exposure, including low family income[132, 139,140,351,403] and low parental education level,[139,268] have also been associated with an increased risk of disease.

Two recent studies have analyzed exposure-related risk factors, including socioeconomic factors, using multivariate analysis to assess the independent effects of each potential risk factor. In one case–control study in Atlanta,[85] household crowding (i.e., $\geq$ 1 person per room) was significantly associated with Hib after controlling for the effects of race, family income, day-care attendance, and breast-feeding. In this multivariate study, a trend toward increased risk was associated with low family income and low maternal education level, although these were not independent risk factors. The second study was conducted in a primarily white population in Colorado.[210] In that study the risk of Hib disease was increased in households with at least one member of elementary school age, suggesting that such children may be sources of introduction of Hib into a household for acquisition by their susceptible younger siblings.

5.11. Influence of Breast-feeding

Based on the results of three case–control studies, breast-feeding appears to be protective against invasive Hib disease in infants under 6 months of age.[85,86,209,250] Lum et al.[250] showed that among Alaskan Eskimos, infants with invasive Hib disease were significantly less likely to have been predominantly breast-fed than controls. Another study, using multivariate analysis, found protection associated with exclusive breast-feeding within the most recent 3-month period among infants under 6 months of age, after controlling for age, day-care attendance, and presence of school-aged household members.[209] The third study, also using multivariate analysis, and controlling for age, day-care attendance, race, household crowding, and family income, found a protective efficacy of 92% associated with breast-feeding as the predominant source of milk.[85,86] Only a trend toward protection existed in infants 6 to 11 months of age. Although the mechanism for protection is not known, it may be due to immune factors or nutritional factors in human milk. These findings are biologically plausible, based on studies demonstrating that human milk contains low levels of secretory antibody to the Hib polysaccharide capsule, which persist for 1 to 6 months after the onset of lactation.[319] Both the colostrum and milk, measured at either 3 or 6 months after delivery, of women immunized at 34 to 36 weeks of gestation with Hib polysaccharide vaccine had an anticapsular antibody titer more than 20 times higher than that observed in nonimmunized women[207] (see Section 9.2.4).

5.12. Underlying Disease

Several hematological and immunological disorders are known to be associated with increased risk for Hib disease. These include sickle-cell anemia,[327,431,470] asplenia or splenectomy,[77] antibody deficiency syndromes, [125,347] complement deficiencies,[348] and malignancies, especially Hodgkin's disease during chemotherapy.[48, 378,445] The precise mechanisms placing such immunocompromised patients at risk have yet to be determined. Reduced reticuloendothelial clearance of bacteria in blood by macrophages in the spleen and liver may be involved. Clearly, complement and antibody are needed to clear bacteremia and to maintain bactericidal activity in blood.

5.13. Genetic Factors

Genetic predisposition to several infectious diseases has been suggested.[219] In particular, selected genetic markers have been associated with invasive Hib disease risk.[15,163,171,173,174,313,406,451,452] However, the results of several of these studies have conflicted. The question of whether genetic factors affect host susceptibility to Hib disease is also clouded by the fact that virtually all studies have found associations in high-risk groups in whom lower socioeconomic status and other risk factors related to exposure to the organism are also disproportionately present.

The NS and NSs blood groups were reported to be more prevalent among patients with Hib epiglottitis, and MNs, NSs, and MSs blood groups more frequent in patients with Hib meningitis.[451,452] However, more recent studies have not confirmed these findings.[163,313] Associations between Hib disease and the HLA-A and -B loci, specifically

Aw28, Bw12, Bw14, and Bw17 antigens, have been reported[406] and refuted.[313] No associations have been reported for HLA-C and HLA-DR. An association between risk for Hib meningitis and absence of the immunoglobulin light chain Km(1) allotype in blacks, but not whites, together with no differences in the frequency of the immunoglobulin heavy chain G2m(n) allotype among patients and controls was reported.[173] However, Ambrosino et al.[15] reported that white children lacking the G2m(n) allotype were at increased relative risk of developing invasive Hib disease, and reduced antibody response to vaccine. Another study failed to show an association in whites of the G2m(n) marker and Hib disease or immune responses to polysaccharide vaccines.[174] Studies in both Eskimos and whites have reported that the combination of two genetic loci—specifically, a Gm immunoglobulin allotype and an HLA antigen—influences susceptibility.[171,313] Selected combinations of Gm allotypes and HLA-B5 were protective, but other combinations of Gm allotypes with HLA-DR3 were associated with increased risk of disease.[313] Lastly, Petersen et al.[312] reported an association between a variant of the enzyme uridine monophosphate kinase (UMPK-3) and Hib disease in Alaskan Eskimos.

Additional studies have evaluated the influence of genetic factors on immune responses to Hib vaccines (see Section 9.2.1). The reports of genetic marker associations with invasive Hib disease risk and responses to vaccines support the view that genetic factors may contribute to disease susceptibility. However, virtually all studies have been subject to potential confounding because cases were not compared with controls who necessarily had similar exposure. Another potential explanation for the varying data on genetic markers may be that earlier studies did not control for multiple cross-comparisons and hence studies of multiple genetic markers may have shown significant results due to chance. Furthermore, even in high-risk Alaskan Eskimos, in whom some genetic factors have been associated with disease risk, the majority of patients with Hib disease still do not possess the genetic marker in question.[312,313] Therefore, it remains to be determined whether genetic factors play a significant role in the risk of population groups, in determining immune response to Hib vaccines, and in the pathogenesis of Hib disease. Admittedly, genetic markers are crude tools with which to identify genes that might influence susceptibility. Even if one assumes that there are genes determining susceptibility, they cannot be identified or characterized by the demonstration of linkage disequilibrium of one or more genetic markers that themselves likely have no influence upon susceptibility.

5.14. Role of Antecedent Viral Respiratory Infection

Viruses have been implicated in the pathogenesis of bacterial infections for many years and respiratory viruses have been shown to increase susceptibility to Hib meningitis in experimental animal models.[271,287] The hypothesis has been advanced that antecedent or concurrent viral respiratory infection may alter mucosal immunity or alter bacterial flora, thereby increasing host susceptibility to invasive Hib disease. Krasinski *et al.*[232] obtained respiratory viral cultures and serology on 131 children hospitalized with Hib meningitis and 30 children with pneumococcal or meningococcal meningitis over a 2½-year period. A recent viral infection could be shown in 40% (63/160) of all bacterial meningitis patients studied by viral isolation, viral serology, or both, while 60% (96/160) had a history of a cold, cough, or rhinorrhea compatible with a viral upper respiratory infection within the previous two weeks. Twenty-two percent (29/131) of patients with Hib meningitis had evidence of recent adenovirus infection. Among the patients with Hib meningitis, however, there was no association between an established viral diagnosis and history of upper respiratory infection. Furthermore, no age-matched control group of children without meningitis was available for comparison. The difficulties and obstacles of conducting prospective studies with appropriate controls have made it diffi-cult to determine conclusively whether antecedent viral respiratory illness predisposes to invasive Hib disease.

5.15. Summary of Risk Factors for Invasive Hib Disease

The development of invasive Hib disease in a given individual is a consequence of the complex interaction of a variety of factors, including events leading to exposure, as well as characteristics of the organism, the environment, and the host, all acting together in a multifactorial interrelationship[137] (Fig. 6). In this discussion, we have enumerated some of those factors. The factors can be divided into those affecting likelihood of exposure to the Hib organism ("exposure factors") and those affecting the host's susceptibility to Hib disease, whether inherently through regulation of the host immune response or because they contribute to a change in the host's ability to defend against the disease ("susceptibility factors"). Some exposure factors that we have described, such as household crowding and day-care attendance, are fairly direct measures of increased exposure to Hib bacteria, while others, such as low family income and low parental education levels, are only indirect measures for increased exposure. Other risk factors cannot be so easily categorized, such as the association of black, Alaskan

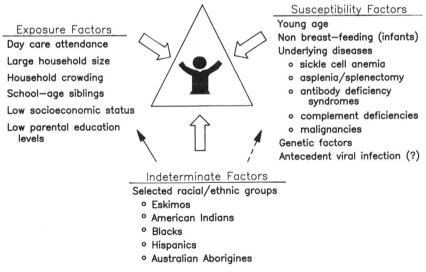

Figure 6. Risk factors for invasive Hib disease.

Eskimo, or Native American race with increased risk for Hib disease. Although abundant evidence suggests that more intense and early exposure to Hib may be the primary factors affecting risk in these populations, other lines of evidence suggest that genetic factors may also affect the antibody response to Hib or other susceptibility factors. Factors not reviewed because of a lack of definitive data include antimicrobial use, altered nasopharyngeal flora, the effects of climate, temperature, and humidity, which may affect survival of the bacteria, and the relative efficiency with which Hib carriers versus persons with clinical Hib disease can transmit the organism.

6. Mechanisms and Routes of Transmission

A great deal remains unknown concerning the mechanisms and routes of transmission of Hib. Although some data would indicate that spread of this organism is relatively slow, there is also impressive evidence that it may be quite contagious for young children exposed to carriers in situations of close contact for prolonged periods of time, such as in household or day-care settings. Existing data on the prevalence and characteristics of the carrier state (Section 5.1.2) and the contagiousness of the organism (Section 5.2) have been reviewed elsewhere and will not be presented here.

Transmission of Hib is presumed to occur by person-to-person spread via respiratory droplets. There are no data that support a role for airborne transmission of the organism. The role of environmental surfaces and fomites in transmission is unknown. Although Hib is generally regarded as a fastidious organism, Murphy and Clements[278] demonstrated that Hib in nasal secretions could survive for up to 18 h on tissue paper, wax paper, and dry gauze. However, they were unable to recover Hib from swab cultures of the cribs and toys of carrier children in day-care settings. This single study raises the possibility that fomites on environmental surfaces may potentially contribute to transmission in circumstances such as the mouthing of toys by young children playing together. It appears unlikely, however, that this is an important mode of transmission.

7. Pathogenesis and Immunity

Hib is usually transmitted asymptomatically from person to person through many transmission cycles before causing disease in a susceptible person. Furthermore, the

organism can be carried in the upper respiratory tract for many months, and it appears that some individuals can carry the organism for a period of time before it becomes invasive. Therefore, it has not been possible to define an incubation period or pattern of transmission in endemic or epidemic settings.

Hib frequently asymptomatically colonizes the upper respiratory tract of humans; invasion occurs when there is dissemination of bacteria from this site to the bloodstream and then elsewhere in the body (Fig. 7).[387] Studies in several animal models have shown that the initial stage of invasive disease involves attachment of the organism to the respiratory epithelium and penetration through the mucosa, leading to invasion of the lymphatics and the bloodstream.[273,298,387] Inflammation of the upper respiratory tissues is generally not apparent and the precise mode of entrance of organisms into the vascular space is not well understood. The bacteremia is initially at a low level, but in a susceptible host this increases quantitatively.[183,273,298,387] When the bacterial concentration in the blood exceeds 10^4–10^5 organisms/ml, seeding of other body sites frequently occurs, especially to the meninges. In the CNS, invasion appears to occur via the choroid plexus[387]; organisms then circulate through the CSF and infect the arachnoid villi and the leptomeningeal membranes. The resulting increased bacterial density, inflammation, edema, cranial nerve damage, and overall increased CSF pressure cause the morbidity and mortality associated with meningitis.[355] Generally, the magnitude of the bacteremia and the degree

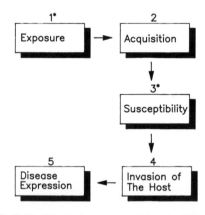

Figure 7. Epidemiological sequence of invasive Hib disease. *, Risk factors

of proliferation of organisms in the CNS correlate with the severity of the clinical illness.[128,349,448,449] Although meningitis is the most severe form of invasive Hib disease, bacteremic seeding of other body sites may also occur, including joint, pleural, or pericardial spaces.[387] However, with pneumonia, cellulitis, and epiglottitis, the exact pathogenesis is less well understood, even though these invasive infections are also usually associated with bacteremia. Presumably, pneumonia occurs following the aspiration of a critical number of virulent organisms, epiglottitis involves the focal infection of the epiglottis, and cellulitis occurs by secondary seeding via the bloodstream of deep subcutaneous tissues. With all forms of invasive Hib disease there is an invasion of the bloodstream, either as a primary or as a secondary event.

The mechanisms that determine which individuals will remain asymptomatically colonized (the vast majority of people) and which will develop invasive disease are undoubtedly related to a multitude of poorly understood factors. Resistance to invasive disease depends upon the successful integration of a wide variety of host defenses, including: (1) mucosal factors that prevent attachment or penetration of organisms through the respiratory epithelium, (2) activation of complement-mediated opsonization, killing, and other mediators of inflammation (including the alternative and classical complement pathways), (3) mucosal and humoral antibody, (4) phagocytosis and killing by macrophages and polymorphonuclear cells, and (5) the poorly understood role of cell-mediated immunity. As discussed, the severity of disease appears to be related in part to the magnitude of the bacteremia, which, in turn, is determined by several factors that influence bacterial proliferation and bacterial clearance. Although antibody is not the sole defense against bacteremia, it has been the immunological basis for the development of vaccines that are designed to induce bactericidal, opsonophagocytic, and ultimately protective antibodies.

Although antibodies to several surface antigens of Hib probably play a role in conferring protective immunity,[28,161,191,208,235,248,376] antibody to the type b capsular polysaccharide appears to be the most important.[342] By 5 years of age most children naturally acquire anticapsular antibody. There is considerable evidence that anticapsular antibody protects humans from invasive disease, in that it: (1) activates complement,[97,332,397,404,415,456] (2) is opsonophagocytic,[197,290] (3) is bactericidal,[25,99,126,133,290,292,399] and (4) protects animals from lethal Hib challenge.[237,288,358] Moreover, passive prophylaxis with serum preparations containing anticapsular antibody pro-

tects agammaglobulinemic patients[339,342,347] and other children at unusual risk for Hib disease.[352] Furthermore, in the preantibiotic era, effective therapy for Hib disease included the administration of hyperimmune type b serum.[2,5,8,136,429] However, perhaps the most compelling evidence for the protective efficacy of anticapsular antibody is the protective immunity induced in older children with PRP vaccine[253,310] and in younger children with newer PRP conjugate vaccines.[122]

Different exposures to the organism, or to vaccines derived from its antigens, will induce variable immune responses, and responses to the capsule are markedly influenced by the age of the individual. In children under 2 years of age with invasive Hib disease (i.e., bacteremia) or in those who have been given the plain polysaccharide vaccine, there is rarely an immune response detected to the type b capsule. In contrast, older children and adults will respond with anticapsular antibody following infection or immunization.[26,27,223,388] There is also some evidence that anticapsular antibody develops after exposure to other bacteria that have immunologically cross-reacting capsular antigens.[340,359] Therefore, the level of antibody is influenced by the type of exposure, duration of exposure, rate of antigen clearance, and most importantly, by the age of the individual.

Estimates of the minimum serum concentration of PRP antibody that provides protection range from 0.05 to 0.15 μg/ml with levels of 1 μg/ml or greater required for long-term protection.[21,221,339,347,364] Unfortunately, these estimates are crude and do not take into account the different functional properties of different immunoglobulins and the contribution of antibodies other than capsular antibody.

Several studies show that IgG, IgM, and IgA antibodies to PRP are induced both by disease and by vaccination[217,220,222,364]; however, the proportion and subclass of IgG antibodies vary by age and type of exposure.[47,53,213,252,302–304,333,338,365,369,370,379] IgG antibody has been shown to be bactericidal, opsonic in the presence of complement, and protective for animals.[364] IgM is equally as protective; however, it is more bactericidal than IgG in the presence of complement, but it opsonizes organisms in the presence of polymorphonuclear leukocytes poorly. In contrast, IgA antibody is not bactericidal, opsonic, or protective in animals.[364] Some have hypothesized that IgA-specific antibody blocks the activity of other more functional antibodies and that this may depress immunity.[184,285,346] Data from experiments in mice and humans suggest that there is also a restrictive IgG subclass response to polysaccharide antigens.[47,53,213,338] In adults this involves predominantly an IgG1 response,[252, 370] but in children both IgG1 and IgG2 predominate following immunization with the purified polysaccharide antigen.[370] However, like proteins, the polysaccharide-conjugate vaccines tend to produce predominantly IgG1 antibodies even in children.[443]

The weak and immature antibody response to the plain polysaccharide vaccine appears to result from limited or absent T-helper-cell activation. These cells are normally involved in the maturation, differentiation, and proliferation of specific B-cell populations. T-helper cells also retain immunological memory, essential to elicit a booster response.[47] Although most of our understanding of the interaction between B cells, T cells, and macrophages derives from extensive research with mice,[47,109,202,213,338] it appears that, based upon the mode of recognition of the antigen, there are T-dependent (thymus-dependent) or T-independent classes of immunogens. Most protein antigens, considered to be T-dependent antigens, induce activation of T-helper cells, which regulate antibody synthesis. Such antigens are recognized and processed by macrophages, T cells, and B cells. The T cells stimulate reactive B-cell subpopulations to proliferate and differentiate specific antibodies and the T cells also retain memory for subsequent booster responses. In contrast, T-independent antigens stimulate little or no T-helper-cell activity. Generally, the plain polysaccharide vaccines appear to elicit predominantly T-independent responses, with little or no antibody responses observed in young children; even in older children the antibody produced is predominantly IgM. Furthermore, there is no booster or anamnestic response with repeat exposures. Activation of T cells is necessary: (1) to regulate the magnitude of the immune response, especially in young infants, (2) to regulate the switch in immunoglobulin classes (IgM to IgG), (3) to enhance the functional activity of antibody, and (4) for booster responses.[342]

In the quest for an Hib vaccine that is both immunogenic and protective in young infants, attempts have been made to convert the capsular polysaccharide (PRP) from a T-independent to a T-dependent immunogen, employing hapten-carrier principles first described by Landsteiner early in this century.[236] To achieve this, the polysaccharide is covalently linked to a T-dependent immunogen (a carrier) to form a conjugate vaccine. As a group, Hib conjugate vaccines demonstrate markedly enhanced immunogenicity, as is described in Section 9.2.3.

Some studies suggest that immune responses are also regulated by genetic factors.[15,17,165,174,305] However, it is not clear whether the degree of variability seen among different populations and among different subjects with different genetic markers (i.e., HLA or immunoglobulin allotypes; see Sections 5.13 and 9.2.1) are clinically relevant. No single genetic relationship has been described that appears to regulate susceptibility or the basic immune response to polysaccharide antigens.

The role of mucosal immunity in killing Hib or inhibiting adhesion or penetration of the mucosa is poorly understood, although studies have been reported of secretory IgA antibody to the type capsule.[36,317,318,320] Moreover, Hib strains produce an IgA protease that may inactivate mucosal antibody.[276] Relatively little is known about direct cell-mediated killing of Hib or other aspects of cellular immunity.[117]

8. Patterns of Host Response

H. influenzae disease can be considered in two major clinical categories, based upon the pathogenesis of disease (Table 7). Invasive disease is characterized by the dissemination of bacteria, almost always Hib, from the pharynx to the bloodstream and subsequently to other body sites. Bacteremia is a common characteristic of all invasive forms of Hib disease and may be the only manifestation of disease in an acutely ill child with high fever and no other recognized focus of infection.

Invasive Hib disease should be distinguished from mucosal infections (Table 7); the latter occur when *H. influenzae* organisms extend from colonized respiratory passages to contiguous body sites. Although mucosal infections occur frequently, they do not result in bacteremia and are therefore rarely life-threatening. The most common infections of this type include otitis media, sinusitis, conjunctivitis, bronchitis, and perhaps urinary tract infections. The microbiological hallmarks of mucosal infections are: (1) they are produced by the same bacteria that normally colonize the pharynx, and (2) they are almost always unencapsulated strains of *H. influenzae* (nontypable).[420] Extension of these organisms into normally sterile body sites is enhanced by compromise in normal defense mechanisms, such as eustachian tube reflux, foreign bodies, antecedent viral infection, or damage to the bronchopulmonary epithelium caused by smoking or selected immune deficiencies.

The clinical separation of invasive and mucosal disease is not absolute, inasmuch as type b strains may cause otitis media or sinusitis.[195] Likewise, other serotypes (nontypable strains and serotypes other than type b) may occasionally cause bacteremia and meningitis. A notable example is disease in neonates that occurs when nontypable strains, presumably acquired from the flora of the mother's genital tract,

Table 7. Spectrum of *H. influenzae* Disease

Invasive disease (predominantly due to type b strains)

Meningitis	Pneumonia	Empyema
Bacteremia	Arthritis	Osteomyelitis
Epiglottitis	Pericarditis	Cellulitis
	Abscesses	

Mucosal disease (predominantly due to nontypable strains)

Otitis media	Bronchitis
Sinusitis	Urinary tract infections
Conjunctivitis	

cause invasive disease (bacteremia and meningitis).[67,428] Most children experiencing invasive *H. influenzae* non-type b infections have underlying predisposing medical conditions.[147] In addition, reports from Nigeria,[382] Papua New Guinea,[177,371] and The Gambia[427] suggest a higher than expected frequency of non-type b pneumonia and meningitis in young children in less developed countries.[180] Whether these differences relate to poor nutrition or concurrent infections that place such children at risk for infections normally considered noninvasive, or whether other unknown factors are involved, requires further study. Nonetheless, the clinical categories of disease described above are useful diagnostically and therapeutically and have important implications regarding strategies for disease prevention.

Hib may produce disease in most organ systems of the body. The organism is virulent for man; however, Hib may exist in the nasopharynx and oropharynx as part of an asymptomatic carrier state. The importance of asymptomatic carriage of Hib is unclear; organisms may be disseminated to other body sites, but may also serve as an antigenic stimulus to the production of antibodies important in host defense. The manifestations of infection with Hib vary depending on the site involved and will be described separately.

8.1. Clinical Features

8.1.1. Spectrum of Disease. The most commonly recognized and most severe clinical manifestation of invasive Hib disease is meningitis, representing 54–67% of all invasive disease in children.[100,170,309,412] Other bacteremic diseases include septicemia, pneumonia, epiglottitis, cellulitis, septic arthritis, osteomyelitis, and pericarditis. Nontypable (unencapsulated) strains of *H. influenzae* commonly colonize the human respiratory tract, and therefore are a major cause of otitis media, sinusitis, and respiratory mucosal infection but rarely result in bacteremic dis-

ease. In contrast, Hib is an uncommon inhabitant of the upper respiratory tract, occurring in the pharynx with a prevalence of only 0.5–3% in normal infants and children and rarely in adults.[269] Hib strains account for only 5–10% of *H. influenzae* causing otitis media.[195]

8.1.2. Mortality and Complications. Despite currently available antimicrobial therapy for invasive Hib disease, about 5% of children die.[1] Neurological sequelae of meningitis are relatively common, occurring in 19–45% of such children.[114,124,129,367,396,405,427] Handicaps include hearing loss, language disorder or delay, mental retardation, motor abnormalities, seizure disorders, and impairment of vision. Deafness is one of the most important and common handicaps associated with Hib meningitis.[91,218,425] During the 1983–1984 school year, an estimated 8.7% of hearing-impaired children under 18 years of age enrolled in special-education programs in the United States had hearing losses attributed to meningitis.[458] Late complications of other forms of invasive Hib disease have generally not been well described, with the exception of functional impairment of joints, including abnormalities in bone growth and limited joint mobility, following septic arthritis.[201,447] Appropriate treatment of empyema caused by Hib has not been associated with functional impairment on long-term follow-up.[262]

8.1.3. Meningitis. The major clinical features of Hib meningitis and the other forms of invasive Hib disease have been thoroughly reviewed elsewhere.[231,263] Most patients with Hib meningitis are less than 3 years of age; however, the disease may occur at any age. The clinical presentation of Hib meningitis is similar to that due to pneumococcus; there are no specific clues to the diagnosis of Hib. Fever, obtundation, and stiff neck are the hallmarks of this illness, although only subtle changes in behavior may be found in infancy. A fulminating course with rapid neurological deterioration may occur.[211]

8.1.4. Epiglottitis. Hib is the most common cause of epiglottitis both in children and in adults.[260] The disease is characterized by rapid progression of sore throat, fever, toxicity, dysphagia with drooling, and upper airway obstruction. On physical examination, the epiglottis is greatly swollen and cherry red. Rapid diagnosis and prompt institution of therapy are necessary to prevent fatalities. Success of treatment depends on the establishment of an adequate airway, often by nasotracheal intubation.

8.1.5. Pneumonia. Hib is the most common cause of the bacteremic form of *H. influenzae* pneumonia. The clinical manifestations are indistinguishable from those of pneumococcal pneumonia, with a lobar or segmental presentation that may be complicated by the development of sterile or infected pleural effusions. Less commonly, patients may present with bronchopneumonia.

8.1.6. Cellulitis. Hib cellulitis usually involves the face, head, or neck (three fourths of all cases). It is characterized by a rapidly progressing skin lesion with indistinct margins, induration, tenderness, and purplish discoloration. The most frequently involved sites are the cheeks and periorbital areas. Buccal cellulitis almost invariably occurs in children under 1 year of age. Hib cellulitis is a bacteremic disease; diagnosis depends on isolation of the organism from blood or the local lesion.

8.1.7. Septic Arthritis. Hib is the second most common cause of septic arthritis in children. In general, the large joints, such as hip or knee, are involved and often a contiguous osteomyelitis is present.

8.1.8. Other Infections. Other clinical manifestations of bacteremic invasive Hib disease include osteomyelitis, pericarditis, endocarditis, epididymitis, endophthalmitis, and peritonitis.

8.2. Diagnosis

Probably the most useful epidemiological feature in arousing suspicion of infection with Hib is the age of the patient. This organism is the most common cause of meningitis in children under 5 years of age and is the most frequent cause of epiglottitis in children and adults. Increasing age is not, however, an absolute barrier to infection with Hib, and clinicians should not ignore this organism in their differential diagnosis in older children and adult patients with meningitis, epiglottitis, and pneumonia.

The primary criterion for the diagnosis of invasive Hib disease is isolation of the organism from a normally sterile body site (e.g., CSF, blood, pleural or joint fluid) that is the focus of infection. The specimens should be processed immediately since the organism is fastidious. Specimens must be placed on primary media that can support the growth of *H. influenzae*, preferably chocolate agar or a semisynthetic medium containing heme and NAD$^+$ (see Section 3.4). Latex agglutination or other rapid antigen detection assays can be used to detect the capsular antigen of Hib in body fluids of infected patients (see Section 4). Such examinations may be particularly useful in the diagnosis of partially treated meningitis or other invasive disease, where the organism may not be viable on culture but PRP capsular polysaccharide antigen may still be detected.

9. Control and Prevention

9.1. Chemoprophylaxis

Chemoprophylaxis has been used as a means to prevent secondary transmission of Hib disease. Because there is usually a high prevalence of colonization with Hib among young household or day-care contacts exposed to a child with Hib disease (see Sections 5.2.1, 5.2.2), attempts have been made to reduce secondary disease risk by eliminating carriage of the organism in close susceptible contacts using antimicrobial prophylaxis. There is no practical value in obtaining pharyngeal cultures in postexposure settings to detect the presence of the organism so as to define persons at risk for Hib disease. First, most secondary cases occur within the first week following diagnosis in the index case; therefore, the time required to detect carriage would delay implementation of prophylaxis. Second, a single culture is an imperfect procedure with less than 100% sensitivity.[269,270] Third, nonselective culture methods are not suitable for detecting Hib carriage; the use of selective antiserum agar medium is expensive and impractical in most situations.[269] Fourth, pharyngeal carriage of the organism may be an important immunizing event such that a positive culture gives no clue as to when the organism was acquired and whether the subject is susceptible to Hib disease.[164,179,267]

The rationale for prophylaxis is to eliminate the carrier state from all contacts of a susceptible child with antimicrobial agents that achieve bactericidal levels in mucosal secretions, saliva, and tears. Presumably, this also eradicates carriage from those who may be at risk for invasive Hib disease and prevents the opportunity for acquisition of the organism by other susceptible children in the contact group. Interestingly, antimicrobials effective in treatment of invasive Hib disease may not be effective in eliminating the carrier state. Continued pharyngeal infection with Hib has repeatedly been documented in patients who have received high-dose parenteral therapy for meningitis with ampicillin[267] or chloramphenicol.[372] Although these agents are bactericidal against the organism and will cure bacteremia, meningitis, and other invasive infections, they are not secreted into the upper airway and do not clear mucosal infection.

9.1.1. Rifampin

a. Eradication of the Carrier State. Rifampin is the most effective antimicrobial for eradicating Hib from the pharynx, primarily because high concentrations of the antimicrobial are secreted into respiratory secretions, saliva, and tears.[113,261] Several studies involving children and adults indicate rifampin in a dosage of 20 mg/kg per dose once daily (maximum daily dose 600 mg) for 4 days will eradicate Hib carriage in 95% or more of household[43,149] or day-care[43,95,144,373] contacts of a case. Rifampin in a dosage of 20 mg/kg once daily for 4 days had an efficacy of 96% in reducing the prevalence of multiply resistant Hib in four different day-care centers.[70] Studies of shorter or lower-dose rifampin regimens demonstrate less successful rates of eradication, including 10 mg/kg twice a day for 2 days with or without trimethoprim,[103,153,467] rifampin 10 mg/kg once daily for 4 days,[465] and rifampin 10 mg/kg twice a day for 4 days.[43,149,153] However, the latter regimen achieved a 96% efficacy in eradicating Hib colonization in one study.[280]

b. Prevention of Hib Disease. In a randomized, placebo-controlled trial, rifampin at a dosage of 20 mg/kg per dose once daily for 4 days administered to all household and day-care classroom contacts, including adults, significantly decreased secondary Hib disease among household and day-care contacts (0 of 303 rifampin-treated contacts less than 4 years of age had secondary disease, compared with 4 of 216 placebo-treated contacts less than 4 years of age; $p = 0.03$).[43] The number of cases in this study was insufficient to evaluate separately the efficacy in the household or day-care setting alone. Because the risk of secondary disease may be different for household and day-care contacts, some have questioned the validity of combining these children together for analysis.[295] A subsequent analysis that stratified the data according to whether each child was a household or a day-care contact revealed that a significant overall effect of rifampin could still be demonstrated.[44]

Two cohort studies have evaluated the efficacy of rifampin prophylaxis in preventing secondary Hib disease in day-care attendees. A retrospective study examined whether routine administration of rifampin in Seattle–King County, Washington; Atlanta, Georgia; and Oklahoma prevented secondary Hib disease in day-care attendees.[130] Among classroom contacts of Hib patients, children 0–23 months of age who received rifampin prophylaxis were at significantly lower risk for secondary disease than children who did not take rifampin [0 of 232, compared with 10 (3%) of 376; $p < 0.02$]. Furthermore, classrooms that did not have secondary disease were found to have achieved more than 75% compliance with rifampin significantly more often than did day-care classes in which secondary disease occurred (47 of 119 classes with only primary Hib disease versus 0 of 10 classes with secondary Hib disease; $p < 0.02$). This demonstrated the importance of achieving a

high rate of compliance with rifampin among the exposed group. Lastly, they found that in those classrooms that experienced secondary disease, administration of rifampin to one or more classroom contacts significantly lengthened the interval between primary and secondary cases.

The second cohort study was a prospective study in Oklahoma.[254] In this study, 5 (1.7%) of 292 classroom contacts under 24 months of age who failed to take rifampin developed secondary Hib disease, compared with 1 (0.3%) of 393 children under 24 months of age who took rifampin. This difference was statistically significant (relative risk = 6.7; 95% confidence interval, 1.1–42.5). As in the retrospective cohort study, rifampin use was significantly less among classroom contacts in day-care facilities in which a secondary case occurred (22%, 41 of 190) compared to day-care facilities where no secondary cases occurred (66%, 1146 of 1748; $p < 0.0001$).

Rifampin prophylaxis is not 100% effective, as evidenced by the rifampin "failure" in the Oklahoma study, and anecdotal reports among both household and day-care contacts.[57,281]

c. Implementation of Prophylaxis. To implement prophylaxis in day-care centers, it is important to ensure that all classroom contacts receive rifampin during the same period. Otherwise, eradication of the organism within the risk group in question cannot be guaranteed because a single untreated carrier can reintroduce it into the group. Some local and state health departments have facilitated the administration of prophylaxis by coordinating rifampin administration following consultation with private physicians and by providing information to parents of day-care contacts. If the health department has the resources and the commitment to assist with implementing rifampin prophylaxis, it is possible to obtain 75% compliance in day-care classroom contacts, even without the health department providing the antimicrobial.[254] "Failures" of prophylaxis will undoubtedly result from lower compliance rates[281,454]; therefore, prophylaxis should only be recommended if it can be carried out correctly.

Rifampin is available in 150- and 300-mg capsules.[1] For those unable to swallow capsules, rifampin may be mixed with several teaspoons of applesauce and eaten, which results in acceptable serum and salivary levels.[261] Alternatively, a suspension of rifampin may be freshly prepared in United States Pharmacopeia syrup; however, the preparation should be vigorously shaken before use.

Side effects of rifampin include nausea, vomiting, diarrhea, headache, or dizziness, which occurred in 20% of those taking rifampin as compared with 11% of placebo recipients. No serious reactions have been reported.[43] Those taking rifampin, including parents and day-care staff, should be informed that orange discoloration of urine, discoloration of soft contact lenses, and decreased effectiveness of oral contraceptives can occur.[385] Rifampin should not be used in pregnant women, as its effect on the fetus has not been established, and it is teratogenic in laboratory animals.[1]

d. Emergence of Rifampin Resistance. Concern over development of Hib resistance to rifampin has arisen from the earlier experience with meningococcal prophylaxis,[119] anecdotal reports of Hib resistance following prophylaxis,[153,279] and *in vitro* studies.[466] However, there is no indication yet that rates of such resistance have become clinically significant.[116]

e. Recommendations. Both the Immunization Practices Advisory Committee (ACIP)[1,330] and the American Academy of Pediatrics Committee on Infectious Diseases[338] agree that there is an increased risk of secondary Hib disease in household contacts under 4 years of age, and therefore in this setting recommend rifampin prophylaxis for contacts and for the index patient. In giving prophylaxis to the index patient, it should be kept in mind that rifampin is a potent inducer of hepatic enzyme activity and theoretically can cause important interactions with other drugs. For example, coadministration of rifampin has been reported to significantly lower serum chloramphenicol concentrations,[226,331] suggesting the need to monitor serum chloramphenicol concentrations in patients during coadministration of rifampin or delay rifampin prophylaxis until the end of chloramphenicol therapy.

There is disagreement about the magnitude of risk for secondary transmission of Hib disease in day-care settings (see Section 5.2.2); consequently, recommendations differ regarding the need for rifampin prophylaxis in this setting.[1,61,101,257,337] Some authorities[1,61,101,257] recommend prophylaxis for day-care classroom contacts under 2 years of age, while others[337] believe that recommendations should be individualized. However, virtually all experts recommend prophylaxis when two or more cases of Hib disease have occurred among attendees within 60 days. We believe that the risk of secondary Hib disease in day-, care attendees can be substantial in many areas, and where the risk has been shown to be substantial, rifampin prophylaxis has been shown to be effective in reducing the risk of secondary disease.

9.1.2. Other Antimicrobials. Ampicillin,[144,151] trimethoprim–sulfamethoxazole,[167,464] erythromycin–sulfisoxazole,[199] and cefaclor[199,465] have been shown to be ineffective agents for antimicrobial prophylaxis, eliminat-

ing Hib carriage in fewer than 70% of culture-positive contacts. These antimicrobials do not get into secretions in adequate concentrations and, therefore, are not recommended for prophylaxis.

9.2. Immunization

9.2.1. PRP Vaccine. This vaccine was licensed in April 1985 as the first vaccine for the prevention of Hib disease. Recently, its role has been supplanted by the subsequent development and licensure of newer second-generation conjugate vaccines (see Section 9.2.3).

a. Composition. PRP vaccine (designated "Haemophilus b polysaccharide vaccine") is composed of the capsular polysaccharide, polyribosyl-ribitol phosphate (PRP) (Fig. 1) from a type b strain of *H. influenzae;* PRP is purified from the supernatant of Hib broth cultures.[24,38,96,345] The currently licensed* commercial products—Hib-VAX[R] (Connaught), Hib-Imune[R] (Lederle), and b-Capsa[R] I (Praxis)—meet minimum physicochemical specifications established by the Food and Drug Administration, including: (1) contamination of < 1% nucleic acid and protein; (2) low levels of endotoxin (< 10 EU/μg); (3) purity (> 32% ribose); and (4) molecular size (exclusion greater than 0.30 kDa on a Sepharose-4B column). Each dose of vaccine contains 25 μg of purified PRP per 0.5 ml when reconstituted in aqueous buffer solution. The vaccine is stabilized with lactose or sucrose, sterilized by filtration, and lyophilized. The lyophilized vaccine is stable for a year when stored at 2–8°C, but it should not be frozen. The vaccines are licensed for administration by either the subcutaneous or the intramuscular route.

b. Immunogenicity. Although antibody to PRP has *in vitro* functional activity and *in vivo* (animals and humans) it confers protection, inducing immunity with a purified PRP vaccine has had limitations. It is not consistently immunogenic in children under 2 years of age (Table 8). In this regard, it has immunological properties similar to some other polysaccharide vaccines (pneumococcal and meningococcal polysaccharide vaccines), which are generally considered to be "T-independent" immunogens. As a result, antibody responses are limited, particularly in young children, and there is no booster response with repeated administrations of the vaccine. Furthermore, the induced antibody may have reduced functional qualities (i.e., primarily IgM, low avidity).[112] Studies have shown no evi-

*Use of trade names is for identification only and does not constitute endorsement by the Public Health Service, U.S. Department of Health and Human Services.

Table 8. Age-Related Immunogenicity to PRP Vaccine[a]

| Age group (months) | Geometric mean anti-PRP antibody levels (µg/ml) | | | | | |
| | Preimmunization | | | Postimmunization | | |
	Study 1	Study 2	Study 3	Study 1	Study 2	Study 3
3–5	0.1 (11)[b]	—	—	0.1 (11)	—	—
6–11	0.11 (40)	—	—	0.25 (40)	—	—
12–17	0.13 (31)	—	—	0.66 (30)	—	—
18–23	0.25 (26)	A: 0.02 (23)	0.63 (34)	3.17 (26)	A: 0.08 (23)	1.88 (34)
		B: 0.05 (19)			B: 0.30 (19)	
24–35	0.38 (68)	A: 0.06 (21)	0.37 (161)	6.96 (68)	A: 0.73 (21)	4.30 (161)
		B: 0.12 (22)			B: 0.96 (22)	
36–47	0.40 (51)	—	0.24 (72)	9.04 (52)	—	12.11 (72)
48–71	0.52 (119)	—	—	11.59 (119)	—	—
Adults	0.99 (49)	—	—	—	—	—

[a] Study 1: Finnish vaccine efficacy trial, 1974. Study 2: Harbor–UCLA Medical Center, 1985. Group A = Praxis PRP, group B = Connaught PRP; age groups 17–19 months, 24–26 months. Study 3: Praxis Biologics, 1984–1985. Age groups 18–20 months, 24–29 months, ≥ 30 months.
[b] Number of persons is shown in parentheses.

dence of immunological tolerance or impairment of immune response with early administration or repeated doses of vaccine,[148,223] despite earlier speculation that this might occur.[102]

It is often difficult to evaluate immune responses to PRP vaccine because many studies group antibody responses of children within broad age groups or specify only the mean responses by age. Other problems in evaluating immunogenicity include differences in antibody assay methods, lack of a consistent definition of immune response, variable preimmunization antibody levels, variable duration of immunity, and differences in PRP vaccines by dose, molecular size, or other characteristics. It has been particularly difficult to analyze and compare antibody levels between different PRP immunogenicity studies because there have been significant variations in the quantitation of antibody levels in different laboratories and within some laboratories over time.[35,118,441] As a result, some studies of children 18–24 months of age show preimmunization geometric mean antibody levels of 0.05 µg/ml and other studies of similar populations report values as high as 0.63 µg/ml, more than 10-fold higher[178,223,329] (Table 8). These preimmunization differences markedly affect the interpretation of postimmunization levels and antibody responses to predetermined levels (i.e., the proportion attaining a protective level or a twofold increase). Nonetheless, within each study, conclusions about relative immunogenicity can be assessed; these are summarized in Table 8.

c. Age-Specific Immune Response. Responsiveness of

children to PRP vaccine is strikingly age-related; infants respond infrequently and with meager levels of antibody (Table 8).[223,253,388] There is a maturation of immune response by 18 months of age, although children 18–23 months of age do not consistently respond and do not respond as well as those 2 years of age or older.[223,253,388] In the Finnish field trial, approximately 75% of children 18–23 months of age ($N = 29$) achieved antibody levels greater than 1 µg/ml, a level that predicted clinical protection for a minimum of 1 year.[221,223,253,310] This compared with 90% of 24- to 35-month-old children ($N = 97$), and less than 45% of 12- to 17-month-old children ($N = 55$).[223,310] The frequency and magnitude of the antibody responses were not equivalent to those of adults until about 6 years of age.[223,310]

Table 8 shows the variability in responses by age as assessed in different studies of PRP vaccines. All studies show an age-related maturation of immune responsiveness to PRP beginning at about 18 months of age to approximately 5 years of age. However, due to marked variability in the studies, one cannot determine an absolute level of protective immunity or a precise age at which children become immunologically responsive to PRP. The age-related nature of the immune response to Hib polysaccharide vaccine has made it difficult to determine the "ideal" age for routine immunization, because the variable estimates must also be balanced against the declining disease risk for children over 12 months of age.

Response to PRP vaccine of children who have previously had invasive Hib disease is also age-dependent. In one study, only 1 of 8 vaccinees under 2 years of age had an antibody response as defined by at least a twofold rise in antibody titer, while 8 of 12 children over 2 years of age responded ($p = 0.02$, Fisher's exact test).[293]

d. Persistence of Immunity. The duration of PRP vaccine-induced antibody is age-dependent. In the Finnish field trial, children vaccinated at 18–23 months of age had a substantial fall in mean antibody titers between 3 weeks and 1½ years after vaccination.[223] The antibody levels 1½ years later were slightly higher than, but not significantly different from, those in unvaccinated controls. A more recent study has shown similar rates of decline in antibody levels,[153] while another study failed to demonstrate a decline 1 year following immunization.[52] In the Finnish group of 24- to 35-month-old children, significantly elevated mean antibody titers persisted for at least 1½ years, but not for 3½ years. Finally, in children 3–4 years of age when vaccinated, the mean serum antibody levels remained elevated for at least 3½ years, and they remained significantly higher than levels of unvaccinated control subjects.[223]

These studies raise important questions about the long-term effectiveness of a single dose of Hib capsular polysaccharide vaccine given to children 18 to 23 months of age. The antibody responses and proportion of responders are appreciably less than in children vaccinated at ≥ 24 months of age; therefore, a greater proportion would be expected to have insufficient antibody 1 or more years after immunization. The length of time after immunization that levels are maintained has not been well defined, and it is doubtful that protective immunity is maintained throughout the entire period of invasive Hib disease risk (i.e., up to 5 years of age).[102,430]

e. Revaccination with PRP. Data on the need to revaccinate with PRP vaccine are limited. Although there is probably no booster effect with repeat doses of the vaccine,[223] the proportion of responders increases with age. Therefore, if the vaccine is given at 18 to 23 months of age, when a poor response might be expected, a subsequent dose at an older age may induce higher levels of immunity in those subjects who did not respond initially. Accordingly, revaccination is recommended by both the American Academy of Pediatrics and the Public Health Service.[1,88,334] Despite a suggestion that disease risk might be increased in very young children (i.e., < 18 months of age) immunized with PRP,[310] neither impairment of immune response nor increased disease risk has been convincingly demonstrated with early administration of PRP vaccine.[175]

A second dose of vaccine for children vaccinated at

less than 24 months of age has been suggested as a means of assuring and sustaining protection.[223,310] A postlicensure study[153] evaluated this question by comparing the antibody responses in two groups of children to a dose of PRP given at 36 months of age; one group was immunized for the first time and the second group had received a prior dose of PRP at 18 months of age. In contrast to the results from the Finnish trial,[223] these investigators found that the geometric mean antibody titer after immunization was significantly higher in the group reimmunized at 36 months compared to that of children immunized initially at 36 months of age. Other investigators have also made this observation.[52] However, no class-specific antibody measurements were made to provide any direct immunological evidence of a true booster response. Reimmunization of children has not been associated with any increase in adverse reactions. Further data would be useful to better define the potential benefit, need for, and timing of a second dose, but the advent of the significantly more immunogenic Hib conjugate vaccines (see Section 9.2.3) has lessened interest in these questions.

f. Molecular Size. There are limited published data to suggest that the molecular size of the PRP polysaccharide polymers correlate with immunogenicity and protective efficacy. A controlled field trial with PRP vaccine that involved approximately 16,000 children 2–71 months of age was conducted in 1974–1975 in Mecklenburg County, North Carolina.[307] In this trial, too few cases of Hib disease occurred to evaluate vaccine efficacy, but substantially poorer immunogenicity was observed. The vaccine used in this study had a significantly smaller molecular size compared with the vaccine used in Finland, and this may have been a reason for the substantially poorer immunogenicity observed. A recent study by Berkowitz *et al.* also showed lesser immune responses with a heat-sized lot of PRP (with lower molecular weight distribution) compared with a non-heat-sized lot.[51] Another study evaluated two high-molecular-weight PRP vaccines and found no significant differences in immunogenicity.[178] It appears that the high-molecular-weight PRP polysaccharide of current vaccines yield maximal immune responses, and reducing the size of the PRP polymer probably reduces immunogenicity, although this effect alone does not appear to be a major determinant of immunogenicity.

g. Simultaneous Administration of Vaccines. Simultaneous administration of PRP concurrently with pneumococcal and meningococcal polysaccharide vaccines has been studied in healthy adult volunteers.[12] These subjects achieved similar concentrations of antibody as did the control group that received only PRP vaccine. Furthermore, antigenic competition has not been observed in children immunized simultaneously with PRP and diphtheria–tetanus–pertussis vaccines.[148,238] No studies have been published evaluating simultaneous administration of PRP with measles–mumps–rubella (MMR) or trivalent oral polio (OPV) vaccines.

h. Underlying Illness. Patients with malignancies who are receiving immunosuppression respond less well to polysaccharide vaccines than healthy controls,[380] and immunosuppression specifically impairs responsiveness to PRP vaccine. It has been shown that in patients with Hodgkin's disease, chemotherapy and radiation treatment results in a selective decrease in serum IgG2 concentrations, and that IgG2 levels correlate with antibody response to PRP.[379] To maximize antibody responses in these patients, it has been recommended that patients with Hodgkin's disease receive PRP vaccine (and pneumococcal vaccine) at least 10 and preferably more than 14 days before splenectomy and the initiation of immunosuppressive therapy.[380] An immunogenicity study of children between 2 and 10 years of age with leukemias and solid tumors who were receiving maintenance chemotherapy suggested that such children did not respond as well as healthy children; however, most achieved postimmunization antibody levels thought to confer protection.[444] Similar results were obtained in children with sickle-cell disease.[138] A clinical syndrome consisting of recurrent sinopulmonary infections associated with an immunodeficiency characterized by a selective absence of IgG antibody response to polysaccharide vaccines has been described.[18] Immunogenicity evaluations in other groups of immunocompromised patients have not been published.

i. Protective Antibody Level. Although a precise protective level of anti-PRP antibody has not been established, data from passive protection of agammaglobulinemic children, challenge experiments in infant rats, and naturally acquired antibody levels in healthy individuals of various ages suggest that an antibody concentration of between 0.05 and 0.15 μg/ml is the minimum level required for protection. However, vaccine-induced antibody levels may decline over time, and therefore a given level does not necessarily predict long-term protection.[21,221,341,389] Because antibody levels decline more rapidly in infants and young children vaccinated with PRP, a peak level 1 month after immunization that is not substantially higher than 0.15 μg/ml would not be expected to protect for a significant length of time. In the Finnish field trial, an antibody level of > 1 μg/ml 1 month after immunization correlated best with clinical protection for a minimum of 1 year.[21,221,310] Recent data on the variability in antibody assays performed in different laboratories suggest that this antibody level, estab-

lished as a predictor of clinical protection in the Finnish field trial, might not be readily extrapolated to immunogenicity data on newer vaccine preparations evaluated in different laboratories[441] (Table 8).

j. Class-Specific Antibody Response. The antibody response to PRP vaccine includes production of antibodies of the IgG, IgM, and IgA classes; however, there appears to be a disproportionate amount of IgM induced.[206,220,222,339,364] Differences in functional activity of anti-PRP antibody by class suggest that IgM is less active than IgG.[339,364] These studies suggest that PRP vaccine induces a relatively immature immune response, which may result in qualitatively less functional antibody than a given level of antibody might suggest. Most IgG is of the IgG1 and IgG2 subclasses, with adults making both subclasses and children primarily IgG1.[252,370]

k. Effect of Immunization on Pharyngeal Hib Colonization. Only a single study has examined the effect of PRP immunization on the Hib colonization rate.[246] Although there was a trend toward lower colonization rates among immunized (22%) as compared to unimmunized (40%) children exposed to a child with invasive Hib disease, this difference was not statistically significant. These data are in keeping with similar studies on the effect of meningococcal and pneumococcal polysaccharide vaccination on subsequent nasopharyngeal carriage, which suggest some reduction in the acquisition of carriage shortly after immunization, but no long-term effect on carriage has been noted.[40,56,58,168,181,182,384,426] For this reason, chemoprophylaxis of household and day-care contacts of children with invasive Hib disease should be given to vaccinated as well as unvaccinated contacts (see Section 9.1.1).

l. Genetic Influences. In addition to the associations of Hib disease with several genetic markers and racial groups (see Section 5.13), other studies have suggested genetic determinants of immune responses to PRP vaccine. It remains to be seen whether these differences have clinical relevance or occur with newer and more immunogenic vaccines.

Siblings of patients with Hib meningitis have been reported to have impaired responses compared with control children, suggesting that a potential genetic factor might influence responsiveness to PRP and susceptibility to invasive Hib disease, although this study evaluated an adjuvant vaccine, PRP–pertussis.[169] Associations of certain immunoglobulin allotypes with the level of immune response to PRP vaccine have also been demonstrated, but the meaning of these findings remains unclear. Immunoglobulin allotypes are genetic markers expressed as antigens on the constant regions of heavy or light chains of immunoglobulins. The first study of immunoglobulin allotype associations with immune response to Hib capsular polysaccharide demonstrated significantly lower responses in white children with Km(1) allotype, a kappa light-chain allotype, but no differences in blacks.[305] A subsequent study predominantly in whites failed to show any association with Km(1).[15] This was confirmed in a third study,[174] but in this later study black children with the Km(1) allotype had significantly higher IgG responses to PRP vaccine than blacks lacking this allotype.[174] Yet another study in white adults demonstrated decreased Hib antibody production of the IgG and IgA classes following PRP immunization in Km(1)-positive persons compared to those lacking the Km(1) allotype.[17]

The other IgG allotype reported to be associated with Hib anticapsular immune response is G2m(n), an IgG2 heavy-chain immunoglobulin allotype. In one study in whites, a higher IgG antibody response was observed in individuals with this marker.[15] However, another study failed to confirm the G2m(n) association.[174]

Host factors, some of which may be genetically regulated, can influence immune responses to vaccines. Perhaps because of their limited immunogenicity or their unique immunological characteristics, the immune response to polysaccharide vaccines may be subject to genetic regulation.

m. Antigenuria Following PRP Immunization. Immunization with PRP vaccine can result in excretion of antigen in urine, which is detectable by latex agglutination for up to 11 days after vaccination.[394,395] The value of antigen detection tests in the evaluation of a recently vaccinated febrile child is, therefore, in doubt.

n. Safety. Purified capsular polysaccharide vaccines are among the safest of all vaccines. Serious systemic adverse events are very rare and may be due to small amounts of endotoxin that were present in earlier vaccine preparations.[234] The current Hib capsular polysaccharide vaccines are highly purified and chemically well defined. Prior to licensure, more than 60,000 doses of the vaccine were administered to infants and children, and the only serious systemic reaction reported occurred in the Finnish study, where a child had an anaphylactic reaction that responded to epinephrine. In that 1974 study,[310] 51% of 363 children studied had local reactions within 24 h after vaccination, but less than 1% had fever $\geq$ 38.5°C (101.3°F). Currently licensed PRP preparations are more purified and exclude endotoxin and other bacterial products, resulting in significantly fewer local and systemic reactions.[54,272] Adverse reactions occurring within 24 h after immunization among 4557 children between 2 and 5 years of age were found in

2.3% with fever $\geq$ 101°F, 4.8% with local erythema, 2.9% with local swelling, and 12.6% with local tenderness.[54]

o. Prelicensure Efficacy. The only prospective study that evaluated the protective efficacy of PRP vaccine prior to its licensure in 1985 was a large clinical trial involving children 3–71 months of age conducted in Finland in 1974[253,310] (Tables 9, 10). This study was originally conducted in response to a nationwide meningococcal epidemic and was designed to evaluate the efficacy of group A meningococcal vaccine. PRP vaccine was used as the control vaccine, and the two vaccines were randomly and blindly administered to approximately 98,000 children, who were then followed for 4 years for Hib disease occurrence. This trial demonstrated impressive efficacy of meningococcal group A vaccine, which led to control of the epidemic.[253] After 4 years of follow-up, the study was analyzed for the effect of PRP in preventing Hib disease, and it was clear that PRP vaccine was protective, but not uniformly effective across the age spectrum studied (Table 10). Although PRP was 90% protective in children 18–71 months of age, a disproportionate number of vaccine failures occurred in children vaccinated before 18 months of age (in this age group, there were more Hib cases in PRP recipients than in the controls). Two cases also occurred in children vaccinated with PRP at 18–29 months of age, although there were fewer cases than in the control group. Therefore, it has been difficult to determine the exact age at which PRP becomes effective. Efficacy estimates in this study necessitated the grouping of children of various ages, which does not provide a definitive answer to the question, "How protective is PRP vaccine in children vaccinated at 18 or 24 months of age?" An 18-month-old vaccine cutoff has often been cited, which groups 18- to 23-month-old vaccine recipients with all older children in the trial and suggests a high degree of efficacy for this younger age group, when there could, in fact, have been none. Unfortunately, the number of cases of Hib disease in children vaccinated at 18 to 23 months of age was insufficient to conclude from this study that the vaccine is effective in this critical age group.

p. Postlicensure PRP Immunogenicity Studies. Based on postlicensure studies in Finland comparing the immunogenicity in 24-month-old children of all three PRP vaccines licensed in the United States and a fourth in France, all preparations appeared to be of equivalent immunogenicity.[225] Antibody measurements in all the vaccinees were done by the same radioimmunoassay and in the same laboratory as in the 1974 Finnish efficacy trial.

q. Postlicensure PRP Efficacy Studies. Subsequent to the licensure of the polysaccharide vaccine in 1985, it became apparent that routine use of the vaccine resulted in

Table 9. Clinical Efficacy of *Haemophilus influenzae* Type b (Hib) PRP Polysaccharide Vaccine, Field Trial, Finland, 1974–1978

Years after vaccination	Vaccinated at 18–71 months		Vaccinated at 3–17 months	
	Hib group (N=37,393)	Men. A group (N=38,431)	Hib group (N=11,584)	Men. A group (N=10,864)
	Cases of bacteremic Hib disease			
1	0	11	7	1
2	2[a]	5	1	3
3	0	2	2	1
4	0	2	0	0
Total cases	2	20	10	5

[a] 1 vaccinated at 24 months, developed meningitis 21 months later; 1 vaccinated at 27 months, developed meningitis 20 months later.

efficacy less than that assessed in the Finnish vaccine trial.[175,310] Some vaccine failures were anecdotally reported both before[430] and after licensure of the vaccine.[175] After licensure of PRP, prospective randomized and controlled trials were no longer possible in the United States, so several investigators resorted to alternative study methods to assess vaccine efficacy and safety: population-based disease surveillance, cohort studies (following a cohort of immunized children), and most importantly, case–control studies.

The results of the five postlicensure case–control studies are summarized in Table 11. The point estimates range from 88% in the multicenter Connecticut/Pittsburgh/Dallas (C/P/D) study, to −55% in the Minnesota study (a negative efficacy implies greater risk for vaccinees than nonvac-

4-Year Follow-up by Age Cohort of Hib Polysaccharide Vaccine Field Trial, Finland, 1974–1978

Age at vaccination (months)	No. of children in vaccine group	
	Hib group	Men. A group
3–5	2,382 (2)[a]	2,046 (1)
6–11	4,825 (4)	4,580 (4)
12–17	4,377 (4)	4,238 (0)
Subtotal	11,584 (10)	10,864 (5)
18–23	4,101 (0)	4,034 (2)
24–29	8,453 (2)	8,573 (8)
30–35	(0)	(2)
36–47	8,526 (0)	8,904 (6)
48–59	8,407 (0)	8,791 (2)
60–71	7,906 (0)	8,129 (0)
Subtotal	37,393 (2)	38,431 (20)
Total	48,977 (12)	49,295 (25)

[a] Number of cases of Hib disease are shown in parentheses.
References: *J. Infect. Dis.* **136**(Suppl. 1):S43–S50 (1977); *Pediatrics* **60**:730–737 (1977); *N. Engl. J. Med.* **310**: 1561–1566 (1984); Peltola–line listing of 2-year follow-up data (unpublished).

Table 10. Efficacy of *Haemophilus influenzae* Type b Polysaccharide Vaccine by Age Group, Finnish Field Trial, 1974

Age (months)	Hib vaccine		Group A meningococcal vaccine (controls)		Vaccine efficacy (95% CI)		*p* value[a]
	No. cases	No. vacc.	No. cases	No. vacc.			
18–23	0	4,101	2	4,034	100%	(−219,100)	0.246
24–35	2	8,453	10	8,573	80%	(5,98)	0.039
36–71	0	24,839	8	25,824	100%	(53,100)	0.0046
18–71 total:	2	37,393	20	38,431	90%	(55,98)	0.00012
24–71 only:	2	33,292	18	34,397	88.5%	(52.1,98.7)	0.0041

[a]FET, two-tailed.

cinees). The finding that the C/P/D and Minnesota studies represent the two extreme estimates may be due to the fact that these areas were split, after the fact, into two separate studies because of a marked heterogeneity in efficacy results between the study sites. If the data from the four areas (C/P/D and Minnesota) had been combined, as originally intended, the efficacy estimate for all four areas would probably be similar to that found in the Harrison and Black studies. The Harrison studies showed an efficacy of 45% in day-care and 62% in non-day-care attendees. Therefore, the only discrepant result was from Minnesota and the weight of the other studies indicates a vaccine efficacy between 45 and 88%. Issues relating to the discrepancy in these studies have been reviewed.[106,277,440]

   r. Postlicensure PRP Safety. More than 10 million doses have been administered in the United States since licensure of PRP in April 1985, and no associations have been established between the vaccine and serious reactions.[175,272] A few serious events have occurred in association with administration of Hib vaccine, and were reported to the FDA, CDC, and the manufacturers, but no cause-and-effect relationship has been convincingly demonstrated.[272] Minor reactions, like fever and local reactions, have been relatively uncommon, occurring in about 5% of vaccinees. The only major concern about safety has been several episodes of Hib disease that occurred within 1 week of Hib polysaccharide vaccination.[55,196,297,374,440] The vaccine is not expected to induce protective immunity until at least 1–2 weeks after immunization. Therefore, the issue is whether the occurrence of disease soon after immunization is greater than what one would expect given the amount of vaccine administered and the natural incidence of dis-

Table 11. Postlicensure Case–Control Efficacy Studies of *Haemophilus influenzae* Type b PRP Polysaccharide Vaccine

Principal investigator	Study location	No. of subjects		% vaccinated		Vaccine efficacy	95% confidence interval
		Cases	Controls	Cases	Controls		
Harrison (day-care)[196]	MO, NJ,OK, TN, WA, Los Angeles	123	286	19%	28%	45%	−1% to 70%
Harrison (no day-care)[196]	MO, NJ, OK, TN, WA, Los Angeles	74	132	12%	23%	62%	7% to 84%
Black[55]	Kaiser–N. California	35[a]	166	11%	23%	69%[a]	−13% to 91%
Shapiro[374]	CT, Pittsburgh, Dallas (C/P/D)	76	152	12%	39%	88%	74% to 96%
Osterholm[297]	MN	65	130	34%	26%	−55%	−238% to 29%

[a]The 35 cases in this study were identified by follow-up of a cohort of approximately 120,000 children. The results of this case–control study were validated by independent analysis of data from the cohort. An analysis of a subset of cases and controls in day-care showed an efficacy of 54% (95% CI 16–92%).

ease. In the studies listed in Table 11, 373 Hib disease cases occurred in children older than 18–24 months; 12 of these cases occurred within 1 week of Hib immunization. Some authors have been concerned that his number may be excessive,[106,277] but to estimate a relative risk for an association between vaccination and disease one must assume that there was no bias toward preferential detection of these unusual cases and that these children are representative of the general population to which they have been compared. However, a disproportionate number of these 12 cases are black, attended day-care facilities, had known recent exposure to Hib disease (a reason for receiving vaccine), or were thought to have increased susceptibility to disease (sickle-cell disease, Down's syndrome, recurrent Hib disease). All of these factors suggest that these children are not strictly comparable to the general population, and that it would be inappropriate to estimate relative risk of vaccine administration by making comparisons with the general population. The best way to assess the true risk for vaccine-induced disease is to use the case–control studies and ask whether there was an association between recent vaccine exposure for Hib cases relative to their healthy matched controls. With such an analysis, there was no significant difference in the Harrison or the Shapiro studies. In the Black study (which had four early cases, in one of whom vaccine was given because of known exposure to Hib disease), there was an estimated 1.4- to 20.1-fold increased risk (95% confidence interval for the odds ratio) for the period 1 week after immunization, but there was no significant association between vaccine use and disease by 3 weeks after immunization. Although one cannot conclusively rule out an association between the vaccine and early onset disease, we conclude that the magnitude of the effect, if any, is small and is outweighed by the potential benefits of the vaccine.

    s. Recommendations for Use of PRP Vaccine. Based on available clinical efficacy, safety, and immunogenicity data, the Immunization Practices Advisory Committee (ACIP) of the United States Public Health Service[1,83,334,335] and the Committee on Infectious Diseases (Red Book Committee) of the American Academy of Pediatrics (AAP)[83,88] have made recommendations for the use of PRP vaccine. Both committees recommended routinely vaccinating all children in the United States against invasive Hib disease at 24 months of age. Although this age was beyond the period of greatest Hib disease risk, this strategy might reduce the incidence of disease by as much as 11–24%, the proportion of disease that occurs in children 24 to 60 months of age (see Fig. 3). These recommendations were supplanted by the availability in January 1988 of a significantly more immunogenic Hib conjugate vaccine (PRP-D),

which was subsequently recommended as the preferred vaccine (see Section 9.2.3).[89,203]

    9.2.2. PRP Adjuvant Vaccines. The limited immunogenicity of PRP vaccine in young infants led to attempts to enhance immunogenicity by combining PRP with adjuvants. These attempts have included combining high-molecular-weight PRP with whole *Bordetella pertussis* organisms ("PRP–pertussis"), mixing PRP with DTP vaccine ("PRP–DTP"), and extracting impure fractions of PRP that included OMPs and other cell-wall constituents of the organism ("PRP complex").[14,93,152,190,230,233,238,274,322,453] PRP complex vaccines have been studied in both animals and adult humans.[22,23,29–31] These vaccines consisted of PRP associated with components of bacterial outer membrane (presumably noncovalently bound) and included some LPS (endotoxin).

    Interest in the "adjuvant" vaccines as a group has been limited because of their poor and inconsistent immunogenicity especially for younger children, lack of T-dependent characteristics in the immune response, lack of efficacy data, difficulty in standardizing vaccine composition, and concern about side effects. Furthermore, concern about the current composition of pertussis vaccines precluded the development of a vaccine with whole pertussis organisms.

    Other vaccines incorporating antigens other than capsule have been evaluated primarily in animals. These include whole killed organisms,[81,463] OMPs[192,229,248,377] and ribosomal or membrane vesicle vaccines.[63,64,194,251,407] The rationale for these vaccines is to include alternative Hib antigens (noncapsular) that might more readily induce protective immunity in young infants and might also provide immunity to non-type b *H. influenzae* organisms that commonly cause otitis media, bronchitis, and sinusitis. With the exception of purified OMPs that might be incorporated in the formulation of future PRP-conjugate vaccines, it is unlikely that the other vaccines will prove to be clinically useful. Much work is yet needed on the OMP vaccines, including the identification of specific proteins common to all or most clinical isolates, purification of these proteins (large scale), demonstration of their immunogenicity, demonstration of the functional activity of the antibodies induced, safety, and decisions about the optimal formulation of a vaccine (e.g., type of conjugate, OMP composition).

    9.2.3. PRP–Protein Conjugate Vaccines. Conjugate vaccines have been developed with the ultimate goal of providing an effective vaccine for infants and young children. Currently, there are at least four PRP-conjugate vaccines undergoing clinical evaluations. As of this writing, three such vaccines have recently been licensed for routine use in children at 18 months of age (see Recommendations, Section 9.2.3e), and these have superseded the use of PRP vaccine. As a group, the conjugate vaccines offer distinct advantages over PRP vaccine.

In attempts to overcome the poor immunogenicity of the plain PRP polysaccharide, particularly in infants, alterations in the antigen have been made to enhance its immunogenicity. The addition of adjuvants alone did not significantly enhance the immunogenicity of PRP because they do not alter the basic recognition of the polysaccharide as a T-independent antigen. However, an important adaptation of the PRP polysaccharide has been the application of carrier–hapten principles to develop PRP–protein conjugate vaccines. These vaccines are novel synthetic modifications of a naturally occurring antigen.

The first successful synthesis of a conjugate bacterial vaccine was accomplished by Avery and Goebel in 1929, [41,154,155] using carrier–hapten principles first defined by Landsteiner in 1924.[236] More recently, Schneerson *et al.*,[361] Gordon,[159] Anderson *et al.*,[20] Tai *et al.*,[401] and Marburg *et al.*[255] have developed PRP–protein conjugate vaccines. Basic to all conjugate vaccines is the use of a protein carrier, which is covalently linked or conjugated to PRP; the PRP acts in this context as the hapten. The protein carrier portion of the vaccine is recognized by macrophages and T cells, thereby eliciting a T-dependent immune response. In principle, the immunological responsiveness of the protein carrier is thereby conferred upon the polysaccharide hapten. This immune response has the following general characteristics: (1) It is quantitatively enhanced, particularly in younger children. (2) Repeat administrations of such vaccines elicit booster responses, thus providing a means of maximizing the level of immunity. This contrasts with the absence of booster responses when repeated doses of the conventional PRP polysaccharide vaccine are administered. (3) There is a maturation of class-specific immunity with a predominance of IgG antibody indicating T-cell modulation of the immune response. (4) The prior or concurrent administration of the carrier protein alone (e.g., diphtheria or tetanus toxoid) enhances T-cell populations responsive to this antigen, thereby maximizing immune responsiveness to the polysaccharide when the conjugate vaccine is administered (so-called "carrier priming").[160]

A variety of studies with mice, rats, rabbits, primates, and humans have confirmed that PRP–protein conjugate vaccines have characteristics of T-dependent immunogens. The evidence of a T-dependent responsiveness includes: the absence of an immune response in athymic nude mice (deficient in T-helper cells), enhanced immunogenicity only when PRP is covalently conjugated to the carrier immu-

nogen, booster responses, a predominance of IgG antibody, and priming of the response by prior administration of the carrier.

As a group, all Hib conjugate vaccines use the same hapten (PRP polysaccharide); however, each conjugate vaccine has important structural and chemical differences that make direct comparisons difficult (Table 12, Fig. 8). For example, the protein carrier, polysaccharide length, configuration of the linkages, proportions of protein and polysaccharide, and other structural characteristics differ. Furthermore, making direct comparisons of immunogenicity among vaccines has been difficult until recently because studies of different conjugates often involve different vaccine doses, routes of administration, schedules, ages of subjects, timings of bleedings, and other differences in study design. In addition, antibody levels in different laboratories have been quantitated by radioimmunoassays that, until recently, have not been standardized. Thus, variability in antibody quantitation has made direct comparisons of immunogenicity of the conjugate vaccines from different studies difficult and only recently have different vaccines been compared in a single study. Therefore, each of the conjugate vaccines will be reviewed separately.

a. PRP–Tetanus Toxoid Conjugate Vaccine (PRP-T). The PRP–tetanus toxoid conjugate vaccine was developed at the National Institutes of Health (NIH),[78,80,342,361-363] and subsequently produced by investigators at Merieux Institute. This vaccine has not yet been licensed by the U.S. Food and Drug Administration (FDA). Initially, several carrier proteins were evaluated at NIH, including tetanus toxoid, diphtheria toxoid, horseshoe crab hemocyanin, bovine serum albumin, human serum albumin, and cholera toxin. The optimal immunogenicity was found with a PRP–tetanus toxoid (PRP-T) conjugate.[363] A schematic of this vaccine is shown in Fig. 8, and an outline of the principal elements involved in its preparation is shown in Table 12.

Immunogenicity. The immunogenicity of this conjugate vaccine was demonstrated in mice [361] and rhesus monkeys,[362] and more recently in humans.[80,363] Preliminary studies showed that a 50-µg dose of the PRP-T conjugate induced maximal increases in anti-PRP antibody levels. The antibody levels were further enhanced by the simultaneous administration of the carrier protein (tetanus toxoid) at a different site. Furthermore, this antibody was shown to be primarily IgG, bactericidal in the presence of complement, and protective when administered passively to infant rats subsequently challenged with Hib organisms.[78,361,362]

In adults who previously were immunized with tetanus toxoid, anticapsular antibody rises of almost 200-fold were

Table 12.   Characteristics of Conjugate Hib Vaccines[a]

Properties	NICHD	Connaught[b]	MSD[b]	University of Rochester	Praxis[b]
Polysaccharide (PS) size	Large	Medium	Large	Variable	Small
PS preparation	Native	Heat-sized	Native	Periodate oxidized	Periodate oxidized
Protein carrier	Tetanus toxoid (+ other proteins)	Diphtheria toxoid	Meningococcal group B OMP	Diphtheria toxoid/CRM$_{197}$	CRM$_{197}$
Linkage					
Activation	PS	Protein	Protein and PS	PS	PS
Reactants	ADH CNBr(PS) carbodiimide-HCl	ADH CNBr (protein)	N-ABC (PS) N-AHC (protein)	Periodate Cyanoboro hydrate	Periodate Cyanoboro hydrate
Linkages	Amide/protein Iminocarbamate/PS	Amide/protein Iminocarbamate/PS	Amide/protein Carbamate/PS Thioester/spacer	Secondary amino	Secondary amino
Spacer	Yes 6-carbon	Yes 6-carbon	Yes "Bigeneric" N-ABC (linked to PS) N-AHC (linked to protein)	No	No
Protein/PS ratio (w/w)	0.4:1	1.2:1	0.16–0.2:1	0.05–0.2:1	0.2–0.6:1

[a] Abbreviations used: NICHD, National Institute of Child Health, NIH; MSD, Merck Sharp & Dohme Laboratories; PS, polysaccharide; meningococcal group B OMP, *Neisseria meningitidis* group B outer membrane protein; CRM$_{197}$, diphtheria toxin mutant protein; ADH, adipic dihydrazide (the completed reaction cleaves both hydrazide moieties leaving a 6-carbon linkage); CNBr, cyanogen bromide; N-ABC, *N*-acetylbutylcarbamate; N-AHC, *N*-acetylhomocysteine.
[b] Currently (January 1990) licensed in the United States.

seen following a single dose of PRP-T conjugate vaccine to levels of 95 to 422 μg/ml.[363] Booster responses were not observed with a second or third dose, presumably because of control mechanisms acting to limit the level of specific antibodies. Antibody was shown to be of the IgM, IgG, and IgA isotypes, but the predominant response was IgG.[363] More recent studies in young children also showed enhanced immune responses.[80]

Safety. One issue in the adult studies was that approximately 75% of subjects had adverse reactions.[363] These were mainly at the injection site and were presumably due to Arthus-type hypersensitivity mediated by preexisting antibodies to tetanus toxoid. None of these reactions were debilitating or long-lasting, and reactions have occurred infrequently in young children who have lower levels of tetanus antitoxin.

b. PRP–Group B Neisseria meningitidis OMP Conjugate Vaccine (PRP–OMP). This PRP–protein conjugate vaccine developed by Merck Sharp & Dohme (MSD)[255] was licensed in December, 1989 by the FDA for routine use in children 18 months of age or older. Although the protective efficacy of this vaccine has not been demonstrated in this age group, licensure was based upon additional safety and immunogenicity data and comparison to plain PRP. The protein carrier is a 40-kDa OMP derived from a type 2 strain of group B *N. meningitidis* (Table 12 and Fig. 8). This protein was selected because of its consistent immunogenicity in young children. Because prior exposure to this protein during infancy is unlikely, the vaccine will not likely have a carrier priming influence. Although it is possible that this vaccine will induce immunity to group B *N. meningitidis,* this has not yet been evaluated. Also, antibody to the type 2 OMP of the organism has not been shown to be protective against *N. meningitidis.*

Immunogenicity. The PRP–OMP vaccine has been evaluated for immunogenicity and safety in children and adults.[120] For adults, the vaccine was uniformly immunogenic after a single dose. For children 8 to 17 months of age there was an impressive response to a single dose, with most subjects developing titers of > 1 μg/ml. A subsequent

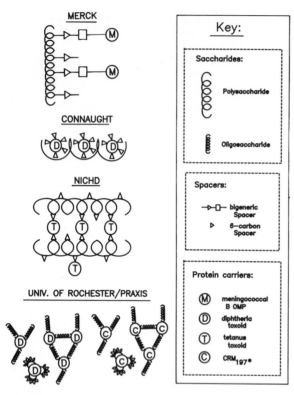

Figure 8. Configurations of PRP–protein conjugate vaccines.

dose of vaccine raised the proportion of responders and the mean level of antibody slightly, but there was no clear demonstration of a booster response.[120] As with all PRP and PRP–protein conjugate vaccines, the degree of immunogenicity correlated with age, with the younger children having lower response rates and lower mean levels of antibody. In children 2 to 6 months of age, a single dose of vaccine elicited antibody in about 75% of subjects, with a mean of approximately 1 μg/ml. These levels rose slightly after a second dose of vaccine, but a significant secondary response was not observed in most subjects.

Safety. Local reactions occurred in all adults and in approximately 25% of children given unadsorbed vaccine. Reactions were not serious and lasted 48 h. The frequency of these reactions was markedly decreased by adsorption of the conjugate vaccine with aluminum hydroxide. With this adjuvant, reactions were observed in 8% of recipients. Presumably the aluminum hydroxide binds endotoxin or slows the local release of vaccine. Although relatively few subjects have been evaluated, there has been no association of reaction rates with age of subject, number of injections, or

dose of vaccine. No serious or lasting reactions have been observed.[120]

c. PRP Oligosaccharide–CRM$_{197}$ Conjugate Vaccine (Oligo-CRM). This vaccine (HibTITER^R—Praxis Biologics) was licensed by the FDA on December 22, 1988, for routine use in children 18 months of age or older. Although the protective efficacy of this vaccine has not been demonstrated in this age group, licensure was based upon additional safety and immunogenicity data and comparison to plain PRP. Several PRP–protein conjugate vaccines of this class have been developed at the University of Rochester and Praxis Biologics.[20,32–34,205,244] These vaccines differ significantly from the other conjugate vaccines described (Table 12). First, they do not employ a spacer; the polysaccharide is linked directly to the protein carrier. Second, the polysaccharide polymer is an oligosaccharide relatively small in length. Coupling of low-molecular-weight oligosaccharides rather than long polymers of PRP to the carrier protein was selected as a potential means for maximizing T-dependent recognition of the antigen and optimizing carrier-specific helper effects. Third, the protein carrier used is either diphtheria toxoid or the nontoxic mutant diphtheria toxin, CRM$_{197}$. Lastly, the PRP oligosaccharide–protein conjugates are prepared with different linkage configurations, ranging from monomeric to highly cross-linked forms (Fig. 8).[34]

Immunogenicity. Several PRP–protein conjugates have been prepared and evaluated for immunogenicity in animals and humans, using varying lengths of oligosaccharide, and either diphtheria toxoid or CRM$_{197}$ as the protein carrier. The different preparations as a group showed evidence of T-dependent immune recognition and response. In children, all were more immunogenic than unconjugated PRP, induced booster responses with repeated vaccine administration, and elicited predominantly IgG antibody. However, in younger subjects, the 20-repeat-unit oligosaccharide with looped linkages proved most immunogenic, and the CRM$_{197}$ protein proved to be the more immunogenic carrier protein.

Diphtheria toxoid conjugated to oligosaccharides of 20 repeat units was given simultaneously with DTP vaccine at 2, 4, and 6 months of age.[34] Mean preimmunization levels were 0.13 μg/ml (indicating maternal antibody), 0.09 μg/ml after one dose, 0.65 μg/ml after two doses, and 3.1 μg/ml at age 9 months after three doses. Approximately 95% of subjects showed an immune response. Better responses were observed in infants immunized at 3, 5, and 7 months of age (geometric mean: 15 μg/ml at age 10 months), due possibly to maturity with age or the effect of prior DTP priming.

Safety. The safety of these PRP–CRM conjugate vaccines is similar to that of other conjugates. The frequency of minor reactions is similar to that with conventional PRP and significantly less than that with DTP. Adverse events were evaluated in 1197 children 1–23 months of age given 2751 doses independent of DTP vaccine, with observations made during the day of vaccination and days 1 and 2 postvaccination. A temperature greater than 38.3°C was recorded at least once during the observation period following 2.4% of the vaccinations. Local erythema, warmth or swelling (≥ 2 cm) was observed following 2.2% of vaccinations. Adverse events in the subset of 268 children 15–23 months of age were as follows: fever greater than 38.3°C, 0.75%; erythema, 1.9%; swelling, 0.75%. Serious systemic reactions have not been observed.

d. PRP–Diphtheria Toxoid Conjugate Vaccine (PRP-D). This conjugate vaccine was developed at Connaught Laboratories[160] using methods similar to those developed at NIH.[361] On December 22, 1987, the PRP-D conjugate vaccine (ProHIBiT[R]—Connaught Laboratories) was licensed by the FDA for routine use in children 18 months of age or older.[89,203] Although the protective efficacy of this vaccine has not been demonstrated in this age group, licensure was based upon additional safety and immunogenicity data and comparison to plain PRP. The vaccine combines a diphtheria toxoid carrier with a moderately sized polymer of PRP polysaccharide (standardized by heat treatment) (see Table 12 and Fig. 8).

Immunogenicity. The PRP-D vaccine has been extensively evaluated in animals (rabbits, mice, monkeys, rats), and more than 120,000 doses were administered to humans prior to its licensure. PRP-D elicits an immune response with the characteristics of a T-dependent immunogen.[160] Furthermore, the antibody induced is bactericidal in the presence of complement, opsonophagocytic, and protective when passively administered to infant rats.[72,73,160,172,239] In adult humans, PRP-D elicits immune responses similar to those of PRP–tetanus toxoid.[172,239] Very high levels of antibody (geometric mean = 200 µg/ml) are elicited by a single dose in nearly all adults. In contrast to conjugate vaccines with tetanus as the carrier, PRP-D causes few reactions in adults.[172,239]

Extensive immunogenicity and safety studies have been carried out with children 2–30 months of age.[51,122,224,240–242,437,469] In a randomized, double-blind study of children 15–24 months of age, more than 90% of children vaccinated with PRP-D responded with antibody levels considered to be protective (≥ 0.15 µg/ml), whereas less than 50% of children vaccinated with PRP had such a response.[415] More than 60% of children vaccinated with PRP-D, but less than 30% of those vaccinated with PRP, produced levels of antibody considered to be indicative of long-term protection (1.0 µg/ml). Postimmunization levels achieved with the PRP-D conjugate vary significantly with age. In the age range of 9 to 15 months, two doses of vaccine were needed to achieve levels grater than 1 µg/ml in the majority of subjects (geometric mean = 4.7 µg/ml).[240] In this age range conventional PRP is neither immunogenic nor does it induce booster responses with repeat administration. In contrast, PRP-D induces a booster response in essentially all subjects. Although immune responses were observed in essentially all subjects, the highest levels of antibody were in older subjects. Antibody responses were primarily IgG, especially in older children. Antibody levels declined significantly in the year after vaccination, but remained significantly higher than those in unvaccinated or PRP-immunized children.[241] Maximum immune responses with the conjugate vaccine were seen with vaccine lots having the greatest proportions of carrier protein to polysaccharide. PRP-D vaccine also boosted antibody levels to diphtheria toxoid.

Several immunogenicity studies have been conducted with PRP-D vaccine given to infants younger than 6 months of age, using a two- or three-dose schedule with 1- to 2-month intervals between doses.[122,224,437,469] The conjugate vaccine is less immunogenic in this age range than it is in older children, but this difference is offset, in part, by responses elicited by a second or third dose. Although most of these studies are not yet published, there have been 12 immunogenicity studies of PRP-D in infants younger than 6 months of age, involving more than 500 subjects, six different lots of vaccine, and various schedules of doses and follow-up bleeds.[122,437,469] With a first dose given at 2 or 3 months of age, there is rarely any measurable antibody response. A second dose at 4 months of age results in moderate response with some lots, but essentially no response with others. Likewise, a second or third dose at 6–7 months of age shows 58–93% of subjects responding with a twofold or greater antibody increase and geometric mean levels of antibody range from 0.18 to 2.20 µg/ml. The most concerning feature of these responses is the marked variability in immunogenicity between vaccine lots, which was not observed when the vaccine was given to older children. Furthermore, the antibody levels declined significantly in the year following vaccination. However, a dose of either PRP-D or conventional PRP induced significant booster responses of antibody when compared to that induced by a primary immunization in children of a similar age. Antibody levels were predominantly IgG, but unlike observations in older children, a significant proportion of young infants who responded did so with IgM antibody. In all studies, none of the infants vaccinated with a control vaccine (PRP or saline) demonstrated immune responses.

Efficacy. The immunogenicity studies demonstrate that PRP antibody can be induced in most young infants and in almost all children over 7 months of age with one to three doses of vaccine; however, it is difficult to extrapolate from these immunogenicity data to predict what the protective efficacy of the vaccine might be. No efficacy study has been performed to date with PRP-D in children 18 months of age or older. However, important information has come from controlled field trials in infants. Two such studies have been conducted, the preliminary results of which have become available in 1987–1988. In Alaska a 4-year prospective, randomized, double-blind trial was carried out to evaluate PRP-D versus a saline placebo concurrent with DTP immunization at 2, 4, and 6 months of age in Native Alaskan infants.[439] Only limited protective efficacy was demonstrated in this population, with an estimated vaccine efficacy of 35% after three doses of vaccine (95% confidence interval: −57 to 73%). This contrasted with another trial conducted in Finland and designed to evaluate the protective efficacy in children vaccinated at 3, 4, and 6 months of age. Approximately 30,000 Finnish infants were given three doses of PRP-D with DTP vaccine and inactivated polio vaccine (IPV) at 3, 4, and 6 months of age, and 30,000 infants did not receive PRP-D. The estimated protective efficacy of PRP-D was 87% (95% confidence interval: 50–96%) during an average follow-up time of 9 months.[123] Further studies are needed to resolve the apparent discrepancy in the vaccine efficacy findings.

Safety. The safety of PRP-D vaccine has been demonstrated in several controlled double-blind clinical trials in humans from 2 months of age to adulthood.[51,72,73,122, 172,224,239–242,437,469] The frequency of adverse events is similar for conventional PRP and PRP-D vaccine. In one study of more than 500 children 15 to 24 months of age, local reactions were noted for 10.3% of children receiving PRP and 12.5% of children receiving PRP-D, while moderate fever $[T > 39.0°C (102.2°F)]$ occurred in 1.4% of children vaccinated with PRP and 0.7% of children vaccinated with PRP-D.[51] PRP-D is associated with significantly fewer adverse events than DTP, and only slightly more than saline placebo (only local erythema was shown to occur more frequently in one study) when evaluated blindly. No serious or lasting adverse effects have been observed with more than 60,000 doses of PRP-D administered through 1986. There have been no associations between reactions and immunity to diphtheria toxoid. Also, there is no evidence of immune tolerance in children immunized at any

age. In the Finnish trial of PRP-D in infants, vaccine reactions were not greater among those given PRP-D with DTP and IPV as compared to those given the latter two vaccines only.[123]

e. Recommendations for Use of Licensed PRP–Protein Conjugate Vaccines. Since antibody production after vaccination with conjugate vaccines in children 18 months of age or older is substantially greater than that after vaccination with PRP vaccine, three conjugate vaccines have been licensed as of this writing for use in these children. The favorable safety and immunogenicity data have led both the Immunization Practices Advisory Committee (ACIP) of the United States Public Health Service and the Committee on Infectious Diseases of the American Academy of Pediatrics to recommend routine use of conjugate vaccines in children at 18 months of age.[89,203] Licensure of conjugate vaccines for use in infants in the United States cannot be considered until efficacy trials already completed or in progress are evaluated.

The licensed conjugate vaccines are now recommended as the preferred vaccines over PRP vaccine for children 18 months of age or older. In this age group, a booster dose of conjugate vaccine has not been recommended because good immune responses are seen in nearly all subjects with a single dose. The duration of immunity is not fully known. The following recommendations for use of the conjugate vaccines were established in 1988:

1. All children should receive a single dose of conjugate vaccine at 18 months of age. In children 19–23 months of age, a single dose of vaccine is recommended regardless of whether the PRP vaccine had previously been given (at least 2 months should elapse between PRP and conjugate vaccinations). Special efforts should be made to immunize children at high risk of disease, such as those in day-care.

2. Children 24–59 months of age should routinely receive a single dose of conjugate vaccine only if they have not previously been given the plain polysaccharide vaccine. Although a booster response and some protective benefit might derive from giving conjugate vaccine to children previously given the PRP vaccine, the degree of benefit does not at this time seem to justify the routine reimmunization of all children. However, there is no contraindication to giving it to these older children.

3. The duration of immunity after a single dose of conjugate vaccine is not known precisely; however, revaccination with conjugate vaccine is not recommended at this time.

4. Children who have had invasive Hib disease when they were less than 24 months of age should receive the vaccine as described above, because adequate immunity rarely follows natural infection, particularly in younger children.

5. Use of conjugate vaccine should not alter use of diphtheria

toxoid (either DT toxoid or DTP vaccine), as immunity to diphtheria is not adequately induced by conjugate vaccines.

6. Immunization with PRP or conjugate vaccine should not alter the need for chemoprophylaxis in appropriate household or day-care contacts of an Hib disease case. Immunization with conjugate vaccine at the time of exposure is unlikely to induce protection quickly enough to be of benefit in contact situations, but is not contraindicated and may be given to previously unvaccinated children of appropriate age to provide protection against future exposure.

7. Simultaneous administration of the conjugate vaccine and DTP, IPV, MMR, or OPV vaccines is acceptable, although serological data on concurrent use of MMR and/or OPV vaccines are lacking.

8. Use of conjugate vaccine in children less than 18 months of age is not recommended at this time.

9.2.4. Passive Immunization. Antibody to PRP provides the immunological basis for both active and passive Hib immunization. As already discussed, there is considerable evidence that antibody to PRP protects against invasive Hib disease; it activates complement, it is opsonophagocytic, and it protects animals from experimental Hib challenge. Moreover, immunoglobulin prophylaxis protects agammaglobulinemia patients from invasive bacterial disease,[347] and before the availability of antimicrobials, immune serum was an effective therapy for Hib disease.[3,4,6] The most compelling evidence for the protective efficacy of PRP antibody is the clinical protection achieved in older children vaccinated with PRP polysaccharide vaccine[253,310] and the PRP-D vaccine[123] in Finland.

Although active immunization is preferred for the control of Hib disease, to date the lack of effective vaccines in young infants has made this goal difficult to achieve. Passive prophylaxis has been proposed as a means of providing protection for selected high-risk groups until effective vaccines are available. Passive prophylaxis could have advantages in the following high-risk settings: (1) to prevent secondary disease in households, day-care centers, or institutions; (2) for selected high-risk racial groups (Eskimos or American Indians); (3) for functionally asplenic patients (those with sickle-cell disease or splenectomized patients); and (4) for immunocompromised patients (Fig. 6).

A human hyperimmune globulin called bacterial polysaccharide immune globulin (BPIG) has been prepared at the Massachusetts Biologic Laboratory.[13,381] This investigational immunoglobulin is prepared from the plasma of adult donors immunized with PRP vaccine, in addition to polyvalent meningococcal and pneumococcal vaccines. The preparation contains approximately 17 times the amount of PRP antibody found in standard immune serum globulin,

and it also has enhanced levels of antibody to selected meningococcal and pneumococcal serotypes. The advantage of hyperimmune globulin is that protection does not depend on inducing an immune response. Pharmacological studies show that high levels of antibody (about 1 μg/ml) can be achieved within 4 days following an intramuscular injection (0.5 cm³/kg), and levels thought to be protective against Hib disease persist for as long as 4 months.[16] Recent studies demonstrate significant protective efficacy against invasive Hib disease in Apache children given three doses during the first year of life.[352] The hyperimmune globulin may be particularly useful in protecting immunocompromised patients and babies in high-risk populations too young to respond to vaccines. Protection lasts for 2–4 months, necessitating repeated administrations; therefore, a more feasible approach may be its use in a combined passive/active immunization schedule. Such an approach has been studied in high-risk Navajo Indian infants who received simultaneous immunization with BPIG and an Hib conjugate vaccine, followed by doses of vaccine at 4 and 6 months of age.[244] Infants who received concurrent passive immunization with BPIG at 2 months had significantly higher anticapsular antibody concentrations than control children who received vaccine alone, maintained antibody concentrations ≥ 0.15 μg/ml before 6 months of age, and appeared to respond similarly to second and third doses of conjugate vaccine as did the control children.

Another theoretical approach to passive prophylaxis for infants is to immunize pregnant women with PRP polysaccharide or newer conjugate vaccines so that newborns might acquire higher levels of antibody transplacentally, thereby protecting them during the first year of life.[19,71] This strategy has been considered as an adjunct to active immunization of infants, but there are three disadvantages: (1) variable immunogenicity of the PRP polysaccharide vaccine, even in adults; (2) a substantial proportion of the antibody induced with this vaccine is IgM, which does not cross the placenta; and (3) questions about the safety and acceptance of vaccinating pregnant women. With recent evidence that new conjugate vaccines induce immunity in infants younger than 6 months of age, interest in maternal immunization has lessened.

Three case–control studies have demonstrated that breast-feeding confers passive protection against invasive Hib disease.[85,210,250] Studies conducted with Alaskan Eskimo infants, children in Atlanta, and children in Colorado all demonstrated a protective influence of breast-feeding at least during the early months of life. However, breast-feeding does not assure protection, and the mechanism for this effect is not understood. Breast milk may provide infants with immune or nutritional factors that reduce the acquisition, attachment, or invasion of Hib organisms.[37] Although this is yet another reason for urging breast-feeding of young infants, it is unlikely to have major public health impact because protection is incomplete and few children are breast-fed throughout the period of disease risk.

Final conclusions about the role of passive prophylaxis must await further clinical studies, efforts to address the high cost of this type of prophylaxis, and the results of studies with the new conjugate Hib vaccines. Development of a safe and protective vaccine for infants and others at high risk would obviate the need for chemoprophylaxis or passive immunization.

10.   Unresolved Problems

In the quest to find ways to prevent invasive Hib disease, investigators have pondered a central enigma—why some individuals become infected but remain asymptomatically colonized while others succumb to invasive disease. In this regard, the analogy drawn with paralytic poliomyelitis, as in the earlier discussion comparing the risks in young children of paralytic poliomyelitis historically and invasive Hib disease in the current era, is again pertinent. Hib is a ubiquitous organism, infecting the upper respiratory tract of essentially all children during their early years of life. Since infection occurs in the vast majority of people without causing any symptoms, it can be considered to be part of the normal bacterial flora of the upper airway. As a control measure, it may never be feasible or necessarily desirable to attempt to eradicate the organism from the population.

From an epidemiological perspective, the research focus has been to define risk factors for disease, whether due to increased exposure or increased host susceptibility. Increased exposure has been defined in households where there is an index case, in day-care facilities, and in certain other population groups. In some of these settings of increased Hib exposure, it has been possible to use antimicrobial prophylaxis to reduce disease risk. To better understand why certain individuals develop disease and to find means to control disease, further characterization of the factors that determine how Hib disease is acquired and what makes an individual susceptible will be important.

From a microbiological perspective, additional characterization of the microbial factors that determine virulence would improve our understanding of disease pathogenesis, and could be useful to define other potential vaccine immunogens. Current vaccines are based on the principle that anticapsular antibody alone is sufficient to prevent disease,

but it is clear that other antigens of the organism also elicit antibody that may be protective. Therefore, conjugate vaccines incorporating OMPs or other antigens of the organism might provide significant additional protective benefit. Lastly, anticapsular vaccines do not address the problem of mucosal disease, due largely to unencapsulated strains. In this regard, the prevention of pneumonia in developing countries may require vaccines active against more than the type b *H. influenzae* strains.

From an immunological perspective, further understanding of the factors that influence immune response to capsule and to capsular derivatives is of considerable importance, not only for the prevention of Hib disease, but also for the prevention of other encapsulated bacterial diseases. Although much is known about hapten–carrier vaccines in animals, relatively little is known about the optimal determinants of immune responses in young humans. The role of mucosal immunity may also be of considerable importance, since the organism resides primarily at the mucosal surface. Although epidemiological evidence clearly shows that age is the most important risk factor for disease, the immunological elements that bring about this unusual susceptibility to disease are not fully understood. Research in the area of developmental immunology might better explain why young infants and children are so uniquely susceptible to numerous encapsulated bacteria.

We have had effective therapy for Hib disease for over 50 years, but it has been only recently that there have been effective means for preventing disease. Three general approaches to the prevention of Hib disease exist: (1) chemoprophylaxis, (2) passive immunization, and (3) active immunization. Although the universal immunization of young infants will ultimately be the means for preventing Hib disease, interim measures that include immunization of older preschool children with "less-than-optimal" vaccines, chemoprophylaxis, and passive immunization have been used.

Chemoprophylaxis with rifampin has been used to prevent secondary transmission of disease in high-risk settings. However, only a small percentage of all Hib cases (probably less than 3%) are due to secondary disease transmission in households and day-care centers. Although the issue of using chemoprophylaxis is of considerable concern for affected families and physicians, the routine use of chemoprophylaxis, even if it were completely effective, could not significantly reduce the overall Hib disease burden.

The development of hyperimmune globulin has provided a passive means of protecting children at defined risk for a limited period of time. This may be useful for prophylaxis of household or day-care contacts of a patient and for immunocompromised patients who have limited responses to active immunization. There may also be a role for passive–active immunization in selected settings.

PRP polysaccharide vaccine was the first vaccine available for the prevention of Hib disease in children older than 18 months of age, although it has proven to be less consistently protective than expected under conditions of routine use. Nonetheless, this vaccine helped to establish that anticapsular antibody, when present, provides protection, and this remains the immunological basis for all newer conjugate vaccines.

The recent development of PRP-conjugate vaccines holds the greatest promise for the prevention of invasive Hib disease. Also, similar vaccines may prove to be of great value in the prevention of other encapsulated bacterial diseases that afflict young children. To date there have been no significant safety problems noted with Hib conjugate vaccines, and their greatly enhanced immunogenicity in young infants holds considerable promise for providing long-term protection. Nonetheless, additional controlled efficacy trials are needed and may define some limitations in protection.

Although many questions still remain to be answered, the prevention of Hib disease, and possibly of disease caused by other polysaccharide-encapsulated bacteria, appears to be within reach. Therefore, one can predict that Hib disease will soon join the list of other diseases that have been virtually eliminated from the United States through vaccination.

Acknowledgments

We would like to acknowledge the helpful comments provided by Stephen Preblud and Walter Orenstein.

11. References

1. ACIP, Update: Prevention of *Haemophilus influenzae* type b disease, *Morbid. Mortal. Weekly Rep.* **35:**170–174, 179–180 (1986).
2. ALEXANDER, H. E., Type "B" anti-influenzal rabbit serum for therapeutic purposes, *Proc. Soc. Exp. Biol. Med.* **40:**313–314 (1939).
3. ALEXANDER, H. E., Experimental basis for treatment of *Haemophilus influenzae* infections, *Am. J. Dis. Child.* **66:**160–171 (1943).
4. ALEXANDER, H. E., Treatment of Haemophilus influenzae infections and of meningococcus and pneumococcic meningitis, *Am. J. Dis. Child.* **66:**172–187 (1943).
5. ALEXANDER, H. E., AND HEIDELBERGER, M., Chemical studies on bacterial agglutination. V. Agglutinin and precipitin content of antisera to *Hemophilus influenzae* type b, *J.*

6. ALEXANDER, H. E., ELLIS, C., AND LEIDY, G., Treatment of type-specific *Hemophilus influenzae* infections in infancy and childhood, *J. Pediatr.* **20:**673–698 (1942).
7. ALEXANDER, H. E., HEIDELBERGER, M., AND LEIDY, G., The protective or curative element in type b *Haemophilus influenzae* rabbit serum, *Yale J. Biol. Med.* **16:**425–440 (1944).
8. ALEXANDER, H. E., LEIDY, G., AND MACPHERSON, C., Production of types a,b,c,d,e, and f *H. influenzae* antibody for diagnostic and therapeutic purposes, *J. Immunol.* **54:**207–211 (1946).
9. ALEXANDER, W. J., AND SHAW, J. F. E., Results of a prospective population-based study of the incidence of invasive *Haemophilus influenzae* disease in children, Abstract 7, Symposium on infectious diseases in day care: Management and prevention, Minneapolis, June 1984.
10. ALPERT, G., CAMPOS, J. M., SMITH, D. R., BARENKAMP, S. J., AND FLEISHER, G. R., Incidence and persistence of *H. influenzae* type b upper airway colonization in patients with meningitis, *J. Pediatr.* **107:**555–557 (1985).
11. ALPERT, G., CAMPOS, J. M., SMITH, D. R., BARENKAMP, S. J., AND FLEISHER, G. R., Incidence and persistence of *Haemophilus influenzae* type b upper airway colonization in patients with meningitis, *J. Pediatr.* **107:**555–557 (1985).
12. AMBROSINO, D. M., AND SIBER, G. R., Simultaneous administration of vaccines for *Haemophilus influenzae* type b, pneumococci, and meningococci, *J. Infect. Dis.* **154:**893–896 (1986).
13. AMBROSINO, D. M., SCHREIBER, J. R., DAUM, R. S., AND SIBER, G. R., Efficacy of human hyperimmune globulin in prevention of *Haemophilus influenzae* type b disease in infant rats, *Infect. Immun.* **39:**709–714 (1983).
14. AMBROSINO, D. M., GLODE, M. P., WILLIAMS, C. L., AND SIBER, G. R., Antibody response of infants to *Haemophilus influenzae* type b capsular polysaccharide combined with *Bordetella pertussis*, *J. Infect. Dis.* **151:**1174 (1985).
15. AMBROSINO, D. M., SCHIFFMAN, G., GOTSCHLICH, E. C., SCHUR, P. H., ROSENBERG, G. A., DELANGE, G. G., VAN LOGHEM, E., AND SIBER, G. R., Correlation between G2m(n) immunoglobulin allotype and human antibody response and susceptibility to polysaccharide encapsulated bacteria, *J. Clin. Invest.* **75:**1935–1942 (1985).
16. AMBROSINO, D. M., LANDESMAN, S. H., GORHAM, C. C., AND SIBER, G. R., Passive immunization against disease due to *Haemophilus influenzae* type b: Concentrations of antibody to capsular polysaccharide in high-risk children, *J. Infect. Dis.* **153:**1–7 (1986).
17. AMBROSINO, D. M., BARRUS, V. A., DELANGE, G. G., AND SIBER, G. R., Correlation of the Km(1) immunoglobulin allotype with anti-polysaccharide antibodies in Caucasian adults, *J. Clin. Invest.* **78:**361–365 (1986).
18. AMBROSINO, D. M. SIBER, G. R., CHILMONCZYK, B. A., JERNBERG, J. B., AND FINBERG, R. W., An immunodeficiency characterized by impaired antibody responses to polysac-

charides, *N. Engl. J. Med.* **316**:790–793 (1987).

19. AMSTEY, M. S., INSEL, R., MUNOZ, J., AND PICHICHERO, M., Fetal–neonatal passive immunization against *Haemophilus influenzae,* type b, *Am. J. Obstet. Gynecol.* **153**:607–611 (1985).

20. ANDERSON, P., Antibody responses to *Haemophilus influenzae* type b and diphtheria toxin induced by conjugates of oligosaccharides of the type b capsule with the nontoxic protein CRM$_{197}$, *Infect. Immun.* **39**:233–238 (1983).

21. ANDERSON, P., The protective level of serum antibodies to the capsular polysaccharide of *Haemophilus influenzae* type b, *J. Infect. Dis.* **149**:1034 (1984).

22. ANDERSON, P., AND INSEL, R. A., A polysaccharide–protein complex from Haemophilus influenzae type b. I. Activity in weanling rabbits and human T lymphocytes, *J. Infect. Dis.* **144**:509–520 (1981).

23. ANDERSON, P., AND SMITH, D. H., Immunogenicity in weanling rabbits of a polyribophosphate complex from *Haemophilus influenzae* type b, *J. Infect. Dis.* **136**(Suppl. 1):S63–S70 (1977).

24. ANDERSON, P., AND SMITH, D. H., Isolation of the capsular polysaccharide from culture supernatant of *Haemophilus influenzae* type b, *Infect. Immun.* **15**:472–477 (1977).

25. ANDERSON, P., JOHNSTON, R. B., JR., AND SMITH, D. H., Human serum activities against *Haemophilus influenzae* type b, *J. Clin. Invest.* **51**:31–38 (1972).

26. ANDERSON, P., PETER, G., JOHNSTON, R. B., JR., WETTERLOW, L. H., AND SMITH, O. H. Immunization of humans with polyribophosphate, the capsular antigen of *H. influenzae* type b, *J. Clin. Invest.* **51**:39–44 (1972).

27. ANDERSON, P., SMITH, D. H., INGRAM, D. L., WILKINS, J., WEHRLE, P. F., AND HOWIE, V. M., Antibody to polyribophosphate of *H. influenzae* type b in infants and children: Effect of immunization with polyribophosphate, *J. Infect. Dis.* **136**(Suppl.):S57–S62 (1977).

28. ANDERSON, P., FLESHER, A. M., SHAW, S., HARDING, A. L., AND SMITH, D. H. Phenotypic and genetic variation in the susceptibility of *H. influenzae* type b to antibodies to somatic antigens, *J. Clin. Invest.* **65**:885–891 (1980).

29. ANDERSON, P., INSEL, R. A., LOEB, M. R., AND SMITH, D. H., A polysaccharide–protein complex from Haemophilus influenzae type b. II. Human antibodies to its somatic components, *J. Infect. Dis.* **144**:521–529 (1981).

30. ANDERSON, P., INSEL, R. A., SMITH, D. H., CATE, T. R., COUCH, R. B., AND GLEZEN, W. P., A polysaccharide–protein complex from *Haemophilus influenzae* type b. III. Vaccine trial in human adults, *J. Infect. Dis.* **144**:530–538 (1981).

31. ANDERSON, P., INSEL, R. A., FARSUD, P., SMITH, D. H., AND PETRUSICK, T., Immunogenicity of "aggregated PRP," "PRP-complex," and covalent conjugates of PRP with a diphtheria toxoid, in: *Haemophilus influenzae* (S. H. SELL AND P. F. WRIGHT, eds.), pp. 275–283, Elsevier, Amsterdam, 1982.

32. ANDERSON, P., PICHICHERO, M. E., AND INSEL, R. A., Immunization of 2-month-old infants with protein-coupled oligosaccharides derived from the capsule of *Haemophilus influenzae* type b, *J. Pediatr.* **107**:346–351 (1985).

33. ANDERSON, P., PICHICHERO, M. E., AND INSEL, R. A., Immunogens consisting of oligosaccharides from the capsule of *Haemophilus influenzae* type b coupled to diphtheria toxoid or the toxin protein CRM$_{197}$, *J. Clin. Invest.* **76**:52–59 (1985).

34. ANDERSON, P. W., PICHICHERO, M. E., INSEL, R. A., BETTS, R., EBY, R., AND SMITH, D. H., Vaccines consisting of periodate-cleaved oligosaccharides from the capsule of *Haemophilus influenzae* type b coupled to a protein carrier: Structural and temporal requirements for priming in the human infant, *J. Immunol.* **137**:1181–1186 (1986).

35. ANDERSON, P., INSEL, R. A., PORCELLI, S., AND WARD, J. I., Immunochemical variables affecting radioantigen-binding assays of antibody to *Haemophilus influenzae* type b capsular polysaccharide in childrens' sera, *J. Infect. Dis.* **156**:582–590 (1987).

36. ANDERSSON, B., PORRAS, O., HANSON, L. A., LAGERGARD, T., AND SVANBORG-EDEN, C., Inhibition of attachment of *Streptococcus pneumoniae* and *Haemophilus influenzae* by human milk and receptor oligosaccharides, *J. Infect. Dis.* **153**:232–237 (1986).

37. ANDERSSON, B., PORRAS, O., HANSON, L. A., LAGERGARD, T., AND SVANBORG-EDEN, C., Inhibition of attachment of *Streptococcus pneumoniae* and *Haemophilus influenzae* by human milk and receptor oligosaccharides, *J. Infect. Dis.* **153**:232–237 (1986).

38. ARGAMAN, M., LIN, T. Y., AND ROBBINS, J. B., Polyribitolphosphate: An antigen of four gram-positive bacteria crossreactive with the capsular polysaccharide of *Haemophilus influenzae* type b, *J. Immunol.* **112**:649–655 (1974).

39. ARPI, M., HONBERG, P. Z., AND FRIMODT-MOLLER, N., Antibiotic susceptibility of *Haemophilus influenzae* isolated from cerebrospinal fluid and blood, *Acta Pathol. Microbiol. Scand.* **94**:167–171 (1986).

40. ARTENSTEIN, M. S., GOLD, R., ZIMMERLY, H. G., WYLE, F. A., SCHNEIDER, H., AND HARKINS, C., Prevention of meningococcal disease by group C polysaccharide vaccine, *N. Engl. J. Med.* **282**:417–420 (1970).

41. AVERY, O. T., AND GOEBEL, W. F., Chemo-immunological studies on conjugated carbohydrate-proteins. II. Immunological specificity of synthetic sugar-protein antigens, *J. Exp. Med.* **50**:533–550 (1929).

42. BACHRACH, S., An outbreak of *Haemophilus influenzae* type b bacteraemia in an intermediate care hospital for children, *J. Hosp. Infect.* **11**:121–126 (1988).

43. BAND, J. D., FRASER, D. W., AND AJELLO, G., Hemophilus Influenzae Disease Study Group, Prevention of *Hemophilus influenzae* type b disease, *J. Am. Med. Assoc.* **251**:2381–2386 (1984).

44. BAND, J. D., FRASER, D. W., HIGHTOWER, A. W., AND BROOME, C. V., Prophylaxis of *Hemophilus influenzae* type b disease, *J. Am. Med. Assoc.* **252**:3249–3250 (1984).

45. BARAFF, L., AND WEHRLE, P. F., Epidemiology of pediatric meningitis: Los Angeles County, 1975 abstracted, *Pediatr.*

Res. **11**:434 (1977).

46. BARENKAMP, S. J., MUNSON, R. S., AND GRANOFF, D. M., Subtyping isolates of *Haemophilus influenzae* type b by outer-membrane protein profiles, *J. Infect. Dis.* **143**:668–676 (1981).

47. BARRETT, D. J., Human immune responses to polysaccharide antigens: An analysis of bacterial polysaccharide vaccines in infants, in: *Advances in Pediatrics* (L. A. Barnes, ed.), Year Book Medical, Chicago, 1958.

48. BARTLETT, A. V., ZUSMAN, J., AND DAUM, R. S., Unusual presentations of *Haemophilus influenzae* infections in immunocompromised patients, *J. Pediatr.* **102**:55–58 (1983).

49. BARTON, L. L., GRANOFF, D. M., AND BARENKAMP, S. J., Nosocomial spread of *H. influenzae* type b infection documented by outer membrane protein subtype analysis, *J. Pediatr.* **102**:820–824 (1983).

50. BELL, S. M., AND PLOWMAN, D., Mechanisms of ampicillin resistance in *Haemophilus influenzae* from respiratory tract, *Lancet* **1**:279–280 (1980).

51. BERKOWITZ, C. D., WARD, J. I., MEIER, K., HENDLEY, J. O., BRUNELL, P. A., BARKIN, R. A., ZAHRADNIK, J. M., SAMUELSON, J., AND GORDON, L., Safety and immunogenicity of *Haemophilus influenzae* type b polysaccharide and polysaccharide diphtheria toxoid conjugate vaccines in children 15 to 24 months of age, *J. Pediatr.* **110**:509–514 (1987).

52. BERKOWITZ, C. D., WARD, J. I., CHIU, C. E., MARCY, S. M., HENDLEY, J. O., MEIER, K., MARCHANT, C. D., McVERRY, P., AND GORDON, L., Persistence of antibody and responses to reimmunization with *Haemophilus influenzae* type b vaccines polysaccharide and polysaccharide diphtheria toxoid conjugate vaccines in children initially immunized at 15 to 24 months, *Pediatrics* 1990; **85**:288–293.

53. BEUVERY, E. C., VAN ROSSUM, F., AND NAGEL, J., Comparison of the induction of immunoglobulin M and G antibodies in mice with purified pneumococcal type 3 and meningococcal group G polysaccharides and their protein conjugates, *Infect. Immun.* **37**:15–22 (1982).

54. BLACK, S. B., AND SHINEFIELD, H. R., b-CAPSA *Haemophilus influenzae* type b, capsular polysaccharide vaccine safety, *Pediatrics* **79**:321–325 (1987).

55. BLACK, S. B., SHINEFIELD, H. R., HIATT, R. A., FIREMAN, B. H., AND THE KAISER PERMANENTE PEDIATRIC VACCINE STUDY GROUP, Efficacy of *Haemophilus influenzae* type b capsular polysaccharide vaccine, *Pediatr. Infect. Dis. J.* **7**:149–156 (1988).

56. BLAKEBROUGH, I. S., GREENWOOD, B. M., WHITTLE, H. C., BRADLEY, A. K., AND GILLES, A. M., Failure of meningococcal vaccination to stop the transmission of meningococci in Nigerian schoolboys, *Ann. Trop. Med. Parasitol.* **77**:175–178 (1983).

57. BOIES, E. G., GRANOFF, D. M., SQUIRES, J. E., AND BARENKAMP, S. J., Development of Haemophilus influenzae type b meningitis in a household contact treated with rifampin, *Pediatrics* **70**:141–142 (1982).

58. BOSMANS, E., VIMONT-VICARY, P., ANDRE, F. E., CROOY, P. J., ROELANTS, P., AND VANDEPITTE, J., Protective efficacy of a bivalent (A + C) meningococcal vaccine during a cerebrospinal meningitis epidemic in Rwanda, *Ann. Soc. Belg. Med. Trop.* **60**:297–306 (1980).

59. BROOME, C. V., Epidemiology of *Haemophilus influenzae* type b infections in the United States, *Pediatr. Infect. Dis. J.* **6**:779–782 (1987).

60. BROOME, C. V., AND SCHLECH, W. F., III, Recent developments in the epidemiology of bacterial meningitis, in: *Bacterial meningitis* (M. A. Sande, A. Smith, and R. D. Root, eds.), pp. 1–10, Churchill Livingstone, Edinburgh, 1985.

61. BROOME, C. V., MORTIMER, E. A., KATZ, S. L., FLEMING, D. W., AND HIGHTOWER, A. W., Use of chemoprophylaxis to prevent the spread of *Haemophilus influenzae* b in day care facilities, *N. Engl. J. Med.* **316**;1226–1228 (1987).

62. BROUGHTON, S. J., AND WARREN, R. E., A review of *Haemophilus influenzae* infections in Cambridge, 1975–1981, *J. Infect.* **9**:30–42 (1984).

63. BURANS, J. P. KRUSZEWSKI, F. H., LYNN, M., AND SOLOTOROVSKY, M., Kinetics of *Haemophilus influenzae* type b infection in normal and ribosome-immunized mice using intraperitoneal and intracerebral routes of inoculation, *Br. J. Exp. Pathol.* **62**:496–503 (1981).

64. BURANS, J. P., LYNN, M., AND SOLOTOROVSKY, M., Induction of active immunity with membrane fractions from *Haemophilus influenzae* type b, *Infect. Immun.* **41**:285–293 (1983).

65. CADOZ, M., PRINCE-DAVID, M., MAR, I. D., AND DENIS, F., Epidemiologie et prognostic des meningites a *Haemophilus influenzae* en Afrique (901 cas), *Pathol. Biol.* **31**:128–133 (1983).

66. CAMPBELL, L. R., ZEDD, A. J., AND MICHAELS, R. H., Household spread of infection due to *Haemophilus influenzae* type b, *Pediatrics* **66**:115–117 (1980).

67. CAMPOGNONE, P., AND SINGER, D. B., Neonatal sepsis due to nontypable *Haemophilus influenzae*, *Am. J. Dis. Child.* **140**:117–121 (1986).

68. CAMPOS, J., GARCIA-TORNEL, S., AND SANFELIU, I., Susceptibility studies of multiply resistant *Haemophilus influenzae* isolated from pediatric patients and contacts, *Antimicrob. Agents Chemother.* **25**:706–709 (1984).

69. CAMPOS, J., GARCIA-TORNEL, S., GAIRI, J. M., AND FABREGUES, I., Multiply resistant *Haemophilus influenzae* type b causing meningitis: Comparative clinical and laboratory study, *J. Pediatr.* **108**:897–902 (1986).

70. CAMPOS, J., GARCIA-TORNEL, S., ROCA, J., AND IRIONDO, M., Rifampin for eradicating carriage of multiply resistant *Haemophilus influenzae* b, *Pediatr. Infect. Dis. J.* **6**:719–721 (1987).

71. CARVALHO, A. D. A., GIAMPAGLIA, C. M. S., KIMURA, H., PEREIRA, O. A., NEVES, J. C., PRANDINI, R., CARVALLO, E. D. S., AND ZARVOS, A. M., Maternal and infant antibody response to meningococcal vaccination in pregnancy, *Lancet* **2**:809–811 (1977).

72. CATES, K. L., Serum opsonic activity for *H. influenzae* type b in infants immunized with polysaccharide–protein conjugate vaccines, *J. Infect. Dis.* **152**:1076–1077 (1985).

73. CATES, K. L., MARSH, K. H., AND GRANOFF, D. M., Serum opsonic activity after immunization of adults with *H. influenzae* type b-diphtheria toxoid conjugate vaccine in adults, *J. Pediatr.* **105:**22–27 (1984).

74. Centers for Disease Control, Ampicillin-resistant *Haemophilus influenzae* meningitis—Maryland, Georgia, *Morbid. Mortal. Weekly Rep.* **23:**77–78 (1974).

75. Centers for Disease Control, Ampicillin-resistant *Haemophilus influenzae*—Texas, *Morbid. Mortal. Weekly Rep.* **23:**99 (1974).

76. Centers for Disease Control, Ampicillin and chloramphenicol resistance in systemic *Haemophilus influenzae* disease, *Morbid. Mortal Weekly Rep.* **33:**35–37 (1984).

77. CHILCOTE, R., BAEHNER, R., HAMMOND, D., Septicemia and meningitis in children splenectomized for Hodgkin's disease, *N. Engl. J. Med.* **275:**709–715 (1966).

78. CHU, C.-Y., SCHNEERSON, R., ROBBINS, J. B., AND RASTOGI, S. C., Further studies on the immunogenicity of *Haemophilus influenzae* type b and pneumococcal type 6A polysaccharide–protein conjugates, *Infect. Immun.* **40:**245–56 (1983).

79. CLAESSON, B., TROLLFORS, B., JODAL, U., AND ROSEN-HALL, U., Incidence and prognosis of *Haemophilus influenzae* meningitis in children in a Swedish region, *Pediatr. Infect. Dis. J.* **3:**35–39 (1984).

80. CLAESSON, B. A., TROLLFORS, B., LAGERGARD, T., TARANGER, J., BRYLA, D., OTTERMAN, G., CRANTON, T., YANG, Y., REIMER, C. B., ROBBINS, J. B., AND SCHREERSON, R., Clinical and immunologic responses to the capsular polysaccharide of Haemophilus influenzae type b alone or conjugated to tetanus toxoid in 18- to 23-month-old children, *J. Pediatr.* **112:**695–702 (1988).

81. CLANCY, R., CRIPPS, A., MURREE-ALLEN, K., YEUNG, S., AND ENGEL, M., Oral immunisation with killed *Haemophilus influenzae* for protection against acute bronchitis in chronic obstructive lung disease, *Lancet* **2:**1395–1397 (1985).

82. CLYMO, A. B. M., AND HARPER, I. A., Ampicillin-resistant *Haemophilus influenzae* meningitis, *Lancet* **1:**453–454 (1974).

83. COCHI, S. L., AND BROOME, C. V., Vaccine prevention of *Haemophilus influenzae* type b disease: Past, present and future, *Pediatr. Infect. Dis. J.* **5:**12–19 (1986).

84. COCHI, S. L., BROOME, C. V., AND HIGHTOWER, A. W., Immunization of U.S. children with *Hemophilus influenzae* type b polysaccharide vaccine: A cost-effectiveness model of strategy assessment, *J. Am. Med. Assoc.* **253:**521–529 (1985).

85. COCHI, S. L., FLEMING, D. W., HIGHTOWER, A. W., LIMP-AKARNJANARAT, K., FACKLAM, R. R., SMITH, J. D., SIKES, R. K., AND BROOME, C. V., Primary invasive *Haemophilus influenzae* type b disease: A population-based assessment of risk factors, *J. Pediatr.* **108:**887–896 (1986).

86. COCHI, S. L., FLEMING, D. W., HIGHTOWER, A. W., AND BROOME, C. V., Does breast-feeding protect infants from *Haemophilus influenzae* infection? [letter], *J. Pediatr.* **110:**162–163 (1987).

87. Committee on Infectious Diseases, Ampicillin-resistant strains of *Haemophilus influenzae* type b, *Pediatrics* **55:**145 (1975).

88. Committee on Infectious Diseases, *Haemophilus* b polysaccharide vaccine, *Pediatrics* **76:**322–324 (1985).

89. Committee on Infectious Diseases, *Haemophilus influenzae* type b conjugate vaccine, *Pediatrics* **81:**908–911 (1988).

90. CONNOR, E. M., AND LOEB, M. R., A hemadsorption method for detection of colonies of *Haemophilus influenzae* type b expressing fimbriae, *J. Infect. Dis.* **148:**855–860 (1983).

91. COOPER, R. F., BAGWELL, C., AND SMITH, T. B., Hearing loss in pediatric meningitis, *Am. Fam. Physician* **35:**133–138 (1987).

92. COULEHAN, J. L., MICHAELS, R. H., WILLIAMS, K. E., LEMLEY, D. K., NORTH, C. Q., WELTY, T. K., AND ROGERS, K. D., Bacterial meningitis in Navajo Indians, *Public Health Rep.* **91:**464–468 (1976).

93. COULEHAN, J. L., HALLOWELL, C., MICHAELS, R. H., WELTY, T. K., LUI, N., AND KUO, J. S. C., Immunogenicity of a *Haemophilus influenzae* type b vaccine in combination with diphtheria–pertussis–tetanus vaccine in infants, *J. Infect. Dis.* **148:**530–534 (1983).

94. COULEHAN, J. L., MICHAELS, R. H., HALLOWELL, C., SCHULTS, R., WELTY, T. K., AND KUO, J. S. C., Epidemiology of *Haemophilus influenzae* type b disease among Navajo Indians, *Public Health Rep.* **99:**404–409 (1984).

95. COX, F., TRINCHER, R., RISSING, J. P., PATTON, M., McCRACKEN, G. H., JR., AND GRANOFF, D. M., Rifampin prophylaxis for contacts of *Haemophilus influenzae* type b disease, *J. Am. Med. Assoc.* **245:**1043–1045 (1981).

96. CRISEL, R. M., BAKER, R. S., AND DORMAN, D. E., Capsular polymer of *Haemophilus influenzae*, type b. I. Structural characterization of the capsular polymer of strain Eagan, *J. Biol. Chem.* **250:**4926–4930 (1975).

97. CROSSON, F. J., JR., WINKELSTEIN, J. A., AND MOXON, E. R., Participation of complement in the nonimmune host defense against experimental *H. influenzae* type b septicemia and meningitis, *Infect. Immun.* **14:**882–887 (1976).

98. CROSSON, F. J., WINKELSTEIN, J. A., AND MOXON, E. R., Enzyme-linked immunosorbent assay for detection and quantitation of capsular antigen of *Haemophilus influenzae* type b, *Infect. Immun.* **22:**617–619 (1978).

99. DAHLBERG-LAGERGARD, T., Target antigens for bactericidal and opsonizing antibodies to *H. influenzae, Acta Pathol. Microbiol. Scand.* **90:**209–216 (1982).

100. DAJANI, A. S., ASMAR, B. I., AND THIRUMOORTHI, M. C., Systemic *Haemophilus influenzae* disease: An overview, *J. Pediatr.* **94:**355–364 (1979).

101. DASHEFSKY, B., WALD, E., AND LI, K., Management of contacts of children in day care with invasive *Haemophilus influenzae* type b disease, *Pediatrics* **78:**939–941 (1986).

102. DAUM, R. S., AND GRANOFF, D. M., A vaccine against *Haemophilus influenzae* type b, *Pediatr. Infect. Dis. J.* **4:**355–357 (1985).

103. DAUM, R. S., GLODE, M. P., GOLDMANN, D. A., HALSEY, N., AMBROSINO, D., WELBORN, C., MATHER, F. J.,

WILLARD, J. E., SULLIVAN, B., MURRAY, M., AND JOHANSEN, T., Rifampin chemoprophylaxis for household contacts of patients with invasive infections due to *Haemophilus influenzae* type b, *J. Pediatr.* **98**:485–491 (1981).

104. DAUM, R. S., GLODE, M. P., GOLDMANN, D. A., HALSEY, N., AMBROSINO, D., WELBORN, C., MATHER, F. J., WILLARD, J. E., SULLIVAN, B., MURRAY, M., AND JOHANSEN, T., Rifampin chemoprophylaxis for household contacts of patients with invasive infections due to *Haemophilus influenzae* type b, *J. Pediatr.* **98**:485–491 (1981).

105. DAUM, R. S., SIBER, G. R., KAMON, J. S., AND RUSSELL, R. R., Evaluation of a commercial latex particle agglutination test for rapid diagnosis of *Haemophilus influenzae* type b infection, *Pediatrics* **69**:406–471 (1982).

106. DAUM, R. S., MARCUSE, E. K., GIEBINK, G. S., HALL, C. B., LEPOW, M. L., McCRACKEN, G. H., PETER, G., PHILLIPS, C. F., WRIGHT, H. T., AND PLOTKIN, S. A., *Haemophilus influenzae* type b vaccines: Lessons from the past, *Pediatrics* **81**:893–897 (1988).

107. DAUM, R. S., MURPHEY-CORB, M., SHAPIR, E., AND DIPP, S., Epidemiology of Rob beta-lactamase among ampicillin-resistant *Haemophilus influenzae* isolates in the United States, *J. Infect. Dis.* **157**:450–455 (1988).

108. DAVEY, P. G., CRUIKSHANK, J. K., McMANUS, I. C., MAHOOD, B., SNOW, M. H., AND GEDDES, A. M., Bacterial meningitis—Ten years experience, *J. Hyg.* **88**:383–401 (1982).

109. DAVIE, J. M., Antipolysaccharide immunity in man and animals, in: *Haemophilus influenzae* (S. H. Sell and P. F. Wright, eds.), pp. 129–134, Elsevier, Amsterdam, 1982.

110. DAVIS, D. J., Influenzal meningitis, *Arch. Intern. Med.* **4**:323–329 (1909).

111. DAWSON, B., AND ZINNEMANN, K., Incidence and type distribution of capsulated *H. influenzae* strains, *Br. Med. J.* **1**:740–742 (1952).

112. DEVEIKIS, A., KIM, K. S., AND WARD, J. I., Prevention of *Haemophilus influenzae* type b in infant rats by human antibody induced by the capsular polysaccharide and polysaccharide-conjugate vaccines, *Vaccines* **6**:14–18 (1988).

113. DEVINE, L. F., JOHNSON, L. F., JOHNSON, D. P., HAGERMAN, C. R., PIERCE, W. E., RHODE, S. L., AND PECKINPAUGH, R. O., Rifampin: Levels in serum and saliva and effect on the meningococcal carrier state, *J. Am. Med. Assoc.* **214**:1055–1059 (1970).

114. DODGE, P. R., AND SWARTZ, M. N., Bacterial meningitis—A review of selected aspects. II. Special neurologic problems, post-meningitis complications and clinicopathological correlations, *N. Engl. J. Med.* **272**:1003–1010 (1965).

115. DOERN, G. V., JORGENSEN, J., THORNSBERRY, C., PRESTON, D. A., AND THE *Haemophilus influenzae* SURVEILLANCE GROUP, Prevalence of antimicrobial resistance among clinical isolates of *Haemophilus influenzae*: A collaborative study, *Diagn. Microbiol. Infect. Dis.* **4**:95–107 (1986).

116. DOERN, G. V., JORGENSEN, J., THORNSBERRY, C., PRESTON, D. A., TUBERT, T., REDDING, J. S., AND MAHER, L. A., National collaborative study of the prevalence of anti-

microbial resistance among clinical isolates of *Haemophilus influenzae*, *Antimicrob. Agents Chemother.* **32**:180–185 (1988).

117. DREXHAGE, H. A., VAN DE PLASSCHE, E. M., KOKJE, M., AND LEEZENBERG, H. A., Abnormalities in cell-mediated immune functions to *Haemophilus influenzae* in chronic purulent infections of the upper respiratory tract, *Clin. Immunol. Immunopathol.* **28**:218–228 (1983).

118. EDWARDS, K. M., DECKER, M. D., PALMER, P., PORCH, C. R., SELL, S. H., AND WRIGHT, P. F., Lack of comparability between commonly used serological assays of immune response to *Haemophilus influenzae* vaccine, *J. Infect. Dis.* **155**:283–291 (1987).

119. EICKHOFF, T. C., In vitro and in vivo studies of resistance to rifampin in meningococci, *J. Infect. Dis.* **123**:414–420 (1971).

120. EINHORN, M. S., WEINBERG, G. A., ANDERSON, E. L., GRANOFF, P. D., AND GRANOFF, D. M., Immunogenicity in infants of *Haemophilus influenzae* type b polysaccharide in a conjugate vaccine with *Neisseria meningitidis* outer-membrane protein, *Lancet* **2**:299–302 (1986).

121. ESKOLA, J., KAYHTY, H., PELTOLA, H., KARANKO, V., MAKELA, P. H., SAMUELSON, I., AND GORDON, L. K., Antibody levels achieved in infants by course of *Haemophilus influenzae* type b polysaccharide/diphtheria toxoid conjugate vaccine, *Lancet* **1**:1184–1186 (1985).

122. ESKOLA, J., PELTOLA, H., TAKALA, A. K., KAYHTY, H., HAKULINEN, M., KARONKO, V., KELA, E., REKOLA, P., RONNBERG, P. R., SAMUELSON, J. S., GORDON, L. K., AND MARKELA, P. H., Efficacy of *Haemophilus influenzae* type b polysaccharide–diphtheria toxoid conjugate vaccine in infancy, *N. Engl. J. Med.* **317**:717–722 (1987).

123. FARRAND, R. J., Recurrent Haemophilus septicemia and immunoglobulin deficiency, *Arch. Dis. Child.* **45**:582–584 (1970).

124. FEIGIN, R. D., TICHMOND, D., HISLER, M. W., AND SHACKELFORD, P. G., Reassessment of the role of bactericidal antibody in *H. influenzae* infection, *Am. J. Med. Sci.* **262**:338–346 (1971).

125. FEIGIN, R. D., STECHENBERG, B. W., CHANG, M. J., *et al.*, Prospective evaluation of treatment of *Haemophilus influenzae* meningitis, *J. Pediatr.* **88**:542–548 (1976).

126. FELDMAN, R., FRASER, D., AND KOEHLER, R., Death certificates as a measure of *Hemophilus influenzae* meningitis mortality in the United States 1962–1968, in: *Haemophilus influenzae* (S. SELL AND E. KARZON, eds.), pp. 221–230, Vanderbilt University Press, Nashville, 1973.

127. FELDMAN, W., Relation of concentrations of bacteria and bacterial antigens in cerebrospinal fluid to prognosis in patients with bacterial meningitis, *N. Engl. J. Med.* **296**:433–435 (1977).

128. FERRY, P. C., CULBERTSON, J. L., COOPER, J. A., SITTON, A. B., AND SELL, S. H., Sequelae of *Haemophilus influenzae* meningitis, in: *Haemophilus influenzae* (S. H. SELL AND P. F. WRIGHT, eds.), pp. 111–116, Elsevier, Amsterdam, 1982.

129. FILICE, G. A., ANDREWS, J. S., JR., HUDGINS, M. P., AND

FRASER, D. W., spread of *Haemophilus influenzae:* Secondary illness in household contacts of patients with *H. influenzae* meningitis, *Am. J. Dis. Child.* **132:**757–759 (1978).

130. FLEMING, D. W., LIEBENHAUT, M. H., ALBANES, D., COCHI, S. L., HIGHTOWER, A. W., MAKINTUBEE, S., HELGERSON, S. D., BROOME, C. V., AND THE CONTRIBUTING GROUP, Secondary *Haemophilus influenzae* type b in day-care facilities: Risk factors and prevention, *J. Am. Med. Assoc.* **254:**509–514 (1985).

131. FLOYD, R. F., FEDERSPIEL, C. F., AND SCHAFFNER, W., Bacterial meningitis in urban and rural Tennessee, *Am. J. Epidemiol.* **99:**395–397 (1974).

132. FORSYTH, K., HANSMAN, D., AND JARVINEN, A., Multiply-resistant *Haemophilus influenzae* type b causing systemic disease in children in Australia, *Pathology* **18:**386–389 (1986).

133. FOTHERGILL, L. D., *Hemophilus influenzae* (Pfeiffer bacillus) meningitis and its specific treatment, *N. Engl. J. Med.* **216:**587–590 (1937).

134. FOTHERGILL, L. D., AND SWEET, L. K., Meningitis in infants and children with special reference to age-incidence and bacteriologic diagnosis, *J. Pediatr.* **2:**696–710 (1933).

135. FOTHERGILL, L. D., AND WRIGHT, J., Influenzal meningitis: The relation of age incidence to the bactericidal power of blood against the causal organism, *J. Immunol.* **24:**273–284 (1933).

136. FRANK, A. L., LABOTKA, R. J., RAO, S., FRISONE, L. R., MCVERRY, P. H., SAMUELSON, J. S., MAURER, H., AND YOGEV, R., *Haemophilus influenzae* type b immunization of children with sickle cell disease, *J. Pediatr.* **82:**571–575 (1988).

137. FRASER, D. W., *Haemophilus influenzae* in the community and in the home, in: *Haemophilus influenzae* (S. H. Sell and P. F. Wright, eds.), pp. 11–22, Elsevier, Amsterdam, 1982.

138. FRASER, D. W., DARBY, C. P., KOEHLER, R. E., JACOBS, C. F., AND FELDMAN, R. A., Risk factors in bacterial meningitis: Charleston County, South Carolina, *J. Infect. Dis.* **127:**271–277 (1973).

139. FRASER, D. W., HENCKE, C. E., AND FELDMAN, R. A., Changing patterns of bacterial meningitis in Olmsted County, Minnesota, 1935–1970, *J. Infect. Dis.* **128:**300–307 (1973).

140. FRASER, D. W., GEIL, C. C., AND FELDMAN, R. A., Bacterial meningitis in Bernalillo County, New Mexico: A comparison with three other American populations, *Am. J. Epidemiol.* **100:**29–34 (1974).

141. FRASER, D. W., MITCHELL, J. E., SILVERMAN, L. P., AND FELDMAN, R. A., Undiagnosed bacterial meningitis in Vermont children, *Am. J. Epidemiol.* **102:**394–399 (1975).

142. GARDNER, J. S., AND SIMONS, B. P., Guideline for isolation precautions in hospitals, *Infect. Control* **4**(Suppl.):245–349 (1983).

143. GESSERT, C., GRANOFF, D. M., AND GILSDORF, J., Comparison of rifampin and ampicillin in day care center contacts of *Haemophilus influenzae* type b disease, *Pediatrics* **66:**1–4 (1980).

144. GILSDORF, J. R., Bacterial meningitis in southwestern Alaska, *Am. J. Epidemiol.* **106:**388–391 (1977).

145. GILSDORF, J. R., Dynamics of nasopharyngeal colonization with *Haemophilus influenzae* b during antibiotic therapy, *Pediatrics* **77:**242–245 (1986).

146. GILSDORF, J. R., *Haemophilus influenzae* non-type b infections in children, *Am. J. Dis. Child.* **141:**1063–1065 (1987).

147. GINSBURG, C. M., MCCRACKEN, G. H., JR., RAE, S., AND PARKE, J. C., JR., *Haemophilus influenzae* type b disease: Incidence in a day-care center, *J. Am. Med. Assoc.* **238:**604–607 (1977).

148. GLODE, M. P., SCHIFFER, M. S., ROBBINS, J. B., KHAN, W., BATTLE, C. U., AND ARMENTA, E., An outbreak of *H. influenzae* type b meningitis in an enclosed hospital population, *J. Pediatr.* **88:**36–40 (1976).

149. GLODE, M. P., DAUM, R. S., GOLDMANN, D. A., LECLAIR, J., AND SMITH, A., *Haemophilus influenzae* type b meningitis: A contagious disease of children, *Br. Med. J.* **1:**899–901 (1980).

150. GLODE, M. P., DAUM, R. S., HALSEY, N. A., JOHANSEN, T. L., GOLDMANN, D. A., AMBROSINO, D., BOIES, E., AND GRANOFF, D. M., Rifampin alone and in combination with trimethoprim in chemoprophylaxis for infections due to *Haemophilus influenzae* type b, *Rev. Infect. Dis.* **5**(Suppl.):S549–S555 (1983).

151. GLODE, M. P., BROGDEN, R. L. B., KUO, J. S. C., AND SCHNEIDER, J., Change in antibody titers to *Haemophilus influenzae* type b in infants immunized at 18 months of age [Abstract], Program and abstracts of the 25th Interscience Conference on Antimicrobial Agents and Chemotherapy, 1985.

152. GLODE, M. P., DAUM, R. S., BOIES, E. G., BALLARD, T. L., MURRAY, M., AND GRANOFF, D. M., Effect of rifampin chemoprophylaxis on carriage eradication and new acquisition of *Haemophilus influenzae* type b in contacts, *Pediatrics* **76:**537–542 (1985).

153. GLODE, M. P., JOFFE, L. S., BROGDEN, R., AND KUO, J., Reimmunization of children immunized at 18 months of age with *Haemophilus influenzae* type b vaccine, *J. Pediatr.* **112:**703–708 (1988).

154. GOEBEL, W. F., Studies on antibacterial immunity induced by artificial antigens. I. Immunity to experimental pneumococcal infection with an antigen containing cellobiuronic acid, *J. Exp. Med.* **69:**353–364 (1939).

155. GOEBEL, W. F., AND AVERY, O. T., Chemo-immunological studies on conjugated carbohydrate-proteins. I. The synthesis of p-aminophenol β-glucoside, p-aminophenol β-galactoside, and their coupling with serum globulin, *J. Exp. Med.* **50:**521–531 (1929).

156. GOLDACRE, M. J., Acute bacterial meningitis in childhood, *Lancet* **1:**28–31 (1976).

157. GOOD, P. G., FOUSEK, M. D., GROSSMAN, M. F., AND BOLSVERT, P. L., A study of the familial spread of *Hemophilus influenzae*, type b, *Yale J. Biol. Med.* **15:**913–918 (1943).

158. GOODMAN, R. A., OSTERHOLM, M., GRANOFF, D. M., AND PICKERING, L. K., Infectious diseases and child day care, *Pediatrics* **74:**134–139 (1984).

159. GORDON, L. K., Characterization of a hapten–carrier conjugate vaccine: *H. influenzae*–diphtheria conjugate vaccine, in: *Modern Approaches to Vaccines* (R. M. CHANOCK AND R. A. LERNER, eds.), pp. 393–396, Cold Spring Harbor Laboratory, Cold Spring Harbor, N.Y., 1984.

160. GOTOFF, S. P., On the surface of *H. influenzae*, *J. Infect. Dis.* **143:**747–748 (1981).

161. GOTSCHLICH, E. C., GOLDSCHNEIDER, I., AND ARTENSTEIN, M. S., Human immunity to the meningococcus: The effect of immunization with meningococcal group C polysaccharide on the carrier state, *J. Exp. Med.* **129:**1385–1395 (1969).

162. GRANOFF, D. M., AND BASDEN, M., *Haemophilus influenzae* infections in Fresno County, California: A prospective study of the effects of age, race, and contact with a case on incidence of disease, *J. Infect. Dis.* **140:**40–46 (1980).

163. GRANOFF, D. M., AND DAUM, R. S., Spread of *Haemophilus influenzae* type b: Recent epidemiologic and therapeutic considerations, *J. Pediatr.* **97:**854–860 (1980).

164. GRANOFF, D. M., AND MUNSON, R. S., JR., Prospects for prevention of *Haemophilus influenzae* type b disease by immunization, *J. Infect. Dis.* **153:**448–461 (1986).

165. GRANOFF, D. M., AND OSTERHOLM, M. T., Safety and efficacy of *Haemophilus influenzae* type b polysaccharide vaccine, *Pediatrics* **80:**590–592 (1987).

166. GRANOFF, D. M., GILSDORF, J., GESSERT, C., AND BASDEN, M., *Haemophilus influenzae* type b disease in a day care center: Eradication of carrier state by rifampin, *Pediatrics* **63:**397–401 (1979).

167. GRANOFF, D. M., GILSDORF, J., GESSERT, C. E., AND LOWE, L., *H. influenzae* type b in a day care center: Relationship of nasopharyngeal carriage to development of anticapsular antibody, *Pediatrics* **65:**65–68 (1980).

168. GRANOFF, D. M., BARENKAMP, S. J., AND MUNSON, R. S., Outer membrane protein subtypes for epidemiologic investigation of *Haemophilus influenzae* type b disease, in: *Haemophilus influenzae* (S. H. Sell and P. F. Wright, eds.), pp. 43–55, Elsevier, Amsterdam, 1982.

169. GRANOFF, D. M., SQUIRES, J. E., MUNSON, R. S., AND SUAREZ, B., Siblings of patients with *Haemophilus* meningitis have impaired anticapsular antibody responses to Haemophilus vaccine, *J. Pediatr.* **103:**185–191 (1983).

170. GRANOFF, D. M., BOIES, E., SQUIRES, J., PANDEY, J. P., SUAREZ, B., OLDFATHER, J., AND RODEY, G. E., Interactive effect of genes associated with immunoglobulin allotypes and HLA specificities on susceptibility to *Haemophilus influenzae* disease, *J. Immunogenet.* **11:**181–188 (1984).

171. GRANOFF, D. M., BOIES, E. G., AND MUNSON, R. S., Immunogenicity of *Haemophilus influenzae* type b polysaccharide–diphtheria toxoid conjugate vaccine in adults, *J. Pediatr.* **105:**22–27 (1984).

172. GRANOFF, D. M., BOIES, E. G., SQUIRES, J. E., PANDEY, J. P., SUAREZ, B. K., OLDFATHER, J. W., AND RODEY, G. E., Histocompatibility leukocyte antigen and erythrocyte MNSs specificities in patients with meningitis or epiglottitis due to *Haemophilus influenzae* type b, *J. Infect. Dis.* **149:**373–377 (1984).

173. GRANOFF, D. M., PANDEY, J. P., BOIES, E., SQUIRES, J., MUNSON, R. S., AND SUAREZ, B., Response to immunization with *Haemophilus influenzae* type polysaccharide–pertussis vaccine and risk of *Haemophilus* meningitis in children with the Km(1) immunoglobulin allotype, *J. Clin. Invest.* **74:**17081714 (1984).

174. GRANOFF, D. M., SHACKELFORD, P. G., PANDEY, J. P., AND BOIES, E. G., Antibody responses to *Haemophilus influenzae* type b polysaccharide vaccine in relation to Km(1) and G2m(23) immunoglobulin allotypes, *J. Infect. Dis.* **154:**257–264 (1986).

175. GRANOFF, D. M., SHACKELFORD, P. G., SUAREZ, B. K., NAHM, M. H., CATES, K. L., MURPHY, T. V., KARASIC, R., OSTERHOLM, M. T., PANDEY, J. P., DAUM, R. S., AND THE COLLABORATIVE GROUP, *Haemophilus influenzae* type b disease in children vaccinated with type b polysaccharide vaccine, *N. Engl. J. Med.* **315:**1584–1590 (1986).

176. GRASSO, R. J., WEST, L. A., HOLBROOK, N. J., HALKIAS, D. G., PARADISE, L. J., AND FRIEDMAN, H., Increased sensitivity of a new coagglutination test for rapid identification of *Haemophilus influenzae* type b, *J. Clin. Microbiol.* **13:**1122–1124 (1981).

177. GRATTEN, M., BARKER, J., SHANN, F., GEREGA, G., MONTGOMERY, J., KAJOI, M., AND LUPIWA, T., Non-type b *Haemophilus influenzae* meningitis, *Lancet* **1:**1343–1344 (1985).

178. GREENBERG, D. P., WARD, J. I., BURKART, K., CHRISTENSON, P. D., GURAVITZ, L., AND MARCY, S. M., Factors influencing immunogenicity and safety of two Haemophilus influenzae type b polysaccharide vaccines in children 18 and 24 months of age, *Pediatr. Infect. Dis. J.* **6:**660–665 (1987).

179. GREENFIELD, S., PETER, G., HOWIE, V. M., PLOUSSARD, J. H., AND SMITH, O. H., Acquisition of type-specific antibodies to *H. influenzae* type b, *J. Pediatr.* **80:**204–208 (1972).

180. GREENWOOD, B. M., The epidemiology of acute bacterial meningitis in tropical Africa, in: *Bacterial Meningitis,* pp. 61–91, Academic Press, New York, 1987.

181. GREENWOOD, B. M., HASSAN-KING, M., AND WHITTLY, H. C., Prevention of secondary cases of meningococcal disease in household contacts by vaccination, *Br. Med. J.* **1:**1317–1319 (1978).

182. GREENWOOD, B. M., BRADLEY, A. K., BLAKEBROUGH, I. S., WALI, S., AND WHITTLE, H. C., Meningococcal disease in the developing world. XIII. Acute bacterial meningitis, *Rev. Infect. Dis.* **6:**374–389 (1984).

183. GREGORIUS, F. K., JOHNSON, B. J., STERN, W. E., AND BROWN, W. J., Pathogenesis of hematogenous bacterial meningitis in rabbits, *J. Neurosurg.* **45:**561–567 (1976).

184. GRIFFISS, J. M., AND BERTRAM, M. A., Immunoepidemiology of meningococcal disease in military recruits. II. Blocking of serum bacterial activity by circulating IgA early in the course of invasive disease, *J. Infect. Dis.* **136:**733–739 (1977).

185. GUERINA, N. G., LANGERMANN, S., CLEGG, H. W., KESSLER, T. W., AND GOLDMANN, D. A., Adherence of piliated

Haemophilus influenzae type b to human oropharyngeal cells, *J. Infect. Dis.* **146:**564 (1982).

186. GUISCAFE, H., SOLORZANO, F., DELGADO, O., AND MUNOZ, O., *Haemophilus influenzae* type b meningitis resistant to ampicillin and chloramphenicol, *Arch. Dis. Child.* **61:**691–707 (1986).

187. GULIG, P. A., PATRICK, C. C., HERMANSTORFER, L., MC-CRACKEN, G. H., JR., AND HANSEN, E. J., Conservation of epitopes in the oligosaccharide portion of the lipooligosaccharide of *Haemophilus influenzae* type b, *Infect. Immun.* **55:**513–520 (1987).

188. GUSTAFSON, T. L., KELLEY, R. A., HUTCHESON, R. H., SCHAFFNER, W., AND SELL, S. H., Statewide survey of the antimicrobial susceptibilities of *Haemophilus influenzae* producing invasive disease in Tennessee, *Pediatr. Infect. Dis. J.* **2:**119–122 (1983).

189. HALL, D. B., LUM, M. K. W., KNUTSON, L. R., HEYWARD, W. L., AND WARD, J. I., Pharyngeal carriage and acquisition of anticapsular antibody to Haemophilus influenzae type b in a high-risk population in southwestern Alaska, *Am. J. Epidemiol.* **126:**1190–1197 (1987).

190. HALSEY, N. A., JOHANSEN, T. L., BOWMAN, L. C., AND GLODE, M. P., Evaluation of the protective efficacy of *Haemophilus influenzae* type b vaccines in an animal model, *Infect. Immun.* **39:**1196–1200 (1983).

191. HANSEN, E. J., FRISCH, C. F., AND JOHNSTON, K. H., Detection of antibody-accessible proteins on the cell surface of H. influenzae type b, *Infect. Immun.* **32:**950–953 (1981).

192. HANSEN, E. J., ROBERTSON, S. M., GULIG, P. A., FRISCH, C. F., AND HAANES, E. J., Immunoprotection of rats against *Haemophilus influenzae* type b disease mediated by monoclonal antibody against a *Haemophilus* outer-membrane protein, *Lancet* **1:**366–368 (1982).

193. HANSMAN, D., HANNA, J., AND MOREY, F., High prevalence of invasive *Haemophilus influenzae* disease in central Australia, 1986, *Lancet* **2:**927 (1986).

194. HARADA, T., SAKAKURA, Y., AND MIYOSHI, Y., Immunological response to outer membrane vesicles of Haemophilus influenzae in patients with acute sinusitis, *Rhinology* **24:**61–66 (1986).

195. HARDING, A. L., ANDERSON, P., HOWIE, V. M., PLOUSSARD, J. H., AND SMITH, D. H., *Haemophilus influenzae* isolated from otitis media, in: *Hemophilus influenzae* (S. H. W. SELL AND D. T. KARZON, eds.), pp. 21–28, Vanderbilt University Press, Nashville, 1973.

196. HARRISON, L. H., BROOME, C. V., HIGHTOWER, A. W., HOPPE, C. C., MAKINTUBEE, S., SITZE, S. L., TAYLOR, J. A., GAVENTA, S., WENGER, J. D., FACKLAM, R. R., AND THE HAEMOPHILUS VACCINE EFFICACY STUDY GROUP, A day care-based study of the efficacy of *Haemophilus* b polysaccharide vaccine, *J. Am. Med. Assoc.* **260:**1413–1418 (1988).

197. HAYASHI, K., LEE, D. A., AND QUIE, P. G., Chemiluminescent response of polymorphonuclear leukocytes to *Streptococcus pneumoniae* and *H. influenzae* in suspension and adhered to glass, *Infect. Immun.* **52:**397–400 (1986).

198. HEIKKILA, R., TAKALA, A., KAYHTY, H., AND LEINONEN, M., Latex agglutination test for screening of *Haemophilus influenzae* type b carriers, *J. Clin. Microbiol.* **25:**1131–1133 (1987).

199. HORNER, D. B., MCCRACKEN, G. H., JR., GINSBURG, C. M., AND ZWEIGHAFT, T. C., A comparison of three antibiotic regimens for eradication of *Haemophilus influenzae* type b from the pharynx of infants and children, *Pediatrics* **66:**136–138 (1980).

200. HOWARD, A. J., HINCE, C. J., AND WILLIAMS, J. D., Antibiotic resistance in *Streptococcus pneumoniae* and *Haemophilus influenzae*, *Br. Med. J.* **1:**1657–1660 (1978).

201. HOWARD, J. B., HIGHGENBOTEN, C. L., AND NELSON, J. D., Residual effects of septic arthritis in infancy and childhood, *J. Am. Med. Assoc.* **236:**932–935 (1976).

202. HUBER, B. R., B cell differentiation antigens as probes for functional B cell subsets, *Immunol. Rev.* **64:**57–79 (1982).

203. IMMUNIZATION PRACTICES ADVISORY COMMITTEE (ACIP), Update: Prevention of *Haemophilus influenzae* type b disease, *Morbid. Mortal. Weekly Rep.* **37:**13–16 (1988).

204. INGRAM, D. L., PEARSON, A. B., OCCHIUTI, A. R., Detection of bacterial antigens in body fluids with the Wellcogen *Haemophilus influenzae* b, *Streptococcus pneumoniae* and *Neisseria meningitidis* (ACYW135) latex agglutination tests, *J. Clin. Microbiol.* **18:**1119–1121 (1983).

205. INSEL, R. A., AND ANDERSON, P. W., Oligosaccharide–protein conjugate vaccines induce and prime for oligoclonal IgG antibody responses to the *Haemophilus influenzae* b capsular polysaccharide in human infants, *J. Exp. Med.* **163:**262–269 (1986).

206. INSEL, R. A., ANDERSON, P., PICHICHERO, M. E., AMSTEY, M. S., EKBORG, G., AND SMITH, D. H., Anticapsular antibody to *Haemophilus influenzae* type b, in: *Haemophilus influenzae* (S. H. Sell and P. F. Wright, eds.), pp. 155–168, Elsevier, Amsterdam, 1982.

207. INSEL, R. A., AMSTEY, M., AND PICHICHERO, M. E., Postimmunization antibody to the *Haemophilus influenzae* type b capsule in breast milk, *J. Infect. Dis.* **152:**407–408 (1985).

208. INZANA, T. J., AND ANDERSON, P., Serum factor-dependent resistance of *H. influenzae* type b to antibody to lipopolysaccharide, *J. Infect. Dis.* **151:**869–877 (1985).

209. ISTRE, G. R., CONNER, J. S., GLODE, M. P., AND HOPKINS, R. S., Increasing ampicillin-resistance rates in *Haemophilus influenzae* meningitis, *Am. J. Dis. Child.* **138:**366–369 (1984).

210. ISTRE, G. R., CONNER, J. S., BROOME, C. V., HIGHTOWER, A., AND HOPKINS, R. S., Risk factors for primary invasive *Haemophilus influenzae* disease: Increased risk from day care attendance and school age household members, *J. Pediatr.* **106:**190–195 (1985).

211. JACOBS, R. F., HSI, S., WILSON, C. B., BENJAMIN, D., SMITH, A. L., AND MORROW, R., Apparent meningococcemia: Clinical features of disease due to *Haemophilus influenzae* and *Neisseria meningitidis*, *Pediatrics* **72:**469–472 (1983).

212. JACOBSON, J. A., MCCORMICK, J. B., HAYES, P., THORNSBERRY, C., AND KIRVIN, L., Epidemiologic characteristics of infections caused by ampicillin-resistant *Haemophilus influenzae*, *Pediatrics* **58**:388–391 (1976).

213. JENNINGS, H. J., Capsular polysaccharides as human vaccines, *Adv. Carbohydr. Chem. Biochem.* **33** (1983).

214. JOHNSTON, R. B., JR., ANDERSON, P., ROSEN, F. S., AND SMITH, D. H., Characterization of human immunity to polyribophosphate, the capsular antigen of *H. influenzae* type b, *Clin. Immunol. Immunopathol.* **1**:234–240 (1973).

215. JOKIPII, L., AND JOKIPII, A. M., Emergence and prevalence of beta-lactamase producing *Haemophilus influenzae* in Finland and susceptibility of 102 respiratory isolates to eight antibiotics, *J. Antimicrob. Chemother.* **6**:623–631 (1980).

216. KALDOR, J., ASZNOWICZ, R., AND DWYER, B., *Haemophilus influenzae* type b antigenuria in children, *J. Clin. Pathol.* **32**:538–541 (1979).

217. KAPLAN, S. L., MASON, E. O., JR., JOHNSON, G., BROUGHTON, R. A., HURLEY, D., AND PARKE, J. C., Enzyme-linked immunosorbent assay for detection of capsular antibodies against *H. influenzae* type b: Comparison with radioimmunoassay, *J. Clin. Microbiol.* **18**:1201–1204 (1983).

218. KAPLAN, S. L., CATLIN, F. I., WEAVER, T., AND FEIGIN, R. D., Onset of hearing loss in children with bacterial meningitis, *Pediatrics* **73**:575–578 (1984).

219. KASLOW, R. A., AND SHAW, S., The role of histocompatibility antigens (HLA) in infection, *Epidemiol. Rev.* **40**:8–15 (1981).

220. KAYHTY, H., JOUSIMIES-SOMER, H., PELTOLA, H., AND MAKELA, P. H., Antibody response to capsular polysaccharides of groups A and C *Neisseria meningitidis* and *H. influenzae* type b during bacteremic disease, *J. Infect. Dis.* **143**:32–41 (1981).

221. KAYHTY, H., PELTOLA, H., KARANKO, V., AND MAKELA, P. H., The protective level of serum antibodies to the capsular polysaccharide of *Haemophilus influenzae* type b, *J. Infect. Dis.* **147**:1100 (1983).

222. KAYHTY, H., SCHNEERSON, R., AND SUTTON, A., Class-specific antibody response to *H. influenzae* type b capsular polysaccharide vaccine, *J. Infect. Dis.* **148**:767 (1983).

223. KAYHTY, H., KARANKO, V., PELTOLA, H., AND MAKELA, P. H., Serum antibodies after vaccination with *Haemophilus influenzae* type b capsular polysaccharide and responses to reimmunization: No evidence of immunological tolerance or memory, *Pediatrics* **74**:857–865 (1984).

224. KAYHTY, H., ESKOLA, J., PELTOLA, H., KARANKO, V., MAKELA, P. H., SAMUELSON, J., AND GORDON, L. K., Antibody levels achieved in infants by a course of H. influenzae type b polysaccharide/diphtheria toxoid conjugate vaccine, *Lancet* **1**:1184–1186 (1985).

225. KAYHTY, H., PELTOLA, H., AND ESKOLA, J., Immunogenicity and reactogenicity of four *Haemophilus influenzae* type b capsular polysaccharide vaccines in Finnish 24-month-old children, *Pediatr. Infect. Dis. J.* **7**:574–577 (1988).

226. KELLY, H. W., COUCH, R. C., DAVIS, R. L., CUSHING, A. H., AND KNOTT, R., Interaction of chloramphenicol and rifampin, *J. Pediatr.* **112**:817–820 (1988).

227. KENNY, J. F., ISBURG, C. D., AND MICHAELS, R. H., Meningitis due to *Haemophilus influenzae* type b resistant to both ampicillin and chloramphenicol, *J. Pediatr.* **66**:14–16 (1980).

228. KHAN, W., ROSS, S., RODRIGUEZ, W., CONTRONI, G., AND SAZ, A. K., *Haemophilus influenzae* type b resistant to ampicillin, *J. Am. Med. Assoc.* **229**:298–301 (1974).

229. KIMURA, A., GULIG, P. A., MCCRACKEN, G. H., JR., LOFTUS, T. A., AND HANSEN, E. J., A minor high-molecular-weight outer membrane protein of *Haemophilus influenzae* type b is a protective antigen, *Infect, Immun.* **47**:253–259 (1985).

230. KING, S. D., RAMLAL, A., WYNTER, H., MOODIE, K., CASTLE, D., KUO, J. S. C., BARNES, L., AND WILLIAMS, C. L., Safety and immunogenicity of a new *Haemophilus influenzae* type b vaccine in infants under one year of age, *Lancet* **2**:705–709 (1981).

231. KLEIN, J. O., FEIGIN, R. D., AND MCCRACKEN, G. H., JR., Report of the Task Force on Diagnosis and Management of Meningitis, *Pediatrics* **78**(Suppl.):S959–S982 (1986).

232. KRASINSKI, K., NELSON, J. D., BUTLER, S., LUBY, J. P., AND KUSMIESZ, H., Possible association of mycoplasma and viral respiratory infections with bacterial meningitis, *Am. J. Epidemiol.* **125**:499–508 (1987).

233. KUO, J. S. C., MONJI, N., AND MCCOY, D. W., Development of *Haemophilus influenzae* type b vaccine: A combined vaccine consisting of the capsular polysaccharide, polyribosyl ribitol phosphate, and *Bordetella pertussis*, in: *Haemophilus influenzae* (S. H. SELL AND P. F. WRIGHT, eds.), pp. 243–252, Elsevier, Amsterdam, 1982.

234. KURONEN, T., PELTOLA, H., NORS, T., HAQUE, N., AND MAKELA, P. H., Adverse reactions and endotoxin content of polysaccharide vaccines, *Dev. Biol. Stand.* **34**:117–125 (1977).

235. LAGERGARD, T., NYLEN, O., SANDBERG, T., AND TROLLFORS, B., Antibody responses to capsular polysaccharide, lipopolysaccharide, and outer membrane in adults infected with *H. influenzae* type b, *J. Clin. Microbiol.* **20**:1154–1158 (1984).

236. LANDSTEINER, K., *The Specificity of Serological Reactions*, rev. ed., Harvard University Press, Cambridge, Mass., 1945; reprinted by Dover Publications, New York, 1962.

237. LEE, C. J., MALIK, F. G., AND ROBBINS, J. B., The regulation of the immune response of mice to *H. influenzae* type b capsular polysaccharide, *Immunology* **34**:149–156 (1978).

238. LEPOW, M. L., PETER, G., GLODE, M. P., DAUM, R. S., CALNEN, G., KNIGHT, K. M., MAYER, D., KUO, J. S. C., AND LUI, N. S. T., Response of infants to *Haemophilus influenzae* type b polysaccharide and diphtheria–tetanus–pertussis vaccines in combination, *J. Infect. Dis.* **149**:950–955 (1984).

239. LEPOW, M. L., SAMUELSON, J. S., AND GORDON, L. K .,

Safety and immunogenicity of *Haemophilus influenzae* type b polysaccharide–diphtheria toxoid conjugate vaccine in adults, *J. Infect. Dis.* **150**:402–406 (1984).

240. LEPOW, M. L., SAMUELSON, J. S., AND GORDON, L. K., Safety and immunogenicity of *Haemophilus influenzae* type b polysaccharide–diphtheria toxoid conjugate vaccine in infants 9 to 15 months of age, *J. Pediatr.* **106**:185–189 (1985).

241. LEPOW, M., RANDOLPH, M., CIMMA, R., LARSEN, D., ROGAR, M., SCHUMACHER, J., LENT, B., GAINTER, S., SAMUELSON, J., AND GORDON, L., Persistence of antibody and responses to booster dose of *H. influenzae* type b polysaccharide diphtheria toxoid conjugate vaccine in infants immunized at 9 to 15 months of age, *J. Pediatr.* **108**:882–886 (1986).

242. LEPOW, M. L., BARKIN, R. M., BERKOWITZ, C. D., BRUNELL, P. A., JAMES, O., MEIER, K., WARD, J., ZAHRADNIK, J. M., SAMUELSON, J., MCVERRY, P. H., AND GORDON, L. K., Safety and immunogenicity of *Haemophilus influenzae* type b polysaccharide–diphtheria toxoid conjugate vaccine (PRP-D) in infants, *J. Infect. Dis.* **156**:591–596 (1987).

243. LERMAN, S. J., KUCERA, J. C., AND BRUNKEN, J. M., Nasopharyngeal carriage of antibiotic-resistant *H. influenzae* in healthy children, *Pediatrics* **65**:287–291 (1979).

244. LETSON, G. W., SANTOSHAM, M., REID, R., PRIEHS, C., BURNS, B., JAHNKE, A., GAHAGAN, S., NIENSTADT, L., JOHNSON, C., SMITH, D., AND SIBER, G., Comparison of active and combined passive/active immunization of Navajo children against *Haemophilus influenzae* type b, *Pediatr. Infect. Dis. J.* **7**:747–752 (1988).

245. LI, K. I., DASHEFSKY, B., AND WALD, E. R., *Haemophilus influenzae* type b colonization in household contacts of infected and colonized children enrolled in day care, *Pediatrics* **78**:15–20 (1986).

246. LI, K. I., WALD, E. R., AND DASHEFSKY, B., Nasal colonization with *Haemophilus* and immunization status, *Pediatr. Infect. Dis. J.* **6**:303–304 (1987).

247. LOEB, M. R., AND SMITH, D. H., Outer membrane protein composition in disease isolates of *Haemophilus influenzae*: Pathogenic and epidemiological implications, *Infect. Immun.* **30**:709–717 (1980).

248. LOEB, M. R., AND SMITH, D. H., Human antibody response to individual outer membrane proteins of *Haemophilus influenzae* type b, *Infect. Immun.* **37**:1032–1036 (1982).

249. LOSONSKY, G. A., SANTOSHAM, M., SEHGAL, V. M., ZWAHLEN, A., AND MOXON, E. R., *Haemophilus influenzae* in the White Mountain Apaches: molecular epidemiology of a high risk population, *Pediatr. Infect. Dis. J.* **3**:539–547 (1984).

250. LUM, M. K., WARD, J. I., AND BENDER, T. R., Protective influence of breast feeding on the risk of developing invasive *H. influenzae* type b disease, *Pediatr. Res.* **16**(Part 2):151A (abstract) (1982).

251. LYNN, M., TEWARI, R. P., AND SOLOTOROVSKY, M., Immunoprotective activity of ribosomes from *Haemophilus influenzae*, *Infect. Immun.* **15**:453–460 (1977).

252. MAKELA, O., MATTILA, P., RAUTONEN, N., SEPPALA, I., ESKOLA, J., AND KAYHTY, H., Isotype concentrations of human antibodies to *Haemophilus influenzae* type b polysaccharide (Hib) in young adults immunized with the polysaccharide as such or conjugated to a protein (diphtheria toxoid), *J. Immunol.* **139**:1999–2004 (1987).

253. MAKELA, P. H., PELTOLA, H., KAYHTY, H., JOUSIMIES, H., PETTAY, O., RUOSLATHI, E., SIVONEN, A., AND RENKONEN, O. V., Polysaccharide vaccines of group A *Neisseria meningitidis* and *Haemophilus influenzae* type b: A field trial in Finland, *J. Infect. Dis.* **136**(Suppl.):S43–S50 (1977).

254. MAKINTUBEE, S., ISTRE, G. R., AND WARD, J. I., Transmission of invasive *Haemophilus influenzae* type b disease in day care settings, *J. Pediatr.* **111**:180–186 (1987).

255. MARBURG, S., JORN, D., TOLMAN, R. L., ARISON, B., MCCAULEY, J., KNISKERN, P. J., HAGOPIAN, A., AND VELLA, P. P., Bimolecular chemistry of macromolecules: Synthesis of bacterial polysaccharide conjugates with *Neisseria meningitidis* membrane protein, *J. Am. Chem. Soc.* **108**:5282–5287 (1986).

256. MARCON, M. J., HAMOUDI, A. C., AND CANNON, H. J., Comparative laboratory evaluation of three antigen detection methods for diagnosis of *Haemophilus influenzae* type b disease, *J. Clin. Microbiol.* **19**:333–337 (1984).

257. MARKS, M. I., AND DORCHESTER, W. L., Secondary rates of *Haemophilus influenzae* type b disease among day care contacts, *J. Pediatr.* **111**:305–306 (1987).

258. MASON, E. O., KAPLAN, S. L., LAMBETH, L. B., HINDS, D. B., KVERNLAND, S. J., LOISELLE, E. M., AND FEIGIN, R. D., Serotype and ampicillin susceptibility of *Haemophilus influenzae* causing systemic infections in children: Three years of experience, *J. Clin. Microbiol.* **15**:543–546 (1982).

259. MASTERS, P. L., BRUMFITT, W., MENDEZ, R. L., AND LIKAR, M., Bacterial flora of the upper respiratory tract in Paddington families, 1952–4, *Br. Med. J.* **1**:1200–1205 (1958).

260. MAYOSMITH, M. F., HIRSCH, P. J., WODZINSKI, S. F., AND SCHIFFMAN, F. J., Acute epiglottitis in adults: An eight-year experience in the state of Rhode Island, *N. Engl. J. Med.* **314**:1133–1139 (1986).

261. MCCRACKEN, G. H., JR., GINSBURG, C. M., ZWEIGHAFT, T. C., AND CLAHSEN, J., Pharmacokinetics of rifampin in infants and children: Relevance to prophylaxis against *Haemophilus influenzae* type b disease, *Pediatrics* **66**:17–21 (1980).

262. MCLAUGHLIN, F. J., GOLDMANN, D. A., ROSENBAUM, D. M., HARRIS, G. B. C., SCHUSTER, S. R., AND STRIEDER, D. J., Empyema in children: Clinical course and long-term follow-up, *Pediatrics* **73**:587–593 (1984).

263. MENDELMAN, P. M., AND SMITH, A. L., *Haemophilus influenzae*, in: *Textbook of Pediatric Infectious Diseases*, 2nd ed. (R. D. FEIGIN AND J. D. CHERRY, eds.), pp. 1142–1163, Saunders, Philadelphia, 1987.

264. MENDELMAN, P. M., DOROSHOW, C. A., GANDY, S. L., SYRIOPOULOU, V., WEIGEN, C. P., AND SMITH, A. L., Plasmid-mediated resistance in multiply resistant *Haemophilus*

influenzae type b causing meningitis: Molecular characterization of one strain and review of the literature, *J. Infect. Dis.* **150:**30–39 (1984).

265. MEYRORITCH, J., FRAND, M., ALTMAN, G., SHOHAT, I., AND BOLCHIS, H., Ampicillin-resistant *Haemophilus influenzae* type b infections in hospitalized pediatric patients, *Isr. J. Med. Sci.* **20:**519–521 (1984).

266. MICHAELS, R. H., Increase in influenzal meningitis, *N. Engl. J. Med.* **285:**666–667 (1971).

267. MICHAELS, R. H., AND NORDEN, C. W., Pharyngeal colonization with *H. influenzae* type b: A longitudinal study of families with a child with meningitis or epiglottitis due to *H. influenzae* type b, *J. Infect. Dis.* **136:**222–228 (1977).

268. MICHAELS, R. H., AND SCHULTZ, W. F., The frequency of *Hemophilus influenzae* infections: Analysis of racial and environmental factors, in: *Hemophilus influenzae* (S. H. W. SELL AND D. T. KARZON, eds.), pp. 243–250, Vanderbilt University Press, Nashville, 1973.

269. MICHAELS, R. H., STONEBRAKER, F. E., AND ROBBINS, J. B., Use of antiserum agar for detection of *H. influenzae* type b in the pharynx, *Pediatr. Res.* **9:**513–516 (1975).

270. MICHAELS, R. H., POZIVIAK, C. S., STONEBRAKER, F. E., AND NORDEN, C. W., Factors affecting pharyngeal *H. influenzae* type b colonization rates in children, *J. Clin. Microbiol.* **4:**413–417 (1976).

271. MICHAELS, R. H., MYEROWITZ, R. L., AND KLAW, R., Potentiation of experimental meningitis due to *Haemophilus influenzae* by influenza virus, *J. Infect. Dis.* **135:**641–645 (1977).

272. MILSTIEN, J. B., GROSS, T. P., AND KURITSKY, J. N., Adverse reactions reported following receipt of *Haemophilus influenzae* b vaccine: An analysis after 1 year of marketing, *Pediatrics* **80:**270–274 (1987).

273. MOXON, E. R., SMITH, A. L., AVERILL, D. R., AND SMITH, D. H., *H. influenzae* meningitis in rats following intranasal inoculation, *J. Infect. Dis.* **129:**154–162 (1974).

274. MOXON, E. R., ANDERSON, P., SMITH, D. H., ADRIANZEN, T. B., GRAHAM, G. G., AND BAKER, R. S., Antibody responses to a combination vaccine against *Haemophilus influenzae* type b, diphtheria, pertussis, and tetanus, *Bull. WHO* **52:**87–90 (1975).

275. MPAIRWE, Y., Observations on the nasopharyngeal carriage of *H. influenzae* type b in children in Kampala, Uganda, *J. Hyg.* **68:**337–341 (1970).

276. MULKS, M. H., KORNFELD, S. J., BRAGIONE, B., AND PLAUT, A. G., Relationship between the specificity of IgA proteases and serotypes in *Haemophilus influenzae*, *J. Infect. Dis.* **146:**266–274 (1982).

277. MURPHY, T. V., Haemophilus b polysaccharide vaccine: Need for continuing assessment, *Pediatr. Infect. Dis. J.* **6:**701–703 (1987).

278. MURPHY, T. V., CLEMENTS, J. F., PETRONI, M., COURY, S., AND STETLER, L., Survival of *Haemophilus influenzae* type b in respiratory secretions, *Pediatr. Infect. Dis. J.* **8:**148–151 (1989).

279. MURPHY, T. V., McCRACKEN, G. H., JR., ZWEIGHAFT, T. C., AND HANSEN, E. J., Emergence of rifampin-resistant *Haemophilus influenzae* after prophylaxis, *J. Pediatr.* **99:**406–409 (1981).

280. MURPHY, T. V., CHRANE, D. F., McCRACKEN, G. H., JR., AND NELSON, J. D., Rifampin prophylaxis v placebo for household contacts of children with *Haemophilus influenzae* type b disease, *Am. J. Dis. Child.* **137:**627–632 (1983).

281. MURPHY, T. V., McCRACKEN, G. H., JR., MOORE, B. S., GULIG, P. A., AND HANSEN, E. J., *Haemophilus influenzae* type b disease after rifampin prophylaxis in a day-care center: Possible reasons for its failure, *Pediatr. Infect. Dis. J.* **2:**193–198 (1983).

282. MURPHY, T. V., DEL RIO, M. A., AND CHRANE, D., Persistent pharyngeal colonization during therapy in patients with meningitis caused by *Haemophilus influenzae* type b, *J. Infect. Dis.* **152:**849 (1985).

283. MURPHY, T. V., CLEMENTS, J. F., BREEDLOVE, J. A., HANSEN, E. J., AND SEIBERT, G. B., Risk of subsequent disease among day-care contacts of patients with systemic *Haemophilus influenzae* type b disease, *N. Engl. J. Med.* **316:**5–10 (1987).

284. MURPHY, T. V., OSTERHOLM, M. T., PIERSON, L. M., WHITE, K. E., BREEDLOVE, J. A., SEIBERT, G. B., KURITSKY, J. N., AND GRANOFF, D. M., Prospective surveillance of *Haemophilus influenzae* type b disease in Dallas County, Texas, and in Minnesota, *Pediatrics* **79:**173–180 (1987).

285. MUSHER, D. M., GOREE, A., BAUGHN, R. E., AND BIRDSALL, H. H., Immunoglobulin A from bronchopulmonary secretions blocks bactericidal and opsonizing, effects of antibody to nontypable *H. influenzae*, *Infect. Immun.* **45:**36–40 (1984).

286. MUSSER, J. M., GRANOFF, D. M., PATTISON, P. E., AND SELANDER, P. K., A population genetic framework for the study of invasive diseases caused by serotype b strains of *Haemophilus influenzae*, *Proc. Natl. Acad. Sci. USA* **82:** 5078–5082 (1985).

287. MYEROWITZ, R. L., AND MICHAELS, R. H., Mechanism of potentiation of experimental *Haemophilus influenzae* type B disease in infant rats by influenza A virus, *Lab. Invest.* **44:**434–441 (1981).

288. MYEROWITZ, R. L., AND NORDEN, C. W., Immunology of the infant rat experimental model of *H. influenzae* type b meningitis, *Infect. Immun.* **16:**218–225 (1977).

289. NELSON, J. D., The increasing frequency of beta-lactamase-producing *Haemophilus influenzae* b [letter], *J. Am. Med. Assoc.* **244:**239 (1980).

290. NEWMAN, S. L., WALDO, B., AND JOHNSTON, R. B., JR., Separation of serum bactericidal and opsonizing activities for *H. influenzae* type b, *Infect. Immun.* **8:**488–490 (1973).

291. NICOLOSI, A., HAUSER, W. A., BEGHI, E., AND KURLAND, L. T., Epidemiology of central nervous system infections in Olmsted County, Minnesota, 1950–1981, *J. Infect. Dis.* **154:**399–408 (1986).

292. NORDEN, C. W., Prevalence of bactericidal antibodies to *H. influenzae,* type b, *J. Infect. Dis.* **130:**489–494 (1974).

293. NORDEN, C. W., MICHAELS, R. H., AND MELISH, M., Effect of previous infection on antibody response of children to vaccination with capsular polysaccharide of *Haemophilus influenzae* type b, *J. Infect. Dis.* **132:**69–74 (1975).

294. OGLE, J. W., RABALAIS, G. P., AND GLODE, M. P., Duration of pharyngeal carriage of *Haemophilus influenzae* type b in children hospitalized with systemic infections, *Pediatr. Infect. Dis. J.* **5:**509–511 (1986).

295. OSTERHOLM, M. T., AND MURPHY, T. V., Does rifampin prophylaxis prevent disease caused by *Hemophilus influenzae* type b? *J. Am. Med. Assoc.* **251:**2408–2409 (1984).

296. OSTERHOLM, M. T., PIERSON, L. N., WHITE, K. E., LIBBY, T. A., KURITSKY, J. N., AND MCCULLOUGH, J. G., Risk of subsequent transmission of *Haemophilus influenzae* type b disease among children in day care, *N. Engl. J. Med.* **316:**1–4 (1987).

297. OSTERHOLM, M. T., RAMBECK, J. H., WHITE, K. E., JACOBS, J. L., PIERSON, L. M., NEATON, J. D., HEDBERG, C. W., MACDONALD, K. L., GRANOFF, D. M., Lack of efficacy of *Haemophilus* b polysaccharide vaccine in Minnesota, *J. Am. Med. Assoc.* **260:**1423–1428 (1988).

298. OSTROW, P. T., MOXON, E. R., VERNON, N., AND KAPKO, R., Studies on the route of meningeal invasion following *H. influenzae* inoculation of infant rats, *Lab. Invest.* **40:**678–685 (1979).

299. OSTROY, P. R., Bacterial meningitis in Washington State, *West. J. Med.* **131:**339–343 (1979).

300. OUNSTED, C., *Haemophilus influenzae* meningitis: A possible ecological factor, *Lancet* **1:**161–162 (1950).

301. OVERTURF, G. D., CABLE, D., AND WARD, J., Ampicillin–chloramphenicol-resistant *Haemophilus influenzae:* Plasmid-mediated resistance in bacterial meningitis, *Pediatr. Res.* **22:**438–441 (1987).

302. OXELIUS, V.-A., Chronic infections in a family with hereditary deficiency of IgG2 and IgG4, *Clin. Exp. Immunol.* **17:**19–27 (1974).

303. OXELIUS, V.-A., Quantitative and qualitative investigations of serum IgG subclasses in immunodeficiency diseases, *Clin. Exp. Immunol.* **36:**112–116 (1979).

304. OXELIUS, V.-A., BERKEL, A. I., AND HANSON, L. A., IgG2 deficiency in ataxia-telangiectasia, *N. Engl. J. Med.* **306:**515–517 (1982).

305. PANDEY, J. P., FUDENBERG, H. H., VIRELLA, G., KYONG, C. U., LOADHOLD, C. B., GALBRAITH, R. M., GOTSCHLICH, E. C., AND PARKE, J. C., JR., Association between immunoglobulin allotypes and immune responses to *Haemophilus influenzae* and meningococcus polysaccharides, *Lancet* **1:**190–192 (1979).

306. PARKE, J. C., JR., SCHNEERSON, R., AND ROBBINS, J. B., The attack rate, age incidence, racial distribution, and case fatality rate of *Haemophilus influenzae* type b meningitis in Mecklenburg County, North Carolina, *J. Pediatr.* **81:**765–769 (1972).

307. PARKE, J. C., JR., SCHNEERSON, R., ROBBINS, J. B., AND SCHLESSELMAN, J. J., Interim report of a controlled field trial of immunization with capsular polysaccharides of *Haemophilus influenzae* type b and group C *Neisseria meningitidis* in Mecklenburg County, North Carolina (March 1974–March 1976), *J. Infect. Dis.* **136**(Suppl.):S51–S56 (1977).

308. PELTOLA, H., Personal communication (1988).

309. PELTOLA, H., AND VIRTANEN, M., Systemic *Haemophilus influenzae* infection in Finland, *Clin. Pediatr.* **5:**275–280 (1984).

310. PELTOLA, H., KAYHTY, H., VIRTANEN, M., AND MAKELA, P. H., Prevention of *Hemophilus influenzae* bacteremic infections with the capsular polysaccharide vaccine, *N. Engl. J. Med.* **310:**1561–1566 (1984).

311. PEPPLE, J., MOXON, E. R., AND YOLKEN, R. H., Indirect enzyme-linked immunosorbent assay for the quantitation of the type-specific antigen of *Haemophilus influenzae* b: A preliminary report, *J. Pediatr.* **97:**233–237 (1980).

312. PETERSON, G. M., SILIMPERI, D. R., SCOTT, E. M., HALL, D. B., ROTTER, J. I., AND WARD, J. I., Uridine monophosphate kinase 3: A genetic marker for susceptibility to *Haemophilus influenzae* type b disease, *Lancet* **2:**417–419 (1985).

313. PETERSON, G. M., SILIMPERI, D. R., ROTTER, J. I., TERASAKI, P. I., SCHANFIELD, M. S., PARK, M. S., AND WARD, J. I., Genetic factors in *Haemophilus influenzae* type b disease susceptibility and antibody acquisition, *J. Pediatr.* **110:**229–233 (1987).

314. PFEIFFER, R., Vorlaufige mitt Heilungen uber die Erreger der Influenzae, *Dtsch. Med. Wochenschr.* **18:**28–34 (1892).

315. PFEIFFER, R., Die Aetiologie der Influenza, *Z. Hyg. Infektionskr.* **13:**357–386 (1893).

316. PHILPOTT-HOWARD, J., AND WILLIAMS, J. D., Increase in antibiotic resistance in *Haemophilus influenzae* in the United Kingdom since 1977: Report of study group, *Br. Med. J.* **284:**1597–1599 (1982).

317. PICHICHERO, M. E., AND INSEL, R. A., Relationship between naturally occurring human mucosal and serum antibody to the capsular polysaccharide of *Haemophilus influenzae* type b, *J. Infect. Dis.* **146:**243–248 (1982).

318. PICHICHERO, M. E., AND INSEL, R. A., Mucosal antibody response to parenteral vaccination with *Haemophilus influenzae* type b capsule, *J. Allergy Clin. Immunol.* **72:**481–486 (1983).

319. PICHICHERO, M. E., SOMMERFELT, A. E., STEINHOFF, M. C., AND INSEL, R. A., Breast milk antibody to the capsular polysaccharide of *Haemophilus influenzae* type b, *J. Infect. Dis.* **142:**694–698 (1980).

320. PICHICHERO, M. E., HALL, C. B., AND INSEL, R. A., A mucosal antibody response following systemic *Haemophilus influenzae* type b infection in children, *J. Clin. Invest.* **67:**1482–1489 (1981).

321. PICHICHERO, M. E., LOEB, M., ANDERSON, P., AND SMITH, D. H., Do pili play a role in pathogenicity of *Haemophilus influenzae* type b? *Lancet* **2:**960–962 (1982).

322. PINCUS, D. J., MORRISON, D., ANDREWS, C., LAWRENCE,

E., SELL, S. H., AND WRIGHT, P. F., Age-related response to two *Haemophilus influenzae* type b vaccines, *J. Pediatr.* **100**:197–201 (1982).

323. PITTMAN, M., Variation and type specificity in the bacterial species *Hemophilus influenzae*, *J. Exp. Med.* **53**:471–495 (1931).

324. PITTMAN, M., The action of type-specific *Hemophilus influenzae* antiserum, *J. Exp. Med.* **58**:683–706 (1933).

325. PORRAS, O., CAUGANT, D. A., GRAY, B., LAGERGARD, T., LEVIN, B., AND SVANBORG-EDEN, C. S., Difference in structure between type b and nontypable *Haemophilus influenzae* populations, *Infect. Immun.* **53**:79–89 (1986).

326. PORRAS, O., CAUGANT, D. A., LAGERGARD, T., AND SVAN-BORG-EDEN, C. S., Application of multilocus enzyme gel electrophoresis to *Haemophilus influenzae*, *Infect. Immun.* **53**:71–78 (1986).

327. POWARS, D., OVERTURF, G., AND TURNER, E., Is there an increased risk of *Haemophilus influenzae* septicemia in children with sickle cell anemia? *Pediatrics* **71**:927–931 (1983).

328. POWELL, M., KOUTSIA-CAROUZOU, C., VOUTSINAS, D., SEYMOUR, A., AND WILLIAMS, J. D., Resistance of clinical isolates of *Haemophilus influenzae* in United Kingdom 1986, *Br. Med. J.* **295**:176–179 (1987).

329. PRAXIS BIOLOGICS, *Haemophilus* b polysaccharide vaccine (package insert), issued April 1985.

330. Prevention of secondary cases of *Haemophilus influenzae* type b disease, *Morbid. Mortal. Weekly Rep.* **31**:672–680 (1982).

331. PROBER, C. G., Effect of rifampin on chloramphenicol levels, *N. Engl. J. Med.* **312**:788–789 (1985).

332. QUINN, P. H., CROSSON, F. J., JR., WINKELSTEIN, J. A., AND MOXON, E. R., Activation of the alternative complement pathway by *H. influenzae* type b, *Infect. Immun.* **16**:400–402 (1977).

333. RAMADAS, K., PETERSON, G. M., HEINER, D. C., AND WARD, J. I., Class and subclass antibodies to *H. influenzae* type b capsule: Comparison of invasive disease and natural exposure, *Infect. Immun.* **53**:468–490 (1986).

334. RECOMMENDATIONS OF THE IMMUNIZATION PRACTICES ADVISORY COMMITTEE (ACIP), Polysaccharide vaccine for prevention of *Haemophilus influenzae* type b disease, *Morbid. Mortal. Weekly Rep.* **34**:201–205 (1985).

335. RECOMMENDATIONS OF THE IMMUNIZATION PRACTICES ADVISORY COMMITTEE (ACIP), Update: Prevention of *Haemophilus influenzae* type b disease, *Morbid. Mortal. Weekly Rep.* **36**:529 (1987).

336. REDMOND, S. R., AND PICHICHERO, M. E., *Haemophilus influenzae* type b disease: An epidemiologic study with special reference to day care centers, *J. Am. Med. Assoc.* **252**:2581–2584 (1984).

337. Report of the Committee on Infectious Diseases, *Haemophilus influenzae Infections*, 20th ed., pp. 169–174, American Academy of Pediatrics, Elk Grove Village, Ill., 1986.

338. RIESEN, W. F., DKVARIL, F., AND BRAUN, D. G., Natural infection of man with group A streptococci: Levels, re-striction in class, subclass, and type, and clonal appearance of polysaccharide-group-specific antibodies, *Scand. J. Immunol.* **5**:383–390 (1976).

339. ROBBINS, J. B., PARKE, J. C., JR., SCHNEERSON, R., AND WHISNANT, J. K., Quantitative measurement of "natural" and immunization-induced *Haemophilus influenzae* type b capsular polysaccharide antibodies, *Pediatr. Res.* **7**:103–110 (1973).

340. ROBBINS, J. B., SCHNEERSON, R., GLODE, M. P., VANN, W., SCHIFFER, M. S., LIV, T. Y., PARKE, J. C., AND HUNTLEY, C., Cross-reactive antigens and immunity to diseases caused by encapsulated bacteria, *J. Allergy Clin. Immunol.* **56**:141–151 (1975).

341. ROBBINS, J. B., SCHNEERSON, R., AND PARKE, J. C., JR., A review of the efficacy trials with *Haemophilus influenzae* type b polysaccharide vaccines, in: *Haemophilus influenzae* (S. H. SELL AND P. F. WRIGHT, eds.), pp. 255–263, Elsevier, Amsterdam, 1982.

342. ROBBINS, J. B., SCHNEERSON, R., AND PITTMAN, M., *H. influenzae* type b infections, in: *Bacterial Vaccines* (R. GERMANIER, ed.), Academic Press, New York, 1984.

343. ROBBINS, J. B., SCHNEERSON, R., AND PITTMAN, M., *H. influenzae* type b infections, in: *Bacterial Vaccines* (R. Germanier, ed.), Academic Press, New York, 1984.

344. ROBERTS, M. C., SWENSON, C. D., OWENS, I. M., AND SMITH, A. L., Characterization of chloramphenicol-resistant *Haemophilus influenzae*, *Antimicrob. Agents Chemother.* **18**:610–615 (1980).

345. RODRIGUES, L. P., SCHNEERSON, R., AND ROBBINS, J. B., Immunity to disease caused by *H. influenzae* type b. I. The isolation, and some physicochemical, serologic and biologic properties of the capsular polysaccharide of *Hemophilus influenzae* type b, *J. Immunol.* **107**:1071–1080 (1971).

346. ROSALES, S. V., LASCOLEA, L. J., JR., AND OGRA, P. L., Development of respiratory mucosal tolerance during *H. influenzae* type b infection in infancy, *J. Immunol.* **132**:1517–1521 (1984).

347. ROSEN, F. S., AND JANEWAY, C. A., The gamma globulins: III. The antibody deficiency syndromes, *N. Engl. J. Med.* **275**:709–715 (1966).

348. ROSS, S. C., AND DENSEN, P., Complement deficiency states and infection: Epidemiology, pathogenesis, and consequences of neisserial and other infections in an immune deficiency, *Medicine* **63**:243–273 (1984).

349. RUBIN, L. G., AND MOXON, E. R., Pathogenesis of bloodstream invasion with *H. influenzae* type b, *Infect. Immun.* **41**:280–284 (1983).

350. SALWEN, K. M., VIKERFORS, T., AND OLCEN, P., Increased incidence of childhood bacterial meningitis: A 25-year study in a defined population in Sweden, *Scand. J. Infect. Dis.* **19**:1–11 (1987).

351. SANTOSHAM, M., KALLMAN, C. H., NEFF, J. M., AND MOXON, E. R., Absence of increasing incidence of meningitis caused by *Haemophilus influenzae* type b, *J. Infect. Dis.* **140**:1009–1012 (1979).

352. SANTOSHAM, M., REID, R., AMBROSINO, D. M., WOLFF, M. C., ALMEIDO-HILL, J., PRIEHS, C., ASPERY, K. M., GARRETT, S., CROLL, L., FOSTER, S., GUIRGE, G., PAGE, P., ZACHER, B., MOXON, R., AND SIBER, G. R., Prevention of *Haemophilus influenzae* type b infections in high-risk infants treated with bacterial polysaccharide immune globulin, *N. Engl. J. Med.* **317:**923–929 (1987).

353. SCHEIFELE, D. W., Ampicillin-resistant *Haemophilus influenzae* in Canada: Nationwide survey of hospital laboratories, *Can. Med. Assoc. J.* **121:**198–202 (1979).

354. SCHEIFELE, D. W., WARD, J. I., AND SIBER, G, Advantage of latex agglutination over countercurrent immunoelectrophoresis in the detection of *Haemophilus influenzae* type b antigen in serum, *Pediatrics* **68:**888–891 (1981).

355. SCHELD, W. M., PARKS, T. S., WINN, H. R., DACEY, R. G., AND SANDE, M. A. J., Clearance of bacteria from cerebrospinal fluid to blood in experimental meningitis, *Infect. Immun.* **24:**102–105 (1979).

356. SCHIFFER, M. S., MACLOWRY, J., SCHNEERSON, R., ROBBINS, J. B., MCREYNOLDS, J. W., THOMAS, W. J., BAILEY, D. W., CLARKE, E. J., MUELLER, E. J., AND ESCAMILLA, J., Clinical, bacteriological, and immunological characterisation of ampicillin-resistant *Haemophilus influenzae* type b, *Lancet* **2:**257–259 (1974).

357. SCHLECH, W. F., BAND, J. D., WARD, J. I., HIGHTOWER, A. W., FRASER, D. W., AND BROOME, C. V., Bacterial meningitis in the United States, 1978–1981: The national bacterial meningitis surveillance study, *J. Am. Med. Assoc.* **253:**1749–1754 (1985).

358. SCHNEERSON, R., AND ROBBINS, J. B., Age-related susceptibility to *H. influenzae* type b disease in rabbits, *Infect. Immun.* **4:**397–401 (1971).

359. SCHNEERSON, R., AND ROBBINS, J. B., Induction of serum *H. influenzae* type b capsular antibodies in adult volunteers fed cross-reacting *Escherichia coli* O75:K100:H5, *N. Engl. J. Med.* **292:**1093–1096 (1975).

360. SCHNEERSON, R., RODRIGUES, L. P., PARKE, J. C., JR., AND ROBBINS, J. B., Immunity to disease caused by *H. influenzae* type b. II. Specificity and some biological characteristics of "natural," infection acquired, and immunization induced antibody to the capsular polysaccharide, *J. Immunol.* **107:**1081–1086 (1971).

361. SCHNEERSON, R., BARRERA, O., SUTTON, A., AND ROBBINS, J. B., Preparation, characterization, and immunogenicity of *Haemophilus influenzae* type b polysaccharide–protein conjugates, *J. Exp. Med.* **152:**361–376 (1980).

362. SCHNEERSON, R., ROBBINS, J. B., CHU, C.-Y., SUTTON, A., VANN, W., VICKERS, J. C., LONDON, W. T., CURFMAN, B., HARDEGREE, M. C., SHILOACH, J., AND RASTOGI, S. C., Serum antibody responses of juvenile and infant rhesus monkeys injected with *Haemophilus influenzae* type b and pneumococcus type 6A capsular polysaccharide–protein conjugates, *Infect. Immun.* **45:**582–591 (1984).

363. SCHNEERSON, R., ROBBINS, J. B., PARKE, J. C., BELL, C., SCHLESSELMAN, J. J., SUTTON, A, WANG, Z., SCHIFFMAN,

G., KARPAS, A., AND SHILOACH, J., Quantitative and qualitative analyses of serum antibodies elicited in adults by *H. influenzae* type b and pneumococcus type 6A capsular polysaccharide–tetanus toxoid conjugates, *Infect. Immun.* **52:**519–528 (1986).

364. SCHREIBER, J. R., BARRUS, V., CATES, K. L., AND SIBER, G. R., Functional characterization of human IgG, IgM, and IgA antibody directed to the capsule of *H. influenzae* type b, *J. Infect. Dis.* **153:**8–16 (1986).

365. SCHUR, P. H., BOREL, H., GELFAND, E. W., ALPER, C. A., AND ROSEN, F. S., Selective gamma-G globulin deficiencies in patients with recurrent pyogenic infections, *N. Engl. J. Med.* **283:**631–634 (1970).

366. SCHWARTZ, R. H., GOLDENBERG, R. I., PARK, C., AND KEIM, D., The increasing prevalence of bacteremic ampicillin-resistant *Haemophilus influenzae* infections in a community hospital, *Pediatr. Infect. Dis. J.* **1:**242–244 (1982).

367. SELL, S. H. W., MERRILL, R. E., DOYNE, E. O., AND ZINSKY, E. P., JR., Long-term sequelae of *Haemophilus influenzae* meningitis, *Pediatrics* **49:**206–217 (1972).

368. SELL, S. H. W., TURNER, D. J., AND FEDERSPIEL, C. F., Natural infections with *H. influenzae* in children: Types identified, in: *Haemophilus influenzae* (S. H. W. SELL AND D. T. KARZON, eds.), Vanderbilt University Press, Nashville, 1973.

369. SHACKELFORD, P. G., GRANOFF, D. M., NAHM, M. H., SCOTT, M. G., SUAREZ, B., PANDEY, J. P., AND NELSON, S. J., Relation of age, race, and allotype to immunoglobulin subclass concentrations, *Pediatr. Res.* **19:**846–849 (1985).

370. SHACKELFORD, P. G., GRANOFF, D. M., NELSON, S. J., SCOTT, M. G., SMITH, D. S., AND NAHM, M. H., Subclass distribution of human antibodies to *Haemophilus influenzae* type b capsular polysaccharide, *J. Immunol.* **138:**587–592 (1987).

371. SHANN, F., GRATTEN, M., GERMER, S., LINNEMANN, V., HAZLETT, D., AND PAYNE, R., Aetiology of pneumonia in children in Goroka Hospital, Papua New Guinea, *Lancet* **2:**537–541 (1984).

372. SHAPIRO, E. D., Persistent pharyngeal colonization with *H. influenzae* type b after intravenous chloramphenicol therapy, *Pediatrics* **67:**435–437 (1981).

373. SHAPIRO, E. D., AND WALD, E. R., Efficacy of rifampin in eliminating pharyngeal carriage of *Haemophilus influenzae* type b, *Pediatrics* **66:**5–8 (1980).

374. SHAPIRO, E. D., MURPHY, T. V., WALD, E. R., AND BRADY, C. A., The protective efficacy of *Haemophilus* b polysaccharide vaccine, *J. Am. Med. Assoc.* **260:**1419–1422 (1988).

375. SHAW, E. D., DARKER, R. J., FELDMAN, W. E., GRAY, B. M., PIFER, L. L., AND SCOTT, G. B., Clinical studies of a new latex particle agglutination test for detection of *Haemophilus influenzae* type b polyribose antigen in serum, cerebrospinal fluid, and urine, *J. Clin. Microbiol.* **16:**1153–1156 (1982).

376. SHENEP, J. L., MUNSON, R. S., JR., AND GRANOFF, D. M.,

Human antibody responses to lipopolysaccharide after meningitis due to *H. influenzae* type b, *J. Infect. Dis.* **145**:181–190 (1982).

377. SHENEP, J. L., MUNSON, R. S., JR., BARENKAMP, S. J., AND GRANOFF, D. M., Further studies of the role of noncapsular antibody in protection against experimental *Haemophilus influenzae* type b bacteremia, *Infect. Immun.* **42**:257–263 (1983).

378. SIBER, G. R., Bacteremias due to *Haemophilus influenzae* and *Streptococcus pneumoniae:* Their occurrence and course in children with cancer, *Am. J. Dis. Child.* **134**:668–672 (1980).

379. SIBER, G. R., SCHUR, P. H., AISENBERG, A. C., WEITZMAN, S. A., AND SCHIFFMAN, G., Correlation between serum IgG-2 concentrations and the antibody response to bacterial polysaccharides, *N. Engl. J. Med.* **303**:178–182 (1980).

380. SIBER, G. R., WEITZMAN, S. A., AND AISENBERG, A. C., Antibody response of patients with Hodgkin's disease to protein and polysaccharide antigens, *Rev. Infect. Dis.* **3**(Suppl.):S144–S159 (1984).

381. SIBER, G. R., AMBROSINO, D. M., McIVER, J., ERVIN, T. J., SCHIFFMAN, G., SALLAN, S., AND GRADY, G. F., Preparation of human hyperimmune globulin to *Haemophilus influenzae* b, *Streptococcus pneumoniae*, and *Neisseria meningitidis, Infect. Immun.* **45**:248–254 (1984).

382. SILVERMAN, M., STRATTON, D., DIALLO, A., AND EGLER, L. J., Diagnosis of acute bacterial pneumonia in Nigerian children, *Arch. Dis. Child.* **52**:925–931 (1977).

383. SIMASATHIEN, S., DHANGMANI, C., AND ECHEVERRIA, P., *Haemophilus influenzae* type b resistant to ampicillin and chloramphenicol in an orphanage in Thailand, *Lancet* **1**:1214–1217 (1980).

384. SIVONEN, A., Effect of *Neisseria meningitidis* group A polysaccharide vaccine on nasopharyngeal carrier rates, *J. Infect.* **3**:266–272 (1981).

385. SKOLNICK, J. L., STOLER, B. S., KATZ, D. B., AND ANDERSON, W. H., Rifampin, oral contraceptives, and pregnancy, *J. Am. Med. Assoc.* **236**:1382 (1976).

386. SMITH, A. L., Antibiotic resistance in *Haemophilus influenzae, Pediatr. Infect. Dis. J.* **2**:352–355 (1983).

387. SMITH, A. L., DAUM, R. S., SCHIEFELE, D., SYRIOPOULOU, V., AVERILL, D. R., ROBERTS, M. C., AND STULL, T. L., Pathogenesis of *H. influenzae* meningitis, in: *Haemophilus influenzae* (S. H. SELL AND P. F. WRIGHT, eds.), Elsevier, Amsterdam, 1982.

388. SMITH, D. H., PETER, G., INGRAM, D. L., HARDING, A. L., AND ANDERSON, P., Responses of children immunized with the capsular polysaccharide of *Haemophilus influenzae*, type b, *Pediatrics* **52**:637–644 (1973).

389. SMITH, D. H., HANN, S., HOWIE, V. M., PLOUSSARD, J. H., HARDING, A. L., AND ANDERSON, P., Studies on the prevalence of antibodies to *Haemophilus influenzae* type b, in: *Haemophilus influenzae* (S. H. SELL AND P. F. WRIGHT, eds.), Elsevier, Amsterdam, 1982.

390. SMITH, E. W. P., JR., AND HAYNES, R. E., Changing incidence of *Haemophilus influenzae* meningitis, *Pediatrics* **50**:723–727 (1972).

391. SMITH, P. F., STRICOF, R. L., SHAYEGANI, M., AND MORSE, D. L., Cluster of *Haemophilus influenzae* type b infections in adults, *J. Am. Med. Assoc.* **260**:1446–1449 (1988).

392. SMITH, W., ANDREWES, C. H., AND LAIDLAW, P. P., A virus obtained from influenza patients, *Lancet* **2**:66–68 (1933).

393. SPANJAARD, L., BOL, P., EKKER, W., AND ZANEN, H. C., The incidence of bacterial meningitis in The Netherlands—a comparison of three registration systems, 1977–1982, *J. Infect.* **11**:259–268 (1985).

394. SPINOLA, S. M., SHEAFFER, C. I., AND GILLIGAN, P. H., Antigenuria after *Haemophilus influenzae* type b polysaccharide vaccination, *J. Pediatr.* **108**:247–248 (1986).

395. SPINOLA, S. M., SHEAFFER, C. I., PHILBIRCK, K. B., AND GILLIGAN, P. H., Antigenuria after *Haemophilus influenzae* type b polysaccharide immunization: A prospective study, *J. Pediatr.* **109**:835–838 (1986).

396. SPROLES, E. T., III, AZERRAD, J., WILLIAMSON, C., AND MERRILL, R. E., Meningitis due to *Haemophilus influenzae:* Long-term sequelae, *J. Pediatr.* **75**:782–788 (1969).

397. STEELE, N. P., MUNSON, R. S., JR., GRANOFF, D. M., CUMMINS, J. E., AND LEVINE, R. P., Antibody-dependent alternative pathway killing of *H. influenzae* type b, *Infect. Immun.* **44**:452–458 (1984).

398. STEPHENSON, W. P., DOERN, G., GANTZ, N., LIPWORTH, L., AND CHAPIN, K., Pharyngeal carriage rates of *Haemophilus influenzae*, type b and non-b, and prevalence of ampicillin-resistant *Haemophilus influenzae* among healthy daycare children in central Massachusetts, *Am. J. Epidemiol.* **122**:868–875 (1985).

399. STULL, T. L., JACOBS, R. F., HAAS, J. E., ROBERTS, M. C., WILSON, C. B., AND SMITH, A. L., Human serum bactericidal activity against *H. influenzae* type b, *J. Gen. Microbiol.* **130**:665–672 (1984).

400. SYRIOPOULOU, V., SCHEIFELE, D., SMITH, A. L., PERRY, P. M., AND HOWIE, V., Increasing incidence of ampicillin resistance in *Haemophilus influenzae, J. Pediatr.* **92**:889–892 (1978).

401. TAI, J. Y., VELLA, P., McLEAN, A. A., *Haemophilus influenzae* type b polysaccharide–protein conjugate vaccine (42460), *Proc. Soc. Exp. Biol. Med.* **184**:154–161 (1987).

402. TAKALA, A. K., VAN ALPHEN, L., ESKOLA, J., PALMGREN, J., BOL, P., AND MAKELA, P. H., *Haemophilus influenzae* type b strains of outer membrane subtypes 1 and 1c cause different types of invasive disease, *Lancet* **2**:647–650 (1987).

403. TARR, P. I., AND PETER, G., Demographic factors in the epidemiology of *Haemophilus influenzae* meningitis in young children, *J. Pediatr.* **92**:884–888 (1978).

404. TARR, P. I., HOSEA, S. W., BROWN, E. J., SCHNEERSON, R., SUTTON, A., AND FRANK, M. M., The requirement of specific anticapsular IgG for killing of *H. influenzae* by the alternative pathway of complement activation, *J. Immunol.* **128**:1772–1775 (1982).

405. TAYLOR, H. G., MICHAELS, R. H., MAZUR, P. M., AND LIDEN, C. B., Intellectual neuropsychological and achievement outcomes in children six to eight years after recovery from *Haemophilus influenzae* meningitis, *Pediatrics* **74:**198–205 (1984).

406. TEJANI, A., MAHADEVAN, R., DOBIAS, B., NANGIA, B., AND WEINER, M., Occurrence of HLA types in *Haemophilus influenzae* type b disease, *Tissue Antigens* **17:**205–211 (1981).

407. TEWARI, R. P., LYNN, M., BIRNBAUM, A. J., AND SOLOTOROVSKY, M., Characterization of the immunoprotective antigen of ribosomal preparations from *Haemophilus influenzae, Infect. Immun.* **19:**58–65 (1978).

408. The Child Day Care Infectious Diseases Study Group, Public health considerations of infectious diseases in child day care centers, *J. Pediatr.* **105:**683–701 (1984).

409. The Meningococcal Disease Study Group, Meningococcal disease: Secondary attack rate and chemoprophylaxis in the United States, 1974, *J. Am. Med. Assoc.* **235:**261–265 (1976).

410. THIRMUMOORTHI, M. C., AND DAJANI, A. S., Comparison of staphylococcal coagglutination, latex agglutination, and counterimmunoelectrophoresis for bacterial antigen detection, *J. Clin. Microbiol.* **9:**28–32 (1979).

411. THOMAS, W. J., MCREYNOLDS, J. W., MOCK, C. R., AND BAILEY, D. W., Ampicillin-resistant *Haemophilus influenzae* meningitis, *Lancet* **1:**313 (1974).

412. TODD, J. K., AND BRUHN, F. W., Severe *Haemophilus influenzae* infections; Spectrum of disease, *Am. J. Dis. Child.* **129:**607–611 (1975).

413. TOLAN, R. W., MUNSON, R. S., AND GRANOFF, D. M., Lipopolysaccharide gel profiles of *Haemophilus influenzae* type b are not stable epidemiologic markers, *J. Clin. Microbiol.* **24:**223–227 (1986).

414. TOMEH, M. O., STARR, S. E., MCGOWAN, J. E., JR., TERRY, P. M., AND NAHMIAS, A. J., Ampicillin-resistant *Haemophilus influenzae* type b infection, *J. Am. Med. Assoc.* **229:**295–297 (1974).

415. TOSI, M. F., KAPLAN, S. L., MASON, E. O., BUFFORE, G. J., AND ANDERSON, O. C., Generation of chemotactic activity in serum by *H. influenzae* type b, *Infect. Immun.* **43:**593–599 (1984).

416. TROLLFORS, B., CLAESSON, B. A., STRANGERT, K., AND TARANGER, J., *Haemophilus influenzae* meningitis in Sweden, 1981–1983, *Arch. Dis. Child.* **62:**1220–1223 (1987).

417. TURK, D. C., Naso-pharyngeal carriage of *H. influenzae* type B, *J. Hyg.* **61:**247–256 (1963).

418. TURK, D. C., Ampicillin-resistant *Haemophilus influenzae* meningitis, *Lancet* **1:**453 (1974).

419. TURK, D. C., An investigation of the family background of acute *Haemophilus* infections in children, *J. Hyg.* **75:**315–332 (1975).

420. TURK, D. C., Clinical importance of *Haemophilus influenzae*—1981, in: *Haemophilus influenzae* (S. H. SELL AND P. F. WRIGHT, eds.), pp. 3–9, Elsevier, Amsterdam, 1982.

421. TURNER, R. B., HAYDEN, F. G., AND HENDLEY, J. O.,

Counterimmunoelectrophoresis of urine for diagnosis of bacterial pneumonia in pediatric outpatients, *Pediatrics* **71:**780–783 (1983).

422. UCHIYAMA, N., GREENE, G. R., KITTS, D. R., AND THRUPP, L. D., Meningitis due to *Haemophilus influenzae* type b resistant to ampicillin and chloramphenicol, *J. Pediatr.* **97:**421–424 (1980).

423. VALMARI, P., KATAJA, M., AND PELTOLA, H., Invasive *Haemophilus influenzae* and meningococcal infections in Finland, *Scand. J. Infect. Dis.* **19:**19–27 (1987).

424. VARAGHESE, P., *Haemophilus influenzae* infection, in Canada, 1969–1985, *Can. Dis. Weekly Rep.* **12:**37–43 (1986).

425. VIENNY, H., DESPLAND, P. A., LUTSCHG, J., DEONNA, T., DUTOIT-MARCO, M. L., AND GANDER, C., Early diagnosis and evaluation of deafness in childhood bacterial meningitis: A study using brainstem auditory evoked potentials, *Pediatrics* **73:**579–586 (1984).

426. WAHDAN, M. H., RIZK, F., EL-AKKAD, A. M., GHOROURY, A. A., HABLAS, R., GIRGIS, N. T., AMER, A., BOCTOR, W., SIPPEL, J. E., GOTSCHLICH, E. C., TRIAV, R., SANBORN, A. R., AND CVETANOVIK, B., A controlled field trial of a serogroup A meningococcal polysaccharide vaccine, *Bull. WHO* **48:**667–673 (1973).

427. WALL, R. A., MABEY, D. C. W., AND CORRAH, P. T., *Haemophilus influenzae* non-type b, *Lancet* **2:**845 (1985).

428. WALLACE, R. J., BAKER, C. J., QUINONES, F. J., HOLLIS, D. G., WEAVER, R. C., AND WISS, K., Nontypable *Haemophilus influenzae* (biotype 4) as a neonatal, maternal, and genital pathogen, *Rev. Infect. Dis.* **5:**123–136 (1983).

429. WARD, H. K., AND FOTHERGILL, L. D., Influenzal meningitis treated with specific antiserum and complement: Report of 5 cases, *Am. J. Dis. Child.* **43:**873–881 (1932).

430. WARD, J. I., Is *Haemophilus influenzae* type b disease preventable? *J. Am. Med. Assoc.* **253:**554–556 (1985).

431. WARD, J., AND SMITH, A. L., *Hemophilus influenzae* bacteremia in children with sickle cell disease, *J. Pediatr.* **88:**261–262 (1976).

432. WARD, J. I., SIBER, G. R., SCHEIFELE, D. W., AND SMITH, D. H., Rapid diagnosis of *Haemophilus influenzae* type b infections by latex particle agglutination and counterimmunoelectrophoresis, *J. Pediatr.* **93:**37–43 (1978).

433. WARD, J. I., TSAI, T. F., FILICE, G. A., AND FRASER, D. W., Prevalence of ampicillin- and chloramphenicol-resistant strains of *Haemophilus influenzae* causing meningitis and bacteremia: National survey of hospital laboratories, *J. Infect. Dis.* **138:**421–424 (1978).

434. WARD, J. I., FRASER, D. W., BARAFF, L. J., AND PLIKAYTIS, B. D., *Haemophilus influenzae* meningitis: A national study of secondary spread in household contacts, *N. Engl. J. Med.* **301:**122–126 (1979).

435. WARD, J. I., LUM, M. K., MARGOLIS, H. S., FRASER, D. W., AND BENDER, T. R., *Haemophilus influenzae* disease in Alaskan Eskimos: Characteristics of a population with an unusual incidence of invasive disease, *Lancet* **1:**1281–1285 (1982).

436. WARD, J. I., LUM, M. K. W., AND BENDER, T. R., *Haemo-*

philus influenzae disease in Alaska: Epidemiologic, clinical, and serologic studies of a population at high risk of invasive disease, in: *Haemophilus influenzae* (S. H. SELL AND P. F. WRIGHT, eds.), pp. 23–34, Elsevier, Amsterdam, 1982.

437. WARD, J., BERKOWITZ, C., PESCETTI, J., BURKART, K., SAMUELSON, J., AND GORDON, L., Enhanced immunogenicity in young infants of a new *Haemophilus influenzae* type b (Hib) capsular polysaccharide (PRP)–diphtheria toxoid (D) conjugate vaccine, *Pediatr. Res.* **18**:287A (1984).

438. WARD, J. I., LUM, M. K. W., HALL, D. B., SILIMPERI, D. R., AND BENDER, T. R., Invasive *H. influenzae* type b disease in Alaska: Background epidemiology for a vaccine efficacy trial, *J. Infect. Dis.* **108**:887–896 (1986).

439. WARD, J. I., BRENNEMAN, G., LETSON, G., HEYWARD, W., AND ALASKA VACCINE EFFICACY TRIAL STUDY GROUP, Limited protective efficacy of an *H. influenzae* type b conjugate vaccine (PRP-D) in Native Alaskan infants immunized at 2, 4, and 6 months of age, Program and abstracts of the 28th Interscience Conference on Antimicrobial Agents and Chemotherapy, Los Angeles, 1988.

440. WARD, J. I., BROOME, C. V., HARRISON, L. H., SHINEFIELD, H. R., AND BLACK, S. B., *Haemophilus influenzae* type b vaccines: Lessons for the future, *Pediatrics* **81**:886–892 (1988).

441. WARD, J. I., GREENBERG, D. P., ANDERSON, P. W., BURKART, K. S., CHRISTENSON, P. D., GORDON, L. K., KAYHTY, H., KUO, J. S. C., AND VELLA, P., Variable quantitation of *H. influenzae* type b anticapsular antibody by radioantigen binding assay, *J. Clin. Microbiol.* **26**:72–78 (1988).

442. WASILAUSKAS, B. L., AND HAMPTON, K. D., Determination of bacterial meningitis: A retrospective study of 80 cerebrospinal fluid specimens evaluated by four in vitro methods, *J. Clin. Microbiol.* **16**:531–535 (1982).

443. WEINBERG, G. A., AND GRANOFF, D. M., Polysaccharide–protein conjugate vaccines for the prevention of *Haemophilus influenzae* type b disease, *J. Pediatr.* **113**:621–631 (1988).

444. WEISMAN, S. J., CATES, K. L., ALLEGRETTA, G. J., QUIN, J. J., AND ALTMAN, A. J., Antibody response to immunization with *Haemophilus influenzae* type b polysaccharide vaccine in children with cancer, *J. Pediatr.* **111**:727–729 (1987).

445. WEITZMAN, S., AND AISENBERG, A. C., Fulminant sepsis after the successful treatment of Hodgkin's disease, *Am. J. Med.* **62**:47–50 (1977).

446. WELCH, D. F., AND HENSEL, D., Evaluation of Bactogen and Phadebact for detection of *Haemophilus influenzae* type b antigen in cerebrospinal fluid, *J. Clin. Microbiol.* **16**:905–908 (1982).

447. WELKON, C. J., LONG, S. S., FISHER, M. C., AND ALBURGER, P. D., Pyogenic arthritis in infants and children: A review of 95 cases, *Pediatr. Infect. Dis. J.* **5**:669–676 (1986).

448. WELLER, P., SMITH, A. L., ANDERSON, P., AND SMITH, D. H., The role of encapsulation and host age in the clearance of *H. influenzae* bacteremia, *J. Infect. Dis.* **138**:427–436 (1978).

449. WELLER, P., SMITH, A. L., SMITH, D. H., AND ANDERSON, P., Role of immunity in the clearance of bacteremia due to *H. influenzae*, *J. Infect. Dis.* **135**:34–41 (1977).

450. WENGER, J. D., HIGHTOWER, A. W., HARRISON, L. H., BROOME, C. F., AND THE HAEMOPHILUS INFLUENZAE STUDY GROUP, Use of discharge codes for detection of *Haemophilus influenzae* disease [abstract], Program and abstracts of the Twenty-eighth Interscience Conference on Antimicrobial Agents and Chemotherapy, Los Angeles, 1988.

451. WHISNANT, J. K., MANN, D. L., ROGENTINE, G. N., AND ROBBINS, J. B., Human cell-surface structures related to *Haemophilus influenzae* type b disease, *Lancet* **2**:895–898 (1971).

452. WHISNANT, J. K., ROGENTINE, G. N., GRALNICK, M. A., SCHLESSELMAN, J. J., AND ROBBINS, J. B., Host factors and antibody response in *Haemophilus influenzae* type b meningitis and epiglottitis, *J. Infect. Dis.* **133**:448–455 (1976).

453. WILLIAMS, C. L., BARNES, L., AND KUO, J. S. C., Clinical studies of an *Haemophilus influenzae* type b PRP vaccine with a *Bordetella pertussis* adjuvant in infants, in: *Haemophilus influenzae* (S. H. SELL AND P. F. WRIGHT, eds.), pp. 285–295, Elsevier, Amsterdam, 1982.

454. WILLIAMS, C. L., LEE, A. C., AND CURRAN, A. S., Prevention of meningitis in a day-care center: Management of an outbreak of *Haemophilus influenzae* type b, *Prev. Med.* **16**:261–268 (1987).

455. WILLIAMS, J. D., AND CAVANAGH, P., Ampicillin-resistant *Haemophilus influenzae* meningitis, *Lancet* **1**:864 (1974).

456. WINKELSTEIN, J. A., AND MOXON, E. R., Role of complement in the host's defense against *H. influenzae*, in: *Haemophilus influenzae* (S. H. SELL AND P. F. WRIGHT, eds.), Elsevier, Amsterdam, 1982.

457. WINSLOW, C. E., BROADHURST, J., BUCHANAN, R. E., KRUMWIEDE, C., JR., ROGERS, L. A., AND SMITH, G. H., The families and genera of the bacteria: Final report of the committee of the Society of American Bacteriologists on characterization and classification of bacterial types, *J. Bacteriol.* **5**:191–229 (1920).

458. WOLFF, A. B., AND BROWN, S. C., Demographics of meningitis-induced hearing impairment: Implications for immunization of children against *Hemophilus influenzae* type b, *Am. Ann. Deaf* **132**:26–30 (1987).

459. WOOD, P. R., MCKEE, K. T., LOHR, J. A., AND HENDLEY, J. O., *Haemophilus influenzae* meningitis in school-aged children, *J. Am. Med. Assoc.* **247**:1162–1163 (1982).

460. World Health Organization, *Weekly Epidem. Rec.* **60**:146–147 (1985).

461. WOTTON, K. A., STIVER, H. G., AND HILDES, J. A., Meningitis in the central Arctic: A 4-year experience, *Can. Med. Assoc. J.* **124**:887–890 (1981).

462. WRIGHT, P. F., Acute bacterial meningitis in developing countries, Unpublished WHO document, EPI/RD/88/WP.5, Geneva (1988).

463. YEUNG, S., PANG, G., CRIPPS, A. W., CLANCY, R. L., AND WLODARCZYK, J. H., Efficacy of oral immunization against non-typable *Haemophilus influenzae* in man, *Int. J. Immunopharmacol.* **9**:283–288 (1987).

464. YOGEV, R., LANDER, H. B., AND DAVIS, A. T., Effect of TMP-SMX on nasopharyngeal carriage of ampicillin-sensitive and ampicillin-resistant *Hemophilus influenzae* type b, *J. Pediatr.* **93:**394–397 (1978).

465. YOGEV, R., LANDER, H. B., AND DAVIS, A. T., Effect of rifampin on nasopharyngeal carriage of *Haemophilus influenzae* type b, *J. Pediatr.* **94:**840–841 (1979).

466. YOGEV, R., MELICK, C., AND GLOGOWSKI, W., In vitro development of rifampin resistance in clinical isolates of *Haemophilus influenzae* type b, *Antimicrob. Agents Chemother.* **21:**387–389 (1982).

467. YOGEV, R., MELICK, C., AND KABAT, K., Nasopharyngeal carriage of *Haemophilus influenzae* type b: Attempted eradication by cefaclor or rifampin, *Pediatrics* **67:**430–433 (1981).

468. YOST, G. C., KAPLAN, A. M., BUSTAMANTE, R., ELLISON, C., HARGRAVE, A. F., AND RANDALL, D. L., Bacterial meningitis in Arizona American Indian children, *Am. J. Dis. Child.* **140:**943–946 (1986).

469. ZAHRADNIK, J. M., AND GORDON, L. K., Augmented antibody (Ab) responses in infants administered a new *H. influenzae* type b capsular polysaccharide (PRP) diphtheria toxoid conjugate vaccine (PRP-D), *Pediatr. Res.* **18:**289A (1984).

470. ZARKOWSKY, H. S., GALLAGHER, D., GILL, F. M., WANG, W. C., FALLETTA, J. M., LANDE, W. M., LEVY, P. S., VERTER, J. I., WETHERS, D., AND THE COOPERATIVE STUDY OF SICKLE CELL DISEASE, Bacteremia in sickle hemoglobinopathies, *J. Pediatr.* **109:**579–585 (1986).

471. ZON, G., AND ROBBINS, J. D., ^{31}P- and ^{13}C-N.M.R.-Spectral and chemical characterization of the end-group and repeating-unit components of oligosaccharides derived by acid hydrolysis of *Haemophilus influenzae* type b capsular polysaccharide. *Carbohydr. Res.* **114:**103–121 (1983).

12. Suggested Reading

Haemophilus influenzae: Epidemiology, Immunology, and Prevention of Disease (S. H. SELL AND P. F. WRIGHT, eds.), Elsevier, Amsterdam, 1982.

MENDELMAN, P. M., AND SMITH, A. L., *Haemophilus influenzae,* in: *Textbook of Pediatric Infectious Diseases,* 2nd ed. (R. D. FEIGIN AND J. D. CHERRY, eds.), pp. 1142–1163, Saunders, Philadelphia, 1987.

Proceedings of a roundtable, *Haemophilus influenzae* type b: The disease and its prevention, *Pediatr. Infect. Dis. J.* **6:**773–807 (1987).

WEINBERG, G. A., AND GRANOFF, D. M., Polysaccharide–protein conjugate vaccines for the prevention of *Haemophilus influenzae* type b disease, *J. Pediatr.* **113:**621–631 (1988).

CHAPTER 15

Legionellosis

David W. Fraser

1. Introduction

Legionellosis is an acute human infection commonly manifested as pneumonia and caused by any of several species of *Legionella*, including *L. pneumophila, L. bozemanii, L. micdadei, L. dumoffii, L. longbeachae, L. jordanis, L. wadsworthii, L. feeleii, L. maceachernii, L. hackeliae, L. gormanii, L. oakridgensis, L. sainthelensi, L. anisa, L. jamestownensis, L. rubrilucens, L. erythra, L. spiritensis, L. parisiensis, L. cherrii, L. steigerwaltii, L. santicrucis,* and *L. israelensis,* all of which are fastidious gram-negative bacilli and the first ten of which have been confirmed by culture to cause disease in humans.[13] Occurring in clusters and sporadically, the long-incubation-period pneumonic form (Legionnaires' disease) is frequently mistaken for "viral pneumonia," which may be a serious error, because specific therapy may prevent death. Nonpneumonic, short-incubation-period legionellosis (Pontiac fever) may also occur in clusters, but this syndrome appears to be self-limited.

2. Historical Background

The Pennsylvania Department of the American Legion held its annual convention in Philadelphia on July 21–24, 1976, with headquarters in the Bellevue-Stratford Hotel. Over the next 4 weeks, 221 persons who had attended the convention or had been in or near this hotel developed pneu-

monia or other febrile respiratory disease, and 34 died.[36] The cause of the explosive outbreak of this disease—which was dubbed Legionnaires' disease—was unknown and remained so for 5 months despite an intensive epidemiological and laboratory investigation. Early in 1977, McDade and co-workers reported using rickettsialogical technique to recover a fastidious gram-negative rod, *Legionella pneumophila*,[14] from lung tissue of patients who had died of the disease and showed that other patients had a specific antibody response to the organism during convalescence.[63] Results of antibody tests on paired serum specimens that had been stored for several years in the Serum Bank at the Centers for Disease Control (CDC) showed that the same organism, or an antigenically similar one, had caused outbreaks in 1965 in a hospital in Washington, D.C.,[101] and in 1968 in a health department building in Pontiac, Michigan,[39] both of which had been investigated intensively at the time but for which no cause had been found. Lung tissue from guinea pigs that had been exposed to air in the health department building in Pontiac in 1968 and developed pneumonia yielded *L. pneumophila* a decade later.[52] A third outbreak that had been investigated inconclusively at the time, in 1957, was shown to be Legionnaires' disease by serological testing of blood from cases and controls redrawn 22 years later.[76] McDade *et al.*[64] also showed that *L. pneumophila* was identical to a "*Rickettsia*-like" organism that had been isolated in 1947 in guinea pigs that had been inoculated with blood of a patient with a febrile illness. In 1978, Morris *et al.*[69] recovered *L. pneumophila* from various environmental specimens in conjunction with investigations of outbreaks that year. Air-conditioning cooling towers and evaporative condensers were implicated as sources of dissemination of *L. pneumophila* in

David W. Fraser · Office of the President, Swarthmore College, Swarthmore, Pennsylvania 19081.

outbreaks in Pontiac in 1968[39] and in Memphis in 1978.[27]

In 1980 Tobin and colleagues isolated the same serogroup of *L. pneumophila* from two people who developed *Legionella* pneumonia after receiving renal homografts in an un-air-conditioned Oxford hospital and from water taken from the shower in their common hospital room.[103] This observation opened up a fruitful line of investigation regarding the role of potable water systems in the dissemination of *Legionella*.

Two of the other 22 recognized *Legionella* species had been isolated but only partially characterized prior to 1976. Tatlock isolated a "rickettsia-like" organism from the blood of a soldier at Fort Bragg, North Carolina, in 1943.[99] Subsequent studies showed that it was identical to the Pittsburgh Pneumonia Agent described by Pasculle *et al.*[78] and it has been named *L. micdadei*.[42] Bozeman isolated a similar organism from lung tissue of a scuba diver in 1959[11]; it has been named *L. bozemanii*.[15]

3. Methodology

3.1. Sources of Mortality Data

Data regarding mortality from legionellosis have been systematically sought in one multicity survey of fatal sporadic nosocomial *L. pneumophila* pneumonia, in several autopsy surveys of one or more hospitals in a city, and in conjunction with several investigations of epidemics. The data from the study of nosocomial pneumonia permit an estimate of disease incidence that is limited by the nonrandom selection of hospitals surveyed and by the broad confidence limits on estimates of the proportion of *L. pneumophila* pneumonia cases that are nosocomial.[21] The search of autopsy material as a case-finding tool in epidemic investigations has been useful only in defining the magnitude of the individual outbreaks. Direct immunofluorescence has been the technique usually used to test postmortem lung tissue, with or without initial screening by routine histopathology to define areas of suspected pneumonia.[20] The fluorescein-labeled antiserum used in direct immunofluorescence testing is specific to the serogroups and species used to immunize donor animals, so the sensitivity of direct immunofluorescence testing is affected by the reagents used. Cherry *et al.*[20] showed that few bacteria cross-react with the *L. pneumophila* serogroup 1 antiserum, and in limited blind testing of lung tissue from persons with serogroup 1 *L. pneumophila* pneumonia or those with pneumonia caused by other gram-negative rods, they easily dif-

ferentiated the serogroup 1 organisms from the others with direct immunofluorescence.

3.2. Sources of Morbidity Data

Only fragmentary data are available on the incidence of legionellosis in the general population. The most reliable information comes from the testing of paired sera obtained in a study that Foy *et al.*[34] carried out on pneumonia patients in a prepaid-medical-care program in Washington. However, that study used reagents for *L. pneumophila* only. Furthermore, the focal nature of legionellosis precludes generalizing these results for the entire country. Results of testing serum pairs submitted to the CDC from patients with pneumonia in many states showed seroconversion to serogroup 1 *L. pneumophila* in 0.3–1.5%[35,63]; however, selection biases that determine which patients will have paired sera drawn and submitted cannot be measured.

One prospective study of nosocomial pneumonia, in the absence of a known outbreak of legionellosis, has been done, although it included only one hospital.[71]

National surveillance of legionellosis has been conducted with varying intensity in different countries. In the United States, formal surveillance began in 1979. The CDC has encouraged state health departments to submit specimens for diagnosis of legionellosis, and has widely distributed diagnostic reagents.

3.3. Surveys

The indirect fluorescent-antibody (IFA) test has been used most widely in serological surveys, although other methods, including hemagglutination, indirect hemagglutination, immune adherence, microagglutination test, and ELISA, have also been used. The existence of at least 12 serogroups of *L. pneumophila* and two serogroups each of *L. longbeachae*, *L. bozemanii*, *L. feeleii*, and *L. hackeliae*,[13,102] the differences in methods of preparing test antigens, the problems of specificity of "antibody" in the IFA test (especially of low titers, i.e., < 1:64), and possible cross-reactions with *Mycoplasma pneumoniae*, rickettsia, and other organisms make the interpretation of serological surveys difficult at this time. Wide variations that may be related to variations in the test procedures have been encountered in the prevalence of antibody in healthy populations from the United States and England.

The prevalence of seropositivity to *L. pneumophila* in the general population has been estimated on the basis of surveying adults participating in A/New Jersey/76 influenza vaccination trials in the District of Columbia, Georgia, Texas, and New York.[97] IFA titers of 128 or higher have tentatively been considered evidence of prior *L. pneumophila* infection, but the specificity of single titers has not been proved.

The possibility of secondary spread of legionellosis has been assessed by interviewing household contacts[36,39] and by serosurveying hospital contacts and controls,[89] as well as by clinical and laboratory investigation of illness in contacts of patients.

The frequency with which legionellosis can occur as an asymptomatic or subclinical infection has been estimated by testing paired serum specimens from well, exposed persons[28,66,116] in conjunction with outbreak investigations.

Case data have been compared with control data in both questionnaire and medical-record surveys to determine host factors and activities that affected the risk of sporadic[96] and epidemic[5,27,36,38,39,41,45,53,90,91,101] disease.

3.4. Laboratory Diagnosis

3.4.1. Isolation and Identification.
Legionellae have been recovered from respiratory secretions, pleural fluid, lung tissue, and blood of patients with pneumonia.[63] Successful techniques have included intraperitoneal inoculation of guinea pigs and direct plating on nonliving media that contain supplementary L-cysteine and ferric salts, such as buffered charcoal–yeast extract (CYE) agar with or without supplemental α-ketoglutarate[84]; growth is best at pH 6.9–7.0. The failure of legionellae to grow on blood agar can help in identifying the bacterium. Inoculated plates should be incubated at 35°C for at least 10 days. On CYE agar, growth of *L. pneumophila* may be evident in 2–4 days and colonies may be as large as 1–2 mm in diameter. Colonies have a ground-glass appearance. The sensitivity of CYE agar in culturing *L. pneumophila* may be 56–80%.[30,117]

L. pneumophila and the other legionellae are weakly staining, gram-negative, aerobic, non-spore-forming unencapsulated rods, commonly 0.3–0.9 μm wide and 2–3 μm long, although filamentous forms 20 μm or more long have been observed.[13] Polar or lateral flagella can be demonstrated except for *L. oakridgensis*. They are oxidase-negative or weakly positive, nitrate-negative, and urease-negative. Most species liquefy gelatin. Carbohydrates are not fermented or oxidized. Branched-chain fatty acids predominate in the cell wall. Legionellae contain major amounts of ubiquinones with more than ten isoprene units in the side chain. Specific identification is made typically by direct immunofluorescence using monoclonal or polyclonal reagents or with a radiolabeled DNA probe.[111] Studying

ribosomal RNA, Brenner has shown legionellae to be related most closely to the purple sulfur bacteria and their relatives, including Enterobacteriaceae, Vibrionaceae, and fluorescent pseudomonads.[13] Twenty-three species of *Legionella* have been described, including five with multiple serogroups: *L. pneumophila*—12, *L. longbeachae*—2, *L. bozemanii*—2, *L. feeleii*—2, and *L. hackeliae*—2.[13,102]

3.4.2. Serological and Immunological Diagnostic Methods.
Serological diagnosis is usually based on results of IFA testing with heat-killed or formalin-treated whole bacterial cells as antigen.[29,30,110] A fourfold or greater rise in titer to 128 or higher to the heat-killed antigen commonly occurs by the 21st day of illness,[63] although seroconversions may not occur until the 6th week.[29] Of the patients with epidemiologically defined cases in the 1976 Philadelphia outbreak, 87% had IFA titers of 128 or higher to the Philadelphia 1 or 2 strains responsible for the outbreak in sera obtained 3 weeks or longer after onset of symptoms.[63] Modification of the IFA since the original report has not much affected sensitivity.[109] IFA titers are often serogroup-specific, although the sera of some patients react more broadly than those of others.[108] Rises of fourfold in immunofluorescence titer to *L. pneumophila* have been observed on single patients with plague, tularemia,[104] and *Bacteroides fragilis* bacteremia, and rises in titer to *L. pneumophila* have been observed in patients with rising titers to *M. pneumoniae*,[39,104] *Rickettsia rickettsii*, and *Leptospira interrogans*. Only 1 of 87 serum pairs from patients ill during outbreaks of tularemia, psittacosis, *Mycoplasma* pneumonia, or Q fever showed a fourfold or higher titer rise to 128 or higher to a polyvalent (serogroups 1–4) *L. pneumophila* antigen.[107] The sensitivity of ELISA for detection of seroconversion to *L. pneumophila* serogroups 1–6 in persons with culture-proven infection has been reported to be 78%, but the specificity is not well defined.[117] The sensitivity and specificity of other serological tests for legionellosis are not well known. It should be stressed that experience with serological testing for legionellae other than *L. pneumophila* serogroup 1 is extremely limited with any method including IFA.

Direct immunofluorescence can be used not only to detect legionellae in lung tissue postmortem as noted in Section 3.1, but also to identify organisms in respiratory secretions or lung tissue obtained by biopsy. Lung-tissue specimens are best prepared by scraping wet, formalin-fixed tissue with a scalpel blade and staining the smeared scrapings,[20] although fresh tissue and paraffin-embedded tissue can be used. The sensitivity of this technique may approach 75% in patients whose respiratory secretions are processed expeditiously,[29] although some have reported much lower sensitivity.[116] Direct immunofluorescence testing is species- and serogroup-specific unless a polyvalent conjugated antiserum is used, and may miss organisms for which corresponding conjugated antisera are not used.

ELISA and radioimmunoassay have been used to detect *Legionella* antigen in patients' urine. Sensitivity of 80% and specificity of 99.6% have been observed.[54] The development of an ELISA that uses a polyvalent antiserum may make urinary antigen detection more broadly useful.[98]

4. Biological Characteristics of the Organism

Ultrastructurally, legionellae resemble typical gram-negative bacilli, with a double envelope of unit membrane and no evident cell wall.[19] Legionellae have several characteristics that may contribute to their pathogenicity. Macrophages readily phagocytose *L. pneumophila*, by a distinctive mechanism,[47] but once inside the bacteria can multiply and kill the macrophage.[48] *L. pneumophila* can multiply in *Tetrahymena* and certain free-living amoebae.[6] In humans, its intracellular location may complicate antibiotic therapy. In nature, its intracellular location may provide it important nutrients.

Several toxins have been demonstrated in *L. pneumophila* including proteases,[24,86] endotoxin, and, shared with *L. micdadei*, a 3400-dalton protein that is lethal to AKR/J mice. Which, if any, of these contributes to the pathogenesis of legionellosis is unknown.

Skaliy and McEachern[93] showed that *L. pneumophila* survives several months in distilled water and over a year in tapwater held at room temperature. On agar, the organism grows most rapidly at 35°C and only very slowly at 25°C. Growth is enhanced by the presence, in moderate concentrations, of iron, zinc, and potassium[95] and by constituents of rubber,[75] as may be found in plumbing systems.

In aerosols, *L. pneumophila* dies rapidly under conditions of low atmospheric humidity; survival is much improved with the addition of an extract of blue-green algae growth medium or of 2,2'-dipyridyl, which sequesters certain cations. Growth on agar is also favored by a high water content.

Several disinfectants in concentrations commonly used in the hospital appear to inhibit growth of *L. pneumophila*, including phenolics, iodophors, quaternary ammonium compounds, glutaraldehyde, formalin, calcium hypochlorite, and ethanol.[107]

5. Descriptive Epidemiology

5.1. Prevalence and Incidence

No firm estimates of the national incidence of legionellosis are available. In a prepaid-medical-care group in Washington, the incidence of *L. pneumophila* pneumonia confirmed as Legionnaires' disease by IFA test using a serogroup 1 antigen was 12/100,000 population per year (1.0% of all patients with pneumonia whose serum pairs were tested).[34] In Nottingham, England, the incidence has been estimated as 2/100,000 per year.[67] Of two catch samples of serum pairs submitted to the CDC from various states for serological diagnosis of pneumonia, seroconversion to *L. pneumophila* was found in 0.3% (from Connecticut, Ohio, Florida, Delaware, New Jersey, and Maryland)[35] and in 1.5% (from all states).[63] To the degree that these pneumonia cases are representative of all those in the United States, which occur at a rate of approximately 1300/100,000 population per year, the incidence of pneumonia due to *L. pneumophila* might be estimated as 4–20 cases/100,000 per year. However, catch samples of sera from pneumonia patients have varied widely in evidencing Legionnaires' disease, making extrapolations imprecise. As an example, Renner *et al.*[85] found that 4.5% of the sera sent to the Iowa State Health Department for testing seroconverted to *L. pneumophila*, third in frequency to *M. pneumoniae* (10.2%) and influenza A (5.8%).

In direct immunofluorescence tests of autopsy tissue, Cohen *et al.*[21] observed that 10 (3.8%) of 263 fatal cases of nosocomial pneumonia were *L. pneumophila* pneumonia of serogroup 1. These included 7.7% in which no other pathogen had been identified, 2.4% in which another pathogen had been identified, and 3.5% in which no attempt had been made to identify another pathogen. They extrapolated that 950 cases of fatal nosocomial *L. pneumophila* serogroup 1 pneumonia occur yearly in the United States. Nosocomial cases appear to occur more commonly among immunosuppressed patients than do community-acquired cases, and the case-fatality rate in immunosuppressed patients is high,[16] making it difficult to extrapolate such a datum to the national mortality or incidence of all legionellosis cases.

As judged by diagnostic specimens tested at CDC, *L. pneumophila* accounts for about 85% of cases of legionellosis, *L. micdadei* 6%, and *L. bozemanii* 3%, with perhaps *L. dumoffii* and *L. longbeachae* next most common.[83] Of *L. pneumophila* cases, the most common causative serogroups are serogroup 1 (61%), serogroup 6 (14%), and serogroup 2 (6%).[83]

The prevalence of antibody to *L. pneumophila* has been measured in many apparently healthy populations. IFA titers of 128 or higher have been found in from less than 1% to more than 30%[10] of those tested. Whether single titers of 128 or higher by the IFA test represent recent or past infection with *L. pneumophila* or reflect antibody to cross-reactive organisms is not known, so it is difficult to estimate the prevalence of *L. pneumophila* infection on the basis of such surveys.

5.2. Epidemic Behavior and Contagiousness

Disease caused by *L. pneumophila* has occurred repeatedly in explosive common-source outbreaks that have continued for a few days or a few weeks.[5,16,27, 33,36,39,53,76,101] Outbreaks of disease caused by *L. micdadei, L. feeleii, L. bozemanii,* and *L. dumoffii* have also been identified.[28,45,50,77] In outbreaks of Legionnaires' disease, attack rates have generally averaged 0.1–5% of those exposed, in sharp contrast to the outbreaks of Pontiac fever, in which the attack rate has been 46–100%.[37,39,45] Pontiac fever also differs from Legionnaires' disease in that the incubation period is short and pneumonia is absent (see Sections 7 and 8.1). In outbreaks of legionellosis, the risk of illness has often been directly associated more with time spent in the area of apparent exposure than with specific activities of people within that area. Outbreaks have ranged in size up to several hundred cases.[91] Many of the outbreaks of legionellosis have been associated with buildings or institutions—including hotels,[5,36,87,90] hospitals,[16,27,28,33,53,77,101] factories,[45,76] and a health department building[39]—but since outbreaks are more likely to be recognized if a large number of people are affected, a selection bias may overemphasize the association with public buildings.

Recurrent outbreaks have been reported in several hotels[7,36,82,87,100] and hospitals,[28,53] suggesting persistence of *L. pneumophila* in some locations. This phenomenon is perhaps best demonstrated by the continuing occurrence of cases of Legionnaires' disease for more than 1 year among patients and staff at a hospital in Los Angeles[91] and at a rate of approximately 0.5%.

There is no convincing evidence that *Legionella* is spread from person to person. Interviews of 193 household contacts of persons with Legionnaires' disease in the 1976 outbreak in Philadelphia disclosed none who developed an illness suggestive of secondary spread (pneumonia or temperature of 102°F or higher and cough) in the subsequent 3 weeks.[36] No secondary clinical cases were observed in hospital staff members in contact with the patients. Since

that time, several anecdotes of illness in case contacts, apparently not exposed to the source of infection of the index case, have been noted, but none have been confirmed serologically. Saravolatz *et al.*[89] reported that the hospital staff members who had direct or indirect contact with persons with Legionnaires' disease had a higher prevalence (9.3%) of serum antibody titers of 128 or higher as measured by hemagglutination than did staff members without known exposure (3.7%), although seropositivity was not related to the intensity of exposure to the patient with Legionnaires' disease. Yu and colleagues found no instances of seroconversion to *L. pneumophila* in 17 household contacts of community-acquired cases or 15 hospital roommates of nosocomial cases.[116] The presence of *L. pneumophila* in respiratory secretions raises the possibility that person-to-person spread may occur, but it must be very rare if it occurs at all.

5.3. Geographic Distribution

Disease caused by *L. pneumophila* has been found essentially wherever it has been sought. Confirmed cases have occurred in every state and the District of Columbia in the United States[57] and in the rest of North America, South America, Europe, Asia, and Oceania. Rates of documented cases by state largely reflect the levels of interest in submitting serum specimens for IFA testing.

The distribution of disease caused by other legionellae is not well defined, although two outbreaks (of disease caused by *L. dumoffii* and *L. feeleii*) have been documented in Canada.[45,50]

5.4. Temporal Distribution

There is no evidence that legionellosis is of recent origin. Although first identified as a cause of human disease in 1976, *L. pneumophila* has retrospectively been shown to be the "*Rickettsia-* like" organism isolated in 1947 by inoculating a guinea pig with blood from a febrile patient.[11,64] *L. micdadei* was first isolated from a patient in 1943[99] and *L. bozemanii* in 1959.[11] No systematic studies have been done to allow the assessment of secular trends in the incidence of disease.

Discrete common-source outbreaks of legionellosis cluster from July to September. This clustering is seen both in outbreaks in which air-conditioning systems are implicated and in those in which such systems are not. Information on the seasonal distribution of sporadic cases is still preliminary, but rates appear to peak from June to October and to be lowest from January to March,[57,115] although cases in Scotland are reported to peak in November.[31] Presumably the seasonality of outbreaks related to air-conditioning systems reflects the usage of air-conditioning, but whether the seasonality of other cases results from changes in the ecology of *L. pneumophila* or from variations in man's interaction with his environment is unknown. In either case, the seasonality differs sufficiently from that associated with many other common bacterial and viral pneumonias that Legionnaires' disease should be suspected any time an adult has pneumonia in the summer or autumn.

5.5. Age

The great majority of confirmed cases of Legionnaires' disease have occurred in middle-aged or elderly adults. The risk of disease appears to increase with age,[36] but this observation may be confounded by the role of underlying medical conditions in predisposing to legionellosis[16,96] (see Section 5.11.3).

Few cases in children have been identified. In the 1976 outbreak in Philadelphia, a 3-year-old boy who attended the convention with his parents developed pneumonia and seroconverted to *L. pneumophila*.[36] A survey of 55 children with pneumonia at St. Jude Children's Hospital, Memphis, Tennessee, showed 1 who seroconverted to *L. pneumophila*—a 2-year-old boy with acute lymphocytic leukemia and community-acquired pneumonia.[88] Seroconversion to *L. pneumophila* occurs frequently during early childhood, but is not often accompanied by notable respiratory disease; whether this represents infection with *L. pneumophila* or some cross-reacting agent is unknown.[1] To date, there is no good information on the percentage of those infected at different ages who develop clinical illness.

5.6. Sex

In confirmed sporadic cases[57] and in most outbreaks,[16,36,100] the attack rate for men has been two to four times that for women, although exceptions have been observed.[87] Serosurveys of well people have generally not shown differences in the prevalences of elevated titers to *L. pneumophila* measured for men and women.[97] The manifestations and severity of the disease have not been shown to differ between the sexes.

5.7. Race

One study suggests that the risk of sporadic, community-acquired *L. pneumophila* pneumonia is 14-fold higher for blacks than for whites,[96] but the proportion of blacks asso-

ciated with sporadic cases of Legionnaires' disease reported to the CDC is 11%, roughly equivalent to the composition of the population.[57] No association of race and risk of legionellosis has been observed in outbreaks.

5.8. Occupation

In a study to compare occupations of persons with sporadic *L. pneumophila* pneumonia with those suspected to have but proved not to have the disease, construction workers were found to be at significantly higher risk of *L. pneumophila* pneumonia.[96] However, serosurveys of construction and other outdoor workers have not shown a higher prevalence of elevated titers to *L. pneumophila*.[61,94] Disease and seropositivity have on occasion been shown to be more common in power plant workers who were exposed to cooling towers.[17,70] As mentioned in Section 5.2, hospital workers who have had direct or indirect contact with patients with Legionnaires' disease have on occasion been shown to have a higher prevalence of elevated antibody titers to serogroup 1 *L. pneumophila* than those not known to have had contact.[89] One epidemic of Pontiac fever occurred in men who had recently cleaned a steam-turbine condenser[37]; apparently that episode was not unique,[26] suggesting that steam-turbine-condenser cleaners may be at increased risk of exposure to *L. pneumophila*. Factory workers were involved in one legionellosis outbreak when grinding fluid became contaminated with *L. feeleii*.[45]

5.9. Occurrence in Different Settings

L. pneumophila pneumonia is widely recognized as a major cause of hospital-acquired pneumonia, occurring both sporadically and in outbreaks.[65] Point-source outbreaks have been associated with excavation,[101] contaminated cooling towers,[27,38,70] and contaminated potable water systems[33,74,77,91] and some cases have been associated with contaminated nebulizers[2] and humidifiers.[51] Most documented cases of *L. micdadei* pneumonia have also been nosocomial. Underlying immune deficiency and duration of hospitalization have been risk factors in outbreaks[16] and in sporadic cases.[96]

5.10. Socioeconomic Factors

Persons with confirmed sporadic legionellosis have been found to have a lower average level of education than those suspected of having the disease but proved not to, but the difference was not statistically significant ($p = 0.09$).[96] Such an association might be largely explained by concomitant cigarette smoking and consumption of large amounts of alcohol, which apparently are more direct contributors to the risk of acquiring Legionnaires' disease[36,96] (see Section 5.11.2).

5.11. Other Factors

5.11.1. Travel. A recent history of travel is strikingly associated with many cases of *L. pneumophila* pneumonia. Several outbreaks have been observed in groups attending conventions and in others in or near convention hotels.[36,100] Several clusters have been observed in tourists in Europe[7,25,59,82,87] and in the Caribbean.[90] For sporadic cases in the United States, travel in the 2 weeks preceding onset of symptoms was a significant risk factor.[96]

5.11.2. Smoking and Drinking. Cigarette smokers have a three- to fourfold higher risk of developing *L. pneumophila* pneumonia than do nonsmokers[36,96]; pipe and cigar smokers do not have a higher risk.[36] People who consume three or more drinks containing alcohol per day have a heightened risk of developing sporadic *L. pneumophila* pneumonia.[96]

5.11.3. Underlying Medical Conditions. Among hospitalized patients, those with cancer or other potentially immunosuppressive underlying diseases were found in one study to have a 2.3-fold higher risk of nosocomial *L. pneumophila* pneumonia.[16] A similar pattern has been observed in several outbreaks.[28,33,56] Corticosteroid treatment has been observed to be a significant risk factor for fatal nosocomial *L. pneumophila* pneumonia.[21] Immunosuppressive therapy commonly is present in pneumonia cases caused by *L. micdadei*[28,78] and *L. bozemanii*.[77] Diabetes mellitus and the use of diuretics were observed in one study[96] to be associated with increased risk of sporadic Legionnaires' disease; in that study, underlying medical problems were found to be associated with Legionnaires' disease no more than with other types of pneumonia suspected but proved not to be Legionnaires' disease.

6. Mechanisms and Routes of Transmission

Legionellae are widespread in unsalty water, which may be able to serve as a vehicle of transmission in several ways. The best documented mode of spread of *L. pneumophila* is airborne, apparently through inhalation of contaminated droplet nuclei.

The source and mechanism of airborne spread of *L. pneumophila* are perhaps illustrated most clearly in the outbreak of Pontiac fever in 1968.[39] In July and August, 144

cases occurred in persons who entered the Pontiac Building of the Oakland County Health Department in Pontiac, Michigan. Nearly everyone who entered the building when the air-conditioning system was operating became ill, although none who entered only when the system was turned off were affected. Unprotected guinea pigs placed in double cages in the building developed a nodular pneumonia, but exposed guinea pigs that were given streptomycin and tetracycline prophylaxis or breathed filtered air were protected to some degree, and those placed in another building did not develop pneumonia. *L. pneumophila* bacilli were recovered 10 years later from frozen lung nodules of the guinea pigs that had developed pneumonia. The air-conditioning system was found to be defective. Defects in the exhaust vent of the evaporative condenser permitted aerosol from the condenser water to enter air-handling ducts; a puddle of water was found in one of those ducts. In laboratory experiments on guinea pigs, the aerosol of evaporative-condenser water from the building caused nodular pneumonia; *L. pneumophila* bacilli were isolated from the guinea pig lung tissue.[52]

Evaporative condensers and cooling towers are designed to dissipate heat to the ambient air.[68] Recirculating water is cascaded over pipes or other materials that break it up into small droplets as air is drawn past, usually by a fan, and expelled to the outside. A small fraction (perhaps 1%) of the water is evaporated, cooling the remainder; an additional 0.1% or so is expelled as aerosol or "drift," small droplets 1–100 μm in diameter, which have roughly the same composition as the water in the evaporative condenser or cooling tower. After they leave the air-conditioning system, these droplets are subject to rapid evaporation down to droplet nuclei of a size (generally < 5 μm) that can be readily inhaled and deposited in pulmonary alveoli. Defects in design or function of air-conditioning systems may permit these droplets and droplet nuclei in the drift to contaminate conditioned air in a building. Several outbreaks of legionellosis have been traced to contaminated evaporative condensers and cooling towers.[5,38,53,70]

Other apparatuses that generate aerosols have also been implicated in spread of *Legionella,* including industrial grinders,[45] nebulizers,[2] mechanical humidifiers,[51] and jets of compressed air.[37]

However, in the large bulk of outbreaks and sporadic cases the mode of spread of legionellae is unknown, although the source is often suspected or proved to be water.[7,33,50,74,77,87,90,91] An instructive example of this phenomenon was the occurrence of more than 200 nosocomial cases of *L. pneumophila* serogroup 1 pneumonia in the 4 years after the Wadsworth Medical Center opened in Los Angeles, California, in 1977. Repeated investigations, including chlorination of the cooling towers, failed to identify the source, until a striking increase occurred to 26 cases in March 1980. This increase occurred a few days after a test of the potable-water pump caused a sharp drop in water pressure and left the hospital's water discolored for several weeks. Cases did not differ from controls in any measurable exposure to hospital potable water, including glasses drunk, use of ice, showers taken, and tooth brushing. However, *L. pneumophila* could be isolated from the potable water, and reproducing the water pressure drop in an isolated segment of the hospital led to a 20- to 36-fold increase in *L. pneumophila* concentration and the recurrence of discoloration of the water. Rechlorination of the hospital's potable water decreased the incidence of legionellosis from 4.5 cases per month in the preceding 41 months to less than 1 per month in the next 20 months.[91]

In one nosocomial outbreak, the rooms of case patients were significantly closer to the hospital's showers than those of control patients,[41] but more often no epidemiological link is found between specific water exposure and illness.[91] Occasional cases have been reported in which contaminated water may have been directly inoculated, as through a whirlpool bath[12] or an enema.[3] The relatively high incidence of *L. pneumophila* pneumonia (0.14% of patients; 29% of those with nosocomial pneumonia) observed in one set of head and neck surgery patients suggests that aspiration may be a route of transmission of *Legionella*.[49]

As indicated in Section 5.2, person-to-person spread has not been proved, although indirect evidence raises the possibility that it may occur under some conditions.[89] Whether or not humans can be asymptomatic carriers of *L. pneumophila* (as in feces or throat) has not been shown.

7. Pathogenesis and Immunity

L. pneumophila pneumonia appears to begin with the inhalation of *L. pneumophila*, which usually induces pneumonia after an incubation period of 2–10 days or possibly longer (mean 5.5 days).[36] Pathologically, the pulmonary infiltrate consists of macrophages and polymorphonuclear leukocytes in alveolar spaces, fibrin, and proliferating alveolar lining cells.[9,112] Terminal and respiratory bronchioles may be involved, but not bronchi or proximal bronchioles. The cellular infiltrate is commonly necrotic, but the underlying pulmonary structure remains intact. Large numbers of bacilli can be demonstrated with Dieterle silver-impregnation stain, but not usually with Brown-Brenn or other tissue modification of the Gram stain.[18] Bacilli are

commonly seen in clusters with macrophages. Grossly, the areas seen in early stages of pneumonia are nodular and commonly bordered by lobular septa[113]; spread to adjacent alveoli appears to occur through the pores of Kohn. The resolution of Legionnaires' disease pneumonia may not be complete; a residual defect in diffusing capacity in some patients may be caused by the deposition of fibrin.[60]

Bacteremia accompanies Legionnaires' disease, but whether involvement of gastrointestinal tract, kidneys, central nervous system, and muscle in the disease results from direct bacterial invasion (which has rarely been demonstrated in extrathoracic organs), toxins, or other indirect effects is not known. No consistent histopathological changes have been demonstrated except in the lungs.

Pontiac fever has an incubation period in most cases of 24–48 h after *L. pneumophila* is inhaled.[39] The pathogenesis of this syndrome is not understood, in part because the disease is not fatal, and no pathological material has been examined. It is also unknown whether proliferation of bacteria is necessary to produce the syndrome and, if it is, where the proliferation occurs. Variations in the pathogenicity of *Legionella* strains in various systems have been observed, but little is known about their relationship to human pathogenicity or the pathogenesis of Pontiac fever.[62]

Cell-mediated immunity is important in defending against these bacteria, which multiply in human blood monocytes and alveolar macrophages.[48,73] *L. pneumophila* elicits from patients' mononuclear phagocytes lymphokines that activate mononuclear phagocytes.[46] Such activated cells inhibit intracellular multiplication of *L. pneumophila*.[73] These and the observations that patients receiving medication that impairs cell-mediated immunity are at increased risk of legionellosis suggest that cell-mediated immunity may play an important role in the host defenses against legionellae.

Serological immunity may play some role also. In the presence of complement and specific antibody, monocytes kill about 0.5 log of *L. pneumophila*, but activation of monocytes does not enhance this modest killing. Passive immunization of mice and guinea pigs by IgG from actively immunized goats is protective.[114]

8. Patterns of Host Response

Two distinct clinical (and epidemiological) syndromes of *L. pneumophila* infection have been identified in epidemic form: Legionnaires' disease and Pontiac fever (Table 1). Each syndrome has its own spectrum of severity. Pa-

**Table 1. Clinical and Epidemiological Characteristics
of Legionnaires' Disease and Pontiac Fever**

Characteristics	Legionnaires' disease	Pontiac fever
Attack rate	0.1–5%	46–100%
Incubation period	2–10 days	1–2 days
Symptoms[a]	Fever, cough, myalgia, chills, headache, chest pain, sputum, diarrhea, (confusion)	Fever, chills, myalgia, headache, (cough), (chest pain), (confusion)
Lung	Pneumonia, pleural effusion	(Pleuritis), no pneumonia
Other organ systems	Kidney, liver, gastrointestinal tract, central nervous system	—
Case-fatality ratio	15–20%	0%

[a]The symptoms in parentheses are less prominent.

tients with sporadic cases of legionellosis have also had a broad range of clinical manifestations, including lung abscess, culture-negative endocarditis, encephalopathy, and diarrhea. Asymptomatic infections (as documented by seroconversion) have been documented in conjunction with epidemic investigations, but they are generally less common than pneumonia.[36,40,66] Most seroconversions in children, however, appear to be asymptomatic.[1]

8.1. Clinical Features

The term *Legionnaires' disease* denotes the syndrome seen in epidemic form in Philadelphia in 1976. It is a multisystem illness characterized by pneumonia, high fever, rigors, cough, myalgia, headache, chest pain, diarrhea, and confusion, with laboratory evidence of mild hepatic involvement and mild renal disease or renal failure necessitating temporary dialysis in 3% of patients.[36,44,105] The white blood cell count is typically normal or slightly elevated, with an increased proportion of young forms. The erythrocyte sedimentation rate is typically markedly elevated. Chest radiographs taken soon after onset of illness show patchy infiltrates that become nodular areas of consolidation and that coalesce in severe cases. Pleural effusions are typically small. In immunosuppressed patients, pneumonia may be associated with cavitation. The pneumonia typically progresses over the first week of illness with daily temperatures of 39.4–40.6°C (103–105°F), and thereafter resolution is gradual. In the absence of specific therapy, mortality averages 15–20%, with death resulting usually from progressive pneumonia with concomitant hypoxemia

or from shock. With erythromycin therapy, the mortality averages 5–10%.[16,36,44] Weakness and shortness of breath may persist for months in a minority of patients. Residual defects in pulmonary diffusing capacity have been observed.[60] Most documented cases of infection with legionellae other than *L. pneumophila* resemble Legionnaires' disease.

Pontiac fever is a syndrome of *L. pneumophila* infection that has been recognized in outbreaks.[37,39,45] It is characterized by high fever, headache, and myalgia. Cough, sore throat, diarrhea, confusion, and chest pain are observed, but are not prominent. One person had a pleural friction rub, but none have had pneumonia. The illness is markedly debilitating for 2–7 days, but all persons have recovered completely.

8.2. Diagnosis

Legionellosis initially appearing as pneumonia must be distinguished from all other common bacterial pneumonias or infections caused by *M. pneumoniae, Chlamydia psittacii, Coxiella burnetii,* influenza virus, or any of several other respiratory viruses.[32]

Epidemiological clues for diagnosing *L. pneumophila* pneumonia include summer–fall season, male sex, middle-aged (or older) patients, history of cigarette smoking or heavy alcohol use, recent history of travel, hospitalization, or exposure to construction or excavation, and occurrence in outbreaks.[36,43,96] Clinical clues that seem to be of differential value include very high fever,[21,67] lack of preceding upper-respiratory symptoms,[43] diarrhea,[92] unexplained impairment of mental function,[43,67,92] hematuria,[43] abnormal liver function,[43,67] lymphopenia,[67] negative routine bacteriological cultures,[21,67] and failure to respond to therapy with antibiotics ineffective in legionellosis.[43,67] The presence of neutrophils and no visible bacteria or weakly staining gram-negative bacilli in well-collected sputum or material obtained by transtracheal aspiration favors the diagnosis of legionellosis.

Specific diagnosis of legionellosis is made by isolating *Legionella* in cultures from blood, pleural fluid, respiratory secretions, or lung tissue[29,117]; demonstrating the presence of *Legionella* in respiratory secretions, lung tissue, pleural fluid, or urine by direct immunofluorescence,[20,29,117] RIA,[55] or ELISA[55,98]; or demonstrating a fourfold or greater rise in antibody titer in paired serum specimens assayed by indirect immunofluorescence or other methods.[29,109,110,117]

9. Control and Prevention

9.1. General Concepts

Legionellosis can be prevented by interrupting transmission of the bacteria from their watery environment to humans. This has been accomplished in the context of disease outbreaks by turning off (or otherwise removing people from exposure to) machinery that generated contaminated aerosols,[27,70] disinfecting that machinery,[38,45,70] or heating or otherwise disinfecting potable water.[8,91]

One can take advantage of certain characteristics of *Legionella* to help control it. *Legionella* grows best at or somewhat above human body temperature and hence is particularly prevalent in warm water.[4,79] However, it grows poorly above 50°C and can be killed by temperatures above 55°C so that maintaining such temperatures on the hot water side of a potable water system has controlled *Legionella*.[8,72,74] Disadvantages of such hot water are cost and the risk of scalding. Growth of *Legionella* in potable water systems is also favored by the presence of rubber washers[22,75] and moderate levels of iron, zinc, and potassium[95] so that eliminating these may help in control.

Legionellae are susceptible to a range of disinfectants, including calcium hypochlorite, quaternary ammonium compounds, dibromonitrilopropionamide, and ozone.[58,72,80] Hyperchlorination (to 2–3 mg free residual chlorine per liter) in particular has successfully controlled legionellosis outbreaks traced to potable water and to cooling towers,[38,91] but corrosion complicates this strategy. Some *L. pneumophila* have been shown to concentrate in foam, so that control of foaming may be useful.[23] Draining, clean-

ing, and regular maintenance of aerosol-generating machinery like cooling towers are likely to be helpful in controlling outbreaks traced to them.[45] The importance of such procedures in the absence of an outbreak has not been conclusively shown.

Using only sterile water in nebulizers and other aerosol-generating apparatus to which hospitalized patients are exposed makes good sense and seems to have helped control some outbreaks.[50]

Routine microbiological surveillance of *Legionella* in potable water systems or machinery does not seem warranted.[81]

Whether secretion precautions for patients with legionellosis would prevent occasional secondary cases is unknown. Person-to-person spread has not been documented, but the organism has been isolated in sputum, and more persons in contact with hospitalized patients with *L. pneumophila* pneumonia than controls have been seropositive.[89]

9.2. Antibiotic and Chemotherapeutic Approaches to Prophylaxis

Erythromycin prophylaxis of immunosuppressed patients has been attempted in one hospital with a high incidence of *L. pneumophila* pneumonia. Although the method of selecting controls was not adequate, the results suggested efficacy.[106] However, if a problem with legionellosis has been identified, it seems wiser to eliminate the source than to rely on chemoprophylaxis of patients.

9.3. Immunization

Immunization of humans has not been attempted.

10. Unresolved Problems

10.1. Legionnaires' Disease versus Pontiac Fever

The striking differences in incubation period, attack rate, and clinical manifestations (see Table 1) suggest a basic difference between infection with *L. pneumophila* that causes Legionnaires' disease and that which causes Pontiac fever. Whether these differences relate to toxins produced by the organism, to the size of the inoculum, or to the viability of the organism is not known. It is unlikely that host factors alone are involved, since a broad range of persons have been affected with each syndrome, and within a given outbreak the syndrome appears to "breed true."

10.2. Spread Other Than Airborne

Although airborne spread of *Legionella* from aerosol-generating machinery has been well demonstrated, for most outbreaks and essentially all sporadic cases the mode of spread is unknown. In particular, the method by which contaminated potable water infects people is largely unknown. Can *Legionella* be spread by ingestion? Does it colonize the pharynx and is it then aspirated? Is it spread by droplets or droplet nuclei, perhaps created in sinks, showers, and toilets?

11. References

1. ANDERSON, R. D., LAUER, B. A., FRASER, D. W., HAYES, P. S., AND MCINTOSH, K., Infections with *Legionella pneumophila* in children, *J. Infect. Dis.* **143:**386–390 (1981).
2. ARNOW, P. M., CHOU, T., WEIL, D., SHAPIRO, E. N., AND KRETZSCHMAR, C., Nosocomial Legionnaires' disease caused by aerosolized tap water from respiratory devices, *J. Infect. Dis.* **146:**460–467 (1982).
3. ARNOW, P. M., BOYKO, E. J., AND FRIEDMAN, E. L., Perirectal abscess caused by *Legionella pneumophila* and mixed anaerobic bacteria, *Ann. Intern. Med.* **98:**184–185 (1983).
4. ARNOW, P. M., WEIL, D., AND PARA, M. F., Prevalence and significance of *Legionella pneumophila* contamination of residential hot tap water systems, *J. Infect. Dis.* **152:**145–151 (1985).
5. BAND, J. D., LAVENTURE, M., DAVIS, J. P., MALLISON, G. F., SKALIY, P., HAYES, P. S., SCHELL, W. L., WEISS, H., GREENBERG, D. J., AND FRASER, D. W. Epidemic Legionnaires' disease: Airborne transmission down a chimney, *J. Am. Med. Assoc.* **245:**2404–2407 (1981).
6. BARBAREE, J. M., FIELDS, B. S., FEELEY, J. C., GORMAN, G. W., AND MARTIN, W. T., Isolation of protozoa from water associated with a Legionellosis outbreak and demonstration of intracellular multiplication of *Legionella pneumophila*, *Appl. Environ. Microbiol.* **51:**422–424 (1986).
7. BARTLETT, C. L. R., SWANN, R. A., CASAL, J., CANADA ROYO, L., AND TAYLOR, A. G., Recurrent Legionnaires' disease from a hotel water system, in: *Legionella* (C. THORNSBERRY, A. BALOWS, J. C. FEELEY, AND W. JAKUBOWSKI, eds.), pp. 237–239, American Society for Microbiology, Washington, D.C., 1984.
8. BEST, M., YU, V. L., STOUT, J., GOETZ, A., MUDER, R. R., AND TAYLOR, F., Legionellaceae in the hospital water supply, *Lancet* **2:**307–310 (1983).
9. BLACKMON, J. A., HICKLIN, M. D., CHANDLER, R. W., AND the Special Expert Pathology Panel, Legionnaires' disease: Pathological and historical aspects of a "new" disease, *Arch. Pathol. Lab. Med.* **102:**337–343 (1978).
10. BOLDUR, L., ERGAZ, M., AND SOMPOLINSKY, D., A prevalence study of antibodies to *Legionella* spp. in geriatric institutions, *J. Hyg.* **92:**37–43 (1984).
11. BOZEMAN, F. M., HUMPHRIES, J. W., AND CAMPBELL, J. M., A new group of rickettsia-like agents recovered from guinea pigs, *Acta Virol.* **12:**87–93 (1968).
12. BRABENDER, W., HINTHORN, D. R., ASHER, M., LINDSEY, N. J., AND LIU, C., *Legionella pneumophila* wound infection, *J. Am. Med. Assoc.* **250:**3091–3092 (1983).
13. BRENNER, D. J., Classification of Legionellaceae: Current status and remaining questions, *Isr. J. Med. Sci.* **22:**620–632 (1986).
14. BRENNER, D. J., STEIGERWALT, A. G., AND MCDADE, J. E., Classification of the Legionnaires' disease bacterium: *Legionella pneumophila*, genus novum, species nova, of the family Legionellaceae, familia nova, *Ann. Intern. Med.* **90:**656–658 (1979).
15. BRENNER, D. J., STEIGERWALT, A. G., GORMAN, G. W., WEAVER, R. E., FEELEY, J. C., CORDES, L. G., WILKINSON, H. W., PATTON, C., THOMASON, B. M., AND SASSEVILLE, K. R. L., *Legionella bozemanii* sp. nov. and *Legionella dumoffii* sp. nov.: Classification of two additional species of *Legionella* associated with human pneumonia, *Curr. Microbiol.* **4:**111–116 (1980).
16. BROOME, C. V., GOINGS, S. A. J., THACKER, S. B., VOGT, R. L., BEATY, H. N., FRASER, D. W., AND Field Investigation Team, The Vermont epidemic of Legionnaires' disease, *Ann. Intern. Med.* **90:**573–577 (1979).
17. BUEHLER, J. W., SIKES, R. K., KURITSKY, J. N., GORMAN, G. W., HIGHTOWER, A. W., AND BROOME, C. V., Prevalence of antibodies to *Legionella pneumophila* among workers exposed to a contaminated cooling tower, *Arch. Environ. Health* **40:**207–210 (1985).
18. CHANDLER, F. W., HICKLIN, M. D., AND BLACKMON, J. A., Demonstration of the agent of Legionnaires' disease in tissue, *N. Engl. J. Med.* **297:**1218–1220 (1977).
19. CHANDLER, F. W., COLE, R. M., HICKLIN, M. D., BLACKMON, J. A., AND CALLAWAY, C. S., Ultrastructure of the Legionnaires' disease bacterium: A study using transmission electron microscopy, *Ann. Intern. Med.* **90:**642–647 (1979).
20. CHERRY, W. B., PITTMAN, B., HARRIS, P. P., HÉBERT, G. A., THOMASON, B. M., THACKER, L., AND WEAVER, R. E., Detection of Legionnaires' disease bacteria by direct immunofluorescent staining, *J. Clin. Microbiol.* **8:**329–338 (1978).
21. COHEN, M. L., BROOME, C. V., PARIS, A., MARTIN, W. T., AND ALLEN, J. R., Fatal nosocomial Legionnaires' disease: Clinical and epidemiologic characteristics, *Ann. Intern. Med.* **90:**611–613 (1979).
22. COLBURNE, J. S., AND ASHWORTH, J., Rubbers, water and Legionella, *Lancet* **2:**583 (1986).
23. COLBURNE, J. S., DENNIS, P. J., LEE, J. V., AND BAILEY, M. R., Legionnaires' disease: Reduction in risks associated with foaming in evaporative cooling towers, *Lancet* **1:**684 (1987).
24. CONLAN, J. W., BASKERVILLE, A., AND ASHWORTH, L. A.

E., Separation of *Legionella pneumophila* proteases and purification of a protease which produces lesions like those of Legionnaires' disease in a guinea pig lung, *J. Gen. Microbiol.* **132:**1565–1574 (1986).

25. COSSAR, J. H., DEWAR, R. D., FALLON, R. J., GRIST, N. R., AND REID, D., *Legionella pneumophila* in tourists, *Practitioner* **226:**1543–1548 (1982).

26. DEUBNER, D. C., AND GILLIAM, D. K., Fever of undetermined origin after cleaning of steam turbine condensers, *Arch. Environ. Health* **32:**116–120 (1977).

27. DONDERO, T. J., JR., RENDTORFF, R. C., MALLISON, G. F., WEEKS, M., LEVY, J., WONG, E. W., AND SCHAFFNER, W., Outbreak of Legionnaires' disease associated with a contaminated air conditioning cooling tower, *N. Engl. J. Med.* **302:**425–431 (1980).

28. DOWLING, J. N., PASCULLE, A. W., FROLA, F. N., ZAPHYR, K., AND YEE, R. B., Infections caused by *Legionella micdadei* and *Legionella pneumophila* among renal transplant recipients, *J. Infect. Dis.* **149:**703–713 (1984).

29. EDELSTEIN, P. H., Laboratory diagnosis of infections caused by Legionellae, *Eur. J. Clin. Microbiol.* **6:**4–10 (1987).

30. EDELSTEIN, P. H., MEYER, R. D., AND FINEGOLD, S. M. Laboratory diagnosis of Legionnaires' disease, *Am. Rev. Respir. Dis.* **121:**317–327 (1980).

31. FALLON, R. J., Legionella infections, *Br. Med. J.* **293:**1175 (1986).

32. FINLAND, M., "Legionnaires' disease": They came, saw, and conquered, *Ann. Intern. Med.* **90:**710–713 (1979).

33. FISHER-HOCH, S. P., BARTLETT, C. L. R., TOBIN, J. O., GILLETT, M. B., NELSON, A. M., PRITCHARD, J. E., SMITH, M. G., SWANN, R. A., TALBOT, J. M., AND THOMAS, J. A., Investigation and control of an outbreak of Legionnaires' disease in a district general hospital, *Lancet* **1:**932–936 (1981).

34. FOY, H. M., BROOME, C. V., HAYES, P. S., ALLAN, I., AND TOBE, R., Legionnaires' disease in a prepaid medical care group in Seattle (1963–1975), *Lancet* **1:**767–770 (1979).

35. FRASER, D. W., Unpublished data.

36. FRASER, D. W., TSAI, T. F., ORENSTEIN, W., PARKIN, W. E., BEECHAM, H. J., SHARRAR, R. G., HARRIS, J., MALLISON, G. F., MARTIN, S. M., McDADE, J. E., SHEPARD, C. C., BRACHMAN, P. S., AND The Field Investigation Team, Legionnaires' disease: Description of an epidemic of pneumonia, *N. Engl. J. Med.* **297:**1189–1197 (1977).

37. FRASER, D. W., DEUBNER, D. C., HILL, D. L., AND GILLIAM, D. K., Nonpneumonic, short-incubation-period legionellosis (Pontiac fever) in men who cleaned a steam turbine condenser, *Science* **205:**690–691 (1979).

38. GARBE, P. L., DAVIS, B. J., WEISFELD, J. S., MARKOWITZ, L., MINER, P., GARRITY, F., BARBAREE, J. M., AND REINGOLD, A. L., Nosocomial Legionnaires' disease: Epidemiologic demonstration of cooling towers as a source, *J. Am. Med. Assoc.* **254:**521–524 (1985).

39. GLICK, T. H., GREGG, M. B., BERMAN, B., MALLISON, G. F., RHODES, W. W., JR., AND KASSANOFF, I., Pontiac fever: An epidemic of unknown etiology in a health department.

Clinical and epidemiologic aspects, *Am. J. Epidemiol.* **107:**149–160 (1978).

40. HALEY, C. E., COHEN, M. L., HALTER, J., AND MEYER, R. D., Nosocomial Legionnaires' disease: A continuing common-source epidemic at Wadsworth Medical Center, *Ann. Intern. Med.* **90:**583–586 (1979).

41. HANRAHAN, J. P., MORSE, D. L., SCHARF, V. B., DEBBIE, J. G., SCHMID, G. P., McKINNEY, R. M., AND SHAYEGANI, M., Community hospital legionellosis outbreak linked to hot-water showers, in: *Legionella* (C. THORNSBERRY, A. BALOWS, J. C. FEELEY, AND W. JAKUBOWSKI, eds.), pp. 224–225, American Society for Microbiology, Washington, D.C., 1984.

42. HÉBERT, G. A., STEIGERWALT, A. G., AND BRENNER, D. J., *Legionella micdadei* species nova: Classification of a third species of *Legionella* associated with human pneumonia, *Curr. Microbiol.* **3:**255–257 (1980).

43. HELMS, C. M., VINER, J. P., STURM, R. H., RENNER, E. D., AND JOHNSON, W., Comparative features of pneumococcal, mycoplasmal, and Legionnaires' disease pneumonias, *Ann. Intern. Med.* **90:**543–547 (1979).

44. HELMS, C. M., VINER, J. P., WEISENBURGER, D. D., CHIU, L. C., RENNER, E. D., AND JOHNSON, W., Sporadic Legionnaires' disease: Clinical observations on 87 nosocomial and community-acquired cases, *Am. J. Med. Sci.* **288:**2–12 (1984).

45. HERWALDT, L. A., GORMAN, G. W., McGRATH, T., TOMA, S., BRAKE, B., HIGHTOWER, A. W., JONES, J., REINGOLD, A. L., BOXER, P. A., TANG, P. W., MOSS, C. W., WILKINSON, H. W., BRENNER, D. J., STEIGERWALT, A. G., AND BROOME, C. V., A new *Legionella* species, *Legionella feeleii* species nova, causes Pontiac fever in an automobile plant, *Ann. Intern. Med.* **100:**333–338 (1984).

46. HORWITZ, M. A., Cell mediated immunity in Legionnaires' disease, *J. Clin. Invest.* **71:**1686–1697 (1983).

47. HORWITZ, M. A., Phagocytosis of the Legionnaires' disease bacterium (Legionella pneumophila) occurs by a novel mechanism: Engulfment within a pseudopod coil, *Cell* **36:**27–33 (1984).

48. HORWITZ, M. A., AND SILVERSTEIN, S. C., Legionnaires' disease bacterium (*Legionella pneumophila*) multiplies intracellularly in human monocytes, *J. Clin. Invest.* **66:**441–450 (1980).

49. JOHNSON, J. T., YU, V. L., WAGNER, R. L., AND BEST, M. G., Nosocomial *Legionella* pneumonia (sic) in a population of head and neck cancer patients, *Laryngoscope* **95:**1468–1471 (1985).

50. JOLY, J. R., DERY, P., GAUVREAU, L., COTE, L., AND TREPANIER, C., Legionnaires' disease caused by *Legionella dumoffii* in distilled water, *Can. Med. Assoc. J.* **135:**1274–1277 (1986).

51. KAAN, J. A., SIMOONS-SMIT, A. M., AND MacLAREN, D. M., Another source of aerosol causing nosocomial Legionnaires' disease, *J. Infect.* **11:**145–148 (1985).

52. KAUFMANN, A. F., McDADE, J. E., PATTON, C. M., BEN-

NETT, J. V., SKALIY, P., FEELEY, J. C., ANDERSON, D. C., POTTER, M. E., NEWHOUSE, V. F., GREGG, M. B., AND BRACHMAN, P. S., Pontiac fever: Isolation of the etiologic agent (*Legionella pneumophila*) and demonstration of its mode of transmission, *Am. J. Epidemiol.* **114**:337–347 (1981).

53. KLAUCKE, D. N., VOGT, R. L., LARUE, D., WITHERELL, L. N., ORCIARI, L. A., SPITALNY, K. C., PELLETIER, R., CHERRY, W. B., AND NOVICK, L. F., Legionnaires' disease: The epidemiology of two outbreaks in Burlington, Vermont, 1980, *Am. J. Epidemiol.* **119**:382–391 (1984).

54. KOHLER, R. B., Antigen detection for the rapid diagnosis of mycoplasma and *Legionella* pneumonia, *Diagn. Microbiol. Infect. Dis.* **4**:47S–59S (1986).

55. KOHLER, R. B., WINN, W. C., JR., AND WHEAT, L. J., Onset and duration of urinary antigen excretion in Legionnaires' disease, *J. Clin. Microbiol.* **20**:605–607 (1984).

56. KUGLER, J. W., ARMITAGE, J. O., HELMS, C. M., KLASSEN, L. W., GOEKEN, N. E., AHMANN, G. B., GINGRICH, R. D., JOHNSON, W., AND GILCHRIS, M. J., Nosocomial Legionnaires' disease: Occurrence in recipients of bone marrow transplants, *Am. J. Med.* **74**:281–288 (1983).

57. KURITSKY, J. N., REINGOLD, A. L., HIGHTOWER, A. W., AND BROOME, C. V., Sporadic legionellosis in the United States, 1970 to 1982, in: *Legionella* (C. THORNSBERRY, A. BALOWS, J. C. FEELEY, AND W. JAKUBOWSKI, eds.), pp. 243–245, American Society for Microbiology, Washington, D.C., 1984.

58. KURTZ, J. B., BARTLETT, C. L. R., NEWTON, V. A., WHITE, R. A., AND JONES, N. L., *Legionella pneumophila* in cooling water systems, *J. Hyg.* **88**:369–381 (1982).

59. L'AGE, M., HORBACH, I., ULMRICH, W., WEYER, H., AND FEHRENBACH, F. -J., Legionerskrankheit bei einer Inland-Reisegruppe, *Dtsch. Med. Wochenschr.* **108**:288–292 (1983).

60. LATTIMER, G. L., RHODES, L. V., III, SALVENTI, J. S., GALGON, J. P., STONEBRAKER, V., BOLEY, S., AND HAAS, G., The Philadelphia epidemic of Legionnaires' disease: Clinical, pulmonary, and serologic findings two years later, *Ann. Intern. Med.* **90**:522–526 (1979).

61. MARKS, J. S., TSAI, T. F., MARTONE, W. J., BARON, R. C., KENNICOTT, J., HOLTZHAUER, F. J., BAIRD, I., FAY, D., FEELEY, J. C., MALLISON, G. F., FRASER, D. W., AND HALPIN, T. J., Nosocomial Legionnaires' disease—Columbus, Ohio, *Ann. Intern. Med.* **90**:565–569 (1979).

62. MCDADE, J. E., AND SHEPARD, C. C., Virulent to avirulent conversion of Legionnaires' disease bacterium (*Legionella pneumophila*)—Its effect on isolation techniques, *J. Infect. Dis.* **139**:707–711 (1979).

63. MCDADE, J. E., SHEPARD, C. C., FRASER, D. W., TSAI, T. F., REDUS, M. A., DOWDLE, W. R., AND The Laboratory Investigation Team, Legionnaires' disease: Isolation of a bacterium and demonstration of its role in other respiratory disease, *N. Engl. J. Med.* **297**:1197–1203 (1977).

64. MCDADE, J. E., BRENNER, D. J., AND BOZEMAN, F. M.,

Legionnaires' disease bacterium isolated in 1947, *Ann. Intern. Med.* **90**:659–661 (1979).

65. MEYER, R. D., Legionnaires' disease: Aspects of nosocomial infection, *Am. J. Med.* **76**:657–663 (1984).

66. MEYER, R. D., SHIMIZU, G. H., FULLER, R., SAYRE, J., CHAPMAN, J., AND EDELSTEIN, P. H., Prospective survey of acquisition of Legionnaires' disease, in: *Legionella* (C. THORNSBERRY, A. BALOWS, J. C. FEELEY, AND W. JAKUBOWSKI, eds.), pp. 218–219, American Society for Microbiology, Washington, D.C., 1984.

67. MILLER, A. C., Early clinical differentiation between Legionnaires' disease and other sporadic pneumonias, *Ann. Intern. Med.* **90**:526–528 (1979).

68. MILLER, R. P., Cooling towers and evaporative condensers, *Ann. Intern. Med.* **90**:667–670 (1979).

69. MORRIS, G. K., PATTON, C. M., FEELEY, J. C., JOHNSON, S. E., GORMAN, G. W., MARTIN, W. T., SKALIY, P., MALLISON, G. F., POLITI, B. D., AND MACKEL, D. C., Isolation of Legionnaires' disease bacterium from environmental samples, *Ann. Intern. Med.* **90**:664–666 (1979).

70. MORTON, S., BARTLETT, C. L. R., BIBBY, L. F., HUTCHINSON, D. N., DYER, J. V., AND DENNIS, P. J., Outbreak of Legionnaires' disease from a cooling water system in a power station, *Br. J. Ind. Med.* **43**:630–635 (1986).

71. MUDER, R. R., YU, V. L., MCCLURE, J. K., KROBOTH, F. J., KOMINOS, S. D., AND LUMISH, R. M., Nosocomial Legionnaires' disease uncovered in a prospective pneumonia study: Implications for underdiagnosis, *J. Am. Med. Assoc.* **249**:3184–3188 (1983).

72. MURACA, P., STOUT, J. E., AND YU, V. L., Comparative assessment of chlorine, heat, ozone, and UV light for killing *Legionella pneumophila* within a model plumbing system, *Appl. Environ. Microbiol.* **53**:447–453 (1987).

73. NASH, T. W., LIBBY, D. M., AND HORWITZ, M. A., Interaction between the Legionnaires' disease bacterium (*Legionella pneumophila*) and human alveolar macrophages. Influence of antibody, lymphokines and hydrocortisone, *J. Clin. Invest.* **74**:771–782 (1984).

74. NEILL, M. A., GORMAN, G. W., GIBERT, C., ROUSSEL, A., HIGHTOWER, A. W., MCKINNEY, R. M., AND BROOME, C. V., Nosocomial legionellosis, Paris, France: Evidence for transmission by potable water, *Am. J. Med.* **78**:581–588 (1985).

75. NIEDEVELD, C. J., PET, F. M., AND MEENHORST, P. L., Effect of rubbers and their constituents on proliferation of *Legionella pneumophila* in naturally contaminated hot water, *Lancet* **2**:180–184 (1986).

76. OSTERHOLM, M. T., CHIN, T. D. Y., OSBORNE, D. O., DULL, H. B., DEAN, A. G., FRASER, D. W., HAYES, P. S., AND HALL, W. N., A 1957 outbreak of Legionnaires' disease associated with a meat packing plant, *Am. J. Epidemiol.* **117**:60–67 (1983).

77. PARRY, M. F., STAMPLEMAN, L., HUTCHINSON, J. H., FOLTA, D., STEINBERG, M. G., AND KRASNOGOR, L. J., Waterborne *Legionella bozemanii* and nosocomial pneumonia

in immunosuppressed patients, *Ann. Intern. Med.* **103:**205–210 (1985).

78. PASCULLE, A. W., MYEROWITZ, R. L., AND RINALDO, C. R., JR., New bacterial agent of pneumonia isolated from renal-transplant recipients, *Lancet* **2:**58–61 (1979).

79. PEEL, M. M., HARKNESS, J. L., COLWELL, J. M., ROUCH, G. J., AND CHRISTOPHER, P. J., *Legionella pneumophila* and water temperatures in Australian hospitals, *Aust. N. Z. J. Med.* **15:**38–41 (1985).

80. POPE, D. H., EICHLER, L. W., COATES, T. F., KRAMER, J. F., AND SORACCO, R. J., The effect of ozone on *Legionella pneumophila* and other bacterial populations in cooling towers, *Curr. Microbiol.* **10:**89–94 (1984).

81. REDD, S. C., AND COHEN, M. L., *Legionella* in water: What should be done. *J. Am. Med. Assoc.* **257:**1221–1222 (1987).

82. REID, D., GRIST, N. R., AND NÁJERA, R., Illness associated with "package tours": A combined Spanish–Scottish study, *Bull. WHO* **56:**117–122 (1978).

83. REINGOLD, A. L., THOMASON, B. M., BRAKE, B. J., THACKER, L., WILKINSON, H. W., AND KURITSKY, J. N., Legionella pneumonia in the United States: The distribution of serogroups causing human illness, *J. Infect. Dis.* **149:**819 (1984).

84. REINHARDT, J. F., NAKAHAMA, C., AND EDELSTEIN, P. H., Comparison of blood culture methods for recovery of *Legionella pneumophila* from the blood of guinea pigs with experimental infection, *J. Clin. Microbiol.* **25:**719–721 (1987).

85. RENNER, E. D., HELMS, C. M., HIERHOLZER, W. J., JR., HALL, N., WONG, Y. W., VINER, J. P., JOHNSON, W., AND HAUSLER, W. J., JR., Legionnaires' disease in pneumonia patients in Iowa: A retrospective seroepidemiologic study, 1972–1977, *Ann. Intern. Med.* **90:**603–606 (1979).

86. ROSENFELD, J. S., KUEPPERS F., NEWKIRK, T., TAMADA, R., MEISSLER, J. J., JR., AND EISENSTEIN, T. K., A protease from *Legionella pneumophila* with cytotoxic and dermal ulcerative activity, *FEMS Microbiol. Lett.* **37:**51–58 (1986).

87. ROSMINI, F., CASTELLANI-PASTORIS, M., MAZZOTTI, M. F., FORASTIERE, F., GAVAZZONI, A., GRECO, D., RUCKDESCHEL, G., TARTAGNI, E., ZAMPIERI, A., AND BAINE, W. B., Febrile illness in successive cohorts of tourists at a hotel on the Italian Adriatic coast: Evidence for a persistent focus of *Legionella* infection, *Am. J. Epidemiol.* **119:**124–134 (1984).

88. RYAN, M. E., FELDMAN, S., PRUITT, B., AND FRASER, D. W., Legionnaires' disease in a child with cancer, *Pediatrics* **64:**951–953 (1979).

89. SARAVOLATZ, L. D., ARKING, L., WENTWORTH, B., AND QUINN, E., Prevalence of antibody to Legionnaires' disease bacterium in hospital employees, *Ann. Intern. Med.* **90:**601–603 (1979).

90. SCHLECH, W. F., III, GORMAN, G. W., PAYNE, M. C., AND BROOME, C. V., Legionnaires' disease in the Caribbean: An outbreak associated with a resort hotel, *Arch. Intern. Med.* **145:**2076–2079 (1985).

91. SHANDS, K. N., HO, J. O., MEYER, R. D., GORMAN, G. W.,

EDELSTEIN, P. H., MALLISON, G. F., FINEGOLD, S. M., AND FRASER, D. W., Potable water as a source of Legionnaires' disease, *J. Am. Med. Assoc.* **253:**1412–1416 (1985).

92. SHARRAR, R. G., FRIEDMAN, H. M., MILLER, W. T., YANAK, M. J., AND ABRUTYN, E., Summertime pneumonias in Philadelphia in 1976: An epidemiologic study, *Ann. Intern. Med.* **90:**577–580 (1979).

93. SKALIY, P., AND MCEACHERN, H. V., Survival of the Legionnaires' disease bacterium in water, *Ann. Intern. Med.* **90:**662–663 (1979).

94. SNOWMAN, W. R., HOLTZHAUER, F. J., HALPIN, T. J., AND CORREA-VILLASENOR, A., The role of indoor and outdoor occupations in the seroepidemiology of *Legionella pneumophila*, *J. Infect. Dis.* **145:**275 (1982).

95. STATES, S. J., CONLEY, L. F., CERASO, M., STEPHENSON, T. E., WOLFORD, R. S., WADOWSKY, R. M., MCNAMARA, A. M., AND YEE, R. B., Effect of metals on *Legionella pneumophila* growth in drinking water plumbing systems, *Appl. Environ. Microbiol.* **50:**1149–1154 (1985).

96. STORCH, G., BAINE, W. B., FRASER, D. W., BROOME, C. V., CLEGG, H. W., II, COHEN, M. L., GOINGS, S. A. J., POLITI, B. D., TERRANOVA, W. A., TSAI, T. F., PLIKAYTIS, B. D., SHEPARD, C. C., AND BENNETT, J. V., Sporadic community-acquired Legionnaires' disease in the United States: A case–control study, *Ann. Intern. Med.* **90:**596–600 (1979).

97. STORCH, G., HAYES, P. S., HILL, D. L., AND BAINE, W. B., Prevalence of antibody to Legionnaires' disease bacterium in middle-aged and elderly Americans, *J. Infect. Dis.* **140:**784–788 (1979).

98. TANG, P. W., AND TOMA, S., Broad-spectrum enzyme-linked immunosorbent assay for detection of *Legionella* soluble antigens, *J. Clin. Microbiol.* **24:**556–558 (1986).

99. TATLOCK, H., A rickettsia-like organism recovered from guinea pigs, *Proc. Soc. Exp. Biol. Med.* **57:**95–99 (1944).

100. TERRANOVA, W., COHEN, M. L., AND FRASER, D. W., 1974 outbreak of Legionnaires' disease diagnosed in 1977: Clinical and epidemiological features, *Lancet* **2:**122–124 (1978).

101. THACKER, S. B., BENNETT, J. V., TSAI, T. F., FRASER, D. W., MCDADE, J. E., SHEPARD, C. C., WILLIAMS, K. H., JR., STUART, W. H., DULL, H. B., AND EICKHOFF, T. C., An outbreak in 1965 of severe respiratory illness caused by the Legionnaires' disease bacterium, *J. Infect. Dis.* **138:**512–519 (1978).

102. THACKER, W. L., WILKINSON, H. W., BENSON, R. F., AND BRENNER, D. J., *Legionella pneumophila* serogroup 12 isolated from human and environmental sources, *J. Clin. Microbiol.* **25:**569–570 (1987).

103. TOBIN, J. O., BEARE, J., DUNNILL, M. S., FISHER-HOCH, S. P., FRENCH, M., MITCHELL, R. G., MORNS, P. J., AND MYERS, M. F., Legionnaires' disease in a transplant unit: Isolation of the causative agent from shower baths, *Lancet* **2:**118–121 (1981).

104. TSAI, T. F., AND FRASER, D. W., The diagnosis of Legionnaires' disease, *Ann. Intern. Med.* **89:**413–414 (1978).

105. TSAI, T. F., FINN, D. R., PLIKAYTIS, B. D., MCCAULEY, W., MARTIN, S. M., AND FRASER, D. W., Legionnaires' disease: Clinical features of the epidemic in Philadelphia, *Ann. Intern. Med.* **90:**509–517 (1979).

106. VEREERSTRAETEN. P., STOLEAR, J. -C., SCHOUTENS-SER-RUYS, E., MAES, N., THYS, J. -P., LIESNARD, C., ROST, F., KINNAERT, P., AND TOUSSAINT, C., Erythromycin prophylaxis for Legionnaires' disease in immunosuppressed patients in a contaminated hospital environment, *Transplantation* **41:**52–54 (1986).

107. WANG, W. L. L., BLASER, M. J., CRAVENS, J., AND JOHNSON, M. A., Growth, survival and resistance of the Legionnaires' disease bacterium, *Ann. Intern. Med.* **90:**614–618 (1979).

108. WILKINSON, H. W., FIKES, B. J., AND CRUCE, D. D., Indirect immunofluorescence test for serodiagnosis of Legionnaires' disease: Evidence for serogroup diversity of Legionnaires' disease bacterial antigens and for multiple specificity of human antibodies, *J. Clin. Microbiol.* **9:**379–383 (1979).

109. WILKINSON, H. W., CRUCE, D. D., AND BROOME, C. V., Validation of *Legionella pneumophila* indirect immunofluorescence assay with epidemic sera, *J. Clin. Microbiol.* **13:**139–146 (1981).

110. WILKINSON, H. W., REINGOLD, A. L., BRAKE, B. J., MCGIBONEY, D. L., GORMAN, G. W., AND BROOME, C. V., Reactivity of serum from patients with suspected legionellosis against 29 antigens of *Legionellaceae* and *Legionella*-like organisms by indirect immunofluorescence assay, *J. Infect. Dis.* **147:**23–31 (1983).

111. WILKINSON, H. W., SAMPSON, J. S., AND PLIKAYTIS, B. D., Evaluation of a commercial gene probe for identification of *Legionella* cultures, *J. Clin. Microbiol.* **23:**217–220 (1986).

112. WINN, W. C., JR., AND MYEROWITZ, R. L., The pathology of the Legionella pneumonias: A review of 74 cases and the literature, *Hum. Pathol.* **12:**401–422 (1981).

113. WINN, W. C., JR., GLAVIN, F. L., PERL, D. P., AND CRAIGHEAD, J. E., Macroscopic pathology of the lung in Legionnaires' disease, *Ann. Intern. Med.* **90:**548–551 (1979).

114. WONG, K. H., MCMASTER, R. B., FEELEY, J. C., ARKO, R. J., SCHALLA, W. O., AND CHANDLER, F. W., Detection of hypersensitivity to *Legionella pneumophila* in guinea pigs by skin test, *Curr. Microbiol.* **4:**105–116 (1980).

115. WOODHEAD, M. A., AND MACFARLANE, J. T., Legionnaires' disease: A review of 79 community acquired cases in Nottingham, *Thorax* **41:**635–640 (1986).

116. YU, V. L., ZURAVLEFF, J. J., GAVLIK, L., AND MAGNUSSEN, M. H., Lack of evidence for person-to-person transmission of Legionnaires' disease, *J. Infect. Dis.* **147:**362 (1983).

117. ZURAVLEFF, J. J., YU, V. L., SHONNARD, J. W., DAVIS, B. K., AND RIHS, J. D., Diagnosis of Legionnaires' disease, *J. Am. Med. Assoc.* **250:**1981–1985 (1983).

12. Suggested Reading

BRENNER, D. J., Classification of *Legionellaceae:* Current status and remaining questions, *Isr. J. Med. Sci.* **22:**620–632 (1986).

EDELSTEIN, P. H., Laboratory diagnosis of infections caused by Legionellae, *Eur. J. Clin. Microbiol.* **6:**4–10 (1987).

FRASER, D. W., TSAI, T. F., ORENSTEIN, W., PARKIN, W. E., BEECHAM, H. J., SHARRAR, R. G., HARRIS, J., MALLISON, G. F., MARTIN, S. M., MCDADE, J. E., SHEPARD, C. C., BRACHMAN, P. S., AND The Field Investigation Team, Legionnaires' disease: Description of an epidemic of pneumonia, *N. Engl. J. Med.* **297:**1189–1197 (1977).

GLICK, T. H., GREGG, M. B., BERMAN, B., MALLISON, G. F., RHODES, W. W., JR., AND KASSANOFF, I., Pontiac fever: An epidemic of unknown etiology in a health department. I. Clinical and epidemiologic aspects, *Am. J. Epidemiol.* **107:**149–160 (1978).

MCDADE, J. E., SHEPARD, C. C., FRASER, D. W., TSAI, T. F., REDUS, M. A., DOWDLE, W. R., AND The Laboratory Investigation Team, Legionnaires' disease: Isolation of a bacterium and demonstration of its role in other respiratory disease, *N. Engl. J. Med.* **297:**1197–1203 (1977).

MUDER, R. R., YU, V. L., AND WOO, A. H., Mode of transmission of *Legionella pneumophila:* A critical review, *Arch. Intern. Med.* **146:**1607–1612 (1986).

THORNSBERRY, C., BALOWS, A., FEELEY, J. C., AND JAKUBOWSKI, W. (eds.), *Legionella,* American Society for Microbiology, Washington, D.C., 1984.

CHAPTER 16

Leprosy

Robert R. Jacobson

1. Introduction

Leprosy (Hansen's disease) is a chronic infectious disease caused by *Mycobacterium leprae* that primarily affects the skin, peripheral nerves, eyes, and mucous membranes. It has been known for well over 2000 years and afflicts more than 11 million people worldwide, mostly in underdeveloped nations. Hansen[31] discovered the etiological agent over 100 years ago, but it has still not definitely been cultured in artificial media, and there is much about the disease process we do not understand. In particular, relatively few good studies on the epidemiology and control of leprosy have been done.

As discussed in Section 8, leprosy may present in several different ways depending upon the resistance of the patient to the infection. The earliest form is referred to as indeterminate. The lesion is usually singular and often self-heals. Where self-healing or treatment does not intervene, the disease may remain localized in relatively resistant patients and evolve into tuberculoid disease, but if resistance is poor, generalized (lepromatous) disease develops. Between these two extremes is borderline leprosy, which may range from relatively localized to generalized skin involvement as one moves across the leprosy spectrum immunologically from the borderline-tuberculoid to borderline-lepromatous forms. Where the disease is uncommon, as in the United States, the diagnosis is often made relatively late. It can be a difficult disease to treat, and an understanding of the clinical aspects and the problems associated with treatment is probably more vital with this than with perhaps

any other infectious disease if one is to understand, for example, the failure of most serious control efforts over the last 40 years. Nevertheless, we have made considerable progress in this interval, and today, if the patient cooperates, we are able to manage nearly all cases satisfactorily and our control efforts are improving. Of equal importance is that we can now counteract most of the fears created by the folklore surrounding this disease so that the patient may retain normal position and repute in society.

2. Historical Background

It is uncertain just where and when the disease first appeared and whether biblical "leprosy" was in fact leprosy as we know it today. However, the opinion of most authorities[9] seems to be that it started in the Far East before 600 B.C. and then spread to the Near East and Africa and later to Europe. The incidence of the disease probably peaked in Europe in the Middle Ages and then gradually declined, ultimately disappearing in most of these countries, though it is still found in those that border the Mediterranean. The reasons for this disappearance are uncertain, but it has been suggested that a general improvement in hygiene and housing played a major role.[9] Leprosy was probably first introduced into the Americas via the early Spanish explorations and later by means of the slave trade. The first definite reference to the disease in the United States, however, was in 1758, in the Floridas,[3] and in the 1760s, cases occurring among the French were isolated near the mouth of the Mississippi River. In 1785, a hospital was established in New Orleans for the treatment of leprosy patients, and over 100 years later (1894), this facility was

Robert R. Jacobson · Clinical Branch, Gillis W. Long Hansen's Disease Center, Carville, Louisiana 70721.

moved to a location near the village of Carville, becoming the Louisiana Leper Home. Because patients from many states began seeking care there, the institution was acquired by the Federal government in 1921, becoming the National Leprosarium. As the Gillis W. Long Hansen's Disease Center (GWLHDC) at Carville, it continues in this function today. Nearly all states have some cases but most are from Hawaii, California, Texas, Louisiana, Florida, and the New York City area. Significant numbers of cases occurred among Scandinavian immigrants residing in and around Minnesota in the 19th century, but this focus has now completely disappeared. A settlement is maintained for Hawaiian patients at Kalaupapa on Molokai. One formerly existed on Penikese Island, Massachusetts, but this was closed in 1921, and the remaining 13 patients were transferred to Carville.

Significant milestones in the history of leprosy would have to include the discovery by Hansen[31] of *M. leprae* as the causative agent of this disease in 1874, the introduction of sulfone therapy in 1941,[23] the development of the mouse-footpad technique for growing the bacillus in 1960,[80] and the discovery that the bacillus grows readily in the armadillo in 1971.[41]

3. Methodology

3.1. Sources of Mortality Data

Leprosy is not, generally speaking, considered a fatal disease. Mortality statistics, therefore, do not reflect incidence.

3.2. Sources of Morbidity Data

Although many countries list leprosy as a reportable disease, existing morbidity data on leprosy are notoriously unreliable. There is still a significant stigma attached to the disease in most countries, so that patients often try to either conceal the diagnosis or seek the care of physicians who will not report it. In addition, even where the incidence is high, few countries have a good case-finding and/or reporting program. The World Health Organization (WHO)[76] considers leprosy "a communicable disease of major public health importance," but presumably because figures on the numbers of cases in member countries are so unreliable, no regular tabulation of data is published. Instead, attempts are periodically made to estimate the size of the problem. The WHO Leprosy Advisory Team surveyed a number of countries in Africa, Asia, and South America, and from their

experience an arbitrary multiplication factor was devised for calculating the total number of cases from registered cases. The factor was based on "an evaluation of the efficacy of case finding and the coverage of the country by health services."[76] The figure obtained probably represents a conservative estimate of the size of the world problem. In 1968, for example, there were 2,831,755 registered cases with an estimated total of 10,786,000 cases worldwide. Recently, the WHO reported[59] the data for 1985, and the number of registered cases had risen to 5,368,202. This represents a 90% increase since 1968, but the WHO believes that the total number of cases in 1985 remains in the 10–12 million range. The WHO recognizes the need for better reporting in this area, however, and is developing a central information system that it is hoped will be generally acceptable and become an integral part of the projected WHO Information System. In the United States, leprosy is a reportable disease in all states except Missouri, Oklahoma, Pennsylvania, South Dakota, and Vermont. National registries are maintained at the GWLHDC at Carville and the Centers for Disease Control (CDC) at Atlanta. Cases are reported on a leprosy surveillance form available from either Carville or the CDC. In the United States as elsewhere, because of attempts to conceal the diagnosis or laxity of physicians, leprosy is undoubtedly underreported, but to what extent is difficult to ascertain. Cases are reported in the *Morbidity and Mortality Weekly Report* under "Summary—Cases of specified notifiable disease, United States," and are periodically summarized in statistical reports issued by the GWLHDC. The Texas State Health Department includes leprosy case-reporting data in its *Texas Morbidity This Week*, but only for cases that occur within the state.

3.3. Serological Surveys and Skin Tests

Lepromin skin testing has been used for survey and classification studies in leprosy for over 60 years. Its preeminence in this area, however, is being challenged by antigen and antibody assays and more direct measures of cell-mediated immunity (CMI) such as the lymphocyte-transformation test (LTT).

Lepromin is prepared by autoclaving a suspension of *M. leprae* separated from human tissue (lepromin H). The separation is incomplete, so variable amounts of tissue are also present in the suspension. "Standard" lepromin H contains 160×10^6 bacilli/ml, but in use wide variations from the "standard" are not uncommon.[52] A 0.1-cm^3 dose of the suspension is injected intracutaneously, and readings are taken at 48 h for the Fernandez and at 3–4 weeks for the Mitsuda reaction. The former is thought to be an indication of preexisting delayed hypersensitivity to *M. leprae*, though its significance is less certain than that of the Mitsuda reaction and correlation between the two is poor. The Mitsuda reaction is read as positive if the induration is 3 mm or more, and doubtful if it is less than 3 mm. The reaction is a measure of the capacity of an individual to respond immunologically to *M. leprae* and will be positive in individuals with preexisting hypersensitivity to *M. leprae* or individuals not previously exposed but capable of developing delayed hypersensitivity to *M. leprae* in the interval between inoculation and the reading of the skin test. The WHO recommends that only the Mitsuda response be read. The test is invariably positive in tuberculoid leprosy cases and negative in lepromatous cases, and may be positive or negative in borderline (dimorphous) and indeterminate cases and in the general population. A more purified preparation, Dharmendra lepromin, is occasionally used. Only the 48-h reaction is generally useful with this, and it is considered equivalent in significance to the responses with integral lepromin. The large quantities of *M. leprae* obtainable from infected armadillos have resulted in the production of similar test preparations with these bacilli such as lepromin A.[52] Some of these are highly purified as with Convit's[16] soluble antigen. Although a considerable body of epidemiological data on whole populations and contacts living in leprosy-endemic areas has been obtained in studies utilizing lepromin testing, the quantities available are still limited and their use in the United States is considered investigational. Furthermore, even though the lepromin test is useful for determining whether an individual can generate an appropriate immune response to an *M. leprae* infection, it is of limited value in surveys of contacts or populations in endemic areas for evidence of infection by this bacillus. A positive Fernandez reaction has been found in up to 22% of those tested in a nonendemic area[84] probably due to cross-reacting antigens shared with other environmental mycobacteria. This same group showed a 100% rate of Mitsuda responsivity. Similar results were obtained elsewhere in the United States,[74] but Waters[93] found considerably lower levels of responsivity. It was hoped that the LTT would prove much more useful for surveys and be a more definitive measure of host response or resistance, or both, than the lepromin test. Overall, the results to date are encouraging. The LTT shows a much higher degree of specificity than the lepromin test for detecting previous exposure to *M. leprae*. It also has little cross-reactivity with *M. tuberculosis*,[27] but a considerable amount of cross-reactivity with bacillus Calmette–Guérin (BCG).[15] An 88% response rate has been found[26] in a subgroup of health personnel with extensive exposure to leprosy patients and without disease, but complete unresponsiveness in those not exposed. Similar findings have been noted among household contacts.[51] Results such as these confirm the usefulness of the test for survey studies and the test has also helped define the immunological spectrum of leprosy,[37] with responsiveness diminishing as one moves from tuberculoid (high-resistance) toward lepromatous (low-resistance) disease. Unfortunately, tests such as the LTT are not readily applicable under field conditions, so greater interest is now focused on antigen and antibody assays.

Two of the earliest assays studied were the fluorescent-leprosy-antibody-absorption (FLA-ABS) test of Abe[1] and a radioimmunoassay (RIA)[33] test for specific and nonspecific *M. leprae* antigens. Both have relatively good sensitivity and specificity in the hands of some investigators, and although studies continue,[2] neither is as yet suitable for large-scale use under field conditions. Much more promising is the use of monoclonal antibodies to detect species-specific antigens of *M. leprae*.[78] Of particular interest is the discovery of the *M. leprae*-specific phenolic glycolipid-I (PGL-I) antigen and the development of an enzyme-linked immunosorbent assay (ELISA) technique to measure PGL-I antibodies.[99] The titers of PGL-I antibodies detected in leprosy patients are proportional to the bacillary load and high titers have also been found in some contacts of multibacillary (MB) patients as well as a portion of the inhabitants of endemic areas.[5] Whether it can reliably detect a major portion of those at high risk for developing leprosy is the focus of current epidemiological studies. It is possible that lepromin testing might have to be combined with assays such as that for PGL-I antibodies if titers are low to define those at greatest risk for developing overt disease. In summary, it is clear that although lepromin testing continues to be the most common approach to survey work, continuing efforts in these areas may eventually result in a reliable serological test for the diagnosis and perhaps follow-up of leprosy patients. Now under development,[5] for example, are tests based on other *M. leprae*-specific antigens or epitopes defined by *M. leprae*-specific monoclonal antibodies, or on peptides defined by the DNA sequences of the corresponding genes. Such tests might be extremely valuable for control programs.

3.4. Laboratory Diagnosis

Only three standard tests are extensively used in leprosy-control work throughout the world: skin scrapings, skin biopsy, and the mouse-footpad cultivation of *M. leprae* for drug-sensitivity studies. Skin scrapings are obtained by pinching the skin to diminish blood flow, wiping the area with an alcohol sponge, and making a small slit with a sterile razor blade or scalpel. The slit is then gently scraped, and the material obtained is smeared on a microscopic slide. The bacillus grows better at cooler temperatures and thus will be more abundant in cool regions such as the earlobes. Selected skin lesions are scraped in all leprosy cases and the ears, elbows, and knees in all newly diagnosed, borderline, and lepromatous patients. Several of the more active sites are then periodically rescraped to follow the clearance of bacilli.

A biopsy should be taken from entirely within the margin of the chosen lesion. Some sections from it are then stained with hematoxylin–eosin for routine histopathology. A Fite–Faraco stain for acid-fast bacilli (AFB) is used on other sections and the skin smears. The number of AFB are then quantitated using a semilogarithmic scale called the bacterial index (BI) as in Table 1. The percentage of bacilli that appear normal with respect to size, shape, and uniformity of staining (1–5% in a typical newly diagnosed case) is also determined and is referred to as the morphological index (MI). This is correlated to some extent with viability in that when the MI becomes 0, the bacillus can no longer be routinely grown in the mouse-footpad system. Shepard[80] first reported that M. leprae will grow to a limited extent in mouse footpads in 1960. In this system, a small biopsy is taken from an active site on a patient. The M. leprae bacilli are separated and put into a suspension, and 5000 bacilli are then routinely injected into one footpad on each mouse. The number of mice used depends on the number of drugs evaluated, but normally 10–20 controls will be injected plus 10 more for each drug concentration to be tested. Typically, treated groups will contain mice fed 0.01, 0.001, and 0.0001% dapsone, 0.001% clofazimine, and 0.01% rifampin. Maximal growth is attained in about 6 months, when the original 5000 bacilli will have increased to about 10^6 if viable M. leprae were present in the inoculum. Lack of growth in the drug-treated group denotes sensitivity to that dietary level of the drug in question.

Table 1. Bacterial Index

0	No	bacilli per	100	OIFs[a]
1+	1–10	bacilli per	100	OIFs
2+	1–10	bacilli per	10	OIFs
3+	1–10	bacilli per		OIF
4+	10–100	bacilli per		OIF
5+	100–1000	bacilli per		OIF
6+	>1000	bacilli per		OIF

[a]OIF, oil-immersion field.

Other laboratory studies are occasionally employed, in particular the measurement of blood sulfone levels. Multiple circulating autoantibodies have been reported,[68] and false-positive serologies are not uncommon.

4. Biological Characteristics of the Organism

M. leprae is considered an obligate intracellular parasite. Our knowledge of it is limited because of the relatively small number of investigators in the leprosy field and inability to culture the organism on artificial media. A report of successful culturing by Skinsnes et al.[87] proved to be a failure, and tissue-culture attempts have also failed. The organism grows readily in the armadillo, however, and this now provides large numbers of relatively tissue-free bacilli for investigation. Although organisms can be isolated and positively identified only from patients with high bacterial counts and the Henle–Koch postulates [see Chapter 1 (Section 13)] have yet to be fulfilled, few would question that M. leprae is the causative agent of leprosy.

M. leprae is an acid-fast bacillus, 0.3–0.4 μm × 2–7 μm. On skin scrapings or biopsy sections, the bacilli are often clustered in oval formations called globi. Over 90% of the bacilli from a typical new patient stain irregularly, appear granular, and have been shown to be nonviable[83] for the mouse footpad. With successful chemotherapy, all bacilli will become granular and disintegrate. Staining is usually done with the Fite-Faraco modification of the Ziehl–Neelsen technique. Although the disintegrating bacilli appear to clear slowly with treatment, this may at least occasionally be due to a loss of acid-fastness by the bacillary remnants. Staining with the Gomori methenamine—silver technique or the Nyka method has demonstrated[43] bacilli in some biopsy sections that had shown none with a Fite-Faraco stain. The substances on which the acid-fastness of M. leprae depends are also extractable with pyridine.[25] The bacilli will survive freezing as low as −80°C for prolonged periods[65] and in dried secretions for up to 9 days in a hot, humid climate.[18] At the temperature of wet ice, they may survive 2 weeks or more. Heating at 45°C for 1 h reportedly[63] kills them, but their antigenic activity persists at temperatures of over 100°C.[85] In the mouse footpad, maximum growth occurs[81] at an average footpad temperature in the 27–30°C range, which corresponds with its growth pattern in humans; i.e., the highest bacterial counts occur in the cooler areas of the body.

Of great importance is the discovery[66] of dihydroxyphenylalanine (dopa) oxidase in suspensions of M. leprae.

Most authorities regard the ability to oxidize dopa as an identifying characteristic of this bacillus, since it has not been found in any other mycobacteria. Dopa oxidase activity has been included in a list[72] of seven criteria that must be met to confirm that bacilli cultured in an artificial medium from human or armadillo leprosy tissues are *M. leprae*. The other six include identity with all known characters of *M. leprae* including drug-sensitivity patterns, identical antigen composition, exclusion of environmental contamination or similarity to other known mycobacteria, similar growth in experimental animals, similar results when used in lepromin testing, and identical chemical composition of the cell-wall skeleton. In this way, bacilli listed in the American Type Culture Collection as *M. leprae* have been shown[40] to be erroneously labeled. Growth in the mouse footpad is very characteristic of *M. leprae* compared to other mycobacteria.[62] The usual sensitivity of *M. leprae* to very low levels of dapsone is also unique.[82] The bacilli have an average generation time of 12.5 days[82] in the mouse footpad, and though there appear to be "fast"- and "slow"-growing strains, this characteristic seems to have no bearing on human disease.

The large numbers of bacilli available from armadillos have allowed the initiation of multiple studies to characterize the bacillus further. The size of the genome in *M. leprae* is about 1.7×10^9 daltons with a guanine + cytosine (G + C) ratio of 54% and homology among bacilli from three different sources.[69] Further advances in molecular biology have led to the construction of genomic libraries of *M. leprae*[14,39] including the cloning and expression of its entire genome in *E. coli*.[100] Likewise, large numbers of nonspecific *M. leprae* antigens are known and some specific antigens have been identified using in particular monoclonal antibodies. The most thoroughly investigated of these is PGL-I,[99] which has yielded a significant serodiagnostic test for leprosy. Obviously, our knowledge of the biological characteristics of *M. leprae* remains limited, but progress in this area has been relatively rapid in the last 5 years and is likely to continue.

5. Descriptive Epidemiology

Statistical data for leprosy are, as noted in Section 3.2, a massive hodgepodge of figures, many of which are inaccurate. What follows is an attempt to ferret out the best available information both for the worldwide leprosy problem and for our relatively limited problem in the United States.

5.1. Prevalence and Incidence

Worldwide figures are meaningless, since the disease occurs only in some countries and often varies markedly within a given country. The estimated prevalence will also be higher than figures based on the actual number of registered cases, and it may not always be clear which figure a given report refers to. Typical prevalences per 1000 population for Southeast Asia,[59] for example, range from 0.67 in Sri Lanka and 4.41 in India to 6.73 in Burma, with some areas of that country having an estimated rate as high as 44/1000.[60] Figure 1 illustrates the prevalence per 1000 population worldwide based on the number of registered cases reported to the WHO. Accurate figures on incidence in these areas are generally not available because of problems in obtaining complete reporting of new cases. In the United States, the total number of known cases for 1986 was about 5500, giving a prevalence of approximately 2.3/100,000 population with an incidence rate of 0.15/100,000 in that year (360 cases). If only "endemic" areas of the United States are considered, incidence ranges from 0.2/100,000 in Louisiana to 3.13/100,000 in Hawaii. The incidence in the United States has been higher in recent years, due mainly to an increase in imported cases particularly from Southeast Asia, Mexico, and the Caribbean,[22] and these cases now outnumber native born cases about 9 to 1. With all these studies, it is important to realize that as Rees and Meade[71] have pointed out, incidence rates in leprosy will tend to be higher with increasing frequency of examination. This occurs because more early lesions are detected, and many of these would have regressed spontaneously and thus have been missed if examinations had been done very infrequently.

5.2. Epidemic Behavior and Contagiousness

It appears from LTT, serological, and epidemiological studies on household contacts and others with extensive exposure that, contrary to older beliefs, leprosy has a very high infectivity, but a low pathogenicity for most individuals. Epidemics in the usual sense of the word do not commonly occur with leprosy. It is true that the spread of leprosy throughout Europe in the Middle Ages is sometimes referred to as an epidemic,[9] but some of these cases were probably not leprosy, the spread was gradual over a period of many years, and we have relatively little accurate information about it. The Nauru epidemic in the 1920s is probably the best-documented occurrence of a true leprosy epidemic.[89] Leprosy was introduced onto this island by a

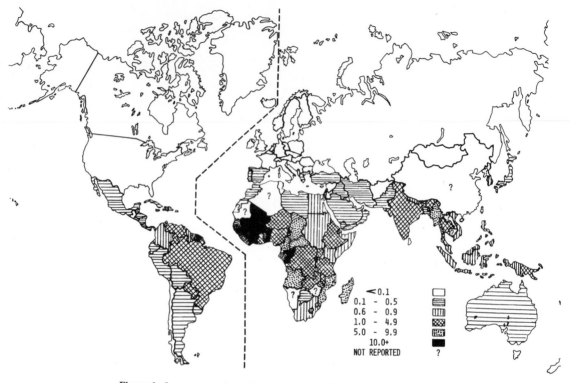

Figure 1. Leprosy prevalence based on registered cases per 1000 population.

woman who arrived there about 1912. In 1920, the first case appeared among the native population, and by 1924, there were 284 cases in the population of 1200–1300. By 1929, 438 cases had been found, and apparently the incidence gradually diminished thereafter. Thus, at the peak of the epidemic, 34% of the population had been afflicted. Over 90% of the cases were the tuberculoid type, and deformities were uncommon. On the basis of the findings in Nauru, New Guinea, and elsewhere, Leiker[45] noted that where leprosy is newly introduced, what is essentially an "epidemic" of tuberculoid leprosy occurs, the disease spreads rapidly, there are no foci of infection, and adults and children are equally susceptible. In old endemic areas, however, there is more lepromatous disease than in the newly infected population, a higher proportion of the cases are among children and young adults, the disease spreads slowly, and there are foci, i.e., particular villages and families with a higher incidence than others. It is evident that the pattern of leprosy in Nauru (an extreme and unprecedented example) and in other newly infected populations does indeed fit Leiker's postulates; however, it does not appear that older foci always behave as he proposed. The incidence of

lepromatous leprosy in much of Africa and India, for example, is rather low (10–20% of all new cases). In the United States, on the other hand,[22] about 50% of cases are classified lepromatous, 15–20% borderline, and 30–35% tuberculoid and indeterminate.

5.3. Geographic Distribution

Leprosy today is found mostly in developing countries, the majority of which are in tropical and semitropical areas. Since it occurred in much of the north temperate zone in the past, however, climate probably has little to do with its present distribution.

5.4. Temporal Distribution

There is no significant variation in occurrence with the seasons.

5.5. Age

It is difficult to make generalizations about the age of onset of leprosy, but several reviews of the topic are worthy of note. A study of childhood leprosy[60] notes that it is uncommon below 2 years of age, though cases below the age of 6 months have been reported. A significant number of cases below 5 years of age will be found in countries with a high or very high prevalence, and prevalence rates rise up to age 14, reaching values as high as and occasionally higher than those for the general population. Guinto[30] states that "it is a fact that children are much more susceptible than adults," but Newell[57] feels that statistics in this regard could be equally well interpreted as indicating only that children have more opportunity for exposure. More recently, the findings in Goa and from several other series in India and throughout the world have been tabulated.[79] These studies emphasize the great variations seen not only from country to country, but also within the same country. Generally speaking, the median age at onset is somewhere between 20 and 30. The most recent data from the United States[22] show about half the cases being below 35 at the time of diagnosis, with the oldest being in their 80s.

5.6. Sex

Sex ratios are generally 1 : 1 for children, but for adults the disease is usually more prevalent among males by a ratio of about 1.5 or 1.6 : 1.[60] In the United States from 1981 to 1987, males predominated by a ratio of 1.6 : 1. The reason for this predominance of adult males is unknown, but it could be due to greater susceptibility or greater exposure outside the household setting in most cultures.

5.7. Race

Although there are wide variations in incidence and prevalence and in the way the disease manifests itself throughout the world, there are no data that indicate any special race-related susceptibility or resistance, all other things being equal.

5.8. Occupation

There is no particular relationship between occupation and the occurrence of leprosy. Some studies[29] have found an increased incidence of leprosy among missionaries working with leprosy patients; however, the prevalence was well below that in the population they were serving and was "increased" only over the prevalence in their homelands. In one study,[49] native hospital workers actually had less chance of contracting the disease than their counterparts in other occupations, and no cases have occurred among the staff at Carville.

5.9. Occurrence in Different Settings

The incidence of leprosy is generally higher in a family with one or more cases than in families with no cases, but considerable variation exists. Guinto[30] notes that in a retrospective study done in the Philippines in 1935, the risk of contracting leprosy was 8 times greater in family contacts of lepromatous patients than in the general population. In a follow-up prospective study (1935–1950), the risk was about 5 times greater, rather than 8 times. A study by Kluth[42] in Texas found that 2.6% of 1522 household contacts of lepromatous patients developed leprosy. On the other hand, after a review of several other series, mostly foreign ones, Filice and Fraser[24] concluded that the long-term risk was such that about 10% of the household contacts of lepromatous patients would ultimately develop the disease. In all these studies, exposure to tuberculoid and probably indeterminate disease had an extremely small effect, i.e., the incidence of leprosy in these families was not significantly higher than in the general population. In United States studies, the risks of exposed adults and children have been about the same, but in other countries, the risk for children is considerably higher.[24] The chance of one spouse's infecting the other has also been evaluated[4] and seems to be about 5%. Institutional exposure can occasionally lead to very high rates. Of 2000 children born in or admitted to Culion Leprosarium in the Philippines in the 1930s without any sign of leprosy, 23% later developed it.[60] Over 75% spontaneously healed, however. Among United States military veterans, the incidence of leprosy has been relatively low. A review[10] of the 240 cases known to have occurred among veterans from 1940 through 1968 reported that only 46 were considered to have service-connected leprosy from exposure outside the United States.

5.10. Socioeconomic Factors

Leprosy today occurs mostly among the poor in underdeveloped countries. Why this is so is uncertain; however, crowded living conditions, poor diet, inadequate medical care, and improper sanitation may all play a role. Protein–calorie malnutrition has been shown,[35] for example, to alter immune responses.

5.11. Genetic Factors

It has long been suspected that a genetic defect determines susceptibility to leprosy and its mode of expression, but definitive proof of this is lacking. Hastings[34] points out that familial clustering of leprosy patients, wide variation in prevalence and type of leprosy within a given population, high concordance rates of leprosy in identical twins, the persistence of anergy to *M. leprae* in inactive lepromatous patients, and the study of Dharmendra and Chatterjee[19] indicating a preexisting immune defect in patients destined to get lepromatous leprosy all favor the existence of a genetic defect, probably in the immune-response (Ir) genes. Although the investigations of leprosy in identical twins[13,53] lend support to the theory, they are not conclusive because the concordance rates, though relatively high, were far from perfect. Multiple studies of histocompatibility antigens in leprosy patients have likewise given mixed results. Recent studies[77,88] have been more fruitful, demonstrating, for example, a possible association between HLA-DR2 and/or HLA-DR3 and a predisposition to tuberculoid leprosy, but further research is needed.

6. Mechanisms and Routes of Transmission

The mechanism by which leprosy is transmitted is unknown, but three possibilities exist. The oldest theory holds that it is the result of prolonged close skin-to-skin-type contact with an active infectious case or through skin via fomites. Since it is unlikely that *M. leprae* could penetrate intact skin, a break such as a cut or an abrasion would seem to be necessary for this to occur. Evidence cited[30] to support this theory includes the appearance of the first leprosy lesion in children at the sites most touched by their infected mothers, the preponderance of initial leprosy lesions on the legs and feet of patients living in rocky areas, and accidental inoculation by tattooing or at surgery. This evidence actually provides relatively little support for transmission via the skin. It would not be surprising that the bacillus might be inoculated via injuries that pierce the skin, and the literature contains a number of studies showing that the site of the first lesion in children is not related to the extent to which an area is touched.[6] Furthermore, over 50% of cases in low- to moderate-endemicity areas give no history of contact with a leprosy case.[22] Thus, "prolonged" or "intimate" contact in these instances seems unlikely. The possible role of the nose and upper respiratory tract in the transmission of leprosy has been studied extensively. Pedley[64] demonstrated that although bacilli may easily be found in the nasal discharge, they are difficult to locate on the skin surface. Davey and Rees[17] demonstrated that a high percentage of bacilli passed out in the nasal discharge are viable and can survive up to 7 days. A single nose blow from 31 patients gave a mean discharge of 1.1×10^8 bacilli with a mean

morphological index of 16.9%. It has also been shown[70] that mice may be infected with *M. leprae* via the respiratory route followed by dissemination of the infection, and many similarities exist[71] between the modes of spread and routes of infection of tuberculosis and leprosy in a population. Of further interest in this regard is a report[12] that 4% of random nasal mucosal biopsies from household contacts showed bacilli and histopathological changes of leprosy.

Reports of acid-fast bacilli (AFB) in the stomachs of insects who had bitten leprosy patients appeared as early as 1912.[30] Proof that transmission by this route is possible has only recently been reported,[54] however. After earlier demonstration that mosquitoes and bedbugs took up viable *M. leprae* when biting untreated patients, it was shown that mosquitoes (*Aedes aegypti*) were capable of transmitting the infection to mouse footpads. This important work demonstrated that arthropod transmission of leprosy is possible, but there is no evidence that it is a probable route in humans, and further studies are needed. The question of how leprosy is transmitted, then, remains undecided, but on the basis of available data, the most likely possibility would seem to be that it is, in the majority of instances, spread by the respiratory route, though insect vectors or the transcutaneous route may occasionally play a role.

Several other possible sources of infection have been suggested. Beginning in 1975, it was reported[91] that uninoculated armadillos caught in Louisiana were infected with AFB ultimately proven to be *M. leprae*. Numerous other surveys have confirmed that this occurs in 2–6.8% of armadillos caught in parts of Texas and Louisiana.[38] The significance of this is uncertain and the problem appears to be confined to the United States. Originally it was felt that this was not a likely source of human infection,[46] but some investigators[48] have found evidence that transmission of the disease from armadillos to humans may at least occasionally occur. Leprosy has also been found in a chimpanzee from Sierra Leone[20] and a sooty mangabey monkey from Nigeria. These animals might have caught it from handlers, but its apparent transmission to a second mangabey monkey kept with the first[28] indicates that monkey-to-monkey spread could occur. Evidence that *M. leprae* may exist free in nature has also been found,[36] raising the possibility that this may be the source of infection in these various animals and perhaps occasionally in man. It is clear that much more research will be needed to resolve these issues. The possibility of a carrier state for leprosy has also been the subject of several studies reviewed by Guinto,[30] but no strong evidence supporting such a condition has been found.

7. Pathogenesis and Immunity

The incubation period of leprosy varies from less than 1 year to decades, but is generally about 3 to 5 years.[4] What determines susceptibility—i.e., who will develop clinically evident leprosy—has been the subject of considerable research over the last 20 years attempting to define the presumed immunological defect in these patients. Our present understanding of the problem is that those who are susceptible have a defect in cell-mediated immunity (CMI) that is relatively specific for *M. leprae*. The etiology of this defect is still not satisfactorily defined, but the most popular view is that the specific depression of CMI results from suppressor T cell activity. This was originally proposed by Mehra[50] who detected *M. leprae*-induced suppressor cells in the blood of lepromatous, but not tuberculoid cases, contacts, or normal controls. It was suggested, but not proven, that these might inhibit the response of helper T cells to *M. leprae* antigens. These findings have recently been duplicated,[56] and a number of arguments for and against this hypothesis and other possibilities are reviewed by Harboe.[32] If this is the source of the defect, it is not yet clear whether it is genetic, acquired, or both. There is also evidence for a moderate general impairment of CMI in untreated lepromatous leprosy patients, in particular such as lack of dinitrochlorobenzene sensitization,[90] reduced numbers of T cells,[47] and diminished response to intradermal skin tests.[11] On the other hand, these patients are capable of handling other infections including mycobacterial ones in a normal fashion, they have no evidence of an increased incidence of cancer,[61] and there is apparently recovery of the generalized CMI impairment with treatment, though the response of lepromatous patients to lepromin does not become positive with elimination of most of the bacterial load. It is apparent that additional research is needed before the immunology of this disease is fully understood.

Two decades ago, it was common to describe the different forms of leprosy as distinct disease entities. While this was satisfactory for clinical purposes, it tended to obscure the fact that these were all merely different manifestations of the same disease. What was needed was a classification that integrated the clinical, immunological, and histopathological findings. It was against this background that the Ridley–Jopling classification[73] was introduced in 1962, and with the addition of a classification for reactions, it has gained relatively widespread acceptance, particularly with all involved in leprosy research. Figure 2 illustrates our current concept of this disease in terms of the five-part Ridley–Jopling classification.

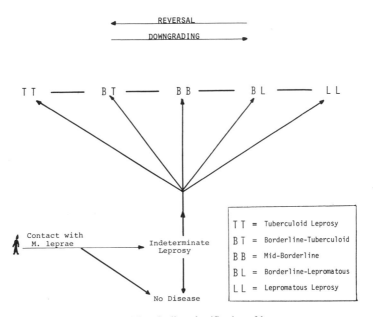

Figure 2. Ridley–Jopling classification of leprosy.

While very important for research purposes and a complete understanding of leprosy, the Ridley–Jopling classification may be difficult to apply under field conditions where the work may be carried out mostly by paramedical help with much less medical training. Therefore, in 1982 the WHO proposed[97] a new classification for use under field conditions that utilizes only two categories, paucibacillary (PB) and multibacillary (MB). PB patients are those with a BI of 0 at all sites and would include indeterminate, TT, and BT patients. MB are those with a BI of 1+ or more at at least one site, and would include those classified BB, BL, and LL. Though now widely used, it has been criticized because occasional MB patients may be misclassified as PB as a result of too few or inadequate skin scrapings. It has also been argued that BT cases with large numbers of lesions might better be classified MB. Thus, it may be modified in the future, but for the present it has greatly simplified classification of patients under field conditions.

When leprosy bacilli are transmitted from a patient to a contact, the overwhelming majority (> 95%) appear able to resist the infection; i.e., their macrophages engulf, destroy, and digest the bacilli with no outward sign of the infection developing. In contacts with the specific CMI defect, on the other hand, the macrophages ingest the bacilli, but in effect fail to fully recognize them as pathogens and, depending on the extent of the defect, allow them to multiply and disseminate to varying degrees. Dissemination is probably hematogenous, since it has been repeatedly demonstrated[21] that *M. leprae* bacilli are readily found within neutrophils and mononuclear phagocytes or occasionally free in the buffy coat of centrifuged blood specimens from untreated lepromatous leprosy cases. Other types also demonstrate this finding, but its frequency diminishes, as one might expect, as one moves from disseminated (lepromatous) to localized (tuberculoid) disease. Because of the long incubation period, finding the source of the infection may be difficult.

As shown in Fig. 2, the earliest lesion in all cases is commonly referred to as indeterminate leprosy. It is usually nothing more than a hypopigmented macule or macules, and biopsy sections will show only a minimal nonspecific chronic inflammatory infiltrate in the upper dermis around nerves, blood vessels, and glands. Only rare bacilli are likely to be present, and locating them may require review of multiple sections. This may be self-healing in up to 75% of the cases,[60] but if diagnosed is always treated. Those lesions that are neither treated nor self-healing will ultimately progress to one of the three common clinical types. Those with the greatest relative degree of resistance keep the infection localized and develop tuberculoid disease, referred to as TT in the Ridley–Jopling classification. Biopsy sections in these cases are characterized by epithelioid-cell granulomas surrounded by lymphocytes. Nerve bundles are invaded and destroyed, often to the point of being unidentifiable, and the nerve involvement is pathognomonic of leprosy. As with indeterminate disease, there are only rare bacilli, and they are difficult to locate.

Those with the least resistance to the infection go on to develop lepromatous disease (LL). Histologically, the infiltrate in these cases initially consists of macrophages around dermal appendages, nerves, and blood vessels. It gradually increases to the point where in advanced cases it may replace most of the dermis. The number of *M. leprae* bacilli in macrophages gradually increases, replacing the cytoplasm, which becomes vacuolated with accumulated lipid, forming foam cells. Bacilli are easily demonstrable [bacterial index (BI) = 4–6+] and lymphocytes are, for practical purposes, absent.

Between these extremes, there is a broad zone referred to as borderline (dimorphous) leprosy. Histologically, lesions in these cases present a varied picture ranging from a tuberculoid appearance on the borderline-tuberculoid (BT) side of the spectrum through the mixed histology of the midborderline (BB) area to a more lepromatous appearance in the borderline-lepromatous (BL) region. The infiltrate consists mostly of lymphocytes and epithelioid and giant cells in BT cases, but as one moves toward BL, the number of lymphocytes steadily diminishes, the infiltrate consists mostly of macrophages, and bacilli increase in numbers (BI = 2–4+). This change in the number of lymphocytes is, of course, consistent with the presumed decrease in immune status from the tuberculoid end of the spectrum to the lepromatous.

While the disease in a patient at either pole (tuberculoid or lepromatous) in the Ridley–Jopling classification tends to be stable, relatively wide shifts in disease type can occur in the broad borderline portion of the spectrum. Without treatment, the tendency is for immunity to diminish with a consequent shift of the disease toward lepromatous. With treatment, on the other hand, the tendency is for the disease to shift in the other direction toward tuberculoid with an enhanced immune response. If reactions (see Section 8) accompany these immunological shifts, they are referred to as downgrading and reversal (type 1) reactions, respectively. Thus, a patient's disease may start out relatively localized (BT), but with time may downgrade with more extensive disease developing and be classified BB or beyond when diagnosed. With treatment, immunological improvement may occur (reversal), moving the patient toward BT again.

8. Patterns of Host Response

The combination of skin lesions and sensory loss is the hallmark of leprosy. Rarely, a combination such as necrobiosis lipoidica diabeticorum with a diabetic polyneuropathy may mimic leprosy, but a skin biopsy will quickly establish the correct diagnosis. In addition to the biopsy, skin scrapings are usually obtained.

Indeterminate leprosy usually presents as one or more hypopigmented, occasionally erythematous macules on the face, extremities, or buttocks. Sensation may be slightly diminished or normal, and diagnosis is confirmed by biopsy. Because of its benign appearance, it is most often diagnosed during contact examinations or case-finding surveys. Tuberculoid leprosy (TT) normally presents as one or two large (up to 30 or more cm) hypopigmented anesthetic lesions that may be macular, with or without a raised margin, or occasionally plaquelike. The surface is generally scaly, and usually only peripheral nerves in the area are involved. Lepromatous leprosy (LL) is usually generalized when diagnosed. It may present as disseminated, faint, erythematous macules, as a generalized papular and nodular eruption, or as diffuse disease with no distinct lesions. In advanced cases, any or all of the following may be seen: loss of eyebrows, nasal stuffiness (occasionally with septal perforation and collapse of the bridge of the nose), epistaxis, hoarseness, and the classic "leonine" facies. Motor loss may produce claw hands, claw toes, or footdrop, or any combination thereof. Sensory loss may affect only the distal extremities or may have progressed to the point of nearly total body anesthesia, sparing only the warmer regions such as the axillae. Borderline disease occupies the broad middle portion of the leprosy spectrum. Skin changes vary from being tuberculoid-like in the BT region to lepromatous-like in BL disease with mixed findings for BB cases. Likewise, sensory loss ranges from being in and around lesions in BT cases to lepromatous-like in BL. Nerve involvement leading to extensive motor loss tends to be more severe in borderline cases than in any of the other types.

Erythema nodosum leprosum [(ENL), or type 2] and reversal (type 1) reactions may develop before diagnosis and treatment, but usually occur afterward and are seen with varying degrees of severity in about 50% of cases. ENL occurs in BL and LL cases and usually presents as fever and erythematous, tender, frequently painful nodules that develop rapidly. Neuritis, malaise, arthralgias, leukocytosis, iridocyclitis, lymphadenitis, pretibial periosteitis, orchitis, and nephritis may also occur. ENL can be controlled with thalidomide, corticosteroids, or clofazimine, or a combination thereof.

Reversal reactions, as noted in Section 7, result from a delayed-type hypersensitivity response to *M. leprae* antigens because a change or "reversal" has apparently occurred in the patient's ability to respond to these. They occur in borderline cases and may produce fever, neuritis, edema, and erythema of preexisting lesions, sometimes progressing to ulceration and new lesions. The neuritis may lead to severe motor or sensory loss, and high doses of corticosteroids must often be used to halt the process and reverse the damage. Other complications of leprosy include iridocyclitis without signs of reaction, which may damage vision if not controlled, and injuries as a result of sensory loss.

9. Treatment, Prevention, and Control

9.1. Treatment

Overall, the results of treatment are very satisfactory for patients who cooperate fully in their care. Further transmission of the disease is eliminated and serious deformities are, for the most part, prevented. However, as noted below there are problems confronting those who treat leprosy patients that must be overcome if overall control efforts are to succeed.

Isolation of patients is not necessary, since all their usual contacts have already received maximal exposure during the incubation period, random contacts are at no significant risk, and treatment rapidly renders them noninfectious. Even the most severe cases of LL, for example, are probably noncontagious within 1–2 weeks of the start of therapy.

The WHO recommends[97] treating all PB patients with dapsone plus rifampin for 6 months and then discontinuing therapy. Many physicians in the United States and elsewhere, however, follow this initial treatment by continuing dapsone as monotherapy for 3–7 years depending on the Ridley–Jopling classification of the patient's disease. MB patients may be given clofazimine in addition to the dapsone and rifampin as recommended by the WHO with therapy continued at least 2 years and preferably to BI negativity. The WHO recommends discontinuing therapy at that point, but in some countries including the United States the patients are often continued thereafter on dapsone monotherapy indefinitely to prevent relapse. Multidrug therapy will hopefully stem the rising tide of primary and secondary dapsone resistance created by the almost universal use of dapsone monotherapy in the past. Whether it will allow the markedly shortened treatment intervals recommended by the WHO is as yet uncertain. Persistent viable bacilli are known to remain in these cases,[94,95] and all trials in the past with dapsone monotherapy invariably had a significant relapse rate.[94] Fortunately, the initial results of multidrug therapy are promising,[5] but long-term follow-up of these patients will be necessary. Obviously, the prolonged treatment required particularly by MB patients, even if the short-term WHO regimens are successful, represents an impediment to leprosy control. Noncompliance thus remains a significant problem and with it may come relapse, perhaps with drug-resistant *M. leprae,* and further transmission of the infection. Thus, research to shorten therapy even further than the intervals recommended by the WHO is a high priority. This would include further improvement of chemotherapy utilizing new drugs such as the fluorinated quinolines[5] and immunotherapy to correct the immune deficit in leprosy patients. Approaches to immunotherapy have included, for example, transfer factor,[34] γ-interferon,[55] and vaccination with a mixture of BCG and heat-killed *M. leprae.*[16] Initial results with all of these have been encouraging, but much more research will be needed before this becomes a practical approach to therapy.

Further complicating therapy are the reversal reactions and ENL mentioned earlier. These will occur with varying degrees of severity in about half the cases and, if not properly treated, can lead to further motor and sensory loss. Therapy should not be discontinued in these cases; instead, the reactive episodes should be suppressed with corticosteroids or other appropriate drugs that will prevent further neural damage and may reverse that which has already occurred. Unfortunately, reactions continue to represent one of the major reasons patients become disillusioned with treatment and discontinue it.

9.2. Prevention

As noted in Section 5, a large portion of new cases occur because of contact within the family; for many cases outside the family setting, no history of contact can be obtained. Thus, preventive measures directed at the household contacts of borderline and LL patients are likely to be the most beneficial. Three approaches are possible: prophylactic dapsone, regular contact examinations, and BCG. Several studies have been reported[58,92] utilizing oral dapsone as a prophylactic measure in doses ranging from 1 mg/kg once weekly to 100 mg three times weekly. All report that prophylactic dapsone reduces the incidence of leprosy in contacts over that in a control group receiving a placebo by about 40–80%. This is not surprising, since if you treat a group of contacts as though they had leprosy, i.e., give them dapsone, there should not be many new

cases showing up in the group while they are treated, and the success rate should theoretically approach 100%. Given the natural history of LL and the effect of interrupted therapy, it would be more important to know what happens when prophylactic dapsone is discontinued; i.e., were, in particular, cases of LL actually prevented, or their onset only delayed? None of these studies answer this question satisfactorily because prolonged (10+ years) follow-up is not reported. Much better in this regard are the trials[75] carried out on two isolated Pacific islands with an incidence rate of $^7/_{1000}$. A moderately successful attempt was made to treat all the population with 15 injections of acedapsone over a 3-year period. This drug is the diacetyl derivative of dapsone and, given in a dose of 225 mg every 11 weeks, maintains a low, relatively stable level of dapsone in the blood throughout the interval. As expected, the incidence of new cases fell to zero during the trial, but cases began appearing again shortly after the trial was discontinued and have continued to appear up to the present, though at a lower rate than before. The authors conclude that the failure of the trial in terms of eliminating leprosy from these islands is due to poor control of preexisting MB (borderline and LL) leprosy cases in the population. However, until the results of at least 10 years' follow-up become available, any conclusions about the effectiveness of 3 years of acedapsone therapy in preventing LL disease in contacts would be premature, though the initial results are encouraging. Furthermore, one possible danger with acedapsone, i.e., that it might encourage the development of sulfone-resistant strains of *M. leprae* because of the low blood levels involved, has not proven to be a problem, but this possibility must be kept in mind by anyone using it.[96] After a review of the available data from these and other trials, the WHO Expert Committee on Leprosy stated in their Fifth Report[96] that they "could not recommend the use of dapsone in large scale control programs," though "in certain circumstances there might be a limited place for the administration of prophylactic dapsone." Nonetheless, a review of the problem by epidemiologists at the CDC[24] concludes that the contacts of untreated LL and borderline cases are at relatively high risk of disease. The reviewers recommend that those up to age 25 should be given therapeutic doses of dapsone for 3 years and that all, regardless of age, should be examined annually for at least 5 years. Though a significant risk exists for up to 12 years, cooperation in follow-up is difficult to maintain for more than 5 years. Contacts should be checked for skin, motor, neural, or sensory changes that suggest the onset of leprosy. Any suspicious findings are followed up with a biopsy and skin scrapings. Figure 3 outlines the CDC's proposals for the management of contacts in the form of a

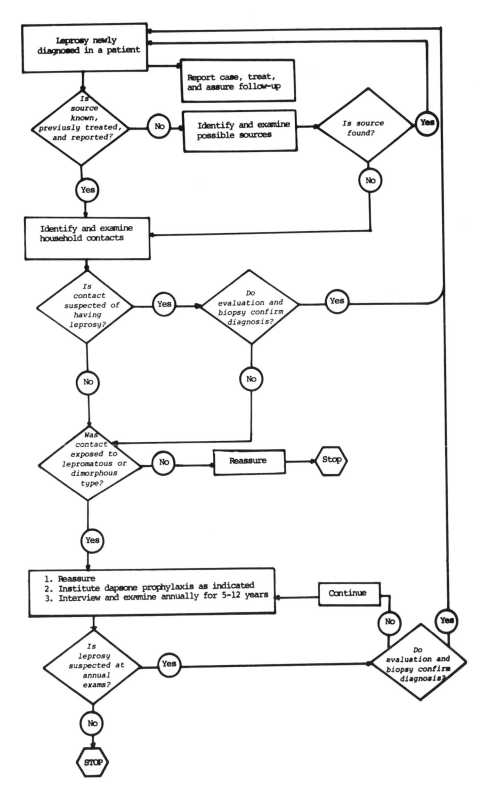

Figure 3. Flow chart of the management of household contacts of leprosy patients.[24]

flow chart. Contacts entering the household after the index case has been placed on treatment are at very little risk because of the "chemical isolation" of the patient[67,98] and need not be given dapsone. The success of chemical isolation has, of course, eliminated whatever justification may have existed for physical isolation. On the other hand, no one has yet addressed the problem of managing contacts of secondary sulfone-resistant cases. The finding of some primary sulfone-resistant cases suggests that sulfone-resistant bacilli are transmissible, and presumably prophylaxis would have to be with rifampin or clofazimine. Random contacts in the United States such as may occur at work, school, socially, or for medical personnel in a hospital setting do not, generally speaking, require follow-up or prophylactic measures.

BCG has been used in several large trials with mixed results. In Uganda,[8] for example, where only 6–8% of cases are LL, there was a reduction in incidence of new cases of over 80% in those receiving the vaccine as compared with controls at up to 6 years' follow-up. In a WHO-sponsored trial in Burma,[7] on the other hand, the protection was about 15% at 9 years. An attempt has been made[86] to explain the failure of BCG in Burma on the basis of much greater previous sensitization to environmental mycobacteria there. Obviously, further trials will be needed to decide whether BCG is, or is not, useful in the prevention of leprosy. The WHO-sponsored[5] vaccine trials comparing BCG alone, killed *M. leprae* alone, and a mixture of killed *M. leprae* and BCG are now under way. Results are several years away but even if a vaccine utilizing killed *M. leprae* proves very immunogenic, obtaining the large numbers of bacilli needed may limit its applicability.

9.3. Control

It is obvious that no easy solution to the problem of leprosy control exists, but its importance might be gauged by the fact that over half the Fifth Report of the WHO Expert Committee deals, directly or indirectly, with this topic. The committee recommends the development of a well-organized national leprosy-control program that sets priorities on the basis of the magnitude of the problem in a particular country as well as availability of the required resources. The whole country should be covered unless prevalence varies widely from region to region. Random sampling surveys provide useful baseline epidemiological data, and school surveys or child surveys are valuable for case-finding in high-prevalence areas. Active case-finding efforts throughout the population are generally carried out

by auxiliary workers. The committee believes that to be successful in terms of reducing the incidence, the program should regularly treat at least 75% of the borderline and LL cases, rendering them bacteriologically negative and giving these and indeterminate cases first priority.[96] These limited goals will not, of course, eliminate the disease. They will merely make the world problem more manageable. How far we are from attaining even these limited goals is shown by the estimate[76] that only 18% of all cases are receiving treatment. Cost is a major factor here, and the extent to which the disease further taxes the various countries' resources is apparent if one considers that perhaps one third of all cases have some disability. An epidemiometric model for leprosy[44] has been developed that predicts the success of various control efforts. Of course, a 100% effective vaccine is the most efficacious, while the other approaches, including segregation, fare little or no better than the methods outlined above. Most control efforts fail because many patients do not maintain treatment, follow-up efforts are often passive rather than active, and funding is frequently inadequate. Further compounding the problem is the fact that outside the United States, many of the necessary drugs are available "over the counter," leading to unsupervised self-medication. However, although it is easy to be pessimistic about the likelihood of leprosy control with methods presently available, success is possible when these methods are diligently applied, as has been demonstrated in Thailand and Burma.[96] In the United States, our goal should be early detection and appropriate treatment of all patients and prevention of the disease in contacts. Because of the limited extent of the problem in this country, however, only household contacts need be examined. It is doubtful that we can eliminate the disease, since most new cases occur among aliens, but the problem should be easily controllable. The efforts of the GWLHDC and the Regional Hansen's Disease Program have made physicians in this country more aware of, and knowledgeable about, leprosy and the multiple clinics of the Regional Hansen's Disease Program operated in 12 cities bring treatment to a majority of patients free of charge.

Health education of patients and their families cannot receive too much emphasis either in the United States or elsewhere. The LL and many borderline cases have a lifetime problem, and they are likely to cooperate with therapy only if they understand it. In this way, they are similar to patients with diabetes, epilepsy, or hypertension. They must be aware of why they are being treated, that they may get worse (reactions) before they get better, how long they will need treatment, and what the long-term benefits of treatment are to them and their families.

10. Unresolved Problems

The discovery nearly half a century ago that the sulfones were effective against this disease is recognized as a major breakthrough in leprosy control. Unfortunately, it led many to believe that the leprosy problem had been solved, and it was not until the large numbers of cases infected with sulfone-resistant bacilli began appearing in the 1960s that the error was recognized. Considerable progress has been made since then, but we have far to go to catch up. As with many other diseases, there are more unresolved than resolved problems in leprosy. The *in vitro* culture of *M. leprae* remains an important goal. Its achievement might significantly accelerate leprosy research and ultimately control by yielding unlimited quantities of pure *M. leprae* to work with.

Although major advances have been made utilizing armadillo-derived *M. leprae,* we still have not reached our goal of a simple, highly sensitive and specific immunological test suitable for patient diagnosis and follow-up under field conditions. The early detection of patients that resulted would help prevent deformities and more effectively interrupt transmission.

Significant improvements in the treatment of this disease have occurred, but even if the short-term WHO regimens prove successful they are probably still too long to allow effective control. Thus, further efforts must be made to shorten treatment and perhaps seek ways to correct the immune deficit that allowed the disease to develop. Likewise, a nonteratogenic form of thalidomide or other nontoxic drugs for use in the control of reactions would markedly reduce the morbidity associated with leprosy and improve compliance.

It would clearly be helpful if the immune defect that allows leprosy to develop could be more precisely defined, thereby increasing our chances of finding a way to correct or even prevent it. Crucial here is the extent to which the defect is genetic or acquired, and we are only just beginning to solve this problem.

An antileprosy vaccine is the most direct approach to prevention of the disease, but even if those now under trial are successful their ultimate usefulness is in doubt because of the large quantities of *M. leprae* that would be required. Thus, the efforts of the molecular biologists to identify species-specific epitopes on *M. leprae* proteins, and their immunogenicity are vital. This might allow the utilization of cloning techniques to develop an inexpensive vaccine, lead to further insights into the immune defect and possible ways to correct it, and increase the chances of developing a better serodiagnostic test.

Finally, all of these efforts will be of little value unless we find ways to markedly improve most control programs without excessive cost. Integration of leprosy control into the general health care scheme as the WHO recommends is the simplest approach, but it is easy for leprosy control to deteriorate under such circumstances. Motivation of health care workers, improving patient compliance, reducing the stigma of leprosy, and obtaining sufficient personnel and funds are vital to a good control program. Clearly, research to develop model programs to solve these problems is important lest we develop the models to control leprosy, but end up without satisfactory means of implementing them.

11. References

1. ABE, M., Fluorescent leprosy antibody absorption (FLA-ABS) test for detecting subclinical infection with *Mycobacterium leprae, Int. J. Lepr.* **47**:379 (1979) (abstract).
2. AMEZCUA, M. E., ESCOBAR-GUTIÉRREZ, A., MAYÉN, E., AND CÁZARES, J. V., Sensitivity and specificity of the FLA-ABS test for leprosy in Mexican populations, *Int. J. Lepr.* **55**:277–285 (1987).
3. BADGER, L. F., Leprosy in the United States, *Public Health Rep.* **70**:525–535 (1955).
4. BADGER, L. F., Epidemiology, in: *Leprosy in Theory and Practice*, 2nd ed. (R. G. COCHRANE AND T. F. DAVEY, eds.), pp. 69–97, John Wright, Bristol, 1964.
5. BAHONG, J., AND NOORDEEN, S. K., Leprosy, in: *Tropical Disease Research: A Global Partnership* (J. MAURICE AND A. M. PEARCE, eds.), pp. 113–124, WHO, Geneva, 1987.
6. BECHELLI, L. M., GARBOJOSA, P. G., GYI, M. M., AND MARTINEZ-DOMINGUEZ, V., Site of early skin lesions in children with leprosy, *Bull. WHO* **48**:107–111 (1973).
7. BECHELLI, L. M., LWIN, K., GARBAJOSA, P. G., GYI, M. M., UEMURA, K., SUNDARESAN, T., TAMONDONG, C., MATEJKA, M., SANSARRICQ, H., AND WALTER, J., BCG vaccination of children against leprosy: Nine-year findings of the controlled WHO trial in Burma, *Bull. WHO* **51**:93–99 (1974).
8. BROWN, J. A. K., STONE, M. M., AND SOUTHERLAND, J., Trial of BCG vaccination against leprosy in Uganda, *Lepr. Rev.* **40**:3–7 (1969).
9. BROWNE, S. G., The history of leprosy, in: *Leprosy* (R. C. HASTINGS, ed.), pp. 1–14, Churchill Livingstone, Edinburgh, 1985.
10. BRUBAKER, M. L., BINFORD, C. H., AND TRAUTMAN, J. R., Occurrence of leprosy in U.S. veterans after service in endemic areas abroad, *Public Health Rep.* **84**:1051–1058 (1969).
11. BULLOCK, W. E., Studies of immune mechanisms in leprosy. I. Depression of delayed allergic responses to skin test antigens, *N. Engl. J. Med.* **278**:298–304 (1968).
12. CHACKO, C. J. G., MOHAN, M., JESUDASAN, K., JOB, C. K.,

AND FRITSCHI, E. P., Primary leprosy involvement of nasal mucosa in apparently healthy household contacts of leprosy patients, *Int. J. Lepr.* **47:**417 (1979) (abstract).

13. CHAKRAVATTI, M. R., AND VOGEL, F., A twin study on leprosy, *Topics in Human Genetics,* No. 1, Thieme, Stuttgart, 1973.

14. CLARK-CURTISS, J. E., JACOBS, W. R., DOCHERTY, M. A., RITCHIE, L. A., AND CURTISS, R., Molecular analysis of DNA and construction of genomic libraries of *Mycobacterium leprae, J. Bacteriol.* **161:**1093–1102 (1985).

15. CLOSS, O., *In vitro* lymphocyte response to purified protein derivative, BCG and *Mycobacterium leprae* in a population not exposed to leprosy, *Infect. Immun.* **11:**1163–1169 (1975).

16. CONVIT, J., ARANZAZU, N., ULRICH, M., PINARDI, M. E., REYES, O., AND ALVARADO, J., Immunotherapy with a mixture of *Mycobacterium leprae* and BCG in different forms of leprosy and in Mitsuda-negative contacts, *Int. J. Lepr.* **50:**415–424 (1982).

17. DAVEY, T. F., AND REES, R. J. W., The nasal discharge in leprosy: Clinical and bacteriologic aspects, *Lepr. Rev.* **45:**121–134 (1974).

18. DESIKAN, K. B., Viability of *Mycobacterium leprae* outside the human body, *Lepr. Rev.* **48:**231–235 (1977).

19. DHARMENDRA AND CHATTERJEE, B. R., Prognostic value of the lepromin test in contacts of leprosy cases, *Lepr. India* **27:**149–158 (1955).

20. DONHAM, K. J., AND LEININGER, J. R., Spontaneous leprosy-like disease in a chimpanzee, *J. Infect. Dis.* **136:**132–136 (1977).

21. DRUTZ, D. J., CHEN, T. S. N., AND LU, W. H., The continuous bacteremia of lepromatous leprosy, *N. Engl. J. Med.* **287:**159–164 (1972).

22. ENNA, C. D., JACOBSON, R. R., TRAUTMAN, J. R., AND STURDIVANT, M., Leprosy in the United States, 1967–1976, *Public Health Rep.* **93:**468–473 (1978).

23. FAGET, G. P., POGGE, R. C., JOHANSEN, F. A., DINAN, J. F., PREJEAN, B. M., AND ECCLES, C. G., The promin treatment of leprosy: A progress report, *Public Health Rep.* **58:**1729–1741 (1943).

24. FILICE, G. A., AND FRASER, D. W., Management of household contacts of leprosy patients, *Ann. Intern. Med.* **88:**538–542 (1978).

25. FISHER, C. A., AND BARKSDALE, L., Elimination of the acid-fastness but not the gram positivity of leprosy bacilli after extraction with pyridine, *J. Bacteriol.* **106:**707–708 (1971).

26. GODAL, T., AND NEGASSI, K., Subclinical infection in leprosy, *Br. Med. J.* **3:**557–559 (1973).

27. GODAL, T., LOFGREN, M., AND NEGASSI, K., Immune response to *Mycobacterium leprae* of healthy leprosy contacts, *Int. J. Lepr.* **40:**243–250 (1972).

28. GORMUS, B. J., WOLF, R. H., BASKIN, G. B., OHKAWA, S. G., WALSH, P. J., MEYERS, W. M., BINFORD, C. H., AND GREER, W. E., A second sooty mangabey monkey with naturally acquired leprosy: First reported possible monkey-to-monkey transmission, *Int. J. Lepr.* **56:**61–65 (1988).

29. GRAY, H. H., AND DREISBACH, J. A., Leprosy among foreign missionaries in northern Nigeria, *Int. J. Lepr.* **29:**279–290 (1961).

30. GUINTO, R. S., Epidemiology of leprosy: Current views, concepts and problems, in: *A Window on Leprosy* (B. R. CHATTERJEE, ed.), pp. 36–53, Statesman Commercial Press, Calcutta, 1978.

31. HANSEN, G. H. A., Undersogelser angaende Spedalskhedens Arsager, *Nor. Mag. Laegevidensk.* **4:**76–79 (1874).

32. HARBOE, M., The immunology of leprosy, in: *Leprosy* (R. C. HASTINGS, ed.), pp. 53–87, Churchill Livingstone, Edinburgh, 1985.

33. HARBOE, M., AND CLOSS, O., A revival of interest in antibody studies in leprosy? *Int. J. Lepr.* **47:**372 (1979) (abstract).

34. HASTINGS, R. C., Transfer factor as a probe of the immune deficit in lepromatous leprosy, *Int. J. Lepr.* **45:**281–291 (1977).

35. Immunological problems in leprosy research (2), *Bull. WHO* **48:**483–492 (1973).

36. INGRENS, L. M., AND KAZDA, J., The epidemiological significance of the occurrence of *M. leprae*-like microorganisms in the environment, *Int. J. Lepr.* **52:**719 (1984).

37. JOB, C. K., CHACKO, C. J. G., TAYLOR, P. M., DANIEL, M., AND JESUDIAN, G., Evaluation of cell mediated immunity in the histopathologic spectrum of leprosy using lymphocyte transformation test, *Int. J. Lepr.* **44:**256–266 (1976).

38. JOB, C. K., HARRIS, E. B., ALLEN, J. L., AND HASTINGS, R. C., A random survey of leprosy in wild nine-banded armadillos in Louisiana, *Int. J. Lepr.* **54:**453–457 (1986).

39. KHANDEKAR, P. S., MUNSHI, A., SINHA, S., SHARMA, G., KAPOOR, A., GAUR, A., AND TALWAR, G. P., Construction of genomic libraries of mycobacterial origin: Identification of recombinants encoding mycobacterial-specific proteins, *Int. J. Lepr.* **54:**416–422 (1986).

40. KIRCHHEIMER, W. F., AND PRABHAKARAN, K., Metabolic and biologic tests on mycobacteria once labeled as leprosy bacilli, *Int. J. Lepr.* **36:**589 (1968).

41. KIRCHHEIMER, W. F., AND STORRS, E. E., Attempts to establish the armadillo (*Dasypus novencintus* Linn.) as a model for the study of leprosy. I. Report of lepromatoid leprosy in an experimentally infected armadillo, *Int. J. Lepr.* **39:**693–702 (1971).

42. KLUTH, F. C., Leprosy in Texas: Risk of contracting the disease in the household, *Tex. State J. Med.* **52:**758–789 (1956).

43. KRIEG, R. E., AND MEYERS, W. M., Demonstration of *Mycobacterium leprae* in tissues from bacteriologically negative treated lepromatous leprosy patients, *Int. J. Lepr.* **47:**367 (1979) (abstract).

44. LECHAT, M. F., BELLUT, C., AND MISSION, C. B., The use and limitations of epidemiometric models in leprosy, in: *A Window on Leprosy* (B. R. CHATTERJEE, ed.), pp. 64–70, Statesman Commercial Press, Calcutta, 1978.

45. LEIKER, D. L., Epidemiological and immunological surveys

in Netherlands New Guinea, *Lepr. Rev.* **31**:241–259 (1960).

46. Leprosy-like disease in wild-caught armadillos, *Morbid. Mortal. Weekly Rep.* **25**:18, 23 (1976).

47. LIM, S. E., KISZKISS, E. F., JACOBSON, R. R., CHOI, Y. S., AND GOOD, R. A., Thymus-dependent lymphocytes of peripheral blood in leprosy patients, *Infect. Immun.* **9**:394–399 (1974).

48. LUMPKIN, L. R., III, COX, G. F., AND WOLF, J. E., JR., Leprosy in five armadillo handlers, *J. Am. Acad. Dermatol.* **9**:899–903 (1983).

49. MATHAI, R., RAO, P. S. S., AND JOB, C. K., Risks of treating leprosy in a general hospital, *Int. J. Lepr.* **47**:322 (1979) (abstract).

50. MEHRA, V., MASON, L. H., FIELDS, J. P., AND BLOOM, B. R., Lepromin induced suppressor cells in patients with leprosy, *J. Immunol.* **123**:1813–1817 (1979).

51. MENZEL, S., BJUNE, G., KRONVALL, G., AND MORROW, R. H., Lymphocyte transformation test in healthy leprosy contacts: Influence of household exposure, *Int. J. Lepr.* **47**:374 (1979) (abstract).

52. MEYERS, W. M., KVERNES, S., AND BINFORD, C. H., Comparison of reactions to human and armadillo lepromins in leprosy, *Int. J. Lepr.* **43**:218–225 (1975).

53. MOHAMED ALI, P., AND RAMANUJAM, K., Leprosy in twins, *Int. J. Lepr.* **34**:405–407 (1966).

54. NARAYANAN, E., SREEVATSA, KIRCHHEIMER, W. F., AND BEDI, B. M. S., Transfer of leprosy bacilli from patients to mouse footpads by *Aedes aegypti, Lepr. India* **49**:181–186 (1977).

55. NATHAN, C. F., KAPLAN, G., LEVIS, W. R., NUSRAT, A., WITMER, M. D., SHERWIN, S. A., JOB, C. K., HOROWITZ, C. R., STEINMAN, R. M., AND COHN, Z. A., Local and systemic effects of intradermal recombinant interferon-γ in patients with lepromatous leprosy, *N. Engl. J. Med.* **315**:6–15 (1986).

56. NELSON, E. E., WONG, L., UYEMURA, K., REA, T. H., AND MODLIN, R. L., Lepromin-induced suppressor cells in lepromatous leprosy, *Cell. Immunol.* **104**:99–104 (1987).

57. NEWELL, K. W., An epidemiologist's view of leprosy, *Bull, WHO* **34**:827–857 (1966).

58. NOORDEEN, S. K., Longterm effects of chemoprophylaxis among contacts of lepromatous cases, *Lepr. India* **49**:504–509 (1977).

59. NOORDEEN, S. K., AND LOPEZ-BRAVO, L., The world leprosy situation, *World Health Stat. Q.* **39**:122–128 (1986).

60. NOUSSITOU, F. M., SANSARRICQ, H., AND WALTER, J., *Leprosy in Children,* WHO, Geneva, 1976.

61. OLEINICK, A., Altered immunity and cancer risks: A review of the problem and analysis of the cancer mortality experience of leprosy patients, *J. Natl. Cancer Inst.* **43**:775–781 (1969).

62. PATTYN, S. R., Comportement de diverses espéces de mycobactéries dans la patte de souris, *Ann. Inst. Pasteur* **109**:309–313 (1965).

63. PATTYN, S. R., Use of the mouse footpad in studying thermoresistance of *Mycobacterium leprae, Int. J. Lepr.* **33**:611–615 (1965).

64. PEDLEY, J. C., The hypothesis of skin to skin transmission, *Lepr. Rev.* **48**:295–297 (1977).

65. PRABHAKARAN, K., HARRIS, E. B., AND KIRCHHEIMER, W. F., Survival of *Mycobacterium leprae* in tissues kept frozen at −80°C, *Microbios Lett.* **1**:193–195 (1976).

66. PRABHAKARAN, K., AND KIRCHHEIMER, W. F., Use of 3,4-dihydroxyphenylalanine oxidation in the identification of *Mycobacterium leprae, J. Bacteriol,* **92**:1267–1268 (1966).

67. RASI, E., CASTELLAZZI, Z., GARCIA, L., QUEVEDO, L., AND CONVIT, J., Evaluation of "chemical isolation" in 1,168 leprosy patients' homes, *Int. J. Lepr.* **43**:101–105 (1975).

68. REA, T. H., Current concepts in the immunology of leprosy, *Arch. Dermatol.* **113**:345–352 (1977).

69. REES, R. J. W., The microbiology of leprosy, in: *Leprosy* (R. C. HASTINGS, ed.), pp. 31–52, Churchill Livingstone, Edinburgh, 1985.

70. REES, R. J. W., AND McDOUGALL, A. C., Airborne infection with *Mycobacterium leprae* in mice, *J. Med. Microbiol.* **10**:63–68 (1977).

71. REES, R. J. W., AND MEADE, T. W., Comparison of modes of spread and incidence of tuberculosis and leprosy, *Lancet* **1**:47–49 (1974).

72. Report of the Workshop on Microbiology of the XI International Leprosy Congress, *Int. J. Lepr.* **47**:291–294 (1979).

73. RIDLEY, D. S., AND JOPLING, W. H., A classification of leprosy for research purposes, *Lepr. Rev.* **33**:119–128 (1962).

74. ROTBERG, A., BECHELLI, L. M., AND KEIL, H., The Mitsuda reaction in a non-leprous area, *Int. J. Lepr.* **18**:209–220 (1950).

75. RUSSELL, D. A., WORTH, R. M., SCOTT, G. C., VINCIN, D. R., JANO, B., FASAL, P., AND SHEPARD, C. C., Experience with acedapsone (DADDS) in a therapeutic trial in New Guinea and the chemoprophylactic trial in Micronesia, *Int. J. Lepr.* **44**:170–176 (1976).

76. SANSARRICQ, H., WALTER, J., AND SEAL, K. S., The World Health Organization in leprosy control, in: *A Window on Leprosy* (B. R. CHATTERJEE, ed.), pp. 12–22, Statesman Commercial Press, Calcutta, 1978.

77. SCHAUF, V., RYAN, S., SCOLLARD, D., JONASSON, O., BROWN, A., NELSON, K., SMITH, T., AND VITHAYASAI, V., Leprosy associated with HLA-DR2 and DQwl in the population of northern Thailand, *Tissue Antigens,* **26**:243–247 (1985).

78. SECKL, M. J., Monoclonal antibodies and recombinant DNA technology: Present and future uses in leprosy and tuberculosis, *Int. J. Lepr.* **53**:618–640 (1985).

79. SEHGAL, V. M., REGE, V. L., AND SINGH, K. P., The age of onset of leprosy, *Int. J. Lepr.* **45**:52–55 (1977).

80. SHEPARD, C. C., The experimental disease that follows the injection of human leprosy bacilli into footpads of mice, *J. Exp. Med.* **112**:445–454 (1960).

81. SHEPARD, C. C., Stability of *Mycobacterium leprae* and tem-

perature optimum for growth, *Int. J. Lepr.* **33**:541–547 (1965).

82. SHEPARD, C. C., Experimental chemotherapy in leprosy, then and now, *Int. J. Lepr.* **41**:307–319 (1973).

83. SHEPARD, C. C., AND MCRAE, D. H., *Mycobacterium leprae* in mice: Minimal infectious dose, relationship between staining quality and infectivity, and effect of cortisone, *J. Bacteriol.* **89**:365–372 (1965).

84. SHEPARD, C. C., AND SAITZ, E. W., Lepromin and tuberculin reactivity in adults not exposed to leprosy, *J. Immunol.* **99**:637–642 (1967).

85. SHEPARD, C. C., WALKER, L. L., AND VANLANDINGHAM, R., Heat stability of *Mycobacterium leprae* immunogenicity, *Infect. Immun.* **22**:87–93 (1978).

86. SHIELD, M. J., STANFORD, J. L., AND ROOK, G. A. W., The reason for the reduction of the protective efficacy of BCG in Burma, *Int. J. Lepr.* **47**:319–320 (1979) (abstract).

87. SKINSNES, O. K., MATSUO, E., CHANG, P. H. C., AND ANDERSSON, B., Cultivation of *Mycobacterium leprae* in hyaluronic acid based medium. 1. Preliminary report, *Int. J. Lepr.* **43**:193–203 (1975).

88. VAN EDEN, W., GONZALEZ, N. M., DE VRIES, R. R., CONVIT, J., AND VAN ROOD, J. J., HLA-linked control of predisposition to lepromatous leprosy, *J. Infect. Dis.* **151**:9–14 (1985).

89. WADE, H. W., AND LEDOWSKY, V., The leprosy epidemic at Nauru: A review with data on status since 1937, *Int. J. Lepr.* **20**:1–29 (1952).

90. WALDORF, D. S., SHEAGREN, J. N., TRAUTMAN, J. R., AND BLOCK, J. B., Impaired delayed hypersensitivity in patients with lepromatous leprosy, *Lancet* **2**:773–776 (1966).

91. WALSH, G. P., STORRS, E. E., BURCHFIELD, H. P., COTTRELL, E. H., VIDRINE, M. F., AND BINFORD, C. H., Leprosy-like disease occurring naturally in armadillos, *J. Reticuloendothel. Soc.* **18**:347–351 (1975).

92. WARDEKAR, R. V., Chemoprophylaxis in leprosy, *Lepr. India* **41**:240–246 (1969).

93. WATERS, M. F. R., Significance of the lepromin test in tuberculin-negative volunteers permanently resident in a leprosy-free area, *Int. J. Lepr.* **41**:563 (1973).

94. WATERS, M. F. R., REES, R. J. W., PEARSON, J. M. H., LAING, A. B. G., HELMY, H. S., AND GELBER, R. H.,

95. WATERS, M. F. R., REES, R. J. W., LAING, A. B. G., FAH, K. K., MEADE, T. W., PARIKSHAK, N., AND NORTH, W. R. S., The rate of relapse in lepromatous leprosy following completion of 20 years of supervised sulfone therapy, *Lepr. Rev.* **57**:101–109 (1986).

96. WHO Expert Committee on Leprosy, Fifth Report, *WHO Tech. Rep. Ser.* No. 607, WHO, Geneva, 1977.

97. WHO Study Group, Chemotherapy of Leprosy for Control Programmes, *WHO Tech. Rep. Ser.* No. 675, WHO, Geneva, 1982.

98. WORTH, R. M., AND WONG, K. O., Further notes on the incidence of leprosy in Hong Kong children living with a lepromatous parent, *Int. J. Lepr.* **38**:745–749 (1971).

99. YOUNG, D. B., AND BUCHANAN, T. M., A serological test for leprosy with a glycolipid specific for *Mycobacterium leprae*, *Science* **221**:1057–1059 (1983).

100. YOUNG, R. A., MEHRA, V., SWEETSER, D., BUCHANAN, T., CLARK-CURTISS, J., DAVIS, R. W., AND BLOOM, B. R., Genes for the major protein antigens of the leprosy parasite *Mycobacterium leprae*, *Nature* **316**:450–452 (1985).

12. Suggested Reading

BAHONG, J., AND NOORDEEN, S. K., Leprosy, in: *Tropical Disease Research: A Global Partnership* (J. MAURICE AND A. M. PEARCE, eds.), pp. 113–124, WHO, Geneva, 1987.

HARBOE, M. (ed.), Immunology of Leprosy: Proceedings of an International Symposium, *Lepr. Rev.* **57**(Suppl. 2):1–308 (1986).

HASTINGS, R. C. (ed.), *Leprosy,* Churchill Livingstone, Edinburgh, 1985.

WHO Study Group, Chemotherapy of Leprosy for Control Programmes, *WHO Tech. Rep. Ser.* No. 675, WHO, Geneva, 1982.

World Health Organization, *A Guide to Leprosy Control,* Publ. No. ISBN 92-4-154147-4, Geneva, 1980.

CHAPTER 17

Leptospirosis

Solly Faine

1. Introduction

Leptospirosis in humans occurs throughout the world as an acute infection ranging in severity from unnoticed and subclinical to fatal.[26,33,92] It is a zoonosis (strictly, an anthropozoonosis) acquired by humans from an animal source. The causal bacterium is *Leptospira interrogans,* of which there are more than 200 serological varieties (serovars), each of which has some special diagnostic, prognostic, or epidemiological significance.[44]

The ultimate reservoir of all leptospirosis is a nonhuman carrier animal that excretes the causal bacteria (leptospires) in its urine. In animals, the leptospires infect primarily young animals, which may become renal carriers and urinary excretors if they survive an acute initial infection. Human-to-human transmission has been recorded extremely rarely, congenital infection has been infrequently reported, and laboratory-acquired infections have been documented.

There are a large number of leptospires identified by serology or by genetic relationships. In general, there is a correlation between animal reservoir, serological type (serovar), and potential severity of the illness. The disease has many local and folk names, frequently originating from historical or clinical features or associated occupations, such as "Weil's disease," "seven-day fever," "hebdomadal fever," "autumnal fever," "pretibial fever," "swineherds' disease," "cane-cutters disease," "mud-fever."[27]

As it is a zoonosis, leptospirosis is most significant for those whose work or leisure brings them into contact with infected animals or their urine. It is highly occupational in societies where animal contact is rare except through work.

In some societies, particularly in tropical areas, it is impossible to avoid direct or indirect contact with feral carrier rodents or with livestock. In others, only those in selected occupations are exposed to significant risks. The public health importance of leptospirosis lies in its occupational, season, sex- and age-related incidence; the acute and sometimes prolonged incapacity for work; loss of human and livestock productivity; costs for medical care, Workers Compensation or other occupational disease insurance payments, and preventive measures. It can be epidemic, sporadic, or endemic.[26]

The geographical distribution of the literature sources cited (references) reflects the inevitable fact that most research on leptospirosis occurs where there is a high morbidity together with a high level of scientific expertise and consequent funding.

2. Historical Background

The early history of leptospirosis is vague because it was not possible to differentiate the different forms of "malignant jaundice," which included hepatitis, yellow fever, leptospirosis, and malaria, until scientific clinical and pathological knowledge had progressed into the 1880s. Nevertheless, an account by Wittman, a British military surgeon, in 1803 may well have been of an epidemic of leptospirosis during the Napoleonic wars in Palestine and Egypt. The clinical entity was described by both Mathieu and Weil in 1886, but Weil's description became the classical reference. The syndrome of fever, hemorrhage, jaun-

Solly Faine · Department of Microbiology, Monash University, Melbourne, Australia.

dice, enlarged liver and spleen, with renal failure, became known as "Weil's disease." Its etiology was unknown until the discovery of pathogenic leptospires, first seen in stained tissue sections of liver from a "yellow fever" patient, and later cultivated independently from Weil's disease patients among coal miners in Japan in 1914 and troops in trenches in Germany during World War I in 1915. It was named *Spirochaeta icterohaemorrhagiae* by the Japanese; *Spirochaeta icterogenes* by the Germans; and later *Leptospira icterohaemorrhagiae* by Noguchi. Both the Japanese and German workers and their associates published quickly much of the basic knowledge of the microorganisms, as well as the pathogenesis, pathology, clinical features and diagnosis, and rodent source of leptospirosis.

Less severe illnesses were soon recognized as forms of leptospirosis, known as "akiyami," "autumnal fever," "hebdomadal or seven-day fever." Dogs were identified as both reservoirs and susceptible animals. Once the wider range of clinical manifestations was recognized, other serovars were isolated from patients and carrier rodents and identified so that by the early 1950s some 45 serovars significant for human leptospirosis and their reservoirs had been identified.

A major discovery was that livestock (pigs, cattle) could be carriers and excrete large numbers of leptospires (up to 10^8 per ml urine). Both primary (rodent–rodent) and secondary (rodent–livestock–rodent) cycles were identified.[26,92] The range of known serovars continued to expand, mainly following research in tropical countries. Although leptospires could be isolated by culturing blood or urine from patients, evidence of leptospirosis was obtained mainly by serological tests on patients' sera. Most culture media required rabbit serum. The use of bovine albumin and oleic acid or polysorbate-linked fatty acids (tweens) to replace rabbit serum was an important advance, facilitating laboratory cultivation and allowing the easier isolation of serovar (sv) *hardjo* from patients and cattle. This serovar, previously isolated from an Indonesian patient, is now recognized as a major cause of human leptospirosis wherever there are dairy cattle. Antibodies to Hebdomadis group leptospires were already known to be prevalent in both humans and cattle.

Vaccines for control of leptospirosis in dogs were introduced in 1939 and in pigs and cattle soon after. These vaccines would also assist in protecting humans by reducing excretion of leptospires by animals. Further developments in knowledge of microbiology of leptospires and of pathology; pathogenesis; immunity; epidemiology and control of leptospirosis are reflected in improved laboratory and diagnostic methods, which are bound to reduce the risk to humans.

3. Methodology

Except where doctors are experienced with leptospirosis, the diagnosis usually depends on laboratory confirmatory tests.[26,28] Laboratory tests may be unavailable or delayed because the diagnosis is not considered at an early stage, or because the patient is not seen until late in the illness. Failure to use appropriate laboratory tests at the proper time can lead to misdiagnosis in both suspected and unsuspected patients. Because of diagnostic deficiencies, mortality, morbidity, and incidence data based on unconfirmed diagnoses or confirmed diagnoses of a few selected patients are fallacious, almost without exception.

3.1. Sources of Mortality Data[26]

Death notifications and autopsy reports have been used. Antemortem diagnosis is required for accurate death notification without an autopsy. Mortality rates may be spuriously high if the diagnosis is made only in advanced cases who are nearly moribund when medical or hospital assistance is sought.

3.2. Sources of Morbidity Data

The World Health Organization has recommended that leptospirosis be a notifiable disease. Notification may be based on hospital admissions and diagnosis, discharge data, notification by private or community practitioners, or laboratory notification of infections diagnosed by isolation of leptospires, or on seroconversion or both. Laboratory notification results in the recording of higher morbidity rates than practitioner notification. This is partly because patients are discharged, or recover, or die before all laboratory results are returned to practitioners, who may then see notification as useless. Follow-up of patient contacts has led to detection of cases, not because of the contagiousness of the disease, but because locally epidemic leptospirosis has been detected as a result of inquiries.

Expression of mortality or morbidity statistics in terms of a total population can give a false index of incidence or prevalence if the disease is not homogeneously distributed in that population, or unless a correction is made for risk of exposure. In a large predominantly urban population, an overall low morbidity rate may mask a very high rate in a selected group of that population, such as sewer workers, abattoir workers, or meat packers. Statistics should be refined and expressed in rates relevant to the size of the population at risk.[27]

3.3. Surveys[26]

Serological surveys have been used frequently in studies of leptospirosis. They can be used on unselected populations to see whether leptospirosis exists at all. In such studies it is necessary to use a battery of antigens in agglutination tests to ensure that representative serovars of all serogroups are included. The initial workload can be reduced by testing against pools of antigens, combining up to five serogroups in one suspension. Reactive sera can be tested against individual serogroups. Alternatively, a broadly *interrogans*-species reacting antigens may be used that will react with antibodies to any serogroup. Members of the nonpathogenic species *L. biflexa* have common antigens with *L. interrogans*. *L. biflexa* sv *patoc* and sv *andamana* have been used as screening antigens to detect antibodies to any type of *L. interrogans*. Unpublished results from the author's laboratory have shown that not all leptospirosis patients develop anti-patoc antibodies, and not all anti-patoc antibodies indicate previous leptospirosis. Broadly cross-reactive antigens have been used in enzyme-linked immunosorbent assays (ELISA) for the same purpose of ascertaining the presence of antibodies to any serovar of *L. interrogans*.

Survey information can be used to show which serovars are likely to be prevalent, by analyzing results of tests on batteries of antigens, or by retesting broadly reactive sera against individual serovars. However, many sera will react with more than one serovar because several serovars have common antigenic factors, and the highest titer is not necessarily against the infecting serovar, especially following recent infections. The fact that leptospirosis may not be distributed homogeneously in the population should be borne in mind when planning surveys. The survey should be properly planned to request necessary information such as age, sex, occupation, travel, previous known leptospirosis or similar undiagnosed illness. Adequate statistical planning beforehand is essential to ensure that an appropriate number of samples is taken in each group and that results can be analyzed by statistical techniques.[26]

Once the presence of leptospirosis is known or detected in a survey, the data may be used to determine the population groups exposed to risk, and once those are delineated, to measure the prevalence of antibodies in one or more selected subgroups. Another important function of surveys is to ascertain prevalence for evaluating control measures, both for a baseline level before their introduction and during and after implementation as part of their evaluation.

Either IgM or IgG or both classes of antibody may be measured in surveys using ELISA with specific antigens or cross-reactive antigens.[3,60,84] IgM antibodies usually indicate relatively recent infections. Survey information can be important for interpretation of diagnostic serology in acute cases, to establish whether the patient is one of a population or subgroup in which there is a known high prevalence of antibodies.

Serological or bacteriological surveys have proved valuable in investigating an epidemic. Information may be obtained retrospectively from serum bank specimens collected from epidemic patients or from patients and their surrounding population in general concurrently with an epidemic. This was seen in the 1984 South Korean epidemic of leptospirosis that was more completely investigated by examination of previously banked sera.

Apart from epidemics, surveys of serum banks have been used to ascertain overall prevalence rates in certain clinical groups, such as patients with jaundice and fever, undiagnosed aseptic meningitis, or pyrexia of unknown origin.

Prospective surveys offer a better chance of understanding incidence of leptospirosis and prevalence of antibodies in selected groups. These may be carried out on selected groups of hospital admissions or patients in primary health care clinics or practices. A suitable protocol is to carry out diagnostic tests for leptospirosis on all clinically suspected patients. If serology is tested, a matched control series, such as nonfebrile patients, must be included.

Ethics of Surveys. The taking of blood or other specimens solely for investigative rather than diagnostic purposes should be done only with the informed consent of the patient or client, or competent relatives. Where surveys are carried out as part of national or international research programs, it is essential that due regard and respect should be paid to the local customs, traditions, and religious practices of the population, and with their cooperation.

3.4. Laboratory Diagnosis[20,26,28,92]

In the absence of clear characteristic clinical features, especially in mild leptospirosis, laboratory diagnosis is essential. Its importance cannot be overstated because it is also the basis of epidemiological statistics and preventive policies and programs. Not only must the diagnosis be established as leptospirosis, but the causal serovar, or at least the serogroup, should be identified for prognosis, management, and prevention.

3.4.1. Isolation and Identification of Leptospires

a. Culture. Culture media containing long-chain fatty acids such as oleic acid or tweens with 1% bovine serum albumin as a detoxicant are used widely. A common formulation is the Ellinghausen–McCullough–Johnson–Harris (EMJH) medium. It is usually used in liquid form in screw-cap containers. In tubes of semisolid media containing 0.1–0.2% agar, growth occurs in one or more zones situated from just below the surface to deep in the medium.[26,45]

In fluid media, growth from inocula of 1–10% of volume can be seen as a birefringent swirl in 3–20 days, depending on the individual strain. Heavier growth, always less than the turbidity seen in cultures of enteric bacteria, may be encouraged by shaking during incubation. Optimum temperature for the cultivation of laboratory strains is 28–30°C. Most strains grow poorly if at all at 37°C.

Cultures of properly collected clinical material cultured shortly after collection are highly sensitive and capable of detecting very small numbers of leptospires in from 2 or 3 days to several weeks. Cultures should be examined at least weekly and incubated for 4 weeks to 2–3 months.

b. Specimens for Culture[26,28] (see Section 8.2.2b). Blood cultures taken during the first few days (up to 10 days, especially in the first week) during the fever are frequently positive. Small volumes of 0.5–1.0 ml in 50 ml of medium are recommended so as to dilute antibacterial blood components. Oxalate or heparin may be used as anticoagulants if bedside cultures cannot be obtained. Addition of a sulfathiazole–neomycin–cycloheximide mixture has been recommended to reduce risks of overgrowth by bacteria from contaminated specimens; however, subculture after a day or two into medium without antibiotic is advisable.

Cultures may also be taken from CSF, urine, and tissue samples, including autopsy specimens. Urine should be alkaline or the patient treated with urinary alkalinizing agents before the specimen is taken, preferably aseptically. The antibiotic medium above, or a selective medium comprising EMJH with 100 μg/ml of 5-fluorouracil is useful for tissues.

c. Microscopy and Examination of Cultures. Microscopy by an experienced person is used to recognize leptospires directly in clinical or pathological specimens and in cultures from them. Leptospires may be seen readily by dark-field microscopy in thin preparations or in direct examination of clinical specimens. Leptospires appear as motile, bright, beaded, rotating, thin rods, usually with one or both ends curved, against a black background. Phase-contrast microscopy is of limited value in diagnostic work because of its strict optical requirements.

d. Staining. Leptospires are poorly stained by conventional microscopic stains. They may be visualized by Giemsa or silver deposition methods. Silver deposition by one of several methods can be used for tissue sections, but flawless technique is required to obtain clean interpretable results. Immunological stains such as immunofluorescence and immunoperoxidase provide a valuable alternative to direct staining methods.[26,34,80] Indirect (antiglobulin) labeled antisera are more practical than direct coupled antisera. Good fluorescence technique will allow the detection of small numbers of approximately 10^3–10^4 leptospires/ml specimen. A major disadvantage of all immunostains is the need for specific antiserum. Although the aim of this test is to seek and allow the recognition of leptospires in the specimen, it cannot work if the test antiserum does not match the serovar, or at least serogroup, antigens of the leptospires in the specimen (see Section 3.4.1e). A secondary result is that a positive reaction also serves to identify at least broadly the serovar or serogroup of the fluorescing leptospires. A battery of antisera may be required if the serovar is unknown or unsuspected. In extreme cases, where the infection is due to a new serovar, only convalescent patients' sera can be used as a source of the primary antibody for the test until the new organism has been isolated and immune sera prepared from it. Results of direct microscopy or immunostaining can be obtained in minutes to a few hours.

e. Serological Typing. If a leptospire is isolated, it must be identified[20,26] by agglutination to titer with reference antisera or serogroup- and serovar-specific monoclonal antibodies. These identification procedures are usually performed only in reference laboratories.[20,26,100]

A list of serogroups recognized currently, with their type serovars and the major serovars in the serogroup, is provided in Table 1. A full list has been published.[49a]

A range of monoclonal murine antibodies has been described reacting with various serovars of *L. interrogans*. Their specificities range from species reactive for all *interrogans* serovars[2] to serogroup reactive for members of serogroups Canicola,[65,66] Icterohaemorrhagiae,[48,51] Pomona,[1] Sejroe[32,86], to highly specific epitopes characteristic of a single serovar.[48] Some of the specific monoclonal antibodies agglutinate leptospires, indicating reaction with a surface epitope. Less serospecific monoclonal antibodies tend to react only with physically, enzymatically, or chemically disrupted leptospires in ELISA. Monoclonal antibodies are obviously useful in allowing rapid pre-

Table 1. Alphabetical List of Serogroups and Main Serovars of *L. interrogans*[a]

Serogroup	Serovar	Serogroup	Serovar
Australis	*australis*		*poi*
	bratislava		*sofia*
	fugis		*sorexjalna*
	jalna	Louisiana	*louisiana*
	lora	Manhao	*lincang*
	muenchen		*manhao 2*
Autumnalis	*autumnalis*		*manhao 4*
	bim	Mini	*beye*
	bulgarica		*georgia*
	erinaceiauriti		*mini*
	fortbragg		*perameles*
	mooris		*szwajizak*
	rachmati	Panama	*cristobali*
Ballum	*arboreae*		*panama*
	ballum	Pomona	*pomona*
	castellonis		*proechimys*
Bataviae	*bataviae*	Pyrogenes	*myocastoris*
	brasiliensis		*pyrogenes*
	paidjan		*robinsoni*
Canicola	*benjamini*		*zanoni*
	broomi	Ranarum	*evansi*
	canicola		*ranarum*
	portlandvere	Sarmin	*sarmin*
	schueffneri		*waskurin*
Celledoni	*celledoni*		*weaveri*
	whitcombi	Sejroe	*balcanica*
Cynopteri	*cynopteri*		*caribe*
	tingomaria		*dikkeni*
Djasiman	*djasiman*		*hardjo*
	sentot		*istrica*
Grippotyphosa	*canalzonae*		*medanensis*
	grippotyphosa		*saxkoebing*
	valbuzzi		*sejroe*
Hebdomadis	*borincana*		*trinidad*
	hebdomadis		*wolffi*
	kremastos	Shermani	*shermani*
Icterohaemorrhagiae	*birkini*	Tarassovi	*atlantae*
	copenhageni		*navet*
	icterohaemorrhagiae		*rama*
	naam		*sulzerae*
	smithi		*tarassovi*
Javanica	*javanica*		*tunis*

[a]Extensively condensed and modified from the official Serovar List of the Taxonomic Subcommittee on *Leptospira*.[49a]

sumptive identification of leptospires without the tedium of agglutination and absorption methods.

f. Gene Probes and Other Methods. Gene probes are capable of detecting about 10^3–10^4 leptospires/ml.[59,85]

Their most useful potential application at present appears to be for detecting leptospires in specimens, and possibly in rapidly identifying large numbers of leptospires in culture isolates.

Chemiluminescence, fluorimetry, and radioactive capture[97,98] have been described. The need for highly specialized equipment must limit their application to selected laboratories, where large numbers of tests will justify the technology.

Alternative nonserological identification, based on analysis and comparison of the electrophoretic banding patterns of DNA after digestion by various restriction endonucleases,[37,57,58,89,90] and characteristic protein banding patterns after electrophoresis in polyacrylamide gel, have also been useful for the characterization and identification of strains of leptospires.[64]

Methods for differentiating *L. biflexa* from *L. interrogans* are described in Section 4.

3.4.2. Serological Methods.[20,26,28,92] Antibodies in sera from patients or survey subjects can be detected and measured directly by agglutination of leptospires either macroscopically or microscopically, or by immunofluorescence of leptospires after reaction with serum followed by fluorescein-conjugated antibodies to human IgG, IgM, or unspecified immunoglobulins. Numerous older indirect methods using carrier particles[26] have been replaced by more recent developments including ELISA using either boiled or sonicated leptospires and immunoblotting of electrophoresed preparations of leptospires (see Section 3.4.2b).

Tests used for diagnosis of acutely ill patients need to be specific and performed rapidly if they are to aid in management and prognosis, as well as for detection of sources common to several patients and for prevention. For epidemiological and survey purposes, there is less urgency for obtaining test results but laboratories should be able to test large numbers of sera rapidly if necessary. Usually, knowledge of the serovar specificity of reacting antibodies is required especially where several serovars are endemic, each with a different reservoir and pattern of transmission.

Almost all laboratories use the microscopic agglutination test (MAT) as their standard test although some use ELISA. Sensitized erythrocyte lysis and complement fixation are still used in a very few centers. These tests and latex agglutination, apparently not used nowadays, will not be discussed further here.

Two milliliters of serum is usually necessary for serological studies. If venous blood is unavailable, capillary blood from an ear, finger, or heel prick may be soaked up on a standard square of absorbent (blotting or filter) paper, and allowed to dry. An approximately 1-cm square will hold about 0.1 ml of blood. The paper is eluted in 0.5 ml of saline. The eluate is treated as a nominal dilution of 1 : 10 of serum for subsequent dilutions, and hemolysis is disregarded.[26] For diagnostic purposes, any blood specimen for serology

should be taken as soon as possible in the illness. It should be followed by two further specimens at intervals of 5 days, to look for a rising titer of antibodies, but the first sample should be tested at once without waiting for a paired sample. Occasionally, late seroconversion has been reported. In clinically characteristic cases, where no other diagnosis is confirmed and seroconversion has not occurred in 15 days, another specimen may be taken after 30 days. Serum may be frozen during transport and storage. Only one specimen is required for epidemiological and prevalence surveys.

a. Agglutination Tests.[20,26] The principle of all agglutination tests is that leptospires are agglutinated by serum antibodies. There are two types of agglutination tests; macroscopic and microscopic (MAT). Macroscopic agglutination tests may be performed on a microscope slide, or a tile, or in a tube. The test is at best semiquantitative but useful for rapid screening to detect high levels of antibody. It is significantly less sensitive than microscopic or tube agglutination and also less serovar-specific because of the greater chance of recording cross agglutinations. A macroscopic tube agglutination test is sometimes used because its endpoint is read easily by the naked eye. Titers are generally lower than for a corresponding MAT and the test is less sensitive than MAT but more sensitive than slide agglutination. A positive reaction is taken as agglutination at a dilution of 1 : 80 or higher.

MAT[20,26,28] remains the basic reference test in leptospirosis. It is extremely sensitive because the endpoint is read microscopically under dark-field. The use of live late-log-phase cultures standardized to 5×10^7 to 10^8 leptospires/ml is recommended, but formalin-killed suspensions may be used where lower sensitivity can be tolerated and in small laboratories or in tropical countries where local production of cultures, transport, and storage free of contamination are problems. They are also safer to handle in the laboratory.

Tests should always be quality controlled by including sera of known high and low specific reactivity as controls. The authenticity of strains used in antigen suspensions should be checked periodically against reference antisera.

The choice of strains of leptospires to be included in tests depends on circumstances. In all cases the use of serologically authenticated, local, recently isolated strains is recommended, but usually standard reference strains obtained from a reference laboratory are used because of their known antigenic composition. Nevertheless, variability of strains of the same reference serovar is known to occur. As a guide to the choice of strains for diagnosis, it should be noted that sera generally react specifically with the infecting serovar, but cross-reactions with other serovars are well known especially early in infection. Frequently the highest titer is recorded against a cross-reacting serovar. Where several serovars from different serogroups are prevalent locally, there is a need to test each patient's serum against each of them, or at least against a representative serovar of each serogroup. This means that in many tropical areas or where the likely infecting serovar is unknown, a battery of up to 30 serovars may be used for each serum. The battery may comprise pools of antigens, or simply two or three serovars where there is a strong likelihood that no others are present. The same considerations apply in epidemiological prevalence surveys.[20,26]

There is no satisfactory single group antigen with which all patients' sera will react. Many laboratories have utilized reported cross-reactions of all patients' sera with sv *patoc* of *L. biflexa*, or *andamana* as a genus reactive screening test. Recent experience in the author's laboratory showed a significant proportion of reactions with *patoc* in nonleptospirosis sera submitted for diagnosis. The reasons for these and previous results are not clear.

Interpretation of MAT depends on the stage of illness, the serovar, and local epidemiology. In an acute infection, a single low titer of under 200 where there is a high prevalence of antibodies to one or more serovars of leptospires may be unrelated to current illness. A rising titer commencing under 400 and either rising fourfold within 1 or 2 weeks, or reaching 400 to 800, is highly suspicious. For diagnostic purposes, an initial low titer of 50 (or 40 depending on the dilution system) in a new patient in a nonendemic area may be an indication to clinicians that the patient has leptospirosis. Subsequent testing 5 to 7 days later may reveal a significant rise. The early low titer is thus diagnostically useful. Some patients fail to seroconvert for several weeks. It is also stated that early penicillin treatment may abort the development of antibodies. In such cases, the positive diagnosis depends solely on culture of the leptospire.

In epidemiological surveys, titers as low as 10 are significant, indicating previous exposure or infection with a leptospire. It is not known for certain how long antibodies persist following clinical or subclinical infection in humans.[10]

It is clear that MAT is rapid, specific, and sensitive but has important disadvantages of subjective endpoint, extreme tedium, and labor-intensive testing leading to observer error and fatigue following prolonged reading of tests, danger due to the use of live cultures, and potential for error if the correct serovars are not chosen: Direct measurement of specific IgM or IgG in MAT is not feasible.

b. Enzyme Immunoassay (ELISA). The main advantages of ELISA currently are clearly precision, objectivity, and instrumentation, adaptability for screening large numbers of sera, cost, and ability to measure specific IgM, IgG, or other immunoglobulin classes. The two main antigens used in diagnosis and epidemiology have been a broadly species-reactive preparation of boiled, formalin-killed leptospiral culture[84] or a sonicated leptospiral suspension.[3,60] In addition, a variety of leptospiral polysaccharides and lipopolysaccharide preparations used experimentally with patients' sera or monoclonal antibodies have potential diagnostic significance.[14,48,51,74] ELISA tests do not measure the same antibodies as those in agglutination, so that there is little correspondence between the optical densities or titers in ELISA and the agglutinating titer in MAT.[60] It was possible to prove that a fetus had a congenital, later fatal infection with sv *hardjo* by using ELISA to demonstrate a titer of anti-*hardjo* IgM in its cord blood (together with detection of *hardjo* in tissues by immunofluorescence).[31] In pigs and cattle, blood levels of IgM reacting in ELISA have been correlated with renal excretion of leptospires.[6,16]

c. Immunoblotting. Patients infected with leptospirosis either recently or some years before testing maintain nonagglutinating antibodies that can be demonstrated by immunoblotting.[14]

4. Biological Characteristics of the Organism

4.1. Morphology

Leptospires are thin, helical, motile, gram-negative bacteria.[30,45] They can be seen by light microscopy only with difficulty after staining because they are so thin. Deposition of Giemsa stain or silver makes them thick enough to see by transmitted light microscopy. They can be seen unstained by phase-contrast or dark-field illumination. The standard method of observation is by dark-field microscopy of a wet preparation on a thin microscope slide under a thin coverslip. Leptospires seen this way rotate rapidly around their long axis and are translationally motile in either direction. One or both ends are usually hooked, imparting a looped appearance to the end of the leptospire when it rotates rapidly. Straight-ended variants occur, and are much less translationally motile. In semisolid agar media, leptospires move like a flexible screw between invisible particles. Within limits of variability for any serovar, all serovars appear the same morphologically.

When seen by electron microscopy, leptospires are made up of a helically wound, protoplasmic cylinder incorporating the cellular contents, surrounded by a cell wall around which a three- or five-layer membrane may be visualized, depending on the methods of preparation and fixation. The whole is enclosed in a trilaminar outer envelope which is easily washed off or damaged in preparation. The cytoplasmic cylinder has a diameter of approximately 0.1 μm and an amplitude of winding of approximately 0.2 μm. Leptospires vary in length from approximately 5 μm after division to more than 20 μm according to age, strain, and culture conditions. The outer envelope, which is an important source of antigens for immunization and the study of immunity, may be separated and purified.[9]

A single flagellum, previously called an "axial filament," is attached close to each end of the leptospire by a characteristic gram-negative-type insertion structure. The flagellum runs down the center of the helix applied to the protoplasmic cylinder and surrounded by outer envelope. Notwithstanding its position, it is presumed to have motor function.[11] In purified preparations, flagella appear to be composed of strands of protein surrounded by a sheath for part of their length. They contain characteristic antigens. Microfibrils arising from the cell wall have been described.

L. interrogans is remarkable for its variable but relatively high lipid content, including unusual long-chained fatty acids.[45]

4.2. Physiology and Growth[45]

L. interrogans is an obligate aerobe or microaerophile with the requisite enzymes for aerobic metabolism. Growth may be accelerated and increased substantially in amount by aeration. Anaerobic growth has not been reported. All *L. interrogans* are inhibited by 8-azaguanine and cannot grow at temperatures below 13–15°C in EMJH medium, in contrast to *L. biflexa*. Leptospires are easily killed by drying; heating above 42–45°C for a few minutes; acid conditions below pH 7.0; alkaline conditions above approximately pH 7.8; and disinfectants such as phenolics, quaternary ammonium derivatives, halogens, and aldehydes (formaldehyde, glutaraldehyde). They may be preserved in media containing protein at −70°C or in liquid nitrogen.

The essential requirements for growth of *L. interrogans* are ammonium ions as a nitrogen source, long-chained fatty acids as a carbon and energy source, and thiamine and cyanocobalamin. There appear to be no major differences in requirements among members of the species. Pyrimidines are not required and carbohydrates are not fermented. A detoxicant, usually 1% bovine serum albumin or whole rabbit serum, is required to bind and detoxify the fatty acids and release them slowly. The optimum pH for growth is in the range 7.2–7.8, and the optimum temperature range is 28–30°C. Large inocula of up to 10% of culture volume are used routinely to initiate growth.

4.3. Antigens

Surface antigens, probably polysaccharide in nature, allow the separation of any strain of *L. interrogans* into serum-sensitive and serum-resistant groups correlating with avirulence and virulence for experimental animals, respectively.[29,46] Antigens on the leptospiral surface are involved in agglutination. Evidence from monoclonal antibody studies suggests that most if not all agglutination results from interaction of surface lipopolysaccharide (LPS) antigens whose determinants and reactive epitopes are polysaccharides or oligosaccharides. Serovar specificity is a property of LPS oligosaccharides and/or glycolipids.

A number of polysaccharide antigens described in the past can now be identified as components or derivatives of LPS, designated by various authors as "specific soluble substance," "erythrocyte sensitizing substance," "fraction 4," and "type-specific main antigen." Leptospiral LPS has many properties similar to those of other gram-negative bacteria but some significant differences, notably much less pyrogenicity and toxicity[41,66,95,96] and an unknown link sugar that in some serovars only partly resembles ketodeoxyoctonate (KDO). Other characteristic antigens are found in flagella, in a glycolipoprotein that had a high level of toxicity for tissue-cultured cells and experimental animals,[96] and in a range of protein antigens of undetermined significance. In addition to their toxic and invasive properties, leptospires are able to adhere to cultured tissue cells by an attachment ligand.[7,43,94] Virulent leptospires were able to attach to the cellular cytoskeleton while avirulent ones were not.[43] Attachment properties have obvious importance for our understanding of the renal carrier state.

4.4. Other Properties

A wide range of antibiotics is effective against leptospires in the laboratory,[12,26] although penicillin and erythromycin are recommended therapeutic antibiotics[26] with doxycycline[82] recommended for chemoprophylaxis. It is relatively easy to select streptomycin-resistant *L. interrogans* in the laboratory following incubation with high concentrations of streptomycin. Strains resistant to antibiotics have not been reported clinically, although antibiotics (especially penicillin) are used widely in treatment.

Isolates of *L. interrogans* have guanosine + cytosine ratios in the range 33–42 mol% GC. Using G + C ratios and DNA homology, it is possible to categorize all *L. interrogans* into four or five major groups.[45,100] These groups do not correspond to classification using serology. New species classifications have been proposed.[100] Methods for study of chromosomal DNA have been described.[53]

Bacterial restriction endonuclease analysis ("BREN-DA") has been used to analyze leptospiral DNA composition in gel electrophoresis. Comparisons of strains have revealed relationships and dissimilarities previously not revealed by serological classification.[37,39,58,89,90] There is obvious epidemiological advantage in better analysis and separation of strains if the strains to be identified correspond with different epidemiological environments.

L. interrogans may persist in body tissues following infection (see Section 7.3.7) in the presence of antibodies. Little is known of the properties of the leptospires or the immunological mechanisms that allow them to live and grow in sequestered sites such as the anterior chamber of the eye, the proximal renal tubules,[26,92] and genital tracts[23] of carrier animals, and possibly in the brain of rodents.

5. Descriptive Epidemiology

5.1. Prevalence and Incidence

Statistics of prevalence and incidence are influenced frequently by the lack of reliability in diagnosis and by failure to recognize the selective risk to population groups. Prevalence figures derived from planned surveys are much more reliable than those based on hospital records or disease notifications. Antibody prevalence rates to local serovars in tropical countries with large feral and peridomiciliary rodent populations are higher, often up to 80–90% of the population, than in temperate climates where leptospirosis tends to be more occupationally segregated. In surveys of dairy farming populations in the state of Victoria in southeastern Australia, antibodies to sv *hardjo* are present in about 25% or 25,000 per 100,000 of the population, and almost zero in the rest of the community. Since dairy farmers and meat workers comprise no more than 20,000 or 1/200th of the 4 million residents of the state, an overall statistic of 125 per 100,000 would be quite erroneous if extrapolated to the whole population, as would be the almost zero figure for the urban population extrapolated to rural areas. Similarly, notifications of approximately 100 cases per year of leptospires among farmers and meat workers result in an incidence rate of 2.5 per 100,000 in the whole population of 4 million but a much more significant rate of 500 per 100,000 among the 20,000 in the population at risk.[26,27] These high rates reflect a high prevalence of antibodies, up to 85% in dairy cattle, a level comparable with that in countries with environments as diverse as Australia, the Netherlands, and the Congo.

Reported statistics are also influenced by technical fac-

tors such as the starting dilution for sera, the interpretation of low titers, and the techniques used for serology. These factors are often not clear from reports. When using prevalence statistics for epidemiological and control policy planning, it should be noted that the duration of persistence of antibodies after infection is variable. It ranged from within 1 year, through a median between 3 and 6 years, to indefinite in some patients[10] in a study where the seroconversion rate in the population was about 4% annually. Second infections with a different serovar have been reported, indicating that there is little immunity between serogroups. Very rare reports of second infections with the same serovar are poorly documented.

In the United States, fewer than 100 cases of leptospirosis are reported each year, representing an incidence of about 0.05 case per 100,000 population. Cases occur throughout the country but are most common in the South Atlantic, Gulf, and Pacific coastal states. Hawaii has the highest annual incidence (1.5 cases per 100,000). Leptospirosis is predominantly a disease of males (80% of cases) between the ages of 10 and 59 (76% of cases). The case-fatality rate averages 5–7%.

In contrast to other countries, slightly fewer than half of U.S. cases are occupation-associated. Patients usually have a history of exposure to animals, mud, or fresh water. Cases occur with a distinct seasonal predominance in the months July through October. In descending order of frequency, infections by members of the Icterohaemorrhagiae, Canicola, Autumnalis, Grippotyphosa, Hebdomadis, Australis, Pomona, and Ballum serogroups are most commonly recognized.

5.2. Epidemic Behavior and Contagiousness

Leptospirosis is considered to be of a low order of contagiousness because spread from human to human is almost unknown and direct inoculation into the body via skin, mucosal, or conjunctival penetration is required for infection. Laboratory infections, a significant occupational problem, have occurred after inoculation into the eye or through the skin. In natural infections an animal source of infection is required,[26,61,92] except for transplacental infection. Animal urine is the most important vehicle of infection for man. Direct contact with infected animals also is an important method of transmission.

Epidemics have occurred apart from sporadic endemic zoonotic infections. The precipitating factors in epidemics have been large buildups of carrier animal populations together with an increase in direct or indirect contact between the animals and humans at risk. Examples of major epi-

demics include an outbreak of primarily nonicteric leptospirosis characterized by severe pulmonary hemorrhages
in Korea in 1984, associated with rice harvesting following
a heavy storm. Urine from a large field rodent population,
attracted by the crop, contributed to heavy contamination of
the rice fields and exposure of harvesters, including many
emergency workers who presumably had little if any immunity. Epidemics of leptospirosis following floods are well
documented in China and elsewhere. Point-source outbreaks have occurred in recent years during military operations and leisure activities such as kayaking, rafting, and
hiking where groups have been exposed simultaneously.[44]
The usual situation in tropical countries and among occupationally exposed risk groups in temperate climates is that
sporadic cases occur according to seasonal and other factors. Precipitating factors are wet conditions, buildup of
rodent populations, or seasonal occupational conditions.
Even where occupation appears to be irrelevant, there is
invariably a history of some contact with animals, as in
hunting, domestic slaughter of livestock, rat catching,
swimming, boating, or cleaning drains or sewers.[26,55,92]

Although leptospirosis is solely a zoonosis, human social factors are most important in epidemiology. The way
people live, their housing, transport, food, livestock and
domestic animals, and social and religious customs will all
contribute positively or negatively to their risks of leptospirosis (see Section 5.10).

5.3. Geographical Distribution

Leptospirosis is distributed worldwide. The most severe clinical forms transmitted via rodent reservoirs are
more commonly diagnosed nowadays in tropical areas. The
anicteric form is the most prevalent. In temperate climates
the pattern tends to less severe types carried by serovars
indigenous to dogs, livestock, or field mice rather than
domestic rats, reflecting as much the influence of social
factors and efficacy of rodent control as a direct geographical effect. There is a direct relationship with soil and geological environment, which can affect the ability of leptospires to survive in surface waters and mud and soil
through their effects on acidity and porosity.[22,92] Changes
to the environment caused by human activities and subsequent changes in the patterns of human life have potential
for profound influence on leptospirosis.[77] Draining of
swamps and waterway control can obviously create drier
conditions. Irrigation and dams can convert desert or dry-
lands to fertile territories into which animals and birds migrate as the environment changes. The increased food avail-

able, moist ground conditions, and ground cover for rodents
protecting them from predators create new ecological conditions in which resident fauna can change quite rapidly. With
these changes come increased risks to humans whose activities take them into the new wet environments.

5.4. Temporal Distribution

The worldwide experience is that leptospirosis is related to wet periods of the year. The wet seasons, be they
monsoon, floods, or spring and summer, are associated with
surface conditions favoring leptospirosis in all parts of the
world. In temperate climates the risks increase with fresh
spring and summer growth of pastures. Risks also increase
for harvest workers for many crops but not wheat and corn.
Well-documented epidemics have been recorded during
rice, sugarcane, and pea harvests.

5.5. Age

Although leptospiral antibodies can be found in people
of all ages, the predominant incidence of acute infection is
found in the 20–50 age range, though in developing countries more cases may be seen in younger people. Pediatric
and congenital infections have been described.[31,36,54] The
age distribution reflects the relative amount of environmental exposure to risk in the age groups concerned.

5.6. Sex

Although some workers have concluded that males and
females are equally affected for equivalent risks of exposure, there are contrary facts that among women engaged
in milking cows in conditions comparable with those for
men the rate in women was considerably lower than in
men.[26,83] The explanation offered is that the women were
more careful about personal occupational hygiene. The
overall predominance of males in statistics reflects the sex
distribution within the occupational or residential populations under review.

5.7. Race

There is no evidence for any risk factors determined by
race. Some statistics showing racial tendencies toward or
against leptospirosis can be explained by social or occupational factors affecting the chances of exposure to risk.
Nothing is known about genetic determinants of susceptibility or resistance to leptospirosis in humans.

5.8. Occupation

There is a strong occupational trend in all areas. Even in tropical climates those whose jobs bring them into indirect contact with animals via rodent urine contamination in such activities as rice planting and harvesting, fish farming, forestry, mining, boating, and military exercises are at special risk. In addition, those in all climates exposed to urine contamination directly or indirectly from livestock and domestic dogs and rodents have a greater risk and increased incidence of infection. Prevalence rates for antibodies to sv *hardjo* in dairy farmers may be as high as 25% or 25,000 per 100,000,[27,60] matched by comparable rates in slaughtermen. In each case the proved infection rate is also high.

Occupational hazards involve special considerations of Workers Compensation and preventive measures to protect workers (see Section 9.1). In turn, these create special social needs and expenses for the workers and the industries involved.

5.9. Occurrence in Different Settings

Leptospirosis poses a special problem in military or civilian emergencies.[47] Rodent infestation may increase and with it risks to humans from leptospirosis as well as other zoonoses. Military, paramilitary, police, or civilian emergency workers may be forced into conditions such as floods and destroyed buildings housing rodents. Frequently, troops have been exposed to leptospirosis in rat-infested trench warfare or in jungle warfare or exercises.

Modern leisure activities have attracted city dwellers to rural settings, sometimes in faraway lands, in search of adventures in canoeing, rafting, caving, and climbing. The risks of contracting leptospirosis on these vacations need to be emphasized.[26,44]

5.10. Socioeconomic Factors

Social class is no barrier to leptospirosis. The only requirement is contact with infected animal urine or animals. Nevertheless, there are social groups whose occupations are more likely to expose them to these risks than others.

An important socioeconomic consideration, however, is the effect of leptospirosis on productivity of animals used for food or burden. Leptospirosis can cause abortions, stillbirths, failure to thrive, retarded growth, milk failure or spoilage for human consumption, and loss of productivity in meat animals among livestock.[26,92] These effects can in themselves place an additional burden of malnutrition on people already threatened by the risk of illness.

It is difficult to calculate the costs of the effects of leptospirosis as a cause of community or individual ill health. Some of the factors to be considered are the costs of labor to replace sick workers; the cost to the self-employed or peasant farmer or villager in money to replace his own inability to produce food for his family, and in pain and sometimes chronic illness; costs of medical attention including hospital and medical services; costs in insurance for lost work, production, and Workers Compensation.[26] The first requirement is adequate diagnosis so that the actual impact of the disease can be assessed. However, costs of special diagnostic facilities and surveillance for leptospirosis are hard to justify if there is an impression that the disease is rare or absent, so that the circular logic leads to continued underdiagnosis and underreporting. Existing mild illnesses have frequently and easily been attributed to numerous other causes including "influenza" or "viral infections" but may well be leptospirosis.

6. Mechanisms and Routes of Transmission[26,61,92]

Leptospirosis is transmitted primarily from its animal host reservoirs by urine. Urine from carrier animals, also sometimes called excretors or shedders, may contain undetectably small numbers of leptospires or as many as about 10^9 per ml urine intermittently in the same animal. The reasons for the variable output are not known. Urine from carriers frequently contains antibodies to the homologous serovar of leptospires; obviously the leptospires are not adversely affected by the urinary immunoglobulins. Carrier animals may shed leptospires constantly or intermittently for short periods or for all of their lives. The intermittent shedding, the difficulties of detecting small numbers of urinary leptospires in livestock, and the potentially enormous load of leptospires excreted into the surface water and soil environment from heavy feral rodent environmental contamination are the main sources of difficulties in control in different situations.

Pathogenic leptospires can survive free in the environment, depending on soil type and geological factors in moist conditions such as in soil, mud, swamps, drains, surface waters, streams, and rivers, as long as conditions are not acid. All of these sites are well known as sources of leptospirosis. The leptospires can infect fresh host animals or humans by penetrating sodden or broken skin or mucosal surfaces.[52] It is not clear whether pathogenic leptospires multiply in these inanimate environments, but credible nutritional models have been described. The nutritional requirements for pathogenic *L. interrogans* serovars for growth in inanimate environments are believed to be sufficiently similar to those of free-living nonpathogenic *L. biflexa* to allow pathogens to grow under these conditions, especially in warm climates.

Food preparation areas can be contaminated by infectious urine from foraging carrier rodents, resulting in infections in food process workers. Urine splash and aerosols can infect milkers, especially in "herringbone"-pattern milking sheds, veterinarians, and animal handlers.

Animal tissues and blood are infrequently causes of leptospirosis. Conception products and autopsy of infected livestock and separated kidneys used for domestic food can transmit leptospirosis to veterinarians, farmers, laboratory workers, and housewives.[38,68] In a bizarre episode, a medical practitioner farmer who resuscitated newborn anemic piglets by mouth-to-mouth resuscitation developed leptospirosis.[35]

Human-to-human transmission is virtually unknown, apart from *in utero* congenital infection.[31,36,81]

Laboratory-acquired infections have usually resulted from accidents involving direct skin penetration with cultures or suspensions of infected tissues via syringe and needle, or broken glass, or splash into an unprotected eye, and from being bitten by infected animals whose urine contaminated the bite.

Leptospires die rapidly when dry. Drying out of surfaces or environments contaminated by infective material prevents spread, even after rehydration. Heating above about 42°C is lethal to leptospires but they survive freezing.[26,44]

Spread of leptospirosis is not known to occur by airborne, respiratory, or gastrointestinal routes. There is evidence for genital infection and venereal transmission in livestock.[23]

7. Pathogenesis and Immunity

7.1. Incubation Period

The incubation period of leptospirosis varies from 2 to 21 days, usually between 3 and 10 days, although longer periods have been reported.[26,33,52,92] It is relatively shorter with larger infective doses or more virulent leptospires. Incubation periods can be calculated from a recognized in-

fection episode[52] but are difficult to define when there is continual or repeated exposure.[19] The relatively sudden onset makes it easier to detect the first clinical symptoms unless they are very mild or unnoticed. In these cases the incubation period may be erroneously dated to the onset of late presenting symptoms such as hemorrhage, meningitis, or renal failure.

7.2. Virulence and Its Attributes

After they penetrate the integument, leptospires must spread, evade body defenses, grow, and produce pathological changes in tissues. In animals destined to become carriers, leptospires must also take up renal tubular residence. The combination of these attributes contributes to the property of pathogenicity, which is the genetically endowed potential for evading and overcoming the resistance of the host and producing lesions or death. Virulence of a defined strain may be measured by the size of the dose or the time taken to produce a lesion or death in a carefully standardized test system. It is difficult to assess accurately in a clinical or epidemiological environment where one or more of the components of virulence, such as surface antigens or toxins, may operate simultaneously in patients or animal reservoir hosts possessing various degrees of natural or acquired immunity. Some serovars of *L. interrogans* such as *icterohaemorrhagiae*, *copenhageni*, and *bataviae* typically produce a more severe clinical picture resembling classical Weil's disease (jaundice, hemorrhages, renal failure) than do other serovars such as *canicola*, *grippotyphosa*, or *hardjo*.[26,92]

The ability to produce lesions following experimental inoculation into animals is lost gradually on cultivation of *L. interrogans* in the laboratory following its isolation from patient or animal tissues. This loss of virulence results from the gradual replacement of the population of leptospires in culture by leptospires better able to grow in laboratory media but less able to damage host tissues.[24,25] The less virulent organisms in culture presumably arise from spontaneous mutants selected by cultural conditions. Frequently the less virulent forms are straight rather than hooked, less translationally motile, and grow in dense small colonies in agar media.[26] Loss of virulence is accompanied by an increase in susceptibility to killing by naturally occurring innate serum IgM antibody acting on a surface polysaccharide antigen.[29,46,63] Nonpathogenic *L. biflexa* are killed by a similar serum leptospiricidal mechanism. Thus, an initial component of virulence, the ability to resist serum killing, is associated with a surface polysaccharide antigen. A virulence-associated antigen has been described recently.[63] Virulence is regained in a single animal passage of a culture, as a result of selection in the host of those members of the inoculated population able to evade leptospiricidal defenses and survive and grow *in vivo*.[25]

There is no information about virulence plasmids or any other mechanism of genetic control of virulence attributes.

7.3. The Course of Events in Infection

7.3.1. Entry. Leptospires gain entry through small abrasions or cuts in the skin or mucosal surfaces. Immersion in water can soften skin to facilitate cutaneous damage. Entry may occur via the conjunctiva or by aerosol into the lungs, as well as by inhalation following immersion in contaminated water. Ingestion into an intact alimentary tract, except for the oral cavity, is not a recognized route of entry. Laboratory infections have occurred through injections, needle-stick injuries and cuts, and eye-splash accidents.

7.3.2. Spread. Leptospires that enter the body spread at once in the lymphatics and bloodstream. There is no initial localizing acute inflammation at the site of entry in natural infection or in models using doses resembling those found in nature, although small abscesses may be produced by local injection of extremely large numbers (e.g., 10^{10} or more) of leptospires intradermally. Leptospires can be found distributed in various tissues within 2 h of infection. Nonpathogenic leptospires (*L. biflexa*) and avirulent *L. interrogans* are opsonized by innate serum IgM. All leptospires may be opsonized by specific immune IgM or IgG in hosts previously immunized by infection or vaccination. Phagocytosis occurs rapidly in reticuloendothelial fixed phagocytes in the liver (Kupffer cells), and lung. These phagocytes later migrate to the spleen. The bloodstream is cleared rapidly following opsonization, which may occur with minimal detectable levels of immunoglobulin recognized as agglutinating antibody at titers as low as 2. Polymorphonuclear and mononuclear phagocytes can be observed to take up leptospires from the tissues following the development of antibody.[24,25]

In the absence of immunity and consequent phagocytosis, leptospires grow in the body in an initial infection as if in culture.[22,23] Nothing is known of specific nutritional requirements *in vivo*. Both virulent and avirulent leptospires have been shown to adhere to fibroblast-derived cells in the laboratory.[6,43,94] Adhesion was enhanced by small amounts of antibody.[94] The adhesion of sv *canicola* to L929 fibro-

blasts and to their cytoskeleton was shown to be a property of virulent strains, and inhibited by antibody.[43]

A threshold level of leptospires is required before lesions occur. The time to reach this level (the incubation period) depends on the number of leptospires in the infecting dose, their rate of growth (possibly related to the fever), the state of the patient's immunity, or the host animal's immunity and genetic makeup.[69] The first and most important lesions to be detected are in small blood vessels throughout the body. Localized endothelial-cell degeneration occurs, followed by small localized extravasations frequently containing leptospires.[18,24]

Fever occurs at an early stage of infection. It is presumably mediated by pyrogenic toxins[41,42,96] released by leptospires following phagocytosis as well as by nonspecific factors associated with all infections.

At this stage it is also possible to demonstrate microscopic focal degeneration of skeletal muscle fibers, notably in the calf muscles. The extreme pain in muscles and acute tenderness found clinically are presumably the result of these lesions.[33] Thus, the main presenting symptoms of severe headache, fever, and muscle pains can be attributed to the effects of leptospires growing in the body to threshold levels sufficient to cause characteristic damage to small blood vessels.

The severity and presenting features of clinical leptospires result from a complex of climactic, social, and geographical factors influencing the animal host and source, vessel damage, local ischemia, and small hemorrhages in most tissues, and eventually to major organ damage. Depending on the serovar of leptospire, there is greater or lesser hepatocellular degeneration, leading to jaundice; renal tubular degeneration similar to that seen in crush injuries or after renal ischemias, leading to an acute, often hemorrhagic interstitial nephritis[17,78,79]; and pulmonary hemorrhages ranging from insignificant to gross and fatal, with hemoptysis. Cholecystitis, symptoms of acute abdominal emergency, meningitis, hemiparesis, myocarditis, adrenal hemorrhage, and placentitis have all been reported. Clearly, there is no single pathognomonic lesion or clinical feature, although typical combinations of lesions with symptoms, associated with particular serovars of leptospires, occur in particular regions and epidemiological circumstances, as in classical severe Weil's disease or the relatively mild sv *hardjo* infections of dairy farmers.

7.3.3. Lesions. Once the infection is fully developed, the typical lesions described in clinical-pathological and postmortem studies of leptospirosis, usually of the severe and fatal types, appear. Hemorrhage is associated with a sudden drop in platelet numbers, possibly as a result of leptospiral toxin action or of adhesion of leptospires.[21] The role of disseminated intravascular coagulopathy syndrome (DIC) is not clear.[21] Anemia is common, not usually solely as a result of hemorrhage. Evidence of nitrogen retention is found almost universally,[33] albeit transitorily, reflecting the renal ischemia occurring even in mild types of leptospirosis. In these cases, patients whose kidneys are functioning poorly and at the limit of compensation due to other causes of renal insufficiency may be precipitated rapidly into renal failure. In severe cases there is very widespread tubular degeneration, which is the usual main cause of death. Other potentially fatal lesions include hepatocellular degeneration, pulmonary hemorrhages, and myocarditis.[17,18,33,71,78,79]

7.3.4. Transplacental Spread. Transplacental infection can occur at any stage of leptospirosis. If the fetus or placenta is severely damaged, abortion will occur.[92] Stillbirth or congenital leptospirosis may follow infection late in pregnancy. Abortion is a well-documented cause of loss of productivity of livestock. In human congenital infection, IgM antibodies can be demonstrated in the fetus and cord blood, and leptospires in the degenerative lesions in tissues.[31,36]

7.3.5. Recovery. Recovery from leptospirosis commences as soon as the patient produces opsonizing antibody leading to rapid phagocytosis of leptospires in the circulation and in the tissues. Mopping up phagocytosis also follows destruction of leptospires by antibiotics. Opsonizing antibody levels can be correlated with agglutinating antibody levels. Virtually any detectable specific agglutinating antibody in MAT can signify opsonic activity. Bacteriological clearance of live leptospires from tissues by antibody does not, however, ensure clinical recovery, especially in severe-type leptospirosis, because lesions in organs and tissue damage may have proceeded to stages where vital functions are almost irreversibly impaired. Clinical supportive measures for renal failure (dialysis), hemorrhage (transfusion), myocarditis, and liver failure may be necessary until the patient's tissues regenerate. Complete recovery is the rule in surviving patients, although rare examples of prolonged asymptomatic renal carriage have been recorded in people. Depressive and psychotic symptoms may persist for many weeks.[4,70]

7.3.6. Carrier State. The carrier state is very rare in humans.[81] In animals it follows recovery from systemic infection, which may be subclinical. Leptospires are attached to the epithelial surface of proximal renal tubule cells, where they grow in the tubular lumen and are excreted in the urine. Homologous antibody may be demonstrated in the urine of carriers. Active excretion may be sporadic or intermittent. The mechanisms of adhesion, immunological events, and nutritional needs of leptospires in renal tubules need to be elucidated. There is no inflammation around affected tubules, which appear to be morphologically intact in electron microscopic studies. In some animals (especially dogs and pigs) there may be considerable scarring in the kidneys where leptospires occupy renal tubules. This scar tissue and inflammation appear to be related more to the recovery and repair processes following renal damage (acute nephritis) and hemorrhage in the acute stage of infection than to the presence of leptospires in the tubules. Leptospires are not found in renal tissue outside renal tubules in carrier animals. Genital carriage of leptospires in livestock has been described.[23]

7.3.7. Autoimmunity and Hypersensitivity. The roles of autoimmunity and hypersensitivity in producing lesions are unclear.[72] The acute nature of infection and absence of chronic infection precludes consideration of these immunopathological mechanisms in the development of initial lesions. However, leptospires may be sequestered in "privileged sites" during acute infection, leading to later allergic reactions to their presence. A notable example is uveitis which has followed either systemic infection or accidental laboratory inoculation into the conjunctiva. Leptospires may be cultured from the anterior chamber of the eye for long periods after infection. Contact with leptospiral antigen can cause an allergic aggravation of the uveitis. A similar condition known as "moon blindness" occurs in horses.[26,67,92]

7.4. Toxins

Numerous toxic properties of leptospirosis have been described. Some have been specific to some serovars, others distributed universally. Hemolysins act on erythrocytes of selected animal species, so that there is a combination of specificity of hemolysin according to serovar and according to animal species. For example, hemolysins produced by sv *pomona*, but not by sv *icterohaemorrhagiae*, are active on bovine, but not on human erythrocytes. Most hemolysins act at 37°C and where they have been characterized have been shown to be phospholipases active on one or more of lecithin, sphingomyelin, phosphatidylcholine, or phosphatidylethanolamine.[49]

The leptospiral phospholipase hemolysins act on the erythrocytes of those animal species whose erythrocyte membranes contain the substrate phospholipid for the phospholipase.[8] Inasmuch as hemolysin activity may be a significant toxin in pathogenesis, this mechanism provides some basis for the range of host specificities seen between leptospiral serovars and animal species. There is electron microscopic evidence for the appearance of holes in erythrocytes of calves infected with sv *pomona,* but the responsible toxin has not been characterized.[91] In addition, lipase and urease have been identified in some serovars, although their pathogenic role is unclear.

Cytopathic effects on various cultured mammalian cell lines have been demonstrated following incubation with leptospires under a bewildering variety of combinations of cell type, cultural and incubation conditions, and leptospiral serovar and virulence. These studies may be summarized by noting that cytopathology can be observed following incubation with cultures of *L. interrogans* that are either virulent or avirulent for animals, and with strains of *L. biflexa,* provided large doses of 10^{10}/ml or more are used. Activity of a toxic leptospiral protein elaborated in hamster blood in leptospirosis was reported but the agent was not characterized.[50] A toxic glycolipoprotein (GLP) is capable of damaging fibroblast cell membranes in culture and is toxic to laboratory animals by virtue of its toxic lipids. These lipids are uniquely leptospiral unsaturated long-chain fatty acids and may act on cell membranes to produce lesions resembling those occurring in the pathogenesis of the essential small blood vessel damage in leptospirosis. The activity of GLP and its fatty acids is neutralized in the presence of serum albumin, which may act as a sponge absorbing the toxic lipid. Presumably the toxin can act in infection once the serum albumin carrying capacity for lipid is saturated.[96]

LPS may be prepared from leptospires by treatment with hot aqueous phenol and extraction from either the phenol or the aqueous phase. Its chemical and physical properties resemble those of LPS from typical gram-negative enteric bacteria but it is very poorly pyrogenic. LPS was found not to be toxic[95] but large amounts may inhibit phagocytosis.[41,42] Antigenic derivatives of LPS are important in diagnosis and immunity (see Section 7.5.3).

7.5. Immunity

There is no evidence for variability in resistance to leptospirosis in humans on the basis of race, gender, genetics, or immunological deficiency, although a genetically endowed relative resistance in certain lines of a breed of pigs has been described.[69] Differences in susceptibility in population groups can be explained on social and cultural epidemiological grounds affecting the magnitude of the risk of exposure.

7.5.1. Specific and Nonspecific Immunity. Low levels of innate antileptospiral IgM antibodies can be found in the serum of humans and other animals not known to have been exposed to leptospirosis. These antibodies may arise from cross-reactions with antigens of *L. biflexa* found in fresh water and soil, or with antigens of intestinal gram-negative bacteria that share antigenic determinants with serovars of *L. interrogans.*[40] These IgM antibodies destroy avirulent *L. interrogans* but are inactive against virulent strains. Nothing is known of nonspecific immunity to leptospirosis stimulated by infection with other bacteria or their LPS.[29,46]

The basic facts about immunity to leptospirosis are that it develops rapidly, within a few days of clinical or subclinical infection. Fully effective immunity can be transmitted passively naturally through the placenta and colostrum and artificially with convalescent or hyperimmune serum. Both IgM and IgG antibodies are protective. Immunity is associated with agglutinating antibodies which are also opsonic; moreover, a very low level of agglutinating antibody (titer 1 : 2) is protective. Immunity to reinfection is specific for the infecting serovar or closely antigenically related serovars, almost exclusively within the same serogroup determined by MAT. Antigenic components of LPS are protective and are involved in agglutination and opsonization as shown in studies with monoclonal murine antibodies.[48,73] Sera from convalescent patients contain antibodies reacting with the same antigens as those revealed in immunoblots with monoclonal antibodies.[14]

Some animal species exhibit relative resistance to leptospiral infection with certain serovars, the basis of which is unknown. It is not known whether humans are incapable of infection with any serovars. Generally, young animals are much more susceptible than old, provided they have no maternally endowed passive immunity. The development of age-related relative resistance to leptospirosis reflects the rate of maturation of the B-cell immune response.

Cell-mediated responses occur following infection[72] but there is no evidence for their operation as determinants of immunity. Thus, all the evidence points to antibody-related (humoral) immunity as the sole significant mechanism for protection from leptospirosis. The duration of immunity in humans is not known. Agglutinating antibodies fall in titer after infection, but the rate is very variable in individuals and there are no studies of the relative rates of fall of IgM and IgG antibodies. Some people known to have had leptospirosis are seronegative in 1 or 2 years, others are still seropositive after more than 10 years, although the possibility cannot be excluded that they have had continued exposure to leptospires during this period.[10] There are no studies of the duration of ELISA-reactive antibodies after infection. Indeed, it is not clear that the loss of detectable agglutinating antibody with time following infection is synonymous with loss of immunity. These deficiencies in knowledge are obviously important for understanding immunity, epidemiology, and planning for vaccines.

7.5.2. Antibodies. Convalescent sera contain specific IgM, IgG, or both. Usually, IgM is elaborated first, within approximately 7–20 days of infection, followed by IgG. In some patients, seroconversion does not occur until 30 days after onset of infection. IgM persists at low levels in certain cases, while in others IgG is sometimes the sole demonstrable immunoglobulin. However, information from this type of retrospective study is necessarily limited in value because one cannot know for certain beforehand the previous history of exposure to leptospirosis.[14] Cross-reactions with related, and occasionally with unrelated serovars occur, especially early in infection. These "paradoxical reactions" occur typically, for example, between svs *icterohaemorrhagiae* and *canicola,* and *icterohaemorrhagiae* and *pomona.*[20,26] IgG antibodies tend to be more specific. In some patients treated very early with penicillin whose infections were proved with blood cultures, seroconversion did not occur at all, or was delayed several weeks.[26]

It is possible to differentiate IgM and IgG activity by any of the serological tests discussed in Section 3.4.2, although this is seldom used for diagnosis in humans. Immunoglobulins that agglutinate usually also opsonize, react with outer envelope in immunofluorescence, and protect. Murine monoclonal antibodies have been prepared to serovars of many serogroups. These have allowed study of classification based on antigens reacting with the monoclonals in ELISA and immunoblots of electrophoresed sonicates of leptospires.[1,32,51,66,86] Use of monoclonal antibodies has allowed the identification of epitopes corresponding to those recognized by immunoglobulin in human convalescent sera.[14]

Antibodies to the infecting serovar may be found in the urine of carrier animals.[26,92]

7.5.3. Antigens Related to Pathogenesis and Immunity. Antibodies reacting with antigens in flagellar, subsurface, and outer-envelope locations have been identified in sera from patients who have been proved to have leptospirosis. Some of the antibodies persist for months and years.[14,75] The only antigens among these for which there is evidence for a role in pathogenesis or immunity are the polysaccharide components of LPS, found in the outer envelope and on the leptospiral surface.[42,48,48a,63,95] Successful experimental immunization has been achieved with purified lipopolysaccharide or polysaccharides.[48a]

7.5.4. Vaccines. Vaccines for leptospirosis were introduced soon after leptospires were identified and could be cultivated. Preparations effective in protecting animals and humans have been made by killing the leptospires in cultures with heat or formalin and injecting doses subcutaneously or intramuscularly.[26,76,92] Outer-envelope preparations have been used to vaccinate animals,[9] and irradiated live cultures rendered avirulent by irradiation have been used experimentally. Formalin-killed cultures are used widely to vaccinate animals[13,56,99] (cattle, pigs, dogs) and are in use in some countries to immunize people. The vaccine is usually given subcutaneously in two doses, and repeated annually. There is a high incidence of painful swellings at the injection site, especially on revaccination.[99] The toxicity is considered to be too great to justify widespread use in many countries.

In countries where leptospirosis is confined to clearly recognized occupational groups whose source of infection is livestock, the vaccination of livestock is recommended and used widely to decrease shedding by carrier animals with the twofold purpose of reducing and eradicating animal leptospirosis and thus increasing productivity, and protecting humans at risk from unavoidable exposure to these animals.[13,56] Considerable improvement has been obtained in New Zealand, where the rate of leptospirosis in dairy farmers milking cows has been reduced to about one third (about 150 cases per year in 1986 compared with over 500 in 1984). However, the vaccinations were accompanied by effective education campaigns to increase awareness and occupational hygiene.

Vaccination of animals requires two doses a month apart and annual revaccination. Serovar-specific vaccines made from leptospires grown in protein-free media are available for use in animals. A common practice is to vaccinate pregnant sows to ensure passive protection to growing piglets. Nevertheless, those piglets may acquire asymptomatic leptospirosis after their passive protection has been lost and may then become shedders and thus a hazard to handlers, slaughtermen, and other abattoir workers.

8. Patterns of Host Response

Several noteworthy epidemiological features of leptospirosis determine the host responses and clinical features. The disease is almost uniquely acquired from carrier animals, which cannot be identified as carriers or shedders without laboratory tests. Furthermore, the tests may miss carriers excreting intermittently or shedding only small numbers of leptospires. Inapparent infections and carriers in humans are not relevant to clinical disease or transmission.[26,92]

The severity and presenting features of clinical leptospirosis result from a complex of climactic, social, and geographical factors influencing the animal host and source, and thus the serovar and the clinical features and in turn the accuracy of diagnosis and notification. Living conditions and social organization, partly dependent on climatic and geographical factors,[27,77] determine the amount and nature of direct or indirect contact with excretor animals of various types (see Sections 5.2–5.10). In general, different leptospiral serovars are associated with characteristic groups of animal species. The nature and severity of leptospirosis in humans depends on the infecting serovar. Living conditions for most people in tropical countries favor contact with rat or related rodent sources of leptospires rather than other animals. Most of the leptospires that clinically result in the very severe leptospirosis of the classical Weil's disease type, which may be fatal following renal failure, hemorrhages, and jaundice, are borne by rats. Serovars of the Icterohaemorrhagiae, Autumnalis, and Bataviae serogroups are examples. Conversely, in temperate climates, in addition to rats there are other carriers of leptospires such as field mice, pigs, dogs, and cattle shedding mainly leptospires of these serovars causing a milder form of illness.[26] The disease also tends to be much more occupationally related and confined to people in contact with these animal sources. Serovars *grippotyphosa*, *hardjo*, *pomona*, and *tarassovi* are examples of this group.

Perceptions and statistics of leptospirosis are influenced by whether the disease is seen as the severe or the mild type. Mild infections of either variety have often been overlooked because the symptoms are not pathognomonic. Usually, seriously ill patients with the severe type who needed hospital treatment or died were accurately diagnosed as leptospirosis. Since they were the only ones in whom the diagnosis was made, the clinical features recorded and reported in textbooks have been those of the severe type emphasizing jaundice, hemorrhages, renal failure, meningitis, and a high case-fatality rate. Overall, these symptoms apply only to a few and late cases of the classical severe Weil's disease type of leptospirosis. Most patients affected with any serovar report initial symptoms as described below. The severe and the mild types differ in their subsequent progress.

8.1. Clinical Features[26,33,92]

Characteristically, leptospirosis commences suddenly with headache, myalgia, fever, and red eyes. Headache develops without warning and may be extremely severe. Myalgia is usually felt in the back and especially in the calf

muscles, which may be excruciatingly tender to touch. The fever is generally greater than 39°C and the red eyes are the result of conjunctival suffusion, reflecting a generalized dilation of blood vessels, rather than a conjunctivitis. There is frequently a macular rash on the trunk, lasting a few hours only. Careful examination of the palate may show a similar petechial rash. In untreated patients with the mild type of leptospirosis, the symptoms usually persist for 3 to 10 days, followed by gradual but complete recovery. Occasionally, further acute symptoms may develop. These include oliguria from renal failure; acute abdominal pain, resembling an acute abdominal emergency and sometimes due to acute cholecystitis; meningism, hemiparesis, or other neurological signs; and cough, sometimes with mild hemoptysis. Jaundice is rare in mild-type leptospirosis. Aseptic meningitis may develop as a later complication, but most patients recover fully within 3 to 6 weeks. In patients with severe-type leptospirosis, the symptoms increase in severity, at times following a 1- or 2-day temporary remission. Delirium and confusion may develop, with increasing evidence of renal failure, together with hemorrhages and jaundice. In addition, the spleen may be enlarged. Pulmonary hemorrhages may be diffuse, resembling multiple infarcts or bronchopneumonia, accompanied by coughing of blood, but in some cases the pulmonary hemorrhages may be gross. As liver and renal failure progress, jaundice and oliguria increase, confusion and delirium give way to unconsciousness, and death occurs through renal and hepatic failure.[26,33,78,79] In patients in whom the disease does not cause fatal renal failure, meningitis may occur. Supportive measures such as renal dialysis can tide patients over renal failure until renal structure is regenerated and function restored, but death from myocarditis may then occur.[18,71] Adult respiratory distress syndrome can also occur and cause death. Final recovery is usually complete unless vital organs are irreparably damaged. The earlier severe phase is described as the septicemic stage and the later the tissue phase.[26]

Death from renal failure may occur at any stage of the illness.[17,78,79] The autopsy appearances will depend on the duration and degree of development of lesions. Usually, there is generalized jaundice and widespread hemorrhage in the skin, muscles, peritoneal surfaces, and lungs. The kidneys are enlarged, bile stained, and have subcapsular hemorrhages. Bleeding into all viscera including the adrenals is common. The liver shows signs of hepatitis and hemorrhages. Death is so rare in mild cases that there is no record of significant and characteristic autopsy appearances.

Uveitis may develop at any time after the second week, and as late as 6 months. It may affect one or both eyes.[26,67]

8.1.1. Congenital Leptospirosis.[31,36,54] Leptospirosis in pregnant women can be transmitted to the developing fetus at any stage of pregnancy. The fetus is actively infected. If it is severely damaged, even by serovars causing the mild type of leptospirosis in the mother, it may die. If infection occurs near the time of birth, the child may develop congenital neonatal leptospirosis, whose manifestations are similar to those of adult leptospirosis. Complete recovery follows satisfactory treatment.[36]

The diagnosis of intrauterine leptospirosis depends on the correct diagnosis in the mother, and evidence that the fetus is infected as shown by fetal distress. Antenatal proof is usually only available if the fetus dies. If the fetus recovers before birth, IgM antibodies will be present in the cord blood. The diagnosis of neonatal congenital leptospirosis involves the same methods used in adults, except that recognition of specific IgM rather than IgG antibodies proves that the fetus was actively infected and that the antibodies were not passively acquired maternal immunoglobulin.[31,36]

8.1.2. Clinical Laboratory Findings.[26,33] Laboratory tests, other than bacteriological or serological, may help support the clinical diagnosis. In the absence of bleeding, the erythrocyte count and hemoglobin may be normal, unless the patient is jaundiced, and then they are both reduced. Leukocytosis of 11–20,000/mm³ (11–20 × 10⁹/liter) is usual in icteric patients. The platelet count is frequently reduced, especially in severely jaundiced patients.[21] The erythrocyte sedimentation rate is generally raised.

Blood urea and creatinine are always raised at least transiently, even in mild cases. Liver function tests are useful diagnostically. The serum aminotransferases are normal or high, while the serum bilirubin level is always raised in icteric or preicteric leptospirosis. The combination of raised blood urea, raised direct bilirubin, and normal or slightly elevated aminotransferases serves to differentiate leptospirosis from hepatitis in which the serum aminotransferases are always significantly elevated.[26]

Proteinurea is a constant but sometimes transient finding, even in mild cases. In severe cases, or wherever there is renal failure, granular and hyaline casts will be found in urine, together with bile.

Examination of CSF reveals increased protein with normal glucose.

8.1.3. Prognosis. Recovery is usually complete within a few weeks in mild-type patients. However, residual depression, irritability, and psychosis have been reported, lasting up to 6 months and preventing a return to normal life and work.[4,70] Occasional reports of prolonged headache and backache following mild leptospirosis are hard to evaluate. Patients who survive the severe type of leptospirosis usually show no further signs of illness within a few weeks of full recovery of function in vital organs. Prolonged neurological symptoms and signs have been recorded, but in some of these patients there is room for doubt about the validity of the original diagnosis.

8.1.4. Treatment. Penicillin (or erythromycin in allergic patients) is the recommended treatment of choice as early as possible in the illness.[26] Given on the first day or two in patients diagnosed in the acute stage of infection, it can abort the symptoms and progress of either the mild or the severe form can be interrupted abruptly, so that the patient is frequently clinically well within 24 h. Antibiotics given in the late ("tissue") stages may make no difference to the outcome because the disease process is then a consequence of established lesions, the leptospires usually having been eliminated by the patient's development of antibodies; nevertheless good results have been reported in late penicillin treatment.[98a]

Symptomatic and supportive systemic treatment is required for hemorrhage; shock; renal, hepatic, or cardiac insufficiency; meningitis and other symptoms, such as headache, fever, and vomiting.[26]

8.2. Diagnosis

8.2.1. Clinical Diagnosis. The clinical features in early leptospirosis of either the mild or the severe type are not pathognomonic and give no indication of the diagnosis to an inexperienced or uneducated clinician.[26] In areas where the disease is common and has been recognized using laboratory confirmation, fresh cases can be diagnosed with a high degree of accuracy. A checklist of symptoms and tests[26] is a valuable aid for primary health workers, especially those not already familiar with clinical leptospirosis. The list provides minimal diagnostic criteria and a point score for likelihood of diagnosis.

Epidemiological factors such as occupational or domestic exposure to risk of infection from carrier animals, or recent travel, will influence the interpretation of clinical findings, pending results of confirmatory laboratory tests.

8.2.2. Laboratory Bacteriological Diagnosis. The principles of diagnosis are cultivation of leptospires from blood, urine, CSF, or other sites in the acute stages, demonstration of leptospires in tissues and body fluids, and serological tests.[24,26]

a. Diagnosis by Direct Microscopy.[26,28] Leptospires can be seen in body fluids by dark-field illumination. The most useful specimens in the acute stage are urine and CSF, although examination of anterior chamber fluid from the eye is indicated in uveitis. Inexpert observers looking at body fluids can mistake fibrin threads for leptospires.

Urine to be examined for leptospires, whether by microscopy or by culture, should be alkaline or alkalinized by medication because leptospires die rapidly in acid.

Leptospires may be found in urine during the first week to 10 days and intermittently thereafter. A negative result for direct microscopy of urine or CSF does not negate the diagnosis.[28]

Leptospires may also be identified directly by immunofluorescence[26] or immunoperoxidase[34,85] staining, or by silver deposition[26,80] in smears or frozen or wax-embedded histological sections of autopsy or biopsy material.[26] Technical problems inherent in silver staining techniques dictate extremely rigorous cleanliness and care.

b. Culture.[26,28] Diagnostic cultures are usually made from specimens, blood, urine, CSF, other body fluids and exudates, and occasionally from tissues obtained at biopsy or autopsy. Tween–albumin fluid culture media such as EMJH are most generally useful because more exacting strains grow better in it on primary isolation. Protein-free culture media are seldom satisfactory for primary cultivation.

Blood cultures are made by inoculating blood drawn aseptically by venipuncture directly into culture media. Multiple inoculation of several tubes each containing 5–10 ml of medium, with one to ten drops of blood, is recommended.[26] Good results can be obtained by adding approximately 0.5 ml of blood to approximately 50 ml of medium, but the volume of medium is not critical. A significant dilution of at least one in ten in culture medium is required to dilute antileptospiral activity in the blood. If blood cannot be inoculated at the bedside, it can be collected in a sterile ammonium oxalate or heparin anticoagulant tube or even as a last resort in a plain tube and transported to a laboratory where the blood or serum can be inoculated into medium. If possible, multiple cultures should be prepared from each specimen. Penicillinase and sodium polyanetholesulfonate (SPS) can be added if required. The inoculated media are incubated at 30°C and examined for growth microscopically daily for the first week and weekly thereafter, up to 2 months, and, ideally, they should be subcultured weekly. The value of blood culture is positive identification of the etiological agent rather than speed. Isolates may be identified serologically.[26] The development of gene probes and other genetic methods should enable further and faster identification of isolates.[59,87,88]

Culture of urine requires an alkalinized fresh midstream or catheter specimen taken with care to minimize contamination. A selective medium containing 100 µg/ml 5-fluorouracil as an inhibitor of contaminant microorganisms is recommended.[26] Media made semisolid with a final 0.1% concentration of agar are preferred by some workers, using at least a tenfold dilution of urine in the medium.[26] Multiple cultures should be prepared from each specimen.

Leptospires may be found in CSF in the first 10 days of illness and can be cultured from it by inoculating 0.1–0.5 ml into 5–10 ml of fluid or semisolid culture medium.

c. Serological Diagnosis (see Section 3.4.2). It can take 14 days or even much longer incubation before cultures become positive. Specimens or media for culture are frequently not available. Furthermore, the diagnosis of leptospirosis is often not suspected, or the patient does not seek medical attention until the illness is well advanced, when leptospires may have been eliminated from the body by antibodies. Thus, serological tests may be the most reliable means by which a retrospective, if not concurrent, diagnosis can be made.

The main test used universally is the MAT in which a small volume of live leptospiral culture of a standard age and density is mixed with a volume of a known dilution of the patient's serum. Agglutination is recorded following observation by dark-field microscopy. A variant, using formalin-killed cultures, gives slower results and lower titers but has advantages in safety and longer shelf life of the antigen suspension. A macroscopic slide agglutination test using a heavy suspension of leptospires is available for rapid screening. It is relatively insensitive and prone to false-positive reactions. Negative results cannot be used to rule out the possible diagnosis of leptospirosis. Sera reacting in slide agglutination tests must be titrated by MAT.

Enzyme immunoassays[3,60,84] are in use at present for experimental and developmental studies but do not supplant MAT for diagnosis because MAT is extremely sensitive and highly specific for the homologous serovar, provided antigenic overlaps within a serogroup are understood. The highest titer recorded is not necessarily to the infecting serovar, especially early in the illness. Both IgM and IgG antibodies can agglutinate leptospires (see Section 7.5.2). IgM antibodies can be detected by immunoblotting in the sera of patients with concurrently proved leptospirosis usually within the first week.[14]

Serum specimens for diagnosis by serological tests should be taken immediately at the outset of investigations, preferably on the 1st day of illness, and tested as soon as possible. A further specimen should be taken on the 5th to 7th days, and further tests if required on the 10th and 12th days (see Section 3.4.2).

In new patients in nonendemic areas, MAT antibodies at titers ≥ 400 in a single specimen may be considered diagnostic (see Section 3.4.2a). Titers of between 100 and 400 are suspicious and are indications for retesting where the clinical picture is consistent with leptospirosis. A fourfold or greater rising titer from an initial level of zero, ≥ 50 or ≥ 100, to $\geq 400-800$ may be considered diagnostic. In an endemic area, or in patients known to have had leptospirosis before, there may be residual background titers of ≥ 10 to ≥ 1000 from previous infections. A fresh infection in such a patient will be indicated by a rise of titer in paired serum specimens. Cross reactivity among serovars is not uncommon.

The level of antibody in MAT will be influenced to some extent by the serovar. Characteristically, very low titers follow sv *hardjo* infections, frequently $\geq 800-3200$, while typically very much higher titers up to $\geq 1000-10,000$ are seen following sv *copenhageni* infections. In patients whose sera cross-react with a heterologous serovar, the higher homologous titer prevails eventually, sometimes after several weeks. MAT antibodies may appear only after a delay of weeks, if at all, in patients in whom leptospirosis has been successfully treated early with penicillin or other antibiotics. Unless the diagnosis was verified by culture of leptospires, it will be impossible to prove that the patient had leptospirosis, leading to possible medicolegal complications in insurance and Workers' Compensation claims, and inaccurate notification and epidemiological statistics.[26]

It is common practice to commence dilutions at 1 : 100 or even greater in screening tests used for antibody prevalence surveys in epidemiological studies. The rationale is that people who have had leptospirosis maintain high antibody levels and lower levels of antibodies are nonspecific, meaning that they may be cross-reactive from infection with other serovars than the one used in the test. This rationale is fallacious in diagnosis of clinical cases, where even a very low titer of antibody may indicate the earliest response to current infection. A further MAT within a few days will show a significant rise. Physicians can use the first low titer in clinically characteristic patients to indicate a need to do a further test soon and perhaps treat as leptospirosis in the meantime. The deciding factor is how one interprets low titers in the epidemiological environment. Where leptospirosis is rarely seen, any titer is significant. Where it is common, low MAT titers, or even a high MAT titer may be irrelevant to a current illness that is not leptospirosis.

Diagnosis by MAT presupposes that the test antigen used is the appropriate infecting serovar of *L. interrogans* or at least a serovar that shares antigens sufficiently to aggluti-nate with the patients' sera. A full range of serovars recommended includes representatives of all 23 serogroups.[26] It is also recommended that local isolates be used, where available, for antigen suspensions.

ELISA tests detect antibodies in patients' sera. The serospecificity depends on the type of antigen used,[3,84] but in general ELISA tests cross-react more widely than MAT. In all ELISA tests, including immunoblots, it is simple to measure reactivity in IgM or IgG separately. The results obtained in ELISA tests using sonicated leptospires correlate with MAT in general qualitatively, but the levels of reaction are often unrelated.[60]

8.2.3. Detection of Leptospires in Urine. Darkfield microscopy is unreliable for small numbers of leptospires. Detection of small numbers of leptospires in carrier animal urine is important. Attempts to improve detection have used radioimmunoassay,[5,15] DNA hydridization and gene probes,[59,88] immunoperoxidase stains,[85] and chemiluminescence[97] although unknown substances in urine can reduce the sensitivity of some tests in field conditions. Fluorescent antibody testing can also be used and cultures (see Section 8.2.2b) can be prepared.

8.2.4. Differential Diagnosis.[26,33,92] At the onset of either mild- or severe-type leptospirosis, there is little to distinguish it from any other acute febrile illness. The very severe headache, fever, and myalgia are characteristic but at this stage may be confused with severe influenza, poliomyelitis, dengue, Q fever, and viral meningitis. The main differentiating criteria in leptospirosis are raised blood creatinine and urea, leukocytosis, and in some cases, an early rise in titer of leptospiral antibodies. At a later stage the main differential diagnoses are with viral meningitis and acute abdominal emergencies in mild-type leptospirosis and with malaria, blackwater fever, viral meningitis, hepatitis, yellow fever, and acute glomerulonephritis in severe-type leptospirosis. The main diagnostic criteria are high serum bilirubin with low or normal levels of serum aminotransferases, with significant and rising titers of specific antileptospiral antibodies. The isolation and identification of leptospires in blood, urine, or CSF confirms the diagnosis positively. At autopsy, differential diagnosis depends on characteristic pathological changes of jaundice and widespread hemorrhages with pale enlarged hemorrhagic kidneys showing histological evidence of renal tubular degeneration and hemorrhage, liver cell degeneration, myocarditis, and pulmonary hemorrhages. Leptospires can be found and stained by immunostaining in tissues up to about 7 to 10 days after onset,[26,34] but are hard to demonstrate thereafter. Postmortem serum specimens may be tested for antibodies.

In all patients, an epidemiological history of occupational or accidental exposure to risk and animal contact, or travel, may elucidate the diagnosis.

9. Control and Prevention

9.1. General Concepts

As is the case in all zoonoses, control of leptospirosis in humans is complex because the primary sources of the disease are in animals, in some of which control is impossible. Regulation if not eradication of leptospirosis may be feasible in livestock and domestic animals even though carriers are clinically normal and shedders hard to detect, but it cannot be envisaged in wildlife. Control is further complicated by the general and nonspecific clinical picture of mild or early severe leptospirosis, indistinguishable from a variety of other incapacitating fevers common in tropical areas, so that an animal source is often not suspected. The essentials of control and prevention lie in awareness and recognition of the disease and in containment in livestock and domestic sources.[26]

Awareness and recognition require a knowledge of epidemiological facts acquired by selected surveillance, reporting, and notification, which in turn need specialized diagnostic laboratory services and education of physicians, veterinarians, administrators, and the public. Although containment of animal sources may be seen as a veterinary public health and hygiene problem, it is essential to the protection of humans. The main measures are veterinary surveillance, treatment, and prevention; occupational hygiene; rodent control; engineering; laboratory safety; and evaluation of preventive measures.[26] In addition, containment extends to the prevention of human disease by the judicious avoidance of risk, by immunization, and by chemoprophylaxis.

9.1.1. Education, Laboratory Services, and Notification. Ordinary routine microbiological diagnostic laboratories are not usually equipped with skilled staff and specialized techniques for leptospirosis. If specialized diagnosis is not available locally, there should be a central leptospirosis laboratory available for referral of specimens and consultation.[26] Reference laboratories staffed by experts are required only on a regional international basis for stock cultures, standard sera, research, education, and consultation.[26]

Evaluation of diagnostic laboratory results provides a useful form of surveillance. In addition, prevalence surveys for antibodies in selected groups can reveal problems or evaluate control measures.[26] The most effective form of information gathering should be notification by health practitioners. Usually, this is of limited value because of inadequate diagnosis, failure to use appropriate laboratory tests, and failure to notify. Statistics of practitioner notifications frequently indicate an incidence much lower than diagnosed by laboratories.

9.1.2. Control Measures in Animals

a. Rodent Control.[26] Removal of rodents from the domestic environment effectively reduces the infection rate of leptospirosis. Standard measures include control of litter and garbage disposal, protecting food sources, trapping, and poisoning. Feral rodents and small marsupials cannot be controlled. When they share the environment with crops, precautions can be taken, such as burning off sugarcane before cutting by hand.

b. Environmental Control. Any measure to reduce the load of leptospires in soil, water, or mud will reduce the risk to humans. Simple drainage can prevent seepage of urine into waterlogged soils or yards where livestock are herded. Environmental engineering can also increase the risk by flooding previously dry areas.[22,26,77]

c. Immunization, Chemotherapy, and Culling of Livestock. Excretor rates in cattle and pig herds frequently reach levels of 65–90%. If shedders can be identified and removed from herds, the risks to the herd and to attendant humans can be reduced, provided the remaining animals are immunized, the herd is restocked with immunized animals, fresh excretor animals are not introduced, and the herd is protected from fresh infection from environmental sources.[55] Immunization alone can reduce both animal and indirectly human leptospirosis, but it is hard to evaluate because most studies have been specially set up under artificial conditions accompanied by education and improvements in occupational hygiene and farming practice. Outer envelope preparations and leptospiral cultures in protein-free media are available as vaccines.[9,56] Immunization of livestock or dogs requires two doses of a killed vaccine a month or so apart followed by annual revaccination. It is relatively expensive and its use by smallholding farmers will depend on the relative values and costs of animals, vaccines, and health (or illness). The associated costs of transport, skilled attention, and equipment may also be relatively high. The control of leptospirosis in stud stock, where leptospires may be found in semen samples used for artificial insemination, requires special methods for testing and transport of semen.[99]

9.1.3. Treatment of the Carrier State. Carrier animals have been cured by streptomycin treatment.[26] The cost is relatively high and the results so hard to evaluate in

field conditions that it is considered impractical for general use.

Humans do not become chronic carriers or excretors for any length of time. Elementary domestic, personal, and hospital hygiene ensures little risk from patients and convalescents still excreting leptospires. Urine specimens from convalescent patients are not recognized sources of laboratory infection but care should be taken nonetheless.

9.1.4. Occupational Hygiene.[26] Preventive measures for people who cannot avoid exposure to risk are centered around methods for physical protection in their work or leisure. Waterproof footwear, watershedding aprons, or other clothing and clear plastic facemasks have all been recommended for milkers and slaughterhouse workers. In hot climates or working conditions, impermeable protective clothing is uncomfortable and poorly accepted. Nevertheless, rubber boots provide obvious protection. Most infections appear to follow penetration of cuts and damaged, abraded, or macerated skin by leptospires. It is therefore important to protect such injuries, but often not practicable to do so in daily working conditions.

Good drainage of floors and herding yards and control of rodent infestation in food preparation areas are important occupational hygienic measures, but no measures will be effective unless people concerned understand the disease, the means of infection, and the need for precautions so that they are prepared to implement recommended practices. The risk for field workers can be reduced by attempting to control the environmental hazards as outlined in Section 9.1.2.

9.2. Antimicrobial Prophylaxis

Chemoprophylaxis with doxycycline has bee used to prevent leptospirosis in soldiers exposed to jungle conditions.[82] It, or prophylactic penicillin, could be used to protect anyone exposed to a significant risk for a brief defined period. People in such categories could include those about to undertake rafting or canoeing trips, cavers, grain farmers and workers at harvest time when risks are serious for a short period only, field ecologists trapping small wild rodents,[55] and people caught in floods. Tetracycline group antibiotics are leptospirostatic rather than leptospiricidal[12] and in any case contraindicated in pregnant women, in children, and in people with renal insufficiency. Prolonged or permanent chemoprophylaxis is not recommended. It is unlikely that antibiotic treatment of humans before or during leptospirosis will lead to leptospirosis from antibiotic-resistant leptospires because human-to-human transmission is almost unrecorded, although leptospires develop resistance to some antibiotics readily in the laboratory.

Antibiotic-resistant leptospirosis has not been recorded in animals, despite some decades of use of streptomycin and penicillin in veterinary medicine. Antibiotic susceptibility tests are not usually performed on leptospires isolated from either human or animal sources.[12] Spontaneous resistance to penicillins, aminoglycosides, tetracyclines, or macrolides, all of which have been used in leptospirosis, is not known. On the other hand, there is a high probability that chemoprophylaxis with any antibiotic will assist in the highly undesirable selection of antibiotic-resistant derivatives of other bacteria including pathogens of the alimentary and respiratory tracts.

9.3. Immunization

Immunization of humans and animals with killed cultures of leptospires has been used almost since leptospires were discovered. Vaccines are serovar specific and currently administered subcutaneously in two or more doses 2 or 4 weeks apart and repeated annually.[99]

Local reactions of pain, redness, and swelling ranging from mild to very severe occur, especially on revaccination. There was always a risk of anaphylaxis or serum sickness from the serum or serum proteins necessarily in the culture media until relatively recently, when protein-free media became available.[76] Some preparations involved washing and resuspending leptospires to reduce the animal protein content, but protein can always be found adherent to the leptospiral surface after washing. Washed or whole culture vaccines have been employed in several countries, mainly in Asia, where the risks to life and health from severe leptospirosis could justify the side effects of the vaccine.[99] There has not been widespread acceptance of an early protein-free vaccine for humans[76,93] although more recent studies showed evidence of effective immunization.[14] Increasing worldwide concern about quality control, safety, pyrogenicity, potential teratogenicity, and efficacy of vaccines ensure that rigorous evaluation will be required before a suitable vaccine can be accepted for human use.

Successful experimental oral immunization of animals has been reported,[62] with obvious potential for use in humans if its efficacy and safety are substantiated.

10. Unresolved Problems

There is a series of interconnected questions that need answers before great improvements in control of leptospirosis can be achieved. Neither the duration of postinfection immunity nor its specificity is known. Conventional wisdom based mainly on animal experimentation states that immunity is specific for antigens that are serovar specific, or at best shared within a serogroup. Is there any underlying genus- or species-specific immunity in humans mediating a level of resistance to all serovars of *L. interrogans?*

Which antigens mediate serospecificity and thus immunity to initial infection following immunization? Are they the same as the antigens mediating immunity to reinfection in nature?

Leptospiral toxins are able to damage host tissues. Is there antitoxic immunity as well as antileptospiral immunity, and if so, is it significant in recovery or protection?

There are genetic differences in the susceptibility of pigs to primary infection.[69] Are there human genetic differences in susceptibility, and if so, are they reflected in the response to particular serovars or to all serovars, and thus to the pathogenicity of particular serovars for humans?

Oral immunization in animals has been described.[62] Would it be effective in humans? If oral immunization were effective in domesticated animals, could it be used to protect and eradicate leptospirosis from wildlife populations, and if it were, what would be the ecological implications of altering a natural population balance achieved by an enzootic disease?

L. interrogans exhibits a large range of antigenic surface characteristics that allow the identification of approximately 200 serovars; new serovars are being described regularly. What is the genetic basis for serovar specificity and variation? A plasmid has yet to be described in *L. interrogans*. What is the basis for genetic exchange in nature? This problem becomes acutely relevant with the recognition that the serovars of *L. interrogans* can be classified into genetic groups by DNA relatedness, and that serovar specificity overlaps the genetic groupings.[100] The effects of these observations on classification of leptospires will have implications for diagnosis, epidemiology, and prognosis.

There are needs for rapid bedside tests that will enable a clinician to identify rapidly whether or not a patient has leptospirosis, and if so, which serovar, often at a time in the illness before antibodies have appeared in blood. Methods explored so far are antigen detection and gene probes. Further development of these or other methods would be invaluable in the early recognition and diagnosis of cases and the institution of appropriate treatment. Direct tests for the leptospira or its antigens would overcome the serious difficulty of evaluating the significance of a positive serological test in a patient in an endemic area where most of the population have antibodies, even residual IgM, to one or more serovars, or where the patient may have residual antibodies from an infection with a serovar unrelated to the present illness. Similar direct diagnostic methods would allow easier and more positive detection or carrier animals than is possible now.

A further problem that cannot be ignored is the fact that most people at risk from leptospirosis live in developing countries without ready access to specialized diagnostic or treatment facilities. There is seldom a capacity for new scientific research into the problems identified here. On the other hand, leptospirosis is rarely diagnosed in urban agglomerations in developed countries where most researchers and institutes capable of high technology are found and there are relatively few among them interested in leptospirosis. Knowledge and research in leptospirosis are thus not available in most developed countries, to which developing countries turn for scientific assistance. The situation is aggravated when inadequate statistics in developed countries indicate a spuriously low rate of leptospirosis, leading to an impression that the disease is nonexistent or unimportant and does not justify allocation of funds for the maintenance of existing research and surveillance or for new studies toward solutions to the problems outlined above.

ACKNOWLEDGMENTS

Original research from the author's laboratory was supported by grants from the Australian National Health and Medical Research Council, Canberra, Australia. The author thanks Dr. A. Kaufmann for the prepublication copy of his manuscript (Ref. 100) and permission to quote from it before publication, and Judith Marks for painstaking care in preparing this manuscript.

11. References

1. ADLER, B., AND FAINE, S., A pomona serogroup-specific, agglutinating antigen in *Leptospira,* identified by monoclonal antibodies, *Pathology* **15**:247–250 (1983).
2. ADLER, B., AND FAINE, S., Species- and genus-specific antigens in Leptospira, revealed by monoclonal antibodies and enzyme immunoassay, *Zentralbl. Bakteriol. Hyg. Abt. 1 Orig. A* **255**:317–322 (1983).
3. ADLER, B., MURPHY, A. M., LOCARNINI, S., AND FAINE, S., Detection of specific anti-leptospiral immunoglobulins M and G in human serum by solid-phase enzyme-linked immunosorbent assay, *J. Clin. Microbiol.,* **11**:452–457 (1980).
4. AVERY, T. L., Leptospirosis and mental illness, *N.Z. Med. J.* **96**:589 (1983).
5. BAHAMAN, A. R., MARSHALL, R. B., AND MORIARTY, K. M., Experimental trials on the use of radioimmunoassay for the detection of leptospiral antigens in urine, *Vet. Microbiol.* **12**:161–167 (1986).
6. BALLARD, S. A., ADLER, B., MILLAR, B. D., CHAPPEL, R. J., JONES, R. T., AND FAINE, S., The immunoglobulin re-

sponse of swine following experimental infection with *Leptospira interrogans* serovar *pomona*, *Zentralbl. Bakteriol. Hyg. Series A* **256**:510–517 (1984).

7. BALLARD, S. A., WILLIAMSON, M., ADLER, B., AND FAINE, S., Interactions of virulent and avirulent leptospires with primary cultures of renal epithelial cells, *J. Med. Microbiol.* **21**:59–67 (1986).

8. BERNHEIMER, A. W., AND BEY, R. F., Copurification of *Leptospira interrogans* serovar *pomona* hemolysin and sphingomyelinase C, *Infect. Immun.* **54**:262–264 (1986).

9. BEY, R. F., AND JOHNSON, R. C., Humoral immune responses of cattle vaccinated with leptospiral pentavalent outer envelopes and whole culture vaccines, *Am. J. Vet. Res.* **39**:1109–1114 (1978).

10. BLACKMORE, D. K., SCHOLLUM, L. M., AND MORIARTY, K. M., The magnitude and duration of titres of leptospiral agglutinins in human sera, *N.Z. Med. J.* **97**:83–86 (1983).

11. BROMLEY, D. B., AND CHARON, N. W., Axial filament involvement in the motility of *Leptospira interrogans*, *J. Bacteriol.* **137**:1406–1412 (1979).

12. BROUGHTON, E. S., AND FLACK, L. E., The susceptibility of a strain of *Leptospira interrogans* serogroup icterohaemorrhagiae to amoxycillin, erythromycin, lincomycin, tetracycline, oxytetracycline and minocycline, *Zentralbl. Bakteriol. Hyg. Series A* **261**:425–431 (1986).

13. BROUGHTON, E. S., AND SCARNELL, J., Prevention of renal carriage of leptospirosis in dogs by vaccination, *Vet. Rec.* **117**:307 (1985).

14. CHAPMAN, A. J., ADLER, B., AND FAINE, S., Immunoblot analysis of antibody responses of vaccinated or naturally infected humans to leptospiral antigens, *J. Med. Microbiol.* **25**:269–278 (1988).

15. CHAPPEL, R. J., ADLER, B., BALLARD, S. A., FAINE, S., JONES, R. T., MILLAR, B. D., AND SWAINGER, J. A., Enzymatic radioimmunoassay for detecting *Leptospira interrogans* serovar *pomona* in the urine of experimentally-infected pigs, *Vet. Microbiol.* **10**:279–286 (1985).

16. COUSINS, D. V., ROBERTSON, G. M., AND HUSTAS, L., The use of the enzyme-linked immunosorbent assay (ELISA) to detect the IgM and IgG antibody response to *Leptospira interrogans* serovars *hardjo*, *pomona* and *tarassovi* in cattle, *Vet. Microbiol.* **10**:439–450 (1985).

17. DE ARRIAGA, A. J. D., ROCHA, A. S., YASUDA, P. H., AND DE BRITO, T., Morpho-functional patterns of kidney injury in the experimental leptospirosis of the guinea-pig (*L. icterohaemorrhagiae*), *J. Pathol.* **138**:145–161 (1982).

18. DE BRITO, T., MORAIS, C. F., YASUDA, P. H., LANCELLOTTI, C. P., HOSHINO-SHIMIZU, S., YAMASHIRO, E., AND FERREIRA ALVES, V. A., Cardiovascular involvement in human and experimental leptospirosis: Pathologic findings and immunohistochemical detection of leptospiral antigen, *Ann. Trop. Med. Parasitol.* **81**:207–214 (1987).

19. DERRICK, E. H., Estimation of the incubation period of canefield leptospirosis from the weekly work pattern, *Pathology* **1**:73–75 (1969).

20. DIKKEN, H., AND KMETY, E., Serological typing methods of leptospires, in: *Methods in Microbiology,* Volume 11 (T. Bergan and J. R. Norris, eds.), pp. 260–294, Academic Press, New York, 1978.

21. EDWARDS, C. N., NICHOLSON, G. D., HASSELL, T. A., EVERARD, C. O. R., AND CALLENDER, J., Thrombocytopenia in leptospirosis: The absence of evidence for disseminated intravascular coagulation, *Am. J. Trop. Med. Hyg.* **35**:352–354 (1986).

22. ELDER, J. K., The influence of environmental factors on the survival of zoonotic bacterial pathogens with special reference to *Leptospirae*, *Aust. Microbiol.* **7**:323–324 (1986).

23. ELLIS, W. A., MCFARLAND, P. J., AND BRYSON, D. G., Isolation of leptospires from the genital tract and kidneys of aborted sows, *Vet. Rec.* **118**:294–295 (1986).

24. FAINE, S., Virulence in Leptospira. I. Reactions of guinea-pigs to experimental infection with *Leptospira icterohaemorrhagiae*, *Br. J. Exp. Pathol.* **38**:1–7 (1957).

25. FAINE, S., Virulence in Leptospira. II. The growth *in vivo* of virulent *Leptospira icterohaemorrhagiae*, *Br. J. Exp. Pathol.* **38**:8–14 (1957).

26. FAINE, S., *Guidelines for the Control of Leptospirosis,* Offset Publ. No. 67, WHO, Geneva, 1982.

27. FAINE, S., Leptospirosis in the western Pacific area, in: "Leptospirosis," Proceedings from the 11th International Symposium of the Korean Academy of Medical Science, June 20, 1985, pp. 18–48 (1986).

28. FAINE, S., Leptospirosis: *Laboratory Diagnosis of Infectious Diseases: Principles and Practice* (A. Balows, W. J. Hausler, and E. H. Lennette, eds.), pp. 344–352, Springer-Verlag, New York, 1988.

29. FAINE, S., AND CARTER, J. N., Natural antibody in mammalian serum reacting with an antigen in some leptospires, *J. Bacteriol.* **95**:280–285 (1968).

30. FAINE, S., AND STALLMAN, N. D., Amended descriptions of the genus *Leptospira* Noguchi 1917 and the species *L. interrogans* (Stimson 1907) Wenyon 1926 and *L. biflexa* (Wolbach and Binger 1914) Noguchi 1918, *Int. J. Syst. Bacteriol.* **32**:461–463 (1982).

31. FAINE, S., ADLER, B., CHRISTOPHER, W., AND VALENTINE, R., Fatal congenital human leptospirosis, *Zentralbl. Bakteriol. Hyg. Series A* **257**:548 (1984).

32. FARRELLY, H. E., ADLER, B., AND FAINE, S., Opsonic monoclonal antibodies against lipopolysaccharide antigens of *Leptospira interrogans* serovar *hardjo*, *J. Med. Microbiol.* **23**:1–7 (1987).

33. FEIGIN, R. D., AND ANDERSON, D. C., Human leptospirosis, *CRC Crit. Rev. Clin. Lab. Sci.* **5**:413–467 (1975).

34. FERREIRA ALVES, V. A., VIANNA, M. R., YASUDA, P. H., AND DE BRITO, T., Detection of leptospiral antigen in the human liver and kidney using an immunoperoxidase staining procedure, *J. Pathol.* **151**:125–131 (1987).

35. GOARD, K. E., Infection by *Leptospira pomona* contracted from pigs by mouth-to-mouth resuscitation, *Med. J. Aust.* **1**:897–898 (1961).

36. GSELL, H. O., OLAFSSON, A., SONNABEND, W., BREER, C., AND BACHMANN, C., Intrauterine leptospirosis pomona, *Dtsch. Med. Wochenschr.* **96**:1263–1268 (1971).

37. HATHAWAY, S. C., MARSHALL, R. B., LITTLE, T. W. A., HEADLAM, S. A., AND WINTER, P. J., Identification by cross-agglutination absorption and restriction endonuclease analysis of leptospires in the Pomona serogroup isolated in the United Kingdom, *Res. Vet. Sci.* **39**:151–156 (1985).

38. HO, H. F., AND BLACKMORE, D. K., Effect of chilling and freezing on survival of *Leptospira interrogans* serovar *pomona* in naturally infected pig kidneys, *N.Z. Vet. J.* **27**:121–123 (1979).

39. HOOKEY, J. V., WAITKINS, S. A., AND JACKMAN, P. J. H., Numerical analysis of *Leptospira* DNA-restriction endonuclease patterns, *FEMS Microbiol. Lett.* **29**:185–188 (1985).

40. IOLI, A., TREDICI, E., AND LOGGINI, F., Studio sulla parentela antigene tra shigelle e leptospire. 1. Parentela antigene tra *Shigella dysenteriae* 1 e *Leptospire sejroe, hardjo* e *sao paulo, Ann. Sclavo* **19**:219–224 (1977).

41. ISOGAI, E., ISOGAI, H., KUREBAYASHI, Y., AND ITO, N., Biological activities of leptospiral lippolysaccharide, *Zentralbl. Bakteriol. Hyg. Series A* **261**:53–64 (1986).

42. ISOGAI, E., KITAGAWA, H., ISOGAI, H., KUREBAYASHI, Y., AND ITO, N., Phagocytosis as a defense mechanism against infection with leptospiras, *Zentralbl. Bakteriol. Hyg. A* **261**:65–74 (1986).

43. ITO, T., AND YANAGAWA, R., Leptospiral attachment to extracellular matrix of mouse fibroblast (L929) cells, *Vet. Microbiol.* **15**:89–96 (1987).

44. JEVON, T. R., KNUDSON, M. P., SMITH, P. A., WHITECAR, P. S., AND BLAKE, R. L., A point-source epidemic of leptospirosis, *Postgrad. Med.* **80**:121–129 (1986).

45. JOHNSON, R. C., AND FAINE, S., Order I. Spirochaetales: Family II. *Leptospiraceae* Hovind-Hougen 1979, 245. Genus I. *Leptospira* Noguchi 1917, 755, in: *Bergey's Manual of Systematic Bacteriology,* Volume 1 (N. R. Krieg and J. G. Holt, eds.), pp. 62–67, Williams & Wilkins, Baltimore, 1984.

46. JOHNSON, R. C., AND MUSCHEL, L. H., Antileptospiral activity of serum. I. Normal and immune serum, *J. Bacteriol.* **91**:1403–1409 (1966).

47. JOHNSTON, J. H., LLOYD, J., MCDONALD, J., AND WAITKINS, S., Leptospirosis: An occupational disease of soldiers, *J. R. Army Med. Corps* **129**(2):111–114 (1983).

48. JOST, B. H., ADLER, B., VINH, T., AND FAINE, S., A monoclonal antibody reacting with a determinant on leptospiral lipopolysaccharide protects guinea pigs against leptospirosis, *J. Med. Microbiol.* **22**:269–275 (1986).

48a. JOST, B. H., ADLER, B., AND FAINE, S., Experimental immunisation of hamsters with lipopolysaccharide antigens of *Leptospira interrogans, J. Med. Microbiol.* **29**:115–120 (1989).

49. KASAROV, L. B., Degradation of the erythrocyte phospholipids and haemolysis of the erythrocytes of different animal species by *Leptospirae, J. Med. Microbiol.* **3**:29–37 (1970).

49a. KMETY, E., AND DIKKEN, H., Revised list of *Leptospira* serovars, published for the Subcommittee on the Taxonomy of *Leptospira,* International Committee on Systematic Bacteriology of the International Union of Microbiological Societies. University Press, Groningen, Netherlands, 1988.

50. KNIGHT, L. L., MILLER, N. G., AND WHITE, R. J., Cytotoxic factor in the blood and plasma of animals during leptospirosis, *Infect. Immun.* **8**:401–405 (1973).

51. KOBAYASHI, Y., TAMAI, T., AND SADA, E., Serological analysis of serogroup icterohaemorrhagiae using monoclonal antibodies, *Microbiol. Immunol.* **29**:1229–1235 (1985).

52. KORTHOF, G., Experimentelles Schlammfieber beim Menschen, *Zentralbl. Bakteriol. Parasitenkd. Infektionskr. Hyg. Abt. 1 Orig. Reihe* **125**:429–434 (1932).

53. LE FEBVRE, R. B., FOLEY, J. W., AND THIERMANN, A. B., Rapid and simplified protocol for isolation and characterization of leptospiral chromosomal DNA for taxonomy and diagnosis, *J. Clin. Microbiol.* **22**:606–608 (1985).

54. LINDSAY, S., AND LUKE, I. W., Fatal leptospirosis (Weil's disease) in a newborn infant. Case of intrauterine fetal infection with report of an autopsy, *J. Pediatr.* **34**:90–94 (1949).

55. LOOKE, D. F. M., Weil's syndrome in a zoologist, *Med. J. Aust.* **144**:597–601 (1986).

56. MACINTOSH, C. G., MARSHALL, R. B., AND BROUGHTON, E. S., The use of a *hardjo–pomona* vaccine to prevent leptospiruria in cattle exposed to natural challenge with *Leptospira interrogans* serovar *hardjo, N.Z. Vet. J.* **28**:174–177 (1980).

57. MARSHALL, R. B., WILTON, B. E., AND ROBINSON, A. J., Identification of *Leptospira* serovars by restriction-endonuclease analysis, *J. Med. Microbiol.* **14**:163–166 (1981).

58. MARSHALL, R. B., WINTER, P. J., AND YANAGAWA, R., Restriction endonuclease DNA analysis of *Leptospira interrogans* serovars *icterohaemorrhagiae* and *hebdomadis, J. Clin. Microbiol.* **20**:808–810 (1984).

59. MILLAR, B. D., CHAPPEL, R. J., AND ADLER, B., Detection of leptospires in biological fluids using DNA hybridisation, *Vet. Microbiol.* **15**:71–78, 1987.

60. MILNER, A. R., JACKSON, K. B., WOODRUFF, K., AND SMART, I. J., Enzyme-linked immunosorbent assay for determining specific immunoglobulin M in infections caused by *Leptospira interrogans* serovar *hardjo, J. Clin. Microbiol.* **22**:539–542 (1985).

61. MINETTE, H. P., Leptospirosis in poikilothermic vertebrates. A review, *Int. J. Zoonoses* **10**:111–121 (1983).

62. NIE, D., ZHU, G., ZHANG, LIU, Y., DOU, G., AND CHENG, W., Experimental studies on oral immunization against leptospirosis in hamsters, *Microbiol. J.* **1**:31–39 (1985).

63. NIIKURA, M., ONO, E., AND YANAGAWA, R., Molecular comparison of antigens on proteins of virulent and avirulent clones of *Leptospira interrogans* serovar *copenhageni* strain Shibaura, *Zentralbl. Bakteriol. Hyg. Series A* **266**:453–462 (1987).

64. Nunes-Edwards, P. L., Thiermann, A. B., Bassford, P. J., and Stamm, L. V., Identification and characterization of the protein antigens of *Leptospira interrogans* serovar *hardjo*, *Infect. Immun.* **48**:492–497 (1985).

65. Ono, E., Naiki, M., and Yanagawa, R., Production and characterization of monoclonal antibodies to lipopolysaccharide antigen of *Leptospira interrogans* serovar *kremastos* and *canicola*, *Zentralbl. Bakteriol Hyg. Abt. I Orig. Reihe A* **252**:414–424 (1982).

66. Ono, E., Takase, H., Naiki, M., and Yanagawa, R., Purification, characterization and serological properties of a glycolipid antigen reactive with a serovar-specific monoclonal antibody against *Leptospira interrogans* serovar *canicola*, *J. Gen. Microbiol.* **133**:1329–1336 (1987).

67. Parma, A. E., Santisteben, C. G., Villalba, J. S., and Bowden, R. A., Experimental demonstration of an antigenic relationship between *Leptospira* and equine cornea, *Vet. Immunol. Immunopathol.* **10**:215–224 (1986).

68. Peet, R. L., Mercy, A., Hustas, L., and Speed, C., The significance of leptospira isolated from the kidneys of slaughtered pigs, *Aust. Vet. J.* **60**:226–227 (1983).

69. Przytulski, T., and Porzeczkowska, D., Studies on genetic resistance to leptospirosis in pigs, *Br. Vet. J.* **136**:25–32 (1980).

70. Ram, P., and Karim, I., Severe psychiatric disturbance in leptospirosis, *Fiji Med. J.* **6**:70–72 (1978).

71. Ramachandran, S., and Perera, M. V. F., Cardiac and pulmonary involvement in leptospirosis, *Trans. R. Soc. Trop. Med. Hyg.* **71**:56–59 (1977).

72. Ratnam, S., Sundararaj, T., Subramanian, S., Madanagopalan, N., and Jayanthi, V., Humoral and cell-mediated immune responses to leptospires in different human cases, *Trans. R. Soc. Trop. Med. Hyg.* **78**:539–542 (1984).

73. Sakamoto, N., Ono, E., Kida, H., and Yanagawa, R., Characterization of a partially purified leptospiral genus-specific protein antigen, *Zentralbl. Bakteriol. Hyg. Series A* **259**:507–519 (1985).

74. Sakamoto, N., Ono, E., Kida, H., and Yanagawa, R., Production of monoclonal antibodies against leptospiral genus specific antigen and localization of the antigen by immunoelectron microscopy, *Zentralbl. Bakteriol., Hyg. Series A* **259**:557–563 (1985).

75. Sakamoto, N., Yanagawa, R., Ono, E., Kida, H., Mori, M., Arimitsu, Y., Akama, K., Yasuda, J., and Too, K., Detection and antibodies to leptospiral genus-specific antigen in human and animal sera by indirect hemagglutination test with a partially purified genus-specific protein antigen, *Zentralbl. Bakteriol. Hyg. Series A* **259**:548–556 (1985).

76. Shenberg, E., and Torten, M., A new leptospiral vaccine for use in man. I. Development of a vaccine from Leptospira grown on a chemically defined medium, *J. Infect. Dis.* **128**:642–646 (1973).

77. Shlyakhov, E., Influence de l'activité humaine sur l'épidémiologie des zooanthroponoses, *Med. Malad. Infect.* **13**:784–787 (1983).

78. Sitprija, V., Renal involvement in leptospirosis, in: *Nephrology* (R. R. Robinson, ed.), pp. 1041–1052, Springer-Verlag, New York, 1984.

79. Sitprija, V., Pipatangaul, V., Mertowidjojo, K., Boonpucknavig, V., and Boonpucknavig, S., Pathogenesis of renal disease in leptospirosis: Clinical and experimental studies, *Kidney Int.* **17**:827–836 (1980).

80. Skilbeck, N. W., and Chappel, R. J., Immunogold silver staining for visualization of leptospires in histologic sections, *J. Clin. Microbiol.* **25**:85–86 (1987).

81. Spinu, I., Topciu, V., Trinh, T. H. Q., and Vo, V. H., L'homme comme réservoir de virus dans une épidémie de leptospirose survenue dans la jungle, *Arch. Roum. Pathol. Exp. Microbiol.* **22**:1081–1100 (1963).

82. Takafuji, E. T., Kirkpatrick, J. W., Miller, R. N., Karwacki, J. J., Kelley, P. W., Gray, M. R., McNeill, K. M., Timboe, H. L., Kane, R. E., and Sanchez, J. L., An efficacy trial of doxycycline chemoprophylaxis against leptospirosis, *N. Engl. J. Med.* **310**:497–500 (1984).

83. Terpstra, W. J., and Bercovich, Z., Dairy farm fever, the leptospirosis of cattlemen, *Ned. Tijdschr. Geneeskd.* **128**:1040–1044 (1984).

84. Terpstra, W. J., Ligthart, G. S., and Schoone, G. J., Serodiagnosis of human leptospirosis by enzyme-linked immunosorbent-assay (ELISA), *Zentralbl. Bakteriol. Hyg. Abt. I Orig. Series A* **247**:400–405 (1980).

85. Terpstra, W. J., Jarboury-Postema, J., and Korver, H., Immunoperoxidase staining of leptospires in blood and urine, *Zentralbl. Bakteriol. Hyg. A* **254**:534–539 (1983).

86. Terpstra, W. J., Korver, H., Van Leeuwen, J., Klatser, P. R., and Kolk, A. H. J., The classification of Sejroe group serovars of *Leptospira interrogans* with monoclonal antibodies, *Zentralbl. Bakteriol. Hyg. Series A* **259**:498–506 (1985).

87. Terpstra, W. J., Schoone, G. J., and Ter Schegget, J., Detection of leptospiral DNA by nucleic acid hybridization with ^{32}P- and biotin-labelled probes, *J. Med. Microbiol.* **22**:23–28 (1986).

88. Terpstra, W. J., Schoone, G. J., Ligthart, G. S., and Ter Schegget, J., Detection of *Leptospira interrogans* in clinical specimens by *in situ* hybridization using biotin-labelled DNA probes, *J. Gen. Microbiol.* **133**:911–914 (1987).

89. Thiermann, A. B., Handsaker, A. L., Moseley, S. L., and Kingscote, B., New method for classification of leptospiral isolates belonging to serogroup pomona by restriction endonuclease analysis; serovar *kennewicki*, *J. Clin. Microbiol.* **21**:585–587 (1984).

90. Thiermann, A. B., Handsaker, A. L., Foley, J. W., White, F. H., and Kingscote, B. F., Reclassification of North American leptospiral isolates belonging to serogroups Mini and Sejroe by restriction endonuclease analysis, *Am. J. Vet. Res.* **47**:61–66 (1986).

91. Thompson, J. C., Morphological changes in red blood cells of calves caused by *Leptospira interrogans* serovar *pomona*, *J. Comp. Pathol.* **96**:517–527 (1986).

92. TORTEN, M., LEPTOSPIROSIS, IN: *CRC Handbook Series in Zoonoses, Section A: Bacterial Rickettsial, & Mycotic Diseases*, Volume 1 (J. H. Steele, ed.), pp. 363–421, CRC Press, Boca Raton, 1979.

93. TORTEN, M., SHENBERG, E., GERICHTER, C. B., NEUMAN, P., AND KLINGBERG, M. A., A new leptospiral vaccine for use in man. II. Clinical and serologic evaluation of a field trial with volunteers, *J. Infect. Dis.* **128:**647–651 (1973).

94. VINH, T., FAINE, S., AND ADLER, B., Adhesion of leptospires to mouse fibroblasts (L929) and its enhancement by specific antibody, *J. Med. Microbiol.* **18:**73–85 (1984).

95. VINH, T., ADLER, B., AND FAINE, S., Ultrastructure and chemical composition of lipopolysaccharide extracted from *Leptospira interrogans* serovar *copenhageni, J. Gen. Microbiol.* **132:**103–109 (1986).

96. VINH, T., FAINE, S., AND ADLER, B., Glycolipoprotein cytotoxin from *Leptospira interrogans* serovar *copenhageni, J. Gen. Microbiol.* **132:**111–123 (1986).

97. WAITKINS, S. A., AND HOOKEY, J. V., The detection of leptospires by chemiluminescent immunoassay, *J. Med. Microbiol.* **21:**353–356 (1986).

98. WAITKINS, S. A., AND HOOKEY, J. V., Time resolved fluorometric detection of leptospires, *J. Med. Microbiol.* **23:**xi (1987).

98a. WATT, G., PADRE, L. P., TUAZON, M. L., CALUBAQUIB, C., SANTIAGO, E., RANOA, C. P., AND LAUGHLIN, L. W., Placebo-controlled trial of intravenous penicillin for severe and late leptospirosis, *Lancet,* **1:**433–435 (1988).

99. World Health Organization, *Report of the WHO Consultation on the Development of National Programmes for the Prevention and Control of Leptospirosis, Sapporo, Japan, 15–16 July 1984* (WhO/CDS/VPH/86.62), WHO, Geneva, 1986.

100. YASUDA, P. H., STEIGERWALT, A. G., SULZER, K. R., KAUFMANN, A. F., ROGERS, F., AND BRENNER, D. J., DNA relatedness between serogroups and serovars in the family *Leptospiraceae* with proposals for seven new *Leptospira* species, *Int. J. Syst. Bacteriol.* **37:**407–415 (1987).

12. Suggested Reading

FAINE, S., *Guidelines for the Control of Leptospirosis*, Offset Publ. No. 67, WHO, Geneva, 1982.

FEIGIN, R. D., AND ANDERSON, D. C., Human leptospirosis, *CRC Crit. Rev. Clin. Lab. Sci.* **5:**413–467 (1975).

JOHNSON, R. C., AND FAINE, S., Order I. Spirochaetales: Family II. *Leptospiraceae* Hovind-Hougen 1979, 245. Genus I. *Leptospira* Noguchi 1917, 755, in: *Bergey's Manual of Systematic Bacteriology*, Volume 1 (N. Kreig and J. G. Holt, eds.), pp. 62–67, Williams & Wilkins, Baltimore, 1984.

MINETTE, H. P., Leptospirosis in poikilothermic vertebrates. A review, *Int. J. Zoonoses* **10:**111–121 (1983).

TORTEN, M., Leptospirosis, in: *CRC Handbook Series in Zoonoses, Section A: Bacterial Rickettsial, & Mycotic Diseases*, Volume 1 (J. H. Steele, ed.), pp. 363–421, CRC Press, Boca Raton, 1979.

CHAPTER 18

Listeria monocytogenes Infections

Donald Armstrong

1. Introduction

Listeria monocytogenes infections resulting in disease occur most often in the immunocompromised host. It is the T-helper cell–mononuclear phagocyte arm of the immune defense that is altered. Disease occurs in the very young and very old as well as in patients with neoplastic disease and in organ transplant patients. Alcoholism and diabetes mellitus are also frequent associated factors. Cases do occur in apparently normal hosts. The types of infections vary. Severe, usually lethal, disseminated, multiorgan disease is seen in neonates following intrauterine infection. In contrast, transient bacteremia resolving without therapy has been documented in a variety of patients. Meningitis and/or cerebritis is the most common disease seen. Focal infection of almost any organ has been described. Table 1 contains a categorization of *L. monocytogenes* infections.

Sporadic cases are the rule, but outbreaks have been well described due to contaminated foods such as cole slaw, cheese, and milk. Pregnant women are those who regularly develop disease and show the highest mortality during out-

Donald Armstrong · Department of Medicine, Memorial Sloan–Kettering Cancer Center, and Cornell University Medical College, New York, New York 10021.

breaks and it can be assumed that many more people are infected than develop disease. Outbreaks have also been described in newborn nurseries and renal transplant units.

The number of outbreaks recorded has been small. It is doubtful that *L. monocytogenes* causes major epidemics even in parts of the world where it might go unrecognized because of problems in isolation and identification. The predilection for severe disease in pregnant women should alert public health officials to the possibility of listeriosis.

2. Background

L. monocytogenes was first isolated from laboratory rabbits and guinea pigs and then from wild gerbils from South Africa in 1926 and 1927, respectively.[38,40] On injection into rabbits, disseminated disease associated with a monocytosis was described, hence the species designation. Early after its discovery, cases of a mononucleosis-like syndrome were described in humans, but these have not been reported in recent years.

An association with pregnancy was described in 1936, and severe disease in the fetus was recognized at the same time.[9]

High carrier rates have been noted among abattoir

Table 1. *Listeria monocytogenes* **Infections**

Host	Illness	Type of infection
Gravid woman	"Flulike" syndrome to meningitis	Bacteremia—source uncertain
Neonate	Disseminated, lethal, septic disease "Granulomatous infantiseptica"	*In utero*, widely disseminated, multiorgan disease
	Sepsis and/or meningitis	Postpartum bacteremia. May or may not progress to meningitis
Adult (often immuno-compromised)	Sepsis and/or meningitis	Bacteremia—source uncertain. May or may not progress to meningitis
	Cerebritis or brain abscess	Subacute cerebritis, usually not progressing to brain abscess
Any age	Focal infection	Resulting from bacteremia, source uncertain or direct inoculation

workers, but outbreaks have not been described in these people nor is it evident that *L. monocytogenes* occurs often as a zoonotic disease.[6,21,22,25,41,45]

The association between *L. monocytogenes* and neoplastic disease was reported by Louria and colleagues in 1967.[31] Since then, confirmatory reports have appeared and extended those at risk to renal and other organ transplant patients, alcoholics, diabetics, and others with conditions resulting in dysfunction of the T-helper lymphocyte and mononuclear phagocyte system.

Foodborne outbreaks were first described in 1961[45] and in 1962.[21] Other well-characterized food outbreaks have been reported more recently,[15,36,43] as well as a multihospital outbreak where the food source was not completely documented.[24] Clusters of cases have occurred in immunocompromised hosts and in a newborn nursery without evidence of a point source.[4,5,14,16,23,26,29,39]

3. Methodology

Since *L. monocytogenes* infections have not been reportable in most countries including the United States, accurate figures on incidence are not available.

The Council of State and Territorial Epidemiologists of the United States recommended in 1986 that listeriosis be made a reportable disease. The most comprehensive U.S. study was recently reported[13] and depended on hospitals participating in the Professional Activities Study (PAS) of the Commission on Professional and Hospital Activities (CPHA), a nonprofit, nongovernmental hospital discharge data system. The data set was made up from the data bank

of the CPHA–PAS participating hospitals using the discharge diagnosis of listeriosis during 1980, 1981, and 1982. The number of hospitals participating in PAS ranged from 1354 (1980) to 1283 (1982) with a mean of 1309 hospitals per year. These hospitals represented 22 to 23% of all short-term, nonfederal hospitals in the United States and included 27 to 29% of all U.S. discharges from such hospitals. Six states with 5% or fewer discharges included in PAS records were excluded. Since these states made up 10% of the population, the values from all the other states were increased by 10%. For each state, total hospitalizations for listeriosis were projected by dividing the number of cases from participating hospitals in a given state by the proportion of all the states' discharges that were from PAS hospitals.

In other reports from the Centers for Disease Control (CDC),[17,18] the investigators of the Listeria Study Group made biweekly contact with all 666 acute-care hospitals in Missouri, New Jersey, Oklahoma, Tennessee, Washington, and Los Angeles County, California during 1986.

3.1. Sources of Mortality Data

Sources of mortality data are case reports, descriptions of outbreaks, reviews, and recent CDC reports detailed above.[13,17,18] Mortality rates vary considerably with the type of host infected. In granulomatous infantiseptica, mortality has ranged from 33 to 100%.[6,22,35] In people with meningitis, mortality has ranged from 12.5 to 43%.[1,8,12,31,39] In foodborne outbreaks, the case-fatality rates were approximately 30%.[13] Overall mortality rates have been estimated as 19.1% with the rate increasing with increasing age.[13]

3.2. Sources of Morbidity Data

Sources of morbidity data are obtained from the few outbreaks that have been recognized and studies done in a number of countries in Europe in addition to those from the United States mentioned above.[6,10,11,22,35,41] Among 27 states participating in The National Bacterial Meningitis Surveillance Study, there were 265 cases of *Listeria* meningitis between 1978 and 1981. In some regions, *Listeria* was reported as the second most common cause of neonatal meningitis (after group B streptococcus) and the second most common cause of meningitis in individuals over 60 years old (after *Streptococcus pneumoniae*).[44]

3.3. Surveys

Carrier rates have been studied by cultures of stools and infection incidence by serological tests, which are difficult to validate (see below). The CDC has initiated a Listeria Study Group, which is actively surveying hospitals for cases.[17,18]

3.4. Laboratory Diagnosis

3.4.1. Isolation and Identification of the Organism.
Isolation and identification of the organism is not difficult as long as laboratory personnel recognize the importance of scrutinizing gram-positive, diphtheroid-like organisms for the possibility of being *L. monocytogenes*.[7,31] Since *L. monocytogenes* is motile and hemolytic unlike any other "diphtheroid," this should not be difficult as long as it is considered and tested. The tumbling motility is best seen at room temperature and the hemolysis may be minimal and enhanced on passage. Presumptive identification can be made on these properties while final identification should take only 24 more hours.

In cases of meningitis, the organism is not seen on Gram stain in up to 90% of cases.[3] The absence of organisms on Gram stain in the presence of a pleocytosis in the appropriate host should strongly raise the possibility of *L. monocytogenes*. It may take 24–36 h to grow, seldom longer. When attempting to isolate the organism from stool or from environmental sources, holding specimens at 4°C has resulted in improved yields. This has been called "cold enrichment" but has not been demonstrated as more efficacious for clinical specimens such as cerebrospinal fluid (CSF), blood, or others.[7]

3.4.2. Serological and Immunological Diagnostic Methods.
Serology has been used for epidemiological purposes, not for diagnosis.[7,46] There are four main serogroups based on agglutination of O and H antigens with at least seven subvarieties.[7,46] Serotypes 1a, 1b, and 4b account for over 92% of all isolates.[7] The epidemiological importance of the various serotypes is not clear. There are other *Listeria* species that have been identified and are not pathogenic for man. These have not posed a problem in clinical specimens since they are not found in them.

4. Biological Characteristics of the Organism

L. monocytogenes lives in the gastrointestinal and genital tract of a variety of animals ranging from shellfish to birds and most mammals including man. Its predilection for the immunocompromised host, including pregnant women and the fetus, attests to its low pathogenicity in immunologically normal individuals. Once infection is established, however, it can be persistent.

5. Descriptive Epidemiology

5.1. Prevalence and Incidence

Listeria is responsible for abortion, mastitis, septicemia, meningitis, and encephalitis in cattle and sheep. The incidence in sheep appears to be increasing in England and Wales.[30] It has been attributed to poor-quality silage.[19,30] In humans, there are a few reports of direct transmission in veterinarians, abattoir workers, and farmers,[30] but these are rare compared to the number of cases in whom there is no evident exposure. Likewise, foodborne outbreaks are rare when the total number of cases without an evident source are considered. Fecal carriage has varied in different studies but has been reported to be as high as 5%[15,30] in normal people in Scandinavia. Poultry workers have been reported to show fecal carriage rates of 29%[30] and *Listeria* has been isolated from more than 50% of chickens before cooking in homes.[26] Carriage rates as high as 77% have been reported in microbiology laboratory personnel who work with the organism.[30] Nevertheless, the attack rate of disease in those regularly exposed or those carrying the organism does not appear especially high. Other sites of isolation in humans, albeit infrequent, have been the genitourinary tract of both women and men.

The immunocompromised host continues to be the main target with or without a history of exposure to a known source. The incidence of perinatal listeriosis reported in

Great Britain in 1978 was 1 per 37,000 births and in 1984, 1 per 18,000 births.[30]

Based on passive surveillance, estimates of the annual incidence have varied from 0.5 to 1.0 case per million.[13] From the CDC discharge summary study[17] using the CPHA–PAS data base from their participating hospitals, there were 234 cases in 1980, 212 in 1981, and 214 in 1982. The female/male ratio was 1.2:1 and 48% of the cases were meningitis, the remainder being septicemias or focal infections. The investigators projected that 800 cases occur annually in the United States for an incidence rate of 3.6 per million per year. The rates reported in Europe—2.0 to 3.0 cases per million population[28,34,37]—are similar. The higher rate of 11.3 cases per million in France[20] may reflect a true difference in incidence or differences in reporting. The total number of deaths projected in the United States was 150 per year without including fetal mortality. The case-fatality ratio was 19.1%. Over age 60 the ratio was 30%. The mortality rate with (19.2%) and without (18.1%) meningitis was essentially the same.

The projected attack rates (Fig. 1) peaked in those less than 1 month of age (568 per million population per year) and in those greater than 60 years of age (about 14 per million). Attack rates for women increased during the reproductive years over those for men (Fig. 1) and in 74% of cases in women between the ages of 10 and 39, they were pregnant. Thirty-three percent or 219 cases occurred in pregnancy.

An increase in the number of cases was evident in the summer in this study,[13] but since considerable year-to-year variation was found the investigators concluded that "a distinct seasonal pattern to human listerial infections was not apparent in this study."

The Listeriosis Study Group of the CDC reported on their study in abstract form[17] and later in the Proceedings of the Epidemic Intelligence Service Conference (April 1988)[18] as follows:

In 1986, 229 culture-positive cases (0.69/100,000) were documented by biweekly contact with 666 acute-care hospitals in Missouri, New Jersey, Oklahoma, Tennessee, Washington, and Los Angeles County, California.

From these data it was estimated that less than 1650 cases occur annually in the United States and result in 450 deaths. Serotyping was done on 137 isolates with the following results: 4b = 47 (33%), 1b = 43 (31%), 1a = 41 (30%), 3b = 4 (3%), and 3a = 2 (1.5%). In 1986 the incidence of listeriosis was similar in all study regions for adults (mean = 0.5/100,000). Perinatal incidence was four times higher in Los Angeles (27.2/100,000) than in other areas (6.8/100,000 births), $p = 10^{-8}$. The perinatal rate in Los Angeles was higher for blacks (51.4/100,000 births) than for whites (20.2/100,000 births) or Hispanics (19.9/100,000 births), $p = 0.03$. The perinatal rate for whites, however, was higher for Los Angeles (20.2/100,000) than in the other regions (5.2/100,000), $p = 0.003$. The higher rates did not reflect maternal age or serotype distribution. Reasons were not found, but there was a well-publicized cheese-borne listeriosis epidemic in Los Angeles in 1985 and this may have stimulated greater efforts aimed at diagnoses.

5.2. Epidemic Behavior and Contagiousness

Epidemics have been foodborne with a few exceptions. Foods have included milk, cheese, and cole slaw. Contamination of the dairy products was the result of direct infection from the cow of the cows' milk. The cole slaw contamination was attributed to sheep manure used to fertilize cabbage. Since the cabbage was kept in silos over the winter, enhancement of growth by cold enrichment was considered as a contributory factor. The attack rate of disease, or those developing disease over those infected, was not determined in the epidemics, but it is likely that the attack rate is low since primarily pregnant women developed disease. Most cases in the foodborne outbreaks have been attributed to the food and not to subsequent person-to-person spread.[15,24,36,43] The outbreaks in nurseries and transplant units have been sluggish at best, suggesting a very low level of contagiousness.[4,14,16,23]

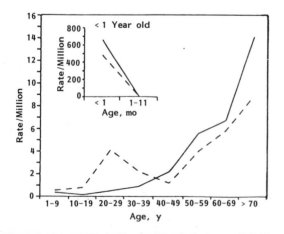

Figure 1. Age-specific incidence of listeriosis, by sex. Solid line indicates male patients; dashed line, female patients. Reprinted with permission from Ciesielski *et al.*[13]

5.3. Geographic Distribution

L. monocytogenes appears to be worldwide in distribution.

5.4. Temporal Distribution

The incidence of listeriosis is generally believed to be higher in humans in the summer. In other animals it appears more often in the winter. There is no apparent explanation for this.

5.5. Age

The very young and very old among normal individuals show a higher attack rate and mortality rate. In the immunosuppressed patient the age varies with the reason for immunosuppression (e.g., pregnancy).

5.6. Sex

There is a predilection for pregnant women.

5.7. Race

There is no apparent racial predilection with the exception of one report[18] of an increased attack rate among perinatal blacks in Los Angeles (see above).

5.8. Occupation

Although people exposed to domestic animals or abattoir workers show a higher incidence of carrier rates, disease is not apparently more common. The same is true of laboratory personnel working with *Listeria*.[30]

5.9. Occurrence in Different Settings

Small outbreaks in organ transplant units and newborn nurseries have been described.

5.10. Socioeconomic Factors

There are no known socioeconomic factors involved in listeriosis.

5.11. Other Factors

The pregnant woman is prone as noted. This association is more striking in relation to *L. monocytogenes* than to any other opportunistic pathogen. The fetus *in utero* is also more prone to severe, disseminated infection than is any other known host.

6. Mechanisms and Routes of Transmission

Since the usual modes of transmission are uncertain and most cases do not occur in clusters, it is assumed that environmental sources such as soil and water form the reservoir. As mentioned before, the organism is passed to humans from other animals and perhaps from human to human by the fecal–oral route. It invades humans from the gastrointestinal and genitourinary tract and has a predilection for the central nervous system during bacteremias.

7. Pathogenesis and Immunity

The incubation period is unknown, but generally it is thought to vary from a few days to 3 weeks though there are cases that suggest that it may be longer. People may carry the organism and only develop invasive infection when T-helper cell function declines. Whether gastrointestinal defects including liver disease can contribute to the dissemination of *Listeria* is uncertain. The organism appears to be protected from activated macrophages by living within nonactivated macrophages and persisting, perhaps protected against antibiotics, which do not penetrate those host cells. *L. monocytogenes* experimentally does not persist through converting to L forms. Persistence is certainly important with regard to therapy and may be important in transmission. In the 1960s the importance of the mononuclear phagocyte in host resistance to *L. monocytogenes* was demonstrated.[32,33] Subsequently, it was shown that antibody, complement, and T-helper lymphocytes were active.[2] It does appear that the nonactivated macrophage may be important in host defenses in listeriosis and may protect even in the absence of activated macrophages (see below).

8. Host Response

8.1. Patterns of Host Response

The response in histopathological studies of both animal models and the human disease varies from the production of a neutrophilic exudate to granulomas. This is reflected in the CSF pleocytosis, which varies from a predominantly neutrophilic to a predominantly mononuclear response. Although in most instances the gastrointestinal tract appears to be the initial site of infection, there is no recognized gastrointestinal lesion. Bacteremias may result in infection at almost any site or organ but most often seed the CNS. The types of illnesses seen in various hosts are summarized in Table 1. It is interesting and presumably important that there have been relatively few cases of listeriosis reported in patients with the acquired immunodeficiency syndrome (AIDS), and that the reported cases were relatively mild.[42] It may be that this reflects a pure defect in AIDS T-helper cell ability to produce macrophage-activating lymphokines that are not so important in resistance against listeriosis as are nonactivated macrophages, monocytes, and neutrophils.[27]

A patient with a meningitis and a CSF pleocytosis with no organisms should be suspected of *Listeria* meningitis. A patient with a clinical cerebritis and a normal CSF should be suspected of *Listeria* cerebritis. In the former, the organism can be expected to be isolated from the CSF even though not seen. In the latter, the bacteria should be isolated from the blood, but may not be isolated from the CSF.

A woman in the third trimester of pregnancy who develops chills and fever with no evident source should be suspected of listeriosis. If the fever is accompanied by signs of a threatened abortion, fetal listeriosis should be considered.

Any spontaneously aborted fetus or stillbirth should be suspected of *Listeria* infection and cultured for it.

A newborn with evidence of sepsis with or without meningitis should be suspected of *Listeria* infection. Unexplained fever with or without meningitis in an individual with a defect in T-helper cell response should suggest listeriosis.

Focal infections usually occur in people with T-helper cell defects.

8.2. Diagnosis

An epidemic of unexplained fever in pregnant women should suggest listeriosis and a common food source should be sought.

The diagnosis should be considered in the settings described above and should be confirmed by isolation and identification of the organism. A presumptive diagnosis can be made by observing gram-positive coccobacillary forms or diphtheroid-like organisms in CSF or purulent specimens.

The differential diagnosis in a patient with meningitis includes the usual causes such as *Streptococcus pneumoniae, Neisseria meningitidis,* or *Haemophilus influenzae* and especially in patients with T-helper cell defects, *Cryptococcus neoformans.* The absence of organisms on Gram stain may suggest partially treated meningitis as well as *Listeria* meningitis. The picture of clinical sepsis without meningitis or other localizing features in the patient with T-helper cell defects may be produced by *Salmonella* species, mycobacteria species, *C. neoformans, Histoplasma capsulatum, Coccidioides immitis,* or cytomegalovirus. Rarely, *Pneumocystis carinii* pneumonia may occur without pulmonary symptoms.

In the pregnant woman the illness resembles influenza and in the neonate the usual causes of neonatal sepsis and meningitis such as *Escherichia coli, Klebsiella pneumoniae,* or group B streptococci, and the enterococci.

Listeria cerebritis appears to be rather unique in that it causes symptoms and bacteremias over a longer period of time before forming a brain abscess than do other organisms. It could be confused with *Toxoplasma gondii* encephalitis in this form.

9. Control and Prevention

9.1. General Concepts

Milk and cheese should be pasteurized although even pasteurized milk has been implicated in one epidemic. Immunocompromised hosts such as those with T-helper cell defects and pregnant women should be educated as to the dangers of improperly processed dairy products and poorly washed raw vegetables such as cole slaw. They should be careful of exposure to farm animals. Since the route of exposure appears to be feces, milk, or birth products to mouth, simple hygiene measures should suffice to protect the pregnant woman.

9.2. Antibiotic and Chemotherapeutic Approaches to Prophylaxis

There is no apparent reason to quarantine individuals, nor to use prophylaxis with the possible exception of a clear-cut exposure in a pregnant woman.

The antibiotic of choice has been ampicillin, but resistant strains have appeared recently. Trimethoprim sulfamethoxazole, generically called co-trimoxazole, may replace ampicillin as the treatment of choice. There are too few cases nationwide to readily do a comparative trial unless a large multicenter study is organized.

9.3. Immunization

A vaccine has not been developed.

10. Unresolved Problems

Cases should be reportable and isolates regularly serotyped so that the epidemiology can be better understood. Obstetricians should be encouraged to culture all spontaneous abortions, stillbirths, or difficult deliveries, and microbiology laboratories should anticipate *L. monocytogenes* in these cultures.

11. References

1. ALBRITTON, W. L., WIGGINS, G. L., AND FEELY, J. C., Neonatal listeriosis: Distribution of serotypes in relation to age at onset of disease, *J. Pediatr.* **88:**481 (1976).
2. ARMSTRONG, D., *Listeria monocytogenes,* in: *Principles and Practice of Infectious Diseases,* 3rd ed. (G. L. MANDELL, R. G. DOUGLAS, AND J. E. BENNETT, eds.), pp. 1587–1592, Churchill Livingstone, New York, 1990.
3. ARMSTRONG, D. (in preparation).
4. ASCHER, N. L., SIMMONS, R. L., MARKER, S., AND NAJARIAN, V. S., Listeria infection in transplant patients, *Arch. Surg.* **113:**90 (1978).
5. BECROFT, D. M. O., FARMER, K., SEDDON, R. J., SOWDEN, R., STEWART, J. H., VINES, A., AND WATTLE, D. A., Epidemic listeriosis in the newborn, *Br. Med. J.* **3:**747 (1971).
6. BOJSEN-MOLLER, J., Human listeriosis, diagnostic, epidemiological and clinical studies, *Acta Pathol. Microbiol. Scand.* (Suppl.) **229:**1–157 (1972).
7. BORTOLUSSI, R., SCHLECH, W. F., III, AND ALBRITTON, W. L., *Listeria: Manual of Clinical Microbiology,* 4th ed., p. 205, American Society for Microbiology, Washington, D.C., 1985.
8. BUCHNER, L. H., AND SCHNEIERSON, S. S., Clinical and laboratory aspects of *Listeria monocytogenes* infection with a report of ten cases, *Am. J. Med.* **45:**904 (1968).
9. BURN, C. G., Clinical and pathological features of an infection caused by a new pathogen of the genus *Listerella, Am. J. Pathol.* **12:**341 (1936).
10. BUSCH, L. A., Human listeriosis in the United States, 1967–1969, *J. Infect. Dis.* **123:**328 (1971).
11. Centers for Disease Control, Zoonosis surveillance, *Listeriosis: Annual Summary, 1969,* Department of Health, Education and Welfare, June 1970.
12. CHERUIK, N. L., ARMSTRONG, D., AND POSNER, J. B., Central nervous system infections in patients with cancer, changing patterns, *Cancer* **40:**268 (1977).
13. CIESIELSKI, C. A., HIGHTOWER, A. W., PARSONS, S. K., AND BROOME, C. V., Listeriosis in the United States: 1980–1982, *Arch. Intern. Med.* **148:**1416–1419 (1988).
14. FILICE, G. A., CANTRELL, H. F., SMITH, A. B., HAYES, P. S., FEELEY, J. C., AND FRASER, D. W., *Listeria monocytogenes* infection in neonates: Investigation of an epidemic, *J. Infect. Dis.* **138:**17–23 (1978).
15. FLEMING, D. W., COCHI, S. L., MacDONALD, K. L., BRONDUM, J., HAYES, P. S., PLIKAYTIS, B. O., HOLMES, M. B., AUDURIER, A., BROOME, C. V., AND REINGOLD, A. L., Pasteurized milk as a vehicle of infection in an outbreak of listeriosis, *N. Engl. J. Med.* **312:**404 (1985).
16. GANTZ, N. M., MYEROWITZ, R. L., MEDEIROS, A. A., CARRERA, G. F., WILSON, R. E., AND O'BRIEN, T. F., Listeriosis in immunocompromised patients: A cluster of eight cases, *Am. J. Med.* **58:**637 (1975).
17. GELLEN, B., BROOME, C. V., WEAVER, R., HIGHTOWER, A., AND The Listeriosis Study Group, Geographic differences in listeriosis in the U.S., Abstract 109, *Proceedings of the Interscience Conference on Antimicrobial Agents and Chemotherapy,* p. 115, 1987.
18. GELLEN, B. G., HIGHTOWER, A. W., WEAVER, R. E., BROOME, C. V., AND The Listeria Study Group, Listeriosis in the United States, Abstract presented at the Epidemic Intelligence Service Conference, April 1988.
19. GITLER, M., Listeria infections in farm animals, *Vet. Rec.* **112:**314 (1983).
20. GOULET, V., LEONARD, J. L., AND CELERS, J., Etude epidemiologique de la listeriose humaine en France en 1984, *Rev. Epidemiol. Sante Publique* **34:**191–195 (1986).
21. GRAY, M. L. (ed.), *Second Symposium on Listeric Infections,* Artcraft Printers, Bozeman, Mont., 1962.
22. GRAY, M. L., AND KILLINGER, A. H., *Listeria monocytogenes* and listeria infections, *Bacteriol. Rev.* **30:**309 (1966).
23. GREEN, H. T., AND MACAULAY, M. B., Hospital outbreak of *Listeria monocytogenes* septicemia: Problems of cross infection, *Lancet* **2:**1039 (1978).
24. HO, J. L., SHANDS, K. N., FRIEDLAND, G., ECHKIND, P., AND FRASER, D. W., An outbreak of type 4b *Listeria monocytogenes* infection involving patients from eight Boston hospitals, *Arch. Intern. Med.* **146:**520 (1986).
25. HOEPRICH, P. D., Infection due to *Listeria monocytogenes, Medicine* **37:**143 (1958).
26. HURLEY, R., Listeriosis in serious infections in the newborn, *Clin. Obstet. Gynecol.* **10:**75 (1983).
27. JACOBS, J. L., AND MURRAY, H. W., Why is *Listeria monocytogenes* not a pathogen in the acquired immunodeficiency syndrome? *Arch. Intern. Med.* **146:**1299 (1986) [editorial].
28. LARSSON, S., Epidemiology of listeriosis in Sweden, 1958–1974, *Scand. J. Infect. Dis.* **11:**47–54 (1979).
29. LEVY, E., AND NASSAU, E., Experience with listeriosis in the newborn. An account of a small epidemic in a nursery ward, *Ann. Paediatr.* **194:**321 (1960).
30. Listeriosis, *Lancet* **1:**364 (1985).
31. LOURIA, D. B., HENSLE, T., ARMSTRONG, D., COLLINS, H. S., BLEVINS, A., KRUGMAN, D., AND BUSE, M., Listeriosis

complicating malignant disease, a new association, *Ann. Intern. Med.* **67:**261–281 (1967).

32. MACKANESS, G. B., Cellular resistance to infection, *J. Exp. Med.* **116:**381 (1962).

33. MACKANESS, G. B., AND HILL, W. C., The effect of antilymphocyte globulin on cell-mediated resistance to infection, *J. Exp. Med.* **129:**993 (1969).

34. MCLAUCHLIN, J., AUDURIER, A., AND TAYLOR, A. G., Aspects of the epidemiology of human *Listeria monocytogenes* infections in Britain, 1967–1984: Use of serotyping and phage typing, *J. Med. Microbiol.* **22:**367–377 (1986).

35. MOORE, R. M., AND ZEHMER, R. B., Listeriosis in the United States—1971, *J. Infect. Dis.* **127:**610 (1973).

36. *Morbid. Mortal. Weekly Rep.,* Epidemiological notes and reports: Listeriosis outbreak associated with Mexican-style cheese—California, **34**(24)**:**357 (1985).

37. MULDER, C. J. J., AND ZANEN, H. C., *Listeria monocytogenes* neonatal meningitis in the Netherlands, *Eur. J. Pediatr.* **145:**60–62 (1986).

38. MURRAY, E. G. D., WEBB, R. A., AND SWANN, M. B. R., A disease of rabbits characterized by a large mononuclear leucocytosis, caused by a hitherto undescribed bacillus, *Bacterium monocytogenes* (n.sp.), *J. Pathol. Bacteriol.* **29:**407–439 (1926).

39. NIEMAN, R. E., AND LORBER, B., Listeriosis in adults: A changing pattern. Report of eight cases and review of the literature, 1968–78, *Rev. Infect. Dis.* **2:**207 (1980).

40. PIRIE, J. H. H., A new disease of veld rodents "Tiger River Disease," *Publ. S Afr. Inst. Med. Res.* **3**(13)**:**163 (1927).

41. Proceedings of the Third International Symposium on Listeriosis, Bilthoven, The Netherlands, July 1966.

42. REAL, F. X., GOLD, J. W., KROWN, S. E., AND ARMSTRONG, D., *Listeria monocytogenes* bacteremia in the acquired immunodeficiency syndrome, *Ann. Intern. Med.* **101:**883 (1984).

43. SCHLECH, W. F., LAVIGNE, P. M., BORTOLUSSI, R. A., ALLEN, A. C., HALDANE, E. V., WORT, A. J., HIGHTOWER, A. W., JOHNSON, S. E., KING, J. H., NICHOLLS, E. S., AND BROOME, C. V., Epidemic listeriosis—Evidence for transmission by food, *N. Engl. J. Med.* **308:**203 (1983).

44. SCHLECH, W. F., III, WARD, J. I., BAND, J. D., HIGHTOWER, A., FRASER, D. W., AND BROOME, C. V., Bacterial meningitis in the United States, 1978 through 1981: The National Bacterial Meningitis Surveillance Study, *J. Am. Med. Assoc.* **253:**1749–1754 (1985).

45. SEELIGER, H. P. R., *Listeriosis,* 2nd ed., Hafner, New York, 1961.

46. SEELIGER, H. P. R., *Listeria monocytogenes,* in: *Medical Microbiology and Infectious Diseases* (A. Braude, ed.), p. 205, Saunders, Philadelphia, 1981.

12. Suggested Reading

ARMSTRONG, D., *Listeria monocytogenes,* in: *Principles and Practice of Infectious Diseases,* 2nd ed., pp. 1177–1182, Wiley, New York, 1985. Third edition in press.

Centers for Disease Control, Listeriosis in the United States—1971, *J. Infect. Dis.* **127:**610–611 (1973).

CIESIELSKI, C. A., HIGHTOWER, A. W., PARSONS, S. K., AND BROOME, C. V., Listeriosis in the United States: 1980–1982, *Arch. Intern. Med.* **148:**1416–1419 (1988).

GELLEN, B. G., AND BROOME, C. V., Listeriosis, *JAMA* **261**(9)**:**1313–1320 (1989).

GRAY, M. L., AND KILLINGER, A. H., *Listeria monocytogenes* and listeria infections, *Bacteriol. Rev.* **30:**309–382 (1966).

LINNAN, M. J., MASCOLA, L., LOU, D. X., GOULET, V., MAY, S., SALMINEN, C., HIRD, D. W., YONEKURA, L., HAYES, P., WEAVER, R., AUDURIER, D., PLIKAYTIS, B. D., FANIN, S. L., KIEKS, A., AND BROOME, C. V., Epidemic listeriosis associated with Mexican-style cheese, *N. Engl. J. Med.* **319:**823–828 (1988).

SEELIGER, H. P. R., *Listeriosis,* 2nd ed., Hafner, New York, 1961.

SEELIGER, H. P. R., Listeriosis—History, and actual developments, *Infection* **16**(Suppl. 2)**:**S80–S84 (1988).

CHAPTER 19

Lyme Disease

Michael T. Osterholm, Kristine L. MacDonald, and Craig W. Hedberg

1. Introduction

Lyme disease is a tickborne multisystem illness caused by the spirochete *Borrelia burgdorferi*. The clinical manifestations of illness are divided into three stages (Table 1). Stage I is predominantly characterized by erythema chronicum migrans (EM), a skin rash that classically begins as a single macule that expands to an annular lesion, frequently with subsequent secondary annular lesions. The occurrence of EM is often associated with minor constitutional symptoms. Stage II is characterized by neurologic involvement (particularly meningoencephalitis) or cardiovascular involvement (endocarditis, endomyocarditis, vasculitis, or fibrinous pericarditis), usually beginning several weeks after the appearance of EM. Stage III is characterized by recurrent migratory arthritis, primarily of the large joints, which occurs several weeks to 2 years after infection. Myositis, fasciitis, and peripheral neuropathies can also be associated with stage III Lyme disease. Patients may develop EM without further sequelae, or they may present with stage II or stage III disease without recalling prior EM or a tick bite. In some instances, Lyme disease can be severely debilitating without appropriate antimicrobial therapy; therefore, accurate diagnosis and treatment are critical to the clinical management and the public health control of this illness.

B. burgdorferi is known to be transmitted by at least two tick vectors in the United States, *Ixodes dammini* and *I. pacificus*. Other tick vectors in the United States have also been suggested. In addition, *B. burgdorferi* is transmitted by *I. ricinus* in Europe. Lyme disease was first described in 1975; since that time the reported incidence has steadily increased (due to either a true increase in cases or an increased physician awareness and diagnosis of the condition). Currently, Lyme disease is the most commonly reported tickborne illness in the United States, with endemic areas in the Northeast (particularly from Massachusetts to Maryland), the upper Midwest (Minnesota and Wisconsin), and the Pacific Northwest (particularly southern Oregon, parts of California, and Nevada).

2. Historical Background

Lyme disease (initially referred to as Lyme arthritis) was first recognized by Steere *et al.* in 1975, following identification of a cluster of children living in Old Lyme, Connecticut, who were diagnosed with juvenile rheumatoid arthritis.[104] Investigation of this cluster demonstrated an exceptionally high prevalence of arthritis in the affected communities. In addition, clustering within families was noted, a majority of affected children had onset of illness in summer or early fall, and a significant proportion of patients recalled the occurrence of an annular skin lesion (originating as a single papule) in the month before onset of arthritis. The skin lesions were typically suggestive of insect bites, and descriptions were compatible with EM. These epidemiologic features supported the hypothesis that this particular cluster of arthritis cases represented a vectorborne

Michael T. Osterholm, Kristine L. MacDonald, and Craig W. Hedberg · Acute Disease Epidemiology Section, Minnesota Department of Health, Minneapolis, Minnesota 55440.

Table 1.   Major Clinical Manifestations of Lyme Disease

Manifestation	Stage I	Stage II	Stage III
Dermatologic	EM[a]	Recurrent EM	Acrodermatitis
	Lymphocytoma cutis	Lymphocytoma cutis	chronica
			atrophicans
Neurologic	Early meningitis	Meningitis	Peripheral
	(Meningismus)	Encephalitis	neuropathies
	Encephalopathy	Cranial neuritis	Chronic
		Radiculoneuritis	meningitis
Cardiovascular		Endocarditis	
		Endomyocarditis	
		Pericarditis	
		Vasculitis	
Rheumatologic	Arthralgias		Arthritis–synovitis
Other	Conjunctivitis	Myositis	Myositis
	Lymphadenopathy	Fasciitis	Fasciitis
	Splenomegaly		
	Hepatitis		
	Pneumonitis		

[a]EM, erythema migrans.

infection. Steere and colleagues subsequently observed that the clinical spectrum of Lyme disease included not only arthritis and EM, but also neurologic and cardiac abnormalities.[82,103,106,108] Early descriptions of Lyme disease correctly identified EM as the clinical hallmark of this disorder.[103]

Although Lyme disease with arthritis as a major manifestation was initially described in the United States in the late 1970s, EM following a tick bite had been previously recognized. The lesion was first described by Afzelius, a Swedish dermatologist, in 1909.[1] Several years later, the lesion was designated as EM.[65] Subsequently, the occurrence of neurologic abnormalities following EM was noted by investigators in France in 1922, in Sweden in 1930, and in Germany in 1941.[4,42,54] Additional descriptions confirmed the systemic nature of the disease and suggested an infectious etiology.[14,55] In Europe, this illness became known as erythema migrans disease (EMD). In 1969, EM was first reported in the United States in a grouse hunter in northwestern Wisconsin, which is an area now recognized as endemic for Lyme disease.[94] In 1975, an additional case of EM was diagnosed in a woman vacationing in northern Minnesota; she reported an arthropod bite 2 days before the development of EM.[96]

Following recognition of Lyme disease as a distinct clinical entity, epidemiologic data indicated that *I. dammini* and *I. pacificus* were the most likely tick vectors for transmission of the etiologic agent in the United States.[101,105]

Other potential tick vectors, including *Amblyomma americanum,* have been suggested.[90] In Europe, cases of EM were recognized in the distribution of an additional tick, *I. ricinus.*

Subsequent to evidence implicating *I. dammini* as a major tick vector for a suspected infectious agent, a spirochete was isolated from *I. dammini* ticks collected in an endemic area.[18] The spirochetal etiology of Lyme disease was then confirmed clinically in two studies.[10,109] One of these studies clearly demonstrated elevated IgG and IgM antibody titers to the newly recognized spirochete.[109] In the other study, the spirochete was isolated from the blood of 2 of 36 patients with characteristic symptoms.[10] This spirochete was subsequently classified as *B. burgdorferi.*[56]

Additional clinical studies have demonstrated that Lyme disease can be effectively treated with penicillin, tetracycline, cephalosporins, and erythromycin.[32,107, 112,115] Furthermore, major late complications (including myocarditis, meningoencephalitis, and arthritis) can be prevented if patients receive appropriate antimicrobial therapy during the early clinical manifestations (when EM and associated constitutional symptoms are present).[110] However, treatment failures have been reported for patients who were promptly treated with recommended antimicrobial therapy.[34] Late manifestations, particularly arthritis, may be relatively refractory to antimicrobial therapy; high-dose intravenous penicillin or ceftriaxone may be efficacious in treating otherwise refractory arthritis and neurologic disease.[32,115]

Currently, Lyme disease occurs predominantly in Europe and the United States. While cases in the United States usually have tick exposures in known endemic areas, increasing numbers of cases are being reported from states outside of endemic areas. Such surveillance data suggest new tick vectors for *B. burgdorferi* or expansion of known vectors, such as *I. dammini,* to new geographic areas.[23]

3. Methodology

3.1. Sources of Mortality Data

Mortality data for Lyme disease are generally lacking. One death due to pancarditis was reported in a patient with concurrent *B. burgdorferi* and *Babesia microti* infections.[73] An additional case, refractory to antimicrobial therapy and associated with fatal adult respiratory distress syndrome, has also been reported.[62] The relative absence of recognized fatal cases of Lyme disease from endemic areas suggests that the case-fatality rate is extremely low.

3.2. Sources of Morbidity Data

In the United States the Centers for Disease Control (CDC) initiated informal national surveillance for Lyme disease in 1980.[89] Cases of Lyme disease reported to the CDC by individual states have been compiled since 1982.[26] Over time, such data have demonstrated the occurrence of Lyme disease in areas of low incidence and areas where Lyme disease had not previously been recognized. However, these data are of limited epidemiologic importance because of a lack of uniform case-definition criteria, changes in case-definition criteria with the introduction of *B. burgdorferi* antibody serology, and differences in reporting requirements among the states. Case ascertainment in most states is by passive surveillance, and verification of reported information may not be routine. Serologic tests for antibody to *B. burgdorferi* performed at private laboratories, state health department laboratories, and the CDC have not been standardized. One study has demonstrated that wide variation in serology can occur.[53] For this reason, previous national recommendations have indicated that use of serology alone for routine disease reporting is not indicated.[24] Due to limitations in interpreting the results of *B. burgdorferi* antibody serology, laboratory-based surveillance for Lyme disease can serve only to identify case-patients for whom clinical information can be collected and

evaluated. Internationally, serologic reference laboratories have served as sources for Lyme disease surveillance data through routine collection of clinical information on patients for whom specimens were submitted for testing. For Lyme disease surveillance to be effective, a reliable and practical clinical case definition that is not dependent on serologic test results is needed. Various investigators from public health departments and academic research centers have developed such case definitions; however, these too have not been standardized.

3.3. Surveys

Several incident surveys of Lyme disease have been conducted in endemic areas. Williams *et al.* reported the annual incidence of Lyme disease over a 2-year period for Westchester County, New York.[120] Case ascertainment involved active surveillance of ten hospitals and medical groups in addition to passive reporting from local physicians, hospitals, and the state health department laboratory. Cases were defined by clinical criteria and did not require the presence of EM. However, 75% of patients identified did have a history of this hallmark skin lesion. Two other prospective surveys have evaluated incidence in defined populations. Hanrahan *et al.* studied a community on Fire Island, New York, for one summer season and Steere *et al.* studied the summertime population of Great Island, Massachusetts, for 4 years.[48,116] In both studies, investigators excluded short-term residents, sought to include all eligible participants, administered multiple questionnaires over time, included a serosurvey for *B. burgdorferi* antibody, and a medical evaluation of incident cases. Thus, case ascertainment in these studies was more complete than for surveillance-based studies.

Investigators in the Fire Island study used a clinical case definition based on the presence of EM and results of an immunofluorescent antibody (IFA) serologic test.[48] Steere *et al.* used a clinical case-definition and results of an ELISA serologic test.[116] Steere *et al.* also demonstrated the focal nature of *B. burgdorferi* activity by the absence of serologic evidence of infection in 44 residents of a nearby town on the mainland end of a peninsula adjoining Great Island.

B. burgdorferi infection has been documented in white-tailed deer (*Odocoileus virginianus*), feral mice (*Peromyscus* species), and ticks in the same geographic areas where Lyme disease occurs in humans.[16,64,68] A serologic survey of dogs in southern Connecticut established the presence of *B. burgdorferi* infection and subsequent lameness in dogs in geographic areas corresponding to the distribution of Lyme disease cases.[69] Serologic and clinical evidence of infection in horses and cows have been reported from New England states, New Jersey, and Wisconsin.[17,21,27,72] *B. burgdorferi* has been isolated from blood samples of horses and cows with lameness and swollen joints and from blood and urine specimens from apparently healthy cows in Wisconsin.[21] Anderson reviewed 31 mammalian and 49 avian host species for *I. dammini* and 15 mammalian species that have been infected with *B. burgdorferi*.[2]

3.4. Laboratory Diagnosis

Selective culture media modified from Kelly medium are available for isolation of *B. burgdorferi*.[60] However, *B. burgdorferi* organisms are difficult to isolate, and, therefore, have been isolated infrequently from blood, skin biopsy specimens of EM, and CSF of patients with Lyme disease.[10,109,112] Visualization of spirochetes with silver stains and immunofluorescence has demonstrated the presence of spirochetes in synovial fluid from a patient with arthritis, in myocardial tissue obtained postmortem from a patient with a fatal case of Lyme disease, and in the remains of a fetus infected *in utero*.[73,87,98] While culture and visualization techniques may aid in defining the pathophysiology of Lyme disease, they are of limited value for routine diagnostic purposes, since the yields are generally low. The low yield from clinical specimens has been attributed to the small number of organisms present in affected tissues.[112] In addition to isolation of *B. burgdorferi* from humans, isolation of spirochetes from ticks and feral rodents has been proposed as a means of identifying endemic areas.[3]

B. burgdorferi antibody serology tests were developed shortly after the spirochete was identified. Craft *et al.* demonstrated an IgM response in 11 of 12 patients who developed severe disease; the response peaked 3–6 weeks following onset of symptoms and persisted in some patients.[28] An IgG response, which was delayed for several weeks in some individuals, was demonstrated for all 12 patients, and titers remained elevated after months of clinical remission.[28] Davis *et al.* reported a seroconversion or fourfold change in *B. burgdorferi* antibody titer in 25 (61%) of 41 patients with EM tested in Wisconsin during 1980–1982.[35] However, treatment with penicillin or tetracycline within 10 days after onset of symptoms resulted in only 8 (44%) of 18 patients with a seroconversion compared to 16 (84%) of 19 patients for whom no antimicrobial therapy was given. No seroconversions were observed in 17 persons whose illness was not compatible with Lyme disease.[35] Osterholm *et al.* found that only 10 (34%) of 29 patients with a history of EM,

reported in Minnesota through a statewide surveillance system for Lyme disease, had either an elevated acute or convalescent *B. burgdorferi* antibody titer.[78] In addition, in a prospective study, Shrestha *et al.* found that only 1 of 10 patients with EM and evidence of localized infection only had an elevated specific IgM response during the acute illness.[95] Eight (36%) of twenty-two patients with EM and evidence of disseminated disease had an elevated specific IgM response during acute illness.[95] Ultimately, 16 (50%) of these 32 patients had at least one elevated IgM or IgG titer either during acute illness or convalescence. Subsequent reevaluation of sera from 30 of these patients by immunoblotting revealed 16 patients (53%) with positive test results in acute-phase sera and 25 patients (83%) with positive test results in convalescent-phase sera.[45] In addition to identification of serum antibody, intrathecal production of antibody has also been demonstrated for patients with neurologic manifestations of Lyme disease.[121]

Availability of serology for antibody to *B. burgdorferi* varies from state to state. Similar antibody responses have been demonstrated with both IFA and ELISA. Although results of serology are being used in the diagnosis of Lyme disease and have been incorporated into the surveillance case definition of Lyme disease by some state health departments, a number of qualifications must be placed on the interpretation of these results. First, currently available serology has not been standardized, and significant variability of results between laboratories has been reported.[53] Second, as noted above, the sensitivity of serology during the acute stages of Lyme disease may be low. Estimates of the sensitivity of *B. burgdorferi* antibody serology vary with respect to the specific test used and the population studied.[28,45,95] Sensitivity has been lower in studies in which patients have been evaluated prospectively[95] than in studies that have evaluated patients retrospectively.[28] In addition, Dattwyler *et al.* concluded that the presence of chronic Lyme disease cannot be excluded by the absence of antibody to *B. burgdorferi*.[34] They found a specific T-cell blastogenic response to *B. burgdorferi* in seronegative patients with clinical indications of chronic Lyme disease. These data suggest that some patients may develop chronic illness as a result of *B. burgdorferi* infection and yet not have detectable antibody to *B. burgdorferi*. Third, false positive results with *B. burgdorferi* antibody serology have been obtained for patients with rheumatoid arthritis and systemic lupus erythematosus.[76] Serologic cross-reactivity has been noted for persons infected with relapsing fever borreliae and various treponeme species, also leading to false-positive test results for Lyme disease.[71] Fourth, although specificity may be improved with the use of monoclonal antibodies, the mere presence of antibody to *B. burgdorferi* in a patient with otherwise nonspecific symptoms and signs may not be diagnostic of Lyme disease. For example, Steere *et al.* found that 12% of residents of Great Island, Massachusetts, with past or present symptoms suggestive of Lyme disease had elevated IgG antibody levels to *B. burgdorferi;* however, 8% of asymptomatic individuals also had high levels.[116] Similarly, one study has shown that immunoblot analysis of sera from dogs in endemic areas failed to distinguish asymptomatic animals from clinically ill animals.[44] In summary, positive results for *B. burgdorferi* antibody serology may be absent during acute disease, preempted by appropriate antimicrobial therapy, found in asymptomatic persons without a history of earlier clinical illness, and need to be distinguished from nonspecific or cross-reacting antibody serology results. For these reasons, the CDC has concluded that *B. burgdorferi* serology should not be used for purposes of routine disease reporting.[24] Similar observations have been made by European investigators.[43]

4. Biological Characteristics of the Organism

B. burgdorferi are helically shaped gram-negative bacteria with cell diameters of 0.18 to 0.25 μm and cell lengths of 4 to 30 μm. On average, seven flagella are inserted subterminally at each end of the cell. *B. burgdorferi* lack the cytoplasmic tubules present in treponemes and the tight coiling characteristic of leptospires. Like other borreliae, they are microaerophilic and do not produce catalase.[56] A lipopolysaccharide has been isolated from the cell wall of *B. burgdorferi* and endotoxinlike activity has been demonstrated in rabbit pyrogen and *Limulus* assays.[41,47] Antigenic differences have been observed among strains of *B. burgdorferi* with respect to two major outer-surface proteins with apparent molecular weights of 31,000 (OspA) and 34,000 (OspB).[8] Wilske *et al.* defined five serotypes of *B. burgdorferi* by antigenic characterization of OspA and OspB from human isolates.[122] Western blot analysis revealed all five serotypes in isolates from CSF of patients in Europe. However, all isolates identified in skin specimens from European patients belonged to a single serotype (serotype 2).[122] Both skin and CSF isolates from patients in North America were serotype 1.[122] The genes encoding OspA and OspB are located on a plasmid.[6] The OspB surface protein has been shown to undergo antigenic change and be lost as a result of serial passage in BSK-II culture medium.[7]

The diagnosis of Lyme disease is primarily based on clinical findings. Proof of causation may be difficult to determine, but in some cases the organisms can be cultured or visualized from skin biopsy tissue, CSF, blood, or other tissue. Also, the diagnosis is supported by a fourfold rise in antibody titer between acute- and convalescent-phase sera, or by the detection of intrathecal production of antibody in CSF of patients with neurologic symptoms compatible with Lyme disease. Detection of an elevated IgM antibody titer in a single serum specimen from a patient with a clinically compatible illness suggests recent infection. However, the absence of an elevated IgM antibody titer does not rule out *B. burgdorferi* infection. Response to appropriate antimicrobial therapy may provide additional support for the diagnosis of Lyme disease.

The susceptibility *in vitro* and *in vivo* of *B. burgdorferi* to several antimicrobial agents has been studied.[13,58,59,66] Using a broth dilution technique to assess *in vitro* susceptibility, Johnson *et al.* measured minimum bactericidal concentrations (MBCs) for the antimicrobials most commonly used to treat Lyme disease.[58] Tests demonstrated the following MBCs: 0.04 μg/ml for ceftriaxone, 0.05 μg/ml for erythromycin, 0.8 μg/ml for tetracycline, and 6.4 μg/ml for penicillin G. In the same report, *in vivo* studies were performed by determining the 50% curative doses of the four antimicrobial agents in Syrian hamsters infected with *B. burgdorferi* by intraperitoneal injection.[58] After a 14-day incubation period, the hamsters were treated with daily subcutaneous injections of the antimicrobials for 5 days. Fourteen days after the last treatment, the hamsters were sacrificed and organs cultured for evidence of *B. burgdorferi* infection. By this method, the 50% curative doses obtained were 240 mg/kg for ceftriaxone, 287 mg/kg for tetracycline, > 1975 mg/kg for penicillin G, and 2353 mg/kg for erythromycin. Results of these *in vivo* and *in vitro* studies correlate with available clinical data on treatment of patients with Lyme disease.[66,110] While some cases of Lyme disease are refractory to antimicrobial therapy,[32,115] *in vitro* antimicrobial resistance has not been reported for *B. burgdorferi*. Thus, treatment failures are more likely due to sequestration of organisms in tissues not well penetrated by antimicrobials used, rather than due to specific antimicrobial resistance.

5. Descriptive Epidemiology

5.1. Prevalence and Incidence

The actual incidence of *B. burgdorferi* infection, including clinically apparent disease and asymptomatic infection, is unknown. In part, this is due to the lack of a sensitive and specific serologic test for *B. burgdorferi* infection or a method for routine isolation of the organisms from infected tissue or blood.

The CDC has described the distribution of Lyme disease in the United States for 1980 through 1986 as determined by the national surveillance system (Table 2).[26,89] Lyme disease is now the most commonly reported tick-

Table 2.   Lyme Disease in the United States by State Where Acquired, 1980–1986[a]

Region	1980	1982	1983	1984	1985	1986
New England						
New Hampshire			1			7
Maine					1	4
Massachusetts	11	15	13	33	69	163
Rhode Island	3	29	20	20	41	57
Connecticut	52	135	78	483	699	6[b]
Mid-Atlantic						
New York	7	170	267	446	5[b]	482
New Jersey	10	57	70	155	175	219
Pennsylvania	1	2		5	29	31
South Atlantic						
Delaware		1	4	1		
Virginia				1	2	7
Maryland	1	1	5	12	21	14
North Carolina			1	16	14	6
South Carolina				1	3	3
Georgia	1			1	1	2
Florida				1	1	1
North Central						
Wisconsin	25	58	69	176	135	162
Minnesota	8	22	55	86	64	94
Michigan			1		1	
Indiana				1		1
Ohio				1	1	1
Illinois					2	
Missouri					2	
Iowa					1	1
South Central						
Arkansas			1	4		1
Alabama						1
Tennessee			1	1	4	1
Texas			1	18	172	8
Oklahoma						2
Mountain Pacific						
Utah		1	1			1
Nevada	1					
Oregon			1	10	5	10
California			11	24	70	107
Unknown	106			4	2	2
Total	226	491	600	1500	1520	1394

[a]Case definition varies by state. Data are provisional. From Ref. 26.
[b]Data not available.

borne illness in the United States. The numbers of cases reported to the CDC for 1984, 1985 and 1986 (1500, 1520, and 1394 cases, respectively) were two to five times higher than the numbers of cases reported for 1980, 1982, and 1983 (226, 491, and 600 cases, respectively).[26] It remains unclear if the increased number of reported cases represents improved clinical recognition of the disease and better surveillance or an actual increased incidence of disease. Therefore, the CDC has indicated that national surveillance data should be used to monitor trends, not to represent the true incidence of Lyme disease in the United States.[26]

In addition to national surveillance, several states and counties have reported surveillance data.[24,35,78] In Minnesota, surveillance for Lyme disease by the Minnesota Department of Health was considered as an epidemiologically defined "passive system" during the period 1980 through 1982.[78] A case was defined as illness with the presence of EM in a patient and a physician's diagnosis of Lyme disease, or a systemic illness characteristic of Lyme disease but without EM in a patient with a positive serology for *B. burgdorferi* antibody. In 1983, the Minnesota Department of Health first publicized the availability of serologic testing for patients with possible Lyme disease to the medical community. During the first 3 years of passive surveillance, a total of 37 cases of Lyme disease were reported (0.3 case per 100,000 residents); however, during 1983 alone, 48 cases were reported (1.5 cases per 100,000 residents). The authors attributed this fivefold increase in the number of cases to increased awareness of Lyme disease by clinicians and not due to an increasing incidence of disease. These results illustrate the difficulty in using surveillance data to comment on the incidence of Lyme disease.

Officials in Connecticut conducted a laboratory-based program of surveillance for Lyme disease from July 1, 1984 to March 1, 1986.[24] Serologic testing was offered without cost to Connecticut physicians for diagnosing Lyme disease. Physicians were requested to include a completed case reported form with serum specimens submitted for testing. Patients were considered to have Lyme disease if they had onset of EM and/or neurologic, cardiac, or arthritic manifestations characteristic of Lyme disease and a positive *B. burgdorferi* serology. From this study, the incidence of Lyme disease for all Connecticut residents in 1985 was estimated to be 22 per 100,000 person-years. Town-specific incidence rates ranged from 0 to 1156 per 100,000 person-years. Eighty-three percent of the patients studied had EM, 24% had arthritis, 8% had neurologic manifestations, and 2% had cardiac involvement. The authors of this study compared their results with those from a similar study by Steere *et al.* conducted in 1977 in the same communities.[105]

They suggested that a 163% increase in the incidence of Lyme disease had occurred from 1977 to 1986 for eight towns studied. In addition, they suggested that the disease had spread inland from the coastal areas. Again, it is unclear if this detected increase reflects an actual increase in the incidence of Lyme disease, or may have resulted from the increased availability of *B. burgdorferi* serology or an increase in the diagnosis of disease as a result of increased physician awareness.

Williams *et al.* reported the annual incidence of Lyme disease in 1982 and 1983 for Westchester County, New York.[120] A case was defined as any person reported by a physician to have symptoms compatible with Lyme disease during that time and to have had at least one of the following disease manifestations: EM, aseptic meningitis, facial nerve palsy, large joint arthritis, or other neurologic manifestations or cardiac findings consistent with the clinical spectrum of Lyme disease. Two-thirds of all the cases resided in ten communities in northern Westchester County, with more than one-fourth of cases from three contiguous census tracts. The highest annual incidence rate for a single census tract was 190 per 100,000 residents, compared with 12 per 100,000 residents for Westchester County as a whole. Although the authors suggested that a "relatively sudden appearance of Lyme disease in Westchester County had occurred," no data were available for comparison of Lyme disease incidence for the same population during previous years.

Two prospective surveys have evaluated the incidence of Lyme disease in defined populations. Hanrahan *et al.* studied a community in Fire Island, New York, for one summer season and Steere *et al.* studied the summertime population of Great Island, Massachusetts, for 4 years.[48,116] Investigators in the Fire Island study used a clinical case definition based on the presence of EM and a positive serologic test for *B. burgdorferi* antibody. They demonstrated an annual incidence rate of 1% and a cumulative frequency of Lyme disease in the community of 7.5%. Steere *et al.* used a clinical case definition that included a history of EM; or a "flulike illness" during the summer followed within 1 year by arthritis; or a series of brief recurrent attacks of oligoarticular arthritis not due to other known causes.[116] The annual detected incidence rate varied from 1.5 to 3.3% during the 4-year study, with a cumulative frequency of 16%. A 1:1 ratio of asymptomatic infection to clinical illness was estimated.

5.2. Epidemic Behavior and Contagiousness

The incidence of Lyme disease in a particular geographic area depends on the population density of the tick vector and the prevalence of *B. burgdorferi* infection in the ticks. In the United States, studies have demonstrated varying rates of *B. burgdorferi* infection in ticks from about 60% in the *I. dammini* population on Shelter Island, New York, to approximately 1.2% in the *I. pacificus* population in the Western states.[19] An additional study identified *I. dammini* ticks near the homes of patients with Lyme disease in Westchester County, New York.[39] In that study, 32 ticks from one lawn were examined; 33% of nymphs and 55% of adult ticks contained spirochetes.

The frequency with which transmission of *B. burgdorferi* occurs following a single bite from an infected tick is unknown.

5.3. Geographic Distribution

In the United States, the number of states where Lyme disease has been acquired has increased annually, from 18 in 1983, to 28 in 1986.[26] As of 1986, Lyme disease had apparently been acquired in 32 (64%) of the 50 states (Table 2). However, the primary endemic area for Lyme disease continues to be the three originally described regions in the United States—coastal areas of the Northeast; the Upper Midwest, including Minnesota and Wisconsin; and the Northwest, including regions in California, southern Oregon, and western Nevada. Specifically, 86% of the 5731 cases reported to the CDC from 1980 through 1986 were acquired in seven states: New York, New Jersey, Massachusetts, Rhode Island, Connecticut, Wisconsin, and Minnesota.

Cases of Lyme disease have been documented from at least 21 countries on four continents.[25,36,88,100] In Europe, the geographic distribution of cases is associated with the known range of *I. ricinus,* the vector of *B. burgdorferi* in Europe (Fig. 1). Clinical observations have suggested that there may be dissimilarities between illnesses occurring in

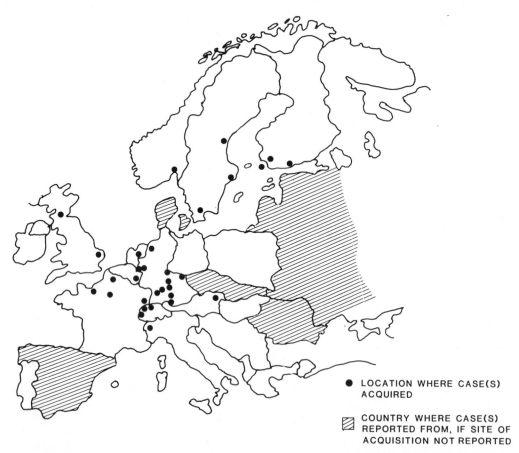

● LOCATION WHERE CASE(S) ACQUIRED

▨ COUNTRY WHERE CASE(S) REPORTED FROM, IF SITE OF ACQUISITION NOT REPORTED

Figure 1. Distribution of cases of erythema migrans in Europe. Reprinted with permission from Ref. 88.

the United States and those occurring in Europe.[88] Lyme disease in European patients may be milder and less likely to have arthritic complications or a relapsing course. However, peripheral nerve involvement appears to be more common in European patients than in patients reported from the United States. Also, multiple secondary EM skin lesions appear to occur more commonly in patients in the United States. Various explanations for the differences in clinical illnesses have been suggested. One explanation is the possibility of strain differences in *B. burgdorferi;* however, data to support this hypothesis are lacking. It is also possible that differences in Lyme disease surveillance methods and case reporting may be responsible for such dissimilarities in epidemiologic observations.

Finally, Lyme disease has been described in areas where none of the currently recognized tick vectors are known to exist including Australia, Japan, and China.[61,88] These reports, and the recent evidence that *A. americanum* and possibly *Ixodes persulcatus* can be infected with *B. burgdorferi,* suggest that cases of Lyme disease in the future may be diagnosed in additional geographic areas throughout the world.[25,88,90]

5.4. Temporal Distribution

Cases of Lyme disease in the United States have been reported with onsets during all 12 months of the year. However, disease incidence is highest in the summer and early fall months as would be expected with a tickborne infection[89] (Fig. 2). Eighty-five percent of patients reported in 1982 through national surveillance in the United States had onset of illness in May, June, July, or August, a period corresponding with peak human outdoor activity and the presence of nymphal ticks seeking blood meals.[89] A similar pattern for disease onset has been documented for cases of EM in Europe.

5.5. Age

Cases of Lyme disease have occurred in individuals of all ages. However, several studies have demonstrated a higher incidence among children. In Connecticut, the age-specific incidence by 5-year groups for patients reported in 1985 ranged from 11 per 100,000 persons for those individuals aged 20 to 24 years, to 39 per 100,000 persons for

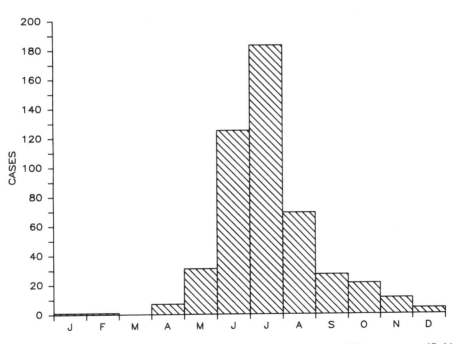

Figure 2. Cases of definite Lyme disease in the United States by month of onset of illness, 1982 (onset not specified in seven cases). Reprinted with permission from Ref. 89.

those aged 5 to 9 years.[24] In Westchester County, New York, two-thirds of all cases of Lyme disease in 1982–1983 occurred in individuals under 40 years of age, with children under 19 comprising almost 43% of the total.[48] In that study, the median age of patients was 27 years. Benach and Coleman documented that 63% of 679 patients reported with Lyme disease to the New York Health Department in 1983 were 19 years of age or younger.[9] A third study by Steere *et al.* demonstrated a different age distribution for patients in Great Island, Massachusetts.[116] The age-specific attack rates in that population suggested that the risk of Lyme disease increased with age; however, cases of arthritis alone occurred predominantly in children.

5.6. Sex

To date, all studies have documented a slight predominance of male patients.[78,89,116,120] This may reflect greater exposure for males due to increased likelihood of engaging in activities out of doors in areas where tick vectors are found.

5.7. Race

The race-specific attack rates for Lyme disease appear to approximate the racial breakdown of the general population in geographic areas with tick vectors. However, further studies are needed to confirm this observation.

5.8. Occupation

Data have been reported by Neubert *et al.* in Bavaria and Smith *et al.* in New York suggesting that outdoor workers in areas with known tick reservoirs of *B. burgdorferi* may have an occupational risk of acquiring Lyme disease.[77,97] In both studies, employees were surveyed regarding exposure and illness histories, blood specimens were collected for serologic determination of antibody to *B. burgdorferi,* and comparisons were made between groups of employees defined as seropositive and seronegative. In addition, Smith *et al.* compared rates of seropositivity in the study group to a group of anonymous blood donors from the same area and to a group of sexually transmitted disease clinic patients who were from a nonendemic area of New York State and whose sera were nonreactive when tested by a reagin test.[97] Neubert *et al.* did not use an external control group; however, 3 years after the original survey they reexamined 53 of 71 workers who were initially seropositive.[77]

Neubert *et al.* found that 71 (34%) of 211 forest workers had reciprocal titers if IgM antibody to *B. burgdorferi* ≥ 10 by IFA.[77] Smith *et al.* found that 27 (7%) of 414 workers had an optical density ≥ 0.2 by ELISA and antibody against polypeptides of *B. burgdorferi* by Western immunoblot assay.[97] Apparent differences in rates of seropositivity between the studies may be due to the different serologic criteria used to define a positive sample. Despite these and other methodologic differences, both studies revealed trends toward associations between the presence of antibody to *B. burgdorferi* and increasing age, history of tick bites, rash compatible with EM, and various heart, joint, and nervous system disorders.[77,97] However, only age, history of tick bites, and history of EM were significantly associated ($p < 0.05$) with being seropositive. Age was believed to be a surrogate for duration of exposure.[77]

In their reexamination of 53 seropositive forest workers, Neubert *et al.* found that 14 (26%) had findings compatible with Lyme disease or a history suggestive of earlier Lyme disease. In addition, 33 (62%) had a fourfold or greater decrease in IgG antibody titer between the initial and subsequent examinations.[77]

Smith *et al.* found only 4 (1%) of 362 blood donors and none of 100 clinic patients were seropositive for antibody to *B. burgdorferi.* Thus, the group of workers with occupational exposure were 5.9 times as likely to be seropositive than were blood donors from the same area.[97] Taken together, these studies suggest that individuals who work outdoors in areas with a high density of the tick vector and a high prevalence of *B. burgdorferi* infection in ticks may be at greater risk for developing Lyme disease than those who do not routinely participate in similar activities.

6. Mechanisms and Routes of Transmission

B. burgdorferi is transmitted to humans by the bite from one of several related species of tick belonging to the genus *Ixodes.* The principal vectors are *I. dammini* in the northeastern and north central United States, *I. pacificus* in the western United States, and *I. ricinus* in northern and western Europe.[101] *A. americanum* has been identified as a potential tick vector in the United States.[90] However, Piesman and Sinsky have shown that larval *A. americanum* are inefficient at acquiring *B. burgdorferi* when allowed to feed on spirochete-infected hamsters. In addition, none of the *A. americanum* examined after molting to nymphs contained spirochetes. Similar laboratory-based studies have shown that *I. scapularis* is an efficient vector of *B. burgdor-*

feri. However, *I. scapularis* collected in the field have not been shown to be infected with spirochetes.[81] *I. persulcatus* has been associated with the first cases of Lyme disease reported from China and Japan.[25,61]

Steere *et al.* first implicated a tick vector for Lyme disease from epidemiologic investigations conducted before the causative organism was identified.[101,105] Ticks had previously been associated with EM in Europe, and the isolation of identical spirochetes from ticks and patients confirmed the etiology and mode of transmission. The nymphal form of the tick is primarily responsible for transmission during the summer months (Fig. 3).[123] Adult females have been implicated in transmission during the early spring and late fall.[91]

Ribeiro *et al.* demonstrated that *B. burgdorferi* organisms are generally restricted to the guts of unfed *I. dammini* nymphs and adults.[85] In their study, infected nymphs produced saliva containing the organisms within 3 days after attachment. For adult female ticks, spirochetes disseminated from the gut to the hemocoel at 4 days after attachment for approximately 50% of the ticks.[85] At that time, approximately one-half of those adult female ticks produced saliva containing spirochetes. Thus, a minimum feeding period for infected ticks (which may be longer for adults than for nymphs) appears to be required before transmission of *B. burgdorferi* to the human host will occur. The smaller size and shorter feeding period of nymphal ticks compared to adults make them more effective vectors of *B. burgdorferi.* This is demonstrated by the seasonal abundance of Lyme disease cases corresponding to periods of nymphal tick activity.[89]

The major reservoir for sustaining *B. burgdorferi* in nature is small rodents, such as the white-footed mouse (*Peromyscus leucopus*).[64] *B. burgdorferi* have also been isolated from raccoons, dogs, and deer.[2] While spirochetemia has been demonstrated in white-tailed deer, larval ticks that feed on deer do not appear to become infected by *B. burgdorferi.*[16,117] Transmission of *B. burgdorferi* from the rodent reservoir to larval ticks occurs when the ticks feed on rodents that harbor the organisms. Transstadial transmission occurs among *I. dammini* and related ticks. The ticks, which acquire infection through a blood meal as larvae, remain infected through their development into nymphal and adult stages. Transstadial transmission is

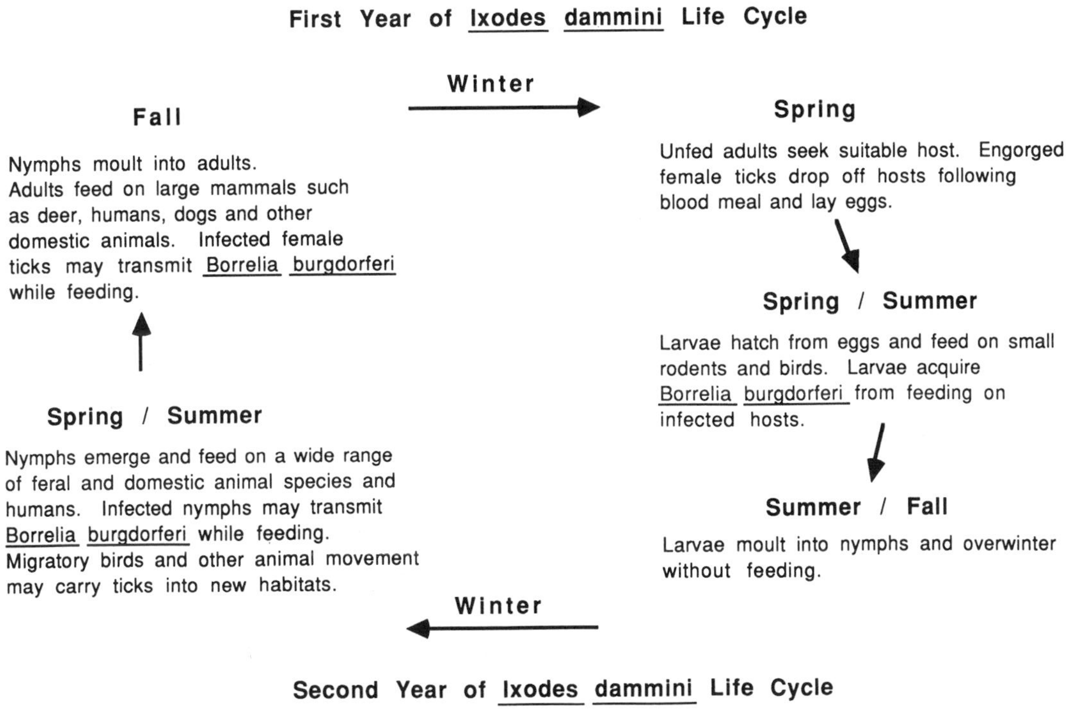

First Year of <u>Ixodes dammini</u> Life Cycle

Winter →

Fall

Nymphs moult into adults.
Adults feed on large mammals such as deer, humans, dogs and other domestic animals. Infected female ticks may transmit <u>Borrelia burgdorferi</u> while feeding.

↑

Spring / Summer

Nymphs emerge and feed on a wide range of feral and domestic animal species and humans. Infected nymphs may transmit <u>Borrelia burgdorferi</u> while feeding. Migratory birds and other animal movement may carry ticks into new habitats.

Spring

Unfed adults seek suitable host. Engorged female ticks drop off hosts following blood meal and lay eggs.

↓

Spring / Summer

Larvae hatch from eggs and feed on small rodents and birds. Larvae acquire <u>Borrelia burgdorferi</u> from feeding on infected hosts.

↓

Summer / Fall

Larvae moult into nymphs and overwinter without feeding.

← **Winter**

Second Year of <u>Ixodes dammini</u> Life Cycle

Figure 3. Representation of the two-year life cycle of *Ixodes dammini* in northern North America.

important to the vectorial capacity of ticks, which may feed on only one host between molts. Ticks such as *Dermacentor variabilis* and *A. americanum,* which appear able to acquire *B. burgdorferi* but are not able to maintain infection through a molt, do not appear to be competent vectors.[81] Nymphs may subsequently infect other rodents, small and large domestic mammals, and humans. Transovarial transmission from one tick generation to the next has been shown to occur in both naturally and experimentally infected *I. dammini.* However, relatively few progeny remain infected, perhaps because eggs infected with *B. burgdorferi* fail to mature or incorporated spirochetes gradually die off during oogenesis.[20] Thus, transovarial transmission does not appear to provide an important mechanism for sustaining *B. burgdorferi* in nature.

Spirochetes have been found in deerflies, horseflies, and mosquitoes.[70] Individual cases have been reported in which EM has developed at the site of mosquito and deerfly bites.[49,70] However, the importance of these isolated reports is difficult to assess when compared to the strong epidemiologic association between the geographic distribution of cases of Lyme disease and vector species of the genus *Ixodes.*[101] Magnarelli and Anderson were not able to transmit *B. burgdorferi* from 11 naturally infected females of two mosquito species to hamsters upon which the mosquitoes were allowed to feed.[67] Thus, the vector potential of these insects for transmission of *B. burgdorferi* remains unproven.

Contact transmission has been demonstrated in the laboratory between mice, and spirocheturic mice have been collected from the wild.[15,22] Contact transmission between animals may help to maintain the organisms in the small rodent reservoir.[22] Currently, there is not evidence to support person-to-person transmission. Transmission of *B. burgdorferi* through transfusion of blood obtained from an infected donor has not been reported; however, bloodborne transmission is theoretically possible. *B. burgdorferi* inoculated into blood samples collected on citrate phosphate dextrose preservative and held at 4°C remained viable in each of nine samples held for 25 days and for 60 days in a tenth sample.[5]

7. Pathogenesis and Immunity

B. burgdorferi spirochetes enter the susceptible host through the skin following a tick bite. The earliest manifestation of Lyme disease, EM, occurs 3 to 30 days following the tick bite. Biopsy specimens of EM lesions reveal a cellular infiltrate around blood vessels and skin appendages

involving all layers of the dermis. The infiltrate consists predominantly of lymphocytes and histiocytes; plasma cells and mast cells may also be present.[103,113] Although generally not identified in examination of biopsy material, *B. burgdorferi* has been cultured from EM lesions, suggesting that the organisms migrate outward in the skin following inoculation at the site of the tick bite.[112]

In addition to migrating locally from the site of inoculation, the spirochetes also disseminate hematogenously, resulting in spread to other organs. Spirochetes have been cultured from the blood of several patients with EM.[10,112] During this phase, diffuse visceral involvement can occur and result in a clinical illness resembling acute mononucleosis. Patients may experience pharyngitis, conjunctivitis, hepatitis, splenomegaly, lymphadenopathy, pneumonitis, myalgias, and fever.[38] Lymphoid hyperplasia of spleen and lymph nodes can occur at this time.

B. burgdorferi can be cultured from the CSF.[112] Thus, it is likely that neurologic manifestations result from direct invasion of the CNS. Many patients with EM have concurrent symptoms of headache or stiff neck; such patients most likely have transient infection of the CNS with *B. burgdorferi.* Most patients apparently clear these infections without subsequently developing symptoms of classic Lyme meningitis; however, approximately 7% of patients with EM go on to develop neurologic involvement.[82] Symptoms of meningitis typically begin a median of 4 weeks after onset of EM.[79] Evaluation of CSF from patients with meningitis generally reveals a lymphocytic pleocytosis with an increased CSF protein.[98] In addition, intrathecal production of antibodies to *B. burgdorferi* has been demonstrated in patients with neurologic involvement through examination of their CSF.[121] Although meningitis likely results from direct CNS infection with *B. burgdorferi,* the pathogenesis of cranial and peripheral neuropathy of Lyme disease is less clear. It is possible that neuropathy results from direct infection with *B. burgdorferi* spirochetes; however, it is also possible that neuropathy is related to inflammation from the contiguous meninges or vasculitis from indirect immune mechanisms.[79]

Cardiac involvement also generally occurs within several weeks after recognition of EM. Evaluations of patients with Lyme carditis generally support diffuse involvement of the conduction system with evidence of mild left ventricular dysfunction and occasional cardiomegaly.[84] Patients with cardiac involvement generally have incomplete (first or second degree) or complete atrioventricular block. Lyme carditis tends to be self-limited, and of relatively short duration (generally less than 6 weeks). The pathogenesis of Lyme carditis is not clearly understood. Some patients with cardiac involvement have evidence of circulating immune complexes, including cryoglobulins and abnormal Clq, suggesting that the immunologic response may be important in the pathogenesis of Lyme carditis.[50,106] Alternatively, Lyme carditis may result from active infection of the myocardium with *B. burgdorferi* spirochetes. This hypothesis is supported by two case reports of Lyme carditis.[73,84] The first case report included an endomyocardial biopsy, which demonstrated a perivascular lymphocytic infiltrate with possible spirochetal organisms present in the myocardium.[84] In an additional case report of fatal myocarditis in a patient with coexistent Lyme disease and babesiosis, pathology findings demonstrated pancarditis with a diffuse bandlike infiltrate of lymphocytes and plasma cells, and the presence of spirochetes within the myocardium.[73]

Arthritis generally occurs later in the course of illness than neurologic or cardiac involvement, and may occur up to several years following an episode of EM. Patients with arthritis also generally have evidence of circulating immune complexes (such as serum cryoprecipitates) early in the course of illness.[51,102] While circulating immune complexes may not be detected at the time of symptomatic arthritis, a study of synovial fluid has demonstrated Clq binding activity, suggesting local production of immune complexes within the joint space.[51] These immune complexes may be formed in response to spirochetal antigens present locally and are likely involved in mechanisms of inflammation that contribute to tissue injury.[50,51] *B. burgdorferi* have been identified in the synovium of patients with Lyme arthritis.[112] Thus, the persistence of infection within the joint space, leading to a localized immune response, may account for the arthritis associated with *B. burgdorferi* infection. The arthritis generally represents a chronic synovitis similar to that seen in patients with rheumatoid arthritis. However, unlike rheumatoid arthritis, patients with Lyme arthritis generally lack evidence of autoantibodies. The proliferative synovitis consists of lymphocytes, plasma cells, macrophages, and mast cells. Investigators have demonstrated that *B. burgdorferi* induces interleukin-1 (IL-1) production by human mononuclear phagocytes *in vitro*.[46] Local production of IL-1 in the joint space may play a role in the pathogenesis of Lyme arthritis. Appropriate antimicrobial therapy, presumably resulting in eradication of persistent foci of infection in the joint spaces and removal of antigenic stimuli, can lead to resolution of symptoms and joint inflammation.[115]

A specific T-cell response to *B. burgdorferi* occurs early in the course of infection, often before a humoral response is detected.[31] Patients also produce IgM antibody to *B. burgdorferi*. Elevated IgM antibody titers are generally not detectable during the first or second week of illness, and peak 3 to 6 weeks after onset of EM.[29] Elevated IgM titers may persist for months or years after disease onset in patients with persistent illness. A second IgM response can occur late in the course of illness. These findings suggest persistent antigenic stimulation secondary to unresolved infection with *B. burgdorferi*.[30] The IgG response generally develops after the occurrence of EM. Evaluation of IgG subclasses has demonstrated that IgG1 and IgG3 are the predominant subclasses that react with *B. burgdorferi*.[52] For patients who develop joint involvement, IgG levels may peak when arthritis is present and may remain elevated for years.[29,30] In addition, a vigorous T-cell proliferative response to whole *B. burgdorferi* has been observed in patients with clinical indications of chronic Lyme disease whose levels of serum antibody to *B. burgdorferi* are no greater than antibody levels from normal controls.[34] The presence of ongoing symptoms, possibly related to persistent antigenic stimulation, in patients with high antibody titers or ongoing T-cell response suggests that patients may remain chronically infected with *B. burgdorferi* following an acute infection.

No studies have been conducted to determine whether past infection or the presence of persistent IgG antibody confers protective immunity in humans. Recurrent infections do not appear to occur commonly; however, recurrent infection may develop in patients who lose their IgG antibody.[80] Also, antimicrobial therapy early in the course of infection may limit the number of organisms producing antigenic stimulation, thereby preventing the development of antibody.[33]

8. Patterns of Host Response

8.1. Clinical Features

The clinical features of Lyme disease can be divided into three stages (Table 1). The first stage involves predominantly dermatologic manifestations, the second stage involves neurologic and/or cardiac manifestations, and the final stage involves arthritis.

8.1.1. Dermatologic Manifestations. Lyme disease typically begins with a characteristic skin lesion, EM. The presence of EM is pathognomonic for stage I Lyme disease. Stage I also includes initial hematologic dissemination of the spirochete.[38] Therefore, stage I may also be associated with constitutional symptoms including fever, chills, malaise, fatigue, headache, and lymphadenopathy. Patients may also develop interstitial pneumonitis, splenomegaly, hepatitis, orchitis, hematuria, and early meningitis.[38] EM begins as a red macule or papule that expands to form an annular lesion, usually with an indurated outer border accompanied by partial central clearing.[113] At times, central clearing does not occur; instead, the initial lesion can become intensely erythematous and indurated or the center can become vesicular and necrotic.[113] Thirty percent of patients recall a tick bite in the previous month at the site of the lesion. The initial lesion occurs most commonly in the thigh, groin, or axilla. Secondary multiple annular lesions generally develop within several days after the onset of EM. In one study, EM persisted for a median of 28 days in 55 patients not treated with antimicrobial agents.[113] With antimicrobial therapy, skin lesions typically resolve within several days. Occasionally, patients who are not treated with antimicrobial agents can have a recurrence of EM lesions months after initial onset. In addition, other dermatologic or mucous membrane abnormalities may be noted including urticaria, conjunctivitis, or a malar rash.

A second dermatologic manifestation of *B. burgdorferi* infection is a spirochetal lymphocytoma and appears as a solitary skin lesion at the site of a tick bite.[118] The lymphocytoma may present as a small nodule or as a plaque several centimeters in diameter; histopathologic examination demonstrates follicles consisting of small lymphocytes and central larger cells are noted. Both B and T lymphocytes are present; macrophages, plasma cells, and eosinophils may also be noted. If untreated, such lesions may last months to years.

A third dermatologic manifestation of *B. burgdorferi* infection is acrodermatitis chronica atrophicans (ACA).[118] ACA has been noted in European patients, but has not been identified in patients diagnosed in the United States. It is a chronic skin disorder that begins with violaceous discoloration of the skin, associated with infiltration and swelling. In later phases, the skin becomes thin and atrophic. ACA is not specific for Lyme disease and may also be seen with other conditions, including hematologic malignancies.

8.1.2. Neurologic Manifestations. Neurologic symptoms are a major hallmark of stage II Lyme disease. However, neurologic involvement can also occur with stage I and stage III Lyme disease. In stage I Lyme disease, patients can experience symptoms suggestive of meningitis (with meningismus) or encephalopathy (with irritability, impairment of memory or concentration) and dizziness. Lumbar punctures performed on such patients are frequently normal.[108]

With stage II Lyme disease, the major neurologic manifestations of *B. burgdorferi* infection include meningitis, encephalitis, cranial neuritis, and radiculoneuritis.[79, 83,86,111] Less commonly, patients may develop dementia or transverse myelitis.[11,12,119] Patients with meningitis frequently complain of headache, photophobia, meningismus, and fever. Evaluation of the CSF generally reveals a lymphocytic pleocytosis associated with increased protein. Patients with meningitis often also have symptoms of encephalitis, including confusion, irritability, poor memory, disorientation, and emotional lability. Cranial neuropathy frequently occurs in the presence of meningitis and may be unilateral or bilateral. Facial nerve palsy is the most common manifestation of cranial neuritis; however, multiple other cranial nerves may be involved and optic neuritis with atrophy can occur.[83,86] Radiculoneuritis is often associated with radicular pain; muscle weakness and sensory loss may also be present. Neurologic complications can frequently be treated successfully with intravenous antimicrobial therapy.[32,111]

In stage III Lyme disease, peripheral sensorimotor neuropathies can occur and are characterized by lymphocytic infiltration of the perineurium.[38] Chronic involvement can result in demyelination and nerve fiber loss.[38] In addition, the meningoencephalitis associated with stage II disease can persist as a chronic syndrome and overlap with arthritis and other symptoms characteristic of stage II disease.

8.1.3. Cardiac Involvement. Cardiac involvement can occur as part of stage II Lyme disease, with onset several weeks after presentation of ECM. The most common abnormality noted is atrioventricular block, including complete heart block. In addition, lymphocytic myocarditis with left ventricular dysfunction has been noted.[84,106] Electrocardiographic findings, including T-wave flattening or inversions, indicative of myocardial involvement are common. The cardiac involvement tends to be of short duration and usually lasts less than 6 weeks. Temporary pacemakers are often indicated for treatment.

8.1.4. Arthritis. Arthritis associated with *B. burgdorferi* infection generally occurs within several months to 2 years after onset of EM.[103] Without initial treatment, investigators have estimated that approximately 60% of patients with EM will go on to develop joint manifestations.[103] Joint involvement generally includes intermittent attacks of joint swelling and pain. Arthritis primarily occurs in large joints, particularly the knees. Occasionally, Lyme disease can mimic rheumatoid arthritis with symmetrical polyarthritis involving smaller joints. Antimicrobial agents have been shown to effectively resolve arthritis in some patients.[115] Involvement of large joints can lead to bone and cartilage erosion in approximately 10% of patients who are not successfully treated.[115]

8.1.5. Other Clinical Manifestations. Several cases involving other clinical conditions have been reported. These include septal panniculitis, panophthalmitis, and possible adverse outcomes of pregnancy with suspected maternal–fetal transmission.[63,74,87,110,114]

8.2. Diagnosis

The diagnosis of stage I Lyme disease (EM with or without constitutional symptoms) is generally made upon clinical recognition of the characteristic skin lesion. Similarly, the diagnosis of stage II or stage III Lyme disease can often be made based on the presence of compatible cardiac, neurologic, or joint signs and symptoms with a history of EM in the past. In the absence of a history of EM, diagnosis of stage II and stage III Lyme disease is more difficult. *B. burgdorferi* antibody serology may be used to support the clinical diagnosis of Lyme disease. However, the positive predictive value of Lyme disease serology may be low, particularly in endemic areas. In addition, the sensitivity of the test is variable, particularly if the patient has received antimicrobial therapy early in the clinical course. *B. burgdorferi* spirochetes have been isolated from some clinical specimens; however, isolation of the spirochete is not routinely performed and serology is the only readily available diagnostic test.

9. Control and Prevention

9.1. General Concepts

Prevention of Lyme disease is currently a matter of personal protection. Commonly recommended measures include: avoiding tick-infested areas during the spring, summer, and fall; taking steps to prevent tick attachment such as using repellents and wearing protective clothing; and performing daily body checks for the presence of ticks. The small size of nymphal ticks, their abundance at times when the larger adults may not be active, and their predilection for attachment sites such as the back of the knee, the groin, the axilla, and behind the ear, indicate the need for constant summertime awareness. Since ticks may need to feed for a day or longer before transmission of the organisms is possible, daily removal of attached ticks should help prevent the disease. However, Smith *et al.* found that outdoor workers who took precautions such as wearing long pants or long-sleeve shirts, tucking pants into socks, using insect repellents on skin or clothing, and checking themselves for ticks were as likely to have antibody to *B. burgdorferi* as were workers who did not take similar precautions.[97] If tick avoidance measures fail, early recognition of signs and symptoms, and appropriate antimicrobial therapy can prevent the later manifestations of Lyme disease.

Several measures to control tick populations also have been evaluated. Wilson *et al.* found acaricidal treatment of deer to be impractical and that removal of 70% of a local deer herd did not markedly reduce the abundance of the tick.[124] However, elimination of the deer herd resulted in reduced abundance of larval ticks the following summer and a more gradual decline in the abundance of nymphs and adults.[125] Mather *et al.* showed that mice will use permethrin-treated cotton as nesting material. The use of this product in wooded sites resulted in a 90% reduction in the number of ticks carried by mice in the treated sites compared to mice captured in an untreated adjacent area.[75] Schulze *et al.* achieved 97 to 100% reductions of adult *I. dammini* with ground applications of insecticide following leaf abscission in the fall; however, this strategy is limited by its lack of effect in immature stages.[92] Destruction of mouse habitat by burning and mowing brush may locally reduce the abundance of questing adult ticks; however, displacement of mice by mowing alone resulted in a short-term increase in the abundance of nymphal *I. dammini* on the freshly mown land.[99] The potential effectiveness of communitywide application of such measures to prevent Lyme disease is unknown.

In the absence of tick control measures, awareness of Lyme disease in endemic areas will remain the primary prevention strategy. Endemic areas can be identified through disease surveillance and through tick surveys or serologic surveys of rodents, other mammals, and humans.

9.2. Prophylaxis

Antimicrobial prophylaxis of persons who are bitten by *Ixodes* ticks has not been formally recommended. Falco and Fish interviewed 71 individuals with documented *I. dammini* bites in Westchester County, New York; an area where approximately half of nymphal and female *I. dammini* have been reported infected with *B. burgdorferi*.[40] Twenty-nine (59%) of forty-nine persons who consulted with a physician regarding the tick bite received some type of prophylactic antimicrobial therapy. None of these and only 2 (5%) of 40 persons who received no prophylactic therapy subsequently developed EM at the site of the tick attachment. Thus, even in highly endemic areas, the likelihood of developing Lyme disease from a single tick bite appears to be relatively low.

9.3. Immunization

No *Borrelia* vaccines are currently available. Johnson *et al.* administered a single dose of whole-cell vaccine of inactivated *B. burgdorferi* to hamsters and found 86 to 100% protection upon subsequent challenge at 30 days.[57] However, protection in an animal model does not predict vaccine efficacy in humans, as was shown by DuPont *et al.* for Rocky Mountain spotted fever (RMSF) vaccine.[37] Lack of protection efficacy led to the withdrawal of RMSF vaccine from commercial production.

Development of a human Lyme disease vaccine may be complicated by several factors. First, antigenic variability of *B. burgdorferi* between strains and during the course of an infection can occur.[6,93,122] Second, designing a clinical trial of Lyme disease vaccine may be difficult. Incidence rates of 1.5 to 3.3% in endemic areas would require enrollment of large numbers of study participants, each of whom must be screened to determine prior exposure to *B. burgdorferi*.[48,116] Also, vaccinating should lead to *B. burgdorferi* antibody production, thereby prohibiting the ability to measure antibody as an endpoint of infection. Thus, vaccine efficacy measurements would need to be based on prevention of certain clinical manifestations, including arthritis and cardiac and neurologic sequelae. Evaluating such endpoints in a large clinical trial poses diagnostic and logistic difficulties. Third, Lyme disease, like RMSF, is a tickborne illness of regional importance. The potential use for a human vaccine would likely be limited to individuals at high risk of exposure (i.e., those in endemic areas). Vaccine manufacturers may determine that a limited market is insufficient to justify vaccine development costs. Finally, the public health impact of a vaccine may be limited, because Lyme disease can frequently be recognized by clinicians and successfully treated with antimicrobial agents in most instances.

10. Unresolved Problems

10.1. Epidemiology

The major impediment to further understanding of the epidemiology of Lyme disease is the lack of objective case-definition criteria. The clinical expression of Lyme disease may develop over several months and needs to be distinguished from other rheumatologic and neurologic disorders. The symptoms and signs of Lyme disease may be nonspecific and may require substantial clinical judgment in the absence of definitive diagnostic tests. Thus, Lyme disease presents problems applicable to both infectious and chronic disease epidemiology.

Currently available serologic tests are neither sufficiently sensitive during the early stages of Lyme disease, nor sufficiently specific during the later stages. If antibody is detected, cross-reacting antibodies need to be ruled out and current infection needs to be distinguished from previous exposure. Additional diagnostic tests, such as antigen detection in tissue or body secretions, are needed.

The impact of *B. burgdorferi* infection on domestic animals, in particular on economically important animals such as cows, needs to be defined. In addition, the potential for transmission of spirochetes between animals by urine, colostrum, or biting insects needs to be evaluated. A major impediment to further understanding Lyme disease in animals is a lack of knowledge about the distribution of other borreliae and of their relatedness to *B. burgdorferi*.

10.2. Control and Prevention

Wide-area tick control has traditionally been difficult to accomplish. Removal of deer herds from endemic landscapes is unlikely to be feasible and the ability of *I. dammini* to utilize other hosts makes the results of such measures unpredictable. Selectively reducing animal hosts could increase the abundance of ticks seeking an alternative human host, thereby temporarily increasing the risk of *B. burgdorferi* transmission to humans. Strategies of local area tick control using insecticides on cotton balls or vegetation need to be evaluated from a clinical perspective. For example, a control method that removed larger, more visible adult ticks from the landscape could lead to a false belief that all ticks had been eliminated, a decreased awareness of the smaller nymphal ticks, less concern for personal tick protection, and ultimately increased risk of exposure to *B. burgdorferi*. Thus, human behavior and response to the environment must be considered in any comprehensive control strategy for Lyme disease.

11. References

1. Afzelius, A., Erythema chronicum migrans, *Acta Derm. Venereol.* **2:**120–125 (1921).
2. Anderson, J., Mammalian and avian reservoirs for *Borrelia burgdorferi*, *Ann. N.Y. Acad. Sci.* **539:**180–191 (1988).
3. Anderson, J., Johnson, R., Magnarelli, L., and Hyde,

F., Identification of endemic foci of Lyme disease: Isolation of *Borrelia burgdorferi* from feral rodents and ticks (*Dermacentor variabilis*), *J. Clin. Microbiol.* **22**:36–38 (1985).

4. BANNWARTH, A., Chronische lymphocytare meningitis, entzundliche polyneuritis und "Rheumatismus". Ein Beitrag zum problem "Allergie und Nervensystem," *Arch. Psychiatr. Nervenkr.* **113**:284–376 (1941).

5. BARANTON, G., AND SAINT-GIBBONS, I., *Borrelia burgdorferi* survival in human blood samples, *Ann. N.Y. Acad. Sci.* **539**:444–445 (1988).

6. BARBOUR, A., AND GARON, C., The genes encoding major surface proteins of *Borrelia burgdorferi* are located on a plasmid, *Ann. N.Y. Acad. Sci.* **539**:144–153 (1988).

7. BARBOUR, A., HEILAND, R., AND HOWE, T., Heterogeneity of major proteins in Lyme disease borreliae: A molecular analysis of North American isolates, *J. Infect. Dis.* **152**:478–484 (1985).

8. BECK, G., HABICHT, G., BENACH, J., AND COLEMAN, J., Chemical and biologic characterization of a lipopolysaccharide extracted from the Lyme disease spirochete (*Borrelia burgdorferi*), *J. Infect. Dis.* **152**:108–117 (1985).

9. BENACH, J., AND COLEMAN, J., Clinical and geographical characteristics of Lyme disease in New York, *Zentralbl. Bakteriol. Mikrobiol. Hyg. A* **263**:477–482 (1986).

10. BENACH, J., BOSLER, E., HANRAHAN, J., COLEMAN, J., HABICHT, G., BAST, T., CAMERON, D., ZIEGLER, J., BARBOUR, A., BURGDORFER, W., EDELMAN, R., AND KASLOW, R., Spirochetes isolated from the blood of two patients with Lyme disease, *N. Engl. J. Med.* **308**:740–742 (1983).

11. BENDIG, J., AND OGILVIE, D., Severe encephalopathy associated with Lyme disease, *Lancet* **1**:681–682 (1987).

12. BENOIT, P., DOURNON, E., DESTEE, A., AND WAROT, P., Spirochaetes and Lyme disease, *Lancet* **2**:1223 (1986).

13. BERGER, B., KAPLAN, M., ROTHENBERG, I., AND BARBOUR, A., Isolation and characterization of the Lyme disease spirochete from the skin of patients with erythema chronicum migrans, *J. Am. Acad. Dermatol.* **13**:444–449 (1985).

14. BINDER, E., DOEPFMER, R., AND HORNSTEIN, O., Experimentelle Übertragung des Erythema chronicum migrans von Mensch zu Mensch, *Hautarzt* **6**:494–496 (1955).

15. BOSLER, E., AND SCHULZE, T., The prevalence and significance of *Borrelia burgdorferi* in the urine of feral reservoir hosts, *Zentralbl. Bakteriol. Mikrobiol. Hyg. A* **263**:40–44 (1986).

16. BOSLER, E., ORMISTON, B., COLEMAN, J., HANRAHAN, J., AND BENACH, J., Prevalence of the Lyme disease spirochete in populations of white-tailed deer and white-footed mice, *Yale J. Biol. Med.* **57**:651–659 (1984).

17. BOSLER, E., COHEN, D., SCHULZE, T., OLSEN, C., BERNARD, W., AND LISSMAN, B., Host responses to *Borrelia burgdorferi* in dogs and horses, *Ann. N.Y. Acad. Sci.* **539**:221–234 (1988).

18. BURGDORFER, W., BARBOUR, A., HAYES, S., BENACH, J., GRUNWALDT, E., AND DAVIS, J., Lyme disease—A tick-borne spirochetosis? *Science* **216**:1319–1320 (1982).

19. BURGDORFER, W., LANE, R., BARBOUR, A., GRESBINK, J., AND ANDERSON, J., The Western black-legged tick, *Ixodes pacificus:* A vector of *Borrelia burgdorferi, Am. J. Trop. Med. Hyg.* **34**:925–930 (1985).

20. BURGDORFER, W., HAYES, S., AND BENACH, J., Development of *Borrelia burgdorferi* in ixodid tick vectors, *Ann. N.Y. Acad. Sci.* **539**:172–179 (1988).

21. BURGESS, E., *Borrelia burgdorferi* infection in Wisconsin horses and cows, *Ann. N.Y. Acad. Sci.* **539**:235–243 (1988).

22. BURGESS, E., AMUNDSON, T., DAVIS, J., KASLOW, R., AND EDELMAN, R., Experimental inoculation of Peromyscus spp. with *Borrelia burgdorferi:* Evidence of contact transmission, *Am. J. Trop. Med. Hyg.* **35**:355–359 (1986).

23. Centers for Disease Control, Update: Lyme disease—United States, *Morbid. Mortal. Weekly Rep.* **33**:268–270 (1984).

24. Centers for Disease Control, Lyme Disease—Connecticut, *Morbid. Mortal. Weekly Rep.* **37**:1–3 (1988).

25. CHENGXU, A., YUXIN, W., YONGQUO, Z., SHAOSHAN, W., QUICHENG, Q., ZHIXUE, S., DEYOU, L., DONGUAN, C., ZIAODUNG, L., AND JIENHUA, Z., Clinical manifestations and epidemiological characteristics of Lyme disease in Hailin County, Heilongjiang Province, China, *Ann. N.Y. Acad. Sci.* **539**:302–313 (1988).

26. CIESIELSKI, C., MARKOWITZ, L., HORSLEY, R., HIGHTOWER, A., RUSSEL, H., AND BROOME, C., The geographic distribution of Lyme disease in the United States, *Ann. N.Y. Acad. Sci.* **539**:283–288 (1988).

27. COHEN, D., BOSLER, E., BERNARD, W., MEIRS, D., EISNER, R., AND SCHULZE, T., Epidemiologic studies of Lyme disease in horses and their public health significance, *Ann. N.Y. Acad. Sci.* **539**:244–257 (1988).

28. CRAFT, J., GRODZICKI, R., AND STEERE, A., Antibody response in Lyme disease: Evaluation of diagnostic tests, *J. Infect. Dis.* **149**:789–795 (1984).

29. CRAFT, J., GRODZICKI, R., SHRESTHA, M., FISCHER, D., GARCIA-BLANCO, M., AND STEERE, A., The antibody response in Lyme disease, *Yale J. Biol. Med.* **57**:561–565 (1984).

30. CRAFT, J., FISCHER, D., SHIMAMOTO, G., AND STEERE, A., Antigens of *Borrelia burgdorferi* recognized during Lyme disease, *J. Clin. Invest.* **78**:934–939 (1986).

31. DATTWYLER, R., THOMAS, J., BENACH, J., AND GOLIGHTLY, M., Cellular immune responses in Lyme disease, *Zentralbl. Bakteriol. Mikrobiol. Hyg. A* **263**:151 (1986).

32. DATTWYLER, R., HALPERIN, J., PASS, H., AND LUFT, B., Ceftriaxone as effective therapy in refractory Lyme disease, *J. Infect. Dis.* **155**:1322–1325 (1987).

33. DATTWYLER, R., VOLKMAN, D., HALPERIN, J., LUFT, B., THOMAS, J., AND GOLIGHTLY M., Seronegative Lyme disease: Specific immune responses in Lyme borreliosis. Characterization of T cell and B cell responses to *Borrelia burgdorferi, Ann. N.Y. Acad. Sci.* **539**:93–102 (1988).

34. DATTWYLER, R., VOLKMAN, D., LUFT, B., HALPERIN, J., THOMAS, J., AND GOLIGHTLY, M., Seronegative Lyme disease: Dissociation of specific T- and B-lymphocyte responses

to *Borrelia burgdorferi*, *N. Engl. J. Med.* **319:**1441–1446 (1988).

35. DAVIS, J., SCHELL, W., AMUNDSON, T., GODSEY, M., SPIELMAN, A., BURGDORFER, W., BARBOUR, A., LAVENTURE, M., AND KASLOW, R., Lyme disease in Wisconsin: Epidemiologic, clinical, serologic, and entomologic findings, *Yale J. Biol. Med.* **57:**685–696 (1984).

36. DEKONENKO, E., STEERE, A., BERARDI, V., AND KRAVCHUK, L., Lyme borreliosis in the Soviet Union: A cooperative US–USSR report, *J. Infect. Dis.* **158:**748–753 (1988).

37. DUPONT, H., HORNICK, R., DAWKINS, A., HEINER, G., FABRIKANT, I., WISSEMAN, C., AND WOODWARD, T., Rocky mountain spotted fever: A comparative study of the active immunity induced by inactivated and viable pathogenic *Rickettsia rickettsii*, *J. Infect. Dis.* **128:**340–344 (1973).

38. DURAY, P., AND STEERE, A., Clinical pathologic correlations of Lyme disease by stage, *Ann. N.Y. Acad. Sci.* **539:**65–79 (1988).

39. FALCO, R., AND FISH, D., Prevalence of *Ixodes dammini* near the homes of Lyme disease patients in Westchester County, New York, *Am. J. Epidemiol.* **127:**826–830 (1988).

40. FALCO, R., AND FISH, D., Ticks parasitizing humans in a Lyme disease endemic area of southern New York state, *Am. J. Epidemiol.* **128:**1146–1152 (1988).

41. FUMAROLA, D., MUNNO, I., MARCUCCIO, C., AND MIRAGLIOTTA, G., Endotoxin-like activity associated with Lyme disease borrelia, *Zentralbl. Bakteriol. Mikrobiol. Hyg. A* **263:**137–141 (1986).

42. GARIN BUJADOUX, C., Paralysie par les tiques, *J. Med. Lyon* **71c:**765–767 (1922).

43. GOUBAU, P., AND BIGGIGNUM, G., Lyme borreliosis: The new face of an old disease, *Acta Clin. Belg.* **42:**1–4 (1987).

44. GREENE, R., WALKER, R., NICHOLSON, W., HEIDNER, H., LEVIN, J., BURGESS, E., WYAND, M., BREITSCHWERDT, E., AND BERKHOFF, H., Immunoblot analysis of immunoglobulin G response to the Lyme disease agent (*Borrelia burgdorferi*) in experimentally and naturally exposed dogs, *J. Clin. Microbiol.* **26:**648–653 (1988).

45. GRODZICKI R., AND STEERE, A., Comparison of immunoblotting and indirect enzyme-linked immunosorbent assay using different antigen preparations for diagnosing early Lyme disease, *J. Infect. Dis.* **157:**790–797 (1988).

46. HABICHT, G., BECK, G., BENACH, J., COLEMAN, J., AND LEICHTLING, K., Lyme disease spirochetes induce human and murine interleukin-1 production, *J. Immunol.* **134:**3147–3154 (1985).

47. HABICHT, G., BECK, G., BENACH, J., AND COLEMAN, J., *Borrelia burgdorferi* lipopolysaccharide and its role in the pathogenesis of Lyme disease, *Zentralbl. Bakteriol. Mikrobiol. Hyg. A* **263:**137–141 (1986).

48. HANRAHAN, J., BENACH, J., COLEMAN, J., BOSLER, E., MORSE, D., CAMERON, D., EDELMAN, R., AND KASLOW, R., Incidence and cumulative frequency of endemic Lyme disease in a community, *J. Infect. Dis.* **150:**489–496 (1984).

49. HARD, S., Erythema chronicum migrans (Afzelii) associated with mosquito bite, *Acta Derm. Venereol.* **46:**473–476 (1966).

50. HARDIN, J., STEERE, A., AND MALAWISTA, S., Immune complexes and the evolution of Lyme arthritis: Dissemination and localization of abnormal Clq binding activity, *N. Engl. J. Med.* **301:**1358–1363 (1979).

51. HARDIN, J., STEERE, A., AND MALAWISTA, S., The pathogenesis of arthritis in Lyme disease: Humoral immune responses and the role of intraarticular immune complexes, *Yale J. Biol. Med.* **57:**589–593 (1984).

52. HECHEMY, K., HARRIS, H., DUERR, M., BENACH, J., AND REIMER, C., Immunoglobulin G subclasses specific to *Borrelia burgdorferi* in patients with Lyme disease, *Ann. N.Y. Acad. Sci.* **539:**162–169 (1988).

53. HEDBERG, C., OSTERHOLM, M., MACDONALD, K., AND WHITE, K., An interlaboratory study of antibody to *Borrelia burgdorferi*, *J. Infect. Dis.* **154:**1325–1327 (1987).

54. HELLERSTROM, S., *Erythema chronicum migrans Afzelii*, *Acta Derm. Venereol.* **11:**315–321 (1930).

55. HOLLSTRÖM, E., Successful treatment of erythema migrans Afzelius, *Acta Derm. Venereol.* **31:**235–243 (1951).

56. JOHNSON, R., SCHMID, G., HYDE, F., STEIGERWALT, G., AND BRENNER, D., *Borrelia burgdorferi* sp. nov.: Etiologic agent of Lyme disease, *Int. J. Syst. Bacteriol.* **34:**496–497 (1984).

57. JOHNSON, R., KODNER, C., AND RUSSELL, M., Active immunization of hamsters against experimental infection with *Borrelia burgdorferi*, *Infect. Immun.* **54:**897–898 (1986).

58. JOHNSON, R., KODNER, C., AND RUSSELL, M., In vitro and in vivo susceptibility of the Lyme disease spirochete, *Borrelia burgdorferi*, to four antimicrobial agents, *Antimicrob. Agents Chemother.* **31:**164–167 (1987).

59. JOHNSON, S., KLEIN, G., SCHMID, G., AND FEELEY, J., Susceptibility of the Lyme disease spirochete to seven antimicrobial agents, *Yale J. Biol. Med.* **57:**99–103 (1984).

60. JOHNSON, S., KLEIN, G., SCHMID, G., BOWEN, G., FEELEY, J., AND SCHULZE, T., Lyme disease: A selective medium for isolation of the suspected etiologic agent, a spirochete, *J. Clin. Microbiol.* **19:**81–82 (1984).

61. KAWABATA, M., BABA, S., IGUCHI, K., YAMAGUTI, N., AND RUSSELL, H., Lyme disease in Japan and its possible incriminated tick vector, *Ixodes persulcatus*, *J. Infect. Dis.* **156:**854 (1987).

62. KIRSCH, M., RUBEN, F., STEERE, A., DURAY, P., NORDEN, C., AND WINKELSTEIN, A., Fatal adult respiratory distress syndrome in a patient with Lyme disease, *J. Am. Med. Assoc.* **259:**2737–2739 (1988).

63. KRAMER, N., RICKERT, R., BRODKIN, R., AND ROSENSTEIN, E., Septal panniculitis as a manifestation of Lyme disease, *Am. J. Med.* **81:**149–157 (1986).

64. LEVINE, J., WILSON, M., AND SPIELMAN, A., Mice as reservoirs of the Lyme disease spirochete, *Am. J. Trop. Med. Hyg.* **34:**355–360 (1985).

65. LIPSCHÜTZ, B., Über eine seltene Erythemform (Erythema

chronicum migrans), *Arch. Dermatol. Syphilol.* **118:**349–356 (1913).

66. LUFT, B., VOLKMAN, D., HALPERIN, J., AND DATTWYLER, R., New chemotherapeutic approaches in the treatment of Lyme borreliosis, *Ann. N.Y. Acad. Sci.* **539:**352–361 (1988).

67. MAGNARELLI, L., AND ANDERSON, J., Ticks and biting insects infected with the etiologic agent of Lyme disease, *Borrelia burgdorferi, J. Clin. Microbiol.* **26:**1482–1486 (1988).

68. MAGNARELLI, L., ANDERSON, J., BURGDORFER, W., AND CHAPPELL, W., Parasitism by *Ixodes dammini* (Acari: Ixodidae) and antibodies to spirochetes in mammals at Lyme disease foci in Connecticut, USA, *J. Med. Entomol.* **21:**52–57 (1984).

69. MAGNARELLI, L., ANDERSON, J., KAUFMAN, A., LIEBERMAN, L., AND WHITNEY, G., Borreliosis in dogs from southern Connecticut, *J. Am. Vet. Med. Assoc.* **186:**955–959 (1985).

70. MAGNARELLI, L., ANDERSON, J., AND BARBOUR, A., The etiologic agent of Lyme disease in deer flies, horse flies, and mosquitoes, *J. Infect. Dis.* **154:**355–358 (1986).

71. MAGNARELLI, L., ANDERSON, J., AND JOHNSON, R., Cross-reactivity in serological tests for Lyme disease and other spirochetal infections, *J. Infect. Dis.* **156:**183–188 (1987).

72. MARCUS, L., PATTERSON, M., GILFILLAN, R., AND URBAND, P., Antibodies to *Borrelia burgdorferi* in New England horses: Serologic survey, *Am. J. Vet. Res.* **46:**2570–2571 (1985).

73. MARCUS, L., STEERE, A., DURAY, P., ANDERSON, A., AND MAHONEY, E., Fatal pancarditis in a patient with coexistent Lyme disease and babesiosis. Demonstration of spirochetes in the myocardium, *Ann. Intern. Med.* **103:**374–376 (1985).

74. MARKOWITZ, L., STEERE, A., BENACH, J., SLADE, J., AND BROOME, C., Lyme disease during pregnancy, *J. Am. Med. Assoc.* **255:**3394–3396 (1986).

75. MATHER, T., RIBEIRO, J., AND SPIELMAN, A., Lyme disease and babesiosis: Acaricide focussed on potentially infected ticks, *Am. J. Trop. Med. Hyg.* **36:**609–614 (1987).

76. MERTZ, L., WOBIG, G., DUFFY, J., AND KATZMANN, J., Ticks, spirochetes and new diagnostic tests for Lyme disease, *Mayo Clin. Proc.* **60:**402–406 (1985).

77. NEUBERT, U., MUNCHHOFF, P., VOLKER, B., REIMERS, C., AND PFLUGER, K., *Borrelia burgdorferi* infections in Bavarian forest workers: A follow-up study, *Ann. N.Y. Acad. Sci.* **539:**476–479 (1988).

78. OSTERHOLM, M., FORFANG, J., WHITE, K., AND KURITSKY, J., Lyme disease in Minnesota: Epidemiologic and serologic findings, *Yale J. Biol. Med.* **57:**677–683 (1984).

79. PACHNER, A., AND STEERE, A., The triad of neurologic manifestations of Lyme disease: Meningitis, cranial neuritis, and radiculoneuritis, *Neurology* **35:**47–53 (1985).

80. PFISTER, H.-W., NEUBERT, U., WILSKE, B., PREAC-MURSIC, V., EINHAUPL, K., AND BORASIO, G., Reinfection with *Borrelia burgdorferi, Lancet* **2:**984–985 (1986).

81. PIESMAN, J., AND SINSKY, R., Ability of *Ixodes scapularis, Dermacentor variabilis,* and *Amblyomma americanum* (Acari: Ixodidae) to acquire, maintain, and transmit Lyme disease spirochetes (*Borrelia burgdorferi*), *J. Med. Entomol.* **25:**336–339 (1988).

82. REIK, L., STEERE, A., BARTENHAGEN, N., SHOPE, R., AND MALAWISTA, S., Neurologic abnormalities of Lyme disease, *Medicine* **58:**281–294 (1979).

83. REIK, L., BURGDORFER, W., AND DONALDSON, J., Neurologic abnormalities in Lyme disease without erythema chronicum migrans, *Am. J. Med.* **81:**73–78 (1986).

84. REZNICK, J., BRAUNSTEIN, D., WALSH, R., SMITH, C., WOLFSON, P., GIERKE, L., GORELKIN, L., AND CHANDLER, F., Lyme carditis: Electrophysiologic and histopathologic study, *Am. J. Med.* **81:**923–927 (1986).

85. RIBEIRO, J., MATHER, T., PIESMAN, J., AND SPIELMAN, A., Dissemination and salivary delivery of Lyme disease spirochetes in vector ticks (Acari: Ixodidae), *J. Med. Entomol.* **24:**201–205 (1987),

86. SCHECHTER, S., Lyme disease associated with optic neuropathy, *Am. J. Med.* **81:**143–145 (1986).

87. SCHLESINGER, P., DURAY, P., BURKE, B., STEERE, A., AND STILLMAN, M., Maternal–fetal transmission of the Lyme disease spirochete, *Borrelia burgdorferi, Ann. Intern. Med.* **103:**67–68 (1985).

88. SCHMID, G., The global distribution of Lyme disease, *Rev. Infect. Dis.* **7:**741–750 (1985).

89. SCHMID, G., HORSLEY, R., STEERE, A., HANRAHAN, J., DAVIS, J., BOWEN, S., OSTERHOLM, M., WEISFELD, J., HIGHTOWER, A., AND BROOME, C., Surveillance of Lyme disease in the United States, 1982, *J. Infect. Dis.* **151:**1144–1148 (1985).

90. SCHULZE, T., BOWEN, G., BOSLER, E., LAKAT, M., ORMISTON, B., AND SHISLER, J., *Amblyomma americanum:* A potential vector of Lyme disease in New Jersey, *Science* **224:**601–603 (1984).

91. SCHULZE, T., BOWEN, G., LAKAT, M., PARKIN, W., AND SHISLER, J., The role of adult *Ixodes dammini* (Acari: Ixodidae) in the transmission of Lyme disease in New Jersey, USA, *J. Med. Entomol.* **22:**88–93 (1985).

92. SCHULZE, T., McDEVITT, W., PARKIN, W., AND SHILSER, J., Effectiveness of two insecticides in controlling *Ixodes dammini* (Acari: Ixodidae) following an outbreak of Lyme disease in New Jersey, *J. Med. Entomol.* **24:**420–424 (1987).

93. SCHWAN, T., AND BURGDORFER, W., Antigenic changes of *Borrelia burgdorferi* as a result of in vitro cultivation, *J. Infect. Dis.* **156:**852–853 (1987).

94. SCRIMENTI, R., Erythema chronicum migrans, *Arch. Dermatol.* **102:**104–105 (1970).

95. SHRESTHA, M., GRODZICKI, R., AND STEERE, A., Diagnosing early Lyme disease, *Am. J. Med.* **78:**235–240 (1985).

96. SMITH, L., BURGDORFER, W., AND KATZ, H., Erythema chronicum migrans, *Cutis* **17(S):**962–964 (1976).

97. SMITH, P., BENACH, J., WHITE, D., STROUP, D., AND MORSE, D., Occupational risk of Lyme disease in endemic areas of New York State, *Ann. N.Y. Acad. Sci.* **539:**289–301 (1988).

98. SNYDMAN, D., SCHENKEIN, D., BERARDI, V., LASTAVICA, C., AND PARISER, K., *Borrelia burgdorferi* in joint fluid in chronic Lyme arthritis, *Ann. Intern. Med.* **104:**798–800 (1986).

99. SPIELMAN, A., Prospects for suppressing transmission of Lyme disease, *Ann. N.Y. Acad. Sci.* **539:**212–220 (1988).

100. STANEK, G., PLETSCHETTE, M., FLAMM, H., HIRSCHL, A., ABERER, E., KRISTOFERITSCH, W., AND SCHMUTZHARD, E., European Lyme borreliosis, *Ann. N.Y. Acad. Sci.* **539:**274–282 (1988).

101. STEERE, A., AND MALAWISTA, S., Cases of Lyme disease in the United States: Locations correlated with distribution of *Ixodes dammini*, *Ann. Intern. Med.* **91:**730–733 (1979).

102. STEERE, A., HARDIN, J., AND MALAWISTA, S., Erythema chronicum migrans and Lyme arthritis: Cryoimmunoglobulins and clinical activity of skin and joints, *Science* **196:**1121–1122 (1977).

103. STEERE, A., MALAWISTA, S., HARDIN, J., RUDDY, S., ASKENASE, P., AND ANDIMAN, W., Erythema chronicum migrans and Lyme arthritis: The enlarging clinical spectrum, *Ann. Intern. Med.* **86:**685–698 (1977).

104. STEERE, A., MALAWISTA, S., SNYDMAN, D., SHOPE, R., ANDIMAN, W., ROSS, M., AND STEELE, F., Lyme arthritis: An epidemic of oligoarticular arthritis in children and adults in three Connecticut communities, *Arthritis Rheum.* **20:**7–17 (1977).

105. STEERE, A., BRODERICK, T., AND MALAWISTA, S., Erythema chronicum migrans and Lyme arthritis: Epidemiologic evidence for a tick vector, *Am. J. Epidemiol.* **108:**312–321 (1978).

106. STEERE, A., BATSFORD, W., WEINBERG, M., ALEXANDER, J., BERGER, H., WOLFSON, S., AND MALAWISTA, S., Lyme carditis: Cardiac abnormalities of Lyme disease, *Ann. Intern. Med.* **93:**8–16 (1980).

107. STEERE, A., MALAWISTA, S., NEWMAN, J., SPIELER, P., AND BARTENHAGEN, N., Antibiotic therapy in Lyme disease, *Ann. Intern. Med.* **93:**1–8 (1980).

108. STEERE, A., BARTENHAGEN, N., CRAFT, J., HUTCHINSON, G., NEWMAN, J., RAHN, D., SIGAL, L., SPIELER, P., STENN, K., AND MALAWISTA, S., The early clinical manifestations of Lyme disease, *Ann. Intern. Med.* **99:**76–82 (1983).

109. STEERE, A., GRODZICKI, R., KORNBLATT, A., CRAFT, J., BARBOUR, A., BURGDORFER, W., SCHMID, G., JOHNSON, E., AND MALAWISTA, S., The spirochetal etiology of Lyme disease, *N. Engl. J. Med.* **308;**733–740 (1983).

110. STEERE, A., HUTCHINSON, G., RAHN, D., SIGAL, L., CRAFT, J., DESANNA, E., AND MALAWISTA, S., Treatment of the early manifestations of Lyme disease, *Ann. Intern. Med.* **99:**22–26 (1983).

111. STEERE, A., PACHNER, A., AND MALAWISTA, S., Neurologic abnormalities of Lyme disease: Successful treatment with high-dose intravenous penicillin, *Ann. Intern. Med.* **99:**767–772 (1983).

112. STEERE, A., GRODZICKI, R., CRAFT, J., SHRESTHA, M., KORNBLATT, A., AND MALAWISTA, S., Recovery of Lyme disease spirochetes from patients, *Yale J. Biol. Med.* **57:**557–560 (1984).

113. STEERE, A., MALAWISTA, S., BARTENHAGEN, N., SPIELER, P., RAHN, D., HUTCHINSON, G., GREEN, J., SNYDMAN, D., AND TAYLOR, E., The clinical spectrum and treatment of Lyme disease, *Yale J. Biol. Med.* **57:**453–461 (1984).

114. STEERE, A., DURAY, P., KAUFFMANN, D., AND WORMSER, G., Unilateral blindness caused by infection with the Lyme disease spirochete, *Borrelia burgdorferi*, *Ann. Intern. Med.* **103:**382–384 (1985).

115. STEERE, A., GREEN, J., SCHOEN, R., TAYLOR, E., HUTCHINSON, G., RAHN, D., AND MALAWISTA, S., Successful parenteral penicillin therapy of established Lyme arthritis, *N. Engl. J. Med.* **312:**869–874 (1985).

116. STEERE, A., TAYLOR, E., WILSON, M., LEVINE, J., AND SPIELMAN, A., Longitudinal assessment of the clinical and epidemiological features of Lyme disease in a community, *J. Infect. Dis.* **154:**295–300 (1986).

117. TELFORD, S., MATHER, T., MOORE, S., WILSON, M., AND SPIELMAN, A., Incompetence of deer as reservoirs of the Lyme disease spirochete, *Am. J. Trop. Med. Hyg.* **39:**105–109 (1988).

118. WEBER, K., SCHIERZ, G., WILSKE, B., AND PREAC-MURSIC, V., European erythema migrans disease and related disorders, *Yale J. Biol. Med.* **57:**463–471 (1984).

119. WEDER, B., WIEDERSHEIM, P., MATTER, L., STECK, A., AND OTTO, F., Chronic progressive neurological involvement in *Borrelia burgdorferi* infection, *J. Neurol.* **234:**40–43 (1987).

120. WILLIAMS, C., CURRAN, A., LEE, A., AND SOUSA, V., Lyme disease: Epidemiologic characteristics of an outbreak in Westchester County, NY, *Am. J. Public Health* **76:**62–65 (1986).

121. WILSKE, B., SCHIERZ, G., PREAC-MURSIC, V., VON BUSCH, K., KUHBECK, R., PFISTER, H., AND EINHAUPL, K., Intrathecal production of specific antibodies against *Borrelia burgdorferi* in patients with lymphocytic meningoradiculitis (Bannworth's syndrome), *J. Infect. Dis.* **153:**304–314 (1986).

122. WILSKE, B., PREAC-MURSIC, V., SCHIERZ, G., KUHBECK, R., BARBOUR, A., AND KRAMER, M., Antigenic variability of *Borrelia burgdorferi*, *Ann. N.Y. Acad. Sci.* **539:**126–143 (1988).

123. WILSON, M., AND SPIELMAN, A., Seasonal activity of immature *Ixodes dammini* (Acari: Ixodidae), *J. Med. Entomol.* **22:**408–414 (1985).

124. WILSON, M., LEVINE, J., AND SPIELMAN, A., Effect of deer reduction on abundance of the deer tick (*Ixodes dammini*), *Yale J. Biol. Med.* **57:**5697–5705 (1984).

125. WILSON, M., TELFORD, S., PRESMAN, J., AND SPIELMAN, A., Reduced abundance of immature *Ixodes dammini* (Acari: Ixodidae) following elimination of deer, *J. Med. Entomol.* **25:**224–228 (1988).

12. Suggested Reading

Lyme Disease and Related Disorders, *Ann. N.Y. Acad. Sci.* **539** (1988).

Proceedings of the First International Symposium on Lyme Disease, *Yale J. Biol. Med.* **54**(4) (1984).

Proceedings of the Second International Symposium on Lyme Disease and Related Disorders, *Zentralbl. Bakteriol. Mikrobiol. Hyg. A.*

CHAPTER 20

Meningococcal Infections

Robert S. Baltimore and Harry A. Feldman†

1. Introduction

The meningococcal diseases* represent a spectrum of illness caused by *Neisseria meningitidis*. Although sporadic endemic cases occur throughout the world, massive, devastating epidemics tend to reflect conditions of crowding, mobilization, and enclosed institutional populations. Such outbreaks tend to be extraordinarily disruptive, especially because of the fear and fright that they induce in the affected populations. Among civilians, children are most often attacked, with mortality rates of 80–90% having been noted in some epidemics that occurred before effective therapeutic agents became available. The disease is also known as "cerebral spinal fever" and "epidemic cerebral spinal meningitis" and by other names. Mobilization for war, with the induction of many young men into crowded military camps, has generally been accompanied by outbreaks. This has been in contrast to the absence of such outbreaks among college freshmen, who also represent a mix from many diverse origins, in dormitories and other sometimes

*In this chapter, the term *case* or *disease* refers to any instance of meningococcal infection other than asymptomatic pharyngeal (carrier).

†Deceased.

Robert S. Baltimore · Departments of Pediatrics and Epidemiology and Public Health, Yale University School of Medicine, New Haven, Connecticut 06510. **Harry A. Feldman** · Department of Preventive Medicine, State University of New York, Upstate Medical Center, Syracuse, New York 13210.

crowded living quarters on many campuses. It should also be stated that generalized outbreaks among the military do not arise *de novo,* but may reflect what is occurring in the associated civilian populations.

2. Historical Background

Clinical meningococcal disease was first described by Vieusseux[102] in 1805 during an outbreak in the vicinity of Geneva, Switzerland. A year later, Danielson and Mann[23] reported a small, probable epidemic of meningococcal meningitis in Medfield, Massachusetts. This paper appeared in a publication known as the *Medical and Agricultural Register* and was entitled "The history of a singular and very mortal disease, which lately made its appearance in Medfield." The nine fatal cases were so similar that only one was fully described; all occurred during March. Weichselbaum[104] identified meningococci in the spinal fluids of patients in 1887.

During the 19th century, possible epidemics occurred in 1805, 1837, 1854, 1876, and 1896. In this century, major outbreaks were noted during World Wars I and II, and subsequent to the latter, there was a massive, lengthy outbreak in sub-Sahara Africa,[72] a more localized one in Morocco,[1] and another affecting more than a quarter of a million people in Brazil,[86] as well as others in Finland[75] and among American military inductees during the Korean and Vietnam mobilizations. Smaller, localized outbreaks have occurred from time to time in various institutions and localities. In the course of the many studies that were conducted during World War I, Gordon[48] identified four serological types of meningococci: I, II, III, and IV. In 1953, Branham,[11] as the result of her very careful, meticulous studies, labeled the different serogroups A, B, C, and D. She believed that organisms of Group A were those principally responsible for epidemics and that sporadic cases tend to be antigenically heterogeneous as the result of infections with Groups B and C. Slaterus[97] subsequently demonstrated three additional meningococcal serogroups (X, Y, and Z), and then Evans *et al.*[31] identified serogroups W-135 and 29-E from U.S. Army isolates.

An enormous step forward was made early in World War II when it was learned not only that sulfadiazine was effective in the treatment of cases, but also that small doses eliminated the organism from the nasopharynx.[17,51,69,90] When sulfadiazine was administered on a mass basis to a closed population, cases of disease disappeared almost instantaneously and the carrier rate was reduced to near-zero levels. Thus was provided an effective, simple, relatively inexpensive control system for preventing meningococcal disease and curtailing epidemics. Unfortunately, this was found to be ineffective in 1963 by Miller *et al.*[79] during several unsuccessful attempts to control the disease among naval recruits in San Diego. It was learned then that many disease-related strains were resistant to large concentrations of sulfadiazine and thus that the sulfonamides could no longer be used effectively for the prevention or control of epidemics.[34] Despite many subsequent trials conducted under the auspices of the Armed Forces Epidemiological Board, no substitute chemotherapeutic agent was found, although the satisfactory treatment of actual cases could be accomplished with large doses of penicillin. The latter was quickly adopted as routine therapy for both military and civilian use. Eventually, in the 1970s, rifampin was adopted as the recommended chemoprophylactic agent for close contacts of cases.[100]

3. Methodology

3.1. Sources of Mortality Data

The principal sources of mortality data on meningococcal diseases are local and federal health agencies such as, in the United States, local and state health departments and the Centers for Disease Control through the *Morbidity and Mortality Weekly Report* (MMWR). In addition, there are publications of the World Health Organization (WHO), and various military sources, but these deal only

with the populations that they serve. By and large, mortality data reflect the incidence of the disease, although they can be affected by a number of variables, especially the level of health care available and the rapidity with which treatment can be instituted. The level of completeness of mortality data is reflected to a great extent by how well public-health reporting is organized and whether adequate laboratory facilities are available for identifying individual disease-causing agents.

3.2. Sources of Morbidity Data

The disease is generally reportable, and because of the fear that it engenders, reporting is reasonably complete and tends to mirror the availability of proper laboratory facilities to identify etiological agents in individual cases. Reporting of meningitis cases is more likely to be complete than if the patient has septicemia, bacteremia, or localized infections such as arthritis, conjunctivitis, urethritis, and others, especially if available laboratory facilities are inadequate.

Prevalence and incidence data are regularly supplied in the CDC MMWRs and in the *Annual Summary* of the same publication. Additional sources of information are the *WHO Weekly Epidemiological Record* and the *Canada Diseases Weekly Report*. Other data may be found in the published reports describing individual outbreaks. The latter generally observe geographic limitations, whereas the MMWR considers the United States as a whole.

Additional data may be found in the reports of various state and local health departments. That of the New York State Department of Health is entitled *Disease Control Newsletter*.

3.3. Surveys

Carrier surveys are often conducted among military populations, whereas among civilians, case contacts are often cultured, especially in schools and families. Carrier surveys are primarily of the posterior nasopharyngeal carrier state. In recent years, carrier surveys have been deemphasized. This is because they generally yield little information about the immune state of the population or the introduction of new, virulent meningococcal strains. This appears to be more predictive of risk for an outbreak. Serological surveys have not been used generally because the available methods do not lend themselves to mass application and, furthermore, because one would have to test for antibodies to all known serogroups.

3.4. Laboratory Diagnosis

3.4.1. Isolation and Identification of the Organism. *N. meningitidis* is a fastidious, gram-negative diplococcus that grows best on enriched media such as blood or chocolate agar and in the presence of increased CO_2. The latter is especially useful for primary isolation. The organism may be isolated from all body areas and orifices. When *N. meningitidis* is sought in places where competing bacteria are prominent, it is best to use Thayer–Martin[99] medium, which consists of chocolate agar to which several antibiotics inhibitory for gram-negative, gram-positive, and yeast-contaminating organisms have been added. This medium is especially useful for the identification of meningococci in nasopharyngeal secretions and cultures from rectal swabs. Organisms may be cultivated frequently from the male urethra, the cervix, the conjunctivae, and in cases of arthritis, from purulent septic joint fluids. In patients with meningococcal bacteremia or meningitis, cultures of the blood are usually positive, as are those of spinal fluid. Meningococci may be demonstrated in Gram-stained smears from petechiae or the buffy coats of those with severe sepsis. Cultures from normally sterile fluids such as blood, CSF, or joint fluid may be cultivated on regular blood or chocolate agar rather than Thayer–Martin medium as inhibition of normal flora is not necessary. The same is true of subcultures of individual colonies from primary isolation media.

The organism ferments glucose and maltose, but not lactose. Sometimes the fermentation of glucose is slow and may require 48 h or more of incubation. More rarely, glucose may not be fermented at all. Meningococci are oxidase-positive, and this reaction may be helpful in the recognition of colonies on plates with mixed flora. The use of Thayer–Martin medium usually removes the latter requirement. The organism does not grow at room temperature or on simple media such as nutrient agar.[35]

3.4.2. Serological and Immunological Diagnostic Methods. While meningococci contain several antigens, the group-specific one is a polysaccharide that is readily detected by slide agglutination.[35]This usually works very well with isolates from body fluids of actual cases. Often, throat and sputum isolates are rough and tend to agglutinate spontaneously in saline. They are also agglutinated in normal rabbit serum and all, or nearly all, group-specific antisera. We usually identify such organisms as "saline agglutinable." Slide agglutination can be performed rapidly, but requires pure cultures and active antisera. These can be done in fairly large numbers on large plates and thus lend themselves well to population studies and epidemiological

investigations. Organisms of serogroups A and C are encapsulated and when freshly isolated, or still in original spinal fluids, may be shown to "quell" with potent antisera. This reaction can be used for rapid identification, especially of organisms in spinal fluid. For serogrouping in a reference laboratory, the hemagglutination inhibition test has been reported to be both highly sensitive and specific.[20]

4. Biological Characteristics of the Organism

Under the special conditions that lead to epidemics, encapsulated (virulent) organisms are transmitted rapidly from person to person, probably in respiratory droplets. They tend to localize primarily in the posterior nasopharynx. Thus, attempts to determine the extent, or degree, of infestation of a population at any given time requires surveys of the posterior nasopharyngeal prevalence of the organism. This is best achieved with a bent wire swab that is passed up behind the uvula, wiped across the posterior nasopharynx, withdrawn, and immediately plated on Thayer–Martin chocolate agar. The warm plates should be placed in an incubator as soon as possible thereafter. If the incubator contains CO_2, no other container need be used. If no CO_2 incubator is available, then the newly inoculated plates should be put into candle jars. The spontaneous extinction of the candle flame will indicate that the CO_2 content is elevated, and when the jar is put at 37 °C, suitable growth for further subinoculation and isolation should appear overnight. Most of the major epidemics of this century have been caused by group A meningococci, although the massive Brazilian epidemic of the 1970s began as a group C outbreak that was then displaced by group A organisms. Localized outbreaks due to meningococci of groups B, C, or Y have been noted, but more often than not, they are present in sporadic cases.

In recent years, at least three systems have been devised for subtyping meningococci. One by Frasch and Chapman[40] utilizes the bactericidal-inhibition technique. Zollinger and Mandrell[105] used both outer-membrane protein and lipopolysaccharide (LPS) to serotype meningococci. Subsequently, Apicella[2] also used LPS to serotype group B meningococci. These techniques are not generally available, but when applied by research laboratories can provide additional information for epidemiological studies of transmission, relationships among cases, or the presence of an epidemic strain in a geographically defined area.

The susceptibility and resistance of meningococci to various chemotherapeutic and antibiotic agents have played a significant role in the treatment of individual patients and, perhaps more important, in the management of epidemics. The new era began in 1941 with a publication by Dingle *et al.*[26] that demonstrated that sulfadiazine was effective in the treatment of meningococcal meningitis. This finding was subsequently supported by others.[38] It was also found during these clinical studies that meningococci were eradicated from the posterior nasopharynx within hours after treatment was initiated. Then came a number of trials in the military in which it was observed that small doses of sulfadiazine given for short periods of time were sufficient to eradicate the carrier state.[17,18,51,69] When 1 g was given twice daily for 2 days to military recruits en masse in a given installation, not only was the carrier rate reduced to negligible levels, but also the effect on disease was almost instantaneous. This simple control measure was instituted as a routine in all military installations as well as in civilian populations with excessive numbers of cases or to prevent secondary cases within households.

All this came to an end in 1963[79] when such control measures seemed to have no impact on the occurrence of cases at the San Diego Naval Training Center. Investigation of this event led to the demonstration by Millar *et al.*[79] that resistance to sulfonamides was widespread throughout the United States in both military and civilian populations. Initially, this seemed to be limited to serogroup B and C meningococci, whereas group A infections that were occurring in Africa and in some parts of the Mediterranean Basin continued to be susceptible. However, in a widespread group A epidemic in Morocco,[1] the causative organisms were found to be significantly resistant to sulfadiazine. This was soon confirmed in other parts of the world and led to the recommendation that cases be treated with large doses of penicillin. This has proven to be successful. No suitable substitute for sulfadiazine has been identified for the control of carriers *and* the *prevention of disease,* although rifampin or minocycline or a combination thereof has been demonstrated to reduce carrier rates[24,27,81,96] (see Section 9.2).

5. Descriptive Epidemiology

5.1. Prevalence and Incidence

Information on prevalence and incidence is complicated by the multiplicity of serogroups of meningococci. Prevalence and incidence are more precisely stated and of greater value when serogroups are identified than when they are categorized under the generic term "meningococci." Jacobson *et al.*[65] reported that in the United States in

1974, there was 0.60 case/100,000 population per year. As noted in Fig. 1, this was a year of low incidence. Yet, despite this low incidence, the rates were 9.47 in infants less than 1 year old and 2.27 in children 1–4 years old.

In an active surveillance program sponsored by the Centers for Disease Control in 1978, the annual incidence of meningococcal meningitis in the United States was estimated to be 0.72 case/100,000 population. The peak age of meningococcal meningitis was 3–8 months (peak incidence 13/100,000). The peak age of meningococcemia was 6–8 months (peak incidence 5/100,000).[13]

5.2. Epidemic Behavior and Contagiousness

Glover,[44] in a classic report, concluded that carrier rates were most affected by "overcrowding" of sleeping arrangements. While "standard" accommodations in the British Army had been defined by a Royal Commission in 1861 as 60 ft² of floor space (600 ft³ of air space and 3-ft spacing between beds) per man, this was reduced to 40 ft² of floor space and 400 ft³ of air space soon after the outbreak of World War I because of mobilization pressures. At the end of the third year of the war, he found the space between beds in a distinguished unit to be less than 6 inches. Glover concluded that distances between beds were so important that he could predict the meningococcal carrier rate in a barracks by computing the distance between its beds. If the distance was 1 ft 4 inches, the carrier rate would be 10%. A slight decrease sent the carrier rate up to between

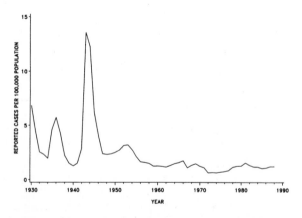

Figure 1. Meningococcal infections: rates by year, United States, 1930–1986. From the CDC.[16a]

10 and 20%. If the beds were closer than 1 ft, 20% was the rate, and if the distance was less than 9 inches, a carrier rate of 28–30% was to be expected. When the recommended distance was maintained, the carrier rate rarely exceeded 5%.

"Overcrowding" (defined as less than 40 ft² per man) was soon followed by a sharp rise in the carrier rate, reaching its maximum in about 2 weeks. The rise was accompanied by an increase in the proportion of epidemic carrier strains. The increase of this rate among noncontact carriers to 20% meant that an outbreak was imminent. The high carrier rates could be reduced, although not as quickly as they had increased, by increasing the space between beds to 2½ ft or more. Thus, he concluded that "to raise the carrier rate by overcrowding was both easier and quicker than to diminish it by spacing out."

In the devastating epidemic of 5885 cases that occurred in Santiago, Chile, during 1941–1942, Pizzi[92] reported that in the area of the city where the epidemic was concentrated, the population density was 7 persons per room and 2.9 per bed. The secondary attack rate overall was 2.5%, but it was 3.9% for those under 15 years of age and 1.5% among those more than 15. This experience tended to support Glover's observations.

Various studies have been reported by other authors in which no cases were seen when carrier rates were high[28] or cases were seen when carrier rates were low. Perhaps a key observation was supplied by Schoenbach,[95] who cultured 200 men in a military unit three times a week for 10 weeks. While the carrier rate averaged 41% during this period, 91% were identified at some time to be carriers. Similar, but unpublished, observations were made by Dr. Harry A. Feldman in conjunction with colleagues at the Fourth Service Command Medical Laboratory at Fort Mc-Pherson, Georgia, during the same period.

A source of great puzzlement for public-health workers, epidemiologists, and microbiologists who have studied epidemics of meningococcal disease over the years has been the apparent discontinuous pattern of disease occurrence. Arkwright,[3] in a truly remarkable albeit much neglected report, concluded:

> The large number and widespread distribution of carriers and the small number of cases of meningitis compared to the population forces upon one the view that for a true understanding of an epidemic of meningitis, the total number of persons who harbour the meningococcus should be looked upon as constituting the true epidemic . . . the carriers constitute the mass of the epidemic, and those who subsequently develop meningitis are only a small

accidental minority. The cases of meningitis, on account of the severity and fatality of this complication, give to the epidemic its importance, and they necessarily bulk largely in the eyes of the clinician . . . a consideration of all the evidence about carriers leads to the conclusion that the statement that cases of meningitis occur when and where carriers of the meningococcus become numerous, is a more correct way of stating the facts than by saying that many carriers occur in the neighbourhood of cases of meningitis.

The meningococcal situation parallels that of poliomyelitis, in which paralytic cases seemed to occur without rhyme or reason until the presence and importance of the nonparalytic individual was established. It was then determined that only about 1 in 100 infected individuals developed paralytic disease.[87] Maxcy[76] concluded that a similar rate occurred in meningococcal infections.

The key to the occurrence of an epidemic is the carrier or acquisition incidence rate. This has to be rapid for an epidemic to happen, since many individuals must acquire the organism for the relatively few cases to occur. It is the concentration of the latter that defines the presence of an epidemic. The key question remains, namely, what initiates the transmission speed-up in a population that results in increased numbers of cases and an epidemic? While the carrier state may persist for months,[52,93] the period of communicability is unknown.

It would seem logical to infer that if there were *no* carriers, there would be no cases. This concept led many to investigate the effectiveness of sulfonamides for the elimination of the carrier state, since it had been observed early in the research on sulfadiazine treatment that organisms disappeared rapidly from the posterior nasopharynx.[17,18,51,69,95] Typical of reports confirming this effective measure was that of Kuhns *et al.*[69] A simple 2-g dose[95] reduced the carrier rate to near zero, but the effect was prolonged when such treatment was maintained for 2–3 days. Cases disappeared just as promptly.

During World War II, an epidemic in the military was defined as the occurrence of 1 or more cases/10,000 per week.[42]

United States rates for the 55 years from 1930 to 1984 are summarized by 5-year averages per 100,000 population in Table 1. The epidemic that accompanied World War II can be readily seen, as can the relative increases noted during the Korean and Vietnam conflicts. The latter two reflect recruit outbreaks primarily, while the World War II increase was noted both in the military and in civilians, worldwide.

Table 1.   Average 5-Year U.S. Rates per 100,000 of Meningococcal Infections[a]

Years	Rate
1930–1934	3.596
1935–1939	3.655
1940–1944	6.308
1945–1949	3.407
1950–1954	2.867
1955–1959[b]	1.602
1960–1964	1.286
1965–1969	1.434
1970–1974	0.8479
1975–1979	0.9369
1980–1984	1.274

[a] Compiled from the CDC.[14,16]
[b] Alaska was included beginning in 1958; Hawaii, beginning in 1959.

5.3. Geographic Distribution

Meningococcal infections are limited to humans and have been noted throughout the world in either small circumscribed concentrations[85] of cases or widespread areas[7,36,54,55,62] involving whole countries (Brazil) or geographically large areas such as sub-Sahara Africa.[72] In 1948–1950, there was an epidemic of 92,964 cases with 14,273 deaths in northern Nigeria.[64]

5.4. Temporal Distribution

Sporadic endemic cases of meningococcal infections are encountered throughout the world at all times. Outbreaks tend to occur in various places for no discernible reason(s). On occasion, epidemics break out almost simultaneously in different places with no apparent connection with each other.

In tropical areas, especially sub-Sahara Africa, cases are most often seen during dry seasons, perhaps because changes in sleeping arrangements accompany the regression of the rainy season. In the cooler temperate zones, outbreaks tend to be clustered in the winter and spring months.[25] In the United States the peak incidence of meningococcal disease is in the late winter and early spring (February through May) and the lowest incidence is from July through October.

5.5. Age

Basically, meningitis is a childhood disease most often seen under age 15.[65,67] Beeson and Westerman,[6] in a study of 3575 British cases, found that 45.5% occurred in children under 15. In the great Detroit epidemic,[84] children under 15 made up 60% of the patients, while in the German epidemic of 1905–1907, 80% were under 15.[6] Recent U.S. data confirm that the age-related predisposition still exists and that the peak incidence is from age 1 month to 1 year (Table 2).

5.6. Sex

As is true of other severe diseases, males are more often subject to meningitis than are females. In the Beeson and Westerman[6] study, the male/female ratio was 6:4, but fatalities were more frequent in females. The excess of males persisted through age 50. This preponderance was also noted in the Detroit civilian outbreak.[84] Since military forces in the past have consisted predominantly of males, an excess prevalence of males is to be expected. Thus, in time of war, one should expect male cases to predominate, especially among recruits.

In a longitudinal study of meningococcal carriage in a population of "normal" families, it was found[52] that males 20 or older were more likely than adult females to become carriers.

Table 2.   Annual Age-Specific Incidence of Meningococcal Meningitis, United States, 1978–1981[a]

Age	Rate[b]
< 1 month	2.0
1–2 months	9.1
3–5 months	11.5
6–8 months	10.6
9–11 months	7.9
1–2 years	3.8
3–4 years	1.8
5–9 years	0.7
10–19 years	0.6

[a] Adapted from Klein et al.[67]
[b] Cases of meningococcal meningitis per 100,000 population.

5.7. Race

Race seems to be of little significance for either the acquisition or the severity of infections, except that those with sickling disease may be more prone to fatal infections, as they are to those caused by other polysaccharide-encapsulated bacteria. In a review of deaths from bacterial meningitis in the United States from 1962 to 1968,[39] it was concluded that excessive deaths from this cause were noted among blacks and American Indians. Race *per se* is not mentioned as a risk factor, but poverty and crowding are. In a population-based study in Charleston County, South Carolina, neither race nor income affected the risk for meningococcal meningitis.[41]

5.8. Occupation

Pike,[91] in an exhaustive review of laboratory-associated infections, records two such fatalities. In 1918, an employee of the State Serum Institute, Copenhagen, Denmark, whose job was concerned with the production of antimeningococcal serum, died of meningococcal meningitis. Another, an employee of the National Institutes of Health, while injecting an animal with meningococci, had some of the syringe's contents sprayed into her eyes as the animal struggled. She became ill 4 days later and died after 4 days of illness.

While these two cases indicate a potential occupational hazard, symptomatic infections with this organism are exceedingly rare. Nonetheless, it is prudent that laboratory personnel receive the available vaccine before taking up their work assignments. Both fatal cases reported above also occurred before the availability of potent therapy. The therapy available currently is so effective that given adequate warning, promptly instituted treatment should be beneficial and favorable.

There are no other identifiable occupational hazards except for military recruits during periods of mobilization, who seem to have a special susceptibility that becomes manifest in outbreaks among them. Despite great fears and expressed anxieties, physicians and nurses tend not to be excessively susceptible either to sporadic cases or during outbreaks. Arkwright[3] stated:

> It is almost universally accepted that doctors and hospital nurses seldom contract the disease. These and similar facts which have been observed in many epidemics are evidence against the spread of the disease being usually due to direct infection from one patient to another.

This concept has been modified in the present era by two new therapeutic procedures. Several cases of meningococcal disease have occurred among physicians who gave mouth-to-mouth resuscitation to patients severely affected by such infections. One of the authors (H.A.F.) was involved in the study of at least one case in which infection was apparently transferred with a kidney transplanted from an undiagnosed fatal case to a susceptible recipient.

5.9. Occurrence in Different Settings

The most predictable outbreaks are those that accompany increased military mobilization and the induction of large numbers of recruits such as were noted in World Wars I and II and the Korean and Vietnamese mobilizations in the United States. The most extensive and largest outbreaks in this century were those in civilians in sub-Sahara Africa and in Brazil. While more than a quarter of a million cases occurred in the latter, even under such conditions, outbreaks are spotty and concentrated in the poor and crowded[81,92]; e.g., during the Vietnamese mobilization, extensive outbreaks occurred among U.S. Army and Navy recruits, while the Air Force and Marines experienced only sporadic cases and were spared the major epidemics that affected the other two services. One would assume that the induction system being what it is, susceptibles would have been distributed more or less equally among all four services. Cases were almost unknown among female recruits, but there were many fewer of them and their housing conditions were relatively uncrowded.

Daniels *et al.*[22] reported that whereas a third of the troops at Fort Bragg, North Carolina, had less than 3 months of service, 59% of all patients with meningococcal infections were in this category. In other places, as many as 90% of cases were reported among recruits with less than 90 days of service. In the military, then, meningococcal infections represent a disease of recruits, whereas among seasoned troops or cadres in training, only sporadic cases are likely to be seen.[42] These are probably the result of specific antibody deficiencies.[47] A similar situation has been noted among South African miners, who represent a young population in whom meningococcal infections tend to occur early in their employment in the mines. Those who reenlist for a second tour of service are seldom troubled by this disease.

Outbreaks may also be noted on occasion in institutions such as jails, mental asylums, residential schools, and other closed populations. They are quite uncommon in day-care centers or other infant-care facilities except when the community at large is involved.

5.10. Socioeconomic Factors

Outbreaks among civilians tend to occur among the poor, especially those overcrowded, ill-housed, and ill-fed.[92] In the great Brazilian epidemic of the 1970s, cases were concentrated in the barrios and typically were unusual among the middle and upper classes. Thus, even within cities, cases are often localized and confined to small areas rather than spread among the community as a whole.

5.11. Other Factors

The principal factors that seem to be related to the occurrence of meningococcal infections are climatic conditions. In the sub-Sahara area, the change from the wet to the dry season tends to lead to an increase in cases. The reason for this relationship is unknown, although Belcher et al.[7] are of the opinion that considerably more population mixing takes place during the dry season, when farming work is reduced and more time is available for socializing and visiting. Also, there is a shift from sleeping outdoors to sleeping indoors in crowded and poorly ventilated rooms. In northern Ghana, the peak occurrence of cases comes during the dry season, when there is little rainfall, low humidity, and cold nights. Since this is the time when food becomes scarcer, it is popularly known as the "hunger season."

Despite much effort, familial and genetic factors have not been found to play a significant role in the acquisition of meningococcal disease except among those who lack one of the terminal complement components.[89] Such persons often have multiple disease episodes.

6. Mechanisms and Routes of Transmission

Transmission of meningococcal infections is usually assumed to be by way of droplets, regardless of the clinical status of the individual. Organisms are present in almost pure culture in the posterior nasopharynx. Thus, direct transmission may occur during mouth-to-mouth resuscitation, by the transfer of infected blood, as an accidental needle puncture from a contaminated syringe, or by organ transplant. Nosocomial transmission, while probably very rare, was documented by Cohen et al.[19] in New Haven, Connecticut. At a time when two patients on a cancer ward developed Group Y meningococcal infections, the preva-

lence of asymptomatic pharyngeal carriage of Group Y strains was 10% among other patients on the ward. The carriage prevalence was significantly lower in ward workers and casual visitors. Spread was presumably due to inhaled aerosols.

Acute, purulent meningococcal urethritis[12] has been reported increasingly in recent years along with more frequent reports of isolations of meningococci from the cervix[9,94] and other unusual areas.[30,32,33,43,56,60,71,80,82] How often these reflect sexual activity, or generalized infection, is unclear. It has been suggested that cervical acquisitions may be related to orogenital sex, or perhaps transmitted by a male with meningococcal urethritis, or the result of generalized dissemination during mild meningococcemia. Whether direct cervical implantation leads to clinical systemic disease is unknown.

6.1. Secondary Attack Rate

Considerable confusion has surrounded the calculation and interpretation of secondary attack rates of meningococcal disease. Norton and Gordon,[84] in their study of the meningococcal epidemic of 1929 in Detroit, found among the 724 cases of meningitis 32 (4.4%) additional cases in households. Among these additional cases, they believed that 2 could be eliminated completely, leading to the conclusion that there had been 30 secondary household cases. In the Santiago, Chile epidemic, Pizzi[92] calculated the secondary attack rate to be 3.9% for those less than 15 years of age and 1.5% for those older than 15. For all ages during this epidemic of 5885 cases, the secondary attack rate was 2.5%. During the massive Brazilian epidemic, a study[66] conducted among classmates of children who had meningococcal disease was interpreted as indicating that classroom exposure to cases did not increase the risk of acquiring meningococcal meningitis. The authors concluded that such exposure was an insufficient indication for prophylactic chemotherapy.

The Meningococcal Disease Surveillance Group[78] analyzed 326 cases reported in the United States from November 1973 through March 1974. Three household members manifested meningococcal disease following initial cases in their homes, a secondary attack rate of approximately 3/1000 household members. Among 293 households for whom follow-up data were available, 4 had two cases and none had more than two. In this study, it seems that the label "coprimary" was applied to cases with onset on the same day. In 107 households in which no chemoprophylaxis was administered to any household members, the secondary attack rate was 2.2/1000. The authors concluded that a secondary attack rate of 2–4/1000 is still a thousand times greater than the overall reported rate of 0.23/100,000 of meningococcal disease in the states with the cases studied. What is not clear here is whether a distinction is drawn between secondary and coprimary cases, as was attempted by Leedom *et al.*[73] in a 3-year study of Los Angeles County cases. There were 290 different families, 3.4% of which had more than one case. From a sample of these cases, it was determined that the average number of people residing in the same household with each patient was 3.71. The risk of multiple cases among household contacts of patients was estimated to be 992/100,000. The 3-year case average (1963–1965) for Los Angeles County was 2.09/100,000. One household had three cases.

The onset of disease was basically simultaneous among all family members except for three in which the cases were separated by 5, 7, and 9 days. The remainder, then, would be considered to have been coprimary cases.

What, then, are the implications of using these different designations, or is it solely a matter of semantics?

The incubation period for meningococcal disease varies from 2 to 10 days, commonly 3–4 days.[8] Bolduan and Goodwin,[10] in a 1905 study in New York City, identified 88 instances where there was more than one case in a house. Among 58 of these, the interval between the index and second case was 7 days in 14 and 2 weeks to 3 months in 16. Norton[83] stated that among 6416 household contacts of 1272 cases, there were 36 homes with more than one case. In 3, two persons became ill the same day, and in another, there were four simultaneous onsets. The latter had a fifth case sometime later. Norton calculated that while 3.6% of homes had additional cases after their first, there were 46 (0.7%) secondary cases among 6416 contacts. Of these 46, 20 had their onsets within 4 days and 14 within the next 5 days, or 34 (74%) within 9 days of the index patient. Thus, with an incubation period up to 10 days, most of these "secondary" cases are really coprimary. In contrast, Jacobson *et al.*[66] defined a secondary case as "the onset of illness more than 24 hours and less than 31 days after onset of another case in the same classroom."

7. Pathogenesis and Immunity

Meningococci are generally transmitted via droplets or through close oral contact. The organisms have a predilection for the posterior nasopharynx and can often be obtained in almost pure culture from that area. It was believed for a long time that the bacteria penetrated to the central nervous system through the cribriform plate, but there is no real evidence for this. Dingle and Finland[25] summarized the evidence for and against this concept and decided, as had most observers, that dissemination from the posterior nasopharynx is via the bloodstream. Once the bloodstream has been entered, a variety of consequences may follow, leading to various clinical expressions.[36] These may run the gamut from mild, self-limited bacteremia—which may or may not be accompanied by low-grade fever, a pinkish, maculopapular rash, arthralgias with malaise, and muscle pains—to overwhelming sepsis with a coalescing, extensive petechial rash that may lead to large areas of necrosis. Disseminated intravascular coagulation (DIC), meningitis, septic arthritis, epididymitis, myocarditis, conjunctivitis, adrenal collapse (Waterhouse–Friderichsen syndrome), and death within an hour or two may follow. Fortunately, it is only the rare individual who falls into this latter category. What there is about such individuals that makes them especially susceptible to such severe disease manifestations is unknown, but they arouse the greatest interest and serve to direct attention to the disease. Probably as many as 90% of those who acquire meningococci have infections that are limited to the posterior nasopharynx with, occasionally perhaps, self-limited bacteremia. Whether infection limited to the posterior nasopharynx leads to clinical signs has been debated for decades and remains unresolved. Unfortunately, most such studies have been performed among military recruits, who are notorious for the amount of bacterial, mycoplasmal, and viral upper-respiratory infections that they support. Each of these agents would have to be excluded before one could conclude that meningococci are producing the reference symptoms. It is the prevalence of posterior nasopharyngeal infections and the paucity of clinical disease that complicate our understanding of the epidemiology of these diseases. That relationship led Arkwright[3] to conclude that epidemics basically affect the nasopharynx and that cases of meningitis and other complications are incidental. This also explains the apparent indiscriminate occurrence of clinical disease and the lack of evidence for direct connections between cases.

Immunity has been studied extensively only during the past two decades. Serum antibodies have been demonstrated by a variety of techniques, including radioimmunoassay (RIA),[59] bactericidal,[47,101] hemagglutination,[50] agglutination,[77,101] and others. Immunity is group-specific and is acquired as the result of infection even when this seems to have been limited to the posterior nasopharynx.[49,101] Thus, the carrier state can induce immunity to the serogroup of the organism carried. The presence of bactericidal antibodies correlates well with protection from disease.[47,49] Since these antibodies are free in the circulation, their protective value supports well the concept that the bloodstream plays the important role in the dissemination of meningococci.

An alternative hypothesis for the role of antibody, in military recruits, has been proposed by Griffiss.[57] He has found antimeningococcal IgA in the acute sera of military recruits who had meningococcal disease. This IgA was able to inhibit the lytic function IgM in sera. Removal of IgA made sera that appeared to lack bactericidal antibody functionally lytic. Thus, it is Griffiss's contention that susceptibility, in addition to being defined by the *absence* of functional antibody, may be due, in some cases, to the presence of blocking IgA.[57] The role of this mechanism, if any, in civilian endemic disease is unknown.

8. Patterns of Host Response

Inapparent infections play an important role in meningococcal disease because they constitute the majority and account for the bulk of carriers. As has been expressed previously, the acquisition of the carrier state leads to immunity[47,101] and thus protection against the disease itself. We have no information as to why, among children, an occasional individual is unable to restrict the acquired meningococci to the posterior nasopharynx and becomes the victim of a life-threatening disease episode. Among adults, deficiency of lytic antibody appears to be the major predisposing factor accounting for biological susceptibility to meningococcal disease. The reason why a small number of adults lack antibody is unknown. Either they were never colonized or colonization did not result in the production of a long-lasting antibody response.

8.1. Clinical Features

Meningococcal infections may manifest themselves clinically by several different syndromes. These may overlap or be noted sequentially in the same patient. The most common occurrence is represented by the asymptomatic acquisition of meningococci in the posterior nasopharynx or the carrier state. While there are some who believe that an acute pharyngitis may be clinically manifest in this stage, this has never really been proven and, while only a possibility, may account for as much as 90% or more of all acquisitions. Thus, disease as such is limited to less than 10% of those who acquire meningococci. The next stage may be that of a mild, self-limited bacteremia that may be accompanied by an evanescent rubellalike rash, arthralgias,

fever, malaise, and myalgias. A blood culture taken at this time is often positive for meningococci. This may regress completely or for several days, only to be followed by an explosive onset of severe illness. This is generally heralded or accompanied by a severe petechial rash that may be very extensive and coalescent, with large areas of necrotic skin and muscle. Similar lesions probably occur in the deeper viscera.

Prostration and shock may follow in short order, with death close behind. Smears made from petechial lesions or from the buffy coat of peripheral blood may contain gram-negative diplococci within or without cells. This is the most devastating form of the infection, in which septicemia is so severe and overwhelming that it often kills before there is localization in the CNS, joints, or other organs.

A less virulent form of septicemia is more common, and while this too is identifiable with a petechial rash, progression is slower and permits other complications to become evident. These patients often are the cases with meningitis, septic arthritis, epididymitis, pneumonitis with pneumonia, conjunctivitis, and myocarditis. All these may occur in a single patient, or in any combination thereof. In infants, "mild" meningococcemia may present with fever as the only symptom. This presentation of meningococcemia is very similar to that of occult pneumococcemia, which occurs more frequently than meningococcemia in ambulatory pediatric patients.[5]

Discrete meningococcal pneumonia has been reported with increasing frequency in recent years, especially from the military. Group Y meningococcus has often been implicated in this form of infection.[68]

Koppes *et al.*[68] reported on 88 cases of Group Y meningococcal disease in Air Force recruits, 68 of whom had primary bacterial pneumonia. All but one did well with penicillin therapy. It is possible that the predominance of Group Y in these cases reflected immunization with Group C polysaccharide vaccine, which had been instituted as a routine procedure in the Air Force.

Other instances of Group Y meningococcal pneumonia have been reported, but whether this indicates a special proclivity of organisms of this serogroup remains questionable because the data are still inadequate. In the study by Koppes *et al.*,[68] 52 of 64 individuals sampled had pure cultures of Group Y meningococci in transtracheal aspirates. In the remainder, growth was due primarily to Group Y meningococci, with relatively small amounts of contaminants such as α streptococci, *Haemophilus influenzae* type b, and others. Primary meningococcal pneumonia, either alone or in concert with other evidence of septic meningococcal infections, has been reported often enough to constitute a disease entity, establishment of the identity of which should be sought in cases of otherwise undefined pneumonia.

Group Y meningococcal infections have also occurred in children.[5,63,98] Pneumonia was reported in one case.[98] Group W-135, which has increased in incidence in the past decade, has also been reported to have a varied presentation in children, similar to other serogroups.[58,61]

There is an unusual and infrequently seen form of the disease that is identified as chronic meningococcemia. This may be a manifestation of subacute bacterial endocarditis or the result of continuous seeding into the bloodstream from an unknown nidus. Such patients may go for weeks or months with recurring fever and evanescent rashes, as either pink macules or small petechiae. They respond rapidly to treatment and are often cured by penicillin administered for other reasons, such as a suspected infectious cause of the fever, malaise, and rash.

Petersen et al.[89] summarized information from various reports of 24 patients who had had *recurrent* episodes of meningococcal or (generalized) gonorrheal infections. Their distinguishing characteristic is that they lack one or more of the late components of the complement system: C6, C7, or C8. Of the 24 patients, 6 were deficient in either C6 or C7 and 8 in C8. In all, 13 of the 24 had had either *N. meningitidis* or *N. gonorrhoeae* bacteremia, and all recovered. The patient with C7 deficiency apparently recovered from four episodes of meningococcal meningitis. The frequency of this abnormality is unknown, but it would seem that while the propensity to have recurrent neisserial infections is present in such individuals, the disease does not appear to be overwhelming or fatal, since so many seem to have recovered. The deficiency is interesting and should be suspected whenever recurrent meningococcal disease is noted.

Ellison et al. studied 20 adults with a *first* episode of meningococcal infection. Six of them had a complement deficiency. Of these six, three had a specific terminal component deficiency and three had multiple component deficiencies due to an underlying illness.[29] In children, the prevalence of underlying complement deficiency in those with one meningococcal infection was 18% in one study.[70]

Corfield[21] may have recorded the first such case in 1945 and suggests another, seen by Boudin, in whom three episodes occurred in 1849, 1850, and 1851. These cases are to be separated from the recurrent disease that was encountered before modern therapy prevented the frequent bacterial relapses common to that era. Patients who have recurrent disseminated neisserial disease should be screened with CH_{50} assays, and if they are positive, specific deficiencies should be sought.

8.2. Diagnosis

As is true of many diseases, the frequency of the diagnosis of meningitis often reflects the observer's index of suspicion. The carrier state is not diagnosable except by culture and is of little importance except under some very special circumstances. In the case of expressed disease, diagnosis generally requires laboratory confirmation. With this in mind, blood cultures should be obtained as quickly as possible. If there are clinical signs of meningitis, an immediate lumbar or spinal puncture is mandatory, followed by prompt examination of the fluid. Its cellular content should be ascertained as to type and number. Sugar and protein should be measured. (It is well to determine the comparative blood sugar at the same time.) A Gram stain should be performed on a smear made from the fluid if the fluid is cloudy, but if it is clear, it should be spun and a thick, stained smear made from the residual drop after the supernate is decanted. Fluid should be cultured on chocolate agar in an atmosphere of increased CO_2. If organisms are visible in the direct smear, it is well to mix a small volume with specific grouping antiserum. Organisms of groups A and C usually have good capsules in spinal fluid, and mixing with specific antiserum may lead to their "Quellung" or swelling. This is a specific reaction that can provide definitive identification. A sensitive modification of this procedure was described by Thomas et al.[101]

Additionally, Gram stains of smears of fluid from petechial lesions or buffy coats of peripheral blood may also yield gram-negative diplococci. If these are present, then they are most likely meningococci. The peripheral white blood count is usually elevated, but in severely ill patients, it may be less than $4000/mm^3$. A culture of the posterior nasopharynx on Thayer–Martin chocolate agar is indicated on admission for all patients with a suspected diagnosis of meningococcal disease.

Because of the nature of the rash and the clinically severe illness, the diagnosis may be confused with Rocky Mountain spotted fever. Less severe cases may be confused with endemic typhus and, when very mild, even with rubella.

9. Control and Prevention

9.1. General Concepts

Because cases of meningococcal disease tend to be distributed indiscriminately in a population and because death may be sudden, the appearance of a case frequently leads to generalized hysteria in the associated population, whether it be open or closed. Outbreaks tend to occur in closed groups such as institutions, recruit military camps, and crowded, impoverished districts of major cities.[86,92] As with poliomyelitis, cases do not seem to lead to other cases, an observation that understandably tends to increase fear and hysteria among the populace in which the cases occur.

Sporadic cases of meningococcal disease occur throughout the year in all places. They often appear as isolated instances for reasons that are not understood. More incomprehensibly, cases may begin to occur in rapid succession in a given population. These are usually closed, institutionalized settings, but numerous cases may be noted in the community at large and constitute an epidemic.

9.2. Antibiotic and Chemotherapeutic Approaches to Prophylaxis: Suggestions for the Management of Outbreaks

Before rational intervention can be instituted or attempted when it is suspected that excessive cases of meningococcal disease are occurring, two important questions must be answered. First, can the affected population be defined; second, what are the characteristics of the causative agent? In respect to the latter, is it of a single serogroup, and most important, is the predominant organism sulfonamide-sensitive or -resistant?

If the affected population can be reasonably well defined, and if only one meningococcal serogroup accounts for most of the cases, and is sulfonamide-sensitive (i.e., susceptible to ≤ 0.1 mg/100 ml of sulfadiazine), then the quickest, simplest, and most effective way to institute control is to provide each member of the population at risk with sulfadiazine for 2 consecutive days. In the case of adults and older children, this should be 1.0 g every 12 h for four doses. For infants and children up to the adult size of 70 kg, the recommended dose is 125–150 mg/kg per day divided into four equal doses on each of 2 consecutive days. In these dosages and with the further precaution that the drug not be administered to individuals with histories of previous sulfonamide reactions, the drug is safe and exceedingly effective. The carrier rate may be expected to drop to near zero almost immediately, slowly rebuilding itself over a period of weeks. Cases also stop occurring as the carrier rate diminishes. It is required, for maximum benefit, that treatment be simultaneous for the total target population.

If the causative organism is sulfonamide-resistant, then there are still two options. One is to attempt chemoprophylaxis with drugs other than sulfonamides; the other is to attempt to immunize the population with a polysaccha-ride vaccine. The latter is feasible only if the causative organisms are of serogroups A, C, Y, or W-135. The licensed vaccine contains the polysaccharides of Groups A, C, Y, and W-135, and only a single dose is required. When the vaccine is used, it must be anticipated that maximum beneficial effects will be noted after 10–14 days, although diminution in the severity of the disease in some cases may be observed by the 7th day.

The other drugs that have been used for meningococcal prophylaxis, and that were alluded to in Section 4, are rifampin and minocycline.[96] In the case of rifampin, the recommended dose for adults is 600 mg twice daily for four doses, but in children 1–12 years of age, this should be reduced to 10 mg/kg for four doses. In infants less than 1 year of age, this dose should be reduced to half, or 5 mg/kg every 12 h, for four doses. For minocycline, the recommended dose is 100 mg every 12 h for 5 days.[96] In several studies with minocycline, vestibular reactions have been an annoying problem,[27,81] sometimes resulting in early withdrawal of the drug. Therefore, prophylaxis of appropriately close contacts has been recommended, using rifampin if the case strain is not known to be susceptible to sulfonamides.[100]

Resistance to rifampin has been noted in as many as one fourth of strains. This proportion increased with each repeated course of the drug. It should be borne in mind that there are no data on the therapeutic effectiveness of either minocycline or rifampin, and thus neither should be used for treatment.[37] In the case of sulfadiazine, part of its effectiveness may be related to its efficiency as a therapeutic agent, so that even small doses may effect cures of mild bacteremias. It cannot be emphasized too much that knowledge of the sulfonamide-resistance pattern of the offending organism(s) and the predominant serogroup present in the target population is an essential requirement for the intelligent management of suspected outbreaks.

9.3. Immunization

Gotschlich, Artenstein, and their colleagues,[47,49,50] in the search for an effective alternative to sulfonamide prevention of meningococcal disease, successfully reopened the investigation of vaccines, an approach that had lain dormant for a quarter of a century. In a series of publications beginning with the demonstration of the importance of serum antibodies in protection against the disease,[47] the effectiveness of pure carbohydrate antigens[49,50] in stimulating specific immunity against infection with organisms of the various serogroups, and finally the value of such antigenic stimulation in providing protection against the disease during epidemic periods was probably the most important contribution to the meningococcal problem in this century. Subsequently, Group A meningococcal vaccine was used in the management of large epidemics of disease in Finland,[75] Brazil,[86] and Egypt.[103]

Greenwood et al.[53] evaluated the effectiveness of Group A vaccine in preventing secondary cases when administered to household contacts of Group A cases and found the secondary attack rate to be 18/1000 among control household contacts who received tetanus toxoid. Among the 520 case contacts who had received Group A meningococcal vaccine, there was only one instance of meningococcal disease. The efficacy of the Group A meningococcal vaccine was clearly demonstrated in the trial of Peltola et al. in Finland in 1974–1975.[88] In two trials conducted during an epidemic of Group A meningococcal disease, 49,295 and 21,007 children, aged 3 months to 5 years, received the vaccine. None developed Group A meningococcal disease. In the first trial there were two control groups that had significantly more cases than the vaccine group.

Despite the Finnish experience, there is good evidence that in children the degree of antibody response to the Group A and C vaccine, measured as the concentration of anticapsular antibody in the serum, is proportional to age. Children under 1 year of age have a poor response and no immunological memory.[45,46] It is not until 2 years of age that there is sufficient maturation of the immune system for there to be a protective antibody response to Group C polysaccharide, although the response to the Group A polysaccharide appears to occur earlier.[45,46]

Initially, meningococcal vaccine was marketed for civilian use as 50 μg of Group A polysaccharide, 50 μg of Group C polysaccharide, or a combination of both. Recently, a quadrivalent vaccine consisting of 50 μg each of Group A, C, Y, and W-135 capsular polysaccharides has been shown to be safe and immunogenic and has been licensed (MenomuneR, manufactured by Connaught Laboratories, Swiftwater, Pa.).[15] After Group B, the commonest, these four are the most common Groups causing meningococcal disease in the United States. No vaccine for Group B has been produced because the B polysaccharide is not immunogenic. Despite extensive research into production of a nonpolysaccharide vaccine or a polysaccharide conjugated with another immunogen, there is no candidate Group B vaccine, at this time.

A single dose of vaccine is sufficient to immunize a child over 2 years of age or an adult. Adverse reactions have not presented a problem, generally being limited to local erythema or soreness or both, usually persisting for no more than 24 h.[74] Reactions are more likely to increase with repeated doses of polysaccharide, which are not required and should be discouraged. While there was some problem originally with stability and persistence of antigenicity, these problems have largely been solved with manufacturing modifications currently in use. One of the difficulties in the production of this vaccine was that it is essentially not immunogenic in animals other than man and therefore must be standardized in humans.

Protection conveyed by vaccines requires about 7 days before noticeable benefits are observed. The initial effect is that of modification of the illness so as to reduce mortality; total protection from disease requires approximately 14 days after inoculation. In various trials, the effectiveness level has been calculated to be in the vicinity of 90%.[4,103] Antibody responses have been found to persist for at least 5 years[4] and may be expected to last much longer in further studies.

9.3.1. Application. Except during World War II, the incidence of meningococcal disease in the U.S. general population has been too low to warrant wide-scale immunization with the available meningococcal vaccines. In the United States, demonstrated Group A infections have been very rare since the end of World War II, while Groups B and C have provided most of the interim cases. Over the past decade, Groups Y and W-135 have emerged as common where previously they had been rare.

On the other hand, the 4-year Brazilian epidemic[86] of the 1970s resulted in more than a quarter of a million cases. In the first 2 years, this was essentially a Group C epidemic that then became a Group A outbreak. A massive countrywide immunization campaign was undertaken, which eventually meant that more than 80 million persons received bivalent A and C, or monovalent A or C, vaccines. This brought the epidemic to a close, and it has not recurred. In Finland, a large outbreak in the military, accompanied by many civilian cases, was also treated with vaccine and was soon brought under control.[75]

When, then, should vaccine be expected to be effective? Meningococcal diseases represent a serious health hazard for military recruits, especially during periods of increased mobilization. Thus, since the early 1970s all recruits entering the United States military have received a single dose of Group C, A/C, or more recently A/C/Y/W-135 vaccine with evident benefit. In the light of extensive past experience, it would seem prudent to continue this policy for recruits entering the military in all its branches.

Usage in civilians is more limited. Since current vaccines are only protective when given at over 2 years of age, and the great majority of civilian cases occur in younger children, routine vaccination is not recommended. Vaccination would seem to be indicated where localized or institutional outbreaks can be defined and the causative strain identified as either Group A, C, Y, or W-135. Usage to prevent secondary cases among close contacts is recommended by the Immunization Practices Advisory Committee of the CDC,[15] but is not recommended by the authors for sporadic cases because the overall risk is low and most such cases occur within less than 6 or at most 9–10 days of the index case. Thus, chemotherapeutic measures should be more effective, especially when the case strains are known to be sulfonamide-susceptible.

In addition, patients with functional or anatomic asplenia such as in sickle-cell disease, or traumatic rupture of the spleen, are prone to severe or fatal infections with polysaccharide-encapsulated bacteria. Individuals with deficiencies of the terminal complement components may also have recurrent meningococcal infections. Patients over 2 years of age who fit any of these categories should receive the current meningococcal vaccine as part of their preventive care.

10. Unresolved Problems

The greatest unresolved problems are the elucidation of the factors that lead to the occurrence of a case; i.e., of the many individuals who acquire meningococci, why do only so few (probably less than 10%) develop meningococcal disease? In parallel with this is the question of which factor or factors lead to the occurrence of an epidemic in a given locality or institution. Such epidemics arise suddenly and for no apparent reason persist for varying periods of time—days, weeks, months, or years—and then either disappear completely or are replaced by meningococci of another serogroup. Are the factors responsible for these fluxes changes in the pathogen, the host, or a combination of the two?

A major problem that has arisen as the result of the vast scientific progress noted during the last few years is that concerned with how best to utilize the available vaccines. This involves questions of optimal timing and the definition of the population that would benefit most from their use, as well as the definition of the conditions under which they achieve maximum effectiveness. Finally, we need new vaccines. Despite immunogenic preparations for adults, we lack vaccines for children under 2 years of age that will protect against the major serogroups, and while a vaccine for Group B *N. meningitidis* may be on the horizon, it is not yet here.

11. References

1. ALEXANDER, C. E., SANBORN, W. R., CHERRIERE, G., CROCKER, W. H., JR., EWALD, P. E., AND KAY, C. R., Sulfadiazine-resistant Group A *Neisseria meningitidis*, *Science* **161**:1019 (1968).
2. APICELLA, M. A., Lipopolysaccharide-derived serotype polysaccharides from *Neisseria meningitidis* Group B, *J. Infect. Dis.* **140**:62–72 (1979).
3. ARKWRIGHT, J. A., Cerebro-spinal meningitis: The interpretation of epidemiological observations by the light of bacteriological knowledge, *Br. Med. J.* **1**:494–496 (1915).
4. ARTENSTEIN, M. S., Control of meningococcal meningitis with meningococcal vaccines, *Yale J. Biol. Med.* **48**:197–200 (1975).
5. BALTIMORE, R. S., AND HAMMERSCHLAG, M., Meningococcal bacteremia: Clinical and serologic studies of infants with mild illness, *Am. J. Dis. Child.* **131**:1001–1004 (1977).
6. BEESON, P. B., AND WESTERMAN, E., Cerebrospinal fever: Analysis of 3,575 case reports with special reference to sulphonamide therapy, *Br. Med. J.* **1**:497–500 (1943).
7. BELCHER, D. W., SHERRIFF, A. C., NIMO, K. P., CHEW, G. L. N., VOROS, A., RICHARDSON, W. D., AND FELDMAN, H. A., Meningococcal meningitis in northern Ghana: Epidemiology and control measures, *Am. J. Trop. Med. Hyg.* **26**:748–755 (1977).
8. BENENSON, A. S., *Control of Communicable Diseases in Man*, 12th ed., p. 206, American Public Health Association, Washington, D.C., 1975.
9. BLACKWELL, C., YOUNG, H., AND BAIN, S. S. R., Isolation of *Neisseria meningitidis* and *Neisseria catarrhalis* from the genitourinary tract and anal canal, *Br. J. Vener. Dis.* **54**:41–44 (1978).
10. BOLDUAN, C., AND GOODWIN, M. E., A clinical and bacteriological study of the communicability of cerebrospinal meningitis and the probable source of contagion: Part I of an investigation of cerebrospinal meningitis carried out under the auspices of the special commission of the Department of Health of New York City, *Med. News* **87**:1222–1228, 1250–1257 (1905).
11. BRANHAM, S. E., Serological relationships among meningococci, *Bacteriol. Rev.* **17**:175–188 (1953).
12. CARPENTER, C. M., AND CHARLES, R., Isolation of meningococcus from the genitourinary tract of seven patients, *Am. J. Public Health* **32**:640–643 (1942).
13. Centers for Disease Control, Bacterial meningitis and meningococcemia—United States, 1978, *Morbid. Mortal. Weekly Rep.* **28**:277–279 (1979).
14. Centers for Disease Control, Reported morbidity and mortality in the United States, annual summary 1979, *Morbid. Mortal. Weekly Rep.* **28**:53–56 (1980).
15. Centers for Disease Control, Recommendation of the Immunization Practices Advisory Committee (ACIP): Meningococcal vaccines, *Morbid. Mortal. Weekly Rep.* **34**:255–259 (1985).

16. Centers for Disease Control, Annual summary 1984: Reported morbidity and mortality in the United States, *Morbid. Mortal. Weekly Rep.* **33**:38 (1986).

16a. Centers for Disease Control, Summary of Notifiable Diseases, United States, *Morbid. Mortal. Weekly Rep.* **35**:30 (1986).

17. CHEEVER, F. S., The control of meningococcal meningitis by mass chemoprophylaxis with sulfadiazine, *Am. J. Med. Sci.* **209**:74–75 (1945).

18. CHEEVER, F. S., BREESE, B. B., AND UPHAM, H. C., The treatment of meningococcus carriers with sulfadiazine, *Ann. Intern. Med.* **19**:602–608 (1943).

19. COHEN, M. S., STEERE, A. C., BALTIMORE, R. S., VON GRAEVENITZ, A., PANTELICK, E., CAMP, B., AND ROOT, R. A., Possible nosocomial transmission of Group Y *Neisseria meningitidis* among oncology patients, *Ann. Intern. Med.* **91**:7–12 (1979).

20. COHEN, R. L., AND ARTENSTEIN, M. S., Hemagglutination inhibition for serogrouping *Neisseria meningitidis*, *Appl. Microbiol.* **23**:289–292 (1972).

21. CORFIELD, W. F., Multiple attacks of cerebrospinal fever, *Lancet* **1**:402–403 (1945).

22. DANIELS, W. B., SOLOMON, S., AND JAQUETTE, W. A., JR., Meningococcic infections in soldiers, *J. Am. Med. Assoc.* **123**:1–9 (1943).

23. DANIELSON, L., AND MANN, E., The history of a singular and very mortal disease, which lately made its appearance in Medfield, *Med. Agric. Register* **1**:65–69 (1806).

24. DEVINE, L. F., JOHNSON, D. P., HAGERMAN, C. R., PIERCE, W. E., RHODE, S. L., III, AND PECKINPAUGH, R. O., The effect of minocycline on meningococcal nasopharyngeal carrier state in naval personnel, *Am. J. Epidemiol.* **93**:337–345 (1971).

25. DINGLE, J. H., AND FINLAND, M., Diagnosis, treatment and prevention of meningococcic meningitis, with a resume of the practical aspects of treatment of other acute bacterial meningitides, *War Med.* **2**:1–58 (1942).

26. DINGLE, J. H., THOMAS, L., AND MORTON, A. R., Treatment of meningococcic meningitis and meningococcemia with sulfadiazine, *J. Am. Med. Assoc.* **116**:2666–2668 (1941).

27. DREW, T. M., ALTMAN, R., BLACK, K., AND GOLDFIELD, M., Minocycline for prophylaxis of infection with *Neisseria meningitidis*: High rate of side effects in recipients, *J. Infect. Dis.* **133**:194–198 (1976).

28. DUDLEY, S. F., AND BRENNAN, J. R., High and persistent carrier rates of *Neisseria meningitidis*, unaccompanied by cases of meningitis, *J. Hyg.* **34**:525–541 (1934).

29. ELLISON, R. T., III, KOHLER, P. F., CURD, J. G., JUDSON, F. N., AND RELLER, L. B., Prevalence of congenital or acquired complement deficiency in patients with sporadic meningococcal disease, *N. Engl. J. Med.* **308**:914–916 (1983).

30. ESCHENBACH, D. A., BUCHANAN, T. M., POLLOCK, H. M., FORSYTH, P. S., ALEXANDER, E. R., LIN, J.-S., WANG, S.-P., WENTWORTH, B. B., MCCORMACK, W. M., AND HOLMES, K. K., Polymicrobial etiology of acute pelvic inflammatory disease, *N. Engl. J. Med.* **293**:166–171 (1975).

31. EVANS, J. R., ARTENSTEIN, M. S., AND HUNTER, D. H., Prevalence of meningococcal serogroups and description of three new groups, *Am. J. Epidemiol.* **87**:643–646 (1968).

32. FALLON, R. J., AND ROBINSON, E. T., Meningococcal vulvovaginitis, *Scand. J. Infect. Dis.* **6**:295–296 (1974).

33. FAUR, Y. C., WEISBURD, M. H., AND WILSON, M. E., Isolation of *Neisseria meningitidis* from the genito-urinary tract and canal, *J. Clin. Microbiol.* **2**:178–182 (1975).

34. FELDMAN, H. A., Sulfonamide-resistant meningococci, *Annu. Rev. Med.* **18**:495–506 (1967).

35. FELDMAN, H. A., Neisseria infections other than gonococcal, in: *Diagnostic Procedures for Bacterial, Mycotic and Parasitic Infections* (H. L. BODILY, E. L. UPDYKE, AND J. O. MASON, eds.), pp. 135–152, American Public Health Association, New York, 1970.

36. FELDMAN, H. A., Meningococcal infections, *Adv. Intern. Med.* **18**:117–140 (1972).

37. FELDMAN, H. A., Editorial comment, in: *Year Book of Pediatrics* (S. S. GELLIS, ed.), p. 81, Year Book Medical, Chicago, 1975.

38. FELDMAN, H. A., SWEET, L. K., AND DOWLING, H. F., Sulfadiazine therapy of purulent meningitis including its use in 24 consecutive patients with meningococcic meningitis, *War Med.* **2**:995–1007 (1942).

39. FELDMAN, R. A., KOEHLER, R. E., AND FRASER, D. W., Race-specific differences in bacterial meningitis deaths in the United States, 1962–1968, *Am. J. Public Health* **66**:392–396 (1976).

40. FRASCH, C. E., AND CHAPMAN, S. S., Classification of *Neisseria meningitidis* Group B into distinct serotypes. III. Application of a new bactericidal-inhibition technique to distribution of serotypes among cases and carriers, *J. Infect. Dis.* **127**:149–154 (1973).

41. FRASER, D. W., DARBY, C. P., KOEHLER, R. E., JACOBS, C. F., AND FELDMAN, R. A., Risk factors in bacterial meningitis: Charleston County, South Carolina, *J. Infect. Dis.* **127**:271–277 (1973).

42. GAULD, J. R., NITZ, R. E., HUNTER, D. H., RUST, J. H., AND GAULD, R. L., Epidemiology of meningococcal meningitis at Fort Ord, *Am. J. Epidemiol.* **82**:56–72 (1965).

43. GIVAN, K. F., THOMAS, B. W., AND JOHNSTON, A. G., Isolation of *Neisseria meningitidis* from the urethra, cervix, and anal canal: Further observations, *Br. J. Vener. Dis.* **53**:109–112 (1977).

44. GLOVER, J. A., Observations of the meningococcus carrier rate, and their application to the prevention of cerebrospinal fever, Medical Research Council of the Privy Council, Special Report Series, No. 50, pp. 133–165, H. M. Stationery Offices, London (1920).

45. GOLD, R., Polysaccharide meningococcal vaccines—Current status, *Hosp. Pract.* **14**:41–48 (1979).

46. GOLD, R., LEPOW, M. L., GOLDSCHNEIDER, I., DRAPER, T. L., AND GOTSCHLICH, E. C., Clinical evaluation of Group A

and Group C meningococcal polysaccharide vaccines in infants, *J. Clin. Invest.* **56:**1536–1547 (1975).

47. GOLDSCHNEIDER, I., GOTSCHLICH, E. C., AND ARTENSTEIN, M. S., Human immunity to the meningococcus. I. The role of humoral antibodies, *J. Exp. Med.* **129:**1307–1326 (1969).

48. GORDON, M. H., Identification of the meningococcus, *J. R. Army Med. Corps* **24:**455–458 (1915).

49. GOTSCHLICH, E. C., GOLDSCHNEIDER, I., AND ARTENSTEIN, M. S., Human immunity to the meningococcus. V. The effect of immunization with meningococcal Group C polysaccharide on the carrier state, *J. Exp. Med.* **129:**1385–1395 (1969).

50. GOTSCHLICH, E. C., LIU, T. Y., AND ARTENSTEIN, M. S., Human immunity to the meningococcus. III. Preparation and immunochemical properties of the Group A, Group B, and Group C meningococcal polysaccharides, *J. Exp. Med.* **129:**1349–1365 (1969).

51. GRAY, F. C., AND GEAR, J., Sulphapyridine, M and B 693, as a prophylactic against cerebrospinal meningitis, *S. Afr. Med. J.* **15:**139–140 (1941).

52. GREENFIELD, S., SHEEHE, P. R., AND FELDMAN, H. A., Meningococcal carriage in a population of "normal" families, *J. Infect. Dis.* **123:**67–73 (1971).

53. GREENWOOD, B. M., HASSAN-KING, M., AND WHITTLE, H. C., Prevention of secondary cases of meningococcal disease in household contacts by vaccination, *Br. Med. J.* **1:**1317–1319 (1978).

54. GREENWOOD, B. M., BRADLEY, A. K., CLELAND, P. G., HAGGIE, M. H. K., HASSAN-KING, M., LEWIS, L. S., MACFARLANE, J. T., TAQI, A., AND WHITTLE, H. C., An epidemic of meningococcal infection at Zaria, northern Nigeria. 1. General epidemiological features, *Trans. R. Soc. Trop. Med. Hyg.* **73:**557–562 (1979).

55. GREENWOOD, B. M., CLELAND, P. G., HAGGIE, M. H. K., LEWIS, L. S., MACFARLANE, J. T., TAQI, A., AND WHITTLE, H. C., An epidemic of meningococcal infection at Zaria, northern Nigeria. 2. The changing clinical pattern, *Trans. R. Soc. Trop. Med. Hyg.* **73:**563–566 (1979).

56. GREGORY, J. E., AND ABRAMSON, E., Meningococci in vaginitis, *Am. J. Dis. Child.* **121:**423 (1971).

57. GRIFFISS, J. M., Epidemic meningococcal disease: Synthesis of a hypothetical immunoepidemiologic model, *Rev. Infect. Dis.* **4:**159–172 (1982).

58. GRIFFISS, J. M., AND BRANDT, M. S., Disease due to W135 *Neisseria meningitidis, Pediatrics* **64:**218–221 (1979).

59. GRUSS, A.D., SPIER-MICHL, I. B., AND GOTSCHLICH, E. C., A method for a radioimmunoassay using microtiter plates allowing simultaneous determination of antibodies to two non cross-reactive antigens, *Immunochemistry* **15:**777–780 (1978).

60. HAMMERSCHLAG, M. R., AND BAKER, C. J., Meningococcal osteomyelitis: A report of two cases associated with septic arthritis, *J. Pediatr.* **88:**519–520 (1976).

61. HAMMERSCHLAG, M. R., AND BALTIMORE, R. S., Infections in children due to *Neisseria meningitidis* serogroup 135, *J. Pediatr.* **92:**503–504 (1978).

62. HASSAN-KING, M., GREENWOOD, B. M., AND WHITTLE, H. C., An epidemic of meningococcal infection at Zaria, northern Nigeria. 3. Meningococcal carriage, *Trans. R. Soc. Trop. Med. Hyg.* **73:**567–573 (1979).

63. HERSH, J. H., GOLD, R., AND LEPOW, M. L., Meningococcal Group Y pneumonia in an adolescent female, *Pediatrics* **64:**222–224 (1979).

64. HORN, D. W., The epidemic of cerebrospinal fever in the northern provinces of Nigeria, 1949–1950, *J. R. Sanit. Inst.* **71:**573–588 (1951).

65. JACOBSON, J. A., WEAVER, R. E., AND THORNSBERRY, C., Trends in meningococcal disease, 1974, *J. Infect. Dis.* **132:**480–484 (1975).

66. JACOBSON, J. A., CAMARGOS, P. A. M., FERREIRA, J. T., AND MCCORMICK, J. B., The risk of meningitis among classroom contacts during an epidemic of meningococcal disease, *Am. J. Epidemiol.* **104:**552–555 (1976).

67. KLEIN, J. O., FEIGIN, R. D., AND MCCRACKEN, G. H., JR., Report of the task force on diagnosis and management of meningitis, *Pediatrics* **78(S):**959–982 (1986).

68. KOPPES, G. M., ELLENBOGEN, C., AND GEBHART, R. J., Group Y meningococcal disease in United States Air Force recruits, *Am. J. Med.* **62:**661–714 (1977).

69. KUHNS, D. M., NELSON, C. T., FELDMAN, H. A., AND KUHN, L. R., The prophylactic value of sulfadiazine in the control of meningococcic meningitis, *J. Am. Med. Assoc.* **123:**335–339 (1943).

70. LAGGIADO, R. J., AND WINKELSTEIN, J. A., Prevalence of complement deficiencies in children with systemic meningococcal infections, *Pediatr. Infect. Dis.* **6:**75–76 (1987).

71. LAIRD, S. M., Meningococcal epididymitis, *Lancet* **1:**469–470 (1944).

72. LAPEYSSONNIE, L., La méningite cérébro-spinale en Afrique, *Bull. WHO* **28** (Suppl.) (1963).

73. LEEDOM, J. M., IVLER, D., MATHIES, A. W., JR., THRUPP, L. D., FREMONT, J. C., WEHRLE, P. F., AND PORTNOY, B., The problem of sulfadiazine-resistant meningococci, in: *Antimicrobial Agents and Chemotherapy, 1966,* pp. 281–292 (1967).

74. LEPOW, M. L., BEELER, J., RANDOLPH, M., SAMUELSON, J. S., AND HANKINS, W. A., Reactogenicity and immunogenicity of a quadrivalent combined meningococcal polysaccharide vaccine in children, *J. Infect. Dis.* **154:**1033–1036 (1986).

75. MÄKELÄ, P. H., PELTOLA, H., KÄYHTY, H., JOUSIMIES, H., PETTAY, O., RUOSLAHTI, E., SIVONEN, A., AND RENKONEN, O.-V., Polysaccharide vaccines of group A *Neisseria meningitidis* and *Haemophilus influenzae* type b: A field trial in Finland, *J. Infect. Dis.* **136:**S43–S50 (1977).

76. MAXCY, K. F., The relationship of meningococcus carriers to the incidence of cerebrospinal fever, *Am. J. Med. Sci.* **193:**438–445 (1937).

77. MAYER, R. L., AND DOWLING, H. F., The determination of meningococcic antibodies by a centrifuge-agglutination test, *J. Immunol.* **51:**349–354 (1945).

78. Meningococcal Disease Surveillance Group, Meningococcal disease: Secondary attack rate and chemoprophylaxis in the United States, 1974, *J. Am. Med. Assoc.* **235:**261–265 (1976).

79. MILLAR, J. W., SIESS, E. E., FELDMAN, H. A., SILVERMAN, C., AND FRANK, P., *In vivo* and *in vitro* resistance to sulfadiazine in strains of *Neisseria meningitidis*, *J. Am. Med. Assoc.* **186:**139–141 (1963).

80. MILLER, M. A., MILLIKIN, P., GRIFFIN, P. S., SEXTON, R. A., AND YOUSUF, M., *Neisseria meningitidis* urethritis: A case report, *J. Am. Med. Assoc.* **242:**1656–1657 (1979).

81. MUNFORD, R. S., SUSSUARANA DE VASCONCELOS, Z. J., PHILLIPS, C. J., GELLI, D. S., GORMAN, G. W., RISI, J. B., AND FELDMAN, R. A., Eradication of carriage of *Neisseria meningitidis* in families: A study in Brazil, *J. Infect. Dis.* **129:**644–659 (1974).

82. MURRAY, E. G. D., Meningococcus infections of the male urogenital tract and the liability to confusion with gonococcus infection, *Urol. Cutaneous Rev.* **43:**739–741 (1939).

83. NORTON, J. F., Meningococcus meningitis in Detroit: 1928–1929. V. Secondary cases, *J. Prev. Med.* **5:**365–367 (1931).

84. NORTON, J. F., AND GORDON, J. E., Meningococcus meningitis in Detroit in 1928–1929. I. Epidemiology, *J. Prev. Med.* **4:**207–214 (1930).

85. OLCÉN, P., BARR, J., AND KJELLANDER, J., Meningitis and bacteremia due to *Neisseria meningitidis:* Clinical and laboratory findings in 69 cases from Orebro County, 1965 to 1977, *Scand. J. Infect. Dis.* **11:**111–119 (1979).

86. Pan American Health Organization, Report of the first hemispheric meeting on meningococcal disease, *Pan. Am. Health Organ. Bull.* **10:**163–174 (1976).

87. PAUL, J. R., *Clinical Epidemiology,* p. 192, University of Chicago Press, Chicago, 1966.

88. PELTOLA, H., MÄKELÄ, H., KÄYHTY, H., JOUSIMIES, H., HERVA, E., HÄLLSTRÖM, K., SIVONEN, H., RENKONEN, O.-V., PÉTTAY, O., KARANKO, V., AHVONEN, P., AND SARNA, S., Clinical efficacy of meningococcal Group A polysaccharide vaccine in children three months to five years of age, *N. Engl. J. Med.* **297:**686–691 (1977).

89. PETERSEN, B. H., LEE, T. J., SNYDERMAN, R., AND BROOKS, G. F., *Neisseria meningitidis* and *Neisseria gonorrhoeae* bacteremia associated with C6, C7, or C8 deficiency, *Ann. Intern. Med.* **90:**917–920 (1979).

90. PHAIR, J. J., SCHOENBACH, E. B., AND ROOT, C. M., Meningococcal carrier studies, *Am. J. Public Health* **34:**148–154 (1944).

91. PIKE, R. M., Laboratory-associated infections: Incidence, fatalities, causes, and prevention, *Annu. Rev. Microbiol.* **33:**41–66 (1979).

92. PIZZI, M., A severe epidemic of meningococcus meningitis in Chile, 1941–1942, *Am. J. Public Health* **34:**231–238 (1944).

93. RAKE, G., Studies on meningococcus infection. VI. The carrier problem, *J. Exp. Med.* **59:**553–576 (1934).

94. REISS-LEVY, E., AND STEPHENSON, J., Vaginal isolation of

Neisseria meningitidis in association with meningococcaemia, *Aust. N. Z. J. Med.* **6:**487–489 (1976).

95. SCHOENBACH, E. B., The meningococcal carrier state, *Med. Ann. D. C.* **12:**417–420 (1943).

96. SIVONEN, A., RENKONEN, O.-V., WECKSTROM, P., KOSKENVUO, K., RAUNIO, V., AND MÄKELÄ, P. H., The effect of chemoprophylactic use of rifampin and minocycline on rates of carriage of *Neisseria meningitidis* in Army recruits in Finland, *J. Infect. Dis.* **137:**238–244 (1978).

97. SLATERUS, K. W., Serological typing of meningococci by means of microprecipitation, *Antonie van Leeuwenhoek J. Microbiol. Serol.* **27:**304–315 (1961).

98. STEPHENS, D. S., EDWARDS, K. M., AND MCKEE, K. T., Meningococcal Group Y disease in children, *Pediatr. Infect. Dis.* **3:**523–525 (1984).

99. THAYER, J. D., AND MARTIN, J. E., JR., A selective medium for the cultivation of *N. gonorrhoeae* and *N. meningitidis,* *Public Health Rep.* **79:**49–57 (1964).

100. The Medical Letter Inc., Preventing the spread of meningococcal disease, *The Medical Letter* **23:**37–38 (1981).

101. THOMAS, L., SMITH, H. W., AND DINGLE, J. H., Investigation of meningococcal infection. II. Immunological aspects, *J. Clin. Invest.* **22:**361–373 (1943).

102. VIEUSSEUX, M., Mémoire sur le maladie qui a regné à Génève au printemps de 1805, *J. Med. Chir. Pharmacol.* **11:**163 (1805).

103. WAHDAN, M. H., RIZK, F., EL-AKKAD, A. M., EL GHOROURY, A. E., HABLAS, R., GIRGIS, N. I., AMER, A., BOCTAR, W., SIPPEL, J. E., GOTSCHLICH, E. C., TRIAU, R., SANBORN, W. R., AND CVJETANOVIC, B., A controlled field trial of a serogroup A meningococcal polysaccharide vaccine, *Bull. WHO* **48:**667–673 (1973).

104. WEICHSELBAUM, A., Ueber die Aetiologie der akuten Meningitis cerebrospinalis, *Fortschr. Med.* **5:**573 (1887).

105. ZOLLINGER, W. D., AND MANDRELL, R. E., Outer-membrane protein and lipopolysaccharide serotyping of *Neisseria meningitidis* by inhibition of a solid-phase radioimmunoassay, *Infect. Immun.* **18:**424–433 (1977).

12. Suggested Reading

ARKWRIGHT, J. A., Cerebro-spinal meningitis: The interpretation of epidemiological observations by the light of bacteriological knowledge, *Br. Med. J.* **1:**494–496 (1915).

DINGLE, J. H., AND FINLAND, M., Diagnosis, treatment and prevention of meningococcic meningitis, with a resume of the practical aspects of treatment of other acute bacterial meningitides, *War Med.* **2:**1–58 (1942).

FELDMAN, H. A., Recent developments in the therapy and control of meningococcal infections, *Dis. Month* (Feb. 1966).

FELDMAN, H. A., Sulfonamide-resistant meningococci, *Annu. Rev. Med.* **18:**495–506 (1967).

FELDMAN, H. A., Meningococcal infections, in: *Adv. Intern. Med.* **18:**117–140 (1972).

GOTSCHLICH, E. C., LIU, T. Y., AND ARTENSTEIN, M. S., Human immunity to the meningococcus. III. Preparation and immunochemical properties of the Group A, Group B, and Group C meningococcal polysaccharides, *J. Exp. Med.* **129:**1349–1365 (1969).

GREENFIELD, S., SHEEHE, P. R., AND FELDMAN, H. A., Meningococcal carriage in a population of "normal" families, *J. Infect. Dis.* **123:**67–73 (1971).

SIVONEN, A., RENKONEN, O.-V., WECKSTROM, P., KOSKENVUO, K., RAUNIO, V., AND MÄKELÄ, P. H., The effect of chemoprophylactic use of rifampin and minocycline on rates of carriage of *Neisseria meningitidis* in Army recruits in Finland, *J. Infect. Dis.* **137:**238–244 (1978).

CHAPTER 21

Mycoplasma pneumoniae

Hjordis M. Foy

1. Introduction

Mycoplasmas are small pliable pleomorph bacteria lacking cell walls, which have been known in veterinary medicine since 1898. They were first called pleuropneumonialike organisms (PPLOs) for the disease they cause in cattle.[22] Their role as human parasites was recognized in the 1950s.[21,143] They belong to the order Mycoplasmatales, family Mycoplasmataceae, and class Mollicutes. *Mycoplasma pneumoniae* is best known as a cause of pneumonitis and of a wide spectrum of milder respiratory symptoms, such as bronchitis, bronchiolitis, and pharyngitis. Because the pneumonia is usually mild and leads to full recovery even without antibiotic treatment, it is frequently called "walking pneumonia." It is often associated with a rise in cold-agglutinin titers. The infection may cause a wide array of complications.

Other mycoplasmas, *M. buccale*, *M. faucium*, *M. orale*, and *M. salivarium*, are commensals in the oral cavity. *M. hominis*, *M. genitalium*, and *Ureaplasma urealyticum* inhabit primarily the genital tract and may act as opportunistic invaders. *M. pneumoniae*, in contrast, is a definite human pathogen that invades the respiratory tract. Before the organism was recognized, the disease was called "primary atypical pneumonia" beginning in 1938.[29,139,143] In

Hjordis M. Foy · Department of Epidemiology, School of Public Health and Community Medicine, University of Washington, Seattle, Washington 98195.

the 1950s, the organism was named Eaton agent after its discoverer.[40] Specific methods for diagnosis of *M. pneumoniae* did not become available until the 1960s.[22,98,99] The organism has been estimated to cause 15–20% of all pneumonia[59] and up to 10% of all pharyngitis[88]; the rate is highest in children and young adults.[31,59,54] *M. pneumoniae* and adenoviruses have been major causes of epidemics of pneumonia in military-recruit populations.[23,41,114,154]

2. Historical Background

The microscopic features of lung specimens obtained as far back as the Civil War suggest that *M. pneumoniae* has been circulating for a long time.[143] In more recent years, *M. pneumoniae* pneumonia has flourished in wartime; cold-agglutinin-positive pneumonia was a frequent diagnosis during World War II.[29,130,132] In the 1930s, almost any pneumonia responded to the newly introduced sulfapyridine derivatives. However, one type of pneumonia was an exception because it failed to respond to the new drugs or to penicillin, and for this reason, as noted in Section 1, was named "primary atypical pneumonia" (PAP).[139] This category was probably made up of pneumonia of several etiologies, including pneumonia caused by viruses. In 1943, cold agglutinins were discovered in the serum of patients with PAP, particularly in the type of PAP occurring in epidemics in the military.[130] The Commission on Acute Respiratory Diseases conducted experiments that showed that the disease agent could be passed to human volunteers by means of bacteria-free filtrates of secretions from ill persons.[29] Thus, this disease-causing organism was first thought to be a virus. However, unlike true viruses, the agent responded to the tetracycline type of antibiotics. As far back as 1944, Eaton et al.[40] reported that the organism caused pneumonia in cotton rats and hamsters and could be passed in egg yolk. It was after this discovery that the organism was named "Eaton agent." Doubt was first cast on this achievement because of the possibility that the agent was indigenous in rats. Liu,[98] using the fluorescent-antibody technique, established that the agent was present in human lung tissue from fatal cases, and also succeeded in isolation, cultivation, and serial passage of the agent in chick embryos. Liu et al.[99] applied immunofluorescent-antibody testing for the serological diagnosis of pneumonia. Retrospective testing of sera from volunteers participating in the earlier transmission studies confirmed an infection with Eaton agent. Also, milder respiratory symptoms and asymptomatic infections following challenge of volunteers came to light with the new methods.[140] Microscopic examinations of tissues revealed coccobacillary bodies on infected bronchial epithelium and colonylike structures in stained preparations, leading to the speculation that they were PPLOs (mycoplasmas).[105] The true character of the organism was confirmed when Chanock et al.[22] grew it on artificial media enriched with serum and yeast extract in 1962. Chanock and co-workers[21,23,85] conducted the first field studies of the agent with the newly developed diagnostic tools. Challenge studies among human volunteers were repeated using agar-grown organisms, confirming that the organism was a human pathogen.

Subsequently, several specific serological tests and isolation methods have been applied on a wider scale. M. pneumoniae was first recognized as a disease that affected military personnel, probably because the incidence was particularly high in recruit training. The Commission on Acute Respiratory Diseases, and subsequently the Armed Forces Epidemiological Board, gave financial support to the original diagnostic and epidemiological studies, focusing first on military populations and later on civilian populations.

3. Methodology

3.1. Sources of Mortality Data

Although national data are available on deaths due to pneumonia and influenza, these statistics do not reflect mortality due to M. pneumoniae pneumonia, since the latter

disease is rarely fatal. Furthermore, the diagnosis cannot be made by autopsy without appropriate microbiological testing, such as fluorescent-antibody staining of tissues or isolation of the agent. Deaths due to this disease have not been reported in the many studies of epidemics among military personnel since the 1950s[23,41,114,130,154] or in the long-term studies of a civilian population in Seattle.[54,59] However, such epidemiological studies often rely on antibody-titer rises between acute and convalescent sera and would not easily detect fatal cases if death occurred early. Back in the 1940s, when the United States appears to have experienced a major wave of M. pneumoniae infections, several deaths due to PAP, diagnosed by the cold-agglutinin test, were described.[130] Since the 1960s, when specific laboratory methods for diagnosis gained general use, many reports of fatalities have appeared in the literature.[1,38,52,87,103,109,118] Although the incidence of the disease is highest in children and adults, most fatal cases have been reported in middle-aged or older persons. All evidence suggests that death is a rare occurrence.

3.2. Sources of Morbidity Data

M. pneumoniae is not reportable, and the Centers for Disease Control do not monitor the disease. WHO has reported on M. pneumoniae infections in its surveillance of neurological disease.[5] Specific diagnostic tools have gained increased use since the 1960s, and public-health laboratories that carry out serological testing of persons with respiratory disease are able to monitor the fluctuations in incidence. So far, this avenue of surveillance has been utilized primarily in Denmark and England.[95,127] In Japan, surveillance of school children has elucidated the epidemiology of the disease.[125] Morbidity data in the United States derive from research funded to carry out in-depth studies in selected representative population samples. The first such studies were conducted at military installations, especially in recruit populations.[23,41,106,114,154]

Subsequently, studies among in- and outpatients at a children's hospital in Washington, D.C., established that M. pneumoniae infections occurred in childhood.[21] Population-based studies have been conducted in pediatric practices in North Carolina,[37,50,64] among families in Tecumseh, Michigan,[116] and in a prepaid-medical-care group in Seattle, Washington.[53,55,57–59] Studies of incidence of the infection and disease have been carried out in children's homes,[32,39,65,145] day-care facilities,[50,155] and schools,[31,55] and among college students[43,44,55,114] and family units[7,13,53,81] (see Section 5.9). Studies of families with an index case of pneumonia have provided information on the secondary attack rates, the spectrum of clinical manifestations, the duration of shedding, and the incubation period. On the other hand, families under continuous observation during both health and illness have provided community infection rates and epidemiological patterns.[30,59,116] Studies of *M. pneumoniae* pneumonia in hospitalized patients in the United States reflect incidence poorly, since only severe cases of pneumonia or its complications are generally hospitalized. In Scandinavia, where the policy for hospitalization is more liberal than in the United States, statistics of hospitalized pneumonia patients reflect seasonal and annual variations of incidence.[78] High proportions (up to 37%) of outpatient pneumonia due to *M. pneumoniae* have been reported in Sweden.[8]

Studies of volunteers inoculated with *M. pneumoniae* have yielded data on immunity and the spectrum of disease manifestations.[34] Ear involvement occurred frequently after artificial inoculation in the nasopharynx by nebulizer.[140]

3.3. Serological Surveys

Serum samples have been collected to compare the prevalence of antibodies in different populations and age groups.[42,106,159] Caution must be exercised in interpreting these data, unless the serological testing is carried out in the same laboratory, because of inherent variability in the tests. Furthermore, knowledge regarding the correlation of immunity and various antibodies and the persistence of antibodies is incomplete. Nevertheless, such studies indicate that the organism is ubiquitous in most parts of the world, and the age distribution of antibody acquisition appears similar in tropical and temperate climates. Prospective serological studies have also been made to measure the incidence of infection (seroconversion) and reinfection rates.[37,39,41,42,106,154]

3.4. Laboratory Diagnosis

3.4.1. Isolation. Because it may take several weeks to grow *M. pneumoniae* in the laboratory, isolation of the organism has more use in epidemiological studies than in clinical decision-making.[67] Isolation of the agent from respiratory specimens usually indicates infection, since prolonged asymptomatic carrier states are rare.[53,64] It is the most conclusive evidence of infection, particularly since false-positive serological tests are a possibility. *M. pneumoniae* pneumonia patients rarely have a productive cough at onset of illness, and throat swabs, but not nasal swabs, are a good substitute for sputum in isolation attempts. A single culture is positive in 65% of cases in the acute stage

(Fig. 1). Especially in children, the organism is often shed for several weeks, although in decreasing amount.[53] Antibiotic therapy at best decreases the amount shed, but does not eliminate the carriage state. The collection medium commonly used contains bovine albumin in trypticase soy broth with penicillin.[83] The SP-4 medium utilized since 1979 appears to enhance growth and to be superior to previously used culture media.[167] Use of monoclonal antibody may also enhance detection.[25] Specimens can be stored refrigerated for several days and withstand transportation and freezing. They are inoculated on special media enriched with fresh yeast extract, peptone, and animal serum. Penicillin is added to suppress bacterial growth; thallium acetate may be used for the same purpose. Both agar plates and broth cultures are utilized. It may take 1–4 weeks for *M. pneumoniae* colonies to become visible under the microscope; most other human *Mycoplasma* species can be detected with magnification within a couple of days. Colonies have a fried-egg appearance, measure 10–150 μm, and are embedded in the agar. Isolates can be presumptively identified by hemolysis of guinea pig red blood cells and fermentation of glucose. In the broth, the organisms cause faint turbidity, but their presence is best demonstrated by pH changes of indicators. Diphasic media, which have an agar base overlaid with a fluid medium and incorporate a pH indicator for glucose fermentation, are especially suited to *M. pneumoniae* isolation, since even small inocula will grow.[67] Subculture is necessary for defi-

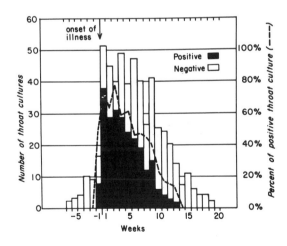

Figure 1. Isolation of *M. pneumoniae* from throat-swab cultures in ill persons by time in relation to onset of illness. Reproduced from Foy *et al*.[53] with permission.

nite identification, which is best carried out by inhibition of specific antisera.

Rapid identification for clinical use has been attempted by use of fluorescent-tagged antisera of throat and sputum specimens, but has not proven successful. DNA probes offer promise, but have had low sensitivity whereas antigen capture enzyme immunoassays have yielded better results.[70]

3.4.2. Serological Tests. The first epidemiological studies of PAP were carried out with cold agglutinins (CAs) as the diagnostic test.[29,132,143] CAs appear 1 week after onset of illness in approximately two-thirds of *M. pneumoniae* pneumonia patients, usually those with more severe disease.[67] Cold agglutination can be used as a rapid presumptive test, since it can sometimes be visualized at the bedside as the blood cools off, but the test is properly carried out at +4°C. However, this test is not specific; it is also positive occasionally in adenovirus pneumonia. A multitude of other conditions are associated with high titers of CAs, particularly in children.[161]

Specific serological tests for *M. pneumoniae* can be separated into those that measure growth inhibition (GI), metabolic inhibition (MI), tetrazolium-reduction inhibition (TRI), and killing and those that measure antibodies with more traditional tests.[83,84,136,163,164]

The first set of tests, which measure GI or killing, all have a dynamic endpoint; that is, titers measured will vary slightly from day to day in the laboratory. The presence of antibiotics in serum can interfere with these tests unless antibiotic-resistant strains are used. These tests appear to correlate with immunity, and also with tests that measure antilipid (membrane) antibody, but in most studies no specific antibody level has been found to be totally protective.[39,42,106,154]

The originally applied indirect fluorescent-antibody technique is specific but cumbersome, and now seldom used.[99] The major antigen in *M. pneumoniae* is found in the lipid fraction of the organism, located in the triple-layer membrane. Most antibody tests measure antibody to the membrane. The original complement-fixing (CF) antibody test for *M. pneumoniae* utilized whole organisms, and the test appears to measure antibody to cytoplasm.[21,23,83] The CF test using lipid antigen, obtained through chloroform–methanol extraction, correlates better with infection than does the original CF test; also, fewer anticomplementary reactions are encountered. This test is widely used to diagnose acute infection. In evaluating the literature regarding serological data, it is worthwhile to note which antigen has been used in the CF test.

Hemagglutination inhibition (HI) and indirect hemag-

glutination (IHA) tests may measure antibodies other than to the lipid membranes.[83,159] The complement-mediated killing test and the radioimmunoassay test are exquisitely sensitive, and low titers may represent cross-reacting antibody to plant antigens.[19,74,83] An additional sensitive technique is the immune-complex-induced platelet-aggregation test.[131] This technique has been used to detect immune complexes in sera of patients with *M. pneumoniae* infection.[12] Enzyme-linked immunosorbent assays (ELISA) have been developed, and measure primarily antibody to protein.[76,138] IgM response has been observed in about 80% of sera collected 9 days or later after onset.[169] Older persons may respond with only IgG.[76] *M. pneumoniae* cross-reacts serologically with *M. genitalium*,[97,170] and false-positive reactions in both CF and ELISA tests occur in patients with bacterial meningitis,[86] and at least in the CF test in those with acute pancreatitis.[92] Concurrent rises to *Legionella pneumophila*[129] and *Chlamydia trachomatis* may also cause confusion as to which is the causative agent.[88] In such cases, polyclonal B-cell activation by *M. pneumoniae* may be the cause of an aberrant antibody response.[11]

Whereas the CF antibody test may be the most practical method to diagnose acute infections, its value in serological surveys to determine immunity is compromised by its relatively fast disappearance, although a few pneumonia patients have measurable CF antibody for up to 5 years after infection.[9,67,120] Antibody in nasal secretions can be measured both with ELISA and with radioimmunoprecipitation.[124]

The clinical and epidemiological experience with all these tests is insufficient to make strong recommendations as to which ones best reflect naturally acquired immunity. Most antibodies appear to decay with time. Also, the great variability in the outcome of tests run in different laboratories jeopardizes comparisons of the prevalence of antibodies among communities unless all testing is done in one laboratory.

4. Biological Characteristics of the Organism

Mycoplasmas are the smallest free-living organisms known; individual organisms measure 300–500 nm. Unlike regular bacteria, they lack a cell wall. This renders them insensitive to antibiotics that interfere with cell-wall synthesis (penicillins and cycloserine). They are sensitive (bateriostatic) to tetracyclines and erythromycin, which act on protein synthesis, but antibiotic treatment does not eradicate the organisms from the host. Lack of a cell wall also allows for pleomorphism and pliability. Morphologically, they resemble cell-wall-defective bacteria (L forms), but the latter revert to normal morphology when cultured on appropriate media. They contain both RNA and DNA and carry out their own reproductive processes. *M. pneumoniae* ferments glucose, produces a hemolysin, and grows under atmospheric conditions.

The organisms have been shown to move on glass surfaces and to react with neuraminic acid receptors.[153] Their ability to agglutinate cells, including erythrocytes and spermatozoa,′ is possibly a virulence factor. They survive drying relatively well, but may be sensitive to small fluctuations in humidity.[71,175] Specimens can be frozen and thawed repeatedly without significant loss of viability. They are vulnerable to treatment with lipid solvents, formalin solutions, and other antiseptics.

The outer triple-layer cell membrane contains glycolipids as major determinants. Antigenically related compounds are found in many animal cells, possibly the cause of cross-reacting antibodies and infection-induced autoimmunity. Information regarding antigenic variability is sparse, but antigenic changes occur after repeated passages in the laboratory, and temperature-sensitive mutants have been developed.[34,68] Antibiotic-resistant strains have been produced in the laboratory and are also found in nature.[126,157] Antigenic drift appears not to occur between epidemics.[170]

5. Descriptive Epidemiology

5.1. Prevalence

True prevalence data, the rate of existing infections at a given time, have rarely been sought for *M. pneumoniae* infections. On the other hand, surveys for throat-culture-positive persons have been carried out among adults and schoolchildren, and these studies have shown a minuscule carriage rate in the community under endemic conditions.[55,64,114] Only three isolates were obtained from 2453 throat swabs from schoolchildren cultured every 6 weeks during the school year 1965–1966, a year before an epidemic in Seattle.[55] When questioned, those who donated positive specimens reported having had respiratory symptoms the week prior to culture. In military populations, the carriage rate can be higher: among U.S. Marine recruits, the carriage rate was estimated as 0 on induction, 1% after 5 weeks, and 9–10% after 9 weeks.[171] With more sensitive culture media now available, a smaller number of *M. pneumoniae* organisms may be recovered so that the carrier rate

may seemingly increase.[167] Thus, in a study of pharyngitis the carriage rate was reported to be 17.6%.[108]

Seroepidemiological studies of prevalence of TRI antibodies show similar antibody patterns among military recruits in Argentina, Colombia, and the United States and among Peace Corps volunteers, with prevalence rates ranging from 49 to 66%.[42]

Using a macrohemagglutination-inhibition test that may measure different antibodies than the more commonly used tests, Suhs and Feldman[159] found increasing antibody levels with increasing age. The prevalence of antibody at Point Barrow, Alaska, was higher than in New York. Prevalence estimates with the highly sensitive radioimmunoprecipitating antibody test suggested that 97% of Americans may have been exposed to the organism by the age of 18.[19] However, the specificity of this test has been questioned, since plant antigens may induce similar antibody.[83]

5.2. Epidemic Behavior and Incidence

M. pneumoniae infections are endemic in larger urban areas, and epidemic increases are observed at 4- to 7-year intervals.[59,78,116,125,127] The spread is slow because of the limited communicability and long case-to-case interval, approximately 3 weeks. Epidemics may last 1–2 years in larger communities. A high incidence is observed among schoolchildren, who often transmit the infection to playmates,[31,55,59,116] but the schoolroom itself appears not to be the focus of spread.[31,55] Neighborhood spread has been observed, and microepidemics occur within the larger community.[55,121] In military recruits, the attack rates vary among platoons,[154] and in institutional settings, the spread can be traced between buildings.[32]

Although most epidemics appear to be propagated person to person, a few common-source outbreaks have been reported. A party at a fraternity house resulted in nearly half the students becoming infected; 7 of 23 required hospitalization for pneumonia.[45] An outbreak in a prosthodontic laboratory may have been transmitted by aerosolization from abrasive drilling of false teeth.[146] In an outbreak on a nuclear submarine, the closeness of the onset dates suggests a common source, and recirculated air could possibly have been the vehicle.[147] An explosive outbreak peaking 1 month after opening was reported from a boys' summer camp.[18] These outbreaks are further discussed in Section 6.

The transmission and the spectrum of symptoms have been studied in detail in family units with index cases of *M. pneumoniae* pneumonia (see further discussion in Section 5.9.1).

The incidence among military-recruit populations can be exceedingly high. Thus, the rate of *M. pneumoniae* pneumonia was 1.5% at Parris Island in 1955, and infection rates regardless of diagnosis were about 30 times higher[23] (see Section 5.9.3 and Fig. 5). Military outbreaks are probably due to the herding of susceptibles together and to behavior patterns that favor transmission.

M. pneumoniae pneumonia was monitored among the 150,000 members of a prepaid-medical-care group in Seattle in 1963–1975.[59] This 10% population sample was considered representative of the total urban–suburban community. The disease was diagnosed by isolation and significant anti-lipid CF-antibody titer rises. The rate of total pneumonia averaged 1200/100,000. *M. pneumoniae* was recognized as the etiological agent in 15%, for an average rate of 180/100,000 per year. It varied between a low endemic rate of 60/100,000 in 1966 and an epidemic rate of 300/100,000 in 1974. However, the rate of recognized *M. pneumoniae* pneumonia constituted only the tip of the iceberg of all infections with this organism. In Seattle schoolchildren who were bled annually, the infection rate was estimated to have been at least 35% during the 1974 epidemic. Since CF antibodies sometimes decay quickly after infection, the rates may have been even higher. Studied with the same CF-antibody test, families who were bled annually in Seattle in 1972–1977 had infection rates averaging 8% for 5- to 9-year-old children and 2% for adults.[59] In Tecumseh, Michigan, where families were bled every 6 months, the annual infection rates were 9 and 4%, respectively, in similar age groups.[116]

5.3. Geographic Distribution

Infection with *M. pneumoniae* is worldwide and has been demonstrated in all continents except Antarctica. It is present in tropical countries as well as in the Arctic.[66,159,160] However, the epidemiology of the infection has been studied primarily in the United States, Europe, and Japan.[7,13,54,78,95,121,125,127] The epidemiology in different climatic entities has not been extensively studied.

So far, the evidence suggests that no geographic differences occur except those due to crowding and other socioeconomic variables.

5.4. Temporal Distribution

Although *M. pneumoniae* infections have been endemic in most civilian communities where the infection has been thoroughly sought, epidemic cyclicity is evident from most long-term population studies (Table 1). In Denmark, centrally located public-health laboratories have monitored infections since 1958 by serological diagnosis of paired sera

Table 1.   Recorded *Mycoplasma pneumoniae* Epidemics by Location, Season, Year, and Population Sampled

Location	Season	Years	Study origins	Ref.
Europe				
Denmark	Winter	1958–1959, 1963, 1967–1968, 1972, 1978, 1987	Public-health laboratories	95, 96
United Kingdom	Winter	1967–1968, 1971–1972, 1975, 1978–1979, 1983, 1986	Public-health laboratories	127, 128, 135
Finland	Winter	1962–1963, 1967–1968, 1973, 1977	Infectious-disease hospital	78, 134
Hamburg, West Germany	Winter	1974–1975	Children's hospital	142
United States				
New Orleans, Louisiana	Late summer–fall	1960, 1961, 1965	Military	114
Madison, Wisconsin	Fall–winter	1954–1955, 1960, 1965	College students	44
Chapel Hill, North Carolina	Fall–winter	1964–1965, 1969, 1972–1973	Pediatric practices	50, 64
Omaha, Nebraska	Fall	1964	Boy's school	145
West Virginia	Winter	1964–1965	Hospital	3
La Crosse, Wisconsin	Fall	1965–1966	In- and outpatients	31
Tecumseh, Michigan	Fall	1968–1969	Community surveillance	116
Seattle, Washington	Winter, summer	1966–1967, 1974, 1981	Prepaid-medical-care group	59, 61
Asia				
Sendai, Japan		1968, 1972, 1976, 1980	School children	125

forwarded from physicians.[95] A cyclicity of approximately 4½ years was observed,[127,135] until the 1980s when the infection became endemic.[71a] Similar studies have been carried out in Great Britain and Japan, where the cycles also took about 4½ years. Epidemic periods lasted for up to 2 years.[125,127] Epidemic periods coincided between these two countries. Epidemic patterns in the Scandinavian countries have been similar, but not identical.[134] However, an epidemic reported from Hamburg, West Germany, in 1974–1975 seems out of step with this European cyclicity.[142]

Epidemic cycles appear not to be synchronized throughout the United States, although epidemics were reported in several areas around 1965 (Table 1). In Seattle, where rates were closely monitored, *M. pneumoniae* pneumonia started to rise in early 1966, but not until January 1967 did the epidemic reach a peak. Rates were low the subsequent year. Slightly increased rates were noticed again in the spring of 1972, but a clear-cut epidemic did not recur until 1974, and

that epidemic peaked in the summer. The subsequent epidemic occurred in 1981.[61] Epidemic increase was noticed in Tecumseh in 1968–1969.[116] Many studies report epidemics in the fall, and this appears to be characteristic of college populations, where epidemics also have recurred at 4- to 5-year intervals.[44] In the military, the highest rates have been observed in late summer, regardless of the influx of new soldiers.[41,114]

Because community rates of pneumonia of other etiologies are at their highest by far in the winter and spring, and *M. pneumoniae* infections are endemic, the proportion of pneumonia due to *M. pneumoniae* is highest in the summer.

5.5. Age

The incidence of all pneumonia regardless of etiology is highest by far in children under the age of 2 and in the elderly. The rates are low among teenagers (Fig. 2). The

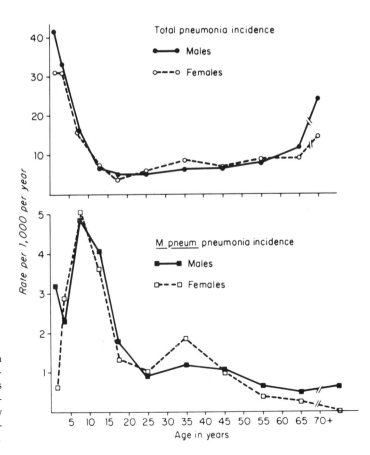

Figure 2. Incidence of *M. pneumoniae* pneumonia by age and sex, Group Health Cooperative, December 1, 1963–February 28, 1975. Infection was determined by isolation or fourfold or greater antilipid CF-antibody rise or both. Reprinted from Foy *et al.*[59] with permission of the University of Chicago Press. © 1979 by the University of Chicago.

incidence of *M. pneumoniae* pneumonia follows a reverse pattern and is highest among school-age children. The Seattle studies of *M. pneumoniae* pneumonia suggested that the incidence in children under the age of 5 was half that in school-age children, and adolescents 15–19 years old had a lower incidence than all younger age groups (Fig. 2). On the other hand, infection rates, regardless of symptoms, are about equal for children of all age groups in family epidemics.[13,53]

It has often been stated that the incidence of *M. pneumoniae* pneumonia is highest among young adults. Such statements probably originate from military studies, where the incidence of *M. pneumoniae* infection can be extraordinarily high.[23,114] But in civilian populations, the incidence declines with age after puberty. The over-40 age group has the lowest incidence, suggesting that immunity builds up over time. Yet, pneumonia in older persons may lead to more severe complications,[5,94,117] and practically all deaths due to *M. pneumoniae* infections have been reported in adults.

Higher *M. pneumoniae* pneumonia rates were observed in Seattle in those 30–39 years old than in slightly younger and older adults.[59] Similar observations were made regarding infection rates in Tecumseh.[116] This age group includes the parents of school-age children, and the high rate is probably a consequence of intensive exposure.

Infection rates, regardless of illness, have been studied through semiannual bleedings of families under continuous surveillance in Seattle and Tecumseh. Infection rates in Seattle in 1965–1968 were estimated at 12% per year for all age groups, based on 4-fold antibody-titer rises or on a rise from no antibody to the lowest detectable titer (1 : 8) as indicators of infection.[30] In Tecumseh, the infection rate was highest, 9%, in the 5- to 9-year age group, being about 2.5% in children under 5 years of age and declining to 4% after the age of 20. Only 4-fold antibody-titer rises were accepted as evidence of infection.[116] In a subsequent study in Seattle (1972–1975), infection rates paralleled those in the Tecumseh studies, possibly because, now, only 4-fold rises were accepted for diagnosis, or because the age composition of the families was now different.[59]

The estimates of proportion of infections expressed in pneumonia vary according to study methods. They have been highest by far (60–70%) in studies of families under intensive surveillance because of an index case with pneumonia.[7,13,53] On the other hand, among families followed continuously with serological testing as the primary means, pneumonia in those infected has only rarely been recorded.[30,116]

The proportion of infections that lead to pneumonia

varies with age and appears highest in the 5- to 14-year age group.[59] Studies among children under the age of 5 have led to diverse findings. Thus, in surveillance in a day-care facility in North Carolina, 5 of 7 children carrying the organisms were totally asymptomatic.[50] The same held true for children with serological rises. In a day-care center in Sweden, 3 of 4 children under the age of 2 with positive throat cultures responded with febrile respiratory disease and cough.[155] Family studies with an index case of *M. pneumoniae* have indicated milder symptoms in children under the age of 5 than in older age groups [7,53] (see further discussion in Section 5.9.1). The low rate of verified pneumonia in children under 5 has led to the theory that the primary infection leads to sensitization and the succeeding infection to pneumonia. This hypothesis has been challenged in hospital studies from outside the United States, which reported high *M. pneumoniae* pneumonia rates in children under the age of 5,[119,156,162] and by a family study in Israel.[69]

In surveillance studies in children's homes, the proportion of *M. pneumoniae* infections leading to pneumonia has been 13–18% in the 5- to 9-year age group.[32,39,145] But in older age groups, this proportion has been lower in most studies: about 2–7% of older teenagers and recruits.[23,32,154]

Figure 3 shows the outcome of isolation from throat swabs and CF-antibody tests in all pneumonia patients in the

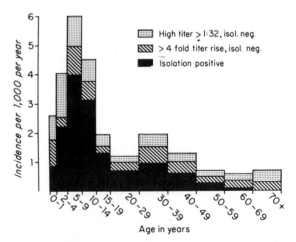

Figure 3. Incidence of pneumonia with evidence of *M. pneumoniae* infection by age measured by different laboratory tests, Group Health Cooperative, December 1, 1963–February 28, 1975. Those who were isolation-positive also had fourfold or higher antibody titers. Reprinted from Foy *et al.*[59] with permission of the University of Chicago Press. © 1979 by the University of Chicago.

Seattle studies. Isolation was more efficient than serological methods in the age group 2–30, but in young children and older adults, about half the infections were diagnosed by CF-antilipid tests. A proportion of pneumonia patients with high antibody titers only probably represented *M. pneumoniae* pneumonia where the initial serum was taken too late for an antibody-titer rise to be demonstrated.

5.6. Sex

The infection rate for *M. pneumoniae* is similar for both sexes, but the rate of *M. pneumoniae* pneumonia is slightly higher in males, except in the age group 30–39, where rates for women were higher (see Fig. 2). Also, infection rates regardless of clinical manifestations were higher in women in the Tecumseh studies.[116] Women may contract the infection by close contact with children. The rate of complications in the form of otitis is higher in males,[53] and most cases of Stevens–Johnson syndrome attributed to *M. pneumoniae* infection have occurred in males.[117]

5.7. Race

The infection probably affects all races equally and with similar symptoms. In the Seattle studies, a large proportion of the *M. pneumoniae* patients were from the Oriental community, which was well represented in the Group Heath Cooperative membership. Sickle-cell anemia, SS or SC hemoglobulinopathy, a congenital disorder of the red blood cells seen among blacks, predisposes to a more severe form of *M. pneumoniae* pneumonia.[133,149]

5.8. Occupation

The high rates observed among military recruits are probably due to crowding and herding during basic training. The disease is frequently observed among physicians and other hospital personnel, although no "hard data" on comparative incidence by occupation are available. The risk associated with being a mother of a school-age child has already been noted.

5.9. Occurrence in Special Settings

5.9.1. Family. Studies of the transmission and symptomatology of *M. pneumoniae* infections in families have contributed substantially to our understanding of the epidemiology of this infection.[7,13,53,69,81] In Seattle, 114 families were under observation after an index case of suspect pneumonia had been identified.[53] Throat cultures were collected weekly, and paired sera when feasible. In 36 of these families, the laboratory results subsequently showed the etiological agent to have been *M. pneumoniae*. Transmission to other family members was demonstrated by isolation in 23 of these 36 families, of whom 84% of the children and 41% of the adults became infected. The case-to-case interval centered around 3 weeks, much longer than for most other acute respiratory diseases. In some families, several cycles of 3- to 4-week intervals passed before all family members were infected.

A typical family episode is illustrated in Fig. 4. The 7-year-old boy became ill with *M. pneumoniae* pneumonia, complicated with otitis, on June 12. He made an uneventful recovery. Despite treatment with tetracycline, his throat cultures remained positive. His 8- and 10-year-old sisters became ill with sore throat, slight fever, and cough at the beginning of July. The mother did not consider their symptoms, which did not interfere with daily activities, severe enough to warrant a visit to the clinic. Only because of our urging were they brought to the clinic, and chest films revealed pneumonitis in one of them. On July 18, the father developed malaise and fever, and was first diagnosed by his physician as having influenza. A subsequent chest film revealed an extensive infiltrate, although physical examination of the chest was almost normal. Figure 4 illustrates negative throat cultures prior to illness, and then intermittent positive throat cultures for several weeks. The mother and oldest child escaped infection despite low CF-antibody titers. Although in this particular family, those who were not treated with antibiotics showed a higher antibody response than those who were, no such relationship between treatment and antibody response has been found when a large number of treated and untreated cases have been compared.

In the Seattle study of families with a suspected index case of pneumonia, asymptomatic infection was seen in 27% of children under the age of 5, in 19% of the age group 5–14, and in 8% of the group 15 years and older.[53] Pharyngitis without cough was the only manifestation in 10% of family cases. The duration of pneumonia illness generally increased with advancing age. Boys had pneumonitis and ear complications more frequently than did girls.

Balassanian and Robbins[7] studied nine families in Cleveland. They observed high infection rates regardless of age, but the rate of pneumonia was lower in those under age 10 than in older persons. Similar family studies were conducted by Biberfeld and Sterner[13] in Sweden. They were able to obtain serological specimens and refer patients for

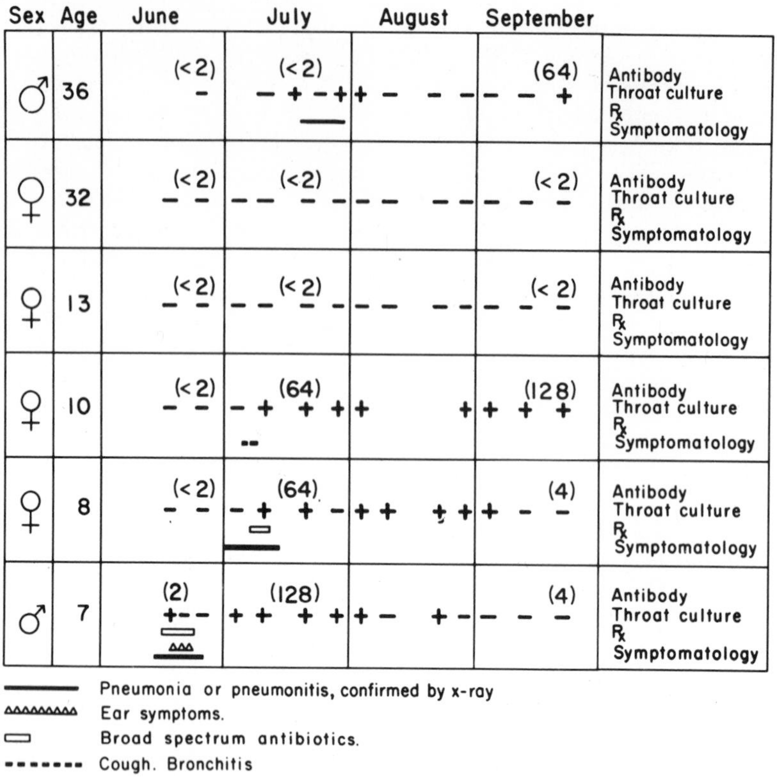

Sex	Age	June	July	August	September	
♂	36	(<2) −	(<2) — + − +	+ − − −	(64) − +	Antibody / Throat culture / Rx / Symptomatology
♀	32	(<2) − −	(<2) — − −	− −	(<2) − −	Antibody / Throat culture / Rx / Symptomatology
♀	13	(<2) − −	(<2) — − −	− −	(<2) − −	Antibody / Throat culture / Rx / Symptomatology
♀	10	(<2) − −	(64) − + + + +	+ +	(128) + + + +	Antibody / Throat culture / Rx / Symptomatology
♀	8	(<2) − −	(64) − + + −	+ + + + +	(4) + − −	Antibody / Throat culture / Rx / Symptomatology
♂	7	(2) + − −	(128) + + + +	+ − + −	(4) − −	Antibody / Throat culture / Rx / Symptomatology

—————— Pneumonia or pneumonitis, confirmed by x-ray
△△△△△△△△ Ear symptoms.
▭ Broad spectrum antibiotics.
▪▪▪▪▪▪ Cough. Bronchitis

Figure 4. Example of a family epidemic with *M. pneumoniae*. Reproduced from Foy *et al.*[53] with permission.

radiological examination to a greater degree than were the American investigators. Transmission was observed in 24 of 25 families. *M. pneumoniae* was isolated from 71% of 45 children and 53% of 62 adults. Chest film demonstrated pneumonia in 13 of 18 infected children and in 27 of 32 adults; only 1 infected person was classified as asymptomatic. A high rate (73%) of pneumonia in children was also reported from a family study in Israel.[69] Jensen *et al.*,[81] when studying the effect of oxytetracycline in transmission of *M. pneumoniae* infection, relied heavily on three serological tests (indirect hemagglutination, CF, and TRI) and reported a higher rate of asymptomatic infections among adults than did the previous investigators.

Whereas the family studies described above started with index cases of *M. pneumoniae* infection, other investigators have observed *M. pneumoniae* infection in families kept under continuous prospective observation.[30,116] In such studies, sera collected at 6-month intervals have yielded information on infection rates (see Section 5.5), but the information on illness becomes sketchy, because of the multitude of intercurrent viral infections.

5.9.2. Hospital. Epidemics of *M. pneumoniae* pneumonia have been encountered in hospital settings.[3,78,142,156] Serologically diagnosed *M. pneumoniae* infections also occurred in 20% of patients undergoing open-heart surgery in one hospital, but no cases of pneumonia were reported, and the mode of transmission was not determined. Serological cross-reaction with myocardial antigen could not be ruled out.[62] At least one nosocomially acquired *M. pneumoniae* pneumonia has been reported.[174] Because the incubation period for *M. pneumoniae* infection is so long, most hospital-acquired *M. pneumoniae* infection may not be manifest until the patient is discharged.

5.9.3. Military. *M. pneumoniae* infections have posed special problems in the military. Probably the most intensive epidemic reported was among Marine recruits at Parris Island, with rates of *M. pneumoniae* pneumonia of 1500/100,000 per training period[23] (Fig. 5). The rate of

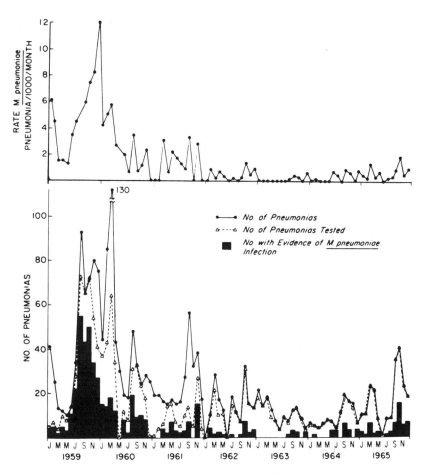

Figure 5. Seven-year surveillance of *M. pneumoniae* pneumonia at Marine Corps Recruit Depot, Parris Island, South Carolina. Reproduced from Chanock *et al.*[23] with permission.

infection was 41% over a 14-week period. The infection spread slowly through the population, and infection rates varied among battalions.[154] Navy recruits were studied prospectively for 4 years at Great Lakes, Illinois, and in Florida.[41] Rates of seroconversion were as high as 45–57%, especially during late summer, but usually rates were lower. They were remarkably similar in the two installations over a 4-year period despite climatic differences; a slight epidemic peak was seen in spring, and a major one in late summer. Similarly, among airmen studied in Mississippi, *M. pneumoniae* rates were highest in late summer, and 44% of all pneumonia could be attributed to *M. pneumoniae*.[114] In all these studies, it is clear that a clinical diagnosis of pneumonia was made in only a small fraction of recruits

who seroconverted. This fraction has been estimated to be 3–5%.[23,154] Pneumonia occurred primarily in those without any or with low antibody titer to the organism.[106,154]

Studies in the Netherlands in the 1960s suggest that *M. pneumoniae* infection is also a problem in recruit training in Europe.[168] In South America, seroconversion rates among Argentinean and Colombian recruits, 17–30% over 1–2 years, are similar to those observed in the United States,[42] suggesting that *M. pneumoniae* infections spread readily during military training in most countries and climates. In susceptible recruits, the infection rate approximated 50%. *M. pneumoniae* is also a leading cause of pneumonia among seasoned troops. Thus, during the Vietnam conflict, 43% of hospitalized pneumonia patients had evidence of *M. pneu-*

moniae infection.[4] However, the total incidence of pneumonia may have been low.

5.10. Socioeconomic Factors

The disease of *M. pneumoniae* pneumonia has been described primarily from economically advanced societies, which suggests that this relatively mild disease is cause for concern primarily among those who can afford to seek medical attention for relatively minor respiratory disease. An alternate explanation is that in a society with high hygienic standards, exposure to the organism is postponed until later childhood, when the disease takes on more severe symptoms. This is in analogy with the relationship of poliovirus infection to age. On the other hand, a high rate of complications was reported among malnourished refugees in a Kampuchean holding center.[160]

5.11. Other Factors

Little is known of the role, if any, of nutritional and genetic factors in *M. pneumoniae* infections. Any relationship to histocompatibility complexes, such as HLA antigens, is not known, but should be explored in severe complications such as hemolytic anemia and Stevens–Johnson syndrome. No difference in antibody prevalence or in the incidence of infection has been found among persons with different blood groups.[42]

Persons with deficiencies of the humoral antibody system are at greater risk of severe *M. pneumoniae* infection.[56,165,166] Children with Down's syndrome also suffer more severe symptoms,[6,32] as do persons with sickle-cell disease[133,149] (see Section 5.7). *M. pneumoniae* infection has also been reported as a severe complication in immunosuppressed patients.[1,63]

Neither smoking nor chronic pulmonary disease has been found to predispose to *M. pneumoniae* pneumonia. However, *M. pneumoniae* infection in persons with impaired pulmonary function may do further damage to the ventilatory capacity, and some exacerbation of chronic pulmonary disease has been associated with rise in *M. pneumoniae* antibody titer, although the organism has rarely been recovered from such patients.[173]

6. Mechanisms and Routes of Transmission

Transmission of *M. pneumoniae* requires close contact such as in the family setting. Several cycles with 3-week

case-to-case intervals are sometimes required before the family epidemic is over.[53] The propagation of epidemics in the community is also exceedingly slow, and epidemics may last 1–2 years.[54] Microepidemics in neighborhoods were identified in studies in Seattle,[55] LaCrosse, Wisconsin,[31] and Japan.[121] The school-age child seemed the most important vector in both intra- and interfamilial spread, yet, as noted in Section 5.2, the school itself appears not to be the focus of spread.[31,55] Introduction of an index case in a school rarely results in classroom epidemics, but the infection spreads, among close playmates. Transmission has been described in an amateur wrestling team.[55] Children carry *M. pneumoniae* longer than do adults, but the potential for an asymptomatic carrier to transmit the infection is not known, and is probably low.

It is not known whether spread is primarily by droplet or direct or indirect contact, or by all these means. The slow community spread makes airborne spread seem unlikely. Nevertheless, airborne transmission was suggested in a prosthodontal laboratory, where dental drilling of false teeth may have aerosolized the organisms.[146] Similarly, the outbreak on a nuclear-powered submarine may have been airborne.[147] In the common-source outbreak that occurred at a fraternity celebration, the exact mode of transmission was not identified, but food, drink, and vomitus were reportedly widely dispersed through the air.[45]

In the hamster model, exposure to small particles (2–3 μm) of *M. pneumoniae* resulted in both upper- and lower-respiratory-tract infection, whereas infection remained limited to the upper respiratory tract when hamsters were given inocula of large-particle aerosol (8 μm).[37] Larger doses of the small-particle (2–3 μm) aerosol resulted in more extensive pneumonia than lower doses[80] suggesting that type and dose of aerosol may affect clinical manifestations of exposure.

7. Pathogenesis and Immunity

7.1. Incubation Period

The incubation period observed in volunteers inoculated with *M. pneumoniae* in the pharynx has been short (6–12 days), probably due to the large infecting dose.[140] In the common-source outbreak related to one single-day exposure, the median incubation period was 13 days.[45] However, the case-to-case interval observed in families and similar settings is considerably longer; the mode was 20 days in one study and 23 in the other.[13,53] This suggests that a person is not infective until after a week of illness, probably when the cough becomes productive.

7.2. Pathogenesis

M. pneumoniae is a surface parasite[28] and has only rarely been isolated from sites other than the respiratory tract. The organisms can be isolated from the pharynx 1 week prior to onset of illness; recovery rates are highest during the first week of illness, and the shedding from the pharynx subsequently decreases, so that very few persons have positive cultures after 6 weeks[53] (see Fig. 1). The organism has been recovered as late as 4 months after the onset of illness[55] and for a much longer period in hypo-gammaglobulinemic patients.[141,166] Healthy controls almost never carry *M. pneumoniae* (see Section 5.1). On the other hand, carriage has not been extensively studied among children under the age of 5, and in surveillance in a day-care center in North Carolina, 11 of 15 infected children (identified by isolation or serological rise) were thought to be asymptomatic.[50]

Many attempts have been made to isolate the organism from sites other than the nasopharynx in *M. pneumoniae* disease. Isolates have been reported from the ear twice,[37,52,152] from CSF at least five times,[1,51,82] from synovial fluid,[36,141,166] pleural fluid,[122] and from skin lesions[101] including blisters from a case of Stevens–Johnson syndrome.[158] Remarkably, the organism has been recovered from heparinized Ficol filtered blood from three patients with neurological sequelae.[110] In the fatal case of a 71-year-old man who had an unusual and severe illness with endocardial lesions and in whom the organism appears to have disseminated, *M. pneumoniae* was recovered from blood in the heart and from the pericardial sac.[118] In another postmortem case, the organism was recovered from spleen, brain, and kidney.[87]

By electron microscopy, the organisms are found embedded between the cilia of the bronchial tree and attached to the respiratory epithelium with a terminal organelle.[28] This attachment is formed by a 165- to 190-kDa protein called P1.[75] Antibody to the P1 protein inhibits adherence.[89] At least five additional protein antigens may be important and may be detected by immunoblotting.[27,170] Some of the proteins may be shared by other organisms.[27,170] The attachment has been studied in detail in the hamster model and in tracheal culture. Ciliary movements ceased after a couple of days; the latter effect is not observed in the case of nonpathogenic mycoplasmas. An infiltrate formed adjacent to the bronchial regions consisted primarily of mononuclear cells and some cells defined as plasma cells.[26,49] A proportion of the cells were rosette-forming, probably leukocytes and T cells. Polymorphonuclear cells increased with time.[26] *M. pneumoniae* rarely invades the alveoli or the interstitial tissues. Tissue damage may be produced by catalase inhibition, allowing the toxicity of hydrogen peroxide to damage the cells.[2] Nonpathogenic strains, recovered through repeated passage in the laboratory, often fail to cause hemolysis[176] and have lost some protein bands as seen by immunoblotting.[89,90] CAs probably constitute cross-reacting autoantibodies to the I antigen on human erythrocytes and the membrane of *M. pneumoniae*.[33] Erythrocyte receptors are sialylated oligosaccharides of the I type.[100]

Although the number of fatalities due to *M. pneumoniae* infection coming to autopsy is small, the postmortem findings are similar to those seen in the hamster model: interstitial infiltrates surround bronchi and bronchioles.[87,103,109] The infiltrates consist primarily of mononuclear cells, especially macrophages, lymphocytes, and plasma cells. The alveolar lining cells are swollen. Exudate, consisting of fibrin and leukocytes, has been observed primarily in the bronchial spaces. The mechanism of death from this disease is often thromboembolism, including disseminated intravascular coagulation.[38,103,109,117] Some patients appear to have died from pulmonary insufficiency.[109]

Interferon is produced during *M. pneumoniae* infection, lasts for a prolonged period, and may be related to prolonged symptomatology.[123,125]

7.3. Immunity

The mechanism of immunity to *M. pneumoniae* is incompletely understood. When previously infected hamsters were rechallenged with *M. pneumoniae* organisms, the immunological response and the development of exudates were accelerated and exaggerated.[26] It was shown that leukocytes played a role in the response.[26] In humans, the presence of most humoral antibodies correlates with immunity. Infection rates and pneumonia rates are low in persons with antibodies.[55,60,106,154] However, serum antibodies, most of which are directed toward the lipid membrane, may constitute only an indirect measure of immunity. Repeated episodes of *M. pneumoniae* pneumonia, 2–7 years after the initial episode, have been documented in children and in young adults by isolation and fourfold titer rises.[58,125] Recurrences were seen only in children under the age of 10 during a 9-month epidemic in two kibbutzim.[91] Yet, the immunity to repeated infection is much better in persons

who have had *M. pneumoniae* pneumonia than in those who
had no infection or only mild infection.[60] Repeated infections have also been observed in persons with naturally
acquired cell-mediated immunity.[10,17] Persons with immunodeficiency in the humoral antibody system suffered prolonged and severe disease,[56,166] but paradoxically, no infiltrates were observed on the chest film.[56] This may
indicate that the pulmonary infiltrate, consisting primarily
of various immune cells, serves a useful purpose in normal
persons.

Children under the age of 5 sometimes appear to suffer
mild or no symptoms when infected with *M. pneumoniae*.[50,53,155] This may support the hypothesis that the
first infection primarily sensitizes the individual and at subsequent exposure, disease develops. However, in some
studies, where children were under close clinical observation, a high rate of pneumonia was observed.[7,13,69,162]
This relationship deserves further study.

M. pneumoniae elicits a variety of immunological responses. The CF antibodies are of both the IgM and the IgG
type.[9,46] Antibodies of the IgA class are induced in nasal
and bronchial secretions after infection with live *M. pneumoniae;* these may be related more to protection than are
humoral antibodies.[14,20,124] An increase in IgG relative to
IgM antibodies has been noticed with time after onset of
illness. Adults respond with a higher IgG antibody ratio
than do children,[14] and may respond with only IgG antibodies. Family studies suggest that persons may be immune
without detectable CF antibody, and the elderly, who appear
to be immune to a high degree, usually lack CF antibody.[53]

The individual variability in response is considerable.
In some cases, antilipid CF antibodies appear to decay
rapidly, particularly in children; in others, especially those
with pneumonia, they may decay slowly over 5
years.[10,17,60,67] The decay of TRI and GI antibodies follows a similar pattern, although they may possibly last
somewhat longer.[17,163]

CAs are of the IgM type and not identical with any of
the *M. pneumoniae*-specific antibodies. Genetic variability
in response is suggested in experiments with different
strains of mice, some of which developed CAs and some of
which did not.[77] Since the I antigens are not completely
developed until the age of 18 months, immunological im-
maturity may partially explain the milder *M. pneumoniae*
infection in infants.

M. pneumoniae patients often develop not only CAs,
but also antibodies that cross-react with various other
human tissues, e.g., brain, liver, heart, and lung.[12,16]
Such antibodies may explain some of the complications of
M. pneumoniae infections, although these antibodies are

found in patients both with and without complications.
Also, circulating antigen–antibody complexes have been
demonstrated in patients both with and without complications.[12,113] *M. pneumoniae* is also a polyclonic B-cell
activator[11] and induces tuberculin anergy after infection,[15,125] suggesting temporary suppression of cell-mediated immunity. Cross-reacting antibodies to streptococcus
MG (*Streptococcus anginosus*) were observed as early as
the 1940s.[143] Rheumatoid factor may develop.[112] This is
also a nonspecific reaction. *M. pneumoniae* patients have
been observed to have positive skin tests for *Micropolyspora faeni* (cause of farmer's lung),[35] and farmers
who had *M. pneumoniae* pneumonia afterwards developed
typical farmer's lung.[107] Patients with sarcoidosis have a
high prevalence of antibodies to *M. pneumoniae,* possibly
reflecting a generalized increase in antibody formation.[137]

Cell-mediated immunity to *M. pneumoniae* following
infection has been shown by lymphocyte stimulation, inhibition of migration of leukocytes, and skin-testing.[10,17,47,111]
Lymphocytes responded to sonicated *M. pneumoniae* antigen up to 10 years after infection. Sensitivity to *M. pneumoniae* skin tests, which is induced by internal (nonlipid)
antigens, increases with advancing age.[11]

In the hamster model, circulating antibody, acquired
by parenteral immunization, did not correlate with protection.[48] GI activity, possibly IgA, was demonstrated in
bronchial washings. Local immune response, whether cell-
mediated or secretory, appears important in immunity.[46]

Based on studies of *in vitro* responses of human lymphocytes to *M. pneumoniae*, Fernald *et al.*[50] postulated
that immunity to *M. pneumoniae* is mediated by circulating
small lymphocytes.

8. Patterns of Host Response

8.1. Clinical Features

The pattern of host response to *M. pneumoniae* infection ranges from asymptomatic infection to pharyngitis,
bronchitis, bronchiolitis, croup, tracheobronchitis, pneumonitis, and pneumonia[23,37,43,53,65,94] (Table 2).

The onset of *M. pneumoniae* pneumonia is usually
insidious, in contrast to the abrupt onset of classic pneumococcal pneumonia. The symptoms include chills (55%),
headache (66%), sore throat (54%), malaise (89%), and
cough (99%).[44,57,114] The disease may mimic any viral
respiratory disease such as influenza or adenovirus infection
and even the common cold. In contrast to most viral respiratory diseases, frank coryza is infrequent, and stuffy nose is
reported in about 30% of cases.[57] Cough is charac-

Table 2. Manifestations of *Mycoplasma pneumoniae* Infections

Pneumonitis/pneumonia
Bronchitis, tracheobronchitis
Bronchiolitis
Tracheobronchitis
Pharyngitis
Croup
Otitis

Common complications
  Otitis, including bullous hemorrhagic myringitis
  Skin rashes, maculopapular or urticarial
  Pleuritis
  Thrombocytopenia
  Meningitis–encephalitis
  Mild anemia

Rare complications
  Hemolytic anemia
  Disseminated intravascular coagulation
  Thromboembolism
  Lung abscess
  Hyperlucent lung syndrome
  Pneumothorax
  Respiratory distress syndrome
  Pericarditis
  Myocarditis, glomerulitis
  Arthritis
  Erythema nodosum
  Stevens–Johnson syndrome

Neurological complications
  Meningitis
  Encephalitis
  Psychosis
  Guillain–Barré syndrome
  Cerebellar ataxia
  Brain-stem syndrome
  Poliomyelitislike syndrome

teristically nonproductive and irritating at onset, and may be paroxysmal. In young children, it may have a staccato character and be exaggerated at night. Although the disease resolves spontaneously even without treatment, relapses occur, convalescence may be prolonged, and patients may keep on coughing for months.

Asthmatic children may be at higher risk of *M. pneumoniae* pneumonia and even normal children may develop wheezing that may persist.[144]

Follow-up studies of *M. pneumoniae* patients have shown a decrease in tracheobronchial clearance that may last for a year or more.[79]

A great variety of complications have been described (Table 2).[117] Otitis,[53,81,152] bullous hemorrhagic myringitis,[140] pleuritis,[122] abscess of the lung,[1,117] and adult respiratory distress syndrome[109] can be considered extensions of the respiratory-tract infections. Complications related to the action of CAs consist of hemolytic anemia, thrombocytopenia, clot formation (thrombosis), and disseminated intravascular coagulation.[38,103,117] It may be speculated that myocarditis,[117] temporary arthritis,[72] and encephalitis and meningitis[73,93] have been due to cross-reacting antibodies or circulating immune complexes.[12] However, the recovery of the organism from CSF[1,51,82] and synovial fluid[166] suggests direct invasion. Skin rashes, usually described as maculopapular or urticarial, occur in about 10–

20% of cases.[24,53,101] Since these manifestations often appear rather late in the disease when the patient has started to improve, they may also be an effect of immune response. Stevens–Johnson syndrome (erythema multiforme major or pluriorificialis) is a rare and sometimes life-threatening complication that mostly affects boys.[117,130,142,156]

Antibody responses to *M. pneumoniae* observed in pancreatitis are probably directed against an antigenic structure revealed during tissue destruction in this disease.[92]

Secondary invasion with bacterial pathogens has not been a major problem in *M. pneumoniae* pneumonia, although superimposed or concurrent *Haemophilus influenzae, Streptococcus pneumoniae,* and *Staphylococcus aureus* infections have been described.[52] Evidence of concurrent viral infection is common, but appears not to aggravate the disease.[57,125]

Based on findings of lipid antibodies in CSF, it has been speculated that *M. pneumoniae* may be a cause of multiple sclerosis.[102]

8.2. Diagnosis

A diagnosis of *M. pneumoniae* pneumonia should be suspected in persons with gradual onset of sore throat, headache, chills, cough, fever, and pneumonitis. The white blood cell count is usually normal or slightly elevated;

eosinophilia has been reported.[3] The sedimentation rate is high.[94,143] Many mild cases escape proper diagnosis even if seen by a physician. Dullness is rarely present on examination of the chest, since consolidation is seldom complete. Only a few rales may be heard despite an extensive infiltrate on the chest film. The radiological infiltrate is more often unilateral (84%) than bilateral.[57] It is often described as segmental and patchy and with punctate mottling. Hilar infiltrates are common and characteristically fan out in a wedge-shaped manner, but any configuration and location of the infiltrate is possible, including upper lobar infiltrates. Attempts are being made to diagnose *M. pneumoniae* infection rapidly with immunofluorescence and with electron microscopy of throat specimens, but these techniques have not found general use.[28] In patients with pneumonia, a high titer of CAs (1 : 32) is highly suggestive of *M. pneumoniae* infection.[94] As noted in Section 3.4.2, the test can sometimes be conducted at the bedside, when agglutination occurs as the blood cools off; placing the tubes in an ice bath will accentuate the effect. The Coombs test, which measures antibody against erythrocytes, is also positive in CA-positive pneumonia. The reticulocyte count may be low.

Epidemiological clues may be helpful: since pneumonia of other etiologies is infrequent among persons 15–29 years of age, a high proportion of pneumonia is due to *M. pneumoniae* in this age group. Likewise, a high proportion of pneumonia encountered in the summer is due to *M. pneumoniae,* because then other respiratory agents are at a low ebb. A history of other family members or contacts having had similar disease about 3 weeks previously is also suggestive.

Isolation of the organism from respiratory secretions is almost diagnostic, since the organism is rarely isolated from healthy individuals.[67] However, it may take 1–4 weeks for the laboratory to grow the organism. In lieu of isolation, which is offered in only a few specialized laboratories, a significant rise in *M. pneumoniae* antibody titer (see Section 3.4.2) between acute and convalescent specimens taken 2–3 weeks apart can be considered diagnostic, as well as presence of specific IgM antibody.[169]

9. Control and Prevention

9.1. Treatment

Controlled double-blind studies have shown that treatment with tetracycline, its derivatives, and erythromycin shortens the duration of illness.[85,148] Josamycin, available outside the United States, is also effective,[172] but clin-

damycin, another macrolide antibiotic similar to erythromycin, is not.[150] The response to treatment is far less dramatic than that to antibiotic treatment of other bacterial infections of the lung. Occasionally, relapses are seen after short duration (5 days) of treatment.[67,151] Despite the patient's clinical improvement, shedding of the organisms continues unabated. Since tetracycline may stain developing teeth, erythromycin is the preferred drug for children. Strains resistant to tetracycline and erythromycin have been isolated.[126,157] Patients with hemolytic anemia may require transfusion of blood, preferably i-erythrocytes, and the blood should be warmed to prevent hemolysis due to CAs in the host.

9.2. Antibiotic Prophylaxis

This has been studied in elegant experiments in the hamster model: early prophylaxis soon after inoculation only postponed the development of pneumonia, which appeared as the antibiotics were stopped.[37] Prophylactic treatment with antibiotics of persons incubating the infection has given mixed results.[81,104] In one such study, it was difficult to distinguish therapeutic and prophylactic effects.[81]

Although antibiotic treatment does not eradicate the organism, it is possible that the number of excreted organisms decreases.

9.3. Vaccines

As early as 1964, Couch *et al.*[34] conducted challenge studies with organisms that had been passed a varying number of times on agar. Challenge with the agar-grown mycoplasmas was followed by less severe illness than was challenge with tissue-grown organisms; furthermore, high-passage-number strains appeared less virulent. A small-scale trial of egg-grown vaccine, in which vaccinated and control subjects were challenged with aerosolized *M. pneumoniae* organisms, showed protection among those who had responded serologically to the vaccine.[151] Those who failed to respond, however, suffered relatively severe disease compared with the total control group. This raised the question of whether low-dose vaccine may sensitize rather than protect. It has been suggested that in this challenge study, only those who had previously undergone natural infection responded serologically to the vaccine and that the nonresponders were a subset of persons without previous natural infection. Comparing this subset with controls composed of persons both with and without natural immunity may have yielded falsely alarming results. Subsequently, two large vaccine trials have been carried out among military personnel using two inactivated vaccines made from organisms grown on glass surfaces.[115,171] The trials showed moderate protection against pneumonia, at most 66–67% in the first year following inoculation. The data on protection from bronchitis are conflicting. Carriage rates were not affected by vaccine, but, as in other military studies, increased from 0 to 10% after 9 weeks of training. In neither trial did vaccinees who contracted pneumonia have more severe disease than controls, although such a phemonemon was diligently sought. Great concern remains about the feasibility of giving vaccines to children, since the response in *M. pneumoniae* pneumonia appears to be immunological in character.[50]

Live vaccine consisting of temperature-sensitive mutants has been tested on a small scale with promising results.[68] This approach has the appeal of inducing local immunity in the respiratory tract. Experiments in the hamster model suggest that this may be the most efficacious method of immunization.[48]

10. Unresolved Problems

A rapid diagnostic test is needed for clinical use. Sensitivity and specificity need to be determined. Why do children under age 5 seem to have milder disease than older children? A similar disease model is seen for rubella and mumps, these being diseases that are also not easily recognized before school age. The hypothesis that a primary infection with *M. pneumoniae* causes asymptomatic infection but sensitizes to more severe disease on second exposure needs to be either verified or refuted. Until this relationship is clarified, attempts to control this infection in children with vaccine, be it live or killed, cannot be carried out because of conjectured adverse reactions. Lack of pulmonary infiltrates in infants infected with *M. pneumoniae* needs to be confirmed by chest film. The duration of immunity and the role of various humoral antibodies, local antibodies, and cell-mediated immunity in protection from illness, possible exaggeration of symptoms, and eradication of the organisms need to be clarified. What exactly is the mode of transmission? Is the mode of transmission (contact or aerosol) important? Is the infecting dose important?

What is the mechanism of certain complications, such as meningoencephalitis, arthritis, skin rash, and Stevens–Johnson syndrome? What role do circulating antigen–antibody complexes and cross-reacting antibodies play in this disease? The rate of serious complications and mortality is unknown and cannot be determined by serologic studies.

To what extent does antigenic variation occur? Does wide use of tetracyclines and erythromycin promote development of resistant strains? Is *M. pneumoniae* pneumonia as easy to treat with these antibiotics nowadays as it was when the antibiotics were first introduced in the 1950s and 1960s?

Why are *M. pneumoniae* antibody titers sometimes high in pancreatitis and sarcoidosis?

A systematic investigation of the role of *M. pneumoniae* in the acute neurological syndromes listed in Table 1 is needed. Current knowledge is based on anecdotal case reports; often the diagnosis is made serologically only.

Clearly, a number of questions concerning the epidemiology, pathogenesis, immunity to, and control of *M. pneumoniae* pneumonia remain as a challenge to further investigation.

11. References

1. ABRAMOVITZ, P., SCHVARTZMAN, P., HAREL, D., LIS I., AND NAOT, Y., Direct invasion of the central nervous system by *Mycoplasma pneumoniae:* A report of two cases, *J. Infect. Dis.* **155:**482–487 (1987).
2. ALMAGOR, M., YATZIV, S., AND KAHANE, I., Inhibition of host cell catalase by *Mycoplasma pneumoniae:* A possible mechanism for cell injury, *Infect. Immun.* **41:**251–256 (1983).
3. ANDREWS, C. E., HOPEWELL, P., BURRELL, R. E., OLSON, N. O., AND CHICK, E. W., An epidemic of respiratory infection due to *Mycoplasma pneumoniae* in a civilian population, *Am. Rev. Respir. Dis.* **95:**972–979 (1967).
4. ARNOLD, K., KILBRIDGE, T. M., MILLER, W. C., JR., SMITH, T. J., AND CUTTING, R. T., Mycoplasma pneumonia: A study on hospitalized American patients with pneumonia in Vietnam, *Am. J. Trop. Med. Hyg.* **26:**743–747 (1977).
5. ASSAAD, F., GISPEN, R., KLEEMOLA, M., SYRUČEK, L., AND ESTEVES, K., Neurological diseases associated with viral and *Mycoplasma pneumoniae* infections, *Bull. WHO* **58:**297–311 (1980).
6. BAERNSTEIN, H. D., JR., TREVISANI, E., AXTELL, S., AND QUILLIGAN, J. J., JR., *Mycoplasma pneumoniae* (Eaton atypical pneumonia agent) in children's respiratory infections, *J. Pediatr.* **66:**829–837 (1965).
7. BALASSANIAN, N., AND ROBBINS, F. C., *Mycoplasma pneumoniae* infection in families, *N. Engl. J. Med.* **277:**719–725 (1967).
8. BERNTSSON, E., LAGERGÅRD, T., STRANNEGÅRD, Ö., AND TROLLFORS, B., Etiology of community-acquired pneumonia in out-patients, *Eur. J. Clin. Microbiol.* **5:**446–447 (1986).

9. BIBERFELD, G., Distribution of antibodies within 19 S and 7 S immunoglobulins following infection with *Mycoplasma pneumoniae*, *J. Immunol.* **100**:338–347 (1968).

10. BIBERFELD, G., Cell-mediated immune response following *Mycoplasma pneumoniae* infection in man. II. Leukocyte migration inhibition, *Clin. Exp. Immunol.* **17**:43–49 (1974).

11. BIBERFELD, G., AND GRONOWICZ, E., *Mycoplasma pneumoniae* is a polyclonal B-cell activator, *Nature* **261**:238–239 (1976).

12. BIBERFELD, G., AND NORBERG, R., Circulating immune complexes in *Mycoplasma pneumoniae* infection, *J. Immunol.* **112**:413–415 (1974).

13. BIBERFELD, G., AND STERNER, G., A study of *Mycoplasma pneumoniae* infections in families, *Scand. J. Infect. Dis.* **1**:39–46 (1969).

14. BIBERFELD, G., AND STERNER, G., Antibodies in bronchial secretions following natural infection with *Mycoplasma pneumoniae*, *Acta Pathol. Microbiol. Scand. Sect. B* **79**:599–605 (1971).

15. BIBERFELD, G., AND STERNER, G., Tuberculin anergy in patients with *Mycoplasma pneumoniae* infection, *Scand. J. Infect. Dis.* **8**:71–73 (1976).

16. BIBERFELD, G., AND STERNER, G., Smooth muscle antibodies in *Mycoplasma pneumoniae* infection, *Clin. Exp. Immunol.* **24**:287–291 (1976).

17. BIBERFELD, G., BIBERFELD, P., AND STERNER, G., Cell-mediated immune response following *Mycoplasma pneumoniae* infection in man, *Clin. Exp. Immunol.* **41**:29–41 (1974).

18. BROOME, C. V., LA VENTURE, M., KAYE, H. S., DAVIS, A. T., WHITE, H., PLIKAYTIS, B. D., AND FRASER, D. W., An explosive outbreak of *Mycoplasma pneumoniae* infection in a summer camp, *Pediatrics* **66**:884–888 (1980).

19. BRUNNER, Z. H., AND CHANOCK, R. M., A radioimmunoprecipitation test for detection of *Mycoplasma pneumoniae* antibody (37261), *Proc. Soc. Exp. Biol. Med.* **143**:97–105 (1973).

20. BRUNNER, H., GREENBERG, H. B., JAMES, W. D., HORSWOOD, R. L., COUCH, R. B., AND CHANOCK, R. M., Antibody to *Mycoplasma pneumoniae* in nasal secretions and sputa of experimentally infected human volunteers. *Infect. Immun.* **8**:612–620 (1973).

21. CHANOCK, R. M., COOK, M. K., FOX, H. H., PARROT, R. H., AND HUEBNER, R. J., Serologic evidence of infection with Eaton agent in lower respiratory illness in childhood. *N. Engl. J. Med.* **262**:648–654 (1960).

22. CHANOCK, R. M., HAYFLICK, L., AND BARILE, M. F., Growth on artificial medium of an agent associated with atypical pneumonia and its identification as a PPLO, *Proc. Natl. Acad. Sci. USA* **48**:41–49 (1962).

23. CHANOCK, R. M., FOX, H. H., JAMES, W. D., GUTEKUNST, R. R., WHITE, R. J., AND SENTERFIT, L. B., Epidemiology of *M. pneumoniae* infection in military recruits, *Ann. N.Y. Acad. Sci.* **143**:484–496 (1967).

24. CHERRY, J. D., HURWITZ, S., AND WELLIVER, R. C., *Mycoplasma pneumoniae* infections and exanthems, *J. Pediatr.* **87**:369–373 (1975).

25. CIMOLAI, N., SCHRYVERS, A., BRYAN, L. E., AND WOODS, D. E., Culture-amplified immunological detection of *Mycoplasma pneumoniae* in clinical specimens, *Diagn. Microbiol. Infect, Dis.* **9**:207–212 (1988).

26. CLYDE, W. A., JR., Immunopathology of experimental *Mycoplasma pneumoniae* disease, *Infect. Immun.* **4**:757–763 (1971).

27. CLYDE, W. A., JR., AND HU, P. C., Antigenic determinants of the attachment protein of *Mycoplasma pneumoniae* shared by other pathogenic *Mycoplasma* species, *Infect. Immun.* **51**:690–692 (1986).

28. COLIER, A. M., AND CLYDE, W. A., Appearance of *Mycoplasma pneumoniae* in lungs of experimentally infected hamsters and sputum from patients with natural disease, *Am. Rev. Respir. Dis.* **110**:765–773 (1974).

29. Commission on Acute Respiratory Diseases, Transmission of primary atypical pneumonia to human volunteers, *J. Am. Med. Assoc.* **127**:146–149 (1945).

30. COONEY, M. K., FOX, J. P., AND HALL, C. E., The Seattle virus watch. VI. Observations of infections with and illness due to parainfluenza, mumps and respiratory syncytial viruses and *Mycoplasma pneumoniae*, *Am. J. Epidemiol.* **101**:532–551 (1975).

31. COPPS, C. J., ALLEN, V. D., SUELTMANN, S., AND EVANS, A. S., A community outbreak of *Mycoplasma pneumonia*, *J. Am. Med. Assoc.* **204**:123–128 (1968).

32. CORDERO, L., CUADRADO, R., HALL, C. B., AND HORSTMANN, D. M., Primary atypical pneumonia: An epidemic caused by *Mycoplasma pneumoniae*, *J. Pediatr.* **71**:1–12 (1967).

33. COSTEA, N., YAKULIS, V. J., AND HELLER, P., The mechanism of induction of cold agglutinins by *Mycoplasma pneumoniae*, *J. Immunol.* **106**:598–604 (1971).

34. COUCH, R. B., CATE, T. R., AND CHANOCK, R. M., Infection with artificially propagated Eaton agent, *J. Am. Med. Assoc.* **187**:442–447 (1964).

35. DAVIES, B. H., EDWARDS, J. H., AND SEATON, A., Cross reacting antibodies to *Micropolyspora faeni* in *Mycoplasma pneumoniae* infection, *Clin. Allergy* **5**:217–224 (1975).

36. DAVIS, C. P., COCHRAN, S., LISSE, J., BUCK, G., DiNUZZO, A. R., WEBER, T., AND REINARZ, J. A., Isolation of *Mycoplasma pneumoniae* from synovial fluid samples in a patient with pneumonia and polyarthritis, *Arch. Intern. Med.* **148**:969–970 (1988).

37. DENNY, F. W., CLYDE, W. A., JR., AND GLEZEN, W. P., *Mycoplasma pneumoniae* disease: Clinical spectrum, pathophysiology, epidemiology, and control, *J. Infect. Dis.* **123**:74–92 (1971).

38. DE VOS, M., VAN NIMMEN, L. V., AND BAELE, G., Disseminated intravascular coagulation during a fatal *Mycoplasma pneumoniae* infection, *Acta Haematol.* **52**:120–125 (1974).

39. DOWDLE, W. R., STEWART, J. A., HEYWARD, J. T., AND

ROBINSON, R. Q., *Mycoplasma pneumoniae* infections in a children's population: A five-year study, *Am. J. Epidemiol.* **85:**137–146 (1967).

40. EATON, M. D., MEIKELJOHN, G., AND VAN HERICK, W., Studies on the etiology of primary atypical pneumonia: A filterable agent transmissible to cotton rats, hamsters, and chick embryos, *J. Exp. Med.* **79:**649–668 (1944).

41. EDWARDS, E. A., CRAWFORD, Y. E., PIERCE, W. E., AND PECKINPAUGH, R. O., A longitudinal study of *Mycoplasma pneumoniae* infections in Navy recruits by isolation and seroepidemiology, *Am. J. Epidemiol.* **104:**556–562 (1976).

42. EVANS, A. S., Serologic studies of acute respiratory infections in military personnel, *Yale J. Biol. Med.* **48:**201–209 (1975).

43. EVANS, A. S., AND BROBST, M., Bronchitis, pneumonitis and pneumonia in University of Wisconsin students, *N. Engl. J. Med.* **265:**401–405 (1961).

44. EVANS, A. S., ALLEN, V., AND SUELTMANN, S., *Mycoplasma pneumoniae* infections in University of Wisconsin students, *Am. Rep. Respir. Dis.* **96:**237–244 (1967).

45. EVATT, B. L., DOWDLE, W. R., JOHNSON, M., JR., AND HEATH, C. W., Epidemic Mycoplasma pneumonia, *N. Engl. J. Med.* **285:**374–378 (1971).

46. FERNALD, G. W., Immunologic aspects of experimental *Mycoplasma pneumoniae* infection, *J. Infect. Dis.* **119:**255–266 (1969).

47. FERNALD, G. W., *In vitro* response of human lymphocytes to *Mycoplasma pneumoniae*, *Infect. Immun.* **5:**552–558 (1972).

48. FERNALD, G. W., AND CLYDE, W. A., JR., Protective effect of vaccines in experimental *Mycoplasma pneumoniae* disease, *Infect. Immun.* **1:**559–565 (1970).

49. FERNALD, G. W., CLYDE, W. A., JR., AND BIENENSTOCK, J., Immunoglobulin-containing cells in lungs of hamsters infected with *Mycoplasma pneumoniae*, *J. Immunol.* **108:**1400–1408 (1972).

50. FERNALD, G. W., COLLIER, A. M., AND CLYDE, W. A., Respiratory infections due to *Mycoplasma pneumoniae* in infants and children, *Pediatrics* **55:**327–334 (1975).

51. FLEISCHHAUER, P., HUBEN, U., MERTENS, H., SETHI, K. K., AND THURMANN, D., Nachweis von *Mycoplasma pneumoniae* im Liquor bei akuter Polyneuritis, *Dtsch. Med. Wochenschr.* **97:**678–682 (1972).

52. FOY, H. M., Pneumonia: *Mycoplasma pneumoniae*, in: *Communicable and Infectious Diseases*, 8th ed. (F. H. TOP, SR., AND P. F. WEHRLE, eds.), pp. 535–549, Mosby, St. Louis, 1976.

53. FOY, H. M., GRAYSTON, J. T., KENNY, G. E., ALEXANDER, E. R., AND McMAHAN, R., Epidemiology of *Mycoplasma pneumoniae* infection in families, *J. Am. Med. Assoc.* **197:**859–866 (1966).

54. FOY, H. M., KENNY, G. E., McMAHAN, R., MANSY, A. M., AND GRAYSTON, J. T., *Mycoplasma pneumoniae* pneumonia in an urban area, *J. Am. Med. Assoc.* **30:**1666–1672 (1970).

55. FOY, H. M., KENNY, G. E., McMAHAN, R., KAISER, G., AND GRAYSTON, J. T., *Mycoplasma pneumoniae* in the community, *Am. J. Epidemiol.* **93:**55–67 (1971).

56. FOY, H. M., OCHS, H., DAVIS, S. D., KENNY, G. E., AND LUCE, R. R., *Mycoplasma pneumoniae* infections in patients with immunodeficiency syndromes: Report of four cases, *J. Infect. Dis.* **127:**388–393 (1973).

57. FOY, H. M., COONEY, M. K., McMAHAN, R., AND GRAYSTON, J. T., Viral and mycoplasmal pneumonia in a prepaid medical care group during an eight-year period, *Am. J. Epidemiol.* **97:**93–102 (1973).

58. FOY, H. M., KENNY, G. E., SEFI, R., OCHS, H. D., AND ALLAN, I. D., Second attacks of pneumonia due to *Mycoplasma pneumoniae*, *J. Infect. Dis.* **135:**673–677 (1977).

59. FOY, H. M., KENNY, G. E., COONEY, M. K., AND ALLAN, I. D., Long-term epidemiology of infections with *Mycoplasma pneumoniae*, *J. Infect. Dis.* **139:**681–687 (1979).

60. FOY, H. M., KENNY, G. E., COONEY, M. K., ALLAN, I. D., AND VAN BELLE, G., Naturally acquired immunity to pneumonia due to *Mycoplasma pneumoniae*, *J. Infect. Dis.* **147:**967–973 (1983).

61. FOY, H. M., NOLAN, C. M., AND ALLAN, I. D., Epidemiologic aspects of *M. pneumoniae* disease complications: A review, *Yale J. Biol. Med.* **56:**469–473 (1983).

62. FREEMAN, R., KING, B., AND HAMBLING, M. H., Infection with *Mycoplasma pneumoniae* after open-heart surgery, *J. Thorac. Cardiovasc. Surg.* **66:**642–644 (1973).

63. GANICK, D. J., WOLFSON, J., GILBERT, E. F., AND JOO, P., *Mycoplasma* infection in the immunosuppressed leukemic patient, *Arch. Pathol. Lab. Med.* **104:**535–536 (1980).

64. GLEZEN, W. P., CLYDE, W. A., JR., SENIOR, R. J., SHEAFFER, C. I., AND DENNY, F. W., Group A streptococci, mycoplasmas, and viruses associated with acute pharyngitis, *J. Am. Med. Assoc.* **202:**455–460 (1967).

65. GLEZEN, W. P., THORNBURG, G., CHIN, T. D. Y., AND WENNER, H. A., Significance of Mycoplasma infections in children with respiratory disease, *Pediatrics* **39:**516–525 (1967).

66. GOVIL, M. K., AGRAWAL, B. D., LAL, M. M., NATH, K., SHARMA, B. K., SAMUEL, K. C., AND GUPTA, B. K., A study of acute respiratory diseases with special references to *Mycoplasma pneumoniae* infections, *J. Assoc. Physicians India* **23:**272–303 (1975).

67. GRAYSTON, J. T., FOY, H. M., AND KENNY, G. E., The epidemiology of Mycoplasma infections of the human respiratory tract, in: *The Mycoplasmatales and the L-Phase of Bacteria* (L. HAYFLICK, ed.), pp. 651–682, Appleton–Century–Crofts, New York, 1969.

68. GREENBERG, H., HELMS, C. M., BRUNNER, H., AND CHANOCK, R. M., Asymptomatic infection of adult volunteers with a temperature sensitive mutant of *Mycoplasma pneumoniae*, *Proc. Natl. Acad. Sci. USA* **71:**4015–4019 (1974).

69. HANUKOGLU, A., HEBRONI, S., AND FRIED, D., Pulmonary involvement in *Mycoplasma pneumoniae* infection in families, *Infection* **14:**1–6 (1986).

70. HARRIS, R., MARMION, B. P., VARKANIS, G., KOK, T., LUNN, B., AND MARTIN, J., Laboratory diagnosis of Mycoplasma pneumoniae infection. 2. Comparison of methods for the direct detection of specific antigen or nucleic acid sequences in respiratory exudates, *Epidemiol. Infect.* **101**:685–694 (1988).

71. HATCH, M. T., WRIGHT, D. N., AND BAILEY, G. D., Response of airborne *Mycoplasma pneumoniae* to abrupt changes in relative humidity, *Appl. Microbiol.* **19**:232–238 (1970).

72. HERNANDEZ, L. A., URQUHART, G. E. D., AND DICK, W. C., *Mycoplasma pneumoniae* infection and arthritis in man, *Br. Med. J.* **2**:14–16 (1977).

73. HODGES, G. R., FASS, R. J., AND SASLAW, S., Central nervous system disease associated with *Mycoplasma pneumoniae* infection, *Arch. Intern. Med.* **130**:277–282 (1972).

74. HU, P. C., POWELL, D. A., ALBRIGHT, F., GARDNER, D. E., COLLIER, A. M., AND CLYDE, W. A., JR., A solid-phase radioimmunoassay for detection of antibodies against *Mycoplasma pneumoniae*, *J. Clin. Lab. Immunol.* **11**:209–213 (1983).

75. HU, P. C., HUANG, C.-H., HUANG, Y.-S., COLLIER, A. M., AND CLYDE, W. A., JR., Demonstration of multiple antigenic determinants on *Mycoplasma pneumoniae* attachment protein by monoclonal antibodies, *Infect. Immun.* **50**:292–296 (1985).

76. JACOBS, E., BENNEWITZ, A., AND BREDT, W., Reaction pattern of human anti-*Mycoplasma pneumoniae* antibodies in enzyme-linked immunosorbent assays and immunoblotting, *J. Clin. Microbiol.* **23**:517–522 (1986).

77. JANNEY, F. A., LEE, L. T., AND HOWE, C., Cold hemagglutinin cross-reactivity with *Mycoplasma pneumoniae*, *Infect. Immun.* **22**:29–33 (1978).

78. JANSSON, E., VON ESSEN, R., AND TUURI, S., *Mycoplasma pneumoniae* pneumonia in Helsinki 1962–1970, *Scand. J. Infect. Dis.* **3**:51–54 (1971).

79. JARSTRAND, C., CAMNER, P., AND PHILIPSON, K., *Mycoplasma pneumoniae* and tracheobronchial clearance, *Am. Rev. Respir. Dis.* **110**:415–419 (1974).

80. JEMSKI, J. V., HETSKO, C. M., HELMS, C. M., GRIZZARD, M. B., WALKER, J. S., AND CHANOCK, R. M., Immunoprophylaxis of experimental *Mycoplasma pneumoniae* disease: Effect of aerosol particle size and site of deposition of *M. pneumoniae* on the pattern of respiratory infection, disease, and immunity in hamsters, *Infect. Immun.* **16**:93–98 (1977).

81. JENSEN, K. J., SENTERFIT, L. B., SCULLY, W. E., CONWAY, T. J., WEST, R. F., AND DRUMMY, W. W., *Mycoplasma pneumoniae* infections in children: An epidemiologic appraisal in families treated with oxytetracycline, *Am. J. Epidemiol.* **86**:419–432 (1967).

82. KASAHARA, I., OTSUBO, Y., YANASE, T., OSHIMA, H., ICHIMARU, H., AND NAKAMURA, M., Isolation and characterization of *Mycoplasma pneumoniae* from cerebrospinal fluid of a patient with pneumonia and meningoencephalitis, *J. Infect. Dis.* **152**:823–825 (1985).

83. KENNY, G. E., Mycoplasmas, in: *Manual of Clinical Microbiology* (E. H. LENNETTE, A. BALOWS, W. J. HAUSLER, JR., AND H. J. SHADOMY, eds.) pp. 407–411, American Society for Microbiology, Washington, D.C., 1985.

84. KENNY, G. E., Serology of mycoplasmal infections, in: *Manual of Clinical Immunology* (N. R. ROSE, H. FRIEDMAN, AND J. L. FAHEY, eds.), pp. 440–445, American Society for Microbiology, Washington, D.C., 1986.

85. KINGSTON, J. R., CHANOCK, R. M., MUFSON, M. S., HELLMAN, L. P., JAMES, W. D., FOX, H. H., MANKO, M. A., AND BOYERS, J., Eaton agent pneumonia, *J. Am. Med. Assoc.* **176**:118–123 (1961).

86. KLEEMOLA, M., AND KÄYHTY, H., Increase in titers of antibodies to *Mycoplasma pneumoniae* in patients with purulent meningitis, *J. Infect. Dis.* **146**:284–288 (1982).

87. KOLETSKY, R. J., AND WEINSTEIN, A. J., Fulminant *Mycoplasma pneumoniae* infection. Report of a fatal case, and a review of the literature, *Am. Rev. Respir. Dis.* **122**:491–496 (1980).

88. KOMAROFF, A. L., ARONSON, M. D., PASS, T. M., ERVIN, C. T., BRANCH, W. T., JR., AND SCHACHTER, J., Serological evidence of chlamydial and mycoplasmal pharyngitis in adults, *Science* **222**:927–929 (1983).

89. KRAUSE, D. C., AND BASEMAN, J. B., Inhibition of *Mycoplasma pneumoniae* hemadsorption and adherence to respiratory epithelium by antibodies to a membrane protein, *Infect. Immun.* **39**:1180–1186 (1983).

90. KRAUSE, D. C., LEITH, D. K., WILSON, R. M., AND BASEMAN, J. B., Identification of *Mycoplasma pneumoniae* proteins associated with hemadsorption and virulence, *Infect. Immun.* **35**:809–817 (1982).

91. LEIBOWITZ, Z. SCHVARTZMAN, P., EPSTEIN, L., LIS, I., AND NAOT, Y., An outbreak of *Mycoplasma pneumoniae* pneumonia in two kibbutzim: A clinical and epidemiologic study, *Isr. J. Med. Sci.* **24**:88–92 (1988).

92. LEINIKKI, P. O., PANZAR, P., AND TYKKA, H., Immunoglobulin M antibody response against *Mycoplasma pneumoniae* lipid antigen in patients with acute pancreatitis, *J. Clin. Microbiol.* **8**:113–118 (1978).

93. LERER, R. J., AND KALAVSKY, S. M., Central nervous system disease associated with *Mycoplasma pneumoniae* infection: Report of five cases and review of the literature, *Pediatrics* **52**:658–668 (1973).

94. LEVINE, D. P., AND LERNER, A. M., The clinical spectrum of *Mycoplasma pneumoniae* infections, *Med. Clin. North Am.* **62**:961–978 (1978).

95. LIND, K., AND BENTZON, M. W., Epidemics of *Mycoplasma pneumoniae* infection in Denmark from 1958 to 1974, *Int. J. Epidemiol.* **5**:267–277 (1976).

96. LIND, K., AND BENTZON, M. W., Changes in the epidemiological pattern of *Mycoplasma pneumoniae* infections in Denmark, *Epidemiol. Infect.* **101**:377–386 (1988).

97. LIND, K., LINDHARDT, B. Ø., SCHÜTTEN, H. J., BLOOM, J., AND CHRISTIANSEN, C., Serological cross-reactions between *Mycoplasma genitalium* and *Mycoplasma pneumoniae*, *J. Clin. Microbiol.* **20**:1036–1043 (1984).

98. LIU, C., Studies on primary atypical pneumonia. I. Localization, isolation, and cultivation of virus in chick embryos, *J. Exp. Med.* **106:**455–456 (1957).

99. LIU, C., EATON, M. D., AND HEYL, J. T., Studies on primary atypical pneumonia. II. Observations concerning the development and immunological characteristics of antibody in patients, *J. Exp. Med.* **109:**545–556 (1959).

100. LOOMES, L. M., UEMURA, K., CHILDS, R. A., PAULSON, J. C., ROGERS, G. N., SCUDDER, P. R., MICHALSKI, J.-C., HOUNSELL, E. F., TAYLOR-ROBINSON, D., AND FEIZI, T., Erythrocyte receptors for *Mycoplasma pneumoniae* are sialylated oligosaccharides of Ii antigen type, *Nature* **307:**560–563 (1984).

101. LYELL, A., GORDON, A. M., DICK, H. M., AND SOMMERVILLE, R. G., Mycoplasmas and erythema multiforme, *Lancet* **2:**1116–1118 (1967).

102. MAIDA, E., Immunological reactions against *Mycoplasma pneumoniae* in multiple sclerosis: Preliminary findings, *J. Neurol.* **229:**103–111 (1983).

103. MAISEL, J. C., BABBITT, L. H., AND JOHN, T. J., Fatal *Mycoplasma pneumoniae* infection with isolation of organisms from lung, *J. Am. Med. Assoc.* **202:**287–290 (1967).

104. MAISEL, J. C., PIERCE, W. E., AND STILLE, W. T., Chemoprophylaxis, *Am. Rev. Respir. Dis.* **97:**366–375 (1967).

105. MARMION, B. P., AND GOODBURN, G. M., Effect of an organic gold salt on Eaton's primary atypical pneumonia agent and other observations, *Nature* **189:**247–248 (1961).

106. McCORMICK, D. P., AND WENZEL, R. P., SENTERFIT, L. B., AND BEAM, W. E., JR., Relationship of pre-existing antibody to subsequent infection by *Mycoplasma pneumoniae* in adults, *Infect. Immun.* **9:**53–59 (1974).

107. McGAVIN, C., Farmer's lung after *Mycoplasma pneumoniae* infection, *Thorax* **41:**68–69 (1986).

108. McMILLAN, J. A., SANDSTROM, C., WEINER, L. B., FORBES, B. A., WOODS, M., HOWARD, T., POE, L., KELLER, K., CORWIN, R. M., AND WINKELMAN, J. W., Viral and bacterial organisms associated with acute pharyngitis in a school-aged population, *J. Pediatr.* **109:**747–752 (1986).

109. MEYERS, B. R., AND HIRSCHMAN, S. Z., Fatal infections associated with *Mycoplasma pneumoniae:* Discussion of three cases with necropsy findings, *Mt. Sinai J. Med.* **39:**258–264 (1972).

110. MICHEL, D., LAURENT, B., GRANOUILLET, R., AND GAUDIN-TERRASSE, O. D., Infections aiguës, récentes, et parfois persistantes à *Mycoplasma pneumoniae*, associées à des manifestations neurologiques, *Rev. Neurol.* **137:**393–413 (1981).

111. MIZUTANI, H., AND MIZUTANI, H., The skin-reactive antigens of *Mycoplasma pneumoniae*, *Jpn. J. Microbiol.* **19:**157–162 (1975).

112. MIZUTANI, H., AND MIZUTANI, H., Immunologic responses in patients with *Mycoplasma pneumoniae* infections, *Am. Rev. Respir. Dis.* **127:**175–179 (1983).

113. MIZUTANI, H., AND MIZUTANI, H., Circulating immune complexes in patients with mycoplasmal pneumonia, *Am. Rev. Respir. Dis.* **130:**627–629 (1984).

114. MOGABGAB, W. J., *Mycoplasma pneumoniae* and adenovirus respiratory illnesses in military and university personnel, 1959–1966, *Am. Rev. Respir. Dis.* **97:**345–358 (1968).

115. MOGABGAB, W. J., Protective efficacy of killed *Mycoplasma pneumoniae* vaccine measured in large-scale studies in a military population, *Am. Rev. Respir. Dis.* **108:**899–908 (1973).

116. MONTO, A. S., BRYAN, E. R., AND RHODES, L. M., The Tecumseh study of respiratory illness. VII. Further observations on the occurrence of respiratory syncytial virus and *Mycoplasma pneumoniae* infections, *Am. J. Epidermiol.* **100:**458–468 (1974).

117. MURRAY, H. W., MASUR, H., SENTERFIT, L. B., AND ROBERTS, R. B., The protean manifestations of *Mycoplasma pneumoniae* infection in adults, *Am. J. Med.* **58:**229–242 (1975).

118. NAFTALIN, J. M., WELLISCH, G., KAHANA, Z., AND DEINGOTT, D., *Mycoplasma pneumoniae* septicemia, *J. Am. Med. Assoc.* **228:**565 (1974).

119. NAGAYAMA, Y., SAKURAI, N., YAMAMOTO, K., HONDA, A., MAKUTA, M., AND SUZUKI, R., Isolation of *Mycoplasma pneumoniae* from children with lower-respiratory-tract infections, *J. Infect. Dis.* **157:**911–917 (1988).

120. NAKAMURA, S., EBISAWA, I., KITAMOTO, O., AND SATO, T., Persistence of serum antibody following *Mycoplasma pneumoniae* infection, *Am. Rev. Respir. Dis.* **101:**620–622 (1970).

121. NAKAO, T., AND UMETSU, M., An outbreak of *Mycoplasma pneumoniae* infection in a community, *Tohoku J. Exp. Med.* **102:**23–31 (1970).

122. NAKAO, T., ORII, T., AND UMETSU, M., *Mycoplasma pneumoniae* pneumonia with pleural effusion, with special reference to isolation of *Mycoplasma pneumoniae* from pleural fluid, *Tohoku J. Exp. Med.* **104:**13–18 (1971).

123. NAKAYAMA, T., URANO, T., OSANO, M., MAEHARA, N., AND MAKINO, S., α interferon in the sera of patients infected with *Mycoplasma pneumoniae*, *J. Infect. Dis.* **154:**904–906 (1986).

124. NAOT, Y., LIS, E., SIMAN-TOV, R., AND BRUNNER, H., Comparison of enzyme-linked immunosorbent assay and radioimmunoprecipitation test for detection of immunoglobulin A antibodies to *Mycoplasma pneumoniae* in nasal secretions, *J. Clin. Microbiol.* **24:**892–893 (1986).

125. NIITU, Y., *Mycoplasma pneumoniae* infections, *Acta Paediatr. Jpn.* **27:**73–90 (1984).

126. NIITU, Y., HASEGAWA, S., SUETAKE, T., KUBOTA, H., KOMATSU, S., AND HORIKAWA, M., Resistance of *Mycoplasma pneumoniae* to erythromycin and other antibiotics. *J. Pediatr.* **76:**438–443 (1970).

127. NOAH, N. D., *Mycoplasma pneumoniae* infection in the United Kingdom: An analysis of reports to the public health laboratory service in England and Wales, *Infection* **4**(Suppl. 1):25–28 (1976).

128. NOAH, N. D., AND URQUHART, A. M., Epidemiology of *Mycoplasma pneumoniae* infection in the British Isles, 1974–9, *J. Infect.* **2:**191–194 (1980).

129. OLDENBURGER, D., CARSON, J. P., GUNDLACH, W. J., GHALY, F. I., AND WRIGHT, W. H., Legionnaires' disease: Association with *Mycoplasma pneumonia* and disseminated intravascular coagulation, *J. Am. Med. Assoc.* **241:**1269–1270 (1979).

130. PARKER, F., JR., JOLLIFFE, L. S., AND FINLAND, M., Primary atypical pneumonia: Report of eight cases with autopsies, *Arch. Pathol.* **44:**581–608 (1947).

131. PATSCHEKE, H., BREINL, M., AND SCHAFER, E., Antibody assay for adenoviruses and *Mycoplasma pneumoniae* by the platelet aggregation test, *Z. Immunitaetsforsch.* **151:**341–349 (1976).

132. PETERSON, D. L., HAM, T. H., AND FINLAND, M., Cold agglutinins (autohemagglutinins) in primary atypical pneumonias, *Science* **97:**167 (1943).

133. PONCZ, M., KANE, E., AND GILL, F. M., Acute chest syndrome in sickle cell disease: Etiology and clinical correlates, *J. Pediatr.* **107:**861–866 (1985).

134. PÖNKÄ, A., Occurrence of serologically verified *Mycoplasma pneumoniae* infections in Finland and in Scandinavia in 1970–1977, *Scand. J. Infect. Dis.* **12:**27–31 (1980).

135. Public Heath Laboratory Service, Report from the PHLS Communicable Disease Surveillance Centre, *Br. Med. J.* **294:**361 (1987).

136. PURCELL, R., CHANOCK, R., AND TAYLOR-ROBINSON, R., Serology of the Mycoplasmas of man, in: *The Mycoplasmatales and the L-Phase of Bacteria* (L. HAYFLICK, ed.), pp. 221–264, Appleton–Century–Crofts, New York, 1969.

137. PUTMAN, C. E., BAUMGARTEN, A., AND GEE, J. B. L., The prevalence of mycoplasmal complement-fixing antibodies in sarcoidosis, *Am. Rev. Respir. Dis.* **3:**364–365 (1975).

138. RÄISÄNEN, S. M., SUNI, J., AND LEINIKKI, P., Serological diagnosis of *Mycoplasma pneumoniae* infection by enzyme immunoassay, *J. Clin. Pathol.* **33:**836–840 (1980).

139. REIMANN, H. A., An acute infection of the respiratory tract with typical pneumonia: A disease entity probably caused by a filterable virus, *J. Am. Med. Assoc.* **111:**2377–2384 (1938).

140. RIFKIND, D., CHANOCK, R., KRAVETZ, H., JOHNSON, K., AND KNIGHT, V., Ear involvement (myringitis) and primary atypical pneumonia following inoculation of volunteers with Eaton agent, *Am. Rev. Respir. Dis.* **85:**479–489 (1962).

141. ROIFMAN, C. M., RAO, C. P., LEDERMAN, H. M., LAVI, S., QUINN, P., AND GELFAND, E. W., Increased susceptibility to Mycoplasma infection in patients with hypogammaglobulinema, *Am. J. Med.* **80:**590–594 (1986).

142. RUHRMANN, G., AND HOLTHUSEN, W., Mycoplasma infection and erythromycin therapy in childhood, *Scott. Med. J.* **22:**401–403 (1977).

143. RYTEL, M. W., Primary atypical pneumonia: Current concepts, *Am. J. Med. Sci.* **247:**118–138 (1964).

144. SABATO, A. R., MARTIN, A. J., MARMION, B. P., KOK, T. W., AND COOPER, D. M., *Mycoplasma pneumoniae:* Acute

145. SALIBA, G. S., GLEZEN, W. P., AND CHIN, T. D. Y., *Mycoplasma pneumoniae* infection in a resident boys' home, *Am. J. Epidemiol.* **86:**409–418 (1967).

146. SANDE, M. A., GADOT, F., AND WENZEL, R. P., Point source epidemic of *Mycoplasma pneumoniae* infection in a prosthodontics laboratory, *Am. Rev. Respir. Dis.* **112:**213–217 (1975).

147. SAWYER, R., AND SOMMERVILLE, R. G., An outbreak of *Mycoplasma pneumoniae* infection in a nuclear submarine, *J. Am. Med. Assoc.* **195:**958–959 (1966).

148. SHAMES, J. M., GEORGE, R. B., HOLLIDAY, W. B., RASCH, J. R., AND MOGABGAB, W. J., Comparison of antibiotics in the treatment of mycoplasmal pneumonia, *Arch. Intern. Med.* **125:**680–684 (1970).

149. SHULMAN, S. T., BARTLETT, J., CLYDE, W. A., JR., AND AYOUB, E. M., The unusual severity of mycoplasmal pneumonia in children with sickle-cell disease, *N. Engl. J. Med.* **287:**164–167 (1972).

150. SMILACK, J. D., BURGIN, W. W., JR., MOORE, W. L., JR., AND SANFORD, J. P., *Mycoplasma pneumoniae* pneumonia and clindamycin therapy: Failure to demonstrate efficacy, *J. Am. Med. Assoc.* **228:**729–731 (1974).

151. SMITH, C. B., FRIEDEWALD, W. T., AND CHANOCK, R. M., Inactivated *Mycoplasma pneumoniae* vaccine: Evaluation in volunteers, *J. Am. Med. Assoc.* **199:**353–358 (1967).

152. SOBESLAVSKY, O., SYRUCEK, L., BRUCKOVA, M., AND ABRAMOVIC, M., The etiological role of *Mycoplasma pneumoniae* in otitis media in children, *Pediatrics* **35:**652–657 (1964).

153. SOBESLAVSKY, O., PRESCOTT, B., AND CHANOCK, R. M., Adsorption of *Mycoplasma pneumoniae* to neuraminic acid receptors of various cells and possible role in virulence, *J. Bacteriol.* **96:**695–705 (1968).

154. STEINBERG, P., WHITE, R. J., FULD, S. L., GUTEKUNST, R. R., CHANOCK, R. M., AND SENTERFIT, L. B., Ecology of *Mycoplasma pneumoniae* infections in Marine recruits at Parris Island, South Carolina, *Am. J. Epidemiol.* **89:**62–73 (1969).

155. STERNER, G., DE HEVESY, G., TUNEVALL, G., AND WOLONTIS, S., Acute respiratory illness with *Mycoplasma pneumoniae:* An outbreak in a home for children, *Acta Paediatr. Scand.* **55:**280–286 (1966).

156. STEVENS, D., SWIFT, P. G. F., JOHNSTON, P. G. B., KEARNEY, P. J., CORNER, B. D., AND BURMAN, D., *Mycoplasma pneumoniae* infections in children, *Arch. Dis. Child.* **53:**38–42 (1978).

157. STOPLER, T., AND BRANSKI, D., Resistance of *Mycoplasma pneumoniae* to macrolides, lincomycin and streptogramin B, *J. Antimicrob. Chemother.* **18:**358–364 (1986).

158. STUTMAN, H. R., Stevens–Johnson syndrome and *Mycoplasma pneumoniae:* Evidence for cutaneous infection, *Clin. Lab. Observ.* **111:**845–847 (1987).

159. SUHS, R. H., AND FELDMAN, H. A., Serologic epidemiologic

illness, antibiotics, and subsequent pulmonary function, *Arch. Dis. Child.* **59:**1034–1037 (1984).

studies with *M. pneumoniae*. II. Prevalence of antibodies in several populations, *Am. J. Epidemiol.* **83:**357–365 (1966).

160. SUKONTHAMAN, A., FREEMAN, J. D., RATANAVARARAK, M., KHAOPARISUTHI, V., AND SNIDVONGS, W., *Mycoplasma pneumoniae* infections—The first demonstration of an outbreak at a Kampuchean holding center in Thailand, *J. Med. Assoc. Thailand* **64:**392–400 (1981).

161. SUSSMAN, S. J., MAGOFFIN, R. L., LENNETTE, E. H., AND SCHIEBLE, J., Cold agglutinins, Eaton agent, and respiratory infections of children, *Pediatrics* **38:**571–577 (1966).

162. SZABO, N., LOOS, T., AND MARTHA, I., Durch *Mycoplasma pneumoniae* verursachte Erkrankungen im Kindesalter, *Z. Erkr. Atmungsorgane* **148:**307–311 (1977).

163. TAYLOR-ROBINSON, D., SHIRAL, A., SOBESLAVSKY, O., AND CHANOCK, R. M., Serologic response to *Mycoplasma pneumoniae* infection. II. Significance of antibody measured by different techniques, *Am. J. Epidemiol.* **84:**301–313 (1966).

164. TAYLOR-ROBINSON, D., SOBESLAVSKY, O., JENSEN, K. E., SENTERFIT, L. B., AND CHANOCK, R. M., Serologic response to *Mycoplasma pneumoniae* infection. I. Evaluation of immunofluorescence, complement fixation, indirect hemagglutination, and tetrazolium reduction inhibition tests for the diagnosis of infection, *Am. J. Epidemiol.* **83:**287–298 (1966).

165. TAYLOR-ROBINSON, D., GUMPEL, J. M., HILL, A., AND SWANNELL, A. J., Isolation of *Mycoplasma pneumoniae* from the synovial fluid of a hypoglobulinaemic patient in a survey of patients with inflammatory polyarthritis, *Ann. Rheum. Dis.* **51:**180–182 (1978).

166. TAYLOR-ROBINSON, D., WEBSTER, A. D. B., FURR, P. M., AND ASHERSON, G. L., Prolonged persistence of *Mycoplasma pneumoniae* in a patient with hypogammaglobulinaemia, *J. Infect.* **2:**171–175 (1980).

167. TULLY, J. G., ROSE, D. L., WHITCOMB, R. F., AND WENZEL, R. P., Enhanced isolation of *Mycoplasma pneumoniae* from throat washings with a newly modified culture medium, *J. Infect. Dis.* **139:**478–482 (1979).

168. VAN DER VEEN, J., AND VAN NUNEN, M. C. J., Role of *Mycoplasma pneumoniae* in acute respiratory disease in a military population, *Am. J. Hyg.* **78:**293–301 (1963).

169. VIKERFORS, T., BRODIN, G., GRANDIEN, M., HIRSCHBERG, L., KROOK, A., AND PETTERSSON, C., Detection of specific IgM antibodies for the diagnosis of *Mycoplasma pneumoniae* infections: A clinical evaluation, *Scand. J. Infect. Dis.* **20:**601–610 (1988).

170. VU, A. C., FOY, H. M., CARTWRIGHT, F. D., AND KENNEY, G. E., The principal protein antigens of isolates of *Mycoplasm pneumoniae* as measured by levels of immunoglobulin G in human serum are stable in strains collected over a 10-year period, *Infect. Immun.* **55:**1830–1836 (1987).

171. WENZEL, R. P., CRAVEN, R. B., DAVIES, J. A., HENDLEY,

J. O., HAMORY, B. H., AND GWALTNEY, J. M., JR., Field trial of an inactivated *Mycoplasma pneumoniae* vaccine. I. Vaccine efficacy, *J. Infect. Dis.* **134:**571–576 (1976).

172. WENZEL, R. P., HENDLEY, J. O., DODD, W. K., AND GWALTNEY, J. M., JR., Comparison of josamycin and erythromycin in the therapy of *Mycoplasma pneumoniae* pneumonia, *Antimicrob. Agents Chemother.* **10:**899–901 (1976).

173. WESTERBERG, S. C., SMITH, C. B., AND RENZETTI, A. D., Mycoplasma infections in patients with chronic obstructive pulmonary disease, *J. Infect. Dis.* **127:**491–497 (1973).

174. WITZLEB, V. W., SPROSSIG, M., ANGER, G., AND HEIDLER, S., Erkrankungen des Respirationstraktes durch *Mycoplasma pneumoniae*, *Dtsch. Med. Wochenschr.* **91:**429–433 (1966).

175. WRIGHT, D. N., AND BAILEY, G. D., Effect of relative humidity on the stability of *Mycoplasma pneumoniae* exposed to simulated solar ultraviolet and to visible radiation, *Can. J. Microbiol.* **15:**1449–1452 (1969).

176. YAYOSHI, M., ARAAKE, M., HAYATSU, E., KAWAKUBO, Y., AND YOSHIOKA, M., Characterization and pathogenicity of hemolysis mutants of *Mycoplasma pneumoniae*, *Microbiol. Immunol.* **28:**303–310 (1984).

12. Suggested Reading

CASSELL, G. H., AND COLE, B. C., Mycoplasmas as agents of human disease, *N. Engl. J. Med.* **304:**80–89 (1981).

CLYDE, W. A., JR., *Mycoplasma pneumoniae* infections of man, in: *The Mycoplasmas*, Volume 2 (M. F. BARILE AND S. RAZIN, eds.), pp. 275–306, Academic Press, New York, 1979.

Current Insights in Mycoplasmology (O. KITAMOTO, W. A. CLYDE, JR., H. KOBAYASHI, AND M. F. BARILE, guest eds.), *Yale J. Biol. Med.* **56:**351–938 (1983).

DENNY, F. W., CLYDE, W. A., JR., AND GLEZEN, W. P., *Mycoplasma pneumoniae* disease: Clinical spectrum, pathophysiology, epidemiology, and control, *J. Infect. Dis.* **123:**74–92 (1971).

FOY, H. M., Pneumonia: *Mycoplasma pneumoniae*, in: *Communicable and Infectious Diseases*, 8th ed. (F. H. TOP, SR., AND P. F. WEHRLE, eds.), pp. 535–549, Mosby, St. Louis, 1976.

KENNY, G. E., Antigenic determinants, in: *The Mycoplasmas*, Volume 1 (M. F. BARILE AND S. RAZIN, eds.), pp. 351–384, Academic Press, New York, 1979.

LEVINE, D. P., AND LERNER, A. M., The clinical spectrum of *Mycoplasma pneumoniae* infections, *Med. Clin. North Am.* **62:**961–978 (1978).

PÖNKÄ, A., The occurrence and clinical picture of serologically verified *Mycoplasma pneumoniae* infections with emphasis on central nervous system, cardiac and joint manifestations, *Ann. Clin. Res.* **11**(Suppl. 24):1–60 (1979).

CHAPTER 22

Nosocomial Bacterial Infections

Walter J. Hierholzer, Jr., and Marcus J. Zervos

1. Introduction

From the combination of Greek *nosos* (disease) with *komein* (to take care of) as *nosokomeion* (hospital) and through Latin *nosocomium* (hospital) comes the English *nosocomial* (pertaining to a hospital). Nosocomial infections, then, are infections that develop and are recognized in patients and personnel in health-care institutions. These infections are not present or incubating on admission, with the exception that a nosocomial infection may be present on admission if it is directly related to or is the residual of a previous admission. Certain nosocomial infections may not be clinically evident until after discharge. It is common to classify all other infections that fail to meet these criteria as "community-acquired" infections.

It is estimated that over 5% of all hospitalized patients fall victim to these infections each year in the United States.[31] Prevalence studies conducted in other countries with collaboration by the World Health Organization (WHO) have found rates from 3 to 20% with a mean of 8.7 infections per 100 patients surveyed.[202] Approximately 90% of reported nosocomial infections are of bacterial etiology, with viral, fungal, protozoal, and other classes of microorganisms associated with a lesser but significant number of cases.[31]

2. Historical Background

Since the use of temples by the Egyptians, there have been documented attempts to provide special care, protection, and segregation for the sick. This collection of the sick has frequently resulted in rapid transmission of infectious agents among patients and personnel and from unrecognized reservoirs within the institution with resultant high morbidity and mortality. Public recognition of hospitals as "pesthouses" was common up to modern times. The role of improved environmental sanitation and the importance of hygienic practices in reducing transmission and infection rates were recognized in the earliest medical traditions and were periodically rediscovered in the following centuries. The medical workers of the middle 1800s were especially productive. Florence Nightingale introduced broad hospital hygiene, transmission of puerperal fever was recognized by Semmelweis and controlled by hand-washing with an antiseptic, and Lister introduced antisepsis to surgery. After Pasteur the putrefaction associated with trauma and surgery was understood as related to transmissible microorganisms, and the importance of aseptic technique became well understood and practiced.[19,203]

The stunning early success of penicillin in controlling gram-positive coccal infections led to the misconception that antibiotics could control and eventually eradicate all

Walter J. Hierholzer, Jr. · Yale University School of Medicine, Department of Hospital Epidemiology and Infection Control, Yale–New Haven Hospital, New Haven, Connecticut 06504. **Marcus J. Zervos** · William Beaumont Hospital, Division of Infectious Diseases, Royal Oak, Michigan 48072.

infectious disease. The carefully learned lessons of the past concerning aseptic technique were no longer given priority and support. The appearance of penicillin-resistant staphylococci in this milieu led to devastating hospital epidemics with these agents.[166] The current resurgent interest in nosocomial infection grew out of the need to control these epidemics.

With the discovery of penicillinase-resistant penicillins, infections by resistant staphylococci became treatable, and associated epidemics decreased in importance. At the same time, the marketing of antibiotics with effectiveness against a broad spectrum of other microorganisms led the unwary to discount the need for other control methods. However, the control of nosocomial infection was not forthcoming. Over the years 1960 to 1980, the place of importance in nosocomial infection was taken over by a new spectrum of agents in which the gram-negative organisms played a major role.[222] More recently, new gram-positive agents, especially resistant staphylococci and enterococci, have assumed increasing significance.[31,80,133,228]

3. Methodology

3.1. Criteria for Infection

Widely accepted criteria for the identification and classification of nosocomial infection have been suggested by the National Nosocomial Infections Study (NNIS) of the Hospital Infections Branch of the Centers for Disease Control (CDC).[150] These criteria satisfy both the need for scientific validity and the practical requirement for easy and uniform recognition necessary to discovery and enumeration. Examples are listed in Table 1. It is common practice

to designate most bacterial infections that appear within the first 48 h of hospital stay as community- and not nosocomially acquired. In these criteria, both infections from endogenous flora and infections transmitted from exogenous sources are included. Since microbiological sampling in clinical situations is neither routine nor uniform, the criteria are not dependent on the laboratory for data for fulfillment. Such clinical definition is mandated by studies indicating that from 16 to 59% of otherwise well-documented nosocomial infections are not supported by microbiological data in that no tests were submitted or tests were invalidated because of poor sampling, inadequate handling, or laboratory error.[21,133,202] Since both preventable and unavoidable infections are included in these criteria, care in assignment of causation and liability must be taken in the individual case (Table 1).

3.2. Sources of Mortality Data

The usual hospital-discharge and death-certificate data rarely include comments on complications of nosocomial infection. Some individual studies[71,72] and an autopsy study[44] have been reported. Autopsy data may provide confirmation or documentation of unsuspected nosocomial infection through gross, microscopic, or microbiological cultural evidence. However, autopsy data are biased for patients dying in the hospital with the most severe, interesting, or puzzling illnesses. These factors are associated with prolongation of hospital stay and other comorbid events predisposing to increased nosocomial infection. The NNIS has reported since 1970 selected mortality and morbidity data from a volunteer group of over 50 hospitals in the United States.[31,94,96] These hospitals range in size from

Table 1.   Sample Criteria for Determination of Nosocomial Infection[a]

Site	Clinical data	Laboratory data
Urinary tract	Back pain, dysuria, frequency, pyuria	Standard quantitative urine culture[b]
Wound	Purulent drainage	Wound culture[b]
Respiratory tract	Physical signs, cough	X ray
	Purulent sputum	Sputum culture[b]
Intravenous	Purulent drainage, pain, erythema	Semiquantitative culture[b]
Gastrointestinal tract	Diarrhea	Stool culture[b]
Skin	Purulent drainage	Culture[b]
	Physical signs	

[a]Modified from the CDC outline.[150]
[b]Combinations of clinical data may be used to document infection in the absence of laboratory microbiological isolation (see the text).

less than 100 beds to over 1000 beds and are geographically an adequate representation of U.S. hospitals. While the system does not represent a probability sample of U.S. hospitals, by stratifying hospitals by size and teaching characteristics, it has provided useful data. The NNIS data have tended to be confirmed by SENIC and other published reports.[82,216] Recent changes in the requirements for participation in the NNIS system and improvements in definitions and methods, including computer-assisted reporting, should improve the quality in the value of this data base as a potential source of national estimates of nosocomial infections in the United States.[95] Prospective data on the role of nosocomial infection in institutional mortality controlled for conditions that predispose to nosocomial infection are lacking.

3.3. Sources of Morbidity Data

Nosocomial bacterial infections are generally not reportable through any routine public-health system. The uniform hospital-discharge summary rarely indicates the complication of a nosocomial infection. In a study of risk factors important in nosocomial infection, Freeman and McGowan[64] found only 59% of nosocomial infections labeled with any diagnosis of infection as a primary or secondary discharge diagnosis and only 2% labeled as clearly indicting infection of a nosocomial origin. In a study conducted after the beginning of the new prospective payment systems in the United States, Massanari *et al.* found that only 57% of nosocomial infections were properly recorded in the discharge abstracts of their university hospital.[135]

The retrospective audit of medical records to determine the frequency of nosocomial infection has been complicated by difficulties in completeness, illegibility, and inaccessibility. However, the results of a large, statistically complex, and well-controlled evaluation of the efficacy of nosocomial infection practice and control, using a measured and highly reliable retrospective medical-record-review methodology, have been reported by the CDC. The methodology and analysis of the SENIC (Study of Efficacy of Nosocomial Infection Control) project have been published in detail.[29,82,83]

The focal point of hospital infection control must be the patient. The most successful acquisition of data on nosocomial infection has been accomplished through a method called nosocomial surveillance. This surveillance method actively acquires data from multiple laboratory and clinical sources and uses it to fulfill criteria set to definitions to confirm the presence of a nosocomial infection at a particular site. These data sources have included concurrent review of the patient's clinical record, review of the medical nursing Kardex and other data sheets for evidence of infection, and coordinated supplement of these clinical sources with radiology reports, pharmacy data, and microbiological laboratory reports.[68,94,113,151,217]

3.4. Surveys

Nosocomial infection data have been collected through a variety of methods. Those frequently reported have centered around either the laboratory[86,92,113,151] or the use of a specially trained individual, the infection control practitioner or nurse epidemiologist.[51,217] In addition to the NNIS and SENIC projects of the CDC, some statewide incidence and prevalence studies have been reported in the United States,[219] and WHO and others have sponsored surveys in other regions of the world.[111,139,149,202]

3.4.1. Microbiological Surveys. Data routinely generated in the hospital bacteriology laboratory have been widely used as a source of information of infections in hospitalized patients, and the increased use of diagnostic tests has been documented to increase the recognition of infectious diseases in acute-care institutions.[81,212] The site of infection (e.g., urinary tract, blood, pulmonary, wound), patient location, causative organism(s), and antimicrobial susceptibility data can be determined and evaluated. Computerized data-processing methods have eased the collation and review of these data for recognition of clusters of infections at specific sites, in geographic locations, or of specific species or strains of bacteria.[86,113,151] Patterns of antibiotic resistance and changes in resistance that may be related to antibiotic use are also conveniently followed by this method.[10,55]

The specificity of the survey of laboratory isolations is low. Isolation does not separate community-acquired from nosocomial infection and does not specify causation in differentiating commensal from infecting bacteria without additional clinical information. Furthermore, the sensitivity of this system is dependent on the uniformity of the collection of specimens and of culturing practices, features of laboratory practice that are known to vary widely. However, when laboratory data are combined with information from other data bases in a highly computerized hospital information system, sensitivities for the identification of nosocomial infection were reported that were equal to or exceeded other methods and at an efficiency that required approximately one third of personnel devoted to routine surveillance.[55]

Routine microbiological surveys of hospitalized patients or the hospital environment are unnecessary and economically unjustifiable. In the absence of epidemic situations, there is no evidence that this type of routine sampling has contributed significantly to detection or prevention of nosocomial infections. The incidence of nosocomial infection has not been related to levels of microbial contamination of air, surfaces, or fomites, and meaningful standards for permissible levels of such contamination do not exist.[74,130,131,196]

The spread of nosocomial organisms in endemic and most epidemic situations is associated with contact transmission or due to contamination of an item that should be sterile. Therefore, the role of environmental microbiological sampling is currently reduced to: (1) assisting in epidemic investigation in selected circumstances, (2) evaluation of new techniques, (3) serving as an important adjunct to educational programs in the support of nosocomial infection control, and (4) quality-control routine monitoring of sterilization, dialysis fluids, infant formula prepared in the hospital, and samples of certain disinfected equipment.

An exception to these limitations has been suggested to determine the presence of certain *Legionella* species in the potable water of hospitals with populations of highly immunocompromised patients known to be at high risk of morbidity and mortality when infected by these agents.[207,225] The CDC and other advisory groups have yet to accept this recommendation.[145]

3.4.2. Prevalence Surveys. A prevalence survey based on application of uniform criteria to all patients in an institution during a single day or time period has provided a rapid, inexpensive, and collaborative means of assessing nosocomial infection risk within an institution. Periodic prevalence data have been used as an evaluative tool in infection control programs,[64] as an estimator of risk across a wide variety of institutions,[20,21] including programs of the WHO,[202] and as an important quality-control feature of other data collection methods.[51] As with all prevalence studies, bias inherent in sampling of a single day's experience as an indicator of typical risk must be recognized.

3.4.3. Surveillance Studies. The currently most widely propagated survey method for the collection of nosocomial infection data employs a trained individual, a nurse epidemiologist, or infection control practitioner.[54,68] This individual concurrently provides a coordinated review of each patient's clinical and laboratory data, recording those instances that satisfy the standard criteria for identification of a nosocomial infection. These data are summarized on a periodic (monthly, quarterly, yearly) basis, collated, analyzed, and reported to a specific multidisciplinary committee within the hospital, and to certain key hospital personnel.[51,150,217]

The importance of the unbiased collection of these data

by a trained professional has been repeatedly documented by studies indicating reduced efficiency and accuracy of reporting by other methods[15,65,201] and by the results of the SENIC project.[83] The presence of the nurse practitioner on the clinical unit is also of value in: (1) reinforcing the importance of infection-control measures, (2) providing early identification of epidemics, (3) providing informal concurrent in-service education, and (4) assisting in providing new information for research efforts in the area of nosocomial-risk control.

The institutional infection control committee recommends appropriate control measures based on the priorities of risk indicated by the data previously collected and evaluated. The continuous collection of nosocomial infection data allows concurrent evaluation of these control efforts. This form of nosocomial infection data collection, evaluation, and recommendation has been termed "a nosocomial infection surveillance and control program."[150] This format has been widely promoted and supported by the Hospital Infections Program of the CDC since the first reports of its successful use in 1969.[51]

Three demonstration projects by the CDC have investigated this format as the prime method with which to investigate and control nosocomial infections in U.S. hospitals. The Comprehensive Hospital Infection Project (CHIP) collected intensive surveillance data in nine community hospitals between January 1970 and June 1973, using definitions and methods suggested by the CDC.[51,150] At 4-month intervals, CDC medical epidemiologists conducted on-site prevalence surveys to evaluate surveillance efficiency.

The NNIS system, while not statistically representative of all U.S. hospitals, does contain community, community teaching, state, local, and university hospitals. Each hospital is required to have an active infection control program, but until recently there was little attempt to evaluate or control the quality of the submitted data. Recently the requirements for membership in the system have been increased, criteria for infection have been improved and focused, and reliable submission of data has been required in an attempt to improve both the scope and the quality of the information submitted. On the basis of selected prevalence surveys comparing NNIS and CHIP methods, it has been suggested that NNIS data be inflated by a factor of 1.5 to compensate for its lower efficiency. The most recent data reported by the NNIS system are from 1984 and are reviewed in Section 5.

In 1974 the CDC initiated the SENIC project, which thereafter collected data in 338 randomly selected U.S. hospitals. The objectives of this study were to estimate the magnitude of the nosocomial infection problem in U.S.

hospitals, to describe the extent of hospitals' infection surveillance and control programs, and to evaluate the efficacy and effectiveness of these programs in reducing nosocomial infection risks. The extensive and complex methodology of the study was reported in 1980 and the results and evaluation in 1985.[29,81-84] The results indicate that in the one third of hospitals supporting the lowest levels of surveillance and control programs, nosocomial infections had increased in the period between 1970 and 1976 by 18%. In the same time period in the 5% of hospitals with the highest levels of surveillance and control, nosocomial infections had decreased by approximately one third.

Of the approximately one third of infections estimated to be reduced by the most intensive surveillance and control programs, surgical wound infections were found to be the risk most amenable to control and the site demonstrating the greatest risk of both increased cost and length of stay. Bacteremias and urinary tract infections were intermediate in reduction by CDC methods, and pneumonias proved most refractory, with nosocomial medical pneumonias not being significantly reduced.

The most effective programs conducted high-level balanced surveillance and control activities, had a trained hospital epidemiologist, supported an infection control practitioner for each 250 beds, and had a system of reporting wound infection rates to individual surgeons. Unfortunately, it was estimated that only 6% of nosocomial infections were being prevented at the end of the study. A follow-up study in 1983 indicated that this figure had risen to 9% or approximately 28% of the potential estimated to be possible by current methods.[85]

3.5. Laboratory Diagnosis

Standard reliable laboratory identification of bacteria in clinical samples from suspected nosocomial infection is important epidemiologically to link sources of transmitted microorganisms. The most important steps in assuring the validity of this process begin at the bedside with sampling of body fluids for testing. Inappropriate collection of specimens magnifies the usual difficulties in differentiation of normal flora of the body from truly infecting microbes.

3.5.1. Isolation and Identification of Organisms. The use of an expectorated sputum in identification of the causal agents of pneumonia typifies this problem. Pulmonary secretions collected through the oropharynx may be heavily contaminated by commensal bacteria. Similarly, urine specimens may become contaminated when not obtained by "clean catch, midstream voiding" or by direct bladder catheterization. Cultures from other normally sterile sites must be obtained only after proper preparation of the location to be sampled for results of cultures to be meaningful.

A delay in transport to the laboratory or transport under inappropriate environmental conditions or in a hostile medium may hinder identification of important infecting bacteria. Urine cultures held at room temperature may allow bacteria therein to multiply beyond the usual criteria for identification of a nosocomial urinary tract infection. A collection of anaerobic organisms in cold medium and carriage at ambient oxygen levels may inhibit subsequent growth to an extent that thwarts laboratory rescue and identification.

Many laboratory findings suggest improper collection or transport of specimens. Isolations of skin flora such as diphtheroids or coagulase-negative staphylococci from normally sterile sites suggest contamination at the time of collection. The recovery of three or more species of bacteria from urine specimens suggests unsatisfactory technique in collection or handling. The inability to recover anaerobes seen on Gram stain suggests inappropriate transport of specimens or culturing technique. Lack of culturing of tuberculosis in patients at high risk may suggest inappropriate sputum collection. If such inappropriate sampling, mishandling, and delay are not recognized by the laboratory, they may result in the unintentional misreporting of no organisms or of microbes of no clinical significance.

3.5.2. Evaluation of Specimens: Initial Screening. The laboratory specialist is guided by the description of the site of sampling and other clinical information forwarded by the requesting physician. The absence of such information accompanying the specimen may lead to serious mishandling or delay in identification in the laboratory. Recording the time of arrival of the specimen in the laboratory as compared to time of collection may be used to determine delays in transport that will result in an inability to culture fastidious organisms. Specimens received in improper collection containers can also be noted at the time of initial evaluation. In these instances, repeat cultures should be requested.

Assessment of specimens at the time they are received in the laboratory by direct microscopic examination is important in evaluating the acceptability of a specimen for further diagnostic testing. The laboratory use of differential cellular characteristics of sputum and saliva has been helpful in clarifying the source of specimens and their acceptability for diagnostic testings.[144] Specimens containing more than ten squamous epithelial cells per low-power ($\times 100$) field suggest contamination with oropharyngeal flora. Material from wounds that do not show polymorphonuclear leukocytes is also unlikely to yield a causative organism when cultured. Smears and other recently developed rapid diagnostic tests that evaluate antigen or antibody detection are of enormous importance in patient management. Smears are also important for detecting organisms of epidemiologic significance, such as *Haemophilus, Legionella,* or tuberculosis that may not be reflected by culture or that may take long periods of time to grow.

Sufficient sophistication in the laboratory is necessary to assure speciation of the common bacteria endemic to the institution. Standard methods are available in many manuals and texts.[60,116] Reference bacteriology should be conveniently available to assist in the identification of more unusual microbes. The degree to which organisms are speciated can also have epidemiologic importance. For example, a report of *Pseudomonas* species may fail to distinguish unrelated organisms such as *P. aeruginosa, P. cepacia,* and *Xanthamonas maltophilia.* Similarly, identifying the organisms as *P. cepacia* has etiologic significance, since *P. cepacia* are associated with outbreaks or pseudoepidemics caused by contaminated water or solutions.[134]

3.5.3. *In Vitro* Susceptibility Testing. Testing of the sensitivity of isolates to a spectrum of antibiotics is a commonly used clinical and epidemiological tool. Standardized Kirby–Bauer disk diffusion testing or the more exacting microdilution minimum inhibitory concentration (MIC) tests provide useful information regarding the susceptibility of the bacterial isolate.[60,116] Disk diffusion testing is performed by measuring the zone of inhibition around an antibiotic-impregnated disk. Zone diameters are interpreted in signifying susceptible, intermediate, or resistant organisms. Microdilution testing provides a quantitative measurement of the MIC, which is defined as the lowest concentration of antibiotic that results in inhibition of growth of the organism.

The results of susceptibility studies provide guidance both to the clinician for appropriate therapy and to the epidemiologist as an inexpensive screen for possible common identity of speciated organisms.[10,212] However, antibiotic sensitivity does not ensure identity of organisms; organisms may have similar antibiotic resistances and yet be epidemiologically unrelated.[8,176,209] Also, modification of resistance under pressure of antibiotic use may take place without other recognized biological changes.[43]

3.5.4. Quality Control in the Laboratory. Quality control is essential to effective microbiology laboratory and infection control programs. Pseudoepidemics due to contamination of specimens in the laboratory by automated laboratory equipment or other routes have occurred.[126,213] New procedures in the laboratory related to susceptibility testing, new culture techniques, new ways of reporting re-

sults, or of naming organisms can also lead to confusion, pseudoepidemics, or lack of recognition of related organisms.

3.5.5. Special Studies for Examining the Relatedness of Isolates. A variety of tests of biological characteristics not generally available in the routine laboratory have proved of value in epidemiological investigation of nosocomial infection. Among those most frequently reported are the following.

a. Phage Typing. The typing of bacteria by their sensitivity to various bacterial phages has been especially important in the investigation of nosocomial outbreaks of *Staphylococcus aureus.*[4,166] The staphylococcal epidemics of the 1950s and 1960s were identified with a number of species types, of which phage type 80/81 was the most notorious. Phage typing of other bacteria such as enteric gram-negatives and *Clostridium difficile* has been reported by research laboratories.[169,182] Many current nosocomial isolates, however, cannot be distinguished by phage typing.[8,176,209]

b. Serotyping. Serotyping of a number of gram-negative bacilli has been reported as a successful epidemiological tool in the investigation of outbreaks of nosocomial infection.[119,156,168,169] Serogrouping has been particularly helpful in evaluating outbreaks of *P. aeruginosa, Klebsiella pneumoniae,* and *Legionella* sp.[119,168]

c. Other Biotyping. Epidemiological identification of bacteria through other biological properties, including sensitivity to bacteriocins, presence of characteristic surface features such as pili, outer-membrane proteins, and distinctive biochemical reactions, has also been useful in selected situations. Bacteriocin susceptibility has been used to differentiate strains of *C. difficilie.*[182] Outer-membrane proteins analyzed by polyacrylamide gel electrophoresis have been used successfully to type strains of *Haemophilus influenzae.*[16] Biotyping and serogrouping also in many instances have been shown to lack the ability to differentiate unrelated strains.[8,176,209]

d. Plasmid Typing. Bacterial DNA has become valuable as a marker for the comparison of strains of nosocomial bacteria. Diverse species of gram-negative and gram-positive bacteria have been studied using this approach.[104,152,153,176,198,209,226,227] The relatedness of strains is evaluated by comparison of the plasmid and/or chromosomal DNA. Plasmids are self-replicating, transferable extrachromosomal DNA elements found in the cytoplasm of prokaryotes. Simplified techniques have been developed for isolating and characterizing bacterial plasmids and chromosomes. Typing is performed by isolation of DNA, restriction enzyme digestion, and comparison of patterns by agarose gel electrophoresis. These techniques have been applied successfully in clinical situations to determine the evolution and spread of antibiotic resistance within hospitals. These techniques have also allowed for differentiation of endemic and epidemic strains. This information is particularly useful in organisms such as citrobacter, enterobacter, non-*Aeruginosa pseudomonas* species, *Staphylococcus epidermidis, Enterococcus faecalis,* and *Branhamella catarrhalis* where other typing systems are not available.

Much of this reference bacteriological testing is available in state and regional public-health laboratories. For many of the research techniques, samples may be referred to regional university research centers or to the CDC in Atlanta.

4. Biological Characteristics of Nosocomial Organisms

The relative frequency of the species of bacteria causing nosocomial infection has changed remarkably over the past 30 years.[14,31,136] Changes in resistance to antimicrobial agents also have been observed. These changes in the development and persistence of resistant strains have been related to the selective pressure of the widespread use and misuse of antimicrobial agents. These patterns appear to be an extremely important phenomenon in local institutions and geographical areas,[52] even though national studies have not been impressive in documenting widespread increases in resistance over the same time period.[10] The biological characteristics important in these resistance changes may be generalized to: (1) the ability of bacteria to survive in the normal flora of the host, (2) the ability of bacteria to survive in the animate and inanimate environments of the health care facility, and (3) the ability of the bacteria to survive antimicrobial stress through acquired resistance.

4.1. Infecting Normal Flora

Bacteria that normally reside as commensals on the internal and external surfaces of the host have been increasingly recognized as causal in nosocomial infections.[103,181,227] In hospitalized patients the normal pharyngeal and intestinal flora may be displaced by antibiotic-resistant strains. The changes brought about by modification in the host by disease and by treatment factors occur within a few days of hospitalization. These bacteria then can serve as sources for infection in the colonized patient or are transmitted between

patients nosocomially. The ability of bacteria to infect is determined by the product of their number and virulence and inversely related to the quality and quantity of host defenses. In this context, the term *normal flora* has become suspect in the recognition that virtually any microorganism that appears in the host may be invasive and disease-causing, given a sufficiently impaired patient.[122]

4.2. Antimicrobial Resistance

The emergence of antibiotic resistance plays a critical role in bacterial nosocomial infections. Epidemic penicillin-resistant staphylococci were controlled by a return to antiseptic techniques and the development of successful penicillinase-resistant antistaphylococcal drugs. Concurrent with these events there began to appear, with increasing frequency, infections with gram-negative bacilli, many of which had been considered nonpathogens heretofore.[14,222] Many of these bacteria are naturally resistant to antibiotics successful in the treatment of gram-positive bacteria. Recently, epidemic staphylococci resistant to methicillin have appeared and spread throughout hospitals worldwide.[41,80,174,200] Multi-drug-resistant enterococci have also emerged as important pathogens.[226,227] Over time, new antibiotics of broader spectrum or of specific usefulness have been developed. In virtually every situation, bacteria in resistant forms equal to the pressure of antibiotic use have emerged.

Epidemiologically important bacterial resistance arises by spontaneous mutation or by the acquisition of plasmids. Spontaneous mutation results in a change in the bacterial chromosome affecting drug resistance. Mutation takes place in approximately every 10^9 cell divisions and appears to be single-drug-specific.

Plasmids are distributed throughout nearly all genera of medically important bacteria. Plasmids that carry antibiotic-resistant genes are termed *R plasmids*. Plasmid-mediated antibiotic resistance was first described in *Shigella* in Japan.[211] Plasmids are responsible for the greatest portion of nosocomial bacterial drug resistance. Plasmids are also responsible for the rapid and widespread development of multidrug resistance. They are frequently composed of two elements: a transfer factor governing intercellular transfer of the plasmid, and genes that mediate antibiotic resistance. Additionally, plasmids often can carry genetic material that assists the cell in surviving or competing in adverse environments. Discrete portions of extrachromosomal DNA, termed *transposons,* may move or "jump" between plasmids, increasing the range of combinations. Plasmids can be conjugative when able to self-initiate and cause their own transfer between bacteria. Conjugative transfer in Enterobacteriaceae takes place through formation of pili. The process of conjugation in gram-positive cocci is quite different and does not involve the synthesis of a sex pilus; yet cell-to-cell transfer does occur.[176] Plasmid transfer across species and genera has been described as an important factor in the rapid appearance of multi-drug-resistant forms in hospitals.[53,56,101,106,175,199] Plasmid-mediated resistance has been reported for most antibiotics as well as for colicins, metals, and ultraviolet light.

While plasmid-associated resistance has been reported in preantibiotic cultures and in antibiotic-free environments, the prevalence of R-factor resistance appears to increase with antibiotic use, hospital stay, and chronicity of institutional contacts.[52,102] It appears that while plasmids are essential to bacterial survival in an antibiotic-containing environment, their maintenance is at some cost to the microbe. In an antibiotic-free environment, plasmid-containing bacteria are at a competitive disadvantage. Plasmid loss, termed *cure*, can occur when bacteria resistant via R factor are transferred and maintained in an antibiotic-free situation. This may explain the reported success in ending multi-drug-resistant epidemics by curtailing the use of antibiotics in the affected units.[6]

5. Descriptive Epidemiology

5.1. Prevalence and Incidence

A large number of studies from the United States and other countries have estimated the magnitude of nosocomial infection by a variety of methods. Examples of data from those that have used criteria for infection compatible with those developed and used by the CDC are presented in Table 2. Based on these criteria, these studies routinely include in their totals infections for which no cultures were done or for which no pathogens were isolated. These infections identified by clinical criteria alone make up from 16 to 59% of the data.[21,29,202]

The nosocomial infection "rate" is commonly determined by citing the number of nosocomial infections per 100, 1000, or 10,000 patient discharges expressed as a ratio.[51,150] A preferred ratio expressed in infection per 1000 or 10,000 patient days of risk[64,91,123,173,208] has begun to appear in reports of incidence data. This latter ratio is especially valuable in considering nosocomial risk in institutions or services with widely varying length of stay and in extended-care facilities.

5.1.1. Mortality Data. Estimates of the role of nosocomial infection in mortality vary widely. The most recently published CDC-NNIS data estimate 0.7% of nosocomial infections directly causing death and 3.1% of infections contributing to death.[31] In an earlier retrospective study of 1000 autopsies from a university hospital in which 75% of patients who died were examined, Daschner *et al.*[44] found an overall nosocomial infection rate of 13.7%. In those individuals with nosocomial infection, 54% of the deaths resulted directly from infection. In a retrospective study of 100 consecutive deaths at each of two hospitals, Gross *et al.*[72] found death causally related to nosocomial infections in 2.5% and contributing in 3.4% of patients without underlying terminal illness. In those with terminal illness on admission, the rates increase to 9.2 and 10.9%, respectively.

5.1.2. Prevalence Studies. Prevalence studies con-

Table 2.   Prevalence and Incidence Rates of Nosocomial Infection[a]

Location	Years	Type of hospitals	Type of study	Rate
United States				
Virginia	1972–1975[216]	University	Incidence	6.7
Utah	1972–1973[21]	Community < 75 beds	Prevalence	7.2
	1977[20]	Community < 75 beds	Incidence	2.0
West Germany	1976[44]	University	Incidence	6.6
United Kingdom	1980[12]	Community	Autopsy	13.7
			Prevalence	9.2
Israel	1975–1976[48]	University	Incidence	12.2
United States	1984[31]	Mixed NNIS-CDC[b]	Incidence	3.4
		Community NNIS-CDC[b]	Incidence	2.2
		University NNIS-CDC[b]	Incidence	4.1

[a] Infections per 100 hospital discharges.
[b] NNIS, National Nosocomial Infections Study.

ducted in U.S. acute-care hospitals, using CDC-NNIS compatible criteria, have reported rates ranging from 7.2% in small, predominantly rural hospitals[21] to as high as 15.5% in a large metropolitan teaching hospital.[14]

A WHO cooperative hospital infection prevalence survey was carried out between 1983 and 1985 in 55 hospitals in 14 countries in the four regions Europe, Mediterranean, Southeast Asia, and western Pacific.[202] Results reported from 47 hospitals and 28,861 patients showed a mean prevalence rate of 8.7% with regional means from 7.7 to 11.8% and individual institutional rates from 3.0 to 20.7%. Since multiple infections were not recorded, an adjusted mean of 9.9% for the total was estimated, suggesting that approximately one patient in ten in these hospitals was infected while under care.

Prevalence data reported from extended-care facilities have ranged from 3 to 18%.[67,185] These studies have used varying criteria and methodology, making comparisons difficult. Studies in these institutions will require special criteria and methods different from those commonly used in acute-care institutions, since the availability of laboratory data, the extent of daily medical record documentation, and the resources available for data collection and analysis are less in this setting.

Prevalence studies have repeatedly yielded values in excess of incidence studies in the same institution. This variance is due to the methodology employed and reflects the association that prevalence approximates incidence times duration.[171]

5.1.3. Incidence Studies. Using definitions and methodologies outlined by the CDC for CHIP and NNIS, a large number of incidence studies have been reported. The most recently reported CDC-NNIS data indicate a mean crude annual nosocomial infection rate of 3.4 for the 51 hospitals contributing data for 1984.[31] The 20 nonteaching hospitals reported a mean rate of 2.2, the 18 small teaching hospitals a mean rate of 3.4, and the 13 large teaching hospitals a rate of 4.4. If CDC-NNIS data are inflated by a factor of 1.5 as suggested (see Section 3.4.3), a mean crude nosocomial infection rate of approximately 5 infections per 100 discharges is observed.[51] Other programs and authors report rates from less than 3 to over 13% (Table 2).

5.1.4. Site–Pathogen Analysis. The site of nosocomial infection and the pathogen(s) reported as responsible for them vary in incidence, relative frequency, morbidity, and mortality. Examples from reported series for site and from the CDC-NNIS data for 1984 for site–service and site–pathogens are illustrated in Tables 3, 4, and 5, respectively. Urinary tract infections, postoperative wound infections, pneumonias, and primary bacteremias make up over 80% of the reported infections. Pediatric services and extended-care facilities report higher comparative rates of cutaneous infections than those reported for other services in acute care. Bacterial infections account for over 85% of those for which an etiology is recognized.

a. Urinary Tract Infections. Infections of the urinary tract are consistently reported in Europe and the United States as comprising 30–45% of the total infections identified.[30,202,216] Over 70% of these infections are caused by

Table 3. Nosocomial Infection by Site[a]

	CDC-NNIS[31] 1984 incidence	WHO[202] 1983–1985 prevalence	University[91] 1978		Small community[21] 1972–1973 prevalence
			Incidence	Prevalence	
Surgical wound	0.56	2.3	1.2	1.4	1.0
	(17%)	(25%)	(18%)	(17%)	(13%)
Lower respiratory tract	0.60	1.8	1.0	1.2	2.5
	(18%)	(21%)	(15%)	(15%)	(33%)
Urinary tract	1.29	1.9	2.4	2.4	2.5
	(38%)	(22%)	(36%)	(30%)	(33%)
Cutaneous	0.29	0.9	0.6	0.9	0.8
	(5.7%)	(11%)	(9%)	(11%)	(10%)
Bacteremia	0.25	—	0.1	0.3	—
	(7.5%)		(2%)	(3.7%)	
Other	0.46	1.7	1.3	1.9	0.9
	(13.8%)	(20%)	(20%)	(23.3%)	(11%)

[a]Infections per 100 hospital discharges; figures in parentheses are the percentages of total nosocomial infection.

Table 4.   Site–Service Nosocomial Infection Rates[a]

Service	UTI	SWI	LRI	BACT	CUT	Other	All sites
				Site			
Nonteaching hospitals							
SURG	12.1	8.5	5.4	1.3	1.4	2.0	30.8
MED	12.6	0.4	5.2	1.9	0.8	2.3	23.3
GYN	5.8	1.6	0.1	0.1	0.1	0.8	8.6
OB	1.1	2.4	0.1	0.1	0.5	1.4	5.6
PED	0.0	0.1	0.1	0.0	0.1	0.9	1.2
NEW	0.5	0.2	1.8	0.6	2.6	2.9	8.6
TOTAL	9.9	3.6	4.2	1.3	1.1	2.0	22.2
Small teaching hospitals							
SURG	17.7	13.6	7.8	1.8	1.6	4.7	47.3
MED	20.1	0.6	7.5	2.8	1.7	5.3	38.1
GYN	19.9	11.1	1.3	0.4	0.2	2.2	35.2
OB	3.8	6.8	0.3	0.2	0.5	3.4	14.9
PED	2.0	0.6	2.0	2.4	2.3	5.2	14.6
NEW	0.6	0.2	1.4	2.0	4.8	5.6	14.7
TOTAL	13.9	6.0	5.4	1.9	1.8	4.7	33.8
Large teaching hospitals							
SURG	19.5	15.0	11.2	4.2	3.3	6.1	59.3
MED	19.5	1.2	10.2	5.7	3.0	7.3	46.9
GYN	14.4	10.2	2.6	0.9	0.6	3.1	31.7
OB	4.2	6.6	0.5	0.9	0.5	7.5	20.3
PED	2.8	1.6	3.9	2.1	1.2	4.9	16.6
NEW	1.0	0.3	2.9	3.6	3.7	5.6	17.1
TOTAL	14.2	6.6	7.7	3.9	2.6	6.4	41.4

[a] From CDC-NNIS Report (1984).[31] Rates are per 10,000 patient discharges.

gram-negative bacilli, with *Escherichia coli* causing approximately one third. Enterococci and *P. aeruginosa* appear next in frequency in hospitals in the United States, while *Proteus* species are more frequently reported in WHO data and in extended-care facilities in the United States. Secondary bacteremia appears in approximately 1% of individuals with nosocomial urinary tract infections, and 30 to 40% of hospital-associated gram-negative bacteremias originate at this site. Platt *et al.*, in a carefully controlled study for other risk factors, have reported a threefold increase in risk of death in patients with nosocomial bacteriuria.[159]

b. Surgical Wound Infections. Postoperative surgical wound infections make up from approximately 15 to 25% of reported nosocomial infections. In some developing areas, up to one third of reported infections have involved surgical wounds.[202] Following a classification system for wounds

(clean, clean contaminated, contaminated, or dirty) used in The National Research Council Study reported in 1964,[163] recent studies usually have reported risk of infection in postoperative wounds based on the probability of wound contamination during surgery. Examples of the results, by wound classification, of several large studies are shown in Table 6. While risk classification and reduction have been thought to be most effective in treating "clean wounds," a simplified multivariate risk index successfully differentiating low, medium, and high risk across all contamination groups has been reported by the CDC, using data gathered during the SENIC project.[84]

Staphylococcus aureus remains the most common isolate from wound infections in the WHO studies[202] and in the CDC-NNIS data,[31] excepting those from gynecology services where *E. coli* is most prominent. *E. coli* is second

Table 5. Relative Frequency of Nosocomial Infection by Site and Selected Pathogens[a]

Pathogen	Site						Total isolates	Percent
	UTI	SWI	LRI	BACT	CUT	Other		
E. coli	30.7	11.5	6.4	10.1	7.0	7.4	5,266	17.8
P. aeruginosa	12.7	8.9	16.9	7.6	9.2	6.7	3,366	11.4
Enterococci	14.7	12.1	1.5	7.1	8.8	7.0	3,063	10.4
S. aureus	1.6	18.6	12.9	12.3	28.9	14.6	3,059	10.3
Klebsiella spp.	8.0	5.2	11.6	7.8	3.8	4.6	2,193	7.4
Coagulase-negative staphylococci	3.4	8.3	1.5	14.9	11.5	11.6	1,868	6.3
Enterobacter spp.	4.8	7.0	9.4	6.3	4.5	3.9	1,748	5.9
Candida spp.	5.4	1.7	4.0	5.6	5.8	14.1	1,620	5.5
Proteus spp.	7.4	5.2	4.2	0.8	3.3	2.1	1,522	5.1
Serratia spp.	1.2	2.1	5.8	3.0	2.2	1.5	691	2.3
Other fungi	2.2	0.4	1.4	1.3	0.9	2.8	496	1.7
Citrobacter spp.	1.8	1.4	1.4	0.7	0.7	0.9	414	1.4
Bacteroides spp.	0.0	3.7	0.2	3.4	1.2	1.4	355	1.2
Group B *Streptococcus*	0.9	1.3	0.7	2.3	1.1	1.9	348	1.2
Other anaerobes	0.0	1.7	0.1	1.8	0.8	4.4	300	1.0
All others[b]	5.2	10.9	22.0	15.0	10.3	15.1	3,253	11.1
Number of isolates	12,218	5,500	4,567	2,264	1,690	3,323	29,562	100.0

[a]From CDC-NNIS report (1984).[31]
[b]No other pathogen accounted for more than 3% of the isolates at any site.

in frequency in most reports but has been exceeded by enterococci on surgical services in the most recent CDC-NNIS report. Other gram-negative bacilli remain important etiologic agents, but coagulase-negative staphylococci have begun to be recognized as an important pathogen in studies reported in the United States. *Bacteroides* and other anaerobes are probably underreported in these data, since many laboratories outside the university setting in the developed world lack sufficient resources and sophistication to collect and process isolates appropriately to identify these agents with sensitivity.

c. Respiratory Infections. Respiratory infections in the form of pneumonias make up a portion equal in importance to wound infections in most reports (approximately 15–25%). *P. aeruginosa* is the most frequently reported pathogen in both the U.S. and WHO reports. Other gram-negative agents and *S. aureus* are also causal agents reported with significant frequency in most studies.[31,165,202] Nosocomial pneu-

Table 6. Postoperative Wound Infection by Class of Operation

Class of operation	Davis, 1984[46]a 1045[b]	Leigh, 1981[115] 29,941	Cruse, 1980[42] 63,939	NRC, 1964[163] 7984
Clean	3.1%	2.9%	1.5%	6.9%
Clean contaminated	7.8	8.6	7.7	11.7
Contaminated	17.0	12.9	15.2	15.1
Dirty	10.0	—	40.0	28.0

[a]Children only.
[b]Number of operations.

monias are the leading cause of death from nosocomial infection. Secondary bacteremias are higher in nosocomial pneumonia than for either urinary or wound infections, and case-fatality rates for nosocomial pneumonias are only exceeded by those for bacteremia.

d. Nosocomial Bacteremia. Nosocomial bacteremias are reported as secondary to another site if there is documented infection at the primary site (in which case they are not included as an additional infection in determining rates) or primary if there is a culture-confirmed septicemia without evidence for an underlying site of infection. Secondary bacteremias are documented in over 5% of infections at all sites and are most commonly associated with cardiovascular, intraabdominal, and intravascular sites of primary infection. Infections with gram-negative organisms, including *Acinetobacter, Bacteroides,* and *Serratia,* have the highest rates of secondary bacteremias but are far exceeded in relative frequency by *S. aureus* and coagulase-negative *Staphylococcus* infections.

Primary bacteremia rates are highest in teaching hospitals in the CDC-NNIS system, making up over 9% of infections in the larger teaching hospitals. The gram-positive organisms of coagulase-negative *Staphylococcus* and/or *S. aureus* have increased to become the most common agents of primary bacteremia in all but gynecology services where *E. coli* and *Bacteroides* species remain the most frequent. This marks a major change from the past 20 years' experience where gram-negative bacteria held preeminence at this site. Bacteremias remain the site with the highest case-fatality rate, exceeding 25% in most reports and 50% or more in many.[136,140,178,183,193]

e. Cutaneous Infection. Cutaneous infections make up approximately 6% of the infections reported from the NNIS system with high rates in the larger university hospitals and on the newborn units. A larger portion of infections in the developing countries and in extended-care facilities in the United States are reported at the cutaneous site.[36,67,208] *S. aureus* is the most frequently reported isolate at this site, with aerobic and anaerobic gram-negative rod organisms of increasing importance at this site in pressure ulcers common to the elderly in extended care.

An important subgroup of infections reported at this site are related to intravascular devices and intravenous therapy. Infections secondary to intravenous fluids,[127] intravenous fluid additives,[128] administration apparatus,[124] infusion devices, and a series of different types of implements have been documented.[191,192,214] These infections are attended by a high rate of continuing secondary bacteremia if the devices are not removed, and case-fatality rates are reported in the 20–40% range. In the United

States, coagulase-negative staphylococci are an important and increasing cause of these infections.[35,140,155]

f. Other Types of Nosocomial Infections. It is common to identify several other sites of nosocomial infection (gynecological, upper respiratory, eye, gastrointestinal),[150] and events including epidemics have been recorded for each. Gastrointestinal infections were especially prominent in data reported from the Southeast Asia and western Pacific areas in the WHO prevalence surveys, apparently indicating important intrahospital endemic transmission of this illness in these predominantly developing countries.[202]

5.2. Epidemic Behavior and Contagiousness

The epidemic form of nosocomial infections has been the most extensively reported. Epidemic behavior is determined by the causal bacteria, the route of transmission, and the characteristics of the host population at risk. These epidemics have mirrored advances in medicine just as the most common causal agents have moved from gram-positive streptococcal wound and puerperal infections, through resistant staphylococcal epidemics, to the present gram-negative bacilli of increasing antibiotic resistance, infecting hosts with decreasing ability to resist.[220] Nosocomial epidemics investigated by the CDC have doubled each 5-year period since 1960.[191] During the period 1970–1975, 42% of the epidemics investigated were associated with some medical device, and 70% were due to gram-negative bacilli.[191] Outbreaks of infection due to methicillin-resistant *S. aureus* have been increasingly reported, especially from large teaching hospitals.[31,80,174] While this experience may represent unusually interesting or difficult outbreaks, it is not unusual for larger medical centers to experience several epidemics per year. The role of the human carrier as either biological or mechanical transmitter has been commented on repeatedly in reports of these outbreaks.

Several pseudoepidemics have been reported.[28,107] A pseudoepidemic is the occurrence of an increased number of isolates of a microorganism misinterpreted as a true epidemic of infection. The main factors in the pseudoepidemics have been improper specimen processing, surveillance artifact, and clinical misdiagnosis.[126]

5.3. Geographic Distribution

Nosocomial infections are not limited by geography (Table 2). Lack of reported nosocomial infection has indicated inadequate study more frequently than an absence of risk. Service (Table 7), organism, and extent of morbidity and mortality vary within and among different institutions. This variation frequently reflects differing case mix (severity of disease, comorbid factors) in the samples admitted from the population served. As a result, it is common for tertiary-care centers to exhibit higher rates than primary-care hospitals.[31] A direct relationship between rates of specific community-acquired infections and nosocomial risk has not been documented. However, the appearance of nosocomial epidemics as extensions of community-acquired and propagated epidemics has been recognized, as has the converse.[60,174]

5.4. Temporal Distribution

An unexplained seasonal variation in certain gram-negative rods, including *Acinetobacter* with summer peaks, has been reported.[2,170] Other common bacteria have not been reported to show a seasonal trend in nosocomial infections.

A direct correlation has been suggested between length of stay in a hospital and the incidence of nosocomial infection, but the confounding variables of disease severity, age, and comorbidity have not been sufficiently separated to confirm this observation.

An analysis of secular trends in nosocomial infections recorded in the NNIS system between 1970 and 1976 has been reported by the CDC as showing a 10% increase over this period.[83] In the one third of hospitals in the SENIC project that had established no infection control programs or ineffective programs between 1970 and 1976, an increase in nosocomial infection rates of 18% was reported. In the 5% of hospitals in the same study with the highest efficacy programs, an overall decrease of 36% was estimated. These

increases would seem to be supported by what is known about changes in length of stay, case mix, and severity in patient populations in acute-care institutions in the United States during the same time period.

5.5. Age

Extremes of age have been reported as directly associated with increasing nosocomial infection rates,[12,73] and the special problems in children[215] and in surgical wound infection[42] have been recorded. Since extremes of age are known to be correlated with host defects resulting in increased susceptibility to infection, this hypothesis seems reasonable and attractive. Unfortunately, most studies have reported only relative frequency of infection by age group and have not been well controlled for frequency of experience, length of exposure, disease severity, treatment, or other conditions that predispose to infection. Daschner *et al.*,[44] in a retrospective autopsy study, found an excess of nosocomial deaths in the 20- to 60-year-old age range. In a controlled study of risk factors for nosocomial infection in a university medical setting, age of 65 years or more increased the risk of nosocomial infection three times.[64]

Morbidity and mortality from nosocomial infection increase directly with age in the elderly, as for most infections, and the special problems of the neonate are similar to other infections in that age group.

5.6. Sex

Incidence of nosocomial infection has been reported to be greater in males than in females, but as with most other variables, these studies have not been well controlled.[12,193] Sex-related morbidity and mortality for

Table 7. Nosocomial Infection Rate by Service[a]

Service	CDC-NNIS[31] 1984 incidence	University[91] 1972–1975 incidence	University[91] 1978		Small community[21] 1972–1973 prevalence
			Incidence	Prevalence	
Medicine	3.7	5	7.7	4.5	5.6
Surgery	4.7	10	6.4	10.2	8.9
Obstetrics	1.5	0.8	5.6	6.6	—
Gynecology	2.8	4	10.3		—
Pediatrics	1.3	4	6.3	9.4	—
All services	3.4	6.0	6.7	8.3	7.2

[a]Infections per 100 hospital discharges.

nosocomial infection seem to parallel the site–pathogen experience for individual diseases.

5.7. Race

No race difference has been suggested or reported for nosocomial infections independent of other disease processes.

5.8. Occupation

Clinical health care professionals, medical laboratory workers, and other support personnel who come into contact with patients or patient specimens have potential increased risk of bacterial infection related to their employment.[154]

While individual cases and outbreaks of a variety of bacterial infectious diseases have been reported,[49,61,187] the only well-documented increased risk for clinical workers appears to be tuberculosis.[11,47] Medical laboratory personnel share this increased risk of tuberculosis and may have increased rates of brucellosis, shigellosis, and other enteric bacterial diseases.[87]

5.9. Occurrence in Different Settings

Nosocomial infections have been reported in both acute- and chronic-care settings. Within acute-care hospitals, several high-risk units for nosocomial infection have been recognized. These include burn units,[11] nurseries,[215] intensive-care units,[45,220] dialysis units,[34,38] transplantation units,[120,172] and oncology units.[99,173] The common denominator in these units appears to be the use of specific hospital procedures and the presence of more severely compromised patients. The high nosocomial infection rates reported for university teaching hospitals may be directly related to the presence of these high-risk units. In one study of 38 U.S. hospitals, 25% of all nosocomial infections reported occurred in intensive-care unit patients.[220]

Information on nosocomial bacterial infections in extended-care facilities is limited.[36,67,117] No data are available on the risk of nosocomial infection related to ambulatory care.

5.10. Socioeconomic Factors

While the importance of socioeconomic factors in infectious disease epidemiology is well recognized, no differential has been reported for nosocomial infections independent of other disease processes.

5.11. Other Host Factors

In addition to age, the genetic and acquired modifications of host defenses usually important in increased susceptibility to infection contribute to nosocomial risk (Table 8). They include metabolic disease, cardiovascular disease, respiratory disease, cutaneous disease, and a spectrum of hematological and immunological abnormalities. Among the host defenses altered by these diseases are modifications in normal flora, changes in anatomical barriers to microorganisms, suppression of inflammatory response, and modifications in the reticuloendothelial system. Among the hematological and immunological factors important in nosocomial infection are those that decrease the number of neutrophils, cause defective function of neutrophils, reduce or cause defective immunoglobulin production, or interfere with cellular immunity.

A single underlying condition may contribute to several defects in host defenses. A solid tumor may cause obstruction, erode a mucosal surface, and metastatically replace bone marrow. The resultant malnutrition, easy portal of entry, and loss of leukocyte function all contribute to infection by opportunistic microorganisms.

The conditions that predispose to such opportunistic infections and the types of organisms involved have been well reviewed elsewhere.[24,205] The epidemic of infections with the human immunodeficiency virus (HIV) and the resultant AIDS has resulted in a major increase in individuals subject to such infections.[97]

5.12. Treatment Factors

5.12.1. Antibiotics.
Antibiotic treatment contributes to the risk of nosocomial infection by several means. In addition to modifying the endogenous microflora of the host, several antibiotics interfere with immune function (chloramphenicol, rifampin) or contribute to renal (aminoglycosides), hepatic (erythromycin, isoniazid), or cutaneous (penicillins) side effects that increase susceptibility to infection.

Under pressure of antibiotic use or abuse, the environmental microbial flora of medical-care institutions increases in antibiotic resistance.[138,142] Patient acquisition of these resistant microbial flora begins shortly after admission and is accelerated by antibiotic treatment or prophylaxis, reaching as much as 60% of the patient population by the third

Table 8. Examples of Factors That Modify Host Defenses

Host defenses	Disease modifiers	Treatment modifiers	Frequent sites of infection	Common organism of infection
Normal flora	Thermal burn	Antibiotic therapy Gastric surgery	Soft tissue Intestine	*Pseudomonas* *Salmonella*
Anatomical barriers	Trauma	Medical devices Surgery	Intravenous site Wound	*Staphylococcus aureus* *S. aureus*
Mucociliary clearance	Cystic fibrosis	Irradiation Tracheostomy	Pulmonary Pulmonary	*S. aureus* *Pseudomonas*
Reticuloendothelial system	Sickle-cell disease, asplenia	Hemodialysis	Bloodstream	*Streptococcus pneumoniae* *Haemophilus influenzae* *Salmonella*
Leukocyte function	Chronic granulomatous disease, Job's syndrome, diabetic ketoacidosis	Corticosteroids Drug-induced neutropenia	Soft tissue Pneumonia	*S. aureus*
Humoral immunity	Agammaglobulinemia, chronic lymphocytic leukemia, multiple myeloma	Immunosuppression Cancer chemotherapy	Soft tissue Pulmonary	*H. influenza* *Streptococcus pneumoniae* Gram-negative aerobes
Cell-mediated immunity	Thymic aplasia, malnutrition, Hodgkin's disease, AIDS	Immunosuppression Corticosteroids	Soft tissue	Gram-negative aerobes *Mycobacterium tuberculosis*

week in some studies.[181] This acquisition is paralleled by an increase in the appearance of these bacteria in the causation of nosocomial infection.

5.12.2. Other Drugs. Those drugs with side effects that decrease normal host defenses have the most profound role in increasing risk of nosocomial infection. Corticosteroids modify inflammatory response, interfere with leukocyte function, and depress cellular and humoral immune responses. Antimetabolites and a variety of other cancer chemotherapy drugs have profound effects on all rapidly proliferating tissue, resulting in hemopoietic side effects that decrease immune function and gastrointestinal side effects that interfere with secretory protection and cause loss of anatomical barriers through ulceration. The patient treated with a combination of intensive chemotherapy, immunosuppressive agents, and antibiotic prophylaxis in an attempt to induce remission of leukemia or in preparation for bone marrow or organ transplantation epitomizes the host at special high risk of nosocomial infection secondary to drug effects.

5.12.3. Device- and Procedure-Related Infections.

Medical implements and devices and the procedures associated with them have assumed a common necessary part of modern medical practice. These devices include intravenous needles and catheters, drains, urinary catheters, indwelling tubes into normally closed body cavities of the peritoneum or the cardiothoracic spaces, prosthesis in the cardiovascular system, the central nervous system, or the skeletal system, as well as a variety of implements in the respiratory system, including nasotracheal, endotracheal, and tracheostomy tubes. Each of these devices provides a route of entry for microorganisms by penetrating host defense mechanisms. One or another of the devices is used in the care of approximately 10% of patients hospitalized in acute-care facilities. It has been estimated that 45% of all nosocomial infections, over 850,000 per year in the United States, are device-related (Table 9). In a CDC report of epidemics investigated between 1970 and 1975, 42% of the epidemics were device-related, and 70% of these were associated with gram-negative bacilli.[191] More recently, coagulase-negative staphylococci have appeared as infections complicating use of central vascular lines, grafts, and other devices.[13,31,35]

Table 9.   Common Device-Related Nosocomial Infections[a]

Device[b]	Hospitalized patients with the device (%)	Most common related infection	Patients developing infection (%)	Case-fatality rate (%)
Urinary catheter	10	Bacteriuria	20	<1
Intravascular infusion	12	Suppurative phlebitis	<0.01	20–40
Scalp vein needle	12	Suppurative phlebitis	<0.01	20–40
Plastic catheter	12	Suppurative phlebitis	0–8	20–40
TPN	0.1	Suppurative phlebitis	0–27	20–40
Arterial catheter	0.2	Suppurative phlebitis	0.2	20–40
Respiratory therapy				
Continuous ventilator	2	Pneumonia	—	40
IPPB	7	Pneumonia	—	40
Hemodialysis		Shunt infection	15–20	5

[a] Modified from Stamm.[190]
[b] TPN, total parenteral nutrition; IPPB, intermittent positive-pressure breathing.

6. Mechanisms and Routes of Transmission

Patients may be infected with bacteria acquired from either endogenous or exogenous sources. Microorganisms from endogenous sources may appear by reactivation of some previous infection, as in tuberculosis, or by invasion of commensal flora, which infect because of some reduction in host defenses.

Transmission from exogenous sources may take place by hands, by the airborne route, through fomites, by insects, or by ingestion of contaminated food or water. While each of these routes, with the exception of insects, has been described in individual outbreaks, transmission by direct and indirect contact remains the common and most significant route in acquiring nosocomial infection.

Exogenous sources are found in three specific reservoirs: (1) within the fixed structures of the facility itself, (2) in devices or equipment used within the institution, and (3) in medical personnel, other patients, or visitors.

6.1. Inanimate Reservoirs

The microenvironment of the hospital, rich in water and nutrient sources, has provided a continuing niche for gram-negative bacilli that have evolved as the most important agents in nosocomial infection. *Enterobacter, Serratia, Acinetobacter, Citrobacter, Flavobacteria, Legionella,* and *Pseudomonas* species have been repeatedly identified as important nosocomial infectors because of their ability to survive in the aqueous and other fluid reservoirs of our institutions.[33,40,59,188,218] Clean environmental surfaces

are not important sources of bacteria-causing nosocomial infections.[130] Extensive reviews of reported inanimate reservoirs are available.[146,218]

6.1.1. Structural or Engineering Reservoirs. The medical-care field is one of rapid change, and this is evident in frequent requirements for modification of structures used for medical care. With limited funding, compromises in terms of structure, space, and function that are less than ideal may be accepted. The result may be crowding, which encourages cross-contamination, or the inconvenient placement of certain fixed equipment (e.g., hand-washing sinks) which makes the use of the equipment problematical. Reconstruction may disguise an inadequate air-conditioning system, resulting in the recirculation of unfiltered air from an "isolated" tuberculosis patient[49] or of air exhausted from microbiological laboratories or other areas of high biohazard.

The airborne spread of staphylococci has been suggested by several studies.[221] Nosocomial Legionnaires' disease has been described either from contaminated cooling towers of air-conditioning systems[88,132] or from construction activity in the vicinity of the hospital.[198]

Airborne transmission has also been implicated in nosocomial aspergillosis.[3,9] Materials used in hospital construction, such as fireproofing materials, have been identified as a source of *Aspergillus* infection in cancer patients.[1]

Reservoirs of nosocomial bacteria within water supplies or plumbing have been a recurrent problem in hospitals caring for high-risk patients.[33,58,59]

6.1.2. Equipment Reservoirs. In addition to the

common medical devices, a wealth of new and increasingly complex equipment attends patient care. Respiratory assistance equipment, cardiovascular assistance pumps, microelectronic monitoring devices, dialysis machinery, and numerous other "black boxes" have reached the bedside. Appropriate use of these instruments is understood by fewer and fewer individuals, and the safe techniques for appropriate disinfection between patients may be overlooked or misunderstood. Portions of this equipment may be expensive, fragile, nondisposable, and unable to withstand the usual harsh but sure techniques of heat sterilization. Alternate methods are often less well understood than classic heat sterilization, and inadequate attention is paid to the detail necessary to assure their full implementation. As a result, residual microorganisms may be transmitted to subsequent patients.[26,157,186] Other problems have arisen when bacterial endotoxins have remained on equipment, causing severe reactions, or residual chemical sterilants themselves have caused toxic effects.[23]

6.2. Animate Reservoirs

Bacteria causing nosocomial infection reside in the animate reservoirs[25,39,177,194,200,227] of the health care worker or of the chronically institutionalized patient. Patients colonized with nosocomial organisms at clinical sites, such as wounds or urine, or colonized in their gastrointestinal, genitourinary tract, or oropharyngeal flora serve as reservoirs for these organisms. Hospital personnel are occasionally personal carriers of nosocomial organisms such as *Salmonella* or staphylococci that are transmitted to hospitalized patients. Of these characteristics, the ability to survive at the time of transmission in mechanical carriage remains the most significant factor in nosocomial infection.

Hospital professionals, medical support workers, and patients provide the animate reservoirs for microorganisms. Biological transmission through symptomatic or asymptomatic carriage of bacteria has led to serious and extensive epidemics.[25,194] While visitors are a potential for microorganisms, they have rarely been implicated in such transmission.

Even more commonly, well but careless individuals mechanically transmit large numbers of bacteria from reservoirs within the facility, from equipment, and from patient to patient during their daily rounds. Hand carriage of microorganisms is recognized as the most important factor in endemic and most epidemic spread of nosocomial infection. In one study in a university neurosurgical unit, 44% of randomly sampled personnel carried gram-negative bacilli, and 11% had *S. aureus* on their hands.[125] More important,

serial culturing demonstrated that all persons at various times carried gram-negative bacilli, and two thirds carried staphylococci. Indirect contact spread via transient hand carriage has been implicated in other nosocomial transmission of staphylococci, enterococci, and gram-negatives.[39,70,200,227] Such carriage is instrumental in the nosocomial colonization that precedes infection in the compromised host.[103,177,181,189,227]

7. Pathogenesis and Immunity

The pathogenesis of nosocomial infection is determined by host and environmental factors that are uniquely combined in health-care institutions.

The susceptible patient is prey to all the conventional pathogens. The compromised host is infected by a much smaller dose of bacteria and by species that are usually considered commensal and "nonpathogenic."[24] Thus, the host with underlying severe disease and impaired host defenses has higher rates of infection, secondary bacteremia, refractory infection, and case fatality.[22,72,178] As in the example of hematological cancers, disease and treatment have so devastated the immune system that response is lethargic or nonexistent, infection is poorly controlled, even by appropriate antibiotic therapy, and case mortality is high.[99,179] Following infection with agents that persist in endogenous sites (e.g., *Mycobacterium tuberculosis*), significant immune depression may result in reactivation and uncontrolled dissemination.

Pathogenicity by nosocomial agents has not been related to the presence of resistant bacteria, but resistance does contribute to difficulty in treatment with conventional drugs. The ecological press of antibiotic use assures the presence of resistant forms available for transmission in the health-care setting. At each site, colonization precedes local multiplication and tissue infection.[66,103] Colonization with nosocomial organisms results from alterations in "normal flora" by broad-spectrum therapy, hospitalization, and instrumentation. Colonization is directly related to the organisms' survival ability, ability to adhere to mucosal surfaces and catheters, and organism virulence.

Special procedures and devices allow bacteria to be delivered past the superficial barriers and to sustain a milieu important to implantation and multiplication. Dissemination through secondary bacteremia occurs in approximately 5.6% of bacteremias reported from the NNIS system.[31] By site, secondary bacteremias are reported following approximately 3% of nosocomial urinary tract infections, 5% of nosocomial wound infections, 5–6% of nosocomial pneumonias, and 8–9% of cutaneous infections.[31] Secondary infections occur with unknown frequency, since the usual reporting methodology excludes their recording.

8. Patterns of Host Response: Clinical Features and Diagnosis

Patterns of host response to nosocomial infection are those classically described with bacterial disease of the sites involved. As with pathogenesis, clinical features and morbidity are determined by the virulence of the agent, the dose and route of transmission, and the character of the host defense mechanisms.

Signs and symptoms in the compromised host may be altered or reduced. Fever may be low or absent. The site of infection may be unusual, as in the predilection to perirectal abscess in cancer patients.[180]

8.1. Urinary Tract Infection

Infections of the urinary tract account for as much as 40% of all nosocomial infections. *E. coli*, *P. aeruginosa*, and *E. faecalis* are the most common causal organisms.[31,202] Almost all nosocomial urinary tract infections are associated with indwelling bladder catheters or instrumentation. The overall risk of bacteriuria in hospitalized patients with indwelling catheters is about 25%. Bacteria gain access to the catheterized bladder by either of two routes. They may migrate from the collection bag or the catheter drainage tube junction, or in the majority of cases bacteria ascend extraluminally within the periurethral space.[66] Fever in a catheterized patient or in a patient with recent urinary tract instrumentation should lead one to suspect urinary tract infection. Greater than 10^5 colony-forming units per milliliter of urine represents significant bacteriuria from a clean catch midstream urine specimen. In catheterized patients, however, a concentration of microorganisms considerably less than 10^5 can be shown to be progressive in the absence of antimicrobial therapy and can be associated with symptomatic infection.[195] The significance of asymptomatic bacteriuria in patients with indwelling bladder catheters remains under discussion.[18,148,159]

8.2. Nosocomial Pneumonia

Pneumonia appears frequently in those patients in whom aspiration has taken place or in whom the upper airway is bypassed by endotracheal intubation. Purulent sputum, pulmonary infiltration on X ray, fever, and hypoxia

indicate the presence of this complication. In individuals with community-acquired pneumonia, a change in microbial flora in the sputum accompanied by a worsening in clinical course usually indicates a pulmonary superinfection. Culture and Gram or other staining of the sputum, transtracheal aspirate, endotracheal aspirate, or percutaneous lung aspirate are essential to the establishment of etiological diagnosis.[165]

Organisms simultaneously isolated from the blood and pleural fluid are strong evidence of pulmonary infection with that agent.

8.3. Surgical Wound Infection

Infection of the wound is suspected in any febrile postoperative patient. Drainage of purulent material or disruption of the wound are considered prima facie evidence of wound infection with or without bacterial isolates. Unfortunately, up to 40% of wound infections are not evident until after the patient is discharged from the hospital. Following certain procedures involving implantation of a prosthesis or other foreign material, infection may not be evident for months.

8.4. Bacteremia

Bacteremia is usually accompanied by fever and a decline in clinical condition. In the absence of evidence of infection at other sites, an intravenous source should be suspected. Intravascular implements in place for more than 48 h should be investigated even in the absence of inflammation. Blood cultures, cultures of infusates, and semiquantitative cultures of the implant itself may establish the diagnosis.[124,129]

8.5. Infection at Other Sites

Nosocomial infection of the skin, soft tissue, gastrointestinal tract, urogenital tract, and other sites is frequently found. A detailed discussion of the appearances, diagnosis, and treatment of the more common and these less common infections has been published.[17]

9. Control and Prevention

9.1. General Concepts

The methods for conducting a successful nosocomial infection control program are outlined in Table 10 and paraphrase the classic scientific method. Identification of

Table 10.   Elements of Nosocomial Infection Control

1. Elaborate criteria for infection
2. Establish surveillance
3. Determine endemic rates
4. Evaluate endemic problems
5. Recognize and control epidemic
6. Effect control program
   a. Orientation
   b. In-service education
   c. Behavior modification
7. Evaluate control programs
8. Evaluate cost benefit

nosocomial infections through application of standard criteria is widely accepted. Routine, continuous collection, collation, evaluation, and reporting of these data by a trained nursing specialist using "surveillance" tools are recommended and have been tested for efficacy by the CDC during the SENIC Project.[83] The presence of one of these infection control practitioners (ICP) for approximately every 250 inpatient beds was important to efficacy as measured by the evaluation models in this study as was the presence of a trained hospital epidemiologist. The expense of this methodology has been of concern, but the SENIC evaluation estimated an approximate 6-to-1 benefit-to-cost ratio in its application, and alternative reporting methods have been of low efficiency, poor specificity, and slow to recognize outbreaks.[15,65,216,217] Evaluation of institutional nosocomial data through these techniques has allowed identification of priority infection problems and planning, implementation, and evaluation of interventions to control them. Control programs usually fall into three areas: preventive engineering, equipment control, and personnel programs.

9.1.1. Preventive Engineering. A careful review of engineering plans for nosocomial risk should be undertaken before construction or reconstruction is begun. Guidelines have been published by some state and national agencies.[37,141] Efficient function follows appropriate form in the hospital, as in other industries. If hand-washing sinks are present and conveniently placed in patient care areas, they will be used. Traffic flow will be determined by design and will be difficult to alter by placing signs thereafter. Control of environmental bacterial contamination will be affected by surface features, air-conditioning, and the convenient presence of housekeeping and other service modules.

9.1.2. Equipment Control. As with structure, the design of equipment is important to its correct use, mainte-

nance, and disinfection. Initially inexpensive devices may multiply future costs by requiring complicated disassembly, cleaning, and time-consuming disinfection in order to render them safe for multiple patient use. Component parts may not tolerate heat sterilization and require gas or chemical sterilization. Gas and chemical sterilization are more demanding in detail and may leave residuals that present toxic problems.[23] The use of disposable equipment has exploded in the hospital industry, contributing to major increases in cost and in problems of waste disposal. Reuse of disposable equipment on individual patients, under strict protocols, has been found acceptable in a few limited situations (e.g., hemodialyzer reuse).[57,74] However, attempts to modify this expense by reuse of disposable equipment on multiple patients have been responsible for several outbreaks of nosocomial infection and are to be decried.[214] Intrinsic contamination of industrially prepared medical devices and supplies has been a rare cause of epidemic nosocomial outbreaks and has usually been associated with and identified by the unique bacteria involved.[125,127] Routine sterility testing of commercially prepared products is tedious, difficult to control, and usually of insufficient benefit-to-cost to be justified.

9.1.3. Personnel Programs. Health care personnel are the common final factor in the transmission of most nosocomial infections. Orientation and in-service education programs are important in gaining staff appreciation of infection control programs and techniques. The direct availability of the ICP during on-the-ward surveillance activities provides important one-on-one education and consultation in support of bedside infection control. Behavior modification through management techniques of observation, retraining, and the use of incentives and penalties is recommended and under expanding use as effective infection control efforts.[100] Occupational health programs, which assure that health care workers are screened for transmissible diseases on employment and have the opportunity to have subsequent illnesses evaluated for potential transmission, are also an important feature of control of animate reservoirs.[5]

9.2. Special Control Programs

9.2.1. Hand-Washing. Routine hand-washing before, between, and after contact with patients is recognized as the most important feature of successful infection control. The use of an antiseptic soap is recommended in high-risk areas but is of little documented improvement over the routine use of a vigorous scrub with soap and running water. Extensive reviews of hand-washing procedures and guidelines have been published.[74,112,197]

9.2.2. Universal Precautions and Isolation Control. Techniques for the recognition and appropriate care of patients with potentially communicable disease have been recommended in a guideline published by the CDC.[75] The recognized inability to identify accurately all such individuals on admission and the rare but real potential for serious health care worker exposure to HIV and other bloodborne disease(s) have led to the recommendation that a modified method of care be used for all patients with whom there is expected to be a medical care worker contact with blood or body fluids. This system of "universal precautions" (UP) or "universal blood and body fluid precautions" recommends the use of gloves in any patient care situation where such contact is expected and the additional use of gown, mask, and eye protection where splashing, aerosolization, or more extensive exposure is common.[32,121]

If appropriately used, UP are reported both to increase patient protection from all nosocomial infection except that transmitted by the airborne route and, at the same time, to protect the medical care worker from dangerous occupational exposure. Major concerns in changing to this new "isolation" system include issues of risk, retraining, efficacy, availability of materials (gloves), and cost. The appropriate and concurrent use of these two barrier systems, in order to optimize both patient care and worker protection, remains under intense discussion.

An important feature of all barrier isolation programs has been the recognition that isolation is frequently overrestrictive, so that it interferes with patient care, and that a significant portion of isolation needs are satisfied by handwashing and very modest geographic groupings. It has been estimated that over 90% of the isolation used in hospitals is inappropriately restrictive, adding significantly to patient hospital costs.[98]

"Protective isolation," a form of isolation designed to protect noninfected patients with seriously impaired resistance to infection from exposure to potentially infective microorganisms, remains a disputed entity in the control of nosocomial infection. Limited protective isolation of the hospitalized immunocompromised patient has not been demonstrated to reduce nosocomial infections significantly. It is estimated that 80–90% of the infections in these patients are from endogenous sources. However, approximately half the bacteria involved in these infections have come from nosocomial colonization. Total protective environments using sterilized food, filtered laminar-flow units, and prophylactic intestinal and systemic antibiotics have been unable to decontaminate the human being effectively.[158] These environments have achieved some reduction in infection in patients, but their contribution to in-

creased longevity has been minimal. These procedures are complicated by high levels of side effects and prohibitive cost.

9.2.3. Epidemic Investigation and Control. The routine collection of surveillance data on nosocomial infections allows one to establish endemic rates by type of nosocomial infection, by organism, and by area and service within the medical facility. This allows rapid recognition of unusual or epidemic events, whether through the appearance of a new or highly resistant microorganism or through a grouping of similar infections. An outline of an epidemic investigation is given in Table 11. The careful documentation and reporting of epidemic investigations are important features in every infection control program.[27]

9.2.4. Nosocomial Urinary Tract Infection. Approximately three quarters of documented nosocomial urinary tract infections are associated with catheter use. The use of a closed sterile drainage system with indwelling catheters provides a significant (50%) short-term reduction in infection related to this device.[110] Appropriate care in the placement and maintenance of these devices is essential to their success in preventing nosocomial infection.[66] Breaks in aseptic technique in placement and disruption and entry into the closed system are the most significant factors in the development of catheter-related urinary tract infection.[210] Guidelines for the control of nosocomial urinary tract infection have been developed and published by the CDC.[76] An outline for catheter use and care is seen in Table 12.[190] In the SENIC project analysis, the combination of high levels of surveillance activity, a modest level of control activity, and the presence of a full-time ICP yielded an estimated 31% reduction of infection in patients at high risk for this event.[83]

9.2.5. Nosocomial Wound Infection. Nosocomial wound infections are usually initiated at the time of surgery.[109,147,160] Guidelines featuring the etiology and control of wound infection have been reviewed and published by

---

Table 11.   Outline of Epidemic Investigation[a]

1. Establish the existence of an epidemic
2. Complete case count
3. Make analysis of pertinent characteristics
4. Form hypothesis
5. Test hypothesis
6. Institute control measures
7. Evaluate control measures
8. Document and report

---

[a]Adapted from a CDC training pamphlet.[27]

Table 12. Guidelines for Urinary-Catheter Use[a]

1. Do not use unless necessary
2. Use correct catheter
3. Use aseptic and gentle techniques
4. Use sterile closed drainage system
5. Maintain system closed
6. Keep bag below level of bladder, but not on floor
7. Culture aseptically
8. Discontinue early
9. Culture at discontinuation
10. Sanitize measuring devices after each use

[a] Modified from Stamm.[190]

the CDC.[30,79] Debate over the importance of airborne bacterial contamination of surgical wounds continues,[93,167] and most modern operating rooms use air-filtration systems. However, a large cooperative study failed to correlate reduction in airborne levels of bacteria with reduced infection rates in most operations.[163] In a more recent cooperative study of certain high-risk operations (e.g., placement of artificial hip joint), improvement in bacterial air quality appeared to be associated with a reduction in wound sepsis.[118] This has led some investigators to advocate even stricter air-quality standards, including the use of special exhaust headgear and laminar-flow air systems.[63]

Cruse and Foord,[42] in a large study of nosocomial wound infections, have reduced their clean wound rates to 1% or less. They report the most important factors in the control of wound infection as being: (1) the length of preoperative stay, (2) the type of preoperative skin care, including avoidance of shaving, (3) meticulous surgical technique, and (4) the dissemination of surgeon-specific nosocomial-wound-infection data to all surgeons. Analyses of the SENIC project by the CDC support these findings, especially the success of reporting wound infection rates to individual surgeons.[83]

The routine use of prophylactic antibiotics just prior to and during selected surgical procedures has been well studied and supported by a growing number of investigations. An excellent review of these recommendations has been published.[7]

9.2.6. Nosocomial Respiratory Infections. Attention to the details of disinfection of various respiratory assistance devices and the use of careful technique and sterile equipment in the suctioning of the endotracheal tree are emphasized as important in the reduction of nosocomial respiratory infection.[26,157,164,165] Prevention of contamination of humidification devices by routine and fre-

quent disinfection and the use of sterile water have contributed to this control.[186,188] Specific details and background for these methods are outlined in another of the CDC Guidelines.[78] Data from the SENIC project suggest that a high level of surveillance and the presence of an ICP were a necessary feature for the 27% reduction in postoperative pneumonia reported. Reductions in medical pneumonia appeared much less successful. Recent studies suggest that specific methods or therapies that maintain or reduce microorganisms to a low level in the stomach are associated with lower risk of nosocomial aspiration and pneumonia.[204]

9.2.7. Nosocomial Intravascular Infection. Proper choice of device, correct placement, and careful maintenance of intravenous systems are important in the control of infections at this site. Needles are associated with lower inflammation and infection rates than are the various catheters.[128] While no improvement in infection rate has been associated with the use of antiseptic or antibiotic creams at the skin site in short-term intravenous use, the effectiveness of a detailed maintenance routine with antibiotic creams has been reported for long-term catheterization for central venous nutrition.[69] Care in prevention of contamination of the delivery system is important, as is the documentation of the appropriate use of additives through dating and labeling.[124] Guidelines for the prevention of nosocomial intravascular infections have been assembled and published by the CDC.[77] Important features for intravenous care are outlined in Table 13.

9.2.8. Antibiotic and Antimicrobial Prophylaxis. The routine prophylactic use of antibiotics has not been demonstrated to control nosocomial infections in most sites

Table 13. Guidelines for Intravenous Use[a]

1. Do not use unnecessarily
2. Choose a low-risk site
3. Routine—use needle
4. Use good technique:
   a. Wash hands
   b. Use aseptic prep and fixation
   c. Date site
   d. Label appropriately
5. Maintain appropriately:
   a. Discontinue emergent site early
   b. Observe daily
   c. Change set every 48 to 72 h
6. Remove early
7. With sepsis, suspect i.v. site

[a] Modified from McGowan.[137]

and situations. In a limited number of surgical procedures, controlled studies of antibiotic prophylaxis have demonstrated a reduction in the rate of wound infection and in subsequent morbidity and mortality.[7,162] Criteria for antibiotic prophylaxis in surgery have been developed.[206] General guidelines for the approach to surgical prophylaxis are reviewed in Table 14.[114]

Routine bathing of the newborn with hexachlorophene-containing soaps for control of staphylococcal colonization and nursery infection is no longer recommended. Cutaneous absorption of hexachlorophene has been demonstrated, especially in the premature infant. Such absorption has been associated with pathological changes in the brain, and in cases of high dosage, permanent neurological damage and death have ensued.[89,108]

Triple dye and a number of other compounds successfully inhibit the colonization of the umbilical stump with staphylococci.[105]

Antibiotic prophylaxis in oncology and burn patients, whose severely compromised host defenses allow repeated endogenous infections, is also in limited use and under continued investigation. Prophylaxis is not recommended in most clinical situations for cancer and burn patients. Early treatment following diagnostic microbiological studies remains the suggested therapeutic program.[223] The recognition of a recurrent infection in a compromised patient with a specific organism may justify the use of continued antibiotic prophylaxis specific to that bacterium.[184]

9.2.9. Immunization. Immunization for the prevention of bacterial nosocomial infection has not been exploited, largely due to the lack of effective vaccines. However, in other institutional situations, pneumococcal and meningococcal vaccines have been tested and found successful. Both passive and active immunization for control of nosocomial *Pseudomonas* infections in oncology and burn units have been investigated.[143,161] Passive immunization

has been reported to provide limited protection. Active immunization has been reported to reduce infection in some high-risk units.[62,224] Side effects, however, have been significant.

9.2.10. Cellular and Transplantation Methods. Granulocyte transfusions have improved the response to infection in some leukemia patients with increased survival. This technique is limited by lack of sources for sufficient cells and recurrent concern about the ability to ensure their safe use in excluding occult microbial agents. Bone marrow transplantation is an increasingly successful technique, but one requiring great sophistication and resources. It remains apparent that further advances in basic immunology and transplantation will be required before wider success with these procedures is achieved.

10. Unresolved Problems

10.1. Efficacy and Cost–Benefit Evaluation: Acute Care

The program of surveillance and infection control recommended by the CDC and mandated by governmental and accreditation agencies has benefited in the support offered in the publication of the results of the SENIC project,[83] indicating a 32% overall reduction in nosocomial infection through application of the program. Since the data on which the study was based were gathered in 1970 and 1975–1976, the applicability to hospital practice a decade later remains open to some question. Medical care continues to change at a rapid pace with new technologies and shifts in practice, which have markedly altered the case mix and intensity of services offered in acute hospital care in the United States. As a result, an even higher portion of nosocomial infections may not be preventable by classic CDC methods, especially those from endogenous sources in highly immunocompromised patients.[180] Continued studies on the characteristics of patients in acute care who are at high risk for preventable nosocomial infection are needed.

The analysis of the SENIC data suggested a 6 : 1 benefit-to-cost ratio for effective CDC-type programs. Changing costs and efficacy in the past decade may have altered this finding, and continued monitoring is important to affirm these data.

The above problems notwithstanding, these programs appear well justified in the competition for resources in acute medical care. These findings must continue to find their way into the medical and administrative discussions that determine program priorities in hospitals.

Table 14. Guidelines for Perioperative Antibiotic Prophylaxis[a]

1. Significant infection risk
2. Significant bacterial contamination
3. Antibiotic spectrum effective
4. Effective concentrations of antibiotic present at incision time
5. Use short regimen—total regimen 48 h
6. Use low-toxicity regimen
7. Avoid antibiotic critical to therapy
8. Benefits should outweigh risk

[a]Modifed from Ledger *et al.*[114]

10.2. Routine Application of Standard Methods

For many infection control procedures (e.g., catheter-care programs), no new information is needed. Uniform, correct implementation of such procedures by all individuals involved in patient care would significantly reduce nosocomial infections at these sites. Responsibility here falls most heavily on the senior professional staff. Whether demonstrating careful surgical technique or simple hand-washing, leadership through role-modeling and monitoring through acceptance of authority are the key to success. Employee health programs are another underused risk-control program in most hospitals.[5] Absence of physician leadership as providers and participants in these programs is frequently responsible for their lack of success.

Where demonstration and persuasion fail to gain compliance, behavior modification through rewards and penalties may be indicated.

10.3. Coordinated Programs

The many common features in nosocomial infection control and other quality assurance programs should be recognized. In U.S. hospitals, the quality assurance programs are commonly thought to include nosocomial infection control, risk management, patient care evaluation, and utilization review. These programs are notable in using common data sources, applying common epidemiologic methods, implementing similar analysis, sharing similar committee structures, and sharing similar goals of improved quality of patient care largely by avoiding increased nosocomial risk.[90] Many institutions are now attempting to coordinate these programs through shared personnel and mutually derived and exploited computerized data bases. The sharing should have a potential for markedly increasing both the efficiencies and effectiveness of these programs.

10.4. Need and Efficacy in Developing Countries

With the exception of the WHO prevalence studies[202] and a few individual reports,[111] data on nosocomial infection risk in the developing countries are not available. Opinions are repeatedly expressed and assumptions made that medical needs in these areas are such that infection control programs are not a potential priority for consideration.

However, the major potential requirement for resources lost to the community in morbidity and mortality from nosocomial illness and in the cost to treat the infectious complications of medical care caused by the relatively inexpensive but often absent tools for sterilization, mate-rials for disinfection, and training in basic aseptic technique, would make the basics of infection control appear even more mandatory in these developing countries.

10.5. Efficacy in Nonacute Care

Most studies of nosocomial infections, including the CDC-NNIS, WHO, and CDC-SENIC projects, have taken place in acute-care hospitals. A small but growing number of investigations are being reported in extended care, but these must be separated by type (e.g., rehabilitation, domiciliary, skilled nursing). Nosocomial infection risk in other care settings, including ambulatory care, physician's office, and home care, is unknown.

10.6. Education

Several professional groups, including the Association of Practitioners in Infection Control, The Hospital Infections Society, and the Society of Hospital Epidemiologists of America, have been organized and are supporting communication and educational efforts in infection control, as has the CDC for several decades. Despite this interest, few medical schools, microbiology training programs, infectious disease training programs, or nursing curricula provide material pertinent to nosocomial infection risk and control. Organizational acceptance of responsibility for these areas of education is important to further program success.[50]

Standards for training ICPs, nurse epidemiologists, infection control committee chairmen, and hospital epidemiologists remain undefined. They continue to be an intense topic of discussion within these professional organizations.

10.7. Technological Standards

Information on standards of construction important to infection control is neither readily available nor widely implemented in hospital architectural planning. Modern facilities are frequently built with no infection control review, resulting in high-risk units that defy or discourage appropriate application of procedures important to the control of nosocomial infection thereafter. Construction standards important to infection control should be formed at a national level and incorporated into planning, much as fire-control standards at present. Special programs for hospital architects may assist in achieving this goal.

Medical equipment design and function frequently provide a reservoir for nosocomial bacteria. Design and manufacturing techniques that allow assembly and disassembly for easy disinfection of critical parts between patients or protection of such parts from contamination should be a part of the engineering of all medical devices. Close cooperation between infectious disease consultants and design engineers will be important to this effort.

11. References

1. AISNER, J., SCHIMPFF, S. C., BENNETT, J. E., YOUNG, V. M., AND WIERNIK, P. H., Aspergillus infection in cancer patients, *J. Am. Med. Assoc.* **235**:411–412 (1976).
2. ALLEN, J. R., HIGHTOWER, A. W., MARTIN, S. M., AND DIXON, R. E., Secular trends in nosocomial infections: 1970–1979, *Am. J. Med.* **70**:389 (1981).
3. ALLO, M. D., MILLER, J., TOWNSEND, T., AND TAN, C., Primary cutaneous aspergillosis associated with Hickman intravenous catheters, *N. Engl. J. Med.* **317**:1105–1108 (1987).
4. ALTEMEIER, W. A., AND LEWIS, S. A., Cyclic variations in emerging phage types and antibiotic resistance of Staphylococcus aureus, *Surgery* **84**:534–540 (1978).
5. American Occupational Medical Association Committee on Medical Center Employee Occupational Health, ROBERT LEWY, Chairman, Committee report: Guidelines for employee health services in health care institutions, *J. Occup. Med.* **28**:518–523 (1986).
6. ANNEAR, D. I., AND GRUBB, W. B., Spontaneous loss of resistance to kanamycin and other antibiotics in methicillin resistant cultures of Staphylococcus aureus, *Med. J. Aust.* **2**:902–904 (1969).
7. Antimicrobial prophylaxis for surgery, *The Medical Letter*, **27**:105–108 (1985).
8. ARCHER, G. L., AND MAYHALL, C. G., Comparison of epidemiological markers used in the investigation of an outbreak of methicillin-resistant *Staphylococcus aureus* infection, *J. Clin. Microbiol.* **18**:395–399 (1983).
9. ARNOW, P. M., ANDERSON, R. L., AND MAINOUS, P. D., Pulmonary aspergillosis during hospital renovation, *Am. Rev. Respir. Dis.* **118**:49–53 (1978).
10. ATKINSON, B. A., AND LORIAN, V., Antimicrobial agent susceptibility patterns of bacteria in hospitals from 1971–1982, *J. Clin. Microbiol.* **20**:791–796 (1984).
11. AYLIFFE, G. A. J., AND LILLY, H. A., Cross-infection and its prevention, *J. Hosp. Infect.* **6**(Suppl. B):47–57 (1985).
12. AYLIFFE, G. A. J., BRIGHTWELL, K. M., COLLINS, B. J., AND LOWBURY, E. J. L., Surveys of hospital infection in the Birmingham region, *J. Hyg.* **79**:299–314 (1977).
13. BANDYK, D. F., Vascular graft infection; epidemiology, bacteriology, and pathogenesis, in: *Complications in Vascular Surgery*, 2nd ed. (V. M. BERNHARD AND J. B. TOWNE, eds.), pp. 471–485, Grune & Stratton, New York, 1985.
14. BARRETT, F. F., CASEY, J. I., AND FINLAND, M., Infections and antibiotic use among patients at Boston City Hospital, *N. Engl. J. Med.* **278**:5–9 (1968).
15. BARTLETT, C. L. R., Efficacy of different surveillance systems in detecting hospital acquired infection, *Chemioterapia* **6**:152–155 (1987).
16. BARTON, L. L., GRANOFF, D. M., AND BAREN-KAMP, S. J., Nosocomial spread of *Haemophilus influenzae*, type B infection documented by outer membrane protein subtype analysis, *J. Pediatr.* **102**:820–824 (1983).
17. BENNETT, J. V., AND BRACHMAN, P. S. (eds.), *Hospital Infections*, 2nd ed., Little, Brown, Boston (1986).
18. BOSCIA, J. A., ABRUTYN, E., AND KAYE, D., Asymptomatic bacteriuria in elderly persons: Treat or do not treat? *Ann. Intern. Med.* **106**:764–766 (1987).
19. BRIEGER, G. H., Hospital infection: A brief historical appraisal, in: *Handbook on Hospital Associated Infections, I: Occurrence, Diagnosis, and Source of Hospital Associated Infections* (W. J. FAHLBURG AND D. GROSCHEL, eds.), pp. 1–12, Dekker, New York, 1978.
20. BRITT, M. R., Infectious diseases in small hospitals, prevalence of infections and adequacy of microbiology services, *Ann. Intern. Med.* **89**(Part 2):757–760 (1978).
21. BRITT, M. R., BURKE, J. P., NORDQUIST, A. G., WILFERT, J. N., AND SMITH, C. B., Infection control in small hospitals: Prevalence surveys in 18 institutions, *J. Am. Med. Assoc.* **236**:1700–1703 (1976).
22. BRITT, M. R., SCHLUEPNER, C. J., AND MATSUMIYU, S., Severity of underlying diseases as a predictor of nosocomial infections: Utility in the control of nosocomial infection, *J. Am. Med. Assoc.* **239**:1047–1051 (1978).
23. BRUCH, C. W., Sterilization of plastics: Toxicity of ethylene oxide residues, in: *Industrial Sterilization* (G. B. PHILLIPS AND W. S. MILLER, eds.), pp. 49–77, Duke University Press, Durham, 1972.
24. BURKE, J. P., AND HILDECK-SMITH, G. Y., *The Infection Prone Hospital Patient*, Little, Brown, Boston, 1978.
25. BURKE, J. P., INGALL, D., KLEIN, J. O., GEZON, H. M., AND FINLAND, M., Proteus mirabilis infections in a hospital nursery traced to a human carrier, *N. Engl. J. Med.* **284**:115–121 (1971).
26. BUXTON, A. E., ANDERSON, R. L., WERDEGAR, D., AND ATLAS, E., Nosocomial respiratory tract infection and colonization with Acinetobacter calcoaceticus, *Am. J. Med.* **65**:507–513 (1978).
27. Centers for Disease Control, Training Pamphlet 00-023, Outline of Procedure in Investigation and Analysis of an Epidemic, CDC, Atlanta, January 1974.
28. Centers for Disease Control, False positive blood cultures related to use of evacuated nonsterile blood collection tubes, *Morbid. Mortal. Weekly Rep.* **24**:387–388 (1978).
29. Centers for Disease Control, Special issue: The SENIC project, *Am. J. Epidemiol.* **111**:465–653 (1980).
30. Centers for Disease Control, Guidelines on infection control, *Infect. Control* **3**(2):187–196 (1982).

31. Centers for Disease Control, Nosocomial Infection Surveillance, 1984, *Morbid. Mortal. Weekly Rep.* **35:**17SS–29SS (No. 1 SS), (1986).

32. Centers for Disease Control, Recommendations for prevention of HIV transmission in health-care settings, *Morbid. Mortal. Weekly Rep.* **36**(Suppl.):3S–18S (1987).

33. CHADWICK, P., The epidemiological significance of Pseudomonas aeruginosa in hospital sinks, *Can. J. Public Health* **67:**323–328 (1976).

34. CHEESBROUGH, J. S., FINCH, R. G., AND BURDEN, R. P., A prospective study of the mechanisms of infection associated with hemodialysis catheters, *J. Infect. Dis.* **154:**579–589 (1986).

35. CHRISTENSEN, G. D., BISNO, A. L., MCLAUGHLIN, B., HEASTER, M. G., AND LUTHER, R. W., Nosocomial septicemia due to multiple antibiotic resistant Staphylococcus epidermidis, *Ann. Intern. Med.* **96:**1–10 (1987).

36. COHEN, E. D., HIERHOLZER, W. J., JR., SCHILLING, C. R., AND SNYDMAN, D. R., Nosocomial infections in skilled nursing facilities: A preliminary survey, *Public Health Rep.* **94:**162–165 (1979).

37. Connecticut Public Health State Code & Other Department Regulations, Chapter 4, Infection Control, pp. 205–206 (Sect. 19-13-D3), January 1983.

38. COPLEY, J. B., Prevention of peritoneal dialysis catheter-related infections, *Am. J. Kidney Dis.* **10:**401–407 (1987).

39. CRAVEN, D. E., REED, C., KOLLISCH, N., DEMARIA, A., LICHTENBERG, D., SHEN, K., AND MCCABE, W. R., A large outbreak of infections caused by a strain of Staphylococcus aureus resistant to oxacillin and aminoglycosides, *Am. J. Med.* **71:**53–58 (1981).

40. CRESPA, J., Dialysis-related infections, *Heart Lung* **11:**111–117 (1982).

41. CROSSLEY, K., LOESCH, D., LANDESMAN, B., MEAD, K., CHERN, M., AND STRATE, R., An outbreak of infections caused by strain of Staphylococcus aureus resistant to methicillin and aminoglycosides, *J. Infect. Dis.* **139:**273–279 (1979).

42. CRUSE, P. J. E., AND FOORD, R., The epidemiology of wound infection: A 10-year prospective study of 62,939 wounds, *Surg. Clin. North Am.* **60:**27–40 (1980).

43. DARLAND, G., Discriminant analysis of antibiotic susceptibility as a means of bacterial identification, *J. Clin. Microbiol.* **2:**391–396 (1975).

44. DASCHNER, F., NADJEM, H., LANGMAACK, H., AND SANDRITTER, W., Surveillance, prevention, and control of hospital acquired infections. III. Nosocomial infection as cause of death; retrospective analysis of 1000 autopsy reports, *Infection* **6:**261–265 (1978).

45. DASCHNER, F. D., FREY, P., WOLFF, G., BAUMANN, P. C., AND SUTER, P., Nosocomial infections in intensive care wards: A multicenter prospective study, *Int. Care Med.* **8:**5–9 (1982).

46. DAVIS, S. D., SOBOCINSKI, K., HOFFMAN, R. G., MOHR, B., AND NELSON, D. B., Postoperative wound infections in a children's hospital, *Pediatr. Infect. Dis.* **3:**114–116 (1984).

47. DOUGLAS, B. E., Health problems of hospital employee, *J. Occup. Med.* **13:**555–560 (1971).

48. EGOZ, N., AND MICHAELI, D., A program for surveillance of hospital-acquired infections in a general hospital: A two-year experience, *Rev. Infect. Dis.* **3:**649–657 (1981).

49. EHRENKRANS, J. J., AND KICKLIGHTER J. L., Tuberculosis outbreak in a general hospital: Evidence for airborne spread of infection, *Ann. Intern. Med.* **77:**377–382 (1972).

50. EICKHOFF, T. C., Standards for hospital infection control, *Ann. Intern. Med.* **89**(Part 2):829–831 (1978).

51. EICKHOFF, T. C., BRACHMAN, P. S., BENNETT, J. V., AND BROWN, J. F., Surveillance of nosocomial infections in community hospitals. I. Surveillance methods, effectiveness, and initial results, *J. Infect. Dis.* **120:**306–316 (1969).

52. ELLNER, P. D., FINK, D. J., NEU, H. C., AND PARRY, M. F., Epidemiologic factors affecting antimicrobial resistance of common bacterial isolates, *J. Clin. Microbiol.* **25:**1668–1674 (1987).

53. ELWELL, L. P., INAMINE, J. M., AND MINSHEW, B. A., A common plasmid specifying tobramycin resistance found in two enterobacteria isolated from burn patients, *Antimicrob. Agents Chemother.* **13:**312–317 (1978).

54. EMORI, T. G., HALEY, R. W., AND STANLEY, R. C., The infection control nurse in US hospitals, 1976–1977, *Am. J. Epidemiol.* **111:**592–607 (1980).

55. EVANS, R. S., LARSEN, R. A., BURKE, J. P., GARDNER, R. M., MEIER, F. A., JACOBSON, J. A., CONTI, M. T., JACOBSON, J. T., AND HULSE, R. K., Computer surveillance of hospital-acquired infections and antibiotic use, *J. Am. Med. Assoc.* **256:**1007–1011 (1986).

56. FALKOW, W., Historical perspectives and the transmission of R factors, in: *Infectious Multiple Drug Resistance* (J. R. LAGNADO, ed.), pp. 4–6, 230–243, Pion Limited, London, 1975.

57. FAVERO, M. S., Dialysis associated diseases and their control, in: *Hospital Infections,* 2nd ed. (J. V. BENNET AND P. S. BRACHMAN, eds.), pp. 267–284, Little, Brown, Boston, 1985.

58. FAVERO, M. S., CARSON, L. A., BOND, W. W., AND PETERSEN, N. J., Pseudomonas aeruginosa: Growth in distilled water from hospitals, *Science* **173:**836–838 (1971).

59. FAVERO, M. W., PETERSEN, N. J., CARSON, L. A., BOND, W. W., AND HINDMAN, S. H., Gram-negative water bacteria in hemodialysis systems, *Health Lab. Sci.* **12:**321–334 (1975).

60. FINEGOLD, S. M., AND BARON, E. J., *Diagnostic Microbiology,* 7th ed., Mosby, St. Louis, 1986.

61. FISHER, B., YU, B., ARMSTRONG, D., AND MAGILL, J., Outbreak of Mycoplasma pneumoniae infection among hospital personnel, *Am. J. Med. Sci.* **271:**205–209 (1978).

62. FISHER, M. W., Development of immunotherapy for infections due to pseudomonas aeruginosa, *J. Infect. Dis.* **130** (Suppl.):S149–S151 (1974).

63. FRANCO, J. A., BAER, J., AND ENNEKING, W. F., Airborne

contamination in orthopedic surgery: Evaluation of laminar air flow system and aspiration suit, *Clin. Orthop.* **122**:231–234 (1977).

64. FREEMAN, J., AND MCGOWAN, J. E., JR., Risk factors for nosocomial infection, *J. Infect. Dis.* **138**:811–819 (1978).

65. FREEDMAN, J., AND MCGOWAN, J. E., JR., Methodological issues in hospital epidemiology, *Rev. Infect. Dis.* **3**:658–667 (1981).

66. GARIBALDI, R. A., BURKE, J. P., DICKMAN, M. L., AND SMITH, C. B., Factors predisposing to bacteriuria during indwelling urethral catheterization, *N. Engl. J. Med.* **291**:215–219 (1974).

67. GARIBALDI, R. A., BIODINE, S., AND MATSUMUYA, S., Infections among patients in nursing homes, *N. Engl. J. Med.* **305**:731–735 (1981).

68. GARNER, J. S., BENNETT, J. V., SCHECKLER, W. E., MAKI, D. G., AND BRACHMAN, P. S., Surveillance of nosocomial infections, in: *Proceedings of the International Conference on Nosocomial Infections,* pp. 277–281, CDC, Atlanta, 1970.

69. GOLDMANN, D. A., AND MAKI, D. G., Infection control in total parenteral nutrition, *J. Am. Med. Assoc.* **233**:1360 (1973).

70. GRAHAM, D. R., ANDERSON, R. L., ARIEL, F. E., EHRENKRANZ, N. J., ROWE, D., BOER, H. R., AND DIXON, R. E., Epidemic nosocomial meningitis due to *Citrobacter diversus* in neonates, *J. Infect. Dis.* **144**:203–209 (1981).

71. GROSS, P. A., AND VAN ANTWERPEN, C., Nosocomial infections and hospital deaths, a case–control study, *Am. J. Med.* **75**:658–662 (1983).

72. GROSS, P. A., NEU, H. C., ASWAPOKEE, P., VAN ANTWERPEN, C., AND ASWAPOKEE, N., Deaths from nosocomial infection: Experience in a university and a community hospital, *Am. J. Med.* **68**:219–223 (1980).

73. GROSS, P. A., RAPUANO, C., ADRIGNOLO, A., AND SHAW, B., Nosocomial infections: Decade-specific risk, *Infect. Control* **4**(3):145–147 (1983).

74. Guidelines for Handwashing and Hospital Environmental Control, 1985, GARNER, J. S., AND FAVERO, M. S., CDC, Atlanta, 1985.

75. Guidelines for Isolation Precautions in Hospitals, GARNER, J. S., AND SIMMONS, B. P., CDC, Atlanta. Reprinted by U.S. Department of Health and Human Services from *Infect. Control* Suppl. **4**:245–325 (1983).

76. Guidelines for Prevention of Catheter-associated Urinary-Tract Infections, WONG, E. S. (HOOTON, T. M., consultants), CDC, Atlanta, October 1982.

77. Guidelines for Prevention of Intravascular Infections, SIMMONS, B. P. (HOOTON, T. M., WONG, E. S., AND ALLEN, J. R., consultants), CDC, Atlanta, 1982.

78. Guidelines for the Prevention of Nosocomial Pneumonia, SIMMONS, B. P., AND WONG, E. S., CDC, Atlanta, 1982.

79. Guidelines for Prevention of Surgical Wound Infections, GARNER, J. S., CDC, Atlanta, 1985.

80. HALEY, R. W., HIGHTOWER, A. W., KHABBAZ, R. F.,

THORNSBERRY, C., MARTONE, W. J., ALLEN, J. R., AND HUGHES, J. M., The emergence of methicillin-resistant Staphylococcus aureus infections in United States hospitals: Possible role of the house staff–patient transfer circuit, *Ann. Intern. Med.* **97**:297–308 (1982).

81. HALEY, R. W., CULVER, D. H., MORGAN, W. M., WHITE, J. W., EMORI, T. G., AND HOOTON, T. M., Increased recognition of infectious diseases in US hospitals through increased use of diagnostic tests, 1970–1976, *Am. J. Epidemiol.* **121**:168–181 (1985).

82. HALEY, R. W., CULVER, D. H., WHITE, J. W., MORGAN, W. M., AND EMORI, T. G., The nationwide nosocomial infection rate: A new need for vital statistics, *Am. J. Epidemiol.* **121**:159–167 (1985).

83. HALEY, R. W., CULVER, D. H., WHITE, J. W., MORGAN, W. M., EMORI, T. G., MUNN, V. P., AND HOOTON, T. M., The efficacy of infection surveillance and control programs in preventing nosocomial infections in US hospitals, *Am. J. Epidemiol.* **121**:182–205 (1985).

84. HALEY, R. W., CULVER, D. H., MORGAN, W. M., WHITE, J. W., EMORI, T. G., AND HOOTON, T. M., Identifying patients at high risk of surgical wound infection: A simple multivariate index of patient susceptibility and wound contamination, *Am. J. Epidemiol.* **121**:206–215 (1985).

85. HALEY, R. W., MORGAN, W. M., CULVER, D. H., WHITE, J. W., EMORI, T. G., MOSSER, J., AND HUGHES, J. M., Update from the SENIC project. Hospital infection control: Recent progress and opportunities under prospective payment, *Am. J. Infect. Control* **13**:97–108 (1985).

86. HANSEN, L., KOLMOS, H. J. J., AND SIBONI, K., Detection of cumulations of infections in hospitals over a three year period using electronic data processing, *Dan. Med. Bull.* **25**:253–257 (1978).

87. HARRINGTON, J. M., AND SHANNON, H. S., Incidence of tuberculosis, hepatitis, brucellosis, and shigellosis in British medical laboratory workers, *Br. Med. J.* **1**:759–762 (1976).

88. HELMS, C. M., MASSANARI, R. M., ZIETLER, R., STREET, S., GILCHRIST, M. J. R., HALL, N., HAUSLER, W. J., JR., SYWASINK, J., JOHNSON, W., WINTERMEYER, L., AND HIERHOLZER, W. J., JR., Legionnaires' disease associated with a hospital water system: A cluster of 24 nosocomial cases, *Ann. Intern. Med.* **99**:172–178 (1983).

89. Hexachlorophene and Newborns, *Food and Drug Administration Bulletin,* December 1971.

90. HIERHOLZER, W. J., JR., The practice of hospital epidemiology, *Yale J. Biol. Med* **55**:225–230 (1982).

91. HIERHOLZER, W. J., JR., STREED, S. A., AND RASLEY, D. A., Comparison of nosocomial infection risk with varying denominators at a university medical center [abstract], 2nd International Conference on Nosocomial Infections, CDC, Atlanta, 1980.

92. HOLZMAN, R. B., FLORNAN, A. L., AND TOHARSKY, B., The clinical usefulness of an ongoing bacteremia surveillance program, *Am. J. Med. Sci.* **274**:13–16 (1977).

93. HOWORTH, F. H., Prevention of airborne infection during surgery, *Lancet* **1**:386–388 (1985).

94. HUGHES, J. M., Nosocomial infection surveillance in the United States: Historical perspective, *Infect. Control* **8**(11):450–453 (1987).

95. HUGHES, J. M., Setting priorities: Nationwide nosocomial infection prevention and control programs in the U.S.A., *Eur. J. Clin. Microbiol.* **6**:348–351 (1987).

96. HUGHES, J. M., CULVER, D. H., WHITE, J. W., JARVIS, W. R., MORGAN, W. M., MUNN, V. P., MOSSER, J. L., AND EMORI, T. G., Nosocomial infection surveillance, 1980–1982, *Morbid. Mortal. Weekly Rep.* **32**(4SS):1SS–15SS (1983).

97. Human immunodeficiency virus infection in the United States: A Review of Current Knowledge, *Morbid. Mortal. Weekly Rep.* **36**(S-6) (1987).

98. HYAMS, P. J., AND EHRENKRANZ, N. J., The overuse of single patient isolation in hospitals, *Am. J. Epidemiol.* **196**:325–329 (1977).

99. INAGAKI, J., RODRIGUEZ, A., AND BODEY, G. P., Causes of death in cancer patients, *Cancer* **33**:568–573 (1974).

100. *Infection Control: An Integrated Approach* (K. J. Axnick and M. Yarbrough, eds.), Mosby, St. Louis, 1984.

101. JAFFE, H. W., SWEENEY, H. M., NATHAN, C., WEINSTEIN, R. A., KABINS, S. A., AND COHEN, S., Identity and interspecific transfer of gentamicin resistance plasmids in Staphylococcus aureus and Staphylococcus epidermis, *J. Infect. Dis.* **141**:738–747 (1980).

102. JAMES, B. O. L., WELLS, D. M., AND GRANT, L. S., Resistance factors in the hospital and non-hospital environment, *Trop. Geogr. Med.* **27**:39–46 (1975).

103. JOHANSON, W. G., JR., PIERCE, A. K., SANFORD, J. P., AND THOMAS, G. D., Nosocomial respiratory infections with gram-negative bacilli: The significance of colonization of the respiratory tract, *Ann. Intern. Med.* **77**:701–706 (1972).

104. JOHN, J. F., JR., AND TWITTY, J. A., Plasmids as epidemiologic markers in nosocomial gram-negative bacilli: Experience at a university and review of the literature, *Rev. Infect. Dis.* **8**:693–704 (1986).

105. JOHNSON, J. D., MALACHOWSKI, N. C., VOSTI, K. L., AND SUNSHINE, P. A., Sequential study of various modes of skin and umbilical care and the incidence of staphylococcal colonization and infection in the neonate, *Pediatrics* **58**:354–361 (1976).

106. JONSSON, M., RUTBURG, L., AND TIMWALL, G., Transferable resistance to antibiotic in gram-negative bacteria isolated in a hospital for infectious disease, *Scand. J. Infect. Dis.* **4**:133–137 (1972).

107. KASLOW, R. A., MACKEL, D. C., AND MALLINSON, G. F., Nosocomial pseudobacteremia: Positive blood cultures due to contaminate benzalkonium antiseptic, *J. Am. Med. Assoc.* **236**:2407–2409 (1976).

108. KIMBROUGH, R. D., Review of recent evidence of toxic effects of hexachlorophene, *Pediatrics* **51**(Suppl.):391 (1973).

109. KLUGE, R. M., CALIA, F. M., MCLAUGHLIN, J. S., AND HORNICK, R. B., Sources of contamination in open heart surgery, *J. Am. Med. Assoc.* **230**:1415–1418 (1974).

110. KUNIN, C. M., AND MCCORMICK, R. C., Prevention of catheter induced urinary tract infections by sterile closed drainage, *N. Engl. J. Med.* **274**:1155–1161 (1966).

111. LARSON, E., Development of an infection control program in Kuwait, *Am. J. Infect. Control* **15**(4):163–167 (1987).

112. LARSON, E., Committee reports: Draft guideline for use of topical antimicrobial agents, *Am. J. Infect. Control* **15**(6):25A–36A (1987).

113. LAXSON, L. B., BLASER, M. J., AND PARKHURST, S. M., Surveillance for the detection of nosocomial infections and the potential for nosocomial outbreaks. I. Microbiology culture surveillance is an effective method of detecting nosocomial infection, *Am. J. Infect. Control* **12**(6):318–324 (1984).

114. LEDGER, W. J., GEE, C., AND LEWIS, W. P., Guidelines of antibiotic prophylaxis in gynecology, *Am. J. Obstet. Gynecol.* **121**:1038–1045 (1975).

115. LEIGH, D. A., An eight year study of postoperative wound infection in two district general hospitals, *J. Hosp. Infect.* **2**:207–217 (1981).

116. LENNETTE, E. H., BALLOWS, A., HAUSLER, W. J., JR., AND SHADOMY, H. J. (eds.), *Manual of Clinical Microbiology*, 4th ed., American Society for Microbiology, Washington, D.C., 1985.

117. LESTER, M. R., Looking inside 101 nursing homes, *Am. J. Nurs.* **64**:111–116 (1964).

118. LIDWELL, O. M., LOWBURY, E. J. L., WHYTE, W., BLOWERS, R., STANLEY, S. J., AND LOWE, D., Effects of ultraclean air in an operating room on deep sepsis in the joint after total hip or knee replacement: A randomised study, *Br. Med. J.* **285**:10–14 (1982).

119. LIV, P. V., MATSUMOTO, H., KUSAMA, H., AND BERGAN, T., Survey of heat-stable, major somatic antigens of *Pseudomonas aeruginosa*, *Int. J. Syst. Bacteriol.* **33**:256–264 (1983).

120. LOBO, P. I., RUDOLF, L. E., AND KRIEGER, J. N., Wound infections in renal transplant recipients—A complication of urinary tract infections during allograft malfunction, *Surgery* **92**:491–496 (1982).

121. LYNCH, P., JACKSON, M. M., CUMMINGS, M. J., AND STAMM, W. E., Rethinking the role of isolation practices in the prevention of nosocomial infections, *Ann. Intern. Med.* **107**:243–246 (1987).

122. MACKOWIAK, P. A., The normal microbial flora, *N. Engl. J. Med.* **307**:83–93 (1982).

123. MADISON, R., AND AFIFI, A. A., Definition and comparability of nosocomial infection rates, *Am. J. Infect. Control* **10**(2):49–52 (1982).

124. MAKI, D. G., Preventing infection in intravenous therapy, anesthesia, and analgesia, *Current Res.* **56**:141–156 (1977).

125. MAKI, D. G., Control of colonization and transmission of pathogenic bacteria in the hospital, *Ann. Intern. Med.* **89**(Part 2):777–780 (1978).

126. MAKI, D. G., Through a glass darkly: Nosocomial pseudoepidemics and pseudobacteremias [editorial], *Arch. Intern. Med.* **140**:26–28 (1980).

127. MAKI, D. G., AND MARTIN, W. T., Nationwide epidemic of septicemia caused by contaminated infusion products. IV. Growth of microbial pathogens in fluids for intravenous infusion, *J. Infect. Dis.* **131**:267–272 (1975).

128. MAKI, D. G., GOLDMANN, D. A., AND RHAME, F. S., Infection control in intravenous therapy, *Ann. Intern. Med.* **79**:867–887 (1973).

129. MAKI, D. G., WEISE, C. E., AND SARAFIN, H. W., A semiquantitative method for identifying intravenous catheter-related infection, *N. Engl. J. Med.* **296**:1305–1309 (1977).

130. MAKI, D. G., ALVARADO, C. J., HASSEMER, C. A., AND ZILZ, M. A., Relation of the inanimate hospital environment to endemic nosocomial infection, *N. Engl. J. Med.* **307**:1562–1566 (1982).

131. MALLISON, G. F., AND HALEY, R. W., Microbiologic sampling of the inanimate environment in U.S. hospitals, 1976–1977, *Am. J. Med.* **70**:941–946 (1981).

132. MARKS, J. S., TSAI, T. F., MARTONE, W. J., BARON, R. C., KENNICOTT, J., HOLTZHAUER, F. J., BAIRD, I., FAY, D., FEELEY, J. C., MALLISON, G. F., FRAZER, D. W., AND HALPIN, T. J., Nosocomial Legionnaires' disease in Columbus, Ohio, *Ann. Intern. Med.* **90**:565–569 (1979).

133. MARPLES, R. R., MACKINTOSH, C. A., AND MEERS, P. D., Microbiological aspects of the 1980 national prevalence survey of infections in hospitals, *J. Hosp. Infect.* **5**:172–180 (1984).

134. MARTONE, W. J., TABLAN, O. C., AND JARVIS, W. R., The epidemiology of nosocomial epidemic Pseudomonas cepacia infections, *Eur. J Epidemiol.* **3**:222–232 (1987).

135. MASSANARI, R. M., WILKERSON, K., STREED, S. A., AND HIERHOLZER, W. J., JR., Reliability of reporting nosocomial infections in the discharge abstract and implications for receipt of revenues under prospective reimbursement, *Am. J. Public Health* **77**:561–564 (1987).

136. McGOWAN, J. E., JR., Bacteremia at Boston City Hospital, occurrence and mortality during 12 selected years with special reference to hospital acquired cases, *J. Infect. Dis.* **132**:316–335 (1975).

137. McGOWAN, J. E., JR., Six guidelines for reducing infections associated with intravenous therapy, *Am. Surg.* **42**:713–715 (1976).

138. McGOWAN, J. E., JR., Antimicrobial resistance in hospital organisms and its relation to antibiotic use, *Rev. Infect. Dis.* **5**:1033–1048 (1983).

139. MEERS, P. D., AYLIFFE, G. A. J., EMMERSON, A. M., LEIGH, D. A., MAYON-WHITE, R. T., MACKINTOSH, C. A., AND STRONGE, J. L., Report on the national survey of infection in hospitals, 1980, *J. Hosp. Infect.* (Suppl.) **2** (December 1981).

140. MILLER, P. J., AND WENZEL, R. P., Etiologic organisms as independent predictors of death and morbidity associated with bloodstream infections, *J. Infect. Dis.* **156**:471–476 (1987).

141. Minimum Requirements of Construction and Equipment for Hospital and Medical Facilities, U.S. Department of Health, Education, and Welfare, Public Health Service, Health Resources Administration, Division of Facilities Utilization, HEW Publ. No. HRA 79-145000, 1979.

142. MOODY, M. M., DEJONGH, C. A., SCHIMPFF, S. C., AND TILLMAN, G. L., Long-term amikacin use: Effects on aminoglycoside susceptibility patterns of gram-negative bacilli, *J. Am. Med. Assoc.* **248**:1199–1202 (1982).

143. MORRISON, A. J., JR., AND WENZEL, R. P., Epidemiology of infections due to Pseudomonas aeruginosa, *Rev. Infect. Dis.* **6**(Suppl. 3):S627–S642 (1984).

144. MURRAY, P. R., AND WASHINGTON, J. A., II, Microscopic and bacteriologic analysis of expectorated sputum, *Mayo Clin. Proc.* **50**:339–344 (1975).

145. MYEROWITZ, R. L., Nosocomial Legionnaires' disease and other nosocomial Legionella pneumonias, *Infect. Control* **4**(2):107–110 (1983).

146. NEWMAN, K. A., AND SCHIMPFF, S. C., Hospital and hotel services as risk factors for infection among immunocompromised patients, *J. Infect. Dis.* **9**(1):206–213 (1987).

147. NICHOLS, R. L., Techniques known to prevent post-operative wound infection, Infect. Control **3**(1):34–37 (1982).

148. NICOLLE, L. E., BJORNSON, J., HARDING, G. K. M., AND MACDONELL, J. A., Bacteriuria in elderly institutionalized men, *N. Engl. J. Med.* **309**:1420–1425 (1983).

149. NYSTROM, B., Hospital infection control in Sweden, *Infect. Control* **8**(8):337–338 (1987).

150. Outline for Surveillance and Control of Nosocomial Infections, Centers for Disease Control, Bureau of Epidemiology, Bacterial Diseases Division, Hospital Infections Branch, Atlanta, November 1976.

151. PARKHURST, S. M., BLASER, M. J., LAXSON, L. B., AND WANG, W. L. L., Surveillance for the detection of nosocomial infections and the potential for nosocomial outbreaks. II. Development of a laboratory-based system, *Am. J. Infect. Control* **13**(1):7–15 (1985).

152. PATTERSON, J. E., MADDEN, G. M., KRISIVNAS, E. P., MASECAR, B., HIERHOLZER, W. J., JR., ZERVOS, M. J., AND LYONS, R. W., A nosocomial outbreak of *Hemophilus influenzae* type B in a geriatric unit, *J. Infect. Dis.* **157**(5):1002–1007 (1988).

153. PATTERSON, T. F., PATTERSON, J. E., MASECAR, B. L., BARDEN, G. E., HIERHOLZER, W. J., JR., AND ZERVOS, M. J., A nosocomial outbreak of *Branhamella catarrhalis* confirmed by restriction endonuclease analysis, *J. Infect. Dis.* **157**(5):996–1001 (1988).

154. PATTERSON, W. B., CRAVEN, D. E., SCHWARTZ, D. A., NARDELL, E. A., KASMER, J., AND NOBLE, J., Occupational hazards to hospital personnel, *Ann. Intern. Med.* **102**:658–680 (1985).

155. PEMBERTON, L. B., LYMAN, B., LANDER, V., AND COVINSKY, J., Sepsis from triple vs single-lumen catheters during total parenteral nutrition in surgical or critically ill patients, *Arch. Surg.* **121**:591–594 (1986).

156. PENNER, J. L., AND HENNESSY, J. N., Application of O-

serogrouping in a study of *Providencia rettgeri* (*Proteus rettgeri*) isolated from human and non-human sources, *J. Clin. Microbiol.* **10:**834–840 (1979).

157. PHILLIPS, J., AND SPENCER, G., Pseudomonas aeruginosa cross-infection due to contaminated respiratory apparatus, *Lancet* **2:**1325–1327 (1965).

158. PIZZO, P. A., AND LEVINE, A. S., The utility of protected environment regimens for the compromised host: A critical assessment, *Prog. Hematol.* **10:**311–332 (1977).

159. PLATT, R., POLK, B. F., MURDOCK, B., AND ROSNER, B., Mortality associated with nosocomial urinary tract infection, *N. Engl. J. Med.* **307:**637–642 (1982).

160. POLK, H. C., Prevention of surgical wound infection, *Ann. Intern. Med.* **89**(Part 2):770–773 (1978).

161. POLLACK, M., Antibody activity against Pseudomonas aeruginosa in immune globulins prepared for intravenous use in humans, *J. Infect. Dis.* **147:**1090–1098 (1983).

162. POLLOCK, A. V., Surgical prophylaxis—The emerging picture, *Lancet* **1:**225–230 (1988).

163. Postoperative Wound Infections: The Influence of Ultraviolet Irradiation of the Operating Room and of Various Other Factors, A Report of an Ad Hoc Committee of the Committee on Trauma, Division of Medical Sciences, National Academy of Sciences–National Research Council, J. M. Howard, Chairman, *Ann. Surg.* Suppl. **160**(2) (1964).

164. Proposed microbiologic guidelines for respiratory therapy equipment and materials, a report of the Committee on Microbial Contamination of Surfaces, Laboratory Science, American Public Health Association, M. S. Favero, Chairman, *Health Lab. Sci.* **15:**177–179 (1978).

165. PUGLIESE, G., AND LICHTENBERG, D. A., Nosocomial bacterial pneumonia: An overview, *Am. J. Infect. Control* **15**(6):249–265 (1987).

166. RAVENHOLT, R. T., History, epidemiology and control of staphylococcal disease in Seattle, *Am. J. Public Health* **11:**1796–1808 (1962).

167. RAVITCH, M. M., AND MCAULEY, C. E., Airborne contamination of the operative wound, *Surg. Gynecol. Obst.* **159:**177–178 (1984).

168. REINGOLD, A. L., THOMASON, B. M., BRAKE, B. J., THACKER, L., WILKINSON, H. W., AND KURITSKY, J. N., *Legionella pneumonia* in the United States: The distribution of serogroups and species causing human illness, *J. Infect. Dis.* **149:**819 (1984).

169. RENNIE, R. P., NORD, C. E., SJOBERG, L., AND DUNCAN, I. B. R., Comparison of bacteriophage typing, serotyping, and biotyping as leads in epidemiological surveillance of Klebsiella infection, *J. Clin. Microbiol.* **8:**638–642 (1978).

170. RETAILLIAU, H. F., HIGHTOWER, A. W., DIXON, R. E., AND ALLEN, J. R., Acinetobacter calcoaceticus: A nosocomial pathogen with an unusual seasonal pattern, *J. Infect. Dis.* **139:**371–375 (1979).

171. RHAME, F. S., AND SUDDERTH, W. D., Incidence and prevalence as used in the analysis of the occurrence of nosocomial infections, *Am. J. Epidemiol.* **113:**1–11 (1981).

172. ROGERS, T. R., Infection complicating bone marrow trans-

plantation: What are the risks and can they be reduced? *J. Hosp. Infect.* **3:**105–109 (1982).

173. ROTSTEIN, C., CUMMINGS, K. M., NICOLAOU, A. L., LUCEY, J., AND FITZPATRICK, J., Nosocomial infection rates at an oncology center, *Infect. Control* **9**(1):13–19 (1988).

174. SARAVOLATZ, L. D., POHLOD, D. J., AND ARKING, L. M., Community-acquired methicillin-resistant staphylococcus aureus infections: A new source for nosocomial outbreaks, *Ann. Intern. Med.* **97:**325–329 (1982).

175. SCHABERG, D. R., AND ZERVOS, M. J., Intergeneic and interspecies gene exchange in gram-positive cocci, *Antimicrob. Agents Chemother.* **30:**817–822 (1986).

176. SCHABERG, D. R., AND ZERVOS, M. J., Plasmid analysis in the study of the epidemiology of gram-positive cocci, *Rev. Infect. Dis.* **8:**705–712 (1986).

177. SCHAFFNER, W., Humans, the animate reservoir of nosocomial pathogens, in: *Infection Control in Health Care Facilities* (K. R. Cundy and W. Ball, eds.), pp. 55–70, University Park Press, Baltimore, 1976.

178. SCHECKLER, W. E., Septicemia and nosocomial infection in a community hospital, *Ann. Intern. Med.* **89**(Part 2):754–756 (1978).

179. SCHIMPFF, S. C., Therapy of infection in patients with granulocytopenia, *Med. Clin. North Am.* **61:**1101–1118 (1977).

180. SCHIMPFF, S. C., YOUNG, V. M., GREENE, W. H., VERMEULEN, G., MOODY, M. R., AND WIERNIK, P. H., Origin of infection in acute nonlymphocytic leukemia, *Ann. Intern. Med.* **77:**707–714 (1972).

181. SELDEN, R., LEE, S., AND WANG, W. L. L., Nosocomial Klebsiella infections: Intestinal colonization as a reservoir, *Ann. Intern. Med.* **74:**657–664 (1971).

182. SELL, T. L., SCHABERG, D. R., AND FEKETY, R. F., Bacteriophage and bacteriocin typing scheme for Clostridium difficile, *J. Clin. Microbiol.* **17:**1148–1152 (1983).

183. SETIA, U., AND GROSS, P. A., Bacteremia in a community hospital, *Arch. Intern. Med.* **137:**1698–1701 (1977).

184. SIEGEL, J. D., Prophylactic antibiotics, *Pediatr. Infect. Dis.* **3:**S37–S41 (1984).

185. SMITH, P. W., Infections in long-term care facilities, *Infect. Control* **6**(11):435–441 (1985).

186. SMITH, P. W., AND MASSANARI, R. M., Room humidifiers as the source of Acinetobacter infections, *J. Am. Med. Assoc.* **237:**795–797 (1980).

187. SMITH, R. T., The role of a chronic carrier in an epidemic of staphylococcal disease in a newborn nursery, *Arch. Dis. Child.* **95:**461–468 (1958).

188. SPAEPEN, M. S., BERRYMAN, J. R., BODMAN, H. A., KINDSIN, R. B., AND TENCL, V., Prevalence and survival of microbial contaminants in heated nebulizers, *Anesth. Analg.* **57:**191–196 (1978).

189. SPECK, W. T., DRISCOLL, J. M., POLIN, R. A., O'NEILL, J., AND ROSENKRANZ, H. S., Staphylococcal and streptococcal colonization of the newborn infant, *Am. J. Dis. Child.* **131:**1005–1008 (1977).

190. STAMM, W. E., Guidelines for prevention of catheter associ-

ated urinary tract infections, *Ann. Intern. Med.* **83**:386–390 (1975).

191. STAMM, W. E., Infection related to medical devices, *Ann. Intern. Med.* **89**(Part 2):764–769 (1978).

192. STAMM, W. E., COLELLA, J. J., ANDERSON, M. S., AND DIXON, R. E., Indwelling arterial catheters as a source of nosocomial bacteremia, *N. Engl. J. Med.* **292**:1099 (1977).

193. STAMM, W. E., MARTINS, S. M., AND BENNETT, J. V., Epidemiology of nosocomial infections due to gram-negative bacilli: Aspects relevant to development and use of vaccine, *J. Infect. Dis.* **136**(Suppl.):S151–S160 (1977).

194. STAMM, W. E., TALEY, J. C., AND FACKLAM, R. R., Wound infections due to group A Streptococcus traced to a vaginal carrier, *J. Infect. Dis.* **138**:287–292 (1978).

195. STARK, R. P., AND MAKI, D. G., Bacteriuria in the catheterized patient: What quantitative level of bacteriuria is relevant? *N. Engl. J. Med.* **311**:560–564 (1984).

196. Statement on microbiological sampling in the hospital, Committee on Infections Within Hospitals, American Hospital Association, *Hospitals* **48**:125–126 (1974).

197. STEERE, A. C., AND MALLISON, G. F., Handwashing practices for prevention of nosocomial infections, *Ann. Intern. Med.* **83**:683–690 (1975).

198. THACKER, S. B., BENNETT, J. V., TSAI, T. F., FRASER, D. W., MCDADE, J. E., SHEPARD, C. C., WILLIAMS, K. H., JR., STUART, W. H., DULL, H. B., AND EICKHOFF, T. C., An outbreak in 1965 of severe respiratory illness caused by Legionnaires' disease bacteria, *J. Infect. Dis.* **138**:512–519 (1978).

199. THOMAS, F. E., JACKSON, R. T., MELLY, A., AND ALFORD, R. H., Sequential hospital-wide outbreak of resistant Serratia and Klebsiella infection, *Arch. Intern. Med.* **137**:581–584 (1977).

200. THOMPSON, R. L., CABEZUDO, I., AND WENZEL, R. P., Epidemiology of nosocomial infections caused by methicillin resistant *Staphylococcus aureus, Ann. Intern. Med.* **97**:309–317 (1982).

201. THORNBURN, R., FEKETY, F. R., CLUFF, L. E., AND MELVIN, V. B., Infections acquired by hospitalized patients: An analysis of the overall problem, *Arch. Intern. Med.* **121**:1–10 (1968).

202. TIKHOMIROV, E., WHO programme for the control of nosocomial infections, *Chemoterapia* **6**:148–151 (1987).

203. TOLEDO-PEREYRA, L. H., AND TOLEDO, M. M., A critical study of Lister's work on antiseptic surgery, *Am. J. Surg.* **131**:736–744 (1976).

204. TRYBA, M., Risk of acute stress bleeding and nosocomial pneumonia in ventilated intensive care unit patients: Sucralfate versus antacids, *Am. J. Med.* **83**(3B):117–124 (1987).

205. VAN GRAVENITZ, A., The role of opportunistic bacteria in human disease, *Annu. Rev. Microbiol.* **31**:447–471 (1977).

206. Veterans Administration Ad Hoc Interdisciplinary Advisory Committee on Antimicrobial Drug Usage, C. KUNIN, Chairman, Audit of antimicrobial usage: Prophylaxis in surgery, *J. Am. Med. Assoc.* **237**:1003–1008 (1977).

207. VICKERS, R. M., LU, V. L., HANNA, S. S., MURACA, P., DIVEN, W., CARMEN, N., AND TAYLOR, F. B., Determinants of Legionella pneumophila contamination of water distribution systems: 15-hospital prospective study, *Infect. Control* **8**(9):357–363 (1987).

208. VLAHOV, D., TENNEY, J. H., CERVINO, K. W., AND SHAMER, D. K., Routine surveillance for infections in nursing homes: Experience at two facilities, *Am. J. Infect. Control* **15**(2):47–53 (1987).

209. WACHSMUTH, K., Molecular epidemiology of bacterial infections: Examples of methodology and investigation of outbreaks, *Rev. Infect. Dis.* **8**:682–692 (1986).

210. WARREN, J. W., PLATT, R., THOMAS, R. J., ROSEN, B., AND KASS, E. H., Antibiotic irrigation and catheter associated urinary tract infection, *N. Engl. J. Med.* **299**:570–573 (1978).

211. WATANABE, T., Infective heredity of multiple drug resistance in bacteria, *Bacteriol. Rev.* **27**:87–115 (1963).

212. WEINSTEIN, R. A., AND MALLISON, G. F., The role of the laboratory in surveillance and control of nosocomial infections, *Am. J. Clin. Pathol.* **69**:130–136 (1978).

213. WEINSTEIN, R. A., AND STAMM, W. E., Pseudoepidemics in hospitals, *Lancet* **2**:862–864 (1977).

214. WEINSTEIN, R. A., STAMM, W. E., KRAMER, L., AND COREY, L., Pressure monitoring devices, overlooked source of nosocomial infection, *J. Am. Med. Assoc.* **236**:936 (1976).

215. WELLIVER, R. C., AND MCLAUGHLIN, S., Unique epidemiology of nosocomial infections in a children's hospital, *Am. J. Dis. Child.* **138**:131–135 (1984).

216. WENZEL, R. P., OSTERMAN, C. A., AND HUNTING, K. J., Hospital-acquired infections. III. Infection rates by site, service, and common procedures in a university hospital, *Am. J. Epidemiol.* **104**:645–651 (1976).

217. WENZEL, R. P., OSTERMAN, C. A., HUNTING, K. J., AND GWALTNEY, J. M., Hospital acquired infections. I. Surveillance in a university hospital, *Am. J. Epidemiol.* **103**:251–260 (1976).

218. WENZEL, R. P., VEAZEY, J. M., JR., AND TOWNSEND, T. R., Role of the inanimate environment in hospital acquired infection, in: *Infection Control in Health Care Facilities* (K. R. CUNDY AND W. BALL, eds.), pp. 71–146, University Park Press, Baltimore, 1977.

219. WENZEL, R. P., OSTERMAN, C. A., TOWNSEND, T. R., VEAZEY, J. M., SERVIS, K. H., MILLER, L. S., CRAVEN, R. B., MILLER, G. B., JR., AND JACKSON, R. S., Development of a statewide program for surveillance and reporting of hospital acquired infections, *J. Infect. Dis.* **140**:741–746 (1979).

220. WENZEL, R. P., THOMPSON, R. L., LANDRY, S. M., RUSSEL, B. S., MILLER, P. J., DE LEON, S. P., AND MILLER, G. B., Hospital-acquired infections in intensive care unit patients: An overview with emphasis on epidemics, *Infect. Control* **4**(5):371–375 (1983).

221. WILLIAMS, R. E. O., Epidemiology of airborne staphylococcal infections, *Bacteriol. Rev.* **30**:660–674 (1966).

222. WILLIAMS, R. E. O., Changing perspectives in hospital infec-

tion, in: *Proceedings of the International Conference on Nosocomial Infections,* pp. 1–10, CDC, Atlanta, 1970.

223. YOUNG, L. S., Empirical antimicrobial therapy in the neutropenic host, *Am. J. Med.* **315:**580–581 (1986).

224. YOUNG, L. S., MEYER, R. D., AND ARMSTRONG, D., Pseudomonas aeruginosa vaccine in cancer patients, *Ann. Intern. Med.* **79:**518–527 (1973).

225. YU, V. L., BEAM, T. R., LUMISH, R. M., VICKERS, R. M., FLEMING, J., McDERMOTT, C., AND ROMANO, J., Routine culturing for Legionella in the hospital environment may be a good idea: A three-hospital study, *Am. J. Med. Sci.* **30:**97–99 (1987).

226. ZERVOS, M. J., DEMBINSKI, S., MIKESELL, T., AND SCHABERG, D. R., High-level resistance to gentamicin in *Streptococcus faecalis:* Risk factors and evidence for exogenous acquisition of infection, *J. Infect. Dis.* **153:**1075–1083 (1986).

227. ZERVOS, M. J., KAUFFMAN, C. A., THERASSE, P. M., BERGMAN, A. G., MIKESELL, T. S., AND SCHABERG, D. R., Nosocomial infection by gentamicin-resistant *Streptococcus faecalis:* An epidemiologic study, *Ann. Intern. Med.* **106:**687–691 (1987).

228. ZERVOS, M. J., TERPENNING, M. S., SCHABERG, D. R., THERASSE, P. M., MEDENDORP, S. V., AND KAUFFMAN, C. A., High-level aminoglycoside-resistant enterococci, *Arch. Intern. Med.* **147:**1591–1594 (1987).

12. Suggested Reading

BENNETT, J. V., AND BRACHMAN, P. S. (eds.), *Hospital Infections,* 2nd ed., Little, Brown, Boston, 1986.

WENZEL, R. P. (ed.), *Prevention and Control of Nosocomial Infections,* Williams & Wilkins, Baltimore, 1987.

CHAPTER 23

Pertussis

Edward A. Mortimer, Jr.

1. Introduction

Bordetella pertussis produces a single disease syndrome in man known as pertussis or whooping cough. Affecting children primarily, it characteristically displays a protracted course measured in weeks with the development of vigorous paroxysmal coughing, often associated with vomiting that sometimes results in inanition and occasionally with brain damage. At the turn of the century, it was a major cause of infant mortality worldwide. To a large extent due to immunization, it is at present of less consequence in developed countries such as the United States, but continues to be a major child health problem in developing nations.

2. Historical Background

The first recorded description of the disease dates from the 16th century.[36] Its absence from prior literature is curiously unexplained for a disease syndrome with such characteristic symptoms. Perhaps it attracted less attention than more devastating epidemic diseases such as plague and smallpox[36] or it may have been a disease of lower animals that became adapted to man.[40]

Identification and isolation on culture of the responsible organism did not occur until the first part of this century. Because the organism is difficult to propagate by culture, attempts to develop vaccines were unsuccessful until the

Edward A. Mortimer, Jr. · Departments of Epidemiology and Biostatistics and Pediatrics, Case Western Reserve University School of Medicine, Cleveland, Ohio 44106.

1930s. In the United States, whole, killed bacterial vaccines appeared to be of sufficient efficacy to warrant licensure and general use in young infants in the 1940s. Current federal regulations for vaccine production were established in 1953.[65]

Mortality from pertussis in the United States and other developed nations has declined throughout this century, even before the development and widespread use of pertussis vaccine and antimicrobial drugs.[25,49,53] Further decreases in death rates have occurred subsequently; the decline prior to the vaccine is unexplained. But the fact that a decrease in mortality rates antedated widespread use of pertussis vaccine caused some authorities to question the necessity for the vaccine as a routine preventive measure for children,[75] particularly since the vaccine displays undesirable reactivity.

3. Methodology

3.1. Sources of Mortality Data

In the United States and other developed nations, the only sources of mortality information are published vital statistics. Case-fatality rates are inaccurate because the disease is underreported.[63] In addition, it is likely that an uncertain proportion of fatal cases are incorrectly diagnosed as other types of bronchopulmonary infections. Nonetheless, mortality rates reflect the occurrence of pertussis more accurately than do other measures currently available.

3.2. Sources of Morbidity Data

Determination of the precise incidence of pertussis in the United States and elsewhere is not presently possible for four reasons. First, the disease is often not reported. Second, the diagnosis may often be missed. Third, it is clear that there are mild unrecognized forms of the disease, especially in older children and adults with waning immunity. Fourth, a syndrome that is clinically indistinguishable from true pertussis may be produced occasionally by two other *Bordetella* species, *B. parapertussis* and *B. bronchiseptica*. Additionally, certain adenoviruses or other viruses may produce the syndrome,[3,42,62] although it is possible that in some way pertussis causes reactivation of these infections. Therefore, except during clear-cut, laboratory-confirmed outbreaks in defined populations, estimates of the prevalence or annual incidence of pertussis are unreliable, because 90% or more cases are not reported.[63] For these reasons, mortality rates, although of less-than-optimum precision, are the best indicators of changes in incidence. It should be recognized, however, that mortality rates may not reflect the true incidence of pertussis in all age groups because of the inverse relationship of case-fatality rates to age.[62]

3.3. Surveys

Surveys to determine proportions of the population immune to pertussis are of limited value for the reasons noted above and, in addition, because of failure to recall the disease or prior immunization and the lack of a practical serological test.[26] In the past, household surveys have been used to determine the incidence during outbreaks.[44]

3.4. Laboratory Diagnosis

Most clinicians consider absolute lymphocytosis of 10,000 or more lymphocytes per mm^3 to be strong circumstantial evidence of pertussis in a child with appropriate symptoms. The magnitude of lymphocytosis roughly parallels the severity of the cough. However, in very young infants lymphocytosis may be absent.

The status of diagnostic tests for pertussis has been reviewed recently.[63] The single, time-tested, unequivocal diagnostic test for pertussis is isolation of the organism on culture from a nasopharyngeal swab. The optimum medium for isolation of this fastidious, slow-growing organism is either modified Bordet–Gengou agar enriched with 15% defibrinated sheep blood or Regan–Lowe medium containing horse blood. Swabs should be inoculated immediately; delay of as little as an hour reduces the likelihood of recovery of the organisms. When inoculation must be delayed, Stuart's transport medium may be employed. The addition of methicillin or cephalexin to the culture medium appears to enhance the likelihood of recovery of *B. pertussis* by

suppressing the growth of other organisms. A more sensitive synthetic medium is currently being assessed.[63]

Cultures should be incubated at 35°C in moist air and examined daily for 5 days, preferably by a bacteriologist skilled in the recognition of *B. pertussis*. Colonies are small and pearly and display a small zone of hemolysis on blood-containing media. Further identification of colonies may be achieved by agglutination with commercially available sera or by direct immunofluorescence.

In experienced hands, identification by culture is nearly 100% specific; unfortunately, the sensitivity of culture methods is far less even in experienced hands. Fresh media are required, and after the fourth week of illness, recovery of the organism is much less likely. Additionally, currently most clinical bacteriology laboratories lack experience in the identification of *B. pertussis* on culture due to the present rarity of the disease.

Examination of direct smears from nasopharyngeal swabs by direct immunofluorescence appears to be approximately as sensitive as culture, but unfortunately lacks optimum specificity. Even experienced professionals may disagree on the interpretation of the same slide,[9] and overdiagnosis by the inexperienced may lead to needless, expensive treatment and prophylaxis and unwarranted concern. It is, however, of maximum utility during outbreaks when false-positives are proportionately less frequent.

Better, though as yet incomplete identification of the antigens present in *B. pertussis* and their relation to disease in man offers promise not only of means for assessment of immunity but also for recognition of infection by serologic methods.[72] For the present, these serologic methods are of utility for pertussis vaccine research but are impractical and too costly for routine use (see Section 4).

4. Biological Characteristics of the Organism

B. pertussis is a small, poorly staining gram-negative organism that appears in coccobacillary form on fresh isolation. Older cultures display pleomorphism, ranging from filamentous forms to larger bacilli. It can be distinguished from *B. parapertussis* and *B. bronchiseptica* by various biochemical characteristics and immunofluorescence.

Colonies of freshly isolated strains of *B. pertussis* comprise morphologically homogeneous coccobacilli ("smooth" colonies) and the organisms display full virulence in experimental animals such as the mouse or in the hamster tracheal tissue culture model. Such virulent strains are designated phase I organisms; on repeated passage in culture, certain biologic characteristics associated with virulence are lost. The so-called "rough" strains are designated as phases II, III, and IV in order of decreasing virulence. For vaccine production, phase I strains are preferred.

A major problem in understanding the disease and its epidemiology and in developing an optimum vaccine has been that the biological anatomy of the organism in relation to man has been difficult to determine precisely. Although a multiplicity of cellular antigens of B. pertussis have been identified, those responsible for the various manifestations of the disease, for clinical immunity, and for the apparent reactivity of the current relatively crude whole-cell vaccine are only now being defined. Indeed, it is not clear whether the immunologically protective and toxic antigens are the same or different. Table 1 lists some of the identified somatic antigens and biologic activities of B. pertussis.

From what is known of the biologic activities of several of these antigens, it is possible to hypothesize about their roles in disease pathogenesis.[45] Of prime interest is what has now been variously called pertussis toxin, pertussigen, or lymphocytosis-promoting factor (LPF). This component of the organism has been shown to be a complex protein that contains LPF, the histamine-sensitizing factor, and the insulin-stimulating factor. Pertussis toxin appears to participate in the pathogenesis of pertussis at several stages by enhancing attachment of the organism to respiratory cilia, interfering with host defenses, and causing cell toxicity. Antibodies to pertussis toxin can be measured serologically following immunization or natural disease.[39]

Filamentous hemagglutinin (FHA) appears to participate with pertussigen in the facilitation of attachment of the organism to respiratory cilia; whether it has other activities in relation to man is unclear. Measurable antibodies to FHA increase following natural infection and immunization.[39]

Strains of B. pertussis can be serotyped and studied epidemiologically by heat-labile K agglutinogens, antibodies to which can be measured serologically in man. Among the three species of the genus Bordetella, 14 such agglutinogens have been identified; those designated 1 through 6 are unique to B. pertussis; agglutinogens 1, 2, and 3 are those most commonly identified.[42] Whether these agglutinogens play a role in disease pathogenesis is uncertain. A question of major importance is whether clinical efficacy of pertussis vaccine may depend on correspondence between the agglutinogens of vaccine strains and those of the strain(s) of B. pertussis circulating in the community.[66]

Adenylate cyclase is a component of the organism, largely somatic, that contributes to overcoming host defenses and, perhaps more importantly, facilitates cellular damage by inducing wasteful cell metabolism.[32] Whether antibodies to adenylate cyclase, which is antigenic, contribute to clinical immunity is unknown.

There are several other components of B. pertussis that may well play roles in disease pathogenesis.[45] Among these are tracheal cytotoxin, which may damage tracheal and bronchial epithelium, and a heat-labile toxin that is dermonecrotic or lethal and cytotoxic for bronchial epithelium in animal models. Antibodies to a recently described outer-membrane protein, designated 69K from its molecular weight, may play a role in clinical immunity.[76] Antibodies to this antigen appear following natural disease and pertussis vaccine. Whether these and other cellular components of the organism participate in disease pathogenesis in humans as well as in the development of immunity is unknown at present.[45]

Table 1. Major Components of *B. pertussis*, Their Actions, and Their Putative Roles in Pertussis

Component	Physiologic actions	Pathogenetic role	Role in immunity
Pertussis toxin (pertussigen, LPF)	Lymphocytosis promotion	Attachment to cilia	Major antigen
	Histamine sensitizatiion	Cell toxicity	
	Insulin stimulation		
	Mitogenicity		
Filamentous hemagglutinin	None known	Probably facilitates attachment to cilia	Probably contributes
Agglutinogens	None known	None known	Possible
Adenylate cyclase	Compromises cell metabolism	Compromises bacterial killing	Possible
Endotoxin	Many	Probably none in pertussis	Probably none
Tracheal cytotoxin	Toxic to respiratory epithelium	Possible cell toxicity	Probably none
Heat-labile toxin	Dermonecrotic and lethal in animals	Unknown	Probably none
69K protein	None known	Unknown	Possible

5. Descriptive Epidemiology

The epidemiology of pertussis has been strikingly modified by immunization. However, even prior to widespread immunization in highly developed countries such as the United States and currently in less developed countries, pertussis has displayed distinctive epidemiological characteristics.

5.1. Prevalence and Incidence

Pertussis is a reportable disease. Because it is associated with high mortality in infants and young children, it is important to make every effort to establish the diagnosis and report probable and proven cases to local health authorities. Pertussis is vastly underreported, for the reasons that the diagnosis is often missed, medical care may not be sought, and some physicians may not be convinced of the importance of reporting. Since the disease is underreported, case-fatality rates have been difficult to determine.

In 1986 approximately 4200 cases of pertussis were reported in the United States.[15] There has been a steady increase in reported cases since 1981; how much this increase is an artifact attributable to augmented reporting because of better diagnostic procedures, enhanced awareness due to the alleged risks of pertussis vaccine being dramatically portrayed in public media, or other factors is unclear. This change in reported cases is remarkable in that the incidence in persons 15 years and older has increased proportionately far more than in young children (Fig. 1).[16] However, mortality from pertussis in the United States has changed little in recent years; during the 10 years 1976–1985, 66 deaths from pertussis were recorded in the United States (4 in 1985).[15,57]

Although it is clear that case-fatality rates from pertussis are inversely related to age, precise rates are difficult to determine, largely because of underreporting of the disease. Moreover, mortality rates in the developed world decreased in this century independent of immunization or any other form of intervention.[5,22,25,53] Direct evidence of the decline in mortality is limited to areas with optimum reporting of cases as well as deaths, such as Providence, Rhode Island,[29] where case-fatality rates steadily declined from 1.36% in 1930–1934 to 0.24% in 1945–1949. Unfortunately, most information related to age-specific case-fatality rates is derived from children hospitalized with pertussis and is thus subject to the biases of such data. However, because almost everyone born in the first half of this century experienced the disease during childhood, the decline in pertussis mortality in the developed world must be attributed to a decrease in case-fatality rates. For example, in

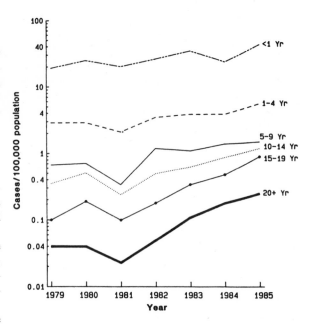

Figure 1. Age-specific incidence of reported cases of pertussis, United States, 1979–1985.[16]

the United States, annual deaths attributed to pertussis in children less than 1 year of age were 4.34/1000 for the years 1900–1904; for 1935–1939, before specific measures such as immunization and antimicrobial therapy were developed, the annual death rate in this age had declined 70% to 1.30/1000.[53] The reasons for this decline are unclear, but may be a consequence of a number of factors. These include better nutrition, the decline of debilitating conditions such as diarrheal diseases that compromised survival, quarantine of recognized cases, better supportive care, and decreasing birth rates that resulted in proportionately fewer children contracting the disease in infancy when case-fatality rates are maximum. There is little doubt that in the last decade the remarkable technology available in intensive care units has resulted in survival of the majority of infants critically ill with pertussis, many or most of whom would have otherwise succumbed. However, in less developed parts of the world, pertussis persists as a major cause of infant mortality. Currently, WHO estimates that 600,000 of the 104 million children born in developing countries die of this preventable disease prior to their fifth birthdays.[30]

5.2. Epidemic Behavior and Contagiousness

In the absence of immunization, essentially no child escapes pertussis.[26] Indeed, during both World War I and World War II, pertussis, in contrast to other childhood contagious diseases, was rarely seen in military personnel.[29] Secondary attack rates in susceptible family members may reach 90% or more,[55] and have been recorded as 100% in some studies.[62] In the United States, pertussis has been both an endemic and an epidemic disease. Since the wide-spread use of vaccine, large-scale outbreaks are unusual, but local or statewide outbreaks continue to occur as in Oklahoma[60] and Seattle.[13]

5.3. Geographic Distribution

The distribution of pertussis is worldwide, though clearly modified by immunization and other poorly defined social, economic, and nutritional factors. The annual number of cases estimated by WHO is 60 million and the reported rates per 100,000 population show great variations for selected countries.[56] The low incidence in some coun-tries may represent poor case-reporting, herd immunity from a preceding outbreak, or high levels of immunization. The highest rates occur in developing countries where im-munization programs are inadequate.

5.4. Temporal Distribution

Outbreaks occur at any time, but are perhaps more frequent in winter. At present in the United States there is a tendency for more cases to be reported in summer months. However, different seasonal patterns have been reported from various countries.[27a] In the past, year-to-year varia-tions occurred, with outbreaks every 2 or 3 years; in isolated areas, intervals of relative freedom from pertussis some-times extended for 5 or 6 years.[29]

5.5. Age

In recent years there has been a noticeable shift in the age distribution of reported cases of pertussis, probably largely due to widespread use of pertussis vaccine and the advent of mandatory immunization before school entry. For the years 1935–1939, prior to the availability of pertussis vaccine, data from ten states indicated that for whites about half of all cases of pertussis were reported in 5- to 14-year-old children.[22] For blacks this proportion was lower (20 to 40%) with the preponderance of cases occurring before 5 years. Less than 15% of cases in whites occurred before 1 year of age, but the proportion of cases in infancy among blacks was nearly twice that in whites, probably for so-cioeconomic reasons.[22] The proportion of reported cases in persons 15 years and older was less than 2% in the late 1930s.[22]

Widespread use of pertussis vaccine during the past four decades has been associated with a marked decline in reported cases and with a striking shift in the proportion of cases in various age groups. For the years 1984–1985, 43% of cases were reported in infants, 23% in children 1 to 4 years old, and about 15% in children 5 to 14 years old.[16] In contrast, 17% of cases were reported in persons 15 years and older. Undoubtedly, the paucity of cases in school-age children reflects the impact of school immunization laws— laws that do not affect younger children. The increased proportion of cases in persons 15 years and older may be relative rather than actual, or an artifact of better diagnosis and enhanced reporting (see Section 7.2).

5.6. Sex

Although both sexes are presumably equally affected, pertussis is unusual in that, inexplicably, the disease is more often reported in females, who also exhibit higher mortality rates. It may be that the smaller larynx of female infants places them at greater jeopardy from the disease.[28]

5.7. Race

Death rates are higher in blacks[22]; it is likely that these higher rates are attributable to socioeconomic and other factors, rather than to race.

5.8. Other Factors

Mortality rates are higher in lower socioeconomic groups, probably because of exposure earlier in life due to crowding and close contact. But case-fatality rates are also inversely related to socioeconomic status for reasons that are unclear, though nutrition may play a role.[42] In contrast to many infectious diseases, mortality from pertussis has been higher in rural than in urban areas.[29]

6. Mechanisms and Routes of Transmission

Pertussis is transmitted via the contact route by drop-lets. It is highly contagious; indeed, up to 90% of suscepti-ble family contacts will develop clinical disease from an index case in the household.[6,20,60,70] There is no evidence of spread by other routes, such as droplet nuclei, fomites, or dust. The disease appears to be most contagious during the catarrhal stage (the first week of symptoms) and declines so that, as the paroxysmal cough begins to wane, infectivity disappears. An important unanswered question is whether pertussis can be transmitted by individuals without overt disease. It is likely that individuals immunized in young childhood ultimately experience a mild, clinically unrecognizable disease in adolescence or young adulthood, and serve as a source of exposure. There is, however, no evidence of a carrier state.

7. Pathogenesis and Immunity

7.1. Pathogenesis

The pathogenesis of the disease, better defined in recent years, comprises attachment of the organism to tracheal and bronchial cilia with loss of function and ultimate destruction. Tissue invasion does not occur. The cough appears to be due to interference with normal mechanisms of bronchial toilet; mucoid secretions accumulate and are responsible for ineffective, repetitive, and paroxysmal coughing and, ultimately, for varying degrees of bronchial obstruction, atelectasis, and bronchopneumonia.[56] Bronchopneumonia is the most frequent serious complication of pertussis. It most often results from invasion by nonspecific respiratory flora; uncommonly, pneumococcal lobar pneumonia or invasion by *B. pertussis* itself may occur. Among 1921 persons in the United States requiring hospitalization for pertussis and its complications during the years 1984–1985, 574 had radiologically diagnosed pneumonia.[16]

A major complication of pertussis is encephalopathy, varying in manifestations from short-lived convulsions to intractable seizures, coma, and permanent cerebral damage.[53] The mechanism of pertussis encephalopathy is unclear. It is likely that anoxia and, in some instances, cerebral hemorrhages are responsible. Whether the effects of one or another of the various toxins elaborated by *B. pertussis,* including the induction of hypoglycemia, contribute is doubtful.

The experience of contagious-disease hospitals and institutions for the handicapped in the past indicate that pertussis encephalopathy is far from rare,[11,68] but few estimates are available. One may be derived from cases reported from the contagious-disease hospital that served residents of Brooklyn, New York, in the 1930s.[43] The childhood population of Brooklyn can be estimated from birth records, and, assuming that every child in Brooklyn experienced pertussis, the incidence of severe encephalopathy was approximately 1 in 22,000 cases. A more precise estimate was made by the British National Childhood Encephalopathy Study (NCES),[50] from which the frequency was about 1 in 11,000 cases. During 1984–1985 in the United States, among 1921 individuals (mostly children)

reported as hospitalized with pertussis, 81 exhibited seizures and 22 were diagnosed as having encephalopathy.[16] However, because of considerable underreporting of the disease, the rates of these complications in the general population cannot be determined at present in the United States.

7.2. Immunity

Clinical pertussis is followed by long-lasting immunity. Although occasional anecdotal reports of second attacks in adults have appeared, it is not clear whether these episodes represented true second attacks because of lack of laboratory confirmation.[29] In recent years, however, several well-documented series of pertussis in adults have been reported.[47,58,73,77] In some instances these illnesses are mild and atypical. It appears, however, that pertussis in adults is more common than formerly appreciated, and may occur not only in persons who experienced the disease in the past but also in those who were actively immunized as children.[77] Whether the disease is more frequently recognized in adults now than in the past or whether there is an actual increase in rates in older persons is uncertain. If there is a true increase, it is tempting to hypothesize that immunity, whether induced by pertussis or by the vaccine, is more apt to wane in recent years due to the present infrequency of exposure to the disease and the consequent lack of repeated, casual "streetcar" boosters.[77] Whatever the reason, it is apparent that pertussis in adolescents and young adults is a problem of some importance, particularly because such persons may constitute a reservoir of infection and a source of transmission to others, including young infants.[53a,73,77]

The mechanisms of clinical immunity to pertussis have escaped definition for many years, and only in the last decade has much progress been made. This progress has resulted from laboratory studies that have defined much better the components of the organism and from new methods of measuring antibodies serologically. Several antigens have been identified that appear to be important in the pathogenesis of pertussis and that, in addition, induce antibodies, one or more of which may provide clinical protection against the illness. One of these is pertussigen (LPF), which appears to be the major antigen that produces immunity in the mouse protection test, long used for laboratory evaluation and standardization of pertussis vaccine. Another antigen that may be important not only in disease pathogenesis but also for induction of clinical immunity is filamentous hemagglutinin (FHA). FHA is thought to facilitate attachment of *B. pertussis* to respiratory cilia; in hamster tracheal explants, antibodies to FHA interfere with such attachment.[46] A third group of antigens that may relate to the induction of clinical immunity are the agglutinogens, of which three appear to be of consequence. Their relation to disease pathogenesis is uncertain, but a number of studies in the past have shown correlation between clinical immunity and levels of antibody against agglutinogens.[46,70] Further, there is some indication that a mismatch between the specific agglutinogens in pertussis vaccine and those of circulating B. pertussis strains is associated with diminished vaccine efficacy.[62]

8. Patterns of Host Response

8.1. Clinical Features

The incubation period of clinical pertussis is usually 7–10 days, and rarely longer than 2 weeks. The first week or two of the illness is called the catarrhal stage, because initial symptoms of the disease are nonspecific, including mild but gradually increasing cough, nasal symptoms suggestive of a cold, slight fever, and some anorexia.

As the catarrhal stage progresses, the cough increases so that severe spells of coughing with the characteristic whoop appear by 2 weeks after onset, marking the beginning of the paroxysmal stage. The paroxysmal cough results from inability to expel tenacious mucus; the whoop is created by vigorous inspiration through the glottis at the end of the paroxysm. Paroxysms may occur repeatedly and may be initiated by eating, drinking, talking, crying, examination of the throat, or even by hearing another individual cough (such as occurs on a hospital division where there are other children with pertussis). During paroxysms, cyanosis may occur. Postparoxysm vomiting may be sufficiently repetitive in young infants to result ultimately in inanition, and tetany in infancy has been attributed to alkalosis from repeated emesis. During the paroxysmal stage, fever is absent or low. Subconjunctival and cerebral hemorrhages and epitaxis may be seen. Convulsions, with or without encephalopathy, and pulmonary complications occur during the paroxysmal stage.

In classic pertussis, the duration of the paroxysmal whooping stage is 4 or more weeks, with increasing frequency of paroxysms for 1 to 2 weeks and gradual subsidence and ultimate disappearance of the whoop thereafter. However, cough may persist for some weeks beyond the paroxysmal stage.

Mortality from pertussis is inversely related to age. The case-fatality rate in very young infants (less than 3 months) may be as high as 50%; after 5 years of age, it is negligible. However, the precise ascertainment of such rates is compromised by underreporting of the disease and by biases introduced by data from hospitalized patients.

The major causes of mortality appear to be pulmonary complications and encephalopathy, but the relative contributions of each are unsatisfactorily defined. In the past in the United States, secondary or intercurrent affections, such as otitis media, mastoiditis, and diarrhea, undoubtedly contributed to mortality and continue to do so in developing countries.

Permanent neurologic sequelae from pertussis, especially in infancy, undoubtedly occur.[11,43,50] More subtle intellectual or behavioral abnormalities may also result in some instances.[10,68] Long-term pulmonary damage has not been described,[7,37] although such might be expected in the future given the success of modern technology in maintaining infants through severe acute pulmonary disease.

8.2. Diagnosis

The diagnosis of the full-blown pertussis syndrome is readily made on clinical grounds by most clinicians who have had experience with the disease. The protracted course, paroxysmal coughing, and whoop are unmistakable. A history of exposure or knowledge of other cases in the area is of help.

Immediate support for the diagnosis of pertussis may frequently be obtained from the leukocyte count. Absolute lymphocytosis, often striking, parallels the severity of the cough, but is said to be less characteristic in young infants.[42]

A definitive diagnosis may be established in two ways: First, a rise in agglutinating or complement-fixing antibodies by testing acute and convalescent sera is of use retrospectively; unfortunately, such serologic testing is not available for routine use. Second, recovery and identification of B. pertussis by culture of respiratory secretions is definitive (see Section 3.4). However, isolation on culture is not easily accomplished. Identification of the organism in respiratory secretions by fluorescent-antibody techniques is difficult because of frequent false-positive tests.[8,63]

9. Control and Prevention

In the absence of widespread immunization, outbreaks of pertussis cannot be prevented and control is difficult.[59] Rates of transmission to susceptible households may be 90% or higher; in classroom situations, up to 50% of susceptible students in the same room may acquire the disease following exposure to an infected child.[42]

9.1. Isolation

Isolation or quarantine of children with clinical whooping cough is of limited value in controlling spread of the disease, for the reason that children in the catarrhal stage, before the diagnostic whoop appears, are quite infectious.

To prevent transmission, recognized cases should be excluded from school and contact with other children for approximately 4 weeks after the onset of the paroxysmal stage. Transmission after that time is very unlikely. The carrier state in pertussis has not been shown definitively to exist; if there is an asymptomatic carrier state, it is doubtful that it plays an important role in transmission. Milder forms of the disease, which occur in partially immune individuals, probably play a role in transmission (see Section 6).

9.2. Antibiotics

Pertussis is relatively insusceptible to antimicrobial therapy clinically. Although the organism is susceptible *in vitro* to various antimicrobial drugs effective against gram-negative organisms, such as ampicillin, streptomycin, chloramphenicol, the tetracyclines, and erythromycin, many studies have indicated that these therapeutic agents are of no use in modifying the full-blown disease. Most of them will reduce the length of time during which the organism can be recovered from patients with clinical pertussis. Erythromycin appears to be the most efficacious of these agents.[4,73]

Erythromycin may prevent or ameliorate the disease in nonimmune, exposed individuals prior to the onset of symptoms[1,4,73] and perhaps has some effect early in the catarrhal stage. The earlier the drug is administered to such individuals, the more likely is success. By the time the patient is well into the catarrhal stage or has begun to whoop, benefit is not expected. Because exposure is often unrecognized and because the disease is rarely suspected during the catarrhal stage, antibiotics do not comprise a satisfactory approach to disease control.

9.3. Passive Immunization

Passive protection of exposed, susceptible individuals was attempted in the past with varying results. In the late 1930s, convalescent and hyperimmune sera were administered to susceptible children exposed within the same household. In one small controlled study, protection appeared to be as high as 70%.[6] More recently, pertussis IgG, prepared from human or rabbit sera, has been employed with negative results.[52] Whether passive immunization is useless or whether there is protective serum antibody in fractions other than IgG is unknown. IgM, IgA, and cellular immunity may play a role in protection. No preparation for passive immunization is currently available in the United States.

9.4. Active Immunization

Studies of active immunization against pertussis were initiated in the 1930s employing a whole-cell killed vaccine, given parenterally. By the mid-1940s in the United States, the vaccine was widely used, and current criteria for standardization of the vaccine were established in 1953 by federal regulation. At present in the United States it is recommended that children receive three doses of pertussis vaccine combined with diphtheria and tetanus toxoids (DPT) adsorbed onto an aluminum salt at 2, 4, and 6 months of age, followed by booster doses of this triple combination at 15 to 18 months and prior to school entry.[12,14]

There is little question that most properly immunized children are protected against pertussis on exposure.[4,8,20,27,46,60,70] However, the proportion of children actually protected when intimately exposed, such as in the home, is probably far less than 100%.[27] Estimates of vaccine efficacy in studies of exposed immunized and unimmunized children vary remarkably because of differences in methods and in ascertainment, particularly in relation to recognition of infection versus clinical disease.[27] Nonetheless, it appears that pertussis vaccine is probably 80 to 95% efficacious in preventing clinical disease following intimate exposure. In spite of this, only 4195 cases of pertussis were reported in the United States in 1986.[16] Even assuming such gross underreporting that the actual number of cases of clinical pertussis is tenfold greater (about 42,000 annually), only about 1% of each birth cohort ultimately experience the disease. Therefore, on a population basis the vaccine is at least 99% efficacious in preventing clinical pertussis. Accordingly, the near disappearance of clinical pertussis in such countries as the United States must be attributed in part to herd immunity.

However, in the past decade concerns have been expressed about universal childhood immunization for two reasons: First, it is well established that mortality from pertussis in the developed world was declining long before development and widespread use of the vaccine (see Section 5.1). Whatever the cause of this decline, some have argued that the low rates of mortality from pertussis observed in recent years in developed countries would have occurred even in the absence of the vaccine, and therefore the vaccine may be superfluous.[74] In contradistinction, several studies have indicated that, although mortality from the disease clearly declined remarkably before the vaccine was extensively used, the decline accelerated significantly in association with its widespread use.[17,53]

Second, concerns have been expressed about the safety of the vaccine itself. Three general types of reactions have been attributed to DTP. The first of these comprises mild local reactions at the site of injection and slight systemic reactions, such as fever and malaise, as observed following receipt of most vaccines. These are usually of no concern. A second group of reactions includes three that are quite disturbing but for which there is no clear explanation or evidence of permanent sequelae. These include excessive sleepiness and incessant, inconsolable crying following injection in young infants, and a strange, shocklike syndrome. The third group of reactions includes those related to the central nervous system. These reactions range from what appear clearly to be simple febrile convulsions without sequelae[34] to severe encephalopathy with permanent brain damage or death. Although it is clear that pertussis vaccine is the antigen in DTP that contributes most to fever and local reactions, it has not been shown that it is the component primarily responsible for the others.

A recent study has provided somewhat more precise information about the frequency of the first two types of side effects.[21] In this study, infants and children who received a total of 15,752 inoculations of DTP and 784 of DT (diphtheria and tetanus toxoids absorbed) were followed for 48 h. Local and systemic reactions, including fever, were considerably more frequent following DTP than DT. Nine children experienced short seizures following DTP; all but one episode was shown to be associated with fever. Nine other children had hypotonic-hyporesponsive episodes. Thus, each of these reactions occurred at a rate of 1 per 1750 injections (95% confidence interval: 1 per 925 to 1 per 3850). However, attribution of these two more worrisome types of reactions solely to the pertussis component of DTP was not feasible because too few immunizations (784) with DT were monitored to permit comparison.

Estimates of rates of post-pertussis-vaccine encephalopathy have ranged from 1/50,000 to 1/300,000 or more[23]; subsequently, a well-designed study that controlled for background rates of encephalopathy suggested that serious neurologic reactions occur following 1/110,000 injections, and that about one-third of children so affected incur permanent sequelae.[48] However, follow-up of the children in this study has cast doubts on the precision of this rate, and it has been concluded by the investigators that the results either fail to show that pertussis vaccine produces permanent brain damage, or, if it does, the rate is too low to measure.[69] Instead, it appears that the majority, if not all,

of the instances of alleged pertussis vaccine encephalopathy represent either coincidence or the precipitation of inevitable manifestations of preexisting disorders by the well-known systemic effects of DTP.[18] Although occasional reports have suggested that DTP may precipitate the sudden infant death syndrome on rare occasions,[78] two large studies have indicated that these events represent simple coincidence.[31,35]

Doubts about the continuing need for pertussis vaccine plus anxiety about its safety, widely publicized in the media, resulted in striking diminutions in pertussis vaccine use in the late 1970s in Britain and Japan because of the concerns not only of parents but also of physicians. In both countries, widespread outbreaks of pertussis with its attendant mortality, particularly in unimmunized infants, ensued.[17,38] In Sweden, pertussis immunization was discontinued in 1979 because of doubts about vaccine efficacy, and, similarly, a recrudescence of the disease occurred.[67] These natural or inadvertent experiments provide strong evidence of the public health merit of widespread immunization against pertussis.

There may be risks, though remote, associated with pertussis vaccine; an important question is whether the risks outweigh the benefits. One analysis has indicated that the benefits outweigh the risks and, additionally, that routine immunization of children is highly cost-effective.[33]

In spite of this, it is clear that it would be advantageous to have an improved pertussis vaccine. Undoubtedly, the current whole-cell vaccine contains antigens and other substances that are not only reactive but also irrelevant to immunity, and contribute to DTP being of concern to physicians and parents and under criticism from the media, whether it produces permanent injury or not. For this reason plus the fact that much better understanding of the biologic anatomy of *B. pertussis* has steadily evolved over the past decade, efforts are being made to develop and evaluate acellular pertussis vaccines. Indeed, acellular vaccines have been licensed and used exclusively in Japan since 1981.[39,71] These Japanese vaccines are combined with diphtheria and tetanus toxoids and adsorbed onto an aluminum salt. The endotoxin content of each is reduced approximately 90%, and other extraneous proteins are removed, although it is not clear as to the exact extent. In terms of antigens believed to participate in the immune process, the composition of these vaccines varies. There are three types. One product, the B type (manufactured by Biken), contains approximately equal amounts of toxoided pertussis toxin and FHA. The Takeda or T-type vaccine, produced by four manufacturers, includes about 90% FHA, 9% toxoided pertussis toxin, and 1% agglutinogens. There is one product that is intermediate between the B and T types in composition. It has been shown that these Japanese acellular vaccines produce antibodies to pertussis toxin and FHA that are comparable to those achieved with the whole-cell vaccine and following natural pertussis.[39,41]

It is also clear that these Japanese acellular vaccines as a group effectively prevent pertussis, as judged by household contact studies.[60] However, three unanswered questions remain regarding efficacy. First, the relative efficacy of these vaccines compared to the whole-cell vaccine is not known for the reason that concomitantly controlled comparative studies have not been conducted. Second, the household contact studies of efficacy in Japan have not included children less than 2 years of age. The reason for this is that the age of initiation of DTP immunization in Japan was changed from infancy to 2 years in 1975 because of the belief that very young infants would be more susceptible to vaccine-induced encephalopathy. When Japan shifted from whole-cell vaccine to acellular vaccines in 1981, this recommendation was not changed. Third, in relation to clinical protection, studies comparing the B-type and T-type preparations are not definitive. One study, limited to children receiving T-type vaccines from several manufacturers, suggests high efficacy.[2]

In Sweden a placebo-controlled prospective trial of two acellular vaccines produced in Japan, one containing only pertussis toxoid and the other containing FHA as well but no agglutinogens (B type), demonstrated that each provided protection against culture-proven pertussis. The efficacy of the monovalent preparation was 54% (95% confidence intervals 26–72%) and that of the bivalent preparation, 69% (95% confidence intervals 47–82%).[1a,61] Both vaccines, however, were 80% effective in preventing pertussis with cough that lasted more than 30 days. However, correlation between antibody levels and clinical protection could not be established. A household contact study of a T-type vaccine produced by a single manufacturer suggested 100% protection against clinical disease (lower 95% confidence interval 94%).[54]

Local and systemic reactions, including fever, appear to be considerably less frequent following receipt of these acellular vaccines than with the whole-cell vaccine. However, studies in Japan comprise comparisons of the acellular vaccines with fluid (unadsorbed) DTP, a preparation known to be more reactive than adsorbed preparations.[39,51,71] However, comparisons of U.S. DTP containing whole-cell pertussis vaccine, adsorbed onto an aluminum salt, indicate that the adsorbed T-type preparation produced in Japan is followed by far fewer local and systemic reactions.[24,41,64]

There is no evidence that these less reactive Japanese acellular vaccines are less apt to produce pertussis vaccine-induced encephalopathy, assuming such occurs. Data from Japan's public recompense system for vaccine injuries show a striking decline in claims for pertussis vaccine injury following the recommendation that the age of initiation of whole-cell DTP be shifted from infancy to 2 years of age. No change of consequence occurred subsequent to 1981 when the acellular preparations replaced the whole-cell vaccine in DTP in Japan.[39] It stands to reason that temporally associated reactions not caused by DTP will continue to occur with DTP containing an acellular pertussis component.[18] However, it is also logical to believe that the induction of inevitable manifestations of underlying CNS disease, such as seizures, will be observed less frequently following administration of the less pyrogenic pertussis vaccine. Thus, less confusion about causation of such events in the minds of the public, physicians, and the media should ensue.

10. Unresolved Problems

Several important unresolved problems regarding pertussis and its control remain.

First, although remarkable progress has been made in understanding the biologic anatomy of *B. pertussis* and its relation to man, the relation of that anatomy to immunity to the disease is not precisely defined. In short, which antigen (or antigens) is (or are) necessary for the production of clinical immunity remains to be determined before an optimum vaccine can be produced. This is not an easy task for several reasons. There is no satisfactory animal model for pertussis. Because the time-tested whole-cell vaccine has nearly eradicated pertussis in the developed world, the number of subjects, the costs and the logistics of such a study in the United States and similar countries present nearly insurmountable problems. Studies in developing countries where pertussis is rife present both ethical dilemmas and enormous difficulties in follow-up. If a vaccine containing two or more components is only fractionally more efficacious than a single-component vaccine, assessment of the relative merits of differently constituted acellular vaccines would require numbers of subjects that stagger the imagination. Thus, the question of the antigenic composition of an optimum acellular pertussis vaccine may not be answerable by field trials in which clinical pertussis is the outcome measure. As a corollary, a serologic surrogate for clinical protection is sorely needed.

Second, although remarkable progress is being made in controlling pertussis in developing nations, achievement of universal, worldwide immunization against pertussis is some years away.

Third, better definition is needed of the role of asymptomatic or atypical pertussis, particularly in partially immune adolescents and young adults. The increasing evidence that such persons comprise a hitherto unrecognized or ignored reservoir for pertussis suggests the need for special attention. It is not unreasonable to predict that, with the anticipated development of a less reactive acellular pertussis vaccine, reinforcing doses will be needed into adolescence and adulthood.[73]

11. References

1. ALTEMEIER, W. A., III, AND AYOUB, E. M., Erythromycin prophylaxis for pertussis, *Pediatrics* **59**:623–625 (1977).
1a. Ad Hoc Group for the Study of Pertussis Vaccines, Placebo-controlled trial of two acellular pertussis vaccines in Sweden—protective efficacy and adverse events, *Lancet* **1**:956–960 (1988).
2. AOYAMA, T., MURASE, Y., GONDA, T., AND IWATA, T., Type-specific efficacy of acellular pertussis vaccine, *Am. J. Dis. Child.* **142**:40–42 (1988).
3. BARAFF, L. J., WILKINS, J., AND WEHRLE, P. F., The role of antibiotics, immunizations, and adenoviruses in pertussis, *Pediatrics* **61**:224–230 (1978).
4. BASS, J. W., Pertussis: Current status of prevention and treatment, *Pediatr. Infect. Dis. J.* **4**:614–619 (1985).
5. BASSILI, W. R., AND STEWART, G. T., Epidemiological evaluation of immunisation and other factors in the control of whooping cough, *Lancet* **1**:471–474 (1976).
6. BRADFORD, W. L., Use of convalescent blood in whooping cough, *Am. J. Dis. Child.* **50**:918–928 (1935).
7. BRITTEN, N., AND WADSWORTH, J., Long term respiratory sequelae of whooping cough in a nationally representative sample, *Br. Med. J.* **292**:441–444 (1986).
8. BROOME, C. V., AND FRASER, D. W., Pertussis in the United States, 1979: A look at vaccine efficacy, *J. Infect. Dis.* **144**:187–190 (1981).
9. BROOME, C. V., FRASER, D. W., AND ENGLISH, W. J., II, Pertussis—Diagnostic methods and surveillance, in: *International Symposium on Pertussis* (C. R. MANCLARK AND J. C. HILL, eds.), pp. 19–22, Washington: U.S. Government Printing Office, 1979, 19–22.
10. BUTLER, N. R., HASLUM, M., GOLDING, J., AND STEWART-BROWN, S., Recent findings from the 1970 child health and education study: Preliminary communication, *J. R. Soc. Med.* **75**:781–784 (1982).
11. BYERS, R. K., AND RIZZO, N. D., A follow-up study of pertussis in infancy, *N. Engl. J. Med.* **242**:887–891 (1950).
12. Centers for Disease Control, Recommendation of the Immunization Practices Advisory Committee (ACIP). Diphtheria,

tetanus, and pertussis: Guidelines for vaccine prophylaxis and other preventive measures, *Morbid. Mortal. Weekly Rep.* **34**:405–414, 419–426 (1985).
13. Centers for Disease Control, Pertussis—Washington, 1984, *Morbid. Mortal. Weekly Rep.* **34**:390–394, 399–400 (1985).
14. Centers for Disease Control, Recommendation of the Immunization Practices Advisory Committee (ACIP). New recommended schedule for active immunization of normal infants and children, *Morbid. Mortal. Weekly Rep.* **35**:577–579 (1986).
15. Centers for Disease Control, Summary of notifiable diseases in the United States, 1986, *Morbid. Mortal. Weekly Rep.* **35**:57 (1987).
16. Centers for Disease Control, Pertussis surveillance—United States, 1984 and 1985, *Morbid. Mortal. Weekly Rep.* **36**:168–171 (1987).
17. CHERRY, J. D., The epidemiology of pertussis and pertussis vaccine in the United Kingdom and the United States: A comparative study, in: *Current Problems in Pediatrics,* Volume 14, No. 2 (J. D. LOCKHART, ed.), Year Book Medical, Chicago, 1984.
18. CHERRY, J. D., AND MORTIMER, E. A., JR., Editorial. Acellular and whole-cell pertussis vaccines in Japan: Report of a visit by U.S. scientists, *J. Am. Med. Assoc.* **257**:1375–1376 (1987).
19. CHERRY, J. D., AND SHIELDS, W. D., Editorial review. Recurrent seizures after diphtheria, tetanus and pertussis immunization. Cause and effect *v* temporal association, *Am. J. Dis. Child.* **138**:904–907 (1984).
20. CHURCH, M. A., Evidence of whooping-cough-vaccine efficacy from 1978 whooping-cough epidemic in Hertfordshire, *Lancet* **2**:188–190 (1979).
21. CODY, C. L., BARAFF, L. J., CHERRY, J. D., MARCY, S. M., AND MANCLARK, C. R., Nature and rates of adverse reactions associated with DTP and DT immunizations in infants and children, *Pediatrics* **68**:650–660 (1981).
22. DAUER, C. C., Reported whooping cough morbidity and mortality in the United States, *Public Health Rep.* **58**:661–676 (1943).
23. Department of Health and Social Security, Committee on Safety of Medicines and Joint Committee on Vaccination and Immunization, Whooping cough, Her Majesty's Stationery Office, London, 1981.
24. EDWARDS, K. M., LAWRENCE, E., AND WRIGHT, P. F., Diphtheria, tetanus, and pertussis vaccine. A comparison of the immune response and adverse reactions to conventional and acellular pertussis components, *Am. J. Dis. Child.* **140**:867–871 (1986).
25. EHRENGUT, W., Whooping cough vaccination: Comment on report from the Joint Committee on Vaccination and Immunisation, *Lancet* **1**:234–237 (1978).
26. FINE, P. E. M., AND CLARKSON, J. A., Distribution of immunity to pertussis in the population of England and Wales, *J. Hyg.* **92**:21–26 (1984).
27. FINE, P. E. M., AND CLARKSON, J. A., Reflections on the

efficacy of pertussis vaccines, *Rev. Infect. Dis.* **9:**866–883 (1987).

27a. FINE, P. E. M., AND CLARKSON, J. A., Seasonal influences on pertussis. *Int. J. Epidemiol.* **15:**237–247 (1986).

28. GERMAK, J., Personal communication (1986).

29. GORDON, J. E., AND HOOD, R. I., Whooping cough and its epidemiological anomalies, *Am. J. Med. Sci.* **222:**333–361 (1951).

30. GRANT, J. P., Immunization leads the way, in: *State of the World's Children 1986*, UNICEF, pp. 1–20, Oxford University Press, London, 1985.

31. GRIFFIN, M. R., RAY, W. A., LIVENGOOD, J. R., AND SCHAFFNER, W., Risk of sudden infant death syndrome (SIDS) following diphtheria–tetanus–pertussis immunization, *N. Engl. J. Med.* **319:**618–623 (1988).

32. HEWLETT, E. L., Biological effects of pertussis toxin and *Bordetella* adenylate cyclase on intact cells and experimental animals, in: *Microbiology—1984* (L. LEIVE AND D. SCHLESSINGER, eds.), pp. 168–171, American Society for Microbiology, Washington, D.C., 1984.

33. HINMAN, A. R., AND KOPLAN, J. P., Pertussis and pertussis vaccine. Reanalysis of benefits, risks and costs, *J. Am. Med. Assoc.* **251:**3109–3113 (1984).

34. HIRTZ, D. G., NELSON, K. B., AND ELLENBERG, J. H., Seizures following childhood immunizations, *J. Pediatr.* **102:**14–18 (1983).

35. HOFFMAN, H. S., HUNTER, J. C., DAMUS, K., PAKTER, J., PETERSON, D. R., VAN BELLE, G., AND HASSELMEYER, E. G., Diphtheria–tetanus–pertussis immunization and sudden infant death: Results of the National Institute of Child Health and Human Development Cooperative Epidemiological Study of sudden infant death syndrome Risk Factors, *Pediatrics* **79:**598–611 (1987).

36. HOLMES, W. H., *Bacillary and Rickettsial Infections*, pp. 395–398. Macmillan Co., 1940.

37. JOHNSTON, I. D. A., BLAND, J. M., INGRAM, D., ANDERSON, H. R., WARNER, J. O., AND LAMBERT, H. P., Effect of whooping cough in infancy on subsequent lung function and bronchial reactivity, *Am. Rev. Respir. Dis.* **134:**270–275 (1986).

38. KANAI, K., Japan's experience in pertussis epidemiology and vaccination in the past thirty years, *Jpn. J. Sci. Biol.* **33:**107–143 (1980).

39. KIMURA, M., AND HIKINO, N., Results with a new DTP vaccine in Japan, *Dev. Biol. Stand.* **61:**545–561 (1985).

40. KLOOS, W. E., MOHAPATRA, N., DOBROGOSZ, W. J., EZZELL, J. W., AND MANCLARK, C. R., Deoxyribonucleotide sequence relationships among *Bordetella* species, *Int. J. Syst. Bacteriol.* **31:**173–176 (1981).

41. LEWIS, K., CHERRY, J. D., HOLROYD, H. J., BAKER, L. R., DUDENHOEFFER, F. E., AND ROBINSON, R. G., A double-blind study comparing acellular pertussis-component DTP vaccine with a whole-cell pertussis-component DTP vaccine in 18-month-old children, *Am. J. Dis. Child.* **140:**872–876 (1986).

42. LINNEMAN, C. C., Host–parasite interactions in pertussis, in: *International Symposium on Pertussis* (C. R. MANCLARK AND J. C. HILL, eds.), pp. 3–18, U.S. Government Printing Office, Washington, D.C., 1979.

43. LITVAK, A. M., GIBEL, H., ROSENTHAL, S. E., AND ROSENBLATT, P., Cerebral complications in pertussis, *J. Pediatr.* **32:**357–379 (1948).

44. LUTTINGER, P., The epidemiology of pertussis, *Am. J. Dis. Child.* **12:**290–315 (1916).

45. MANCLARK, C. R., AND COWELL, J. L., Pertussis, in: *Bacterial Vaccines* (R. GERMANIER, ed.), pp. 69–106, Academic Press, New York, 1984.

46. Medical Research Council, Vaccination against whooping-cough. The final report to the Immunization Committee of the Medical Research Council and to the medical officers of health for Battersea and Wandsworth, Bradford, Liverpool, and Newcastle, *Br. Med. J.* **1:**994–1000 (1959).

47. MERTSOLA, J., RUUSKANEN, O., EEROLA, E., AND VILJANEN, M. K., Intrafamilial spread of pertussis, *J. Pediatr.* **103:**359–363 (1983).

48. MILLER, D. L., ROSS, E. M., ALDERSLADE, R., BELLMAN, M. H., AND RAWSON, N. S. B., Pertussis immunisation and serious acute neurological illness in children, *Br. Med. J.* **282:**1595–1599 (1981).

49. MILLER, D. L., ALDERSLADE, R., AND ROSS, E. M., Whooping cough and whooping cough vaccine: The risks and benefits debate, *Epidemiol. Rev.* **4:**1–24 (1982).

50. MILLER, D., WADSWORTH, J., DIAMOND, J., AND ROSS, E., Pertussis vaccine and whooping cough as risk factors for acute neurological illness and death in young children, *Dev. Biol. Stand.* **61:**389–394 (1985).

51. MILLER, E., Progress towards a new pertussis vaccine, *Br. Med. J.* **292:**1348–1350 (1986).

52. MORRIS, D., AND MCDONALD, J. C., Failure of hyperimmune gamma globulin to prevent whooping cough, *Arch. Dis. Child.* **32:**236–239 (1957).

53. MORTIMER, E. A., JR., AND JONES, P. K., An evaluation of pertussis vaccine, *Rev. Infect. Dis.* **1:**927–932 (1979).

53a. MORTIMER, E. A., JR., Perspectives. Pertussis and its prevention: A family affair. *J. Infect. Dis.* **161:**473–479 (1990).

54. MORTIMER, E., DEKKER, C., MIYAMOTO, Y., HAYASHI, R., KIMURA, M., SAKAI, H., KATO, T., ISOMURA, S., AOYAMA, T., KAMIYA, H., NOYA, J., SUZUKI, E., TAKEUCHI, Y., STOUT, M., AND CHERRY, J., Protection against pertussis provided by a 3 antigen acellular pertussis vaccine combined with diphtheria and tetanus toxoids (APDT): A household contact study in Japan (Abstract), *Pediatr. Res.* **23:**367A (1988).

55. MULLER, A. S., LEEUWENBURG, J., AND PRATT, D. S., Pertussis: Epidemiology and control, *Bull. WHO* **64:**321–331 (1986).

56. MUSE, K. E., FINDLEY, D., ALLEN, L., AND COLLIER, A. M., In vitro model of Bordetella pertussis infection: Pathogenic and microbicidal interactions, *International Symposium on Pertussis: Report of a Conference* pp. 41–50 (1979).

57. National Center for Health Statistics, Advance Report of Final

Mortality Statistics, 1985, Monthly Vital Statistics Report **36**(5), Suppl. 28 (1987).

58. NELSON, J. D., The changing epidemiology of pertussis in young infants. The role of adults as reservoirs of infection, *Am. J. Dis. Child.* **132**:371–373 (1978).

59. NKOWANE, B. M., WASSILAK, S. G. F., MCKEE, P. A., O'MARA, D. J., DELLAPORTAS, G., ISTRE, G., ORENSTEIN, W. A., AND BART, K. J., Pertussis epidemic in Oklahoma. Difficulties in preventing transmission, *Am. J. Dis. Child.* **140**:433–437 (1986).

60. NOBLE, G. R., BERNIER, R. H., ESBER, E. C., HARDEGREE, C., HINMAN, A. R., KLEIN, D., AND SAAH, A. J., Acellular and whole-cell pertussis vaccines in Japan. Report of a visit by U.S. scientists, *J. Am. Med. Assoc.* **257**:1351–1356 (1987).

61. OLIN, P., Status of acellular pertussis vaccines—Swedish trial update, Presented at the combined meeting of NIAID, FDA, CDC, and USAID, National Institutes of Health (February 1988).

62. OLSON, L. C., Pertussis, *Medicine* **54**:427–469 (1975).

63. ONORATO, I. M., AND WASSILAK, S. G. F., Laboratory diagnosis of pertussis: The state of the art, *Pediatr. Infect. Dis. J.* **6**:145–151 (1987).

64. PICHICHERO, M. E., BADGETT, J. T., RODGERS, G. C., JR., MCLINN, S., TREVINO-SCATTERDAY, B., AND NELSON, J. D., Acellular pertussis vaccine: Immunogenicity and safety of an acellular pertussis vaccine *vs.* a whole cell pertussis vaccine combined with diphtheria and tetanus toxoids as a booster in 18- to 24-month old children, *Pediatr. Infect. Dis. J.* **6**:352–363 (1987).

65. PITTMAN, M., The concept of pertussis as a toxin-mediated disease, *Pediatr. Infect. Dis. J.* **3**:467–486 (1984).

66. PRESTON, N. W., Effectiveness of pertussis vaccines, *Br. Med. J.* **2**:11–13 (1965).

67. ROMANUS, V., JONSELL, R., AND BERGQUIST, S. E., Pertussis in Sweden after the cessation of general immunization in 1979, *Pediatr. Infect. Dis. J.* **6**:364–371 (1987).

68. ROSENFELD, G. B., AND BRADLEY, C., Childhood behavior sequelae of asphyxia in infancy with special reference to pertussis and asphyxia neonatorum, *Pediatrics* **2**:74–83 (1948).

69. ROSS, E., AND MILLER, D., Risk and pertussis vaccine. Correspondence, *Arch. Dis. Child.* **61**:98–99 (1986).

70. SAKO, W., Studies on pertussis immunization, *J. Pediatr.* **30**:29–40 (1947).

71. SATO, Y., KIMURA, M., AND FUKUMI, H., Development of a pertussis component vaccine in Japan, *Lancet* **1**:122–126 (1984).

72. STEKETEE, R. W., BURSTYN, D. G., WASSILAK, S. G. F., ADKINS, W. N., JR., POLYAK, M. B., DAVIS, J. P., AND MANCLARK, C. R., A comparison of laboratory and clinical methods for diagnosing pertussis in an outbreak in a facility for the developmentally disabled, *J. Infect. Dis.* **157**:441–449 (1988).

73. STEKETEE, R. W., WASSILAK, S. G. F., ADKINS, W. N., JR., BURSTYN, D. G., MANCLARK, C. R., BERG, J., HOPFENSPERGER, D., SCHELL, W. L., AND DAVIS, J. P., Evidence for a high attack rate and efficacy of erythromycin prophylaxis in a pertussis outbreak in a facility for the developmentally disabled, *J. Infect. Dis.* **157**:434–440 (1988).

74. STEWART, G. T., Vaccination against whooping-cough. Efficacy versus risks, *Lancet* **1**:234–237 (1977).

75. STEWART, G. T., Pertussis vaccine: The United Kingdom's experience, in: *International Symposium on Pertussis* (C. R. MANCLARK AND J. C. HILL, eds.), pp. 262–278, U.S. Government Printing Office, Washington, D.C., 1979.

76. THOMAS, M. G., REDHEAD, K., AND LAMBERT, H. P., Human serum antibody responses to *Bordetelle pertussis* infection and pertussis vaccination, *J. Infect. Dis.* **159**:211–218 (1989).

77. TROLLFORS, B., AND RABO, E., Whooping cough in adults, *Br. Med. J.* **283**:696–697 (1981).

78. WALKER, A. M., JICK, H., PERERA, D. R., THOMPSON, R. S., AND KNAUSS, T. A., Diphtheria–tetanus–pertussis immunization and sudden infant death syndrome, *Am. J. Public Health* **77**:945–951 (1987).

12. Suggested Reading

American Academy of Pediatrics, Report of the Task Force on Pertussis and Pertussis Immunization—1988. 81(Suppl 2):939–984.

MORTIMER, E. A., JR., Pertussis and pertussis vaccine: 1990. In: *Advances in Pediatric Infectious Diseases*, pp. 1–33, Chicago: Year Book Medical Publishers, 1990.

WARDLAW, A. C., AND PARTON, R., *Pathogenesis and Immunity in Pertussis*. John Wiley & Sons, London, 1988.

CHAPTER 24

Plague

W. D. Tigertt

1. Introduction

Plague is a zoonotic disease of rodents and their fleas caused by *Yersinia pestis*. Fleas infected by feeding on a diseased rodent may transfer the infection to other rodents and to man. Commonly, the initial response, in man and in rodent, is a lymphadenitis, adjacent to the site of the bite. If not contained at this level, there is bloodstream invasion, and a frequent complication is involvement of the lungs. This can result in direct patient-to-person transfer of *Y. pestis*. There can be either a few sporadic secondary cases or devastating epidemics. In the flea-transferred form (bubonic) prior to 1940, the death rate was 50–70%. In the pneumonic transfer form, practically all patients were expected to die. The disease was greatly feared, and this fear continues, despite the ability of today's drugs to control the disease.

2. Historical Background

Some students of this disease consider that the severe illness described in Ist Samuel was plague. In the succeeding centuries, there were a variety of outbreaks termed pestilences or plagues.[15] Many of these are not accepted as *Y. pestis* infections. Little purpose would be served by a detailed review of the many articles that have been written in efforts to settle the true nature of these epidemics.

It is generally agreed that the Great Plague of Justinian in the 6th century was true plague, appearing first in Egypt

and then extending through Syria, North Africa, and much of Europe. The historian Procopius wrote[22] that the initial sign of illness is a

> . . . languid fever . . .

and

> . . . on the same day in some cases, in others on the following day, and in the rest not many days later, a bubonic swelling developed; and this took place not only in the particular part of the body which is termed bubon [groin], that is below the abdomen, but also inside the armpit, and in some cases behind the ears, and at different points on the thighs.

He then describes the associated suffering and delirium and continues:

> Death came in some cases immediately, in others after many days, and with some the body broke out with black pustules about as large as a lentil and these did not survive even one day, but all succumbed immediately. With many a vomiting of blood came without visible cause and straightway brought death.

According to some reports, half the population of the Roman Empire died.

In the 14th century, plague again appeared in Europe. It is said that the epidemic began in Cathay and upper India and then moved along trade routes to the Crimea and the Levant. From these points, movement was by ship to Sicily and Sardinia, and to Italy in 1346, and onward to England in 1348. Two writers who are often quoted in their description of this epidemic, Gabriel de Mussis on Crimea and Giovanni Boccaccio on Florence, apparently did not have firsthand knowledge of their subject.[12,51]

W. D. Tigertt · *American Journal of Tropical Medicine and Hygiene,* Baltimore, Maryland 21201.

The description of the plague in Avignon, by Guy de Chauliac, physician to the Pope, was set down many years after the fact.[51] The fatality rates ranged from 40 to 80% in population groups living in areas where the disease occurred, and the epidemic was termed "The Great Mortality" with good reason.[15] The often-used term "Black Death" was coined several hundred years later.[37] Whatever may have been the true number of deaths, the outcome was to produce far-reaching social changes.

Plague recurred or was reintroduced into Europe repeatedly during each succeeding century. The "Great Plague" of London was in 1665. In a population of 500,000, deaths during August and September were reported to be 7000 per week. Plague gradually disappeared from Europe during the following decades, with the entire continent apparently being free by 1840.[15] Zinsser[52] considered that this disappearance ". . . presents one of the unsolved mysteries of epidemiology . . ." and Pollitzer[39] notes that ". . . this has been the subject of much debate and few conclusions." Others[15] attribute this freedom from disease to a replacement of the black rat in European homes by a less efficient transmitter, *Rattus norvegicus*.

The disease reappeared in the last years of the 19th century, apparently originating in China and reaching Hong Kong in 1894. From this seaport, it was spread by cargo vessels throughout most of the world. India experienced epidemics that recurred for more than 20 years with thousands of deaths. It was in Hong Kong that Yersin first isolated the causative organism, and it was in India that the association of rat deaths (rat-falls) and subsequent human illness was noted. These early studies in India also proved the indispensable role of fleas in the transmission of the bacilli.[15]

Various types of vaccines were made and tested, and antisera received extensive study. Effective therapy was found in the 1950s with chloramphenicol, streptomycin, and the broad-spectrum antibiotics.[30]

During the last 20 years, much of the world has known only sporadic plague, although plague infection is widespread as a zoonosis. In one of these known foci, Vietnam, human plague appeared in 1961 and in subsequent years, and with the associated disruption of war, many hundreds of cases occurred.[3,39]

3. Methodology

3.1. Sources of Mortality Data

International agreements require that telegraphic notification be made to the World Health Organization (WHO) of the first transferred or first nonimported case of plague in any area previously free of the disease. This information is published in the *Weekly Epidemiological Record,* in the *Weekly Epidemiological Report* of the Pan American Health Organization, and in the *Morbidity and Mortality Weekly Report* from the Centers for Disease Control of the U.S. Public Health Service. Currently available worldwide figures are considered to be approximately correct. Frequently, there is underreporting at the onset of an epidemic and overreporting during the course of the epidemic. Sporadic cases may go unrecognized. While these few missed cases are of much possible import epidemiologically, they do not influence the total disease incidence or fatality rates.

In addition to all the problems associated with the recognition and reporting of plague in the developing countries, bureaucratic decrees may also contribute to underreporting. For instance, in some parts of the world, to be officially recorded, cases of plague must be confirmed by animal inoculation, but often no effort is made to perform such studies.

3.2. Sources of Morbidity Data

Much of the information in Section 3.1 is applicable here. Governments have been slow to admit the existence of a new case or cases of plague in an effort to prevent panic in their peoples or to avoid the problems associated with a possible quarantine. The response to broad-spectrum antibiotics and streptomycin is such that scattered cases may be treated effectively early in their course, fail to develop a recognizable clinical picture, and thus go unreported.

3.3. Surveys

Methods for the isolation of *Y. pestis* and for the serological evidence of experience with this organism by humans, rodents, and other carnivores are available. In addition to confirming overt cases, these procedures permit recognition of cases treated early and of "inapparent" infections. They also provide information essential for the institution of control measures and for the evaluation of such procedures. Details are given in subsequent sections.

3.4. Laboratory Diagnosis

In view of common misconceptions, it is appropriate to emphasize that the proper collection of laboratory specimens from plague patients does not place the collector at more risk than does the examination of the patient. Likewise, the laboratory manipulation of plague specimens for initial bacteriological or serological procedures does not require precautions beyond those needed for good laboratory work in general, including the prohibition of mouth pipetting and the use of tightly sealed tubes for centrifugation or vortex mixing.

Animal inoculations and dissections should be performed only by appropriately trained personnel in properly equipped quarters. The same is true for examination of trapped rodents or those found dead.

3.4.1. Presumptive Diagnosis.

A presumptive diagnosis of plague can be made by the direct microscopic examination of films prepared from material aspirated from the bubo or from sputum. This is of particular importance in the often-unrecognized sporadic cases. It is the diagnostic procedure that should lead to the institution of effective therapy and of public-health procedures appropriate for the protection of others.

For bubo aspiration, a small sterile syringe containing a few milliliters of sterile saline should be used. After the skin is cleansed, the needle is inserted into the central part of the suspect bubo. Then an attempt should be made to aspirate fluid. If this is not successful, the saline is injected and aspirated. Films on glass slides are prepared from a portion of the aspirate, care being taken not to produce an aerosol when expelling the fluid. Films from buboes or from sputum should be air-dried and then fixed by immersion in pure methanol for 5 min. After being dried, one film should be stained by Weyson's method* and the second by a Gram stain. From most human or animal sources, *Y. pestis* is a gram-negative plump bacillus that with Weyson's stain shows a typical bipolar (safety-pin) configuration.

3.4.2. Definitive Bacteriology.

Material from buboes and from sputum should be inoculated at the time of collection onto deoxycholate agar (Difco), peptone agar (Difco), and brain–heart infusion broth (Difco); alternately, specimens may be placed in Cary–Grant transport medium. Blood from plague suspects should be inoculated into brain–heart infusion broth (Difco) and kept at room temperature. Certain presumptive procedures (e.g., morphology, fermentation reactions, motility) can be performed in any good laboratory. Whenever the diagnosis of plague is considered in the United States, contact should be made with the Zoonosis Section, Ecological Investigation Program, Centers for Disease Control, Post Office Box 551, Fort Collins, Colorado 80521 for completion of the definitive diagnosis.

3.4.3. Serological and Immunological Diagnostic Methods.

Three procedures are available. The best is the passive hemagglutination (HA) test utilizing *Y. pestis* Fraction 1 antigen (see Section 4.1.1). The second is a complement-fixation (CF) test with the same antigen. As is true of all such tests, the results can be altered by the quality of the available sera. Agglutination tests have also been used, but the specificity is questionable even after absorption with *Y. pseudotuberculosis*.[1,18] A monoclonal antibody to F1 antigen in an enzyme-linked immunosorbent assay (ELISA) to detect the F1 antigen in serum or blood clot is useful. This procedure does not recognize all blood culture-positive patients.[10,50] Care is essential, since the early sample may contain viable organisms. CF and HA antibodies appear a few weeks after the onset of infection and persist for months. Prior vaccination or maternal transfer of antibodies may confuse the picture.

4. Biological Characteristics of the Organism

4.1. Virulence

There seems to be general agreement that there are at least five determinants of virulence of *Y. pestis* in guinea pigs and in mice, and there is the presumption that these are of importance in man.[4]

4.1.1. Fraction 1 Antigen.

This material has been called the diffusible envelope or the capsule of the organism. Maximum production is at 37 °C, and it is associated with protection against phagocytosis.

4.1.2. Virulence or V and W Antigens.

These are recognized by the use of gel-diffusion plates. One is a protein and the other is a lipoprotein. They are associated with the ability of the organism to survive and to multiply within phagocytes.

4.1.3. Pesticidin I.

This is a product of the virulent organism that inhibits the growth of *Y. pseudotuberculosis*. The capacity of cultures to produce pesticidin has been correlated with the production of a fibrinolytic factor and a coagulase.

4.1.4. Pigmentation.

Some cultures have the ability to utilize exogenous hemin as manifested by the appearance of pigmented colonies. This suggests a role in the utilization of iron, but no satisfactory explanation has been offered.

4.1.5. Purine Independence.

The capacity to synthesize purines is a component of virulence in *Y. pestis,* as it is in a variety of other organisms.

4.2. Avirulence

For many years, it was said that plague bacilli recovered in nature were remarkably constant in character.[31]

---

*To prepare Weyson's stain, dissolve 0.2 g basic fuchsin and 0.7 g methylene blue each in 10 ml absolute methanol. Then mix the two and add to 200 ml 5% phenol in distilled water. Dispense and store in dark bottles.[1]

Recent studies indicate diversity.[49] For example, drug-resistant organisms have been recovered, a strain deficient in Fraction 1 antigen production has been reported from a fatal case in the United States, pesticidin was not produced from an isolate from a case in Arizona, and a culture that did not produce pigment was recovered from a mild case of plague in South Africa. Similar organisms, lacking the capacity to produce pigment, have been reported from Vietnam and from fleas and rabbits in New Mexico. From central Java, isolates from infected fleas lack V and W antigen, making them comparable to certain of the "avirulent" strains that have been used as vaccines. While definitive associations cannot be made yet, these observations must be examined carefully in light of the reports of mild and asymptomatic plague noted in later sections.

4.3. Geographic Biotypes

These are not known to be related to virulence, but are of some possible importance to epidemiologists. The *Y. pestis* organism, spread over much of the world at the beginning of this century and termed variety *orientalis*, can form NO_2^- from NO_3^-, but cannot ferment glycerol. Variety *mediaevalis*, which occurs around the Caspian Sea, does not form NO_2^-, but ferments glycerol. Variety *antigua*, present in southeast Russia, central Asia, and parts of Africa, can form NO_2^- and ferment glycerol.[4]

5. Descriptive Epidemiology

Plague in humans occurs as the result of their intrusion into the zoonotic (also termed sylvatic or rural) transmission cycle or by the entry of man's habitat by infected animals and their infected fleas. Certain species of fleas and rodents play major roles in the transfer of this infection. These species are considered briefly below; other fleas and rodents, to the extent that they lack the attributes of these species, are less efficient in the transmission of plague.

Fleas are small, wingless, bloodsucking ectoparasites of warm-blooded animals that will leave a dead host as the body temperature drops and seek another host, preferably similar to the one abandoned. A principal vector of plague is *Xenopsylla cheopis*. Other important fleas are *X. astia, X. braziliensis, X. vexhabilis,* and *Nosophyllus fasciatus.*[1]

X. cheopis has a wide distribution, can live in urban environments, and will take blood from many species of rodents and from man. If the blood of the rodent host contains *Y. pestis*, the organisms will multiply in some fleas

and completely block the alimentary canal. Such hungry "blocked" fleas make repeated attempts to feed, but are able to suck only a small amount of blood into the esophagus. Here, it mixes with the masses of plague bacilli and is then regurgitated into the wound. Blocking is common in *X. cheopis* and in the other fleas noted above. Other vectors can be of importance in transmitting the infection to man if the level of septicemia in the host is high.

Of the more than 200 species of rodents that may carry plague, only a few are responsible for most direct infection of humans. *Rattus rattus*, the domestic black rat, is of prime importance in this role. It has been said that in the absence of *R. rattus*, plague is never transmitted to man to any serious extent.[32] The black rat lives in close association with man in both urban and rural areas, is a vigorous breeder, is a host highly acceptable to *X. cheopis,* and will develop fulminating fatal septicemic plague. These rats ordinarily become infected by a transfer of infected fleas as a result of contact with diseased or recently dead field rodents, such as *R. norvegicus*, a rat having most of the characteristics listed above except for association with enzootic plague foci. Other species of rats can replace *R. norvegicus,* or in some instances, more than one species may be active in this intermediate transfer activity. In the enzootic plague foci, several rodent species may coexist. In addition to rats, these include marmots and ground squirrels in central Asia[15,17]; prairie dogs, rabbits, and ground squirrels in the United States[32]; gerbils and multimammate mice in Africa; cavies in South America[15]; and shrews in Vietnam.[25] In theory, any infected animal or the associated fleas could serve as the source of infection of humans.

When flea-transmitted plague is introduced into an area where the infection has not occurred for several years, there may follow an extensive rat epizootic with many dead rats in evidence. One suitable flea (such as *X. cheopis*) per rat, in an appropriate climatic environment, is sufficient to maintain the transmission. The mixing of wandering outdoor rats with house rats may transfer the infection to humans. In some of the urban areas with massive rodent populations studied in Vietnam, plague infection in rodents was continuous and rat-falls did not precede the appearance of human cases. Three rodent species were of importance. All were infected, all had fleas, and probably all had contact with humans.[25] *R. exulans*, living in both fields and houses, may have been the most important link.[1]

5.1. Prevalence and Incidence

WHO figures show 483 cases of human plague reported in 1985.[17] This is the lowest reported incidence in recent years and essentially all were from known endemic areas. In 1984 there were 908 cases reported and in 1983, 715. The registered cases of human plague from Vietnam continued to decline. In 1985 there were 137 cases and 6 deaths. In the rest of Asia, only China notified 6 cases, all resulting from the skinning of infected marmots. There were no reports of disease in Europe. In 1985 in Africa there was continued activity with 85 cases in Madagascar (85 cases in 1985) and 125 in Tanzania. In the Americas, for the first time in recent years there were no cases recorded in Bolivia. There was continued activity in Brazil and Peru.

In the United States during this 3-year period (1983–1985), the number of reported cases were 40, 31, and 17 with a total of 8 deaths. It was uncommon for more than a single case to appear in a given area, with the individual cases being widely distributed in the western states. The infection was usually of sylvatic origin and bubonic in type.

5.2. Epidemic Behavior and Contagiousness

Since plague epitomizes our classic concepts of pestilence and contagiousness, statements under this rubric must be made with care. It should be emphasized that most patients with bubonic plague are not a significant source of infection for their family, contacts, or attendants. To quote Hirst,[15] describing the early 1900s, ". . . . it soon became well-known saying in India that a plague hospital was one of the safest places to be in a plague epidemic."

Chronic plague, characterized by the persistence of organisms after infection, or by the presence of *Y. pestis* in the throats of "healthy" individuals, has been described repeatedly.[19,24,33] The duration may be for days to months. There are no sound data to suggest that such "carriers" play any significant role in the transmission of the infection. Problems associated with other forms of plague are noted in Section 6.

5.3. Geographic Distribution

Countries reporting disease in 1983–1985 are noted in Section 5.1. Europe and Australia have been free for many years. The classic foci in Asia are active.

5.4. Temporal Distribution

Outbreaks of bubonic plague usually occur in temperature ranges of 10–26 °C associated with a high relative humidity.[15] These conditions, in which flea survival is favored, represent winter in India and summer in England.

Very high temperatures may be associated with unblocking of the infected fleas, while low relative humidities can cause flea deaths. Cavanaugh and Marshall,[8] in an 8-year study in Vietnam, examined the role of climate and concluded that "slight variations in temperature, relative humidity, and vapor pressure deficits either permit an epidemic to flourish or cause a decline in its intensity."

Pneumonic plague has often occurred in winter temperatures with a maximum relative humidity. Under other circumstances, the airborne organisms have only a short survival period. It must be appreciated that pneumonic plague can occur whenever a patient has primary or secondary plague pneumonia and there is close contact with a susceptible individual. The California outbreaks in 1919 and 1924 are examples of pneumonic plague in moderate temperatures.[32]

5.5. Age

Plague has been said to be rare in children, but during an outbreak in Madagascar, over 3% of the patients were under 2 years of age.[32] In Vietnam, plague in children was not uncommon. It may be that this alleged immunity in children is a function of the amount of disease occurring in a population. In the Norway rat (*R. norvegicus*), there is passive transfer of antibody to Fraction 1 antigen of the plague bacillus from the immunized dam by both placental and lacteal routes. The offspring were afforded protection against challenges that killed all controls.[48] Thus, if extrapolation is permitted, children born of immunized mothers may have some degree of protection.

5.6. Sex

There is no evidence of any difference in susceptibility between males and females. Any apparent differences in attack rates can usually be explained by examination of occupations and habits.

5.7. Race

It is generally stated that all races seem to be equally susceptible.[32]

5.8. Occupation

Certain occupations and habits produce an increased risk of exposure to infected fleas or rodents. This infection is seen in hunters, trappers, naturalists, pet owners,[47] and campers, in at least one golfer, in those who live on or adjacent to sylvatic foci, in those who attend pneumonic-plague patients, pathologists, and funeral attendants, and in stevedores, seamen, and grain handlers. Finally, mention should be made of the several investigators of this zoonosis who became infected and died.

5.9. Occurrence in Different Settings

As noted in Section 5.2, a case of bubonic plague in a family generally does not place the other members at risk, although obviously some may have been exposed to the same lot of infected fleas. When multiple cases occur, the dates of onset are often nearly identical.

Pneumonic-plague patients obviously are a threat. In addition to transmission to family members, such patients traveling to their homes with intermediate stops have been responsible for multiple infected contacts.[32] Transmission occurs only when there is a productive cough.

Plague epidemics have often been associated with the disruption of wars. Invading or retreating troops have introduced the disease. Emergency shipments of grain to supply food have often carried infected rats or fleas.[25] Crowding of refugees provides the opportunity for preexisting plague to become epidemic.[19] Under such circumstances, conventional methods of disease control may be impossible to apply.

5.10. Socioeconomic Factors

Historically, the lower income groups have had a higher incidence of plague than the more affluent. Factors involved include housing likely to harbor rats, locations near docks, warehouses, or granaries, plus crowding of occupants. During major epidemics in India, British subjects were rarely infected, presumably due to their higher living standards.[16]

6. Mechanisms and Routes of Transmission

The sources of *Y. pestis* for infection of man in order of frequency are infected fleas, fomites of pneumonic-plague cases, tissues of infected animals including carnivores from plague-infected areas, laboratory cultures, and flea feces. From these sources, infection can occur through the skin, the respiratory tract, the conjunctiva, and the digestive tract.

While flea bites constitute the most common route of

infection via the skin, transmission may also occur through abrasions or wounds in those who handle infected animals.

Mention was made in Section 1 of the entry of the organisms through the respiratory tract. Bacilli contained in large-particle aerosols lodge in the oropharynx with a resultant "tonsillar" plague, while smaller particles travel to the lower respiratory tract to enter the lymphatics with or without the production of pneumonia.[32] Tonsillar plague has also been associated with the practice of killing fleas by the affected subject having crushed them between his teeth.[32]

Infection through the conjunctiva may occur. This is of primary importance to those handling infected animals or engaged in laboratory activities without proper safeguards.

Finally, entry of *Y. pestis* through the digestive tract has been demonstrated in animals, and presumably the use of infected rodents for food in certain societies could produce a similar result.

7. Pathogenesis and Immunity

7.1. Pathogenesis

Following the bite of an infected flea, *Y. pestis* may be retained at the site, and in a few instances, a local skin lesion termed a phlyctenule appears. It is a small papule in the center of which there is a clear vesicle containing plague bacilli. Individuals with this lesion are considered to have a favorable prognosis.

With or without the cutaneous response, the organisms travel by way of the lymphatics to the nearest lymph nodes. The disease may be contained at this level (pestis minor), or there follows a bloodstream invasion. This septicemia may occur in the absence of any apparent local lymphatic involvement. As a result of septicemia, a percentage of bubonic-plague patients develop pneumonia. The factors that control this are not known, nor is there firm information concerning the efficiency of such individuals in the transmission of the disease to others by aerosols produced by the act of coughing. In some instances, many contacts become ill, and in other cases of pneumonic plague, without treatment, close family contacts remain healthy.

7.2. Incubation Period

For the main forms of plague, the incubation period is probably dose-dependent. The usual elapsed time between exposure and the appearance of overt bubonic plague is believed to be 3–6 days. For pneumonic plague, the period is from 1 to 10 days, with an average of 5 days.[20] In a vaccinated laboratory worker in the United States, the interval was 5 days[5]; in a vaccinated American in Vietnam, the interval was at least 8 days[23]; and in an unvaccinated South African exposed to a pneumonic-plague case, the incubation period was between 3 and 6 days.[20] In a well-studied epidemic in Vietnam, the initial case had an illness of 3 days' duration.[46] Six contacts were infected from this man. Three of these incubation periods could have been 3–6 days, two periods could have been 4–7 days, and the last could have been 5–8 days.

7.3. Immunity

Almost any statement regarding immunity to plague must be qualified. Rats trapped from areas where plague has occurred will survive challenge doses of *Y. pestis* that kill the same species taken from an area free of plague.[32] McCoy[28] believed that some rats had an innate resistance. Chen and Meyer[11] have studied this natural resistance in rats from a plague-free area. They found that the survivors of a small challenge inoculum (approximately an LD_{50}) might or might not show an antibody response. On rechallenge with a similar or larger inoculum, some animals with an antibody response survived, while most of those that had not shown evidence of antibodies died.

Humans show antibody responses to both clinical and subclinical infection. The first evidence of subclinical disease came in 1956 when it was demonstrated that some humans in Madagascar had plague antibodies and no history of illness.[38] In a group of Montagnards, living in a fortified village in Vietnam in 1967, 27 suspect cases of plague occurred in 5 weeks. With one exception, all were confirmed bacteriologically or by a rise in antibody titers. Of 37 unvaccinated asymptomatic contacts of these patients, 10 showed at least a fourfold rise in plague-antibody titers in bloods collected some 2 weeks apart. Another 8 contacts had significant titers in the initial sample. Antibodies were present in single samples from 8 of 21 contacts.

The significance of plague-antibody responses in human remains in question. For example, Butler and Hudson[7] described two plague patients in Vietnam who had recovered from bacteriologically confirmed plague 4 and 6 years previously and who began their second plague attacks with high titers of antibody to Fraction 1 antigen. These titers fell during convalescence. No explanation was attempted.

The problem of immunity also will be noted in Section 10.

8. Patterns of Host Response

The host response to *Y. pestis* is very diverse, ranging from an inapparent infection to pneumonia and death.

8.1. Clinical Features

For the typical case of bubonic plague, the description written in the 6th century by Procopius (see Section 2) is as applicable today as when it was written. Along with the tender, swollen mass of lymph nodes, fever may or may not be present. Prostration, headache, and malaise are common. During the course of the next 3–5 days, evidence of septicemia may appear, associated with mental confusion, subcutaneous hemorrhages, and shock in fatal cases. In patients who survive, there may or may not be suppuration of the bubo. Mild and severe cases may occur in the same epidemic.

In pneumonic plague, the onset may often be with a chill followed by fever, cough, and splinting of the chest, with the production of sputum that soon becomes bloody. Focal lung lesions are present, as manifested by dullness, decreased breath sounds, and roentgenographic evidence of infiltration. Mediastinal lymphadenopathy may be evident.[43] Without effective therapy, progress of the disease is rapid, with extensive lung consolidation, septicemia, prostration, mental confusion, subcutaneous hemorrhages due to intravascular coagulation,[6] and shock, with death ensuing in 2 or 3 days.

So-called cases of septicemic plague may occur in which the original portal of entry of the organism is unclear. Meningeal involvement is well known, but is an uncommon presenting picture.

8.2. Diagnosis

When plague occurs in epidemic form, recognition is usually not a problem. Conversely, the isolated case is often missed. Plague should be considered in any individual with adenopathy and a history of having been in an area known or suspected to harbor plague-infected animals. Bubonic plague has been confused with tularemia.[44] The latter is more likely to have an associated skin lesion. The mistake is not too serious, since both respond to the same therapy. Granuloma venereum and lymphogranuloma inguinale have been considered in the differential diagnosis, although neither has the rapidly progressive course of many cases of bubonic plague. In a nonepidemic case of bubonic plague, the diagnoses of incarcerated hernia and lymphoma were entertained.[13] In Vietnam in 1965, both plague and typhoid fever were epidemic, and *Salmonella typhosa* was isolated on several occasions from bubo aspirates or blood cultures from patients with plague.[23]

Pneumonic plague may be confused with any pneumonic involvement with a sudden onset, but again, a history of exposure to a patient or in a laboratory should be available to guide the physician.

As noted in Section 3.4.1, the presumptive diagnosis of plague can be made by finding the characteristic bipolar stained organisms in the bubo aspirate or in the sputum. Such a finding should result in starting specific therapy for plague. Should culture prove that an organism other than *Y. pestis* was present, the error is acceptable.

Plague is a reportable disease. Under international law, it is also a quarantinable disease. Prior to departure from an area where pneumonic plague is occurring, exposed personnel may be placed in isolation for 6 days. On arrival at their destination, international travelers may be held in surveillance for 6 days reckoned from the day of arrival.[3] These regulations antedate the use of prophylactic drugs. Contacts on drugs, as specified in Section 9.2, constitute little, if any, hazard to others, although they should be kept under supervision to ensure appropriate drug intake. The last confirmed plague case introduced into the United States was in 1924. A suspect case came from Vietnam in 1966.[13]

9. Control and Prevention

9.1. General Concepts

The major method of control is reduction of the likelihood of bites by infected fleas.

Known areas of sylvatic plague should be avoided by humans and their pets to the extent possible. Obviously, the use of such locales as campsites is unwise. Animals, alive or dead, are not to be handled.

When permanent habitations are located adjacent to areas of sylvatic plague, or when plague-infected rodents are in urban areas, the floors, walls, and roofs should be solid to avoid rat harborages. Accumulation of trash and the use of open food containers should not be permitted.

During epidemics of bubonic plague, it is mandatory that the initial control efforts be directed to the reduction of the flea population. Insecticides to which the fleas are susceptible should be applied to rodent burrows, nests, and trails. This should be done under the supervision of a qualified sanitarian. Concurrent tests must be set up to determine the presence or absence of resistant fleas. After reduction of the flea population, trapping or poisoning of rodents may be appropriate in limited areas.[1]

When first seen, bubonic-plague patients may still be carrying infected fleas, and for this reason their clothes should be sterilized or destroyed and the patient rid of fleas by the use of appropriate insecticides. If the site of exposure and of treatment are the same, such as the home, insecticide application to protect those providing care may be desirable.

To reduce the interhuman transfer risk, suspect pneumonic-plague patients should be placed in strict isolation, whether treated at home or in a hospital, contacts being limited to those necessary to provide proper care. The sputum of pneumonic-plague patients contains very large numbers of organisms, but appropriate therapy causes a prompt and marked decrease in a matter of hours. All excreta and bed linens should be sterilized before disposal. Persons in contact with pneumonic-plague patients should wear face masks and glasses or goggles, and all are to be maintained on a prophylactic drug until 7 days after the last case has been cured or has died.[1]

9.2. Antibiotic and Chemotherapeutic Approaches to Prophylaxis

Drug prophylaxis is advisable for all immediate associates of a patient with bubonic plague who may have been exposed at the same time. This includes members of the household, visitors, and hunting companions.

Drug prophylaxis is essential for all contacts of patients with pneumonic plague. This is for the welfare of the individuals concerned and for the successful control of the epidemic. Those who refuse drug prophylaxis should be placed in custody for 7 days.

Recommended chemoprophylaxis is 15 mg tetracycline/kg body wt daily in divided doses for a week after exposure. Alternatively, 40 mg of a sulfonamide/kg body wt on a similar schedule may be used.[1] It is necessary to emphasize that in some areas of the world, individuals with malaria or trypanosomiasis or some other febrile illnesses may become ill with plague.

Streptomycin resistance of laboratory strains of *Y. pestis* is known, and such strains appear to be fully virulent for animals. A streptomycin-resistant strain of *Y. pestis* was isolated from a rat spleen pool in Vietnam in 1965.[23] During 1965–1966, two more such strains were isolated from humans in Vietnam.[21] In the same time period, nine tetracycline-resistant strains were isolated from Vietnamese patients.

9.3. Immunization

Since 1895, a variety of vaccines have been used. The protective value of any of these is still a matter of debate. After vaccination and after recovery from plague, antibodies to many antigens are present.[4]

Some indirect evidence may be noted. Serum from animals immunized by the administration of killed *Y. pestis* provided some protection when administered to test animals or to humans with plague. Sokhey[45] (cited from Hirst[15]) in India reported a case mortality of 25% of 94 serum-treated cases as compared to 82% among the controls.

In some countries, living "avirulent" *Y. pestis* organisms have been used as a vaccine. Studies in the United States have confirmed that such preparations are effective in experimental animals, but they were not considered safe for use in man.[35,36]

Since 1942, the vaccine licensed for use in the United States has been a formalin-killed suspension of whole virulent plague bacilli with phenol added as a preservative. Different strains of *Y. pestis* have been used, the quantity of organisms per dose has been varied, and the dose schedule has been altered repeatedly.[26] All workers seem to agree that sequential inoculations are necessary. In World War II, vaccinated Americans had no plague despite documented exposure.[34] In Vietnam during 1961–1971, there were eight cases in vaccinated Americans while thousands of cases occurred in the indigenous peoples.[9,10]

In 117 laboratory workers who received from 10 to 51 injections of a killed plague vaccine over a 20-year period, there were 10 who failed to produce antibody levels deemed to be protective, while 23 had intermediate responses and 84 had high levels. Persistence of antibody for as long as 6 years after the last vaccination was noted. Following several episodes in which it was believed that some of these vaccinees had been exposed to virulent *Y. pestis,* an abrupt rise in antibody titer was observed.[27]

In Vietnam in 1969, rats were found to be infected with *Rickettsia mooseri* and with *Y. pestis.* Acute and convalescent sera were collected from 59 Americans who had received killed plague vaccine and who were suffering from clinical and serologically proved murine typhus. Fraction 1 antibody was found in the initial sera of 39 individuals, and this was attributed to prior vaccination. Tests on convalescent sera showed a greater than fourfold rise in 4 patients with preexisting titers, and in 3 instances antibodies were present when there had been none in the original samples. This was interpreted as evidence of a dual infection, with plague being subclinical as a result of prior vaccination.[10] This conclusion must be tempered in light of the large number of inapparent infections in unvaccinated individuals elsewhere in Vietnam.[19]

A 1973 report describes the serological response in Americans initially receiving 2×10^9 organisms followed by 4×10^8 bacilli on days 90 and 270. Of 29 subjects, 2 did not develop antibodies at a level considered to be protective.[2] Whether the lack of response is evidence of immunity or susceptibility is unknown.

In typhoid fever and in tuleremia,[16,29] carefully controlled studies in volunteers have shown that vaccinated individuals have some protection against small inocula of virulent challenge organisms, but that large numbers of such challenge organisms will override this "protection" and produce overt disease. It seems not unlikely that a comparable level of protection exists after vaccination against plague. In an effort to sum up the value of killed *Y. pestis* vaccine, one can best quote the late Dr. K. F. Meyer, who, in a lecture at the Walter Reed Army Institute of Research in 1950, indicated that in his opinion, the killed vaccine favorably altered the susceptibility of the recipients to infection with plague bacilli.

10. Unresolved Problems

Little is known about the components of *Y. pestis* that are responsible for "virulence," and there is a similar lack with respect to the significant antigens of this organism. Obviously, information on both subjects would be highly desirable.

Human "inapparent" infections are well known in some parts of the world. Whether these are due to host characteristics or to a decreased virulence of the organisms is unknown. Continued studies of atypical organisms deserve priority. The relative rarity of the disease in the world today may be a barrier to research on the pathogenesis and response in the human host.

Enzootic foci are widespread and readily available for examination. The persistence or nonpersistence of enzootic plague seems to be based on a complex interplay between susceptible and resistant rodents, their fleas, the habitations of the people, and climate. Thus, in this century, plague has been introduced repeatedly into the British Isles,[42] Ghana,[41] and Malaya,[14] but has failed to become an established problem. If this zoonosis is as complex and as delicately balanced as is suggested, perhaps continued investigation would allow protection of man by reduction or elimination of the enzootic cycle.

11. References

1. BAHMANYAR, M., AND CAVANAUGH, D. C., *Plague Manual,* World Health Organization, Geneva, 1976.
2. BARTELLONI, P. J., MARSHALL, J. D., JR., AND CAVANAUGH, D. C., Clinical and serological responses to plague vaccine U.S.P., *Mil. Med.* **138:**720–722 (1973).
3. BENENSON, A. S. (ed.), *Control of Communicable Diseases in Man,* 13th ed., American Public Health Association, Washington, D.C., 1981.
4. BRUBAKER, R. R., The genus *Yersinia:* Biochemistry and genetics of virulence, *Curr. Top. Microbiol. Immunol.* **57:**111–158 (1972).
5. BURMEISTER, R. W., TIGERTT, W. D., AND OVERHOLT, E. L., Laboratory-acquired pneumonic plague, *Ann. Intern. Med.* **56:**789–800 (1962).
6. BUTLER, T., A clinical study of bubonic plague: Observations of the 1970 Vietnam epidemic with emphasis on coagulation studies, skin histology, and electrocardiograms, *Am. J. Med.* **53:**268–276 (1972).
7. BUTLER, T., AND HUDSON, B. W., The serologic response to *Yersinia pestis* infection, *Bull. WHO* **55:**39–42 (1977).
8. CAVANAUGH, D. C., AND MARSHALL, J. D., JR., The influence of climate on the seasonal prevalence of plague in the Republic of Vietnam, *J. Wildl. Dis.* **8:**85–94 (1972).
9. CAVANAUGH, D. C., DANGERFIELD, H. G., HUNTER, D. H., JOY, R. J. T., MARSHALL, J. D., JR., QUY, D. V., VIVANO, S., AND WINTER, P. E., Some observations on the current plague outbreak in the Republic of Vietnam, *Am. J. Public Health* **58:**742–752 (1968).
10. CAVANAUGH, D. C., ELISBERG, B. L., LLEWELLYN, C. H., MARSHALL, J. D., JR., RUST, J. H., WILLIAMS, J. E., AND MEYER, K. F., Plague immunization. V. Indirect evidence for the efficacy of plague vaccination, *J. Infect. Dis.* **129**(Suppl.):S37–S49 (1974).
11. CHEN, T. H., AND MEYER, K. F., Susceptibility and antibody response of *Rattus* species to experimental plague, *J. Infect. Dis.* **129**(Suppl.):S62–S71 (1974).
12. CHUBB, T. C., *The Life of Giovanni Boccaccio,* p. 161, Albert and Charles Boni, New York, 1930.
13. DICKERSON, M. S., Suspected case of imported bubonic plague—Texas, *Morbid. Mortal.* **15:**377–378 (1966).
14. GREEN, R., Plague, in: *Studies from the Institute for Medical Research* (J. W. FIELD, R. GREEN, AND F. E. BYRON, eds.), pp. 243–252, Government Press, Kuala Lumpur, Malaysia, 1951.
15. HIRST, L. F., *The Conquest of Plague,* Oxford University Press, London, 1953.
16. HORNICK, R. B., GRIESMAN, S. E., WOODWARD, T. E., DAWKINS, A. T., AND SNYDER, M. J., Typhoid fever: Pathogenesis and immunologic control, *N. Engl. J. Med.* **283:**686–691, 739–746 (1970).
17. Human plague in 1985, *WHO Weekly Epidemiol. Rec.* **61:**273–274 (1987).
18. LEGTERS, L. J., COTTINGHAM, A. J., JR., AND HUNTER, D. H., Comparison of serological and bacteriological methods in the confirmation of plague infections, *Bull. WHO* **41:**859–863 (1969).
19. LEGTERS, L. J., COTTINGHAM, A. J., AND HUNTER, D. H., Clinical and epidemiological notes on a defined outbreak of plague in Vietnam, *Am. J. Trop. Med. Hyg.* **19:**639–652 (1970).
20. LEWIN, W., BECKER, B. J. P., AND HORWITZ, B., Two cases of pneumonic plague: Recovery of one case treated with streptomycin, *S. Afr. Med. J.* **22:**699–703 (1948).
21. LOUIS, J., Sensibilité "in vitro" de *Yersinia pestis* à quelques antibiotiques et sulfamides, *Med. Trop.* **27:**313–317 (1967).
22. MARKS, G., AND BEATTY, W. K., *Epidemics,* pp. 44–48, Scribner's, New York, 1946.
23. MARSHALL, J. D., JR., JOY R. J. T., AI, N. V., QUY, D. V., STOCKARD, J. L., AND GIBSON, F. L., Plague in Vietnam 1965–1966, *Am. J. Epidemiol.* **86:**603–616 (1967).
24. MARSHALL, J. D., JR., QUY, D. V., AND GIBSON, F. L., Asymptomatic pharyngeal plague infection in Vietnam, *Am. J. Trop. Med. Hyg.* **16:**175–177 (1967).
25. MARSHALL, J. D., JR., QUY, D. V., GIBSON, F. L., DUNG, T. C., AND CAVANAUGH, D. C., Ecology of plague in Vietnam. I. Role of *Suncus murinus, Proc. Soc. Exp. Biol. Med.* **124:**1083–1086 (1967).
26. MARSHALL, J. D., JR., BARTELLONI, P. J., CAVANAUGH, D. C., KADULL, P. J., AND MEYER, K. F., Plague immunization. II. Relation of adverse clinical reactions to multiple immunizations with killed vaccine, *J. Infect. Dis.* **129**(Suppl.):S19–S25 (1974).
27. MARSHALL, J. D., JR., CAVANAUGH, D. A., BARTELLONI, P. J., AND MEYER, K. F., Plague immunization. III. Serologic response to multiple inoculations of vaccine, *J. Infect. Dis.* **129**(Suppl.):S26–S29 (1974).
28. MCCOY, G. W., Immunity of wild rats (*Mus norvegicus*) to plague infection, *Public Health Bull.* **53:**12–14 (1912).
29. MCCRUMB, F. R., JR., Aerosol infection of man with *Pasteurella tularensis, Bacteriol. Rev.* **25:**262–267 (1961).
30. MCCRUMB, F. R., JR., MERCIER, S., ROBIC, J., BOUILLAT, M., SMADEL, J. E., WOODWARD, T. E., AND GOODNER, K., Chloramphenicol and Terramycin in the treatment of pneumonic plague, *Am. J. Med.* **14:**284–293 (1953).
31. MEYER, K. F., Pneumonic plague, *Bacteriol. Rev.* **25:**249–261 (1961).
32. MEYER, K. F., *Pasteurella and Francisella,* in: *Bacterial and Mycotic Infections of Man* (R. J. DUBOS AND J. G. HIRSCH, eds.), pp. 659–697, Lippincott, Philadelphia, 1965.
33. MEYER, K. F., CONNOR, C. L., SMYTH, F. S., AND EDDIE, B., Chronic relapsing meningeal plague, *Arch. Intern. Med.* **59:**967–980 (1937).
34. MEYER, K. F., AND MCCOY, O. R., Plague, in: *Preventive Medicine in World War II* (J. B. COATES, JR., ed.), Volume 7, pp. 79–100, U.S. Government Printing Office, Washington, D.C., 1964.
35. MEYER, K. F., CAVANAUGH, D. C., BARTELLONI, P. J., AND

MARSHALL, J. D., JR., Plague immunization. I. Past and present trends, *J. Infect. Dis.* **129**(Suppl.).:S13–S18 (1974).

36. MEYER, K. F., SMITH, G., FOSTER, L., BROOKMAN, M., AND SUNG, M., Live, attenuated *Yersinia pestis* vaccine: Virulent in nonhuman primates, harmless to guinea pigs, *J. Infect. Dis.* **129**(Suppl.):S85–S120 (1974).

37. *Oxford English Dictionary,* Volume III, p. 73, Oxford University Press, London, 1933.

38. PAYNE, F. E., SMADEL, J. E., AND COURDURIER, J., Immunologic studies on persons residing in a plague endemic area, *J. Immunol.* **77**:24–33 (1956).

39. POLLITZER, R., Plague, *WHO Monogr. Ser.* **22**:14 (1954).

40. Reports of the U.S. Army Medical Research Team, Walter Reed Army Institute of Research, Saigon, Vietnam, 1961–1971.

41. SCOTT, D., *Epidemic Disease in Ghana, 1901–1960,* pp. 1–25, Oxford University Press, London, 1965.

42. SHREWSBURY, J. F. D., *A History of Bubonic Plague in the British Isles,* Cambridge University Press, London, 1970.

43. SITES, V. R., AND POLAND, J. D., Mediastinal lymphadenopathy in bubonic plague, *Am. J. Roentgenol. Radium Ther. Nucl. Med.* **66**:567–570 (1972).

44. SITES, V. R., POLAND, J. D., AND HUDSON, B. W., Bubonic plague misdiagnosed as tularemia: Retrospective serologic diagnosis, *J. Am. Med. Assoc.* **222**:1642–1643 (1972).

45. SOKHEY, S. S., *Report of the Haffkine Institute for 1938,* Bombay Government Central Press, 1939.

46. TRONG, R., NHU, T. Q., AND MARSHALL, J. D., JR., A mixed pneumonic bubonic plague outbreak in Vietnam, *Mil. Med.* **132**:93–97 (1967).

47. WERNER, S. B., WEIDMER, C. E., NELSON, B. C., NYGAARD, G. S., GOETHALS, R. N., AND POLAND, J. D., Primary plague pneumonia contracted from a domestic cat at South Lake Tahoe, Calif., *J. Am. Med. Assoc.* **252**:929–931 (1984).

48. WILLIAMS, J. E., MARSHALL, J. D., JR., SCHABERG, D. M., HUNTLEY, R. F., HARRISON, D. N., AND CAVANAUGH, D. C., Antibody and resistance to infection with *Yersinia pestis* in the progeny of immunized rats, *J. Infect. Dis.* **129**(Suppl):S72–S77 (1974).

49. WILLIAMS, J. E., HARRISON, D. N., QUAN, T. J., MULLINS, J. L., BARNES, A. M., AND CAVANAUGH, D. C., Atypical plague bacilli isolated from rodents, fleas, and man, *Am. J. Public Health* **68**:262–264 (1978).

50. WILLIAMS, J. E., ARNTZEN, L., TYNDAL, G. L., AND ISAACSON, M., Application of enzyme immunoassays for the confirmation of clinically suspect plague in Namibia, 1982, *Bull. WHO* **64**:745–752 (1986).

51. ZIEGLER, R., *The Black Death,* p. 15, John Day, New York, 1969.

52. ZINSSER, H., *Rats, Lice and History,* p. 91, Little, Brown, Boston, 1935.

12. Suggested Reading

BAHMANYAR, M., AND CAVANAUGH, D. C., *Plague Manual,* World Health Organization, Geneva, 1976. (This manual is an absolute requirement for any physician or laboratorian who must deal with or consider the problems of plague.)

BALTAZARD, M., Séance spéciale consacrée à la mémoir de Georges Blanc: Étude de l'épidémiologie de la peste dans le Kurdistan Iranien, *Bull. Soc. Pathol. Exot.* **56**:1101–1246 (1963). (This paper is a summary of investigations on plague in the Middle East.)

GREEN, R., Plague, in: *Studies from the Institute for Medical Research* (J. W. FIELD, R. GREEN, AND F. E. BYRON, eds.), pp. 243–252, Government Press, Kuala Lumpur, Malaysia, 1951.

HIRST, L. F., *The Conquest of Plague,* Oxford University Press, London, 1953. (This book is recommended reading to learn of the activities in the Indian subcontinent in the early years of this century, presented by a very astute student of plague.)

LINK, V. B., *A History of Plague in the United States,* U.S. Public Health Service Monogr. No. 26, Washington, D.C., 1955.

Plague in the Americas, Pan American Health Organization, Washington, D.C., 1965.

POLLITZER, R., Plague, *WHO Monogr. Ser.* **22** (1954).

POLLITZER, R., *Plague and Plague Control in the Soviet Union: History and Bibliography through 1964,* Fordham University, New York, 1966.

SHREWSBURY, J. F. D., *A History of Bubonic Plague in the British Isles,* Cambridge University Press, London, 1970. (The author's primary interest is in the impact of plague on the social structure of the country.)

WILSON, G. S., AND MILES, A., *Principles of Bacteriology, Virology and Immunity,* Volume II, pp. 2120–2138, Williams & Wilkins, Baltimore, 1975. (This readily accessible text contains an excellent review of the early studies of plague in the Indian subcontinent.)

WU LIEN TEH, *A Treatise on Pneumonic Plague,* League of Nations, Geneva, 1926. (This treatise is the classic description of plague.)

CHAPTER 25

Pneumococcal Infections

Robert S. Baltimore and Eugene D. Shapiro

1. Introduction

The pneumococcus (*Streptococcus pneumoniae*) is a major cause of pneumonia and meningitis worldwide. In his classic book entitled *The Biology of the Pneumococcus* published in 1938, Benjamin White[162] listed 19 different names applied to the pneumococcus between 1897 and 1930, the year when the 4th edition of *Bergey's Manual*[15] approved the designation *Diplococcus pneumoniae* Weichselbaum. In a more recent (8th) edition of *Bergey's Manual*,[26] it is listed as *Streptococcus pneumoniae*, the designation now generally accepted.

Although any of a large number of microorganisms may cause acute inflammation of the lungs (pneumonia),[51] typical (primary) lobar pneumonia is nearly always caused by the pneumococcus, which is also the most frequent cause of bronchopneumonia. Pneumococcal pneumonia of either variety is generally preceded by a simple acute infection of the upper respiratory tract such as the common cold and may also occur as a complication of influenza. It has been called "captain of the men of death" and "the friend of the aged" because it had long been the

principal immediate cause and most frequent contributing cause of death in the aged and infirm and in those with otherwise fatal diseases. Since public-health statistics of morbidity and mortality are usually reported by diseases and not by etiological agents, most of the references are to data on "pneumonia," of which the majority are presumed to be due to the pneumococcus, except during unusual epidemics due to other organisms.

The pneumococcus is also the most frequent cause of acute bacterial meningitis over age 15, being exceeded in frequency only by the meningococcus during periods of epidemic prevalence.[53] The pneumococcus is also the most frequent cause of purulent empyema of the pleura[54] (usually as a complication of primary pneumonia) and of otitis media at all ages.[83] Less frequently, it may cause focal infections at other sites in the body. It is also the most common organism cultured from the blood of patients with acute febrile illness, usually pneumonia or meningitis, but not infrequently also from infants and young children with no demonstrable localized site of infection.[97,148]

2. Historical Background

The early history of the discovery of the pneumococcus and its pathogenic potentials for animals and man was presented chronologically and in some detail by White,[162] subsequently by Finland,[49] and recently and more concisely by Austrian[8] in 1981. According to the latter, the pneumococcus was probably first visualized in pulmonary

Robert S. Baltimore and Eugene D. Shapiro · Departments of Pediatrics and Epidemiology and Public Health, Yale University School of Medicine, New Haven, Connecticut 06510. The first edition of this chapter was written by the late Maxwell Finland. In this chapter, significant parts of the background and epidemiologic data come from Dr. Finland's manuscript.

tissues by Klebs in 1875, later by Eberth in 1880, and then by Koch in 1881. However, the organism was first isolated in the laboratory independently by Pasteur in France and Sternberg in the United States and reported by both in 1881; both these workers had injected saliva subcutaneously in rabbits, who died and were shown to have the organisms in large numbers in their blood. Pasteur used saliva of an infant that died of rabies; Sternberg injected his own saliva. Both thus demonstrated the occurrence of pneumococcus in the pharynges in carriers without relation to disease.

During the next few years, a considerable controversy resulted from the descriptions and characterizations of the bacteria seen in pneumonic lungs by Friedlander, Weichselbaum, and Freinkel (quoted by Austrian[8]); this was eventually resolved by the application of the Gram stain described in 1884. The stain permitted the differentiation of Friedlander's bacillus, now known as *Klebsiella pneumoniae,* which was decolorized by the Gram method (gramnegative), from the pneumococcus, which was not decolorized (gram-positive).

During the late 1880s, reports were published of the presence of pneumococci in focal infections other than those of the lung, including valvular lesions of cases of endocarditis, purulent meningitis, otitis, arthritis, sinusitis, conjunctivitis, and from other organs and sites.

At the turn of the century, Neufeld[103] reported on the solubility of pneumococci in bile, which became a useful tool in the differentiation of pneumococci from other streptococci, especially the viridans variety. Most important were the demonstrations of the development of antibodies against the homologous pneumococcus following infection or vaccination, which protected animals against subsequent infection with that organism, and the description of the specific agglutination and Quellung reactions in homologous antisera by Neufeld[104] in 1902. The agglutination reaction led to the more definite segregation of pneumococci into specific types in 1913 by Lister[88] in South Africa and by Dochez and Gillespie[42] at the Rockefeller Institute in New York. Some partially successful attempts were made to protect the highly susceptible workers in the gold and diamond mines in South Africa by vaccination with mixtures of these pneumococcal types.[89,110] This also led to the development of specific antisera for therapy and the use of the agglutination reaction to identify the causative type before administering the therapeutic antisera. It was not until 1931, however, that Armstrong[6] in England first reported the clinical use of the Quellung reaction for the rapid typing of pneumococci, which was then popularized in the United States by Sabin.[127] By 1932, Cooper *et al.*[38] in New York City had segregated more than 30 specific types;

subsequently, workers in the United States and in Denmark increased that number to the more than 80 types known at present.[93] The typing of pneumococci and the type-specific antibody response to infection or to immunization, first with whole organisms[165] and later with type-specific capsular polysaccharides,[80] proved to be potent tools that enhanced the capabilities for epidemiological studies of pneumococcal infections[128] and offered the possibility of control of infections in individuals and in susceptible population groups.

Meanwhile, progress was being made, notably at the Rockefeller Institute, in delineating the biology of the pneumococcus and its biochemical constituents and immunogenic properties. Most important was the demonstration that the type specificity, pathogenicity (virulence), and eventually also its immunogenicity resided in the specific chemical composition of its capsular polysaccharide. When purified, this component proved to be essentially nontoxic when injected in humans and capable of inducing typespecific antibodies in varying quantities. When it was also shown that 80% of all serious and life-threatening pneumococcal infections, bacteremia, meningitis, endocarditis, and infections of normally sterile body cavities were caused by only 14 of the known 80 or more types, a vaccine incorporating these 14 types was made available,[80] and early trials showed it to be effective in many circumstances. Its effects on the control of pneumococcal infections are a major subject of contemporary investigation of pneumococcal disease. A separate section of this chapter is devoted to pneumococcal vaccine.

3. Methodology

3.1. Sources of Epidemiological Data

In introducing his chapter on the epidemiology of pneumonia, Heffron[74] indicated that the absolute frequency of its occurrence is unknown. Statistics from various health organizations throughout the world provide information on the total number of deaths from all causes, including pneumonia, but in many instances, especially in Africa, where the disease is widely prevalent, deaths are frequently unreported and inaccurate. In the United States, pneumonia and influenza deaths from 121 cities are reported in MMWR but are generally regarded as an index of influenza mortality. In 1934, Collins and Gover[35] reported that acute infections of the respiratory tract caused more deaths and a higher morbidity in the United States than did any other group of diseases. However, it is impossible in the United

States or elsewhere to obtain exact figures on morbidity or mortality because pneumonia has not been a reportable disease in most states; it is estimated that even in those states wherein it is reportable, only about half the cases are actually reported. Also, there is no uniform method of reporting cases (as lobar pneumonia, bronchopneumonia, or both). In temperate zones, lobar pneumonia, but not bronchopneumonia, has a definite seasonal incidence, but their differentiation is often impossible. In the United States, the best estimate of the incidence of pneumococcal pneumonia has come from special surveys (see Section 3.2). Pneumococcal meningitis, while also not a reportable disease, has been included in special meningitis surveys.[30]

3.2. Surveys

A number of surveys have been carried out to estimate the incidence of pneumonia. These include a population study of 2,602,000 people conducted by the federal government for 1935–1963, data from the Cleveland family study reported in 1936, health records from the Kaiser-Permanente Health Center, and reports from hospitals such as the large retrospective regional study performed in Sweden 1964–1980.[28] These have been summarized by Mufson,[100] Austrian,[8] and the CDC[31] and are presented in Section 5.1. Antibody surveys have not been reported except when associated with vaccine trials. The assays are not sufficiently specific to use in establishing estimates of incidence.

3.3. Laboratory Diagnosis

3.3.1. Isolation and Identification of the Organism. Growth of pneumococci requires suitable media such as nutrient broth to which serum or defibrinated blood, preferably rabbit's or sheep's, is added. For epidemiological purposes, however, reliance is placed on three methods: (1) direct culture on solid media (blood agar); (2) mouse inoculation, particularly of materials that may contain mixed cultures, such as sputum or broth-moistened swabs of environmental materials; mouse peritoneal exudate may be withdrawn by capillary pipette after 3 or 4 h, mixed with specific sera, stained, and examined for type-specific agglutination[126]; (3) application of the Neufeld Quellung method to cultures or to fresh materials (sputum, exudate, blood cultures) for specific typing of pneumococci. Use of the Quellung test has the advantage of being type-specific for the pneumococcus; it can rapidly diagnose the type and also detect multiple types of pneumococci in the same specimen (e.g., in sputum, mouse peritoneal exudate, environmental swab, or any purulent materials). Currently, ag-

glutination of antibody-coated latex beads has replaced the Quelling test in many laboratories and can be used for rapid identification in the laboratory by testing culture supernates. For cultures of materials from air, dust, skin, or fomites, broth-moistened swabs of the material or surfaces may be streaked directly on blood agar, and characteristic colonies of pneumococci are easily recognized after incubation for 12–24 h (as are those of hemolytic or viridans streptococci and staphylococci). The swab may then be placed in blood broth and pneumococci identified from subcultures on blood agar or by mouse inoculation or both. Initiation of growth of pneumococci may be enhanced by incubation in 5% carbon dioxide or in a candle jar. Additional cultures in broth and mouse inoculation enhance the yield. Nasal or pharyngeal swabs may be plated directly on blood agar, or cultivated in broth and some of the latter inoculated into mice after incubation for 3–4 h. Prior exposure to sulfonamides or antibiotics (during prophylaxis or therapy) markedly reduces or may eliminate the chance of growing pneumococci from the nose and throat.

3.3.2. Serological Methods. Serological tests for demonstrating type-specific antibodies include opsonic or pneumococcidal tests in fresh defibrinated or heparinized whole blood, the mouse protection test on serum, macroscopic or microscopic agglutination of heat- or formalin-killed suspensions of organisms, or precipitin and diffusion tests with supernatant fluids of cultures or exudates or with type-specific polysaccharides. These tests differ in sensitivity and also somewhat in specificity. Specific antibody has been quantitated with specific polysaccharides and used in surveys for susceptibility in relation to immunization and to measure the response to polysaccharide vaccines.[128] A highly type-specific radioimmunoassay (RIA) and enzyme-linked immunoassay (ELISA) can also be used to derive similar data,[123,129] and most recent information on responses to pneumococcal vaccine is based on this method.

4. Biological Characteristics of the Organism

Morphologically, the pneumococcus typically appears as an ovoid or spherical, coccoidlike form of 0.5–1.25 μm, in pairs, the distal ends of which tend to be pointed or lancet-shaped, and surrounded by a distinguishable capsule that contains a polysaccharide [soluble specific substance (SSS)]. The diplococci may occur in chains, particularly in liquid medium, hence the designation streptococcus. The chemical composition of the SSS determines its specific serological type, of which there are now at least 83, including several that are closely related serologically. The diplococci usually stain gram-positive, but may decolorize and appear gram-negative in old cultures or after exposure to antibacterial agents. When grown on blood agar, pneumococci form clear, round, mucoid, colorless, umbilicated colonies surrounded by an area of green hemolysis. Heavily capsulated organisms, such as those of type 3, grow in dome-shaped, clear, mucoid colonies.

Resistance of pneumococci to chemotherapeutic agents was recognized as emerging during therapy with ethylhydrocupreine (optochin) in 1918, the first chemical to receive extensive clinical trials in pneumonia.[99] Resistance to sulfapyridine was also recognized as a possible cause of failure of that drug in the treatment of pneumococcal pneumonia in 1938.[92,161] Although significant resistance of pneumococci to penicillin has been infrequent and limited in geographic distribution, resistance to other antibacterial agents has been reported from many areas and has accounted for therapeutic failures. Reports have included resistance to sulfonamides, tetracycline, erythromycin, lincomycin, and chloramphenicol in addition to β-lactam antibiotics.[4,159] Pneumococci are also relatively resistant to aminoglycosides, and some are highly resistant to streptomycin. Multiantibiotic-resistant pneumococci have been reported from South Africa and in occasional strains isolated in the United States (see Section 5.1.1). Drug-resistant organisms, especially those isolated from individuals undergoing treatment with effective antibiotics, are often reduced in virulence for mice.

5. Descriptive Epidemiology

5.1. Prevalence and Incidence

In the United States, a federal government survey over a 12-month period in 1935 that involved over 2.6 million people in 83 widely scattered cities and 24 rural counties suggested an incidence rate of 558 cases of pneumonia per 100,000.[9] Data from several centers reported for 1920–1928 indicated that deaths from pneumonia generally accounted for 7.4–8.3% of deaths from all causes. On the basis of recent data from various sources, Austrian[9] estimated ("with limited confidence") that the attack rate of pneumococcal pneumonia in the United States lies somewhere in the range of 1.5–10 (more likely between 2 and 5)/1000 man-years of exposure.

The Cleveland study of illness in middle-class families comprising 292 adults and their school-aged children reported in 1953, has been summarized by Austrian.[9] There

were three illnesses diagnosed as pneumococcal over a 3-year period, 1974–1976, an attack rate of 10.3/1000 man-years. At the Kaiser-Permanente Health Center, the estimated attack rate of pneumococcal pneumonia of all types was 1.4/1000 among Californians 45 years of age or older. However, among institutionalized patients, the attack rate was calculated to be 12.5/1000 for pneumonia due to all pneumococcal types.[9]

Data on incidence of pneumococcal infections has come from the CDC[31] and from a detailed review of morbidity and mortality by Mufson.[100] Table 1 depicts the CDC estimates in the early 1980s of the rates per 100,000 of pneumococcal pneumonia of 68–260, of pneumococcal meningitis of 1.2–2.8, and of pneumococcal bacteremia of 7–25; the case-fatality rates of these syndromes have been 5–7, 32, and 20%, respectively.[31] Mufson's estimates of incidence, converted to rates per 100,000, were 100–200 for pneumonia and 0.3–4.9 for pneumococcal meningitis based on published studies from the mid-1970s. Higher rates of pneumococcal infection were observed in patients with sickle-cell anemia, congenital asplenia, renal transplants, Hodgkin's disease, and multiple myeloma than in subjects without these preexisting conditions.[100]

The importance of *S. pneumoniae* in different clinical syndromes and at different ages has been reviewed by Klein[83] in infants and children and by Mufson[100] in the general population. On the basis of recent cooperative studies, the pneumococcus was shown to be the most common pathogen cultured from the respiratory tract in infants (other than neonates) and children, and it is also the most frequent cause of serious infections, including pneumonia and bacteremia.[83]

In the general population of nine cities, *S. pneumoniae* was the most common cause of community-acquired pneumonia requiring hospitalization: pneumococcal pneumonia accounted for 26–78% of all pneumonia cases in the nine areas and in most studies exceeded 50%.[100] The mortality

Table 1. Estimated Occurrence of Serious Pneumococcal Disease, United States[a]

Pneumococcal disease	Estimated cases (thousands per year)	Estimated incidence per 100,000	Case-fatality rate (%)
Pneumonia	150–570	68–260	5–7
Meningitis	2.6–6.2	1.2–2.8	32
Bacteremia	16–55	7–25	20

[a]Data derived from limited surveys, research reports, and several community-based studies as summarized in the MMWR.[31]

rate varied from 6 to 19%, but was 2–5 times higher in the 20% of adults who developed bacteremia. Indeed, this organism is the most common cause of bacteremia in adults, as well as in children over 1 month old.[100]

Pneumococcal meningitis occurs at a rate of about 0.3–4.9 persons/100,000, with children under age 5 at higher risk.[100] In a summary from the CDC reviewing reports of meningitis from 38 states in 1978, the incidence per 100,000 of *S. pneumoniae* meningitis was 0.30.[30] It was exceeded by *H. influenzae* meningitis and *Neisseria meningitidis* meningitis, with rates per 100,000 of 1.24 and 0.72, respectively. The incidence of pneumococcal meningitis was highest in the first year of life (age-specific rate of 8.0/100,000). While the absolute incidence is much less in older age groups (0.1–0.4/100,000), its *relative* importance increases, and this organism is the most common cause of meningitis for elderly individuals in the United States. *S. pneumoniae* is also the most common aerobic organism grown from blood of febrile infants and children in whom no focus of infection is determined. The highest rate of pneumococcal carriage in the United States is also among preschool children; it is somewhat lower in older children and is about the same in adolescents as in adults, but in the last two groups, carriers are more frequent in households with preschool children.

About one-third of all pneumococcal disease affects the respiratory tract, another one-third is associated with focal infections (mostly otitis media), and one-third is associated with fever and bacteremia without a discernible focus.[97,148] The pneumococcus is the most frequent organism grown from middle-ear fluid; the most common types in such fluid are 3, 9, 19, and 23, the same as in healthy carriers. The most frequent types in bacteremia and meningitis are 6, 15, 18, 19, and 23. Healthy carriers may harbor the same serotypes as are encountered in invasive infections but carrier strains are often the higher-numeral types rarely associated with disease.

5.1.1. Occurrence of Penicillin-Resistant Pneumococci. Since penicillin has been the antibiotic of choice for most severe and milder cases of pneumococcal infections, there has been monitoring of pneumococci worldwide for susceptibility to this agent. Pneumococci have generally been inhibited by less than 0.05 μg/ml of penicillin. In the literature there are sporadic reports of strains relatively resistant, with minimum inhibitory concentrations (MIC) of 0.1 to 1.0 μg/ml of penicillin. Strains with this range of susceptibility have been termed relatively or intermediately resistant strains because they are clearly less susceptible than are usual strains, but in the absence of meningitis, infections due to these strains are often successfully treated

with high doses of penicillin.[159] In a case–control study of 18 patients from whom relatively resistant strains of pneumococci were isolated, there was no difference in prior antibiotic treatment or other infectious disease in the household, compared with matched patients from whom susceptible strains were isolated.[125] Response to antibiotic therapy was less prompt but the number of patients was too small for this to be statistically evaluated. These strains have been reported with low-frequency prevalence worldwide since 1967 when a well-documented case of respiratory infection due to a pneumococcal strain with an MIC of 0.6 μg/ml of penicillin G was reported from Sydney, Australia.[71] The patient involved was a 25-year-old with hypogammaglobulinemia and bronchiectasis who had received many courses of antibiotic treatment in the past. Since then there have been many reports of such isolates. Pneumococcal serotype does not appear to correlate with intermediate or relative resistance.[40,159]

Beginning in South Africa in 1977,[5,78] there have been reports of pneumococcal isolates resistant to penicillin with MICs at 2–10 μg/ml. These strains generally had resistance to multiple antibiotics including tetracyclines, streptomycin, chloramphenicol, erythromycin, clindamycin, and sulfonamides. In a recent study of patients with pneumococcal pneumonia from whom resistant strains were isolated, it appeared that only strains with an MIC of penicillin of > 2 μg/ml were resistant to treatment with high-dose penicillin *in vivo*.[111] Only a small number of pneumococcal serotypes have been associated with high-level resistance. Generally the level of resistance to penicillin correlates with resistance to all semisynthetic penicillins and cephalosporins.[159] Resistance of pneumococci has not been associated with the production of β-lactamases but with the alteration in cell membrane-associated enzymes that are responsible for cell wall assembly and that bind penicillin. Alteration of these penicillin-binding proteins has been associated with high resistance[166] and more recently low-level resistance too.[70]

The outbreak of multiply resistant pneumococci that began in Johannesburg, South Africa, in 1977 deserves special mention. The first isolate was a Danish type 19A from the sputum of a hospitalized 3-year-old with pneumonia. Additional isolates were recovered by screening patients and hospital personnel from the same hospital using an agar–disk diffusion method for screening pneumococcal respiratory isolates. It was clear that these were virulent strains as there was considerable morbidity and some deaths attributable to invasive infection due to these pneumococci. These isolates were resistant to penicillin concentrations of 0.12 to 4 μg/ml and were found in 29% of 543 pediatric patients and 2% of 436 hospital staff members. The year 1977 appeared to be a watershed year as resistant pneumococcal strains were reported from Durban, South Africa; Minneapolis, Minnesota; and London, England.[78] The report from Durban involved five cases of meningitis or sepsis in children from 3 months to 2 years of age. Each had severe malnutrition with recent courses of antibiotic treatment. Three occurred while hospitalized and receiving antibiotics. The isolates were serotype 19A and had MICs of 4–8 µg/ml of penicillin and exhibited resistance to other β-lactams, aminoglycosides, and chloramphenicol. The three with meningitis died and the two with septicemia responded to treatment with alternative antibiotics.[5] While early reports were of infections that were acquired nosocomially, in patients who had previously received penicillin, more recent reports indicate that there can be community acquisition in previously healthy individuals.[47]

A cluster of serotype 19A isolates was reported to have been isolated in Brooklyn, New York. Of nine isolates with penicillin MICs of 1.0 to 2.0 µg/ml, six came from asymptomatically colonized adults and three from patients with lower-respiratory-tract infections. These isolations were made in 1983–1984 as part of a vaccine-related pneumococcal surveillance program. These strains were also resistant to other penicillins, cephalosporins, tetracycline, chloramphenicol, and trimethoprim/sulfamethoxazole. No common source for the strains was discovered. At the time of this report (1985), the CDC had confirmed six other isolations of fully resistant pneumococci (MIC 2–4 µg/ml) from 1979 to 1984 but 3.7% of 3400 strains sent to them through a monitoring program were intermediately resistant (MIC 0.1–1.0 µg/ml).[136,138]

There has been an increase in worldwide surveillance of pneumococcal susceptibility due to the well-documented epidemics. Substantial numbers of strains resistant to 0.1 µg/ml of penicillin have been reported from all continents and individual reports of highly resistant strains continue. While in clinical medicine, susceptibility of pneumococcal isolates was the rule and was not monitored, it is now recommended that isolates from significant foci of infection be tested for susceptibility.[4]

5.1.2. Distribution of Pneumococcal Types. The importance of pneumococcal types and their distribution in various populations need to be stressed. In the past, when immunotherapy with type-specific serum was used, typing of organisms and provision of the proper sera required knowledge of the prevalent serotypes. Since the introduction of the pneumococcal polysaccharide vaccine, which induces type-specific immunity, it is now necessary to know the prevalence of pneumococcal serotypes in a multivalent

vaccine. Because the frequency of the different serotypes varies with time and with different clinical syndromes,[52] constant monitoring continues to be a necessity for inclusion of the appropriate types in vaccine formulations.

The occurrence of specific types of pneumococci in pneumonia, bacteremia, focal infections, and carriers has been reported from various locations, including South Africa,[108,109] Boston City Hospital,[50,52,53] Denmark,[93] Germany,[94] Britain,[113] and worldwide.[74] Essentially all known types have been identified, but in different orders of frequency, with lobar pneumonia, bronchopneumonia, otitis media, and other focal infections, as well as in healthy carriers. However, the type distribution in bronchopneumonia and in focal infections is similar to that in carriers, but in roughly inverse relationship to that in lobar pneumonia. The distribution of types in infected individuals and healthy carriers among infants and children[27,100,101] is different than in adults. Multiple types of pneumococci can be isolated from infected patients and carriers at the same time or at different times and may persist for varying lengths of time, continuously or intermittently in carriers as well as after recovery from pneumonia. The role of these types of infections in the individual patient may be surmised from the clinical findings of the demonstration of antibodies to the homologous types during the infection or convalesence. They may also account for recrudescences, recurrences, and reinfections by those types.[50,58,146] The serotypes present in the current vaccine and those most commonly encountered in bacteremic pneumococcal diseases of adults and children are summarized in Tables 2 and 4 from several sources. These change with time and place, so that individual reports may vary from the data shown. Tables 2 and 4 demonstrate that: (1) the vaccine includes the types most commonly responsible for bacteremic disease in children and adults; (2) there is broad overlap in the serotypes seen in children and adults but some differences exist; (3) bacteremic diseases are largely due to serotypes with lower numbers; the higher-numbered serotypes are more commonly found in the pharynges of healthy carriers.

5.1.3. Occurrence in Carriers. Pneumococci are present in the nose or throat or both of about one-fourth of all healthy persons at any given time; they are more prevalent in the winter months, and nearly all individuals carry them transiently or intermittently in the course of a year. In young infants, they are usually found only if they occur in the mother, but in older infants, they are more frequent. The presence of upper-respiratory infections is not ordinarily a determinant in the individual, but epidemics of respiratory infections tend to increase the spread of disease-producing types of pneumococci, particularly in families of cases.

Table 2. Serotypes Most Commonly Associated with Bacteremic Pneumococcal Infections in Children and Adults

American serotype designation		Danish serotype designation
Adults	Children	
1	1	1
	2	2
3	3	3
4	4	4
6	6	6A
8	8	8
9	9	9N
12	12	12F
14	14	14
19	19	19F
23	23	23F
	25	25
	51	7F
	56	18C

The epidemiology of pneumococcal infections was discussed in some detail at a symposium on the *Pneumococcus*[117] in 1980 in which Riley and Douglas from Papua, New Guinea, likened the situation in their country to that in the New World at the turn of the century.[119] Acquisition of pneumococci in the nasopharynx begins there in infancy, reaches the highest rates in preschool children, and then declines in advancing age groups. The rates in New Guinea, as elsewhere, are generally related to the amount, degree, and duration of contact with cases or other carriers. There is an inverse ratio of case-rates and carrier-rates of the common invasive types. The findings in Papua confirm the general well-known epidemiological principles developed and established in South Africa in 1914,[165] among recruits in military camps in 1918[34,140] and 1921,[105] and from the classic studies on experimental epidemiology in 1928 by Greenwood *et al.*[69] and by Webster.[160]

5.2. Epidemic Behavior and Contagiousness

As early as 1888, Netter[102] presented evidence, mostly on clinical grounds, for the contagiousness of pneumonia and for the part played by the pneumococcus. He described family outbreaks of pneumonia and other pneumococcal infections even in the same household. He and others[39,79] traced cases to direct or close contact with other cases or convalescents. He found that pneumococci sur-

vived in dried sputum for many months and recovered the organisms from the dust of hospital rooms.

Epidemics involving multiple cases in families[24,57] or in institutions[141,142] were described in which direct contagion was traced either separately or during outbreaks in small communities. In some of them, the pneumococcus was identified by culture or mouse inoculation.[154] Outbreaks of focal pneumococcal infections have been recorded both in association with pneumonia and independently. Pneumonia acquired in foundling homes was early recognized as an important cause of high death rates in infant asylums and as a frequent cause of deaths in babies who were healthy on arrival. Direct contagion was also recognized as the cause of the spread of pneumonia among workers in mining camps in South Africa[108–110] as well as during the construction of the Panama Canal[67,74] in which overcrowding, especially in sleeping quarters, and high attack rates soon after arrival were the two most important features.

Although pneumonia was the leading cause of death in army camps during World War I,[34,105,112,140] it occurred mostly in relation to epidemics of measles and influenza associated with hemolytic streptococci, but the majority of cases and deaths after and even during such epidemics were typical pneumococcal lobar pneumonia. In 1919, epidemics of type I pneumomoccal pneumonia were reported from Camp Jackson[112] and Camp Upton[149] and of type II from Camp Grant.[75] New draftees and southern blacks were the most susceptible. Direct contagion was later demonstrated when typing was used. In 1940, spread of pneumococcal pneumonia could also be traced in some hospitals from bed to bed.[76] In 1937, Harris and Ingraham[72] described an epidemic of type II pneumonia in the Civilian Conservation Corps confirmed in many cases by serological studies; these involved primarily members of the corps in the same barracks and only two officers who had the most contact with the men. Recent reports have stressed smaller epidemics and nosocomial spread of resistant strains,[5,78,138] the association of pneumococcal disease with influenza,[100] and conditions responsible for greater susceptibility to pneumococcal infection (see Section 7.1). Epidemics of meningitis separate from pneumonia have not been described.

5.3. Geographic Distribution

As already noted, reliable information on the geographic distribution, prevalence, and incidence of pneumonia and particularly of other pneumococcal infections is unknown because of lack of adequate reporting in most parts of the world and the unreliability of those reports that are available. It may be said, however, that such infections are ubiquitous, worldwide, and endemic and, under some conditions, may occur in well-circumscribed epidemics. Although usually thought to be particularly prevalent in temperate zones, they also occur in warmer regions and in the tropics.[74]. Temperature and humidity appear to influence the prevalence of pneumonia, and in countries where the most abrupt and severe changes occur in winter, the incidence of the disease is correspondingly high during such times.[68,122]

Among admissions to the Boston City Hospital, the incidence of pneumococcal bacteremia[98] and meningitis[53] decreased after 1935 and again after 1941 with the general use of sulfonamides and penicillin, but has fluctuated within a moderate range after that. The case-fatality rate after 1941, however, still remained high in cases of meningitis and varied with age in other bacteremic cases, being highest in infants and in persons 70 or older.

5.4. Age

Pneumococcal infections occur at all ages. They are most frequent in the first year of life, decrease rapidly to a low between 10 and 15 years, and then increase in incidence steadily in advancing age groups. Deaths from such infections are also most frequent in the first year of life, least frequent between 15 and 20 years, and rise with advancing age groups more steeply than do the case rates.[74] The estimates of incidence for invasive pneumonococcal infection in Goteborg, Sweden, which are typical, are

25.8/100,000 in the first year of life, falling to 2/100,000 in the second decade, then rising by decade and peaking in the eighth decade at 16.4/100,000[28] (see Fig. 1). The case-fatality rate from pneumonia and meningitis increases with each decade from under 10% in the young to over 50% in the eighth decade. The age distribution of cases of pneumococcal meningitis followed the same trend among patients at Boston City Hospital during 12 selected years between 1935 and 1972, but the case-fatality rates were higher, about 60%, for those in the first decade of life, 50% in the second decade, and increased with each decade thereafter to 81% in patients 70 years old or older.[53] In addition to age, another major risk factor for increased mortality rate from pneumococcal pneumonia is the development of a nonpneumococcal superinfection. The use of high doses of antibiotics and prolonged administration of broad-spectrum antibiotics predisposes to superinfection.[152]

5.5. Sex

Among cases of lobar pneumonia occurring in Massachusetts between 1921 and 1930, males predominated over females (58/42) in all age groups, but male predominance was less among infants and young children.[74] Among bacteremic patients at Boston City Hospital in 1972, the ratio was 51.7% males and 48.3% females for all patients.[98] The ratio of males to females among cases of pneumococcal meningitis for the 12 selected years between 1935 and 1972[53] was much higher and averaged 65% male for all ages, but varied in different age groups: 67% males among infants (< 1 year old), 78% males in those 1–9 years

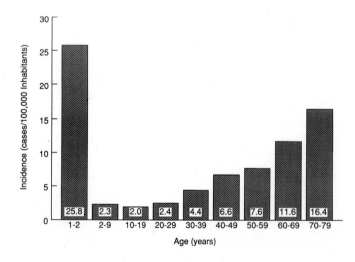

Figure 1. Age-specific incidence (cases/100,000 inhabitants per year) of invasive pneumococcal disease in Goteborg, Sweden, 1970–1980. From Ref. 28.

old, 100% males among the small number 10–19 years, dropping steadily with each decade to 50% males among patients 70 or older.

5.6. Race

It has long been recognized that the black race is peculiarly susceptible to pneumonia when residing in cold climates, especially when moved from warm tropical regions. Under certain conditions, there is also a pronounced susceptibility in blacks to pneumonia and pneumococcal infections in general even in warm climates. For example, high rates were encountered among the construction workers, who were predominantly blacks, during the building of the Panama Canal and among pneumonia patients elsewhere in Central America and tropical Africa.[74] Death rates from lobar pneumonia in various widely scattered states in this country are also considerably higher in blacks, sometimes twice as high as among whites. Thus, while true genetic susceptibility has not been separated from socioeconomic factors, blacks are most likely to be subject to crowding in occupational as well as residential life (which is related to risk of infections), may have a higher incidence of certain life-style risks[9,100] and reduced availability of medical care.

5.7. Occupation

Pneumonia has been known to be unusually prevalent in certain mining and milling industries.[25] In some mills, this has been associated with a high carrier rate that has been followed by an outbreak of pneumonia in the community.[65] In certain mining regions, the living conditions of the workers themselves, rather than the circumstances surrounding the work, may be the determining factor in spread of the disease. This was true in a group of steel workers crowded into small shanties in 1917,[147] among workers and their families during the construction of the Panama Canal in 1913,[67] among miners in South Africa,[91,106,107,110] and among plantation workers.[44]

5.8. Occurrence in Families

The occurrence and spread of pneumococcal infections among members of the households of patients admitted to Boston City Hospital with lobar pneumonia were reported by Finland and Tilghman[57] and by Brown and Finland.[24] They included multiple cases of infections with the same type as the index case; some had lobar pneumonia and others had empyema, primary pneumococcal meningitis, otitis media, simple upper-respiratory infections, bronchopneumonia, or were carriers without evidence of infection. Some cases admitted with lobar pneumonia were traced to contacts with other cases already in the hospital, but not from the same household. Serologic studies demonstrated the presence or development of antibodies to the same types. The appearance and spread of additional new types among members of the household were also noted; these were also associated with pneumonia or focal infections or mild upper-respiratory infection and with the development of specific antibodies to the homologous types in a large percentage of members of these households.

5.9. Occurrence in Animals

The occurrence of pneumococcal carriers and of widespread epidemics of pneumococcal infections among animals was reviewed by Finland.[49] They probably play very little or no part in infections and outbreaks in humans beyond causing occasional cases among animal handlers and will not be considered here.

5.10. Laboratory Infections

Cases of pneumonia acquired in the laboratory are not frequent. They have been associated with exposure to aerosols[121] or droplets or with handling of sputum.[14] They are of interest in delineating the incubation periods of pneumonia in man, since the clinical evidence of infection was manifest from 36 h to 3 days after a single exposure. Various types, including 1, 2, 7, and 18, were involved, and the same individual has been subject to more than one attack, but with different types and at different times.

5.11. Nutrition

The effect of specific nutritional deficiencies in predisposing to pneumonia is not known. Undernutrition, particularly of calories and proteins, is recognized as predisposing to infectious diseases in general. Deficiencies and abnormality in cellular (phagocytes) and circulating immune factors (e.g., complement) may play a role.[156] Alcoholism has been regarded as a major predisposing factor for invasive pneumococcal infections. In a Swedish study it was the most important risk factor in adults.[28] In a U.S. study, alcoholics also had a higher fatality rate from pneumococcal sepsis than did nonalcoholics, but only when accompanied by leukopenia.[116]

6. Mechanisms and Routes of Transmission

The most common route of transmission of pneumococci is by droplets from cases and carriers. In hospitals, the most frequent spread is from the patient to the one in the adjacent bed, the disease rarely skipping a distance of more than two beds. Physicians, nurses, attendants, and others with frequent and close contact with patients are subject to colonization or infection from the patients unless they take special precautions to avoid or reduce exposure to the patients' droplets (coughing and sneezing), such as by masking the patient or themselves or both. Although pneumococci may be cultured from the air or from the dust on the floors or in the rooms of patients with pneumonia and remain viable in dried secretions for long periods, documented infections from such sources are rare.

In cases of pneumococcal meningitis following fractured skulls, the infecting organism comes from the patient's own nasopharynx or accessory sinuses, and these foci are probably the sources of "primary" pneumococcal meningitis. The route by which the organism reaches the meninges in "primary" cases can often be traced to previous head trauma involving small fractures in the cribiform plate, difficult to recognize even by X ray. Such fractures may be associated with recurrent pneumococcal (and other bacterial) meningitis that no longer recurs after the defect in the cribiform plate has been repaired.

Otitis media in the acute form, and probably also acute sinusitis, usually occurs during or after simple upper-respiratory-tract infections and is caused by the same type of pneumococcus found in the nose and/or pharynx or both. Experimentally, inflammation associated with occlusion of the eustachian tube (produced by influenza virus) is required to produce otitis media in the chinchilla after colonization of the nasopharynx with pneumococcus.[59,63]

7. Pathogenesis and Immunity

7.1. Pathogenesis

The incubation period for pneumococcal pneumonia is not known. Most sources state that it is 1–3 days. Heffron[74] suggests "in the neighborhood of a few hours to about 48 hours." This would be infection from an exogenous source. Endogenous infection in an asymptomatic carrier can occur with an "incubation period" of weeks.

While significant details of human immunity to the pneumococcus are known, the exact mechanisms by which it can multiply in tissues and produce local inflammation or

invasive disease are not known. The mouse, rabbit, rat, and dog, and probably also man, can remove large numbers of inhaled virulent pneumococci. This is done in part by the ciliary epithelium of the trachea and bronchi but in greater measure by the phagocytic cells, predominantly the pulmonary macrophage system, and is effected with or without the mediation of humoral antibodies.[81] It is known that damage to the ciliary system, particularly to the macrophages, by alcohol or other inhaled toxic substances or by minor viral respiratory infections is necessary to establish pulmonary infection by pneumococci. In experimental animals, intrabronchial inoculation of pneumococci in a gelatin or starch plug is necessary to establish the pneumonia, which extends out from the local alveoli to other parts of the lung.[37] In the dog, infection occurs in the local alveoli, and the pneumococci appear very rapidly in the local lymphatics, then in the hilar lymph nodes, thence in the thoracic duct and subclavian vein, and finally in the peripheral blood.[43,150] The healthy mouse, in which a single virulent (e.g., type I) pneumococcus injected intraperitoneally produces a lethal infection, can inhale a large number of the same organism from an aerosolized culture without ill effect, but the same aerosol will produce bronchopneumonia, bacteremia, and death if inhaled after the mouse has been anesthetized or alcoholized to unconsciousness. Intranasal instillation of the broth culture will also produce pneumonia and death in the mouse[145] and in the rabbit.[144] A dermal pneumococcal infection has been produced by intradermal inoculation in rabbits; this lesion can be prevented by previous immunization and terminated by specific antiserum.[66] The same is true of experimental infections in the mouse and the dog. The importance of inflammation and obstruction of the eustachian tube for the establishment of pneumococcal otitis media was mentioned in Section 6. A counterpart to this in human pneumococcal pneumonia is the increased susceptibility of acutely alcoholic patients and the higher mortality among those who develop bacteremic pneumococcal infections.[151]

In humans, host defenses against the pneumococcus can be divided into natural and acquired. Some of the natural host defenses have been deduced from experimental studies but to a large extent they have been inferred from high rates of disease in people with underlying (predisposing) abnormalities.

The natural defenses in individuals with normal lungs include the production of an inflammatory response and the transport of bacteria out of the lungs by coordinated motion of the cilia. Damage to the lungs by previous infections, smoking, occupational exposure to lung toxins, or chronic obstructive pulmonary disease, is associated with defective clearance by these mechanisms and therefore susceptibility to infection by *S. pneumoniae*.

Humoral immunity is of considerable importance in acquired resistance to infection with the pneumococcus. Individuals whose B-cell function is abnormal are predisposed to infection on this basis. This includes infants, children, and adults who have congenital B-cell deficiency and hypogammaglobulinemia. This predisposition is ameliorated by treatment with intramuscular or intravenous gammaglobulin every 3–4 weeks. Acquired dysgammaglobulinemias including multiple myeloma and the acquired immunodeficiency syndrome (AIDS) are associated with unusual susceptibility to infection by the pneumococcus. Children with AIDS are highly susceptible to pneumococcal infections[16] and they are often prophylactically treated with gammaglobulin.

The presence of a normal spleen is important in containing pneumococcemia. In persons with anatomical or functional asplenia, there is a high risk of overwhelming sepsis. Congenital asplenia is often part of a complex of midline defects and is termed Ivemark syndrome.[77] Individuals with this syndrome frequently die from severe cardiac disease in infancy. Of those who survive past 6 months of age, sepsis is a frequent occurrence and *S. pneumoniae* is most frequently the cause of sepsis.[157] Of those who have a splenectomy in later life, overwhelming pneumococcal sepsis is a significant threat. Posttraumatic splenectomy may be associated with a lower risk than is elective surgical splenectomy because splenic rupture is often associated with splenosis; implantation of functioning spleen cells in the abdominal cavity. In the absence of splenosis, susceptibility to overwhelming pneumococcal sepsis is lifelong.

The condition most clearly associated with acquired hypofunction of the spleen and hypersusceptibility to pneumococcal infection is in sickle-cell anemia. In this disease the spleen is normal in the early months of life and then develops progressive autoinfarction due to stasis of sickled red cells. Finally there is loss of splenic function even though the spleen may be anatomically present. This is the time of maximum susceptibility to life-threatening pneumococcal infection. The threat of pneumococcal sepsis and meningitis may be decreased by the use of prophylactic penicillin, or in those over 2 years of age, pneumococcal vaccine.[115]

Recent research has focused on the important role of the complement system in the pathogenesis of pneumococcal infections. Using animal models it has been possible to demonstrate that opsonization of pneumococci, which is necessary for eradication of bacteremia, requires participation of the complement system.[23] Pneumococci can acti-

vate the terminal complement components via the classical or alternative complement pathways. The alternative complement pathway can be activated by pneumococci and immunoglobulin that does not have to be specific for pneumococcal antigens. This pathway is responsible for "natural immunity" in nonimmune individuals and activates opsonic C3b. Activation of the classical complement pathway is more efficient and occurs in immune individuals who have specific antipneumococcal antibody in the serum. It also involves activation of C3b. Hypersusceptibility to pneumococcal infection may be a consequence of dysfunction of either system. With congenital absence of any of the early components of the complement cascade, there is frequently recurrent infection, especially with pneumococci. In sickle-cell disease there is abnormally low function of the alternative complement system and this appears to be part of the susceptibility to overwhelming pneumococcal infections.[163]

The pneumococcal specific capsular substances (referred to as SSS in the past) are complex polysaccharides, and the chemical structures of many have been elucidated in detail. These polysaccharides are responsible for the type specificity of protective antibodies that are elicited during infection[55] and the serological classification of which can be determined by the Quellung reaction. The presence of the capsule is required for a strain to be pathogenic, and a larger amount of capsule production is associated with increased pathogenic potential. Other than the antiphagocytic property of the capsular polysaccharide, no role for other antigens or toxins liberated by pneumococci has been definitely established.[56] A "purpura-producing principle" has been described in experimental animal studies, but no toxin has been demonstrated in humans, even those with overwhelming infections. There is some clinical and laboratory evidence that when the concentration of free polysaccharide antigen in the blood is very high, there is spontaneous activation of complement that could result in disseminated intravascular coagulation and shock.[61,124]

7.2. Immunity

Type-specific anticapsular antibody appears about the 5th or 6th day of illness in untreated patients and promotes the ingestion of bacteria by leukocytes. The antibody appears to be protective and long-lasting and is specific for the pneumococcal capsular type. Recurrent systemic infection due to the same serotype is rare except in patients with impaired defenses or persistent foci of infection. However, the pneumococcus may persist in the upper respiratory tract for days or weeks in the presence of humoral antibody.

Type-specific capsular antibodies also appear about 11 days after immunization, peak in 3–4 weeks, and persist at protective levels for at least 5 years.[129] Numerous studies have demonstrated that antibody production in response to pneumococcal vaccine is poor below the age of 2 years and is probably not effective in preventing infection in children of that age.[41,132]

8. Patterns of Host Response

8.1. Clinical Features

Pneumococcal infections in man are manifested in various ways (Table 3). These range from the healthy carrier state or minor respiratory infection to pneumonia and meningitis, otitis media, conjunctivitis, and other focal purulent infections. Bacteremia may occur in association with manifestations ranging from simple pharyngitis and fever without a demonstrably localized lesion[97,148] to fulminating septicemia with purpura and adrenal hemorrhage (Waterhouse–Friderichsen syndrome), which may be rapidly lethal in the immunocompromised or asplenic patient.[158] Pneumococcal meningitis is most commonly a complication of skull fracture, sinusitis, mastoiditis, or pneumonia. Pneumococcal empyema of the pleura is the most frequent complication of lobar pneumonia, with vegetative endocarditis generally a late complication.

Clinically, "primary" pneumococcal lobar pneumonia begins characteristically, most often after a few days of mild upper-respiratory symptoms and bronchitis, with a sudden severe chill or pleuritic pain or both. This is accompanied by a hacking cough, with production of small amounts of orange-, rust-, or prune-juice-colored sputum, and followed by fever and the appearance of physical and X-ray signs of moisture and consolidation of the lung(s). If the condition is untreated, the organism invades the bloodstream (bacteremia), and the consolidation spreads to involve an entire lobe. It may spread to other parts of the lung, with a stormy course that ends in death or in recovery by rapid drop in fever and cessation of symptoms (crisis) or by slow resolution of fever, symptoms, and signs over several days (lysis).

8.2. Diagnosis

The diagnosis may be made by demonstrating the specific type of pneumococcus (by the Quellung reaction) in the sputum or in the blood culture if obtained before effective chemotherapy is instituted. Meningitis, otitis media, and other focal pneumococcal infections are diagnosed by characteristic physical signs and by demonstrating the organism in a similar manner in the purulent spinal fluid or local exudate. Serologic tests have not been used routinely for the diagnosis of pneumococcal infections. Counterimmunoelectrophoresis and latex agglutination using latex beads coated with pneumococcal antisera both detect free antigen in body fluids. They can be used in clinical situations for rapid diagnosis of sepsis, meningitis, and other focal infections. Agglutination of antibody-coated latex beads can be used for rapid identification of S. pneumoniae from colonies picked off of primary isolation plates in the diagnostic laboratory.

9. Control and Prevention

9.1. Prevention

Although controversy about the efficacy of active immunization with a polyvalent vaccine persists, it has been the mainstay for the prevention of invasive pneumococcal infections. More recently, investigators have used passive immunization with specific immune intravenous immunoglobulin preparations to attempt to prevent invasive infections in selected patients.

9.2. Pneumococcal Vaccine

Because of the extremely high incidence of serious pneumococcal infections among South African goldminers,[96] in 1911 Wright and his co-workers[165] immunized miners with a crude whole-cell pneumococcal vaccine. Subsequently, a number of other investigators conducted clinical trials of the safety and efficacy of polysaccharide vaccines against pneumococci of various serotypes.[45,48,90] However, the validity of the results of

Table 3. Clinical Spectrum of Pneumococcal Infections

Minor respiratory infections	Meningitis
Conjunctivitis	Focal infections
Otitis media	Bacteremia with:
Sinusitis	Pharyngitis
Lobar pneumonia	Fever
Bronchopneumonia	Septicemia
Empyema of pleura	Purpura
Endocarditis	Adrenal hemorrhage

many of these trials was questionable because of such methodologic flaws as nonrandomization, inadequacies in the clinical follow-up of subjects, and inadequacies in the bacteriologic confirmation of the outcomes. However, controlled trials of bivalent, trivalent, and quadravalent polysaccharide vaccines that were conducted in the 1940s provided stronger evidence that vaccines were efficacious.[82,95] Two different hexavalent vaccines subsequently were commercially produced and marketed. At about the same time, antimicrobials that were effective against pneumococci became available and the outcomes of patients with pneumococcal infections improved substantially. Interest in the vaccines rapidly diminished and they were eventually withdrawn from the market.

However, in 1964 Austrian reported a mortality rate of 25% in adults with bacteremic pneumococcal pneumonia.[11] Many of these patients died despite early treatment with appropriate antibiotics. Furthermore, most of the patients were either elderly or had a chronic illness that represented a population at increased risk of serious pneumococcal disease. This population could be targeted for immunization if an effective vaccine could be developed. Accordingly, Austrian and others worked together to develop a polyvalent vaccine.[155] The vaccine was tested with prospective double-blind randomized controlled trials in young South African goldminers. This group of subjects was chosen because of the extraordinarily high incidence of pneumococcal disease they experienced, which enabled these trials to be conducted expeditiously and at a relatively low cost.[12] These well-designed trials produced conclusive evidence of the efficacy of these vaccines in this population (the estimates of protective efficacy ranged from 76 to 92%).[12,143]

Two large clinical trials were conducted to try to assess the vaccine's efficacy in the populations at high risk of serious pneumococcal disease in the United States.[7] These trials were conducted among 13,600 ambulatory patients over 45 years of age at the Kaiser-Permanente Health Plan in San Francisco and among 1300 subjects at a chronic-care facility in North Carolina. Despite the relatively large number of subjects, these studies were inconclusive because of the low incidence of invasive pneumococcal infections and the consequent poor statistical power of these trials.[7,131] A small clinical trial conducted among patients with sickle-cell disease found excellent efficacy for these patients, but the study was flawed because the trial was neither randomized nor blinded.[2]

Despite these equivocal results, a quadradecavalent vaccine that contained 50 μg each of the polysaccharide antigen of 14 serotypes of pneumococci was licensed by the FDA in 1977 (Table 4). This vaccine was replaced in 1983 by one containing polysaccharide antigens of 23 capsular types. The vaccine was recommended for use in persons over 2 years of age with a variety of chronic conditions that placed them at increased risk of serious pneumococcal infection.[118] These conditions included anatomical or functional asplenia and chronic pulmonary, cardiac, or renal diseases. The recommendations for the exact target population were rather vague, in part because of a lack of firm data on the magnitude of the increased risk of serious pneumococcal infections associated with various chronic conditions. These original recommendations about whom to vaccinate have been updated several times.[31,32,32a,73] The most recent recommendations from the Immunization Practices Advisory Committee (ACIP) of the CDC are as follows[31,32a]:

> Despite conflicting findings, the data continue to support the use of the pneumococcal vaccine for certain well defined groups at risk:

Table 4. Antigenic Serotypes of Pneumococcal Polysaccharides Contained in Pneumococcal Vaccine

14-valent vaccine		23-valent vaccine	
Danish system	American system	Danish system	American system
1	1	1	1
2	2	2	2
3	3	3	3
4	4	4	4
6A	6	5	5
7F	51	6B	26
8	8	7F	51
9N	9	8	8
12F	12	9N	9
14	14	9V	68
18C	56	10A	34
19F	19	11A	43
23F	23	12F	12
25	25	14	14
		15B	54
		17F	17
		18C	56
		19A	57
		19F	19
		20	20
		22F	22
		23F	23
		33F	70

Adults

1. Immunocompetent adults who are at increased risk of pneumococcal disease or its complications because of chronic illnesses (e.g., cardiovascular disease, pulmonary disease, diabetes mellitus, alcoholism, cirrhosis, or cerebrospinal fluid leaks) or who are $\geq$ 65 years old.
2. Immunocompromised adults at increased risk of pneumococcal disease or its complications (e.g., persons with splenic dysfunction or anatomic asplenia, Hodgkin's disease, lymphoma, multiple myeloma, chronic renal failure, nephrotic syndrome, or conditions such as organ transplantation associated with immunosuppression).
3. Adults with asymptomatic or symptomatic HIV infection.

Children

1. Children $\geq$ 2 years old with chronic illnesses sporadically associated with increased risk of pneumococcal disease or its complications [e.g., anatomic or functional asplenia (including sickle cell disease), nephrotic syndrome, cerebrospinal fluid leaks, and conditions associated with immunosuppression].
2. Children $\geq$ 2 years old with asymptomatic or symptomatic HIV infection.
3. The currently available 23-valent vaccine is not indicated for patients having only recurrent upper respiratory tract disease, including otitis media and sinusitis.

Special Groups

Persons living in special environments or social settings with an identified increased risk of pneumococcal disease or its complications (e.g., certain Native American populations).

Adverse Reactions

Approximately 50% of persons given pneumococcal vaccine develop mild side effects, such as erythema and pain at the injection site. Fever, myalgia, and severe local reactions have been reported in < 1% of those vaccinated. Severe systemic reactions, such as anaphylaxis, rarely have been reported.

Precautions

The safety of pneumococcal vaccine for pregnant women has not been evaluated. Ideally, women at high risk of pneumococcal disease should be vaccinated before pregnancy.

Timing of Vaccination

When elective splenectomy is being considered, pneumococcal vaccine should be given at least 2 weeks before the operation, if possible. Similarly, for planning cancer chemotherapy or immunosuppressive therapy, as in patients who undergo organ transplantation, the interval between vaccination and initiation of chemotherapy or immunosuppression should also be at least 2 weeks.

Revaccination

In one study, local reactions after revaccination in adults were more severe than after initial vaccination when the interval between vaccinations was 13 months. Reports of revaccination after longer intervals in children and adults, including a large group of elderly persons revaccinated at least 4 years after primary vaccination, suggest a similar incidence of such reactions after primary vaccination and revaccination.

Without more information, persons who received the 14-valent pneumococcal vaccine should not be routinely vaccinated with the 23-valent vaccine, as increased coverage is modest and duration of protection is not well defined. However, revaccination with the 23-valent vaccine should be strongly considered for persons who received the 14-valent vaccine if they are at highest risk of fatal pneumococcal infection (e.g., asplenic patients). Revaccination should also be considered for adults at highest risk who received the 23-valent vaccine $\geq$ 6 years before and for those shown to have rapid decline in pneumococcal antibody levels (e.g., patients with nephrotic syndrome, asplenia, or sickle cell anemia who would be $\leq$ 10 years old at revaccination).

Strategies for Vaccine Delivery

Recommendations for pneumococcal vaccination have been made by the ACIP, the American Academy of Pediatrics, the American College of Physicians, and the American Academy of Family Physicians. Recent analysis indicates that pneumococcal vaccination of elderly persons is cost-effective. The vaccine is targeted for approximately 27 million persons aged $\geq$ 65 years and 21 million persons ages < 65 years with high-risk conditions. Despite Medicare reimbursement for costs of the vaccine and its administration, which began in 1981, annual use of pneumococcal vaccine has not increased above levels observed in earlier years. In 1985, < 10% of the 48 million persons considered to be at increased risk of serious pneumococcal infection were estimated to have ever received pneumococcal vaccine.

Opportunities to vaccinate high risk persons are missed both at time of hospital discharge and during visits to clinicians' offices. Two thirds or more of patients with serious pneumococcal disease had been hospitalized at least once within 5 years before their pneumococcal illness, yet few had received pneumococcal vaccine. More effective programs for vaccine delivery are needed, including offering pneumococcal vaccine in hospitals (at the time of discharge), clinicians' offices, nursing homes, and other chronic-care facilities. Many patients who receive pneumococcal vaccine should also be immunized with influenza vaccine.

Based upon systematic surveillance of the serotypes of pneumococci that caused serious invasive disease, the vaccine was formulated to include serotypes that were responsible for approximately 80% of the cases of systemic pneumococcal infections in the United States.[20,21] However, soon after the vaccine was licensed and distributed, reports of clinical failures of the vaccine began to appear.[1,62] Furthermore, studies suggested that some high-risk patients had poor antibody responses to the vaccine.[3,64,85] In addition, surveillance data from the CDC suggested that the vaccine's efficacy was poor for many high-risk patients.[19,22] Thus, there was considerable uncertainty about the vaccine because it was shown to be effective in a very select population (young goldminers) but there were serious questions about its efficacy for the population in the United States that was at increased risk of serious pneumococcal infections. However, because of the low incidence of bacteremic pneumococcal infections in developed countries, even in high-risk patients, there are formidable logistical and financial obstacles to conducting a randomized clinical trial in the United States.[33] Furthermore, because the vaccine was licensed (and presumably is efficacious), it may be unethical to allocate high-risk patients randomly to receive placebo, as would be necessary in a randomized trial.

Alternatives to randomized clinical trials to assess the vaccine's efficacy were necessary.[33] Shapiro and Clemens conducted a case–control study that found the vaccine's efficacy to be 67% (95% confidence interval: 13–87%) in high-risk patients.[134] Although there were too few subjects to assess the vaccine's efficacy accurately in immunocompromised patients, its efficacy in high-risk patients with chronic conditions such as diabetes mellitus or chronic pulmonary, cardiac, or renal disease was 77% (95% confidence interval: 27–93%). Bolan and her colleagues[17] from the CDC extended their estimates of the vaccine's efficacy based on their surveillance data of reports of serotypes of pneumococci that caused bacteremic disease from 1978 to 1984. They found the vaccine's efficacy against bacteremic disease to be 64% (95% confidence interval: 47–76%). Based on these results, experts have concluded that the vaccine is cost-effective and that it is underutilized.[10,31,84,114,139]

Despite the serious obstacles to such a study, Sim-berkoff and his colleagues[137] conducted a randomized clinical trial of the protective efficacy of the 14-valent vaccine at several different Veterans Administration Medical Centers. Although they were unable to demonstrate that the vaccine was efficacious, there were a number of serious flaws in their methodology that compromise the validity of their conclusions.[133] Many of the events that the investigators counted as episodes of pneumococcal infection were really of uncertain cause since their definition of pneumococcal infection included patients with a cough and isolation of pneumococci from their sputa (even in the absence of an abnormal chest X ray). Because it is known that immunization with pneumococcal vaccine will not affect colonization of the respiratory tract with pneumococci, the definitions of pneumococcal infection used in this study limit its usefulness. By the investigators' own criteria, there were only two subjects who had proved (bacteremic) pneumococcal infection. As a result, the statistical power of the study to assess the vaccine's efficacy against proved pneumococcal infections was extraordinarily poor (only 6%).

Shapiro has conducted a multicenter case–control study of the vaccine's efficacy in Connecticut from 1984 to 1987. Preliminary results of data from nearly 400 case–control pairs indicate that the vaccine's type-specific efficacy was 67% (E. D. Shapiro, unpublished data).

In July 1983 the 14-valent vaccine was replaced by a new vaccine that contains 25 μg each of the polysaccharides of 23 different serotypes of pneumococci (Table 4). These serotypes were included in the vaccine after extensive examination of data on the serotypes that had been isolated from the blood or CSF of infected individuals, as well as data on the cross-reactivity of antibodies against the different serotypes.[120] As was true of the 14-valent vaccine, serious adverse reactions to the 23-valent vaccine are extremely rare.[73]

Despite the recommendations of official bodies such as the Advisory Committee on Immunization Practices[31] and the American Academy of Physicians[73] that pneumococcal vaccine be administered to high-risk patients, physicians have been slow to implement these recommendations. Studies have indicated that fewer than a quarter of the eligible patients have received the vaccine.[46,134] Consequently, one of the major issues in maximizing the full potential benefit of this vaccine is to find a strategy to increase its utilization among high-risk patients. Fedson and others[46] have found that a large majority of the patients who develop pneumococcal bacteremia had been hospitalized in the preceding several years. Consequently, he suggests a strategy of immunizing with pneumococcal vaccine hospitalized patients who have indications for the vaccine.[46] This strategy would specifically target the group at highest risk of serious invasive pneumococcal disease and thus enhance the efficiency of an immunization program.

The type-specific pneumococcal polysaccharide appears to be a T-cell-independent antigen. Booster (anamnestic) responses to repeated exposure to the polysaccharide antigen are not observed.[18] Although the attack rate of invasive pneumococcal infection is very high in young children, most of the serious infections occur in children under 2 years of age. Unfortunately, children under 2 years of age have a poor immunological response to T-cell-independent antigens such as those in pneumococcal vaccine. Consequently, universal immunization of children with pneumococcal vaccine has not been recommended, since most cases of serious disease occur among young children who are unlikely to respond to the vaccine.[60] The vaccine has also not been effective in preventing otitis media in young children.[60] Pneumococcal vaccine is indicated for children 2 years of age or older with chronic conditions that place them at increased risk of serious pneumococcal infections.[36,60]

Studies have indicated that if the polysaccharide antigen is conjugated to a protein, the immune response to the antigen may be transformed into a T-cell-dependent immune response that even young infants may mount. Efforts are under way to perfect conjugate pneumococcal vaccines that may hold the promise of providing protection against pneumococcal disease for young children and others who are unable to respond to the conventional simple polysaccharide vaccine.[87,130]

9.3. Passive Immunization

Recent studies have shown that commercial preparations of immunoglobulins contain substantial concentrations of antibodies against specific serotypes of pneumococci.[164] These preparations, administered on a regular basis, may prove to be useful in preventing pneumococcal infections in certain very high-risk patients.[29,164] An experimental preparation of a hyperimmune globulin against pneumococci, prepared from the serum of adult volunteers who were immunized with pneumococcal vaccine, may also be useful for certain patients.[135]

10. Unresolved Problems

The detailed studies of the pneumococcus have been the basis of modern molecular biology and immunochemistry. Probably more is known about the biology of the pneumococcus than about that of any other bacterium. However, the exact mechanism(s) whereby this organism is able to multiply in animal and human tissue and produce its more or less unique type of inflammation in the lung is not fully known. Some progress has been made in the elucidation of the function of various chemical and morphological constituents of the pneumococcus other than the capsular polysaccharide.[153] Although many of the defects in cellular and humoral immunity that predispose to pneumococcal infections have been revealed, there are still others that need to be elucidated. Also, the exact mechanism whereby viral infection and chemical irritants predispose local pulmonary tissues to pneumococcal disease needs further elucidation. The reasons for the predominance of infection in males need to be clarified, as does the peculiar increased susceptibility of blacks, apart from environmental factors. The chemical basis for the cross-reactions between some types has been clarified,[86] but for others it is not known. The basis for virulence of pneumococci needs further study. Transformation of types has been shown to be mediated by DNA,[13] but whether transformation occurs under natural conditions is not known. The significance of skin reaction to various fractions of pneumococcus other than SSS [56] also remains unknown. Finally, while a pneumococcal vaccine is currently in use, the extent of its use in target populations is too low, and a vaccine for use in infants and children under 2 years of age is only now being developed.

11. References

1. AHONKHAI, V. I., LANDESMAN, S. H., FIKRIG, S. M., SCHMALZER, E. A., BROWN, A. K., CHERUBIN, C. E., AND SCHIFFMAN, G., Failure of pneumococcal vaccine in children with sickle-cell disease, *N. Engl. J. Med.* **301**:26–27 (1979).

2. AMMANN, A. J., ADDIEGO, J., WARA, D. W., LUBIN, B., SMITH, W. B., AND MENTZER, W. C., Polyvalent pneumococcal-polysaccharide immunization of patients with sickle-cell anemia and patients with splenectomy, *N. Engl. J. Med.* **297**:897–900 (1977).

3. AMMANN, A. J., SCHIFFMAN, G., ADDIEGO, J. E., WARA, W. M., AND WARA, D. W., Immunization of immunosuppressed patients with pneumococcal polysaccharide vaccine, *Rev. Infect. Dis.* **3**(Suppl.):S160–S167 (1981).

4. APPLEBAUM, P. C., World-wide development of antibiotic resistance in pneumococci, *Eur. J. Clin. Microbiol.* **6**:367–377 (1987).

5. APPLEBAUM, P. C., BHAMJEE, A., SCRAGG, J. N., HALLETT, A. F., BOWEN, A. J., AND COOPER, R. C., Streptococcus pneumoniae resistant to penicillin and chloramphenicol, *Lancet* **2**:995–997 (1977).

6. ARMSTRONG, R. R., A swift and simple method for deciding pneumococcal "type," *Br. Med. J.* **1**:214–215 (1931).

7. AUSTRIAN, R., Surveillance of pneumococcal infection for field trials of polyvalent pneumococcal vaccine, Report DAB-VDP-12-84, pp. 1–84, *National Institutes of Health*, Bethesda, 1980.

8. AUSTRIAN, R., Pneumococcus, the first hundred years, *Rev. Infect. Dis.* **3**:183–189 (1981).

9. AUSTRIAN, R., Some observations on the pneumococcus and on the current status of pneumococcal disease and its prevention, *Rev. Infect. Dis.* **3**(Suppl.):S1–S17 (1981).

10. AUSTRIAN, R. A reassessment of pneumococcal vaccine [Editorial], *N. Engl. J. Med.* **310**:651–653 (1984).

11. AUSTRIAN, R., AND GOLD, J., Pneumococcal bacteremia with especial reference to bacteremic pneumococcal pneumonia, *Ann. Intern. Med.* **60**:759–776 (1964).

12. AUSTRIAN, R., DOUGLAS, R. M., SCHIFFMAN, G., COETZEE, A. M., KOORNHOF, H. J., HAYDEN-SMITH, S., AND REID, R. D. W., Prevention of pneumococcal pneumonia by vaccination, *Trans. Assoc. Am. Physicians* **89**:184–194 (1976).

13. AVERY, O. T., MacLEOD, C. M., AND McCARTY, M., Studies on the chemical nature of the substance inducing transformation of pneumococcal types: Induction of transformation by a desoxyribonucleic acid fraction isolated from pneumococcus type III, *J. Exp. Med.* **79**:137–158 (1944).

14. BENJAMIN, J. E., RUEGSEGGER, J. M., AND SENIOR, F. A., Cross-infection in pneumococcic pneumonia, *J. Am. Med. Assoc.* **112**:1127–1130 (1939).

15. BERGEY, D. H., A key to the identification of organisms of the class Schizomycetes, in: *Bergey's Manual of Determinative Bacteriology*, 4th ed., p. 48, Williams & Wilkins, Baltimore, 1934.

16. BERNSTEIN, L. J., KRIEGER, B. Z., NOVICK, B., SICKLICK, M. J., AND RUBINSTEIN, A., Bacterial infection in the acquired immunodeficiency syndrome of children, *Pediatr. Infect. Dis.* **4**:472–475 (1985).

17. BOLAN, G., BROOME, C. V., FACKLAM, R. R., PILKAYTIS, B. D., FRASER, D. W., AND SCHLECH, W. F., III, Pneumococcal vaccine efficacy in selected populations in the United States, *Ann. Intern. Med.* **104**:1–6 (1986).

18. BORGONO, J. M., McLEAN, A. A., VELLA, P. P., WOODHOUR, A. F., CANEPA, I., DAVIDSON, W. L., AND HILLEMAN, M. R.,Vaccination and revaccination with polyvalent pneumococcal polysaccharide vaccines in adults and infants, *Proc. Soc. Exp. Biol. Med.* **157**:148–154 (1978).

19. BROOME, C. V., Efficacy of pneumococcal polysaccharide vaccines, *Rev. Infect. Dis.* **3**(Suppl.):S82–S83 (1981).

20. BROOME, C. V., AND FACKLAM, R. R., Epidemiology of clinically significant isolates of *Streptococcus pneumoniae* in the United States, *Rev. Infect. Dis.* **3**:277–281 (1981).

21. BROOME, C. V., FACKLAM, R. R., ALLEN, J. R., FRASER, D. W., AND AUSTRIAN, R., Epidemiology of pneumococcal serotypes in the United States, 1978–79, J. Infect. Dis. **141**:119–123 (1980).

22. BROOME, C. V., FACKLAM, R. R., AND FRASER, D. W.,

Pneumococcal disease after pneumococcal vaccination: An alternative method to estimate the efficacy of pneumococcal vaccine, *N. Engl. J. Med.* **303**:549–552 (1980).

23. BROWN, E. J., HOSEA, S. W., AND FRANK, M. M., The role of antibody and complement in the reticuloendothelial clearance of pneumococci from the blood stream, *Rev. Infect. Dis.* **5**:S797–S805 (1983).

24. BROWN, J. W., AND FINLAND, M., A family outbreak of type V pneumococcus infections: Clinical, bacteriological and immunological studies, *Ann. Intern. Med.* **13**:394–401 (1939).

25. BRUNDAGE, D. K., RUSSELL, A. E., JONES, R. R., BLOOMFIELD, J. J., AND THOMPSON, R., Frequency of pneumonia among iron and steel workers, *Public Health Bulletin* No. 202, U.S. Government Printing Office, Washington, D.C., 1932.

26. BUCHANAN, R. E., AND GIBBONS, W. E. (co-eds.), *Bergey's Manual of Determinative Bacteriology*, 8th ed., pp. 499–500, Williams & Wilkins, Baltimore, 1974.

27. BULLOWA, J. G. M., *The Management of the Pneumonias for Physicians and Medical Students*, Oxford University Press, New York, 1937.

28. BURMAN, A., NORRBY, R., AND TROLLFORS, B., Invasive pneumococcal infections: Incidence, predisposing factors and prognosis, *Rev. Infect. Dis.* **7**:133–142 (1985).

29. CALVELLI, T. A,. AND RUBINSTEIN, A., Intravenous gammaglobulin in infant acquired immunodeficiency syndrome, *Pediatr. Infect. Dis.* **5**:S207–S210 (1986).

30. Centers for Disease Control, Surveillance summary: Bacterial meningitis and meningococcemia, *Morbid. Mortal. Weekly Rep.* **28**:277–279 (1979).

31. Centers for Disease Control, Recommendations of the Immunization Practices Advisory Committee (ACIP): Pneumococcal polysaccharide vaccine, *Morbid. Mortal. Weekly Rep.* **30**:410–419 (1981).

32. Centers for Disease Control, Recommendations of the Immunization Practices Advisory Committee (ACIP) update: Pneumococcal vaccine usage—United States, *Morbid. Mortal. Weekly Rep.* **33**:273–281 (1984).

32a. Centers for Disease Control, Recommendations of the Immunization Practices Advisory Committee (ACIP): Pneumococcal polysaccharide vaccine, *Morbid. Mortal. Weekly Rep.* **38**:64–76 (1989).

33. CLEMENS, J. D., AND SHAPIRO, E. D., Resolving the pneumococcal vaccine controversy: Are there alternatives to randomized clinical trials? *Rev. Infect. Dis.* **6**:589–600 (1984).

34. COLE, R., AND MacCALLUM, W. G., Pneumonia at a base hospital, *J. Am. Med. Assoc.* **70**:1146–1156 (1918).

35. COLLINS, S. D., AND GOVER, M. Age and seasonal incidence of minor respiratory attacks classified according to clinical symptoms, *Am. J. Hyg.* **20**:533–554 (1934).

36. Committee on Infectious Diseases, American Academy of Pediatrics, Recommendations for using pneumococcal vaccine in children, *Pediatrics* **75**:1153–1158 (1985).

37. COONROD, J. D., AND YONEDA, K., Complement and opsonins in alveolar secretions and serum of rats with pneu-

monia due to *Streptococcus pneumoniae, Rev. Infect. Dis.* **3**:310–322 (1981).

38. COOPER, G., ROSENSTEIN, C., WALTER, A., AND PEIZER, L., The further separation of types among the pneumococci hitherto included in group IV and the development of therapeutic antisera for these types, *J. Exp. Med.* **55**:531–554 (1932).

39. CRUICKSHANK, R., PNEUMOCOCCAL INFECTIONS (Milroy Lectures), *Lancet* **1**:563–568, 621–626, 680–685 (1933).

40. DAJANI, A. S., Antibiotic-resistant pneumococci, *Pediatr. Infect. Dis.* **1**:143–144 (1982).

41. DAVIES, J. A. V., The response of infants to inoculation with type 1 pneumococcus carbohydrate, *J. Immunol.* **33**:1–7 (1937).

42. DOCHEZ, A. R., AND GILLESPIE, L. J., A biological classification of pneumococci by means of immunity reactions, *J. Am. Med. Assoc.* **61**:727–730 (1913).

43. DRINKER, C. K., AND FIELD, M. E., *Lymphatics, Lymph and Tissue Fluid*, Williams & Wilkins, Baltimore, 1933.

44. EBGERT, J. H., Epidemic pneumonia in the tropics, *N.Y. Med. J.* **103**:1125 (1916).

45. EKWURZEL, G. M., SIMMONS, J. S., DUBLIN, H., AND FELTON, L. D., Studies of immunizing substances in pneumococci. VIII. Report on field test to determine the prophylactic value of a pneumococcus antigen, *Public Health Rep.* **53**:1877–1893 (1938).

46. FEDSON, D. S., Improving the use of pneumococcal vaccine through a strategy of hospital-based immunization: A review of its rationale and implications, *J. Am. Geriatr. Soc.* **33**:142–150 (1985).

47. FELDMAN, C., KALLENBACH, J. M., MILLER, S. D., THORBURN, J. R., AND KOORNHOF, H., Community-acquired pneumonia due to penicillin-resistant pneumococci, *N. Engl. J. Med.* **313**:615–617 (1985).

48. FELTON, L. D., Studies on immunizing substances in pneumococci. VII. Response in human beings to antigenic pneumococcus polysaccharides, type I and II, *Public Health Rep.* **53**:2855–2877 (1938).

49. FINLAND, M., Recent advances in the epidemiology of pneumococcal infections, *Medicine* **21**:307–344 (1942).

50. FINLAND, M., The present status of the higher types of antipneumococcus serums, *J. Am. Med. Assoc.* **120**:1294–1307 (1942).

51. FINLAND, M., Pneumonia and pneumococcal infections, with special reference to pneumococcal pneumonia: The 1979 J. Burns Amberson Lecture, *Am. Rev. Respir. Dis.* **120**:481–502 (1979).

52. FINLAND, M., AND BARNES, M. W., Changes in occurrence of capsular serotypes of *Streptococcus pneumoniae* at Boston City Hospital during selected years between 1935 and 1974, *J. Clin. Microbiol.* **5**:154–166 (1977).

53. FINLAND, M. AND BARNES M. W., Acute bacterial meningitis at Boston City Hospital during 12 selected years, 1935–1972, *J. Infect. Dis.* **136**:400–415 (1977).

54. FINLAND, M., AND BARNES, M. W., Changing ecology of

acute bacterial empyema: Occurrence and mortality at Boston City Hospital during twelve selected years from 1935 to 1972, *J. Infect. Dis.* **157**:274–291 (1978).

55. FINLAND, M., AND SUTLIFF, W. D., Specific cutaneous reactions and circulating antibodies in the course of lobar pneumonia. I. Cases receiving no serum therapy, *J. Exp. Med.* **54**:637–652 (1931).

56. FINLAND, M., AND SUTLIFF, W. D., Specific antibody response of human subjects to intracutaneous injection of pneumococcus products, *J. Exp. Med.* **55**:853–865 (1932).

57. FINLAND, M., AND TILGHMAN, R. C., Bacteriological and immunological studies in families with pneumococcic infections: The development of type-specific antibodies in healthy contact carriers, *J. Clin. Invest.* **15**:501–508 (1936).

58. FINLAND, M., AND WINKLER, A. W., Recurrences in pneumococcus pneumonia, *Am. J. Med. Sci.* **188**:309–320 (1934).

59. GIEBINK, G. S., The pathogenesis of otitis media in chinchillas and the efficacy of vaccination on prophylaxis, *Rev. Infect. Dis.* **3**:342–352 (1981).

60. GIEBINK, G. S., Preventing pneumococcal disease in children: Recommendations for using pneumococcal vaccine, *Pediatr. Infect. Dis.* **4**:343–348 (1985).

61. GIEBINK, G. S., GREBNER, J. V., KIM, Y., AND QUIE, P. G., Severe opsonic deficiency produced by *Streptococcus pneumoniae* and by capsular polysaccharide antigens, *Yale J. Biol. Med.* **51**:527–538 (1978).

62. GIEBINK, G. S., SCHIFFMAN G., KRIVIT, W., AND QUIE, P. G., Vaccine-type pneumococcal pneumonia after vaccination in an asplenic patient, *J. Am. Med. Assoc.* **241**:2736–2737 (1979).

63. GIEBINK, G. S., BERZINS, J. K., MARKER, S. C., AND SCHIFFMAN, G., Experimental otitis media after nasal inoculation of *Streptococcus pneumoniae* and influenza A in chinchillas, *Infect. Immun.* **30**:445–450 (1980).

64. GIEBINK, G. S., LE, C. T., COSIO, F. G., SPIKA, J. S., AND SCHIFFMAN, G., Serum antibody responses of high-risk children and adults to vaccination with capsular polysaccharides of *Streptococcus pneumoniae, Rev. Infect. Dis.* **3**(Suppl.): S168–S178 (1981).

65. GILMAN, B. B., AND ANDERSON G. W., Community outbreak of type I pneumococcus infection, *Am. J. Hyg.* **28**:345–358 (1938).

66. GOODNER, K., Development and localization of dermal pneumococcic infection in the rabbit, *J. Exp. Med.* **54**:847–858 (1931).

67. GORGAS, W. C., Sanitation on the Panama Canal, *J. Am. Med. Assoc.* **40**:953–955 (1913).

68. GREENBERG, D., Relation of meteorological conditions to the prevalence of pneumonia, *J. Am. Med. Assoc.* **72**:252–257 (1919).

69. GREENWOOD, M., NEWBOLD, E. M., TOPLEY, W. N., AND WILSON, J., On the mechanism of protection against infectious disease, *J. Hyg.* **28**:117–132 (1928).

70. HANDWERGER, S., AND TOMASZ, A., Alterations in pen-

icillin-binding proteins of clinical and laboratory isolates of pathogenic *Streptococcus pneumoniae* with low levels of penicillin resistance, *J. Infect. Dis.* **153**:83–89 (1986).

71. HANSMAN, D., AND BULLEN, M. M., A resistant pneumococcus, *Lancet* **2**:264–265 (1967).

72. HARRIS, A. H., AND INGRAHAM, H. S., Study of carrier condition associated with type II pneumonia in camp of Civilian Conservation Corps, *J. Clin. Invest.* **16**:41–48 (1937).

73. Health and Public Policy Committee, American College of Physicians, Pneumococcal vaccine, *Ann. Intern. Med.* **104**:118–120 (1986).

74. HEFFRON, R., *Pneumonia with Special Reference to Pneumococcus Lobar Pneumonia, p. 268,* Commonwealth Fund, New York, 1939; reprinted by Harvard University Press (1979).

75. HIRSCH, E. F., AND MCKINNEY, M., An epidemic of pneumococcus bronchopneumonia, *J. Infect. Dis.* **24**:594–617 (1919).

76. HOLLE, H. A., AND BULLOWA, J. G. M., Pneumococcal cross-infections in home and hospital, *N. Engl. J. Med.* **223**:887–890 (1940).

77. IVEMARK, B., Implications of agenesis of the spleen on the pathogenesis of cono-truncal anomalies in children, *Acta Pediatr. Scand.* (Suppl. 104) **44**:590 (1955).

78. JACOBS, M. R., KOORNHOF, H. J., ROBINS-BROWN, R. M., STEVENSON, C. M., VERMAAK, Z. A., FREIMAN, I., MILLER, G. B., WITCOMB, M. A., ISAÄCSON, M., WARD, J. I., AND AUSTRIAN, R., Emergence of multiply resistant pneumococci, *N. Engl. J. Med.* **299**:735–740 (1978).

79. JOHNSTON, H., Pneumonia as contagious disease, *Can. Med. Assoc. J.* **38**:270–271 (1938).

80. KASS, E. H. (ed.), Assessment of the pneumococcal polysaccharide vaccine: A workshop held at the Harvard Club of Boston, Boston, Massachusetts, October 6, 1980, *Rev. Infect. Dis.* **3**(Suppl.):S1–S197 (1981).

81. KASS, E. H., GREEN, G. M., AND GOLDSTEIN, E., Mechanism of antibacterial action in the respiratory tract, *Bacteriol. Rev.* **30**:488–496 (1966).

82. KAUFMAN, P., Pneumonia in old age. Active immunization against pneumonia with pneumococcus polysaccharides; results of a six year study, *Arch. Intern. Med.* **79**:518–531 (1947).

83. KLEIN, J. O., The epidemiology of pneumococcal disease in infants and children, *Rev. Infect. Dis.* **3**:246–253 (1981).

84. LaFORCE, F. M., AND EICKHOFF, T. C., Pneumococcal vaccine: The evidence mounts, *Ann. Intern. Med.* **104**:110–112 (1986).

85. LAZARUS, H. M., LEDERMAN, M., LUBIN, A., HERZIG, R. H., SCHIFFMAN, G., JONES, P., WINE, A., AND RODMAN, H. M., Pneumococcal vaccination: The response of patients with multiple myeloma, *Am. J. Med.* **69**:419–423 (1980).

86. LEE, C.-J., FRASER, B. A., SZU, S., AND LIN, K.-T., Chemical structure of and immune response to polysaccharides of *Streptococcus pneumoniae*, *Rev. Infect. Dis.* **3**:323–331 (1981).

87. LIN, K.-T., AND LEE, C.-J., Immune response of neonates to pneumococcal polysaccharide–protein conjugate, *Immunology* **46**:333–342 (1982).

88. LISTER, F. S., Specific serological reactions with pneumococci from different sources, *Publ. S. Afr. Inst. Med. Res.* **1**:1–14 (1913).

89. LISTER, F. S., An experimental study of prophylactic inoculation against pneumococcal infection in the rabbit and in man, *Publ. S. Afr. Inst. Med. Res.* **1**:231–287 (1916).

90. LISTER, F. S., Prophylactic inoculation of man against pneumococcal infections, and more particularly against lobar pneumonia, *Publ. S. Afr. Inst. Med. Res.* **10**:304–322 (1917).

91. LISTER, S., AND ORDMAN, D., Epidemiology of pneumonia on the Witwatersrand goldfields and prevention of pneumonia and other acute respiratory diseases in native laborers in South Africa by means of vaccine, *Publ. S. Afr. Inst. Med. Res.* **7**:1–124 (1935).

92. LOWELL, F. C., STRAUSS, E., AND FINLAND, M., Observations on the susceptibility of pneumococci to sulfapyridine, sulfathiazole and sulfamethoxazole, *Ann. Intern. Med.* **14**:1001–1023 (1940).

93. LUND, E., Types of pneumococci found in blood, spinal fluid and pleural exudate during 15 years (1954–1969), *Acta Pathol. Microbiol. Scand. Sect. B* **78**:333–336 (1970).

94. LUND, E., PULVERER, G., AND JELJASZEWICZ, J., Serological types of *Diplococcus pneumoniae* strains isolated in Germany, *Med. Microbiol. Immunol.* **159**:171–178 (1974).

95. MACLEOD, C. M., HODGES, R. G., HEIDELBERGER, M., AND BERNHARD, W. G., Prevention of pneumococcal pneumonia by immunization with specific capsular polysaccharides, *J. Exp. Med.* **82**:445–465 (1945).

96. MAYNARD, G. D., An enquiry into the etiology, manifestations and prevention of pneumonia amongst natives on the Rand from tropical areas, *Publ. S. Afr. Inst. Med. Res.* **1**:1–101 (1913).

97. MCGOWAN, J. E., JR., BRATTON, L., KLEIN, J. O., AND FINLAND, M., Bacteremia in febrile children in a "walk-in" pediatric clinic, *N. Engl. J. Med.* **288**:1309–1312 (1973).

98. MCGOWAN, J. E., JR., BARNES, M. W., AND FINLAND, M., Bacteremia at Boston City Hospital: Occurrence and mortality during 12 selected years 1935–1972, with special reference to hospital-acquired cases, *J. Infect. Dis.* **132**:316–335 (1975).

99. MOORE, H. F., AND CHESNEY, A. M., A further study of ethyl-hydrocupreine (optochin) in the treatment of acute lobar pneumonia, *Arch. Intern. Med.* **21**:659–681 (1918).

100. MUFSON, M. A., Pneumococcal infections, *J. Am. Med. Assoc.* **246**:1942–1948 (1981).

101. NEMIR, R. L., ANDREWS, E. T., AND VINOGRAD, J., Pneumonia in infants and children: Bacteriologic study with special reference to clinical significance, *Am. J. Dis. Child.* **51**:1277–1295 (1936).

102. NETTER, Contagion de la pneumonie, *Arch. Gen. Med. (Paris)* **21**:530–544, 699–718; **22**:42–59 (1888).

103. NEUFELD, F., Ueber eine specifische bakteriolytische Wirkung der Galle, *Z. Hyg. Infektionskr.* **34**:454–464 (1900).

104. NEUFELD, F., Ueber die Agglutination der Pneumokokken und Ueber die Theorien der Agglutination, *Z. Hyg. Infektionskr.* **40**:54–72 (1902).

105. OPIE, E. L., BLAKE, F. G., SMALL, J. C., AND RIVERS, T. M., *Epidemic Respiratory Disease: The Pneumonias and Other Infections of the Respiratory Tract Accompanying Influenza and Measles,* Mosby, St. Louis, 1921.

106. ORDMAN, D., Pneumonia in the native mine workers of the Witwatersrand goldfields: A bacteriological and epidemiological study, *J. Med. Assoc. S. Afr.* **5**:108–116 (1931).

107. ORDMAN, D., Pneumonia in the native mine labourers of northern Rhodesia copperfields with an account of an experiment in pneumonia prophylaxis by means of a vaccine at the Roan Antelope Mine, *Publ. S. Afri. Inst. Med. Res.* **7**:1–124 (1935).

108. ORDMAN, D., Pneumococcus typing: Its value in pneumonia, *S. Afr. Med. J.* **11**:569–573 (1937).

109. ORDMAN, D., Pneumococcus types in South Africa: A study of their occurrence and the effect thereon of prophylactic inoculation, *Publ. S. Afr. Inst. Med. Res.* **9**:1–27 (1938).

110. ORENSTEIN, A. J., Vaccine prophylaxis in pneumonia: A review of fourteen years' experience with inoculation of native mine workers on the Witwatersrand against pneumonia, *J. Med. Assoc. S. Afr.* **5**:339–346 (1931).

111. PALLARES, R., GUDIOL, F., LIÑARES, J., ARIZA, J., RUFI, G., MURGUI, L., DORCA, J., AND VILADRICH, P. F., Risk factors and response to antibiotic therapy in adults with bacteremic pneumonia caused by penicillin-resistant pneumococci, *N. Engl. J. Med.* **317**:18–22 (1987).

112. PARK, J. H., JR., AND CHICKERING, H. T., Type I pneumococcal lobar pneumonia among Puerto Rican laborers of Camp Jackson, South Carolina, *J. Am. Med. Assoc.* **73**:183–186 (1919).

113. PARKER, M. T., Type distribution of pneumococci isolated from serious diseases in Britain, in: *Pathogenic Streptococci* (M. T. Parker, ed.), pp. 191–192, Redbooks, Chertsey, England, 1979.

114. PATRICK, K. M., AND WOOLLEY, F. R., A cost–benefit analysis of immunization of pneumococcal pneumonia, *J. Am. Med. Assoc.* **245**:473–477 (1981).

115. PEARSON, H. A., Splenectomy: Its risks and its roles, *Hosp. Pract.* **August**:85–94 (1980).

116. PERLINO, C. A., AND RIMLAND, D., Alcoholism leukopenia and pneumococcal sepsis, *Am. Rev. Respir. Dis.* **132**:757–760 (1985).

117. QUIE, P. G., GIEBINK, G. S., AND WINKELSTEIN, J. A. (guest eds.), *The Pneumoncoccus:* A symposium held at the Kroc Foundation Headquarters, Santa Ynez Valley, California, February 25–29, 1980, *Rev. Infect. Dis.* **3**:183–371 (1981).

118. Recommendation of the Public Health Service Advisory Committee on Immunization Practices: Pneumococcal polysaccharide vaccine, *Morbid. Mortal. Weekly Rep.* **27**:25–31 (1978).

119. RILEY, I. D., AND DOUGLAS, R. M., An epidemiologic approach to pneumococcal disease, *Rev. Infect. Dis.* **3**:233–245 (1981).

120. ROBBINS, J. B., AUSTRIAN, R., LEE, C.-J., RASTOGI, S. C., SCHIFFMAN, G., HENRICHSEN, J., MAKELA, P. H., BROOME, C. V., FACKLAM, R. R., TIESJEMA, R. H., AND PARKE, J. C., JR., Considerations for formulating the second-generation pneumococcal capsular polysaccharide vaccine with emphases on the cross-reactive types within groups, *J. Infect. Dis.* **148**:1136–1159 (1983).

121. ROBERTSON, O. H., Instance of lobar pneumonia acquired in the laboratory, *J. Prev. Med.* **5**:221–224 (1931).

122. ROGERS, L., Relationship between pneumonia incidence and climate in India, *Lancet* **1**:1173–1177 (1925).

123. RYTEL, M. W., Pneumococcal pneumonia, in: *Rapid Diagnosis in Infectious Disease* (M. W. Rytel, ed.), pp. 91–103, CRC Press, Boca Raton, 1979.

124. RYTEL, M. W., DEE, T. H., FERSTENFELD, J. E., AND HENSLEY, G. T., Possible pathogenic role of capsular antigens in fulminant pneumococcal disease with disseminated intravascular coagulation, *Am. J. Med.* **57**:889–896 (1974).

125. SAAH, A. J., MALLONEE, J. R., TARPAY, M., THORNSBERRY, C. T., ROBERTS, M. A., AND RHOADES, E. R., Relative resistance to penicillin in the pneumococcus, *J. Am. Med. Assoc.* **243**:1824–1827 (1980).

126. SABIN, A. B., "Stained slide" microscopic agglutination test: Application to (1) rapid typing of pneumococci, (2) determination of antibody, *Am. J. Public Health* **19**:1148–1150 (1929).

127. SABIN, A. B., Immediate pneumococcus typing directly from sputum by the Neufeld reaction, *J. Am. Med. Assoc.* **100**:1584–1586 (1933).

128. SCHIFFMAN, G., Immune response to pneumococcal polysaccharide antigens: A comparison of the murine model and the response in humans, *Rev. Infect. Dis.* **3**:224–231 (1981).

129. SCHIFFMAN, G., DOUGLAS, R. M., BONNER, M. J., ROBBINS, M., AND AUSTRIAN, R., A radioimmunoassay for immunologic phenomena in pneumococcal disease and for the antibody response to pneumococcal vaccines. 1. Methods for the radioimmunoassay of anticapsular antibodies and comparison of other techniques, *J. Immunol. Methods* **33**:133–144 (1980).

130. SCHNEERSON, R., ROBBINS, J. B., CHU, C., SUTTON, A., VANN, W., VICKERS, J. C., LONDON, W. T., CURFMAN, B., HARDEGREE, M. C., SHILOACH, J., AND RASTOGI, S. C., Serum antibody responses of juvenile and infant rhesus monkeys injected with *Haemophilus influenzae* type b and pneumococcus type 6A capsular polysaccharide–protein conjugates, *Infect. Immun.* **45**:582–591 (1984).

131. SCHWARTZ, J. S., Pneumococcal vaccine: Clinical efficacy and effectiveness, *Ann. Intern. Med.* **96**:208–220 (1982).

132. SELL, S. H., WRIGHT, P. F., VAUGHAN, W. K., THOMPSON,

J., AND SCHIFFMAN, G., Clinical studies of pneumococcal vaccine in infants. 1. Reactogenicity and immunogenicity of two polyvalent polysaccharide vaccines, *Rev. Infect. Dis.* **3**:S97–S107 (1981).

133. SHAPIRO, E. D., Pneumococcal vaccine failure [letter], *N. Engl. J. Med.* **316**:1272–1273 (1987).

134. SHAPIRO, E. D., AND CLEMENS, J. D., A controlled evaluation of the protective efficacy of pneumococcal vaccine for patients at high risk for serious pneumococcal infections, *Ann. Intern. Med.* **101**:325–330 (1984).

135. SIBER, G., Immunoprophylaxis and therapy of *Haemophilus influenzae* and pneumococcal infections, Program and Abstracts of the Twenty-Seventh Interscience Conference on Antimicrobial Agents and Chemotherapy, p. 63, American Society for Microbiology, Washington, D.C., 1987.

136. SIMBERKOFF, M. S., RICHMOND, A., LUKASZEWSKI, M., CROSS, A. P., BALTCH, A., NADLER, J., AL-IBRAHIM, M., AND GEISLER, P. J., Isolation of multiply antibiotic-resistant pneumococci, New York, *Morbid. Mortal. Weekly Rep.* **34**:545–546 (1985).

137. SIMBERKOFF, M. S., CROSS, A. P., AL-IBRAHIM, M., BALTCH, A. L., GEISLER, P. J., NADLER, J., RICHMOND, A. S., SMITH, R. P., AND VAN EECKHOUT, J. P., Efficacy of pneumococcal vaccine in high-risk patients: Results of a Veterans Administration cooperative study, *N. Engl. J. Med.* **315**:1318–1327 (1986).

138. SIMBERKOFF, M. S., LUKASZEWSKI, M., CROSS, A., AL-IBRAHIM, M., BALTCH, A. L., SMITH, R. P., GEISLER, P. J., NADLER, J., AND RICHMOND, A. S., Antibiotic isolates of *Streptococcus pneumoniae* from clinical specimens: A cluster of serotype 19A organisms in Brooklyn, New York, *J. Infect. Dis.* **153**:78–82 (1986).

139. SISK, J. E., AND RIEGELMAN, R. K., Cost effectiveness of vaccination against pneumococcal pneumonia: An update, *Ann. Intern. Med.* **104**:79–86 (1986).

140. SMALL, A. A., Pneumonia at a base hospital: Observations in one thousand and one hundred cases at Camp Pike, Ark., *J. Am. Med. Assoc.* **71**:700–702 (1918).

141. SMILLIE, W. E., Study of an outbreak of type II pneumococcus pneumonia in Veterans' Administration Hospital at Bedford, Massachusetts, *Am. J. Hyg.* **24**:522–535 (1936).

142. SMILLIE, W. E., WARNOCK, G. H., AND WHITE, H. J., Study of a type I pneumococcus epidemic at the State Hospital at Worcester, Mass., *Am. J. Public Health* **28**:293–302 (1938).

143. SMIT, P., OBERHOLZER, D., HAYDEN-SMITH, S., KOORNHOF, H. J., AND HILLEMAN, M. R., Protective efficacy of pneumococcal polysaccharide vaccines, *J. Am. Med. Assoc.* **238**:2613–2616 (1977).

144. STILLMAN, E. G., Susceptibility of rabbits to infection by the inhalation of type II pneumococcus, *J. Exp. Med.* **52**:215–224 (1930).

145. STILLMAN, E. G., AND BRANCH, A., Experimental production of pneumococcus pneumonia in mice by inhalation method, *J. Exp. Med.* **40**:733–742 (1924).

146. STRAUSS, E., AND FINLAND, M., Further studies on recur-

rences in pneumococcic pneumonia with special reference to the effect of specific treatment, *Ann. Intern. Med.* **16**:17–32 (1942).

147. SYDENSTRICKER, V. P. W., AND SUTTON, A. C., An epidemiological study of lobar pneumonia, *Bull. Johns Hopkins Hosp.* **38**:312–315 (1918).

148. TEELE, D. W., PELTON, S. I., GRANT, M. J. A., HERSKOWITZ, J., ROSEN, D. J., ALLEN, C. E., WIMER, R. S., AND KLEIN, J. O., Bacteremia in febrile children under 2 years of age: Results of cultures of blood in 600 consecutive febrile children in a "walk-in" clinic, *J. Pediatr.* **87**:227–230 (1975).

149. TENNY, C. F., AND RIVENBURGH, W. T., A group of 68 cases of type I pneumonia occurring in 30 days at Camp Upton, *Arch. Intern. Med.* **24**:545–552 (1919).

150. TERRELL, E. E., ROBERTSON, O. H., AND COGGESHALL, L. T., Experimental pneumococcus lobar pneumonia in the dog. I. Method of production and course of disease, *J. Clin. Invest.* **12**:393–432 (1933).

151. TILGHMAN, R. C., AND FINLAND, M., Clinical significance of bacteremia in pneumococcal pneumonia, *Arch. Intern. Med.* **59**:602–619 (1937).

152. TILLOTSON, J. R., AND FINLAND, M., Bacterial colonization and clinical superinfection of the respiratory tract complicating antibiotic treatment of pneumonia, *J. Infect. Dis.* **119**:597–624 (1969).

153. TOMASZ, A., Surface components of *Streptococcus pneumoniae, Rev. Infect. Dis.* **3**:190–211 (1981).

154. TOMFORDE, Eine Endemie von croupöser Pneumonie im Dorfe Laumuhlen, Kreis Neuhaus an der Oste, Januar 1902, *Dtsch, Med. Wochenschr.* **28**:577–579 (1902).

155. U.S. Congress, Office of Technology Assessment, A Review of Selected Federal Vaccine and Immunization Policies, U.S. Government Printing Office, Washington, D.C., 1979.

156. VERHOEF, J., Effects of nutrition on antibiotic action, in: *Action of Antibiotics in Patients* (L. D. Sabath and G. G. Grassi, eds.), Huber, Bern, 1982.

157. WALDMAN, J. D., ROSENTHAL, A., SMITH, A. L., SHURIN, S., AND NADAS, A. S., Sepsis and congenital asplenia, *J. Pediatr.* **90**:555–559 (1977).

158. WARA, D. W., Host defense against *Streptococcus pneumoniae:* The role of the spleen, *Rev. Infect. Dis.* **3**:299–309 (1981).

159. WARD, J., Antibiotic-resistant *Streptococcus pneumoniae:* Clinical and epidemiologic aspects, *Rev. Infect. Dis.* **3**:254–266 (1981).

160. WEBSTER, L. T., Mode of spread of Friedlander's bacillus-like respiratory infection in mice, *J. Exp. Med.* **47**:685–712 (1928).

161. WHITBY, L., Chemotherapy of bacterial infections (Bradshaw Lecture), *Lancet* **2**:1095–1103 (1938).

162. WHITE, B. (with the collaboration of ROBINSON, E. S., AND BARNES, L. A.), *The Biology of Pneumococcus: The Bacteriological, Biochemical and Immunological Characters and Activities of Diplococcus pneumoniae,* Commonwealth Fund, New York, 1938; reprinted by Harvard University Press (1979).

163. WINKELSTEIN, J. A., The role of complement in the hosts' defense against *Streptococcus pneumoniae, Rev. Infect. Dis.* **3:**289–298 (1981).

164. WOOD, C. C., MCNAMARA, J. G., SCHWARZ, D. F., MERRILL, W. W., AND SHAPIRO, E. D., Prevention of pneumococcal bacteremia in a child with AIDS-related complex, *Pediatr. Infect. Dis. J.* **6:**564–566 (1987).

165. WRIGHT, A. E., MORGAN, W., COLBROOK, L., AND DODGSON, R. W., Observations on prophylactic inoculations against pneumococcus infection, and on the results which have been achieved by it, *Lancet* **1:**1–10, 87–95 (1914).

166. ZIGHELBOIM, S., AND TOMASZ, A., Multiple antibiotic resistance in South African strains of *Streptococcus pneumoniae:* Mechanism of resistance to β-lactam antibiotics, *Rev. Infect. Dis.* **3:**267–276 (1981).

12. Suggested Reading

APPLEBAUM, P. R. World-wide development of antibiotic resistance in pneumococci, *Eur. J. Clin. Microbiol.* **6:**367–377, 1987 (131 refs.).

FINLAND, M., Recent advances in the epidemiology of pneumococcal infections, *Medicine* **21:**307–344 1942 (332 refs.).

HEFFRON, R., *Pneumonia with Special Reference to Pneumococcal Lobar Pneumonia,* Commonwealth Fund, New York, 1939; reprinted by Harvard University Press, 1979 (1471 refs.).

KASS, E. H. (ed.), Assessment of the pneumococcal polysaccharide vaccine: A workshop held at the Harvard Club of Boston, Boston, Massachusetts, October 6, 1980, *Rev. Infect. Dis.* **3**(Suppl.):S1–S197, 1981 (213 refs.).

MUFSON, M. A., Pneumococcal infections, *J. Am. Med. Assoc.* **246:**1942–1948 1981 (132 refs.).

QUIE, P. G., GIEBINK, G. S., AND WINKELSTEIN, J. A. (guest eds.), *The Pneumococcus:* A symposium held at the Kroc Foundation Headquarters, Santa Ynez Valley, California, February 25–29, 1980, *Rev. Infect. Dis.* **3:**183–371 (1981) (197 refs.).

WHITE, B. (with the collaboration of ROBINSON, E. S., AND BARNES, L. A.), *The Biology of Pneumococcus: The Bacteriological, Biochemical and Immunological Characters and Activities of Diplococcus pneumoniae,* Commonwealth Fund, New York, 1938; reprinted by Harvard University Press, 1979 (1593 refs.).

CHAPTER 26

Q Fever

Paul Fiset and Theodore E. Woodward

1. Introduction

Q fever is an acute infectious disease caused by *Coxiella burnetii*. The infection has been reported from all continents and occurs in sporadic and epidemic forms. Human infection is usually acquired by inhalation of the organisms from the tissues of infected domestic animals or their contaminated environment. In its classic form, Q fever has a sudden onset with fever, chills, malaise, weakness, and a severe headache. There is frequently a pneumonitis and, in some cases, signs of hepatic involvement. Infection with *C. burnetii,* however, is usually mild and clinically unrecognized. In contrast to the other rickettsioses, there is no rash and *Proteus* agglutinins do not develop. Chloramphenicol and the tetracyclines are highly effective except in cases of endocarditis.

2. Historical Background

In 1935, Derrick investigated an outbreak of a febrile illness that occurred in abattoir workers in Brisbane, Australia. The disease was characterized by a sudden onset with fever, chills, and an intractable headache. His first report[33] included nine cases. Respiratory signs and symptoms were not prominent; one patient had signs of hepatic involvement. All attempts to isolate bacterial pathogens failed.

Paul Fiset · Department of Microbiology and Immunology, University of Maryland School of Medicine, Baltimore, Maryland 21201. **Theodore E. Woodward** · Department of Medicine, University of Maryland School of Medicine, Baltimore, Maryland 21201.

Lacking a better name, Derrick called the disease Q (for query) fever. Although the etiology is now well known, the term Q fever has been retained.

Burnet and Freeman[19] isolated an organism from specimens received from Derrick that were passaged in mice. It was characterized as a rickettsia unrelated to any other rickettsia known at that time. Derrick[34] suggested that the organism be called *Rickettsia burnetii*. Working on the principle that rickettsiae had natural vertebrate hosts and were transmitted by specific arthropod vectors, Derrick and Smith[37] conclusively demonstrated that bandicoots and their ticks were involved in the natural life cycle of *R. burnetii*. This observation did not help in popularizing Q fever abroad. It was considered merely as another Australian oddity.

Meanwhile, halfway across the world, Davis and Cox,[30] during their studies on the ecology of Rocky Mountain spotted fever in western Montana, isolated an agent from *Dermacentor andersoni* that they characterized as a rickettsia. It was unrelated to any other known rickettsiae and, because of its filterability through Berkfeld candles, they named it *R. diaporica*.[25] Its potential as a human pathogen was unknown until several laboratory infections occurred. The clinical picture was similar to that of Q fever, and the organism isolated from these patients was identical to *R. diaporica* and *R. burnetii*.[14,20,40]

Emulsions of rickettsiae extracted from infected mouse spleens were specifically agglutinated by sera of patients convalescing from Q fever.[20] Parker and Davis[87] demonstrated that *R. diaporica* could be transmitted to laboratory animals by *D. andersoni*. However, neither the role of ticks in natural transmission nor the broad prevalence of infection in animals and man was known at the time. Although Q fever had been shown to exist outside Australia in the late

1930s, its importance as a cause of human disease outside the abattoirs of Brisbane or the laboratories of the National Institutes of Health was not fully appreciated. These observations were overshadowed by the onset of World War II.

Until 1944, Q fever was generally considered an Australian disease. By this time, Derrick[35] had reported 176 cases occurring among abattoir and farm workers in Queensland. During the winter of 1944–1945, however, Q fever emerged as a serious infectious disease of military significance. There were several outbreaks of severe respiratory infections with systemic manifestations among American and British troops in Italy. The disease was recognized as Q fever, and approximately 1000 cases were identified. One outbreak merits a brief description since its study led to a better understanding of the epidemiology of Q fever. The 3rd Battalion of the 362nd Infantry was withdrawn from the front and billeted in the Apennine Mountains north of Florence, for rest and recuperation. Headquarters were established in a farmhouse; troops were settled in tents, and a barn was used as a makeshift cinema where training and recreational films were shown. Much dust was created by the movement of men in the barn. Between April 7 and 29, 1945, of 900 men stationed on the base, 269 came down with Q fever. At the 15th Medical General Laboratory in Naples, where specimens from the outbreaks were processed, 20 cases occurred among the personnel.[95,96]

Study of the 1944–1945 outbreak led to the following important epidemiological conclusions: (1) arthropod vectors were not involved in transmission; (2) infection seemed to be associated with the respiratory route through contaminated dust; (3) although there was a high morbidity rate, Q fever was not a lethal illness; (4) Q fever, as it occurred among the troops, was unknown in the local population; and (5) the local population showed a high incidence of specific antibodies.

It was learned that German troops, during 1943–1944, in Bulgaria, Greece, Italy, and the Crimea had experienced an illness called "Balkan grippe."[32] During an outbreak of "Balkan grippe," Caminopetros in Athens isolated an organism that was maintained through passages in guinea pigs. Blood samples obtained from Caminopetros by Zarafonetis were transported unrefrigerated for several weeks to Washington. *R. burnetii* was isolated from the specimens, which established it as the etiological agent of "Balkan grippe."[24] The observation demonstrated the amazing stability of the agent. Q fever was then recognized as a disease with considerable epidemic potential.

Because the agent of Q fever differed markedly from other rickettsiae (no rash, no Weil–Felix reaction, relatively more resistant to chemical and physical agents, no requirement for arthropod vectors), Philip[89] proposed a new genus, *Coxiella*. *Coxiella burnetii* is the only member of the genus.

3. Methodology

The intensive study of the outbreaks of Q fever among Allied troops in Europe in 1944–1945 resulted in a greater ability on the part of the medical profession to recognize outbreaks of the disease in other areas of the world.

Investigation of the wartime outbreaks among Allied troops was greatly facilitated by the observation of Cox[26] that rickettsiae of Rocky Mountain spotted fever, typhus, and Q fever groups grew profusely in the yolk sac of chick embryos. This simple methodology, unavailable to German scientists at the time, resulted in the production of excellent antigens for agglutination and complement-fixation (CF) reactions. This methodology also led to the production of an effective typhus vaccine.

Experience acquired from the investigation of the outbreaks of Q fever among Allied troops in Europe was, undoubtedly, instrumental in the recognition of several outbreaks that occurred in the United States shortly after World War II.

3.1. Sources of Mortality Data

Q fever is rarely fatal and has a mortality of under 1%, even untreated. Furthermore, the diagnosis requires laboratory confirmation. Thus, mortality data are not useful for assessing the importance of the disease.

3.2. Sources of Morbidity Data

Q fever is not a reportable disease in the United States, so incidence rates are not available. Infection is often mild or subclinical. The data on recognized cases come from investigation of epidemics, studies of high-risk exposure groups, and public-health and veterinary-hospital laboratories where the diagnosis is made. The laboratory information is probably the most reliable source of morbidity data and is periodically reported in national health reports and the *WHO Weekly Epidemiological Record*.

3.3. Surveys

With the use of isolation procedures and the CF reaction for serosurveys, it became quite obvious that infection of man and domestic animals with *C. burnetii* occurred frequently without recognizable clinical manifestations. It was also evident that death following Q fever was rare.

The CF test with Phase II antigen (see Section 4) has been most commonly used in serological surveys but since Phase II antibody disappears in 2–3 years, it reflects only more recent infection (see Section 3.4.2).

A skin test for detecting hypersensitivity to *C. burnetii* has been very useful in epidemiological surveys because skin positivity persists longer than detectable antibody. Aziz *et al.*,[4] in Egypt, clearly demonstrated the superiority of the skin test over serological procedures as an epidemiological tool. They showed that 26% of young army recruits were skin-test-positive, whereas only 10% were seropositive.

3.4. Laboratory Diagnosis

3.4.1. Isolation Procedures. *C. burnetii* is readily isolated from the blood of patients during the febrile period; it has been recovered also from urine. Milk, birth fluids, urine, and tissues of infected domestic animals yield *C. burnetii*. The guinea pig is exquisitely sensitive to experimental infection, although large inocula are usually required to cause death. Infection can be recognized by serological conversion 21–28 days after inoculation. *C. burnetii* will also grow profusely in the yolk sac of chick embryos. With strains adapted to chick embryos, yields are on the order of 10^{11} rickettsiae/g yolk sac,[84] which is considerably more than that achieved with other rickettsiae.

Because of the high risk of infection, attempts at isolation of *C. burnetii* from human or animal specimens should be made only in laboratories with proper skills and facilities.

3.4.2. Serological Procedures. In the past the most commonly used serological procedure for diagnosis and epidemiological surveys was the CF test carried out with yolk-sac-grown *C. burnetii* in Phase II (see Section 4). The antigen is available commercially, and the procedure was carried out by most state health department laboratories.

Phase I CF antibodies (see Section 4) rarely develop following acute Q fever; however, they reach high titers and are considered pathognomonic of chronic infections, i.e., hepatitis and endocarditis.[76]

Phase II CF antibodies usually become detectable by about 7 days after onset of illness, reach a peak at 21–28 days, and slowly decline thereafter. By 24–36 months after onset, antibody titers have usually dropped to levels that, on random serological surveys, would be considered insignificant (< 1:8).[80,110]

Over the years, many agglutination tests have been

devised. Burnet and Freeman[20] used suspensions of infected mouse spleens. Lennette *et al.*[67] and Ormsbee[72,81] used rickettsiae extracted from yolk sacs. These procedures require large amounts of antigen. Microscopic techniques have been developed to overcome this problem.[8,50] Although these latter procedures have been quite useful, they are time-consuming and do not lend themselves to the processing of large numbers of sera. A capillary agglutination test (CAT) was developed by Luoto[68] and was shown to be useful for detecting antibodies in milk. An agglutination reaction was adapted to the microtiter technique[47] for the measurement of rickettsial antibodies. It is simple to perform, rapid, and economical of reagents, and seems to be as sensitive and specific as the CF reaction. Although it is gaining general acceptance by laboratories around the world involved in rickettsial diagnosis and research, it has certain limitations. The antigens must be highly purified and are not at present commercially available. It should be noted that Phase II agglutinins appear at about the same time as Phase II CF antibodies. Although Phase I CF antibodies are rarely detected after acute Q fever in man, Phase I agglutinins usually are detectable after the appearance of Phase II antibodies.[46]

An indirect fluorescent-antibody (IFA) technique is available.[91] It has the distinct advantage that highly purified antigen is not required and that immunoglobulin classes of specific antibody can be identified. This procedure is now considered the method of choice and is carried out in most state health laboratories with antigens provided by CDC.

Although ELISA technology has been developed, its application has been limited mainly to research and has not yet been extensively adapted to diagnosis or serosurvey.

3.4.3. Skin-Testing Procedure. A skin test for the detection of hypersensitivity to *C. burnetii* was first introduced by Giroud and LeGac[52] and Giroud and Jadin.[50] They observed positive skin reactions in individuals who had serologically confirmed Q fever. The skin reactivity appears later than circulating antibodies, but also persists after antibodies are no longer detectable. The procedure has limited diagnostic value, but is an important epidemiological tool. Early reports on the use of a skin test indicated that local necrosis and sometimes systemic reactions occurred. These reactions were believed to be due to a toxic factor associated with the rickettsiae.[50,51] Although there are those who still believe this theory, it is more likely that the local and systemic reactions are immunological in nature and that their severity in previously sensitized individuals resulted from the large antigenic mass administered as a skin test dose.

The need to identify hypersensitive individuals became

obvious as a consequence of field trials of experimental Q fever vaccines. Q fever vaccines developed for military use proved to be highly effective in protecting against experimental Q fever.[13,114] However, there was a high incidence of local and systemic reactions that were more likely to occur in individuals receiving repeated injections of vaccine.[12]

Lachman *et al.*[62] developed a skin-test antigen that was initially standardized in CF units but subsequently standardized in term of dry weight of highly purified Phase I antigen. It contains 0.02 µg of organisms per dose (Ormsbee, personal communication). At the Rocky Mountain Laboratory of the National Institutes of Health, Hamilton, Montana, this skin-test antigen has been used on all incoming personnel for about 25 years. Only skin-test-negative individuals receive Q fever vaccine. After the introduction of this practice, no reactions to the vaccine occurred, and only a few laboratory-acquired infections have been reported (Ormsbee, personal communication).

4. Biological Characteristics of the Organism

C. burnetii possesses the general properties of the other rickettsiae, i.e., it is an obligate intracellular parasite with a cell wall similar to that of gram-negative bacteria. It is pleomorphic, ranging from coccobacillary forms measuring 0.2 by 0.5 µm to forms measuring 0.25 by 1.5 µm. Tiny spheres about 0.2 µm in diameter also exist, hence its early name, *R. diaporica*. It is considerably more resistant to hostile environmental conditions than are other rickettsiae. For instance, *C. burnetii* will survive a temperature of 60°C (140°F) for 30–60 min, while other rickettsiae are inactivated following exposure to 50°C (122°F) for 15 min. *C. burnetii* will survive exposure to 0.5% formalin for 4 days, whereas the other rickettsiae are inactivated following exposure to 0.1% formalin for less than 24 h.[94] Babudieri and Moscovici[7] demonstrated that *C. burnetii* is much more resistant to UV inactivation than are the other rickettsiae. These resistant characteristics allow *C. burnetii* to survive for weeks or even months in dust, which contributes markedly to its epidemiological potential. It can be stored at freezer temperatures for years without any loss of infectivity.[82] McCaul and Williams[78] have shown the presence of sporelike structures inside *C. burnetii*. Whether these structures are similar to the small spheres that led to the early designation of *R. diaporica*[25] is not clear nor is it clear whether these structures have anything to do with the unusual resistance of *C. burnetii* to hostile environmental conditions.

C. burnetii undergoes an antigenic phase variation

very similar to that of the rough–smooth variation of bacteria.[42,105] In nature, *C. burnetii* is found only in Phase I, the smooth phase, whereas Phase II is a laboratory artifact obtained after adaptation to growth in chick embryos. Phase I organisms possess a cell-wall-associated surface antigen[59] that behaves as a capsule masking the Phase II antigenic component.[43,44,46,105] The Phase I antigen is antiphagocytic[18,119] and appears related to virulence.[44,46] Phase II organisms lack the surface Phase I antigen, are of lesser virulence than the parent strains,[92] and are readily phagocytized in the absence of specific antisera. The phenomenon is reversible. Phase II organisms revert to Phase I by passage in animals (guinea pigs, mice, hamsters).[105] Ormsbee *et al.*[85] have demonstrated that repeatedly plaque-purified Phase II organisms are completely avirulent for guinea pigs in which they do not seem to replicate and therefore do not revert to Phase I. Repeatedly plaque-purified Phase I organisms, on the other hand, are fully virulent for guinea pigs and, when serially passed in developing chick embryos, revert to Phase II.

Experimental infection of guinea pigs with either Phase I or Phase II or vaccination with killed Phase I leads to a similar antibody response. Phase II CF antibodies and agglutinins appear early, within 7–10 days after inoculation, reach a peak by about 20 days, and decline thereafter. Phase I agglutinins appear about a week after Phase II antibodies. Phase I CF antibodies are not detectable until 40–60 days after inoculation. Vaccination of guinea pigs or rabbits with thoroughly egg-adapted killed Phase II organisms leads to a Phase II antibody response only.[43,46] The significance of the phase variation in relation to the epidemiology of Q fever is not clear except that in nature, *C. burnetii* is found only in Phase I.

High titers of Phase I antibodies rarely develop in man following acute Q fever.[105] High Phase I titers are considered pathognomonic of chronic disease, i.e., hepatitis and endocarditis.[76] Peacock *et al.*[88] have refined this observation by demonstrating that elevated levels of IgA Phase I antibodies are indicative of Q fever endocarditis. There seems to be only one serotype of *C. burnetii*.[48] The antigenic differences observed by early investigators can be explained, for the most part, on the basis of the phasevariation phenomenon.[44] However, Hackstadt[55] in his studies of the lipopolysaccharide (LPS) of several strains of *C. burnetii* Phase I by PAGE and immunoblotting techniques has demonstrated that strains isolated from cases of endocarditis have an LPS that is different from that of other strains isolated from cases of acute Q fever or Q fever hepatitis. The important implication of this observation is that only certain strains of *C. burnetii* are likely to cause endocarditis. Also there is some suggestive evidence that a plasmid is associated with certain strains involved in endocarditis.[98]

5. Descriptive Epidemiology

Q fever is a zoonosis. There is probably no other organism pathogenic for man with a host range as broad as that of *C. burnetii*. It has been isolated from over 40 species of ticks, from about a dozen species of chiggers,[6,27,121] from lice,[51] and from flies.[90] It has been isolated from a large variety of animals including wild and domestic mammals and birds.[6,27]

5.1. Prevalence and Incidence

Since Q fever is not on the list of nationally notifiable diseases in the United States and in many other countries, the information concerning its epidemiology has been acquired either from investigations of defined outbreaks, from serosurveys in human and animal populations conducted in various countries, or from public-health-laboratory data.

In the United States, Q fever is not a disease reportable to CDC. It is, however, reportable in some states.[28] Between 1948 and 1977, 1169 cases have been optionally reported to CDC from 26 states. Of these cases, 67% (785) were reported from California. Between 1948 and 1977 there have been an average of 39 cases per year reported to CDC, with peaks of 105 in 1953 and 106 in 1954.[28] Between 1978 and 1986, 228 cases were reported to CDC.[99]

In the United Kingdom, the public-health laboratories reported between 48 and 78 cases annually between 1967 and 1974, averaging about 59 cases a year. In 1976 and 1977, there were 215 reported cases.[116] Although we do not have more recent data for the incidence, there is no reason to believe that the situation has changed significantly in recent years.

The prevalence of infection has been determined by serological surveys. A serological survey carried out on 12,000 human sera collected in Los Angeles and vicinity[11] yielded the following: (1) A first group (5000 individuals) were selected as representatives of the general population of Los Angeles without any particular association with livestock. In this population, 1.4% had CF antibodies at significant titers. Considering the fairly rapid decay of CF antibodies after Q fever, 2–3 years,[80] these results would imply that within the past few years, there had been 50,000 cases of Q fever in the Los Angeles area. (2) In groups

selected because of their association with livestock, the incidence varied depending on the closeness of the association. In packing plants where few or no dairy cows were slaughtered, the incidence was 4.0%. In plants where dairy cows or young calves were slaughtered, it was 11%. Among dairy workers, it was 23%. (3) Of raw-milk drinkers, 12% were seropositive, as opposed to 1.2% of non-raw-milk drinkers.

The incidence and prevalence of infection in animals are also relevant to human exposure. Important observations that led to a better understanding of the epidemiology of Q fever were that dairy cows frequently have a recrudescent infection during pregnancy, that *C. burnetii* can be recovered from the placentas and birth fluids in extremely large numbers [10^8 guinea pig infective doses ($GPID_{50}$)/g], and that the organism is excreted in the milk over a long period.[70] Such massive infections seemed to have no deleterious effect on gestation, parturition, or the newborn. The excretion of such massive numbers of organisms into the environment and the unusual resistance of *C. burnetii* to desiccation indicated that effective transmission to man and domestic animals could occur by inhalation. A serosurvey of the dairy cattle in Los Angeles County revealed that 10% were constantly infected. When uninfected cows were introduced into the enzootic area, 40% became infected within 6 months.[57] Several serosurveys were carried out on dairy cattle in Los Angeles County over the subsequent 25 years. By 1960, 62% were seropositive,[69] and by 1967, 98%.[54] By 1973, 92% were positive and 62% were shedding *C. burnetii* in their milk.[16] Gross et al.[54] suggest that the insignificant increase of prevalence of evidence of Q fever infection in the human population from 1.3% in 1949 to 2.3% in 1967, despite an increase of prevalence in cattle from 10% to 90%, is probably due to: (1) a requirement for a higher temperature for pasteurization of milk; (2) a drop in the consumption of raw milk from 20,196 gallons/day to 4400 while the population doubled in the same time; and (3) a 55% decrease in the number of dairy farms in the area (from 595 to 268).

The involvement of domestic animals as a source of infection for man has been confirmed by numerous other serosurveys carried out in various parts of the world in the last three decades. There are, however, some different epidemiological patterns conditioned by different cultural factors and life-styles. For example, in a serosurvey carried out in Egypt in the 1950s, Taylor et al.[108] demonstrated that 18.3% of the sera were positive. However, there was great variation form one area to another. For instance, in the rural Sinbis Sanitary District, about 30 km north of Cairo, the incidence was 37.4%, with the highest incidence (47%) and highest titers found in children under the age of 2. Thereafter, there was a decline to about 25% in the age group 5–9 years, with a leveling off at this figure in the adult population. The evidence of infection was slightly higher in females than in males. Approximately 60% of sheep and goats had serological evidence of infection. The high incidence of infection in this rural population, particularly in the young, could be explained by the intimate and constant contact of people with their livestock. It was customary for a family and its domestic animals to be housed under the same roof. Despite evidence for widespread infection with *C. burnetii,* Q fever, in its classic form, had never been recognized in the native Egyptian population. However, of 55 Americans residing in Egypt and observed for approximately 2 years, 11 had a serological conversion, of whom 7 had clinically recognized Q fever.

There have been several other epidemiological surveys carried out in other parts of the world. They all have provided strong evidence for incriminating domestic animals as a source of human infection, directly (by contact with infected animal tissues or excretions) or indirectly (by contaminated dust). They also clearly indicate that human infection is usually mild and clinically unrecognized.

5.2. Epidemic Behavior and Contagiousness

The first major outbreak recognized in the United States occurred in Amarillo, Texas, in 1946. There were 55 cases with two deaths among 136 employees of three packing houses.[112] In the same year, another outbreak occurred in a Chicago packing house, where 33 of 81 employees acquired Q fever.[100]

In 1947, several cases of Q fever were identified among patients in Artesia, a dairy community located in Los Angeles County.[120] The clinical diagnosis was "viral pneumonia." The observation that Q fever seemed to be endemic in California led to extensive investigations conducted by Huebner and his co-workers in southern California[57] and by Lennette and his co-workers in northern California.[63] Most of the current knowledge of the epidemiology of Q fever and the ecology of *C. burnetii* stems from these studies.

In northern California in 1947–1948, there were 350 confirmed cases of Q fever.[23] The epidemiological investigation that followed these observations demonstrated that sheep and goats were the main source of infection.[65] Serosurveys of sheep, goats, and cattle indicated that in areas where Q fever occurred, a high percentage of animals were seropositive.[66] It was also shown that sheep, whether naturally or experimentally infected, undergo a recrudescence during pregnancy and shed enormous amounts of *C. burnetii* in their birth fluids, placentas (10^8 $GPID_{50}/g$), milk, feces, and urine.[2,3] Although most animals shed *C. burnetii* only following their first lambing, about one third shed the organisms twice, and a few shed them during three consecutive paturitions.[11]

DeLay *et al.*[31] and Lennette and Welsh[64] demonstrated that *C. burnetii* could be isolated from the air of premises harboring infected animals.

The California studies clearly showed that *C. burnetii* infection of domestic animals is not a veterinary problem. Infection does not lead to loss of weight, does not affect gestation or parturition, and has no deleterious effect on the young. Infection is clinically inapparent. The studies also showed that most human infections are either completely asymptomatic or so mild that the diagnosis of Q fever is seldom considered. Classic Q fever, as described by Derrick, seems to be a rare event, whereas silent, inapparent infection seems to be common.

Over the years there have been several outbreaks of Q fever in different parts of the world. All of them have been associated with direct or indirect contact with domestic animals. Suffice it to consider, as an example, an outbreak that occurred in Switzerland in 1983. In the Valais (at Val de Bagnes, population 4642), between mid-October and the first week of December there were 191 symptomatic and 224 asymptomatic cases of serologically confirmed Q fever. The outbreak began suddenly 3 weeks after herds of sheep, returning from alpine pasture, were led through the village.[117] Several similar outbreaks have occurred in Slovakia over the years as herds of sheep or cattle are led through small villages.[86]

5.3. Geographic Distribution

Q fever has a worldwide distribution and has been reported from all continents.[61,72,109]

5.4. Temporal Distribution

Most of the infections in California occurred in adult males (ratio of 10:1), suggesting occupational exposure.[63] In northern California, most of the cases occurred in March, April, and May, coinciding with the lambing season, when contamination of the environment was at its maximum.[1] In southern California, where dairy cattle produce milk the year around and where calving is not seasonal, cases occurred through the year.[11] In the United Kingdom, they tended to occur in the summer months.[116]

5.5. Age

The age of infection and disease is related to the opportunity for exposure to infected animals and their products. In Egypt, serosurveys have shown that infection without classic disease occurs in some districts in persons under the age of 2.[108] Clinical cases are most common in adults. In the United Kingdom, the age distribution of 215 clinical cases was as follows: 0–10 years, 4.1%; 11–20 years, 14.0%; 21–40 years, 44.6%.[116]

5.6. Sex

Males are more commonly involved than females. In the United Kingdom, 72% of 215 cases were males and 28% females. The higher rate in males is related to greater exposure.

5.7. Race

There is no known difference by race except as related to exposure in different geographic areas or by occupation.

5.8. Occupation

Persons whose occupations directly or indirectly involve them in exposure to infected sheep, goats, cattle, and other animals, to the contaminated products of conception, or to airborne particles from such contaminated sources are at highest risk. This includes sheep and goat herders, dairy farmers, dairy and slaughterhouse workers, and workers in plants that process wool and hair. Laboratory personnel working with the agent are also at risk, especially via the airborne route.[60,79,102–104] Sheep used for medical research have been responsible for several outbreaks of Q fever in recent years.[79,102–104]

5.9. Occurrence in Different Settings

Enclosed environments containing infected animals or their products of parturition have been the source of many outbreaks. This includes packing houses,[100] wool and hair processing plants,[101] and soldiers' billets in many different areas. Any time susceptible individuals are exposed to infected animals, outbreaks of Q fever are likely to occur.

Over the past 10 years there have been several outbreaks of Q fever associated with sheep used for perinatal research. The scenarios of these outbreaks were remarkably similar. Pregnant ewes were held on a farm or some similar

facility at some reasonable distance from the research laboratory to which they were transported at an appropriate time for experimental manipulations. The animals were carted to their destination, in a hospital environment, through elevators and corridors, passing by various secretarial and laboratory personnel not involved with sheep. A major outbreak occurred in 1979 at the University of California at San Francisco where 600 sheep were used annually for perinatal research. Between March and June 1979, 88 clinical and subclinical cases of Q fever were identified.[103,104] Another outbreak occurred at the University of Colorado School of Medicine, where 65 clinical and 72 subclinical cases were identified between April and October 1980.[79] An outbreak occurred at The Hospital for Sick Children of the University of Toronto where, between July and October 1982, 12 clinical and 47 subclinical cases of Q fever were diagnosed.[102] Another laboratory outbreak of Q fever acquired from sheep occurred at the University of Bristol, England, where, in April and May 1981, there were 28 clinical and subclinical cases.[56]

5.10. Socioeconomic Factors

No relationship other than through occupation has been noted.

5.11. Other Factors

The presence of infected cattle, goats, sheep, and other animals and that of the appropriate vector for spread among the animals is the most important determinant as to whether human infection will occur. This is discussed in detail in Section 6.

6. Mechanisms and Routes of Transmission

Human infection with *C. burnetii* is usually acquired by inhalation. Whether milk-associated infection is acquired by ingestion or by aerosolization in the process of drinking is still not known. Although there is a possibility that infection may be acquired from ticks or tick feces, this is unlikely to be a frequent occurrence. The overwhelming evidence incriminates domestic animals as a primary source of human infection. The massive contamination of the environment at time of parturition and the unusual resistance of *C. burnetii* to desiccation are important factors in transmission to other domestic animals and to man. Derrick[36] has calculated that an infected bovine placenta weighing 4 kg, powdered and dispersed on the ground, would provide enough coxiellae to dust each square millimeter of a 100-acre field with one organism, which is sufficient to infect one guinea pig. It is easy to understand that during dry periods, wind can blow contaminated dust thus exposing to infection individuals living in proximity to infected animals. Outbreaks can also occur at a considerable distance from the original focus through contaminated straw used as packing material, wool, hides, clothing, and other materials.[6]

It should be stated that the infective dose of *C. burnetii* for man is less than ten organisms.[111]

Person-to-person transmission, if it occurs, seems to be a rare event. There have been outbreaks associated with the performance of autopsies.[73]

The role of arthropods in the overall maintenance of *C. burnetii* in nature is not fully understood; their role may be significant. In some species of ticks, transovarial and transstadial transmission have been demonstrated. In some species of ticks, *C. burnetii* has been shown to persist for as long as 1000 days[29] and propagate in tick tissues to extraordinary numbers. One gram of feces from infected *Rhipicephalus sanguineus* (brown dog tick), for example, may contain as many as 10^8 GPID$_{50}$.[6] Although several ecological systems have been described in various parts of the world whereby *C. burnetii* seems to be efficiently maintained in wild animals and their ectoparasites, they seem to have no significant bearing on human infection.

Domestic animals are far more important as a source of human infection. Derrick *et al.*[38] suspected cattle as a source of human infection, but assumed that ticks were the vectors of transmission. Caminopetros[21] demonstrated that sheep and goats in Greece were infected and concluded that they were the probable source of human infection. Huebner and Bell[57] demonstrated a close association between infected cattle and human cases in southern California. Lennette and Clark[63] demonstrated a similar association with infected sheep and goats in northern California. Several studies carried out in other parts of the world in the last three decades have confirmed the California findings.[16,75,106,108,115]

It became evident from the California studies and others that infection of domestic animals was benign, clinically unrecognizable, did not lead to unthriftiness, and did not interfere with good husbandry.

A study of 300 cases of Q fever in Los Angeles and vicinity investigated in 1947–1948[9] indicated that human infections were related to association with cattle. More than half the patients either worked in the dairy or livestock industries, resided close to dairies or livestock yards, or

consumed raw milk. Huebner *et al.*[58] recovered *C. burnetii* from 40 of 50 milk samples from serologically positive cows obtained from five dairies in the Los Angeles area. Infected milk may contain as many as 10^5 GPID/g.[10]

7. Pathogenesis and Immunity

The mechanisms by which *C. burnetii* causes infection and illness are not known. It is assumed that the surface Phase I antigen is a virulence factor.[46] It is antiphagocytic,[18,119] and organisms that lack this component (Phase II organisms) are considerably less virulent than the parent Phase I.[84,92] Ormsbee *et al.*[85] demonstrated that a pure Phase II strain obtained by repeated plaque purification was unable to infect guinea pigs.

Immunity following infection, whether overt or inapparent, seems to be solid and long-lasting. However, it seems to be a nonsterile immunity maintained by persistence of the organism in the host. This immunity seems to be able to prevent disease but not recrudescence of infection. Luoto and Huebner[70] have demonstrated such recrudescence in cattle, and Abinanti *et al.*[2,3] reported recrudescence during successive gestations in sheep. Recrudescence also occurs in women. Babudieri[5,6] reported that a woman who had contracted Q fever in the laboratory gave birth, 6 months later, to a healthy child. *C. burnetii* was isolated from her placenta and, 1 month after delivery, from her milk. Syrucek *et al.*[107] isolated *C. burnetii* from the placentas of three women and from the curettage material of another in whom pregnancy was interrupted in the 3rd month. All four women had had Q fever 2–3 years previously. None of these women, at time of recrudescence, had any clinical manifestation of Q fever. The mechanisms, probably immune, that allow massive infections of the host and yet protect the host from disease are unknown.

8. Patterns of Host Response

As noted several times previously, most infections of man with *C. burnetii* are probably mild and not recognized as Q fever. The situation encountered in Egypt by Taylor *et al.*[108] indicated that there was widespread infection in children without evidence of Q fever. It is likely that in this setting, *C. burnetii* was responsible for a mild febrile illness clinically indistinguishable from that caused by a multitude of other microbial agents.

The patterns of host response may thus be grouped into (1) inapparent infection, (2) acute febrile illness, (3) pneumonic forms, and (4) forms with extrapulmonary localization (hepatitis and endocarditis).[6]

8.1. Clinical Features

Q fever in its classic form as first described by Derrick[33] and subsequently by others [22,35,93] does not pose a difficult diagnostic problem, particularly if the appropriate epidemiological background is present.

The most accurate data on the incubation period were obtained by Tigertt and his colleagues[110,111] from experimental aerosol infection of young, healthy adult volunteers. The duration of the incubation period was clearly dose-dependent and varied from 18 days to 9 days with aerosol challenges ranging from 10 $GPID_{50}$ to 1.5×10^5. Onset of disease is usually sudden, with headache, chilly sensations, fever, and malaise, followed by myalgia and anorexia. For several days, the temperature ranges from 101 to 104°F; the entire course rarely exceeds 2 weeks and usually lasts from 3 to 6 days. There may be wide fluctuations in the fever. During the early stages, respiratory symptoms are not conspicuous. A dry cough and chest pain occur after about 5 days, when rales are usually audible. The cough usually produces a small amount of mucoid sputum that is occasionally streaked with blood. *C. burnetii* has been recovered from the sputum, but not visualized directly. Although pneumonitis may be prominent in some cases, it must be emphasized that Q fever is a systemic disease, and serious illness may occur in the absence of pneumonitis (see below).

Respiratory symptoms and physical findings produced by the lung lesion of Q fever are often minimal. During the peak of illness, fine crepitant rales may be heard after deep inspiration. Dullness to percussion is occasionally elicited and may indicate consolidation or the presence of pleural effusion. *C. burnetii* has been isolated from pleural fluid. Other clinical signs are relative bradycardia, hepatomegaly, and splenomegaly.

The roentgen lung findings are often indistinguishable from those of viral atypical pneumonia and may, at times, closely resemble those of pneumococcal pneumonia. Infiltration is usually present by day 3 or 4 of disease, first as patchy areas of consolidation involving a portion of one lobe giving a homogeneous ground-glass appearance. The lesions tend to occur in the peribronchial and alveolar areas, rather than the hilar regions, and often in the lower lobes. These manifestations persist beyond the febrile period and may appear in patients who are unaware of pulmonary in-

volvement. Segmental or lobar infiltrations occur more commonly in Q fever than in many atypical pneumonias. The sputum of patients with pneumococcal lobar pneumonia differs significantly from that of Q fever patients. In Q fever, there are small amounts of mucoid sputum occasionally streaked with blood and a few mononuclear cells; frequently in pneumococcal pneumonia, there is rusty mucoid sputum with leukocytes, erythrocytes, and identifiable *Streptococcus pneumoniae*.

The incidence of pneumonia in Q fever varies considerably from one series of reports to another. Powell[93] recognized only 3 in a series of 72 cases of Q fever reported from Brisbane. Clark *et al.*[22] observed it in about one third of 180 cases, Marmion *et al.*[74] in 25 of 30 cases (83%), and in a report from Britain,[116] it was observed in 111 of 215 cases (52%).

Complications are rare, and coincident with defervescence, the appetite begins to return. Convalescence progresses slowly for several weeks, during which time the principal disability is weakness. It is not uncommon for patients to lose 15–20 lb during the active stages of disease. The disease may be protracted in approximately 29% of cases, with fever persisting for longer than 4 weeks, particularly in elderly patients. Occasionally, relapse occurs, especially in patients treated with antibiotics during the first days of disease.

Hepatitis, with the development of clinically detectable icterus, occurs in approximately one third of patients with the protracted form. This form of Q fever is characterized by fever, malaise, absence of headache or respiratory signs, and hepatomegaly with right upper quadrant pain. Liver biopsy specimens show diffuse granulomatous changes with multinucleated giant cells and scattered infiltrations of polymorphonuclear leukocytes, lymphocytes, and macrophages. *C. burnetii* may be demonstrated in such specimens with the fluorescent-antibody technique. Therefore, Q fever must be in the differential diagnosis of liver granulomas such as tuberculosis, sarcoidosis, histoplasmosis, brucellosis, tularemia, syphilis, and others.[39]

Endocarditis has also been reported, and *C. burnetii* has been identified by smear and isolation from vegetations on the heart valves obtained at operation or autopsy. The aortic valve is most commonly involved, often with large vegetations. It is important, therefore, to suspect the possibility of Q fever in cases of apparent subacute bacterial endocarditis with persistently negative blood cultures. Because antibiotics seem unable to penetrate the valvular vegetations, they are ineffective in treating Q fever endocarditis. Surgical valve replacement is required.

As mentioned earlier, high Phase I titers are indicative

of chronic Q fever, hepatitis, or endocarditis. High IgA Phase I titers, however, are characteristic of endocarditis.[76,88,113,118]

8.2. Diagnosis

The clinical diagnosis of Q fever, in its classic form, is easy. The sudden onset of chills, severe headache, fever, and signs of pneumonitis are fairly characteristic. Q fever should be considered in the differential diagnosis of atypical pneumonias. If, along with signs and symptoms suggestive of the disease, there is a history of association with domestic animals, a tentative diagnosis can be made. The diagnosis should be confirmed by demonstrating a rise in specific antibodies by CF, microagglutination, or indirect immunofluorescence tests. However, since most infections with *C. burnetii* do not manifest themselves as Q fever, the diagnosis is rarely made. To get an estimate of the incidence of *C. burnetii* infection, it might be necessary to carry out specific serological tests on all cases of unidentified febrile illnesses.

C. burnetii infection should be considered in the differential diagnosis of granulomatous hepatitis and in the differential diagnosis of subacute endocarditis when repeated blood cultures are negative. In these instances, there is usually a high Phase I titer (Section 8.1). Attempts at isolation of the organism should be made only in laboratories that have the facilities and expertise to do so.

9. Control and Prevention

Livestock are the main source of human infection. In some parts of the world, most of the livestock are infected and shedding *C. burnetii* in massive quantities in milk, birth fluids, urine, and feces. These infections, however, are of little importance to the livestock industry, since they do not result in significant economic loss. Dairy cattle do not have reduced milk production. Abortion does not seem to be a serious problem, although abortions have been reported in goats and cattle. In the case of meat animals, there is no unthriftiness or food wastage.[53] There certainly is no economic justification for massive slaughtering to control infection. There is good evidence that vaccination of cattle with Phase I vaccine will prevent infection.[17,71,97] Whether the livestock industry can be convinced that this should be done is another question.

Prevention of human infection can be achieved, to a certain degree, by pasteurization of milk. Standard pasteurization at 143°F for 30 min is not adequate, whereas,

remarkably, pasteurization at 145°F for 30 min or flash pasteurization at 161°F for 15 s is sufficient.[41] Effective vaccines for human use have been developed over the years.[13,45,114] Ormsbee *et al.*[83] demonstrated that a Phase I vaccine was approximately 300 times more effective than the corresponding Phase II. Such a vaccine has been used for over 25 years at the Rocky Mountain Laboratory with excellent results. To avoid side reactions, it is important that the vaccine be administered only to individuals who are skin-test-negative.[77] Such a vaccine would be of benefit to laboratory, slaughterhouse, and dairy workers, and others at risk, though one is not yet commercially available.

Laboratory personnel working with *C. burnetii* are aware of the risks and usually take appropriate precautions to avoid infection. The situation is different, however, with researchers who, unknowingly, carry out experimental surgery on *C. burnetii*-infected sheep. There is a potential for serious problems if one considers that, in the United States alone, in fiscal year 1987–1988, the National Institutes of Health funded 328 projects in which sheep were used for research. Investigators working with sheep should abide by the recommendations set forth by CDC.[15]

10. Unresolved Problems

As noted in Section 6, Q fever can be induced in man by aerosol administration of one to ten organisms,[111] and the infective dose for guinea pigs is about one organism.[84] Given the efficacy with which experimental disease can be induced, how can one explain the high incidence of inapparent, subclinical infection in endemic areas? It was suggested that milkborne, opsonized *C. burnetii* might lead to a passive–active immunization without overt disease. There is no experimental proof to support this concept, and even if there were, it would account for only a small number of infections.

Phase I organisms are the only forms found in nature, their Phase II counterparts having little survival value outside chick embryos and tissue cultures. The Phase I surface antigen seems to endow *C. burnetii* with antiphagocytic activity and is therefore assumed to be a virulence factor. However, Ormsbee *et al.*[83] have demonstrated that a pure Phase II immune response can protect guinea pigs from a Phase I challenge. The biological significance of phase variation and its involvement in pathogenesis and immunity are unknown. It was suggested that the Phase I surface antigen may behave as an adjuvant for the Phase II antigenic component.[46]

The most baffling problem is the recrudescence of infection during gestation. What are the mechanisms that allow such massive infections to occur without any evidence of pathological changes? What modulates the immune response in such a way that immunopathological changes do not develop? How can the mammary gland excrete 10^5 $GPID_{50}$/g milk in the presence of high levels of antibody for long periods without the stimulation of an inflammatory reaction? What inhibits the host from reacting violently to the presence of 10^8 infective organisms/g placenta?

Although there is evidence that human fetal infections occur,[49] there is, at present, no evidence that such infections lead to neonatal or early childhood pathology. By what mechanism is the fetus protected from damage?

11. References

1. ABINANTI, F. R., The varied epidemiology of Q fever infections: Symposium on Q fever, *Med. Sci. Publ. Walter Reed Army Inst. Res.* **6**:8–14 (1959).
2. ABINANTI, F. R., LENNETTE, E. H., WINN, J. F., AND WELSH, H. H., Q fever studies. XVIII. Presence of *Coxiella burnetii* in the birth fluids of naturally infected sheep, *Am. J. Hyg.* **58**:385–388 (1953).
3. ABINANTI, F. R., WELSH, H. H., LENNETTE, E. H., AND BRUNETTI, O., Q fever studies. XVI. Some aspects of the experimental infection induced in sheep by the intratracheal route of inoculation, *Am. J. Hyg.* **57**:170–184 (1953).
4. AZIZ, A. A., EL TAYEB, E., AND EL BATAWI, Y., Field studies of Q fever in U.A.R.: (1) Serological investigation of human and animal populations. *J. Egypt. Public Health Assoc.* **43**:329–341 (1968).
5. BABUDIERI, B., La febbre Q o rickettsiosi burnetii, *G. Mal. Infett. Parassit.* **6**:449–476 (1954).
6. BABUDIERI, B., Q fever: A zoonosis, *Adv. Vet. Sci.* **5**:81–181 (1959).
7. BABUDIERI, B., AND MOSCOVICI, C., Ricerchi sul comportamento di *Coxiella burneti* di fronte ad alcuni agenti fisici e chimici, *Rend. Ist. Super Sanita* **13**:739–748 (1950).
8. BABUDIERI, B., AND SECCHI, P., La reazione di agglutinazione nella serodiagnosi dell'infezione da *Coxiella burneti, Rend. Ist. Super. Sanita (Ital. Ed.)* **15**:584–608 (1952).
9. BECK, M. D., BELL, J. A., SHAW, E. W., AND HUEBNER, R. J., Q fever studies in southern California. II. An epidemiological study of 300 cases, *Public Health Rep.* **64**:41–56 (1949).
10. BELL, E. J., PARKER, R. R., AND STOENNER, H. G., Q fever: Experimental Q fever in cattle, *Am. J. Public Health* **39**:478–484 (1949).
11. BELL, J. A., BECK, M. D., AND HUEBNER, R. J., Epidemiologic studies of Q fever in southern California, *J. Am. Med. Assoc.* **142**:868–872 (1950).
12. BELL, J. F., LACKMAN, D. B., MEIS, A., AND HADLOW, W. J., Recurrent reaction at site of Q fever vaccination in a sensitized person, *Mil. Med.* **129**:591–595 (1964).
13. BENENSON, A. S., Q. fever vaccine: Efficacy and present status, Symposium on Q fever, *Med. Sci. Publ. Walter Reed Army Inst. Res.* **6**:47–60 (1959).
14. BENGTSON, I. A., Immunological relationship between the rickettsiae of Australian and American Q fever, *Public Health Rep.* **56**:272–281 (1941).
15. BERNARD, K. W., PARHAM, G. L., WINKLER, W. G., AND HELMICK, C. G., Q fever control measures: Recommendations for research facilities using sheep, *Infect. Control* **3**:461–465 (1982).
16. BIBERSTEIN, E. L., BUSHNELL, R., CRENSHAW, G., RIEMANN, H. P., AND FRANTI, C. E., Survey of Q fever (*Coxiella burnetii*) in California dairy cows, *Am. J. Vet. Res.* **35**:1577–1582 (1974).
17. BIBERSTEIN, E. L., RIEMANN, H. P., FRANTI, C. E., BEHYMER, D. E., RUPPANNER, R., BUSHNELL, R., AND CRENSHAW, G., Vaccination of dairy cattle against Q fever (*Coxiella burnetii*): Results of field trials, *Am. J. Vet. Res.* **38**:189–193 (1977).
18. BREZINA, R., AND KAZAR, J., Phagocytosis of *Coxiella burnetii* and the phase phenomenon, *Acta Virol.* **7**:476 (1963).
19. BURNET, F. M., AND FREEMAN, M., Experimental studies on the virus of Q fever, *Med. J. Aust.* **2**:299–305 (1937).
20. BURNET, F. M., AND FREEMAN, M., A comparative study of rickettsial strains from an infection of ticks in Montana (USA) and from Q fever, *Med. J. Aust.* **1**:887–891 (1939).
21. CAMINOPETROS, J., La "Q fever" en Grece: Le lait source de l'infection pour l'homme et les animaux, *Ann. Parasitol. Hum. Comp.* **23**:107–108 (1948).
22. CLAKR, W. H., LENNETTE, E. H., RAILSBACK, O. C., AND ROMER, M. S., Q fever in California. VII. Clinical features in 180 cases, *Arch. Intern. Med.* **88**:155–167 (1951).
23. CLARK, W. H., LENNETTE, E. H., AND ROMER, M. S., Q fever studies in California. XI. An epidemiologic summary of 350 cases occurring in northern California in 1948–1949, *Am. J. Hyg.* **54**:319–330 (1951).
24. Commission on Acute Respiratory Diseases, Identification and characteristics of the Balkan grippe strain of *Rickettsia burneti, Am. J. Hyg.* **44**:110–122 (1946).
25. COX, H. R., Studies of a filter passing infectious agent isolated from ticks. V. Further attempts to cultivate it in cell-free media: Suggested classification, *Public Health Rep.* **54**:1822–1827 (1939).
26. COX, H. R., Cultivation of rickettsiae of the Rocky Mountain spotted fever, typhus and Q fever groups in embryonic tissues of developing chicks, *Science* **94**:399–403 (1941).
27. CRACEA, E., AND POPOVICI, V., *Fevra Q la Om si Animale*, Editura Ceres, Bucharest, 1975.
28. D'ANGELO, J. L., BAKER, E. F., AND SCHLOSSER, W., Q

fever in the United States, 1948–1977, *J. Infect. Dis.* **139:**613–615 (1979).

29. Davis, G. E., American Q fever: Experimental transmission by the argasid ticks *Ornithodoros moubata* and *O. hermsi, Public Health Rep.* **58:**984–987 (1943).

30. Davis, G. E., and Cox, H. R., A filter passing infectious agent isolated from ticks. I. Isolation from *Dermacentor andersoni,* reactions in animals and filtration experiments, *Public Health Rep.* **53:**2259–2267 (1938).

31. DeLay, P. D., Lennette, E. H., and DeOme, K. B., Q fever in California. II. Recovery of *Coxiella burnetii* from naturally infected airborne dust, *J. Immunol.* **65:**211–220 (1950).

32. Dennig, H., Q Fieber (Balkangrippe)3, *Dtsch. Med. Wochenschr.* **72:**369–371 (1947).

33. Derrick, E. H., Q fever, a new fever entity: Clinical features, diagnosis and laboratory investigation, *Med. J. Aust.* **2:**281–299 (1937).

34. Derrick, E. H., *Rickettsia burnetii;* The cause of Q fever, *Med. J. Aust.* **1:**14 (1939).

35. Derrick, E. H., The epidemiology of Q fever, *J. Hyg.* **43:**357–361 (1944).

36. Derrick, E. H., The epidemiology of Q fever: A review, *Med. J. Aust.* **1:**245–253 (1953).

37. Derrick, E. H., and Smith, D. J. W., Studies in the epidemiology of Q fever. 2. The isolation of three strains of *Rickettsia burneti* from the bandicoot *Isoodon torosus, Aust. J. Exp. Biol. Med. Sci.* **18:**99–102 (1940).

37. Derrick, E. H., Smith, D. J. W., and Brown, H. E., Studies on the epidemiology of Q fever. 9. The role of the cow in the transmission of human infection, *Aust. J. Exp. Biol. Med. Sci.* **20:**105–110 (1942).

39. Dupont, H. L., Hornick, R. B., Levin, H. S., Rapoport, M. I., and Woodward, T. E., Q fever hepatitis, *Ann. Intern. Med.* **74:**198–206 (1971).

40. Dyer, R. E., Similarity of Australian Q fever and a disease caused by an infectious agent isolated from ticks in Montana, *Public Health Rep.* **54:**1229–1237 (1939).

41. Enright, J. B., Sadler, W. W., and Thomas, R. C., Thermal inactivation of *Coxiella burnetii* and its relation to pasteurization of milk, *Public Health Rep.* **72:**947–948 (1957).

42. Fiset, P., Antigenic variation of viruses and rickettsiae with particular reference to *Rickettsia burneti,* Ph.D. thesis, Cambridge University (1955).

43. Fiset, P., Phase variation of *Rickettsia (Coxiella) burneti:* Study of the antibody response in guinea pigs and rabbits, *Can. J. Microbiol.* **3:**435–445 (1957).

44. Fiset, P., Serological diagnosis, strain identification and antigenic variation: Symposium on Q fever, *Med. Sci. Publ. Walter Reed Army Inst. Res.* **6:**28–37 (1959).

45. Fiset, P., Vaccination against Q fever, 1st International Conference on Vaccines against Viral and Rickettsial Diseases of Man, Sci. Publ. No. 147, PAHO/WHO, pp. 528–531 (1967).

46. Fiset, P., and Ormsbee, R. A., The antibody response to

antigens to *Coxiella burnetii, Zentralbl. Bakteriol. Parasitenkd. Infektionskr. Hyg. Abt. 1 Orig.* **206:**321–328 (1968).

47. Fiset, P., Ormsbee, R. A., Silberman, R., Peacock, M. G., and Spielman, S. H., A microagglutination technique for detection and measurement of rickettsial antibodies, *Acta Virol.* **13:**60–66 (1969).

48. Fiset, P., Wike, D. A., Pickens, E. G., and Ormsbee, R. A., An antigenic comparison of strains of *Coxiella burnetii, Acta Virol.* **15:**161–166 (1971).

49. Fiset, P., Wisseman, C. L., Jr., and El Batawi, Y., Immunologic evidence of human fetal infection with *Coxiella burnetii, Am. J. Epidemiol.* **101:**65–69 (1975).

50. Giroud, P., and Jadin, J., Comparison entre différents tests pour le diagnostic de la fièvre Q: Réactions allergiques, fixation du complément et agglutination des rickettsies, *C.R. Acad. Sci.* **230:**2347–2348 (1950).

51. Giroud, P., and Jadin, J., Infection latente et conservation de *Rickettsia burneti* chez l'homme: Le rôle du pou, *Bull. Soc. Pathol. Exot.* **45:**764–765 (1954).

52. Giroud, P., and LeGac, P., Test d'hypersensibilité à l'antigène de la fièvre Q chez des sujets d'Oubanghi-Chari ayant presenté une affection exanthématique s'accompagnant d'adénopathie et de signes de stase pulmonaire, *C.R. Acad. Sci.* **230:**1803–1805 (1950).

53. Gochenour, W. S., Veterinary importance of Q fever: Symposium on Q fever, *Med. Sci. Publ. Walter Reed Army Inst. Res.* **6:**20–22 (1959).

54. Gross, P. A., Portnoy, B., Salvatore, M. A., Kogan, B. A., Heidbreder, G. A., Schroeder, R. J., and McIntyre, R. W., Q fever in Los Angeles County: Serological survey of human and bovine populations, *Calif. Med.* **114:**12–15 (1971).

55. Hackstadt, T., Antigenic variation in the phase I lipopolysaccharide of *Coxiella burnetii* isolates, *Infect. Immun.* **52:**337–340 (1986).

56. Hall, C. J., Richmond, S. J., Caul, E. O., Pearce, N. H., and Silver, I. A., Laboratory outbreak of Q fever acquired from sheep, *Lancet* **1:**1004–1006 (1982).

57. Huebner, R. J., and Bell, J. A., Q fever studies in southern California: Summary of current results and a discussion of possible control measures, *J. Am. Med. Assoc.* **145:**301–305 (1951).

58. Huebner, R. J., Jellison, W. L., Beck, M. D., Parker, R. R., and Shepard, C. C., Q fever studies in southern California. I. Recovery of *Rickettsia burneti* from raw milk, *Public Health Rep.* **63:**214–222 (1948).

59. Jerrells, T. R., Hinrichs, D. J., and Mallavia, L. P., Cell envelope analysis of *Coxiella burnetii,* Phase I and phase II, *Can. J. Microbiol.* **20:**1465–1470 (1974).

60. Johnson, J. E., and Kadull, P. J., Laboratory acquired Q fever: A report of fifty cases, *Am. J. Med.* **41:**391–403 (1966).

61. Kaplan, M. M., and Bertagna, P., The geographical distribution of Q fever, *Bull. WHO* **13:**829–860 (1955).

62. Lackman, D. B., Bell, E. J., Bell, J. F., and Pickens, E.

G., Intradermal sensitivity testing in man with a purified vaccine for Q fever, *Am. J. Public Health* **52**:87–93 (1962).

63. LENNETTE, E. H., AND CLARK, W. H., Observations on the epidemiology of Q fever in northern California, *J. Am. Med. Assoc.* **145**:306–309 (1951).

64. LENNETTE, E. H., AND WELSH, H. H., Q fever in California. X. Recovery of *Coxiella burnetii* from the air of premises harboring infected goats, *Am. J. Hyg.* **54**:44–49 (1951).

65. LENNETTE, E. H., CLARK, W. H., AND DEAN, B. H., Sheep and goats in the epidemiology of Q fever in northern California, *Am. J. Trop. Med.* **29**:527–541 (1949).

66. LENNETTE, E. H., DEAN, D. H., ABINANTI, F. R., CLARK, W. H., WINN, J. F., AND HOLMES, M. A., Q fever in California. V. Serologic survey of sheep, goats and cattle in three epidemiology categories from several geographic areas, *Am. J. Hyg.* **54**:1–15 (1951).

67. LENNETTE, E. H., CLARK, W. H., JENSEN, F. W., AND TOOMB, C. D., Q fever studies. XV. Development and persistence in man of complement fixing and agglutinating antibodies to *Coxiella burnetii*, *J. Immunol.* **68**:591–598 (1952).

68. LUOTO, L., A capillary agglutination test for bovine Q fever, *J. Immunol.* **71**:226–231 (1953).

69. LUOTO, L., Report on the nationwide occurrence of Q fever infections in cattle, *Public Health Rep.* **75**:135–140 (1960).

70. LUOTO, L., AND HUEBNER, R. J., Q fever studies in southern California. IX. Isolation of Q fever organisms from parturient placentas of naturally infected dairy cows, *Public Health Rep.* **65**:541–544 (1950).

71. LUOTO, L., WINN, J. F., AND HUEBNER, R. J., Q fever studies in southern California. XIII. Vaccination of dairy cattle against Q fever, *Am. J. Hyg.* **55**:190–202 (1952).

72. MARMION, B. P., Worldwide Q fever, *Lancet* **2**:616–617 (1953).

73. MARMION, B. P., AND STOKER, M. G. P., Q fever in Great Britain: Epidemiology of an outbreak, *Lancet* **2**:611–616 (1950).

74. MARMION, B. P., STOKER, M. G. P., McCOY, J. H., MALLOCH, R. A., AND MOORE, B., Q fever in Great Britain, *Lancet* **1**:503–510 (1953).

75. MARMION, B. P., STOKER, M. G. P., WALKER, C. B. B., AND CARPENTER, R. G., Q fever in Great Britain: Epidemiological information from a serological survey of healthy adults in Kent and East Anglia, *J. Hyg.* **54**:118–140 (1956).

76. MARMION, B. P., HIGGINS, F. E., BRIDGES, J. B., AND EDWARDS, A. T., A case of acute rickettsial endocarditis with a survey of cardiac patients with this infection, *Br. Med. J.* **11**:1264–1268 (1960).

77. MARMION, B. P., ORMSBEE, R. A., KYRKOU, M., WRIGHT, J., WORSWICK, D., CAMERON, S., ESTERMEN, A., FEERY, B., AND COLLINS, W., Vaccine prophylaxis of abattoir-associated Q fever, *Lancet* **2**:1411–1414 (1984).

78. McCAUL, T. F., AND WILLIAMS, J. C., Developmental cycle of *Coxiella burnetii:* Structure and morphogenesis of vegetative and sporogenic differentiations, *J. Bacteriol.* **147**:1063–1076 (1981).

79. MEIKLEJOHN, G., REIMER, L. G., GRAVES, P. S., AND HELMICK, G., Cryptic epidemic of Q fever in a medical school, *J. Infect. Dis.* **144**:107–113 (1981).

80. MURPHY, A. M., AND FIELD, P. R., The persistence of complement fixing antibodies to Q fever (*Coxiella burnetii*) after infection, *Med. J. Aust.* **1**:1148–1150 (1970).

81. ORMSBEE, R. A., An agglutination resuspension test for Q fever antibodies, *J. Immunol.* **92**:159–166 (1964).

82. ORMSBEE, R. A., Q fever rickettsia, in: *Viral and Rickettsial Diseases of Man* (F. L. HORSFALL AND T. TAMM, eds.), pp. 1144–1160, Lippincott, Philadelphia, 1965.

83. ORMSBEE, R. A., BELL, E. J., LACKMAN, D. B., AND TALLENT, G., The influence of phase on the protective potency of Q fever vaccine, *J. Immunol.* **92**:404–412 (1964).

84. ORMSBEE, R. A., PEACOCK, M., GERLOFF, R., TALLENT, G., AND WIKE, D., Limits of rickettsial infectivity, *Infect. Immun.* **19**:239–245 (1978).

85. ORMSBEE, R. A., PEACOCK, M. G., AND TALLENT, G., Dynamics of phase I to phase II antigenic shift in populations of *Coxiella burnetii*, Proceedings of IIIrd International Symposium on Rickettsiae and Rickettsial Diseases (J. Kazar, ed.), pp. 146–149, Publishing House of the Slovak Academy of Sciences, 1985.

86. PALANOVA, A., REHACEK, J., AND BREZINA, R., Epidemiology of Q fever in Slovakia, in: *Rickettsiae and Rickettsial Diseases* (J. KAZAR, R. A. ORMSBEE, AND I. N. TARASEVICH, eds.), Veda, Bratislava, 1978.

87. PARKER, P. R., AND DAVIS, G. E., A filter passing agent isolated from ticks. II. Transmission by *Dermacetor andersoni*, *Public Health Rep.* **53**:2267–2270 (1938).

88. PEACOCK, M. G., WILLIAMS, J. C., AND FAULKNER, R. S., Serological evaluation of Q fever in humans: Enhanced Phase I titers of immunoglobulins G and A are diagnostic for Q fever endocarditis, *Infect. Immun.* **41**:1089–1098 (1983).

89. PHILIP, C. B., Comments on the name of the Q fever organism, *Public Health Rep.* **63**:58 (1948).

90. PHILIP, C. B., Observations on experimental Q fever, *J. Parasitol.* **34**:457–464 (1948).

91. PHILIP, R. M., CASPER, E. A., ORMSBEE, R. A., PEACOCK, M. G., AND BURGDORFER, W., Microimmunofluorescence test for the serological study of Rocky Mountain spotted fever and typhus, *J. Clin. Microbiol.* **3**:51–61 (1976).

92. PINTO, M. R., Alguns aspects da biologia da *Coxiella burnetii*, Proceedings of the Seventh International Congresses of Tropical Medicine and Malaria, Volume III, pp. 261–262, Rio de Janeiro, September 1963.

93. POWELL, O., Q fever: Clinical features in 72 cases, *Aust. Ann. Med.* **9**:214 (1960).

94. RANSOM, S. E., AND HUEBNER, R. J., Studies on the resistance of *Coxiella burnetii* to physical and chemical agents, *Am. J. Hyg.* **53**:110–119 (1951).

95. ROBBINS, F. C., AND RUSTIGIAN, R., Q fever in the Mediterranean area: Report of its occurrence in Allied troops. IV. A laboratory outbreak, *Am. J. Hyg.* **44**:64–71 (1946).

96. ROBBINS, F. C., GAULD, R. L., AND WARNER, F. B., Q

fever in the Mediterranean area: Report of its occurrence in Allied troops. II. Epidemiology, *Am. J. Hyg.* **44:**23–50 (1946).

97. SADECKY, E., BREZINA, R., KAZAR, J., SCHRAMEK, S., AND URVOLGYI, J., Immunization against Q fever of naturally infected dairy cows, *Acta Virol.* **19:**486–488 (1975).

98. SAMUEL, J. E., FRAZIER, M. E., AND MALLAVIA, L. P., Correlation of plasmid type and disease caused by *Coxiella burnetii, Infect. Immun.* **49:**775–779 (1985).

99. SAWYER, L. A., FISHBEIN, D. B., AND McDADE, J. E., Q fever in patients with hepatitis and pneumonia: Results of laboratory-based surveillance in the United States, *J. Infect. Dis.* **158:**497–498 (1988).

100. SHEPARD, C. C., An outbreak of Q fever in a Chicago packing house, *Am. J. Hyg.* **46:**185–192 (1947).

101. SIGEL, M. M., SCOTT, T. F. M., HENLE, W., AND JANTON, O. H., Q fever in a wool and hair processing plant, *Am. J. Public Health* **40:**524–532 (1950).

102. SIMOR, A. E., BRUNTON, J. L., SALIT, I. E., VELLEND, H., FORD-JONES, L., AND SPENCE, L. P., Q fever: Hazard from sheep used in research, *Can. Med. Assoc. J.* **130:**1013–1016 (1984).

103. SPINELLI, J. S., Managing the Q fever crisis: How UCSF made bureaucracy work fast, *Lab Anim.* **10:**29–38 (1981).

104. SPINELLI, J. S., ASCHER, M. S., BROOKS, D. L., DRITZ, S. K., LEWIS, H. A., MORRISH, R. H., ROSE, L., AND RUPPANNER, R., Q fever crisis in San Francisco: Controlling a sheep zoonosis in a lab animal facility, *Lab. Anim.* **10:**24–27 (1981).

105. STOKER, M. G. P., AND FISET, P., Phase variation of the Nine Mile and other strains of *Rickettsia burneti, Can. J. Microbiol.* **2:**310–321 (1956).

106. STOKER, M. G. P., AND MARMION, B. P., The spread of Q fever from animals to man: The natural history of a rickettsial disease, *Bull. WHO* **13:**781–806 (1955).

107. SYRUCEK, L., SOBESLAVSKY, O., AND GUTVIRTH, I., Isolation of *Coxiella burnetii* from human placentas, *J. Hyg. Epidemiol.* **2:**29–35 (1958).

108. TAYLOR, R. M., KINGSTON, J. R., AND RIZK, F., Serological (complement-fixation) surveys for Q fever in Egypt and the Sudan, with special reference to its epidemiology in areas of high endemicity, *Arch. Inst. Pasteur Tunis* **36:**529–556 (1959).

109. THIEL, N., *Das Q-Fieber und seine geographische Verbreitung,* Dunker & Humbolt, Berlin, 1974.

110. TIGERTT, W. D., Studies on Q fever in man: Symposium on Q fever, *Med. Sci. Publ. Walter Reed Army Inst. Res.* **6:**39–46 (1959).

111. TIGERTT, W. D., BENENSON, A. S., AND GOCHENOUR, W. S., Airborne Q fever, *Bacteriol. Rev.* **25:**285–293 (1961).

112. TOPPING, N. H., SHEPARD, C. C., AND IRONS, J. V., Q fever in the United States. I. Epidemiologic studies of an outbreak among stock handlers and slaughterhouse workers, *J. Am. Med. Assoc.* **133:**813–821 (1947).

113. TURCK, W. P., HOWITT, G., TURNBERG, L. A., FOX, H., LONGSON, M., MATTHEWS, M. B., AND DASGUPTA, R., Chronic Q fever, *Q. J. Med.* **178:**193–217 (1976).

114. VIVONA, S., LOWENTHAL, J. P., BERMAN, S., BENENSON, A. S., AND SMADEL, J. E., Report of a field study with Q fever vaccine, *Am. J. Hyg.* **79:**143–153 (1964).

115. WAGSTAFF, D. J., JANNEY, J. H., CRAWFORD, K. L., DIMIJIAN, G. G., AND JOSEPH, J. M., Q fever studies in Maryland, *Public Health Rep.* **80:**1095–1099 (1965).

116. *WHO Weekly Epidemiol. Rec.*, Q fever, **54:**45–46 (1979).

117. *WHO Weekly Epidemiol. Rec.*, Q fever, **60:**121–122 (1985).

118. WILSON, H. G., NEILSON, G. H., GALEA, E. G., STAFFORD, G., AND O'BRIEN, M. F., Q fever endocarditis in Queensland, *Circulation* **53:**680–684 (1976).

119. WISSEMAN, C. L., JR., FISET, P., AND ORMSBEE, R. A., Interaction of rickettsiae and phagocytic host cells. V. Phagocytic and opsonic interactions of phase I and phase II *Coxiella burnetii* with normal and immune human leukocytes and antibodies, *J. Immunol.* **99:**669–674 (1968).

120. YOUNG, F. W., Q fever in Artesia, California, *Calif. Med.* **6:**10–16 (1948).

121. YUNKER, C. E., BRENNAN, J. M., HUGHES, L. E., PHILIP, C. B., PERALTA, C. H., AND VOGEL, J., Isolation of viral and rickettsial agents from Panamanian acarina, *J. Med. Entomol.* **12:**250–255 (1975).

12. Suggested Reading

BABUDIERI, B., Q fever: A zoonosis, *Adv. Vet. Sci.* **5:**81–181 (1959).

BACA, O. G., AND PARETSKY, D., Q fever and *Coxiella burnetii:* A model for host–parasite interactions, *Microbiol. Rev.* **47:**127–149 (1983).

LEEDOM, J. M., Q fever: An update, in: *Current Clinical Topics in Infectious Diseases,* Volume 1 (J. S. REMINGTON AND M. N. SWARTZ, eds.), pp. 304–331, McGraw-Hill, New York, 1980.

ORMSBEE, R. A., Q fever rickettsia, in: *Viral and Rickettsial Diseases of Man* (F. L. Horsfall and I. Tamm, eds.), pp. 1144–1160, Lippincott, Philadelphia, 1965.

SAWYER, L. A., FISHBEIN, D. B., AND McDADE, J. E., Q fever: Current concepts, *Rev. Infect. Dis.* **9:**935–946 (1987).

CHAPTER 27

Rocky Mountain Spotted Fever

Theodore E. Woodward

1. Introduction

Rocky Mountain spotted fever is an acute febrile illness transmitted to man by ticks infected with *Rickettsia rickettsii*. Usually sudden in onset, it is characterized by chills, headache, and fever lasting 2 or more weeks. A characteristic rash appears on the extremities on about the 4th febrile day and, later, on the trunk. The exanthem and other anatomical manifestations result from focal areas of endangitis scattered throughout the body. Central nervous system manifestations of delirium and coma as well as shock and renal failure occur in the severely ill. Serum antibodies to *Proteus* organisms and specific rickettsial antigens appear during the 2nd and 3rd weeks of illness. Chloramphenicol and the tetracyclines are highly specific therapeutically.

2. Historical Background

Idaho physicians described a form of "black measles" in the Snake River Valley as early as 1873. In 1899, Maxcy described a febrile illness with delirium and a blotchy-skin, red-purple-black rash that appeared first on the ankles, wrists, and forehead, with rapid general body spread. This was the "spotted fever of Idaho." It was noted to be sporadic and more common in the spring, and local opinion attributed

---

Theodore E. Woodward · Department of Medicine, University of Maryland School of Medicine, Baltimore, Maryland 21201.

it to the drinking of water from melted snow or inhalation of sawdust.[1] Dr. Earl Strain, a practicing physician in Great Falls, Montana, first suspected the role of ticks, having noted a relationship between death and a history of a tick bite. Wilson and Chowning[31] concurred with this relationship and concluded that the disease was transmitted by a local wood tick and the ground squirrel (gopher) as a possible reservoir.

They proposed *Piroplasma hominis,* an erythrocyte parasite, as the causative agent. In a series of brilliant studies carried out from 1906 to 1909, usually during the spring and summer months, Howard Taylor Ricketts successfully transmitted the disease to guinea pigs and monkeys by inoculation of blood from patients with spotted fever, incriminated the wood tick, *Dermacentor andersoni,* as vector by feeding experiments on animals, and demonstrated the occurrence of naturally infected ticks. He observed bacterialike bodies in smears prepared from tick tissues and showed the transovarial transmission of infection to offspring of infected female ticks. Ticks were shown to be infected throughout their life span. Studies of immunity showed that blood from animals that survived the infection protected other animals if blood was administered several days before infection.[20,21] Wilder and Ricketts showed through cross-immunity studies that spotted fever and typhus were distinct entities. Ironically, the Montana legislature in 1909 allocated for Rickett's research studies the sum of $6000, which the board of examiners failed to appropriate.[1] In July 1909, Ricketts proceeded to Mexico to study typhus fever; there, his life was cut short by this disease, which is closely related to Rocky Mountain spotted fever. In 1916, Dr. da Rocha Lima, another pioneer in this field, gave the name *Rickettsia* to those agents that cause the typhus and spotted fever disorders. An independent study conducted by McCalla and Brereton of Boise, Idaho, in 1905, unknown to Ricketts, showed that the bite of a tick removed from one of their patients transmitted spotted fever to two human subjects, a healthy prisoner and a woman, in whom a moderate and a mild attack, respectively, of Rocky Mountain spotted fever occurred. This work was not published until 1908.[13]

Wolbach[32] was the first to detail the microscopic lesions of Rocky Mountain spotted fever with descriptions of the classic focal lesions of blood vessels. He distinguished between pathogenic and nonpathogenic organisms in ticks and demonstrated the intranuclear multiplication of rickettsiae in tick tissues.

Much knowledge was added by Spencer and Parker,[27] who showed that guinea pigs could be infected readily by intraperitoneal injection of macerated tick tissue. Ticks obtained in the Bitter Root Valley during early spring failed to cause illness in guinea pigs. Ticks fed on infected goats killed inoculated animals. These workers demonstrated "reactivation" by showing that unfed ticks immunized animals despite their inability to cause demonstrable infection and that virulence could be revived by providing ticks a blood meal (see Section 4). Also, phenolyzed tick juice effectively afforded protection in guinea pigs. Vaccinated humans developed neutralizing antibodies, and their sera protected guinea pigs from experimental infection. Inactivated infected tick-tissue vaccine for man became a reality.[27]

Cox[3] provided an additional milestone by showing that rickettsiae propagated well in chick-embryo yolk sacs, particularly after death of the embryo. The yolk-sac vaccine was simpler to produce and gave fewer reactions.

Therapeutically, immune serum did not prove to be really effective in patients with Rocky Mountain spotted fever. This is principally because rickettsiae are localized intracellularly at the time when the clinical diagnosis becomes apparent, on about the 5th or 6th day. The first effective and specific treatment was paraaminobenzoic acid, which did reduce mortality and morbidity, but it proved awkward to use.[22]

In 1948, first with chloramphenicol and later with the tetracyclines, specific treatment was placed on a firmer basis, and therapy for Rocky Mountain spotted fever became readily available.[34]

It is quite likely that Rocky Mountain spotted fever was prevalent in the eastern Atlantic states before its reported recognition in 1930. Zachary Taylor is said to have died of typhus on July 9, 1850, after 16 months in the presidency. The illness lasted about 5 days, and one wonders whether this was not Rocky Mountain spotted fever, which occurs on either bank of the Potomac. Most of the cases in the East probably masqueraded as endemic typhus or were called Brill's disease. Pinkerton and Maxcy[18] reported a case in Charlottesville that was undoubtedly Rocky Mountain spotted fever. Dyer *et al.*[7] noted in 1930 that patients whose illness occurred in the spring and summer along the Eastern Seaboard states closely resembled Rocky Mountain spotted fever. One of these patients was recognized in Maryland by Maurice C. Pincoffs[17]; Dr. Pincoffs's case was published by Dyer *et al.*[7]

3. Methodology

3.1. Sources of Mortality Data

The mortality from Rocky Mountain spotted fever has been variable, especially after the introduction of antibiotics, so that mortality data are not a reliable indicator of incidence. Prior to specific antibiotic usage, the overall mortality rate annually averaged about 20% for all ages. In the mountain and eastern states, where occupational pursuits exposed adults to infected feces, fatality exceeded 50% in those persons aged 40 or older. It was appreciably lower in children and young adults. Two developments have drastically improved treatment, reduced fatality, and shortened the clinical course of infection. The broad spectrum antibiotics, first chloramphenicol and later the tetracyclines, were introduced in 1948. When they were given early during the course of Rocky Mountain spotted fever, when the rash was noted, usually on the 3rd–6th day of illness, recovery ensued rapidly. Of equal importance was the elucidation of the pathophysiological abnormalities responsible for the severe manifestations and complications that occur during the 2nd febrile week. Properly applied supportive measures and antibiotic treatment led to recovery in patients who did not come under medical care until late in the illness.

3.2. Sources of Morbidity Data

Rocky Mountain spotted fever is a reportable disease; in patients whose illness is not detected early and treated properly, serious sequelae and a long hospitalization often follow. The Centers for Disease Control (CDC) publish the number of cases that occur weekly in various states under the category of typhus fever ("Tick-borne RMSF"). The data are published in an annual supplement. Criteria for diagnosis are reliable, since confirmatory serological tests, including either the Weil–Felix reaction or the complement-fixation (CF) reaction and isolation and identification of *Rickettsia*, are utilized.

3.3. Laboratory Diagnosis

Several types of confirmatory laboratory tests are useful for diagnosis of Rocky Mountain spotted fever: (1) serological tests to detect the presence and increase of specific antibodies in the patient's blood during illness[15]; (2) isolation and identification of *R. rickettsii* from blood or tissues; and (3) identification of the agent in skin or other tissues by immunofluorescence techniques.

3.3.1. Serological Tests. Serological tests, to be useful, require three serum samples: during the 1st, 2nd, and 4th–6th weeks of illness.[24] Certain of the serological tests such as the CF and immunofluorescent-antibody (IFA) reactions are useful in surveys to detect convalescents of Rocky Mountain spotted fever. Antibodies of these types persist for indefinite periods after the acute infection, in contrast to the Weil-Felix reaction, which becomes negative in several months.

a. Weil–Felix Reaction. Strains of *Proteus* OX-19 and OX-2 are agglutinated by sera of patients with Rocky Mountain spotted fever, but they provide no specificity for this disease or typhus fever. A single convalescent serum titer of 1:320 is usually diagnostic, but demonstration of a rise in titer is of greater value. *Proteus* agglutinins may appear as early as the 5th day and are generally present by the 12th febrile day. A maximum titer is generally reached in early convalescence and declines rapidly to nondiagnostic levels in several months. In approximately 10% of cases, OX agglutinins fail to appear. When antibiotics are given early during the 1st week of illness, the titer may be delayed but usually reaches the same level.

b. Complement-Fixation Reaction. Utilization of group-specific soluble rickettsial antigens permits differentiation of the various rickettsial diseases, i.e., spotted fevers, the typhus fevers, and Q fever. Various member diseases of the spotted-fever group such as Rocky Mountain spotted fever, rickettsialpox, fièvre boutonneuse, North Asian tick-borne rickettsiosis, and Queensland tick typhus may be distinguished by use of type-specific washed rickettsial-body antigen. Antibodies during response to a primary infection of Rocky Mountain spotted fever are usually 19 S globulins. CF antibodies appear during the 2nd and 3rd weeks of Rocky Mountain spotted fever and later in those treated with antibiotics within the first 3–5 days of illness. Under these circumstances, a later convalescent specimen should be taken at 4–6 weeks.

c. Other Serological Tests. Utilizing better antigens, other serological procedures for rickettsiosis not only distinguish among the specific rickettsial infections but also help the clinician and epidemiologist determine the type of immunoglobulin in acute (IgM) and late or recurrent (IgG) illnesses such as recurrent typhus fever. The Weil–Felix and CF tests are useful for routine diagnoses; microagglutination (MA), IFA, and hemagglutination (HA) reactions are valuable for identification. These are developing as standard procedures.[15]

3.3.2. Isolation and Identification of *R. rickettsii.* If isolation is attempted, blood should be obtained from the febrile patient prior to antibiotic treatment. Male guinea pigs are inoculated intraperitoneally with 2–4 ml of defibrinated blood or emulsified clot. Details of how to establish infection may be found in standard texts.[34] Primary isolation of rickettsiae by inoculation in the yolk sac of the chick embryo or tissue-culture cells usually fails because of the small numbers of organisms in patients' blood. Rickettsiae have been identified in stained cultured monocytes of infected monkeys[5] and by direct or indirect immunofluorescence (IF) of tissues of animals infected with *R. rickettsii.*[16]

3.3.3. Identification of *R. rickettsii* in Tissues. IF techniques are useful for detection of *R. rickettsii* in tissues of chick embryos, guinea pigs, and vector ticks.[2,16] Identifiable rickettsiae have been visualized in skin lesions of patients with Rocky Mountain spotted fever as early as the 4th day of illness or as late as the 10th day.[35] Rickettsiae may be stained by the IF technique in formalinized tissues.[29]

3.3.4. Antigenic Composition. Two types of CF antigens are derived from the spotted fever rickettsiae. One is soluble and is released by ether treatment; it is common to all members of the group and specifically differentiates them from rickettsiae of the typhus group, scrub typhus, and Q fever. Suspensions of purified organisms are type-specific, and although there are cross-reactions between different type-specific antigens and antisera, the serum titer with homologous-strain antigen is usually higher. With these two types of CF antigens, it is possible to distinguish between all rickettsiae of the spotted fever group in North, Central, and South America and the various tick typhus fevers of the Eastern Hemisphere.

4. Biological Characteristics of the Organism[15,34]

R. rickettsii, which possesses the general properties of other rickettsiae, is an obligate intracellular, parasitic pleomorphic organism with tapered ends that resemble pneumococci. They are minute coccoid and bacillary organisms averaging 0.6–1.2 µm that stain purple with Giemsa, light blue with Castaneda, red with Macchiavello, and bright red with Gimenez techniques.[15] These rickettsiae grow in the nucleus and cytoplasm of infected cells of ticks, mammals, and embryonated eggs. Electron micrographs reveal the organisms to have limiting membranes enclosing protoplasmic substance with dense granules. They divide by a process analogous to binary fission.[8,34]

Biochemically, *R. rickettsii* simulate other rickettsiae in chemical composition, metabolic consistency, and nutritional requirements. They contain both RNA and DNA and oxidize certain intermediates of the Krebs cycle.[8,19]

The agent is relatively labile and readily inactivated by heat and chemical agents. Suspensions of infected tissues are inactivated within 24 h by 0.1% formaldehyde U.S.P. or 0.5% phenol. They remain viable for long periods when stored at −70°C. When carefully lyophilized from buffered sucrose–glutamate media' and stored at 5°C, they remain viable for years.[34]

R. rickettsii exist in ticks in a nonvirulent immunizing phase that can be "reactivated" to a virulent infection-producing phase of ticks with a fresh blood meal or when incubated at 37°C for 24 h. This phenomenon probably accounts for the failure of infected ticks, after winter hibernation, to transmit illness to humans in the early spring until they have attached and fed for several hours. Later, during spring and summer, when natural reactivation has presumably occurred, ticks may infect humans after shorter exposure. Virulence of *R. rickettsii* is altered by the metabolic state.[8,34]

R. rickettsii elaborate a toxin that is lethal for mice when given intravenously. It is neutralized by sera of convalescent humans and animals or after their immunization with spotted fever vaccine.[8,34]

5. Descriptive Epidemiology

5.1. Prevalence and Incidence

The annual number of patients with Rocky Mountain spotted fever in the United States during the years 1950–1986 is shown in Fig. 1. In 1981, there were 1176 cases, which exceeded the number of cases reported in any other of these years. For many years, approximately 500 cases occurred annually in the United States; then, after the introduction of specific therapy in 1948, the number of infected cases decreased to a low of about 200 in 1959, 1960, and 1961. This decrease was primarily, however, an artifact of

the widespread use of broad-spectrum antibiotics early in the illness, which led to underreporting and the use of pesticides.

Beginning in 1969, there has been a gradual increase in annual incidence in the United States. There were approximately 900 cases reported in 1975 and 1976 and cumulative totals of 1115 in 1977, 1011 in 1978 (see Fig. 1), and 1067 in 1979.[9,15] The average annual death rate was 7.0%.[9] Transformation of farms into housing developments and recreation of children and adults in wooded areas probably account for the added exposure to infected ticks, particularly in the southeastern Atlantic states, where the largest number of cases occur. The cumulative totals for 1980, 1981, 1982, 1983, 1984, 1985, and 1986 were 1163, 1176, 976, 1126, 836, 700, and 755, respectively. The lowered incidence during the past 3 years is unexplained but could relate to a cyclic reaction involving vector and parasite (see Fig. 1).

Rocky Mountain spotted fever in the United States and São Paulo typhus in Brazil are the most significant and clinically severe types of the tick-borne group. In the Eastern Hemisphere and elsewhere, the tick-borne rickettsioses are milder and are known variably as fièvre boutonneuse, South African, North Asian, Indian, Siberian, Queensland tick typhus, and others. Mite-borne rickettsialpox with its rodent reservoir is meddlesome rather than important.

5.2. Epidemic Behavior and Contagiousness

The epidemiology of spotted fever is associated with the biology of the ticks that transmit this disease. Man is entirely an accidental victim and is in no way responsible for the maintenance of the infection in nature, which is due largely to ticks and the animals on which they feed. A number of species of ticks are found infected with *R. rickettsii* in nature. Four species of ixodid ticks have been recognized as natural carriers of *R. rickettsii*: the Rocky Mountain wood tick, *Dermacentor andersoni*; the American dog tick, *D. variabilis*; the Lone Star tick, *Amblyomma americanum*; and the rabbit tick, *Haemaphysalis leporis-palustris*.[4,11] *D. andersoni* is the principal vector in the West and *D. variabilis* in the East. Infected adult female ticks transmit the agent transovarially to many of their offspring. Ticks that become infected, either through the egg or by feeding on an infected mammal at one of the stages during their developmental cycle, harbor the rickettsiae throughout their life span, which may be as long as several years. Usually, cases occur sporadically within an endemic area, although there appears to be an increasing clustering

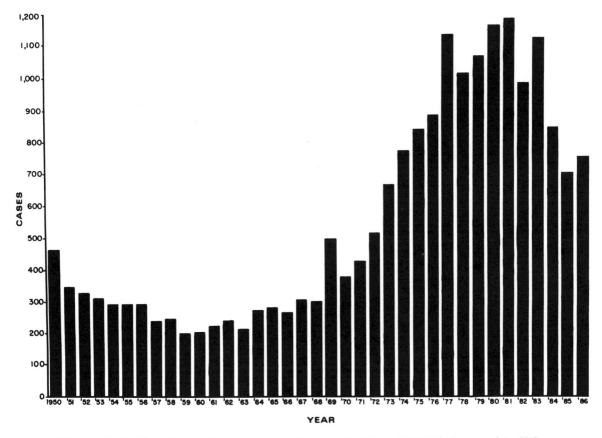

Figure 1. Rocky Mountain spotted fever: cases reported in the United States, 1950–1986. Courtesy of the CDC.

of patients within families, which have numbered up to four. Person-to-person infection does not occur. Thus, the tick probably serves as a reservoir in addition to being a vector. Small wild animals and puppies may play an important role in spreading rickettsiae in nature by infecting those new ticks that feed on them during the period of disease when rickettsemia is occurring. Most of the natural hosts show only inapparent infections with no diagnostic gross lesions.[34]

5.3. Geographic Distribution

Spotted fever caused by *R. rickettsii* is limited to the Western Hemisphere. During the latter 19th century, the first reports were in Idaho and Montana, which led to the name Rocky Mountain spotted fever. The disease has been recognized throughout the United States except in Vermont. It

occurs in Canada, Mexico, Panama, Colombia, and Brazil (see Fig. 2).

5.4. Temporal Distribution

There are seasonal variations in the incidence of cases of spotted fever. Most cases occur during the period of maximal tick activity, usually during the late spring and summer; however, confirmed cases are reported in every month of the year, particularly from the southeastern and south-central states.[9,34]

5.5. Age, Sex, and Occupational Factors

Differences in age and sex distribution of cases relate to exposure to ticks. In the western United States, a relatively higher proportion of adult males contract the disease

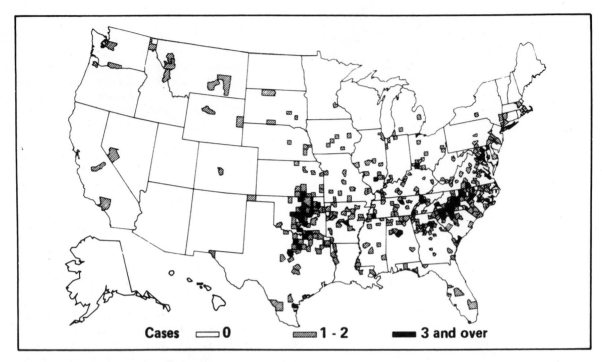

Figure 2. Geographic distribution of Rocky Mountain spotted fever in the United States for 1984, by county. Note the heavy localization in the southeastern Atlantic states. Courtesy of the CDC.

because of occupational pursuits, whereas in the East, children and women are infected. This distribution is undoubtedly influenced by occupational propinquity to wood and dog ticks and is not due to variations in susceptibility of various ages or sexes.[9,34]

For the years 1970–1974, the age and sex distributions were virtually the same for confirmed and unconfirmed cases. Nearly two-thirds of the cases were in persons less than 15 years of age, and 61% were in males. The case-fatality rates were significantly higher for nonwhites (13.9%) than for whites (5.8%), higher for male patients (8.2%) than for female patients (4.5%), and higher for persons older than 30 (13.9%) than for persons younger than 30 (5.4%).[9]

6. Mechanisms and Routes of Transmission

Man is generally infected by the bite of an infected tick. The need for ticks to "reactivate" their infection from a nonvirulent immunizing phase in unfed adult ticks to a virulent infection-producing phase brought about by the ingestion of fresh blood probably explains why ticks do not

cause illness unless they have attached and have fed for several hours. Infection may also be acquired through abrasions in the skin or through mucous membranes that become contaminated with infected tick feces or tissue juices. Hence, there is a hazard associated with crushing ticks between the fingers when removing them from persons or animals.[34] Quantitative studies conducted to test the efficacy of vaccines in volunteers showed that a very small number of viable rickettsiae given intradermally cause illness in man, i.e., 0.1 $GPIPID_{50}$ (50% guinea pig intraperitoneal infectious dose), which is about one rickettsial organism.[6]

7. Pathogenesis and Immunity

7.1. Pathogenesis

Rocky Mountain spotted fever in man follows infection through the skin or respiratory tract. The bite of a tick usually transmits *R. rickettsii* after the tick has been attached for several hours. Infection may be acquired through an abrasion in the skin contaminated with infected tick feces or juices. Local lesions (eschars) develop with considerable rapidity at sites of arthropod attachment and initial multiplication of rickettsiae in scrub typhus, the tick-borne rickettsioses of the Eastern Hemisphere, and rickettsialpox. A primary lesion occurs occasionally at the site of tick attachment in Rocky Mountain spotted fever (Fig. 3). An eschar also occurs as an initial lesion in tick-borne tularemia, which may confuse the diagnostic picture.[33,34]

After infection, illness occurs within a period varying from 3 to 12 days, the mean being about 7 days. A short incubation period usually indicates a more serious infection. Studies in volunteers have shown that patients with scrub typhus and Q fever have rickettsemia late in the incubation period prior to onset of fever.[12,28]

Similar events probably occur in all rickettsial diseases; circulating rickettsiae can be detected during the early febrile period in practically all patients. Little is known about the pathogenesis of infection during the midportion of the incubation period. Presumably, during this time in patients with Rocky Mountain spotted fever, a transient low-grade rickettsemia results from release of organisms multiplying at the initial site of infection, which then seeds infection within endothelial cells of the vascular tree. The mechanism of entry into the endothelial cell is unknown. Vascular lesions that develop at such sites account for the pathological changes, including the rash. There is a report of a patient with Rocky Mountain spotted fever who contributed blood as a donor during his late incubation period. The blood, stored for about 9 days, transmitted the disease to the recipient.[30]

Rickettsiae apparently invade and proliferate in the endothelial cells of small blood vessels. Endothelial-cell proliferation often leads to eventual disruption. Rickettsiae may exert a toxic effect on endothelial cells; in mice, the

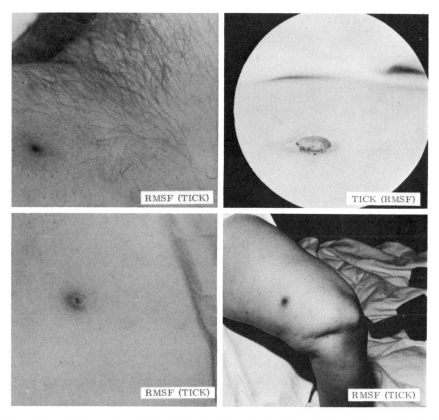

Figure 3. Rocky Mountain spotted fever primary lesions (eschars) at sites of tick attachment. *Upper right:* attached female engorged tick.

rickettsial toxin causes a remarkable increase in capillary permeability independent of proliferation. Later manifestations in rickettsial diseases may result from immunopathological mechanisms, since humoral antibodies are present during the 2nd febrile week, when increases in capillary permeability and vascular thrombosis and ecchymosis are greatest.[34] Also, a delayed type of hypersensitivity occurs during infection. The cause of the toxic febrile state that characterizes Rocky Mountain spotted fever and other rickettsioses is unknown. Studies by various investigators have shown a specific toxic action in the capillaries of animals resulting in vasoconstriction, plasma leakage, hemoconcentration, and the unusual finding of an unaltered reactivity to epinephrine.[8] Cortisone is antitoxemic for humans and suppresses the febrile response, but does not prevent death of mice injected with rickettsial toxins.

Rickettsemia occurs usually until the end of the 2nd week of illness; occasionally, it is demonstrable longer. *R. rickettsii* do not appear in sputum or feces in sufficient amounts to permit isolation in animals. They are said to have been isolated from the spinal fluid of patients.

Neutralizing-type antibodies, which favorably halt the rickettsemia, are detected in the patient's serum by the end of the 2nd week. The various types of antibodies that make their appearance during the 2nd week include MA, CF, and IF antibodies, and others of lesser importance. Interferon is produced during Rocky Mountain spotted fever, highest titers being detected within the first several days.

7.2. Immunity

Second attacks of Rocky Mountain spotted fever have not been reported, although recurrent infection has developed in patients treated with antibiotics very early in illness. These are really continuing infections and not true recurrences.[6]

A recurrent type of Rocky Mountain spotted fever such as Brill–Zinsser epidemic louse-borne type has not been reported. Clinicians should be alert to this possibility. Studies of cross-immunity in susceptible animals show protection among the various rickettsiae of the tick-borne group and rickettsialpox. Always, the protection with homologous antigens is more significant.

8. Patterns of Host Response

A history of tick bite is elicited in approximately 80% of patients. In a recent report, this was said to be 58%.[9,33,34]

8.1. Common Clinical Features

The onset is usually abrupt in nonvaccinated persons, with severe headache, a shaking chill, prostration, generalized myalgia, especially in the back and leg muscles,[34] nausea with occasional vomiting, and fever that reaches 102–104°F within the first several days. Onset in children and adults may be mild, accompanied by lethargy, anorexia, headache, and low-grade fever. These symptoms are similar to those of many infectious diseases and make specific diagnosis difficult during the first several days. It is doubtful whether many human inapparent infections occur.

Fever: In severe cases, fever continues for approximately 15–20 days; the febrile course in children may be shorter. Usually, the fever maintains a high continuous course with morning remissions that do not reach normal. Hyperpyrexia of 105°F or greater is usually an unfavorable sign, although death may occur when the patient is hypopyrexic with associated vasomotor collapse. Defervescence usually occurs by lysis over several days; rarely, there is a crisis. Recurrent fever is unusual except in the presence of pyogenic complications.

Headache: Headache is usually general and severe, with frontal intensity. It persists during the 1st and 2nd weeks of illness in untreated cases; occasionally, it is mild. Malaise and muscle pain continue during the 1st week. Irritability is common, and the patient shows distraction in such circumstances as during questioning and examination.

Rash: One of the most characteristic and helpful diagnostic signs is the rash, which usually appears on the 4th febrile day; the range is 2–6 days. Initial lesions are on the wrists, ankles, soles, palms, and forearms. They are macular, pink, nonfixed, and irregularly defined, and measure 2–6 mm. A warm compress on the extremities may accentuate a faint rash, and the rash is more prominent with elevated temperature. After about 12–24 h, the rash extends centrally to the legs, buttocks, arms, axillae, trunk, neck, and face. In epidemic typhus fever, the rash spreads from the trunk to the extremities. In about 2–3 days, the rash becomes maculopapular and assumes a deeper red hue. After 4 days or so, the rash is petechial and fails to fade on pressure. Often, the hemorrhagic lesions coalesce to form large ecchymoses. These lesions often form over bony prominences and may slough to form indolent, slow-healing ulcers. In convalescence, the petechiae fade to form brown-pigmented discolorations for several weeks. In mild cases, the rash does not become petechial or purpuric and may disappear within several days. Antibiotic treatment may abort the early exanthem; the late fixed lesions fade slowly with specific therapy. In some patients, particularly dark-skinned patients, a rash does not occur or is unnoticed.

When tourniquets are applied to the extremities for several minutes or when the blood pressure is taken, additional petechiae may appear (Rumpel–Leade phenomenon); this is further evidence of capillary abnormalities. Photophobia and redness of the peripheral conjunctivae are often present.

Cardiovascular and Respiratory Signs: In severe cases, the pulse is rapid and the blood pressure lowers. Circulatory failure with shock is an ominous sign and is an indication of the peripheral vascular atonicity and collapse. Ecchymotic skin lesions, cyanosis, and gangrene of the fingers, toes, genitalia, and buttocks are all unfavorable signs. The electrocardiogram shows changes indicative of myocardial involvement, and arrhythmias of various types indicate myocarditis, which may lead to cardiac arrest and death. In severely ill patients, edema of the arms, legs, and face indicates vascular decompensation and capillary abnormalities.

Respiration is usually rapid, and a nonproductive cough with pulmonary rales is indicative of a form of rickettsial pneumonitis. Lung consolidation is rare.

Unwarranted use of intravenous fluids may provoke pulmonary edema.

Hepatic and Renal Signs: Hepatomegaly occurs; usually, there is no jaundice. Hypoalbuminemia results from leakage of albumin into subcutaneous tissues and abnormal hepatic function. Oliguria, anuria, and azotemia are indicators of vascular decompensation and renal involvement.

Gastrointestinal Signs: Abdominal distension is frequent and occasionally some degree of intestinal ileus is observed. Constipation is usual. More acute manifestations with abdominal pain may suggest the presence of either appendicitis or cholecystitis.

Neurological Signs: Headache, restlessness, insomnia, and back stiffness are common neurological manifestations. Coma, muscular rigidity, athetoid movements, convulsive seizures, and hemiplegia (rare) are grave signs and indicate the presence of encephalitis. Deafness during the acute illness and in convalescence is common. Most of the CNS signs abate with time.

8.2. Clinical Course and Complications

In mild and moderately severe cases, the illness abates in about 2 weeks. Convalescence is rapid. If death occurs, it is usually during the latter part of the 2nd week as a result of toxemia, vasomotor weakness, and shock or renal failure with azotemia. In a few patients, the course is rapidly fulminant with death, outdistancing treatment, occurring as early as the 6th day of illness.[9,34]

In vaccinated persons who contract the disease, the illness is usually milder, with a short febrile course and a sparse pink rash.

8.3. Diagnosis

During the early stages of infection before the rash has appeared, differentiation from other acute infections is difficult. History of tick bite while living or traveling in a high endemic area is helpful. The rash of meningococcemia resembles that of Rocky Mountain spotted fever in certain aspects, since it is macular, maculopapular, or petechial in the chronic form, and petechial, confluent, or ecchymotic in the fulminant type. The meningococcic skin lesion is tender and develops with extreme rapidity in the fulminant form, whereas the rickettsial rash occurs on about the 4th day of disease and gradually becomes petechial. High blood leukocyte counts are common in meningococcal infections. The exanthem of rubella rapidly becomes confluent, while that of rubeola almost never becomes petechial. The exanthem of varicella or variola is first erythematous and later becomes vesicular. The rose spots of typhoid fever are usually on the lower chest or abdomen and remain delicate, without hemorrhagic character. Rocky Mountain spotted fever skin lesions, in contrast to those of typhoid, begin on the periphery of the skin and later become petechial. The rash of infectious mononucleosis is usually morbilliform on the trunk and rarely becomes petechial. Angina, lymphadenopathy, and atypical lymphocytes in the blood are differentiating features. Murine typhus is a milder disease than Rocky Mountain spotted fever; the rash is less extensive and is nonpurpuric and nonconfluent; renal and vascular complications are uncommon. Not infrequently, differentiation of these two rickettsial infections must await the results of specific serological tests. Epidemic typhus fever is capable of causing all the pronounced clinical, physiological, and anatomical alterations seen in cases of Rocky Mountain spotted fever, i.e., hypotension, peripheral vascular failure, cyanosis, skin necrosis, and gangrene of digits, renal failure with azotemia, and neurological manifestations. However, the rash of classic typhus is noted initially in the axillary folds and on the trunk and later extends peripherally, rarely involving the palms, soles, or face. The serological patterns in these two diseases are distinctive when specific rickettsial antigens are employed in tests. Moreover, louse-borne typhus is not recognized in the United States except in the form of Brill–Zinsser disease (recurrent typhus fever). Recently, the agent has been isolated from flying squirrels and human cases have occurred. Rickettsialpox, although caused by a member of the spotted-fever group of organisms, is usually readily differentiated from Rocky Mountain spotted fever by the initial lesion, the relative mildness of the illness, and the early vesiculation of the maculopapular rash. The Weil–Felix reaction is positive in Rocky Mountain spotted fever and in murine and epidemic typhus, but negative in rickettsialpox. Agglutinins against *Proteus* OX-19 and OX-2 appear in the serum of patients with spotted fever, but only those against OX-19 are found in murine and epidemic typhus.[34]

9. Control and Prevention

9.1. Vector Control

Avoiding or reducing the chance of contact in tick-infested areas of known endemicity is the principal preventive measure. When this is impractical, area control of spotted fever ticks may include the following prophylactic measures:

1. Spraying the ground with dieldrin or chlordane for tick control. Although there are environmental objections to the use of residual insecticides, such procedures may be warranted under special conditions.
2. Application of repellents such as diethyltoluamide or dimethylphthalate to clothing and exposed parts of the body, or in very heavily infected areas, the wearing of clothing that interferes with the attachment of ticks, i.e., boots and a one-piece outer garment preferably impregnated with repellent.[34]
3. Daily inspection of the entire body, particularly of children, including the hairy parts, to detect and remove attached ticks. Care should be taken in removing attached ticks to avoid crushing the arthropod, which will contaminate the bite wound. Touching the tick with gasoline or whiskey encourages detachment, but gentle traction with small forceps applied close to the mouth parts allows ready extraction. The skin area should be disinfected with soap and water or other antiseptics such as alcohol. These precautions should be employed in removing engorged ticks from dogs and other animals because infection through minor abrasions in the hands is possible.

9.2. Immunization

Spencer and Parker[27] were aware that infected ticks, when they first come out of hibernation, produce either no or low-grade infections in guinea pigs. They found that one infected egg from an infected female tick produced spotted fever in a guinea pig and that suspensions of infected ticks treated with phenol protected guinea pigs against virulent challenge. Spencer and Parker[25–27] tested the new vaccine

on themselves and showed that a sample of their blood, taken after vaccination, mixed with virulent rickettsiae protected guinea pigs against infection. They developed a tick-derived vaccine, inactivated and preserved with 1.6% phenol and 0.4% formalin. The vaccine was difficult to produce and expensive, originally costing $20.00 per injection. Studies of efficacy were carried out over a number of years. Although no carefully controlled experimental trials were conducted, it appeared, on the basis of differences of attack rates in small groups of vaccinees and control volunteers, that the vaccine prevented the mild type of spotted fever and sharply reduced the mortality in the highly fatal type.[14]

The vaccine was moderately reactive, producing malaise, nausea, slight fever, arthralgia, myalgia, and serum sickness in about 1% of recipients.

Cox developed an inactivated vaccine prepared from rickettsiae grown in yolk sacs of fertile hens' eggs. This was the standard preparation for a number of years.[23] Immunization consisted of a course of three injections of 1.0 ml each given subcutaneously at weekly intervals. Vaccination was preferably performed in the spring before the advent of the spotted fever season, and a 1.0-ml stimulating dose was recommended each year for those at risk. There was little reaction from the vaccine. This chick-tissue vaccine produced commercially (Lederle) was not conclusively tested in the field and, furthermore, the relationship between the immunity demonstrated in guinea pigs and that induced in man following administration of vaccine was inconclusive.

A quantitative trial of inactivated vaccines made from infected tissue and embryonated hens' eggs was conducted in volunteers followed by a challenge with virulent (viable) *R. rickettsii*.[6] Humoral antibodies appeared in a low percentage of vaccinees after use of either available vaccine. It was noted in the vaccinated group that when they were injected with a few virulent rickettsiae 3–6 months after a full course of vaccination, the incubation period was prolonged and the frequency of early clinical relapse was lessened. Vaccinated volunteers were not protected (when compared with controls) against development of clinical illness. In vaccinees, the clinical illness appeared to be shortened,[6] which coincided with the earlier findings of Parker.

There is no currently available licensed commercial vaccine. An inactivated vaccine that is prepared using tissue-culture techniques is now under development. This has permitted the preparation of a vaccine consisting of rich suspensions of purified whole rickettsiae. A new vaccine should be available for use in those exposed to great risk, namely, persons who frequent highly endemic areas and laboratory workers exposed to the agent.

9.3. Antibiotic Prophylaxis

The question is often raised whether antibiotics should be given prophylactically after human exposure to virulent *R. rickettsii*. In guinea pigs, a single dose of oxytetracycline prevented the disease when the antibiotic was given shortly before expected onset. However, relapses occurred when treatment preceded expected onset by 48 h or more.[10] This regimen is not recommended. After a tick bite in a known endemic area, an exposed person should be observed for signs of fever, headache, prostration, and rash; therapy is very effective at the early stage of illness.

10. Unresolved Problems

Specific chemotherapy of the rickettsial diseases was achieved in 1948, which advance inadvertently diverted attention from pursuit of studies aimed at elucidating pathogenesis, pathophysiological abnormalities, and control by vaccines. Some unanswered puzzles awaiting solution are:

1. What is the nature of the increased capillary permeability and the cause of the characteristic vascular lesion? Are the changes a result of direct effects by rickettsiae within endothelial cells, an action of their toxins, a combination of both, or an immunopathological reaction? Evidence does not permit the exclusion of any one mechanism.
2. Hematological findings in severely ill patients with spotted fever and typhus show a disseminated intravascular-coagulation defect late in illness. Its mechanism and the relationships of complement abnormalities merit study. Whether heparin treatment is indicated is not clear.
3. Therapy for early cases is simple and effective. For seriously ill patients during later stages, there is a need for better antitoxemic measures, which will evolve only when the nature of the pathological lesions and the toxic manifestations is understood. Short-term high-dose steroid treatment for several days combined with antibiotics is helpful and is unassociated with sequelae.
4. Spotted and typhus fever rickettsiae persist indefinitely within human cells, presumably within macrophages; Brill–Zinsser disease is a recurrence of epidemic typhus years after the initial infection. This is a remarkable example of microbial persistence. Conceivably, there is a Brill–Zinsser pattern for other rickettsial diseases such as spotted fever, murine and scrub typhus, and Q fever. An understanding of the intracellular growth requirements might provide leads to complete inactivation of rickettsiae. An important lead will be the cultivation of rickettsiae on artificial media.
5. There is need for better biological vaccines for prevention of typhus, spotted, and Q fevers. Inactivated Q fever vaccine is effective, but causes reaction on repeated inocula-

tion. A tissue-culture-derived inactivated vaccine for spotted fever is under development and appears promising. This system may be useful for production of better epidemic typhus vaccines. Live strain E vaccine for typhus is effective but reactive. There are no effective vaccines for scrub typhus. Whether the threat of certain of the rickettsial diseases for humans warrants research directed toward developing attenuated viable vaccines is a major concern.
6. The interrelationships of rickettsiae in animal hosts, vectors, and other environmental factors for epidemic and murine typhus, Rocky Mountain spotted fever, and Q fever are really underdeveloped. For example, there may be a significant reservoir of *R. prowazekii* other than man, such as flying squirrels. Fleas or lice may serve as vectors.

Current work by several investigators is directed to these questions.

11. References

1. AIKAWA, J. K., *Rocky Mountain Spotted Fever,* Thomas, Springfield, Ill., 1966.
2. BURGDORFER, W., Evaluation of the fluorescent antibody technique for the detection of Rocky Mountain spotted fever rickettsia in various tissues, *Pathol. Microbiol.* **24**(Suppl.):27–39 (1961).
3. COX, H. R., Use of yolk sac of developing chick embryo as medium for growing rickettsiae of Rocky Mountain spotted fever and typhus groups, *Public Health Rep.* **53**:2241–2247 (1938).
4. COX, H. R., The spotted fever group, in: *Viral and Rickettsial Diseases of Man,* 3rd ed. (T. M. RIVERS AND F. L. HORSFALL, JR., eds.), pp. 828–868, Lippincott, Philadelphia, 1959.
5. DESHAZO, R. D., BOYCE, J. R., OSTERMAN, J. V., AND STEPHENSON, E. H., Early diagnosis of Rocky Mountain spotted fever: Use of primary monocyte culture technique, *J. Am. Med. Assoc.* **235**:1353–1355 (1976).
6. DUPONT, H. L., HORNICK, R. B., DAWKINS, A. T., HEINER, G. G., FABRIKANT, I. B., WISSEMAN, C. L., JR., AND WOODWARD, T. E., Rocky Mountain spotted fever: A comparative study of the active immunity induced by inactivated and viable pathogenic *Rickettsia rickettsii, J. Infect. Dis.* **128**:340–344 (1973).
7. DYER, R. E., RUMREICH, A. S., AND BADGER, L. F., The typhus Rocky Mountain spotted fever group in the United States, *J. Am. Med. Assoc.* **97**:589 (1931).
8. FULLER, H. S., Biologic properties of pathogenic rickettsiae, *Arch. Inst. Pasteur Tunis* **36**:311–338 (1959).
9. HATTWICK, M. A., O'BRIEN, R. J., AND HANSON, B. F., Rocky Mountain spotted fever: Epidemiology of an increasing problem, *Ann. Intern. Med.* **84**:732–739 (1976).
10. KENYON, R. H., WILLIAMS, R. G., OSTER, C. N., AND PEDERSEN, C. E., JR., Prophylactic treatment of Rocky Mountain spotted fever, *J. Clin. Microbiol.* **8**:102–104 (1978).

11. KOHLS, G. M., Vectors of rickettsial diseases, in: *Rickettsial Diseases of Man* (F. R. MOULTON, ed.), pp. 83–96, American Association for the Advancement of Science, Washington, D.C., 1948.

12. LEY, H. L., JR., DIERCKS, F. H., PATERSON, P. Y., SMADEL, J. L., WISSEMAN, C. L., JR., AND TRAUB, R., Immunization against scrub typhus. IV. Living Karp vaccine and chemoprophylaxis in volunteers, *Am. J. Hyg.* **56:**303–312 (1952).

13. McCALLA, L. P., Direct transmission from man to man of the Rocky Mountain spotted (tick) fever, *Med. Sentinel* **16:**87 (1908).

14. PARKER, R. R., Rocky Mountain spotted fever: Results of fifteen years of prophylactic vaccination, *Am. J. Trop. Med.* **21:**369 (1941).

15. PEDERSON, C. E., JR., Rocky Mountain spotted fever: A disease that must be recognized, *J. Am. Med. Technol.* **39:**190–198 (1977).

16. PEDERSON, C. E., JR., BAGLEY, L. R., KENYON, R. H., SAMMONS, L. S., AND BURGER, G. T., Demonstration of *Rickettsia rickettsii* in the rhesus monkey by immune fluorescence microscopy, *J. Clin. Microbiol.* **2:**121–125 (1975).

17. PINCOFFS, M. C., Personal communication.

18. PINKERTON, H., AND MAXCY, K. F., Pathological study of a case of endemic typhus in Virginia with demonstration of rickettsia, *Am. J. Pathol.* **7:**95–103 (1931).

19. PRICE, W. H. The epidemiology of Rocky Mountain spotted fever: The characterization of strain virulence of *Rickettsia rickettsii*, *Am. J. Hyg.* **58:**248–268 (1953).

20. RICKETTS, H. T., The study of "Rocky Mountain spotted fever" (tick fever) by means of animal inoculations, *J. Am. Med. Assoc.* **47:**358 (1906).

21. RICKETTS, H. T., The role of the wood-tick (*Dermacentor occidentalis*) in Rocky Mountain spotted fever, and the susceptibility of local animals to this disease, *J. Am. Med. Assoc.* **49:**24 (1907).

22. ROSE, H. M., DUANE, R. B., AND FISCHELL, E. E., The treatment of spotted fever with para-aminobenzoic acid, *J. Am. Med. Assoc.* **129:**1160–1163 (1945).

23. SMADEL, J. E., Rocky Mountain spotted fever vaccine, in: *Symposium on the Spotted Fever Group,* Med. Sci. Publ. No. 7 WRAIR 55-61, U.S. Government Printing Office, Washington, D.C., 1960.

24. SMADEL, J. E., AND JACKSON, E. B., Rickettsial infections, in: *Diagnostic Procedures for Viral and Rickettsial Disease,* 3rd ed., pp. 743–771, American Public Health Association, New York, 1964.

25. SPENCER, R. R., AND PARKER, R. R., Rocky Mountain spotted fever: Infectivity of fasting and recently fed ticks, *Public Health Rep.* **38:**33 (1923).

26. SPENCER, R. R., AND PARKER, R. R., Studies on Rocky Mountain spotted fever: Vaccination of monkeys and man, *Public Health Rep.* **40:**2159 (1925).

27. SPENCER, R. R., AND PARKER, R. R., Studies in Rocky Mountain spotted fever, National Health Service, Hygienic Library Bull. No. 154, U.S. Government Printing Office, Washington, D.C., 1930.

28. TIGERTT, W. D., Studies on Q fever in man, in: *Symposium of Q Fever,* Med. Sci. Publ. Walter Reed Army Inst. Res., No. 6, pp. 39–46, U.S. Government Printing Office, Washington, D.C., 1959.

29. WALKER, D. H., AND CAIN, B. G., A method for specific diagnosis of Rocky Mountain spotted fever on fixed, paraffin-embedded tissues by immunofluorescence, *J. Infect. Dis.* **137:**206 (1978).

30. WELLS, G. M., WOODWARD, T. E., FISET, P., AND HORNICK, R. B., Rocky Mountain spotted fever caused by blood transfusion, *J. Am. Med. Assoc.* **239:**2763–2765 (1978).

31. WILSON, L. B., AND CHOWNING, W. M., Studies in pyroplasmosis hominis ("spotted fever" or "tick fever" of the Rocky Mountains), *J. Infect. Dis.* **1:**31 (1904).

32. WOLBACH, S. B., Studies on Rocky Mountain spotted fever, *J. Med. Res.* **41:**1–97 (1919).

33. WOODWARD, T. E., Rickettsial diseases in the United States, *Med. Clin. North Am.* **43:**1507–1535 (1959).

34. WOODWARD, T. E., AND JACKSON, E. B., Spotted fever rickettsiae, in: *Viral and Rickettsial Infection of Man,* 4th ed. (F. L. HORSFALL, JR., AND T. TAMM, eds.), pp. 1095–1129, Lippincott, Philadelphia, 1965.

35. WOODWARD, T. E., PEDERSEN, C. E., JR., OSTER, C. N., BAGLEY, L. R., ROMBERGER, J., AND SNYDER, M. J., Prompt confirmation of Rocky Mountain spotted fever: Identification of rickettsiae in skin tissues, *J. Infect. Dis.* **134:**293–301 (1976).

12. Suggested Reading

HARRELL, G. T., Rocky Mountain spotted fever, *Medicine* **28:**333–370 (1949).

HATTWICK, M. A. W., O'BRIEN, R. J., AND HANSON, B. F., Rocky Mountain spotted fever: Epidemiology of an increasing problem, *Ann. Intern. Med.* **84:**732–739 (1976).

HECHEMY, K. E., Laboratory diagnosis of Rocky Mountain spotted fever, *N. Engl. J. Med.* **300:**859–860 (1979).

PHILIP, R. N., CASPERIE, A., MacCORMACK, J. N., SEXTON, D. K., THOMAS, L. A., ANACKER, R. L., BURGDORFER, W., AND VICK, S., A comparison of serologic methods for diagnosis of Rocky Mountain spotted fever, *Am. J. Epidemiol.* **105:**56 (1977).

SONESHINE, D. E., BOZEMAN, M. F., WILLIAMS, M. S., MASIELLO, S. A., CHADWICK, D. P., STOCKS, N. I., LAUER, D. M., AND ELISBERG, B. I., Epizootiology of epidemic typhus (*Rickettsia prowazeki*) in flying squirrels, *Am. J. Trop. Med. Hyg.* **27:**339–349 (1978).

WOODWARD, T. E., Section 10, The Rickettsioses, *Harrison's Principles of Internal Medicine,* 9th ed., pp. 746–759, McGraw-Hill, New York, 1980.

WOODWARD, T. E., AND JACKSON, E. B., Spotted fever rickettsiae, in: *Viral and Rickettsial Infections of Man,* 4th ed. (F. L. HORSFALL, JR., AND I. TAMM, eds.), pp. 1095–1129, Lippincott, Philadelphia, 1965.

CHAPTER 28

Salmonellosis: Nontyphoidal

Andrew T. Pavia and Robert V. Tauxe

1. Introduction

Nontyphoidal salmonellosis refers to disease caused by any serotype of organisms in the genus *Salmonella,* other than *Salmonella typhi,* the causative agent of typhoid fever (see Chapter 39). The most common manifestation of non-typhoidal salmonellosis is acute enterocolitis, but the organism can cause focal infection, bacteremia, meningitis, as well as "enteric fever" that may be clinically indistinguishable from that caused by *S. typhi.* Nontyphoidal salmonellosis is a disease of considerable clinical and public health importance. An estimated 2 to 4 million cases of salmonellosis occur each year in the United States, of which a small fraction are cultured and reported. The direct patient-care costs alone have been estimated to exceed $2 billion annually, but when one considers the added costs of plant closings, product recalls, and losses of food production, the true economic impact of salmonellosis is likely to be substantially greater.[25]

Over 2000 serotypes of *Salmonella* have been described.[54] The nomenclature of *Salmonella* has undergone considerable evolution over recent years, which has led to some confusion. By DNA hybridization, six subgroups have been identified. Most *Salmonella* serotypes associated with human diseases belong to subgroup 1, but strains in subgroup 3, referred to as the Arizona group, are occasionally isolated.[30] Previously, the genus *Salmonella* was classified into three primary species: *S. typhi, S. cholerae-suis,* and *S. enteritidis;* Arizona organisms were in a separate genus. The species *S. typhi* and *S. cholerae-suis* consisted of a single serotype each; the remaining 2000 serotypes were in the species *S. enteritidis.* Thus, the formal designation of a serotype might be *S. enteritidis* serotype *typhimurium,* or *S. enteritidis* serotype *enteritidis.* To avoid the awkwardness present in either system of nomenclature, we will refer to each serotype as if it were a species, which is a common convention. Thus, *S. enteritidis* serotype *typhimurium* is written as *S. typhimurium, S. enteritidis* serotype *enteritidis* as *S. enteritidis.*

Salmonellae are pathogens in many lower animals, but some serotypes have a narrow range of hosts. For example, clinically important infections due to *S. typhi* occur only in humans, and humans are the only known reservoir for this organism. The primary reservoir of *S. pullorum, S. gallinarum,* and *S. heidelberg* is chickens, the reservoir of *S. cholerae-suis* is pigs, for *S. bovis-morbificans* it is cows, and *S. java, S. urbana,* and *S. litchfield* are predominantly turtle-associated. Nonetheless, all serotypes should be considered potentially pathogenic for humans and animals. In addition to distinctive host ranges, many serotypes exhibit unique patterns of virulence, antibiotic resistance, and geographic distribution that make the epidemiology of *Salmonella* particularly fascinating and complex.

Andrew T. Pavia · Department of Medicine, Division of Infectious Diseases, University of Utah Medical Center, Salt Lake City, Utah 84132. **Robert V. Tauxe** · Enteric Diseases Branch, Division of Bacterial Diseases, Center for Infectious Diseases, Centers for Disease Control, Atlanta, Georgia 30333.

2. Historical Background

Salmon and Smith reported the isolation of "hog cholera bacillus," later named *S. cholerae-suis,* from diarrheic swine in 1885.[76] Three years later, Gaertner reported the first foodborne outbreak of nontyphoidal salmonellosis, in which 58 persons fell ill after eating raw meat from an ill cow; "Gaertner's bacillus," later named *S. enteritidis,* was isolated from the meat, and from the spleen of a man who died in the outbreak.[43] In 1889, Loeffler isolated *S. typhimurium* during an outbreak of diarrheal illness in a laboratory mouse colony; the same organism was demonstrated among victims of a meat-associated outbreak in Aertrycke, Belgium, in 1899.[44,49] By the turn of the century, the pathogenic potential of *Salmonella* for humans was widely appreciated in Europe, and following World War I, salmonellosis emerged as a common public health problem on that continent. Between 1923 and 1938, 374 outbreaks due to 11 different serotypes of nontyphoidal salmonellae were reported in the United Kingdom.[44] In 1941, Kauffmann presented an expanded version of White's approach to the great antigenic diversity of *Salmonella.*[44] The Kauffmann–White schema defined the antigenic formula of each serotype, and provided the widely used nomenclature that we have followed here.

In the United States, nontyphoidal salmonellosis did not emerge as a public health problem until after World War II. The number of reported clinical cases increased from 502 in 1942, the first year that the condition was made nationally reportable, to 49,984 in 1986 (Fig. 1). Over the same time, typhoid fever, caused by *S. typhi,* became rare. In 1962, following a large multistate outbreak of egg-associated *S. derby* infections, a second national surveillance system for *Salmonella* was instituted, based on reports of laboratory isolates, which thus includes serotype. This surveillance system, coupled with intensive epidemiologic investigations, has helped to clarify our understanding of the complex routes of *Salmonella* transmission. As a result of this improved understanding, specific control measures have been implemented, including the Egg Product Inspection Act of 1970, the ban on the sale of small pet turtles in 1975, improvements in the methods used to produce precooked roast beef in 1978 and 1981, and the ban on interstate shipments of raw milk in 1987. The reported incidence of salmonellosis, however, continues to increase in the United States and in other industrialized countries, indicat-

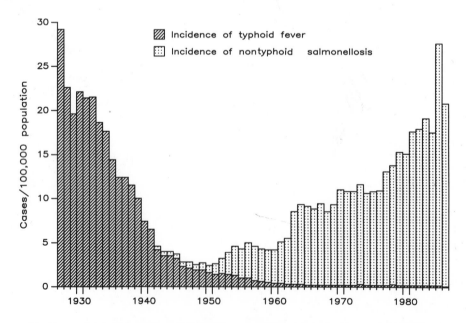

Figure 1. Reported incidence of typhoid fever and nontyphoidal salmonellosis in the United States, 1927–1986. Disease reports from Refs. 17 and 88. Population data from U.S. Census Bureau.

ing the need for further improvements in our efforts to control this pathogen of the modern era.

3. Methodology

3.1. Sources of Mortality Data

Data are limited on the mortality resulting from salmonellosis in the United States. Deaths due to salmonellosis are not routinely reported to the CDC surveillance systems. Mortality can be estimated from periodic nationwide surveys of sentinel counties (see Section 3.3), from death certificates, and from epidemiologic investigations. The surveys of sentinel counties probably give the most reliable overall estimate of mortality, since all reported cases are actively investigated. These studies yielded a mortality rate of 1.4% during 1979–1980, which is identical to that found in 16 years of surveillance in Massachusetts,[50] but lower than the 4.1% mortality rate observed in New York between 1939 and 1955.[77] In outbreaks, the typical case-fatality rate is 0.1% of affected persons.[17] This is lower than the mortality for reported cases because outbreak investigations identify many milder cases that would not be cultured, diagnosed, or reported had they occurred as sporadic cases. Sixty to one hundred deaths per year due to salmonellosis are identified from death certificate data.[16,18] Death certificates may not reflect the bacteriologic diagnosis in patients dying of gastroenteritis, dehydration, sepsis, or meningitis if appropriate cultures are not obtained or culture results are not available at the time of death. Deaths due to *Salmonella* may be hidden in those attributed to septicemia, meningitis, or cardiopulmonary arrest.

3.2. Sources of Morbidity Data

Since 1962, the laboratory-based National *Salmonella* Surveillance Program has been conducted by the Centers for Disease Control (CDC) working jointly with the Association of State and Territorial Epidemiologists, State Public Health Laboratory Directors, the U.S. Department of Agriculture, and the U.S. Food and Drug Administration. This program is based on weekly reports of *Salmonella* isolations from 49 states and from the District of Columbia, and regular summaries of nonhuman isolates from the Food and Drug Administration and the U.S. Department of Agriculture. All laboratories are requested to forward clinical isolates of *Salmonella* to the state or regional laboratory for serotyping, and the results are reported along with information on sex, age, county of residence, and site of isolation.

The purpose of this surveillance program is to define patterns of endemic salmonellosis in the United States, to identify trends in disease transmission, and to monitor control efforts. The predecessor to this system, based on physicians' reports of cases, began in 1942 when nontyphoidal salmonellosis became a notifiable disease, and continues to function in parallel. The clinical case-reporting system yields comparable numbers of cases, but because case definitions vary from state to state and the reports do not include serotype, it is of limited epidemiologic use.

Limitations and biases exist in the laboratory-based data as well. The reports do not discriminate between symptomatic and asymptomatic cases, and cases of salmonellosis without laboratory confirmation are not included. Several factors influence whether a case of salmonellosis will be reported to the *Salmonella* surveillance system, including the following: the severity of illness, access to medical care, and the association with a recognized outbreak. Physicians may be more likely to obtain stool cultures from infants and elderly persons with gastroenteritis than from young adults, and illness in these age groups may be oversampled. By comparing the number of cases detected in outbreak investigations with the number of outbreak-related cases that are reported to the *Salmonella* surveillance system, it is possible to estimate the sensitivity of the system. Reviewing a series of outbreaks in the 1960s, Aserkoff estimated that 1% symptomatic infections were reported to the laboratory-based surveillance system.[4] Using a variety of methods, including extrapolation from the carrier rate, estimating sequential error in the reporting system, and reviewing recent outbreaks, Chalker and Blaser estimated that between 1 and 5% of infections are reported.[19] Laboratory-based incidence rates can also be obtained from limited defined populations such as health maintenance organizations.

3.3. Surveys and Investigations

Because of the inherent limitations of nationwide surveillance, other studies have been performed to obtain a more detailed picture of the epidemiology of salmonellosis. In 1979–1980, CDC performed a survey of all persons from whom *Salmonella* was isolated in a randomly selected, stratified sample of counties.[66] Patients were administered a detailed epidemiologic questionnaire concerning exposures, symptoms, and complications, and the isolates were examined for antimicrobial resistance. A similar survey was repeated in the same sentinel counties in 1984–1985.[51]

The most detailed information on the epidemiology of salmonellosis has come from outbreak investigations. These investigations provide the opportunity to determine vehicles of transmission, the spectrum of illness, and risk factors for infection and for poor clinical outcomes. Case–control methods and molecular biologic techniques for precisely defining the strains involved have made the outbreak investigation an occasion for extraordinarily fruitful research,[89] and outbreak investigations have in turn spawned systematic studies. Examples include studies of the decline of turtle-associated serotype[26] and studies of the dissemination of chloramphenicol-resistant *S. newport* following an outbreak in California.[60]

3.4. Laboratory Diagnosis

3.4.1. Isolation and Identification. Members of the *Salmonella–Arizona* group are gram-negative, flagellated, nonsporulating, aerobic bacilli. *Salmonella* can usually be directly isolated from primary plates inoculated with stool or rectal swabs from persons with *Salmonella* enterocolitis. The diagnostic yield may be slightly higher if one uses an aliquot of 5–10 g of feces rather than a rectal swab, particularly when attempting to identify *Salmonella* carriers, who may be shedding only small numbers of organisms. As carriers may shed *Salmonella* intermittently, culturing specimens on two or more occasions may increase the likelihood of detection. In clinical laboratories, an enrichment broth is also recommended to increase the isolation of *Salmonella* from stool specimens.[31] Three selective enrichment media are in widespread use to isolate *Salmonella*: tetrathionate broth, tetrathionate broth with brilliant green, and selenite F broth. Many microbiologists prefer to use either selenite or tetrathionate without the brilliant green dye because neither inhibits *S. typhi,* in contrast to tetrathionate brilliant green broth. Numerous selective plating media, varying from low to high selectivity, have been used to isolate *Salmonella* from fecal specimens. The purpose of these selective media is to suppress the growth of other Enterobacteriaceae. Mac-Conkey, eosin–methylene blue (EMB), and deoxycholate agar are media of low selectivity. *Salmonella–Shigella* (SS), Hektoen enteric (HE), and xylose–lysine–desoxycholate–citrate (XLD) agars are widely used to screen for *Salmonella* and *Shigella* because they support the growth of both organisms and are considered moderately selective media. When laboratory resources permit the use of an additional plate, highly selective media such as brilliant green or bismuth sulfite agar may be superior to the less selective media. Bismuth sulfite agar is the preferred medium for isolating *S. typhi.* For specimens obtained from a normally sterile source such as blood or CSF, using selective media has no advantage.

Colonies that are suspicious for *Salmonella* should be further identified by a chemical test. At least two representatives of each type of suspicious colony should be selected and transferred to either triple sugar iron (TSI) or Kliger's iron (KI agar). Lysine iron agar (LIA) indicates the decarboxylation or deamination of lysine and the production of hydrogen sulfide, and is particularly helpful when used in conjunction with TSI agar for the presumptive identification of *Salmonella*. The usual reaction of *Salmonella* on TSI or KI will be an alkaline slant and acid butt, and they will produce gas and H_2S. Lactose-positive strains may occasionally occur that will produce an acid slant and do not produce H_2S or gas. On LIA, the usual reaction is an alkaline slant and alkaline butt with production of H_2S. Isolates can be screened for *Salmonella* antigens using a polyvalent O or H antiserum. Colonies with typical TSI and LIA reactions that react to polyvalent O and H antisera are presumptively considered to be *Salmonella.*

If stool specimens must be transported, as is often necessary in epidemiologic investigations, a swab coated with feces should be placed in a transport medium and held refrigerated until it can be examined. Commonly used transport media include Stewart's, Amies, Cary Blair, and buffered glycerol saline. Of these, Cary Blair is probably the most suitable general transport medium.[31]

Rapid diagnostic tests using enzyme immunoassay, latex agglutination, or other immunologic methods to detect *Salmonella* in feces and in foods are under development.

3.4.2. Serologic Diagnostic Methods. Salmonellae, as do other Enterobacteriaceae, possess somatic (O) and flagellar (H) antigens. The O antigenic determinants define the serogroup, and the H antigens further break these down into more than 2000 serotypes, according to the Kauffmann–White schema. Each serogroup has a major determinant and one or more minor somatic antigens. Serogroups A through I have been identified; most serotypes that cause human disease fall into serogroups A through E. Many clinical laboratories can readily identify serogroup using commercial polyvalent group antisera. Further identification of specific serotype is usually performed by a public health laboratory or other reference laboratory. Serotype determination is extremely useful in epidemiologic investigations since many serotypes have specific reservoirs, host ranges, virulence, and age specificity.

Since the ten most common serotypes account for 70% of human isolates in the United States, laboratory techniques for further subtyping a common serotype are often useful for epidemiologic purposes.[89] Antimicrobial resistance patterns are the simplest method of further characterizing an epidemic strain. Plasmid profiles have proved useful in defining outbreak strains.[38,64,79,83] Phage-typing schemes for *S. typhimurium* and other serotypes have been used extensively for epidemiologic purposes in England and Canada. Isoenzyme typing is also under investigation as a tool for answering specific epidemiologic questions.

The antibody response to human *Salmonella* infection has not been useful for serodiagnosis. *Salmonella* enterocolitis does not always provoke a measurable serologic response. The Widal reaction, used historically to diagnose *S. typhi* infection, measures agglutinating antibodies to O and H antigens of *S. typhi*. The usefulness of this test has been severely hampered by nonspecific cross-reactivity with other *Salmonella* antigens, elevated titers due to nonspecific inflammatory disease, antibodies due to typhoid vaccination, and the suppression of O and H agglutinins by early treatment.[75]

4. Biological Characteristics of the Organism

Salmonellae are a hardy and resourceful group of organisms. They successfully parasitize a broad variety of hosts including insects, reptiles, amphibians, birds, and mammals. Although not true spore-formers, they are resistant to drying and freezing and may survive for long periods in a nutrient-poor environment. The organism can survive for over 200 days in contaminated soil, 10 months in dust, more than 5 months in roach and rodent feces, and more than 4 years in dried whole egg. They multiply in food at temperatures ranging from 44 to 114°F (7 to 46°C) and can survive at a pH as low as 4.5.[13,55]

After more than a century of study, the virulence mechanisms of these organisms remain less than perfectly understood. Salmonellae have several virulence factors that contribute to pathogenicity. It appears likely that different serotypes and strains rely to varying degrees on individual virulence and invasiveness factors, accounting for the marked variation in virulence, host specificity, and clinical manifestations. The O-specific side-chain portion of lipopolysaccharide (LPS) has been associated with invasiveness of *Salmonella*, and rough mutants with incomplete O side chains have markedly diminished virulence.[67] The lipid A portion of LPS is responsible for many of the endotoxin-mediated effects of *Salmonella* infections.[56]

Other virulence factors include adherence pili, flagella, enterotoxin, and cytotoxin (see Section 7).

Antimicrobial Resistance

The resistance of *Salmonella* to antimicrobial agents has been a matter of increasing concern. Antimicrobial resistance is important for clinical and epidemiologic reasons. Although antimicrobial treatment is not necessary in uncomplicated *Salmonella* enterocolitis, and appears to prolong carriage,[3] antimicrobial treatment is essential in extraintestinal infections. The emergence of multiply resistant strains can lead to treatment failures in this setting and may require the use of new and more expensive antibiotics. Antimicrobial resistance in *Salmonella* also has several important epidemiologic ramifications because prior exposure to antimicrobials is associated with an increased risk of infection with resistant *Salmonella*. In one outbreak, 12 of 18 persons infected with the outbreak strain of multiply resistant *S. newport* had taken a penicillin derivative in the week before the onset of their illness, compared to 0 of 11 persons infected with sensitive strains of *S. newport*.[38] In most cases, illness began within 3 days after taking the antibiotic, suggesting that the antibiotic provided a selective advantage for the resistant organism and converted asymptomatic colonization to overt infection. Exposure to antimicrobials can also lower the infectious dose for a resistant strain. This was demonstrated in a massive outbreak of multiply resistant *S. typhimurium* infections in 1985.[71] In that outbreak, two brands of milk were contaminated, and the amount of implicated milk that persons reported drinking was an index of the dose of *Salmonella* they had received. Some persons affected by the outbreak had taken an antimicrobial to which the outbreak strain of *S. typhimurium* was resistant just before becoming ill with salmonellosis. These persons reported drinking smaller volumes of implicated milk than ill persons not taking such antimicrobials, suggesting that a smaller dose of *Salmonella* caused illness in the former group.

At any given moment, some fraction of the population is taking antimicrobials for a variety of reasons. Because those persons appear to have heightened susceptibility to resistant strains of *Salmonella*, an outbreak due to a resistant strain may produce a somewhat larger number of cases than would an outbreak due to a sensitive strain. From 16 to 64% of cases in outbreaks of resistant *Salmonella* infections can be called "excess cases," occurring as a result of this interaction between resistance and prior or concurrent use of antimicrobials.[24]

The overall level of antimicrobial resistance of *Salmonella* isolates appears to be increasing. In the sentinel county survey of *Salmonella* isolates conducted by the CDC in 1984–1985, 24% of isolates were resistant to at least one antimicrobial, a significant increase over the 16% resistance demonstrated in a similar survey in 1979–1980.[51] The number of multiply resistant strains rose from 12% to 15%. The most frequent resistance was to streptomycin, an antibiotic seldom used to treat humans (Table 1). Nine percent of isolates were resistant to ampicillin, 2% to chloramphenicol, 7% to sulfamethoxazole, and 0.6% to trimethoprim-sulfamethoxazole. Resistance to nalidixic acid rose significantly, as did resistance to tetracycline.

Antimicrobial resistance in *Salmonella* may result from exposure to antimicrobials used to treat human illness, or exposure of food animals to antimicrobials. Resistance genes may be transferred between *Salmonella* and other Enterobacteriaceae via plasmids or other transposable genetic elements. Considerable evidence has accumulated that points to the major role of antimicrobial use in food animals that become a source of human infections with antimicrobial-resistant *Salmonella* in the United States. In the 1984 sentinel county survey, the drugs to which *Salmonella* were likely to be resistant were frequently ones that are seldom used in treating human infections, including streptomycin, nitrofurantoin, and kanamycin, yet these drugs are frequently used in animal husbandry.[24] This increase in tetracycline resistance noted above occurred despite the fact that the number of prescriptions dispensed for human use of tetracycline decreased 61% between 1973 and 1984. During that period, tetracyclines continued to be used extensively as growth enhancers, particularly among cattle. More compelling evidence comes from outbreak investigations in which resistant strains have been traced from ill persons back through the food distribution chain to the farm. In one outbreak a multiply resistant strain of *S. newport* was traced from ill persons in one state back through supermarket distribution and the meat processing plant to a farm where the beef cattle had been fed nontherapeutic doses of chlortetracycline.[38] In another outbreak, almost 1000 persons in California became infected with a strain of chloramphenicol-resistant *S. newport* with a unique plasmid profile. The chain of transmission was followed from ill persons, to hamburger, to beef from meat packers, to slaughterhouses, and, finally, to cows and calves on farms where chloramphenicol had been used.[79] At each stage, the unique epidemic strain of *S. newport* was isolated. Experience in other countries and preliminary evidence in the United States suggest that decreased use of antimicrobials in animal feed may result in a decrease in antimicrobial-resistant strains of *Salmonella* causing human infection. Between 1979 and 1984, the percentage of *S. heidelberg* isolates from humans that were antimicrobial-resistant decreased significantly. Surveillance data suggest that most *S. heidelberg* infections are due to poultry, and during that time the use of antimicrobials used to treat humans decreased substantially in the poultry industry.[51]

5. Descriptive Epidemiology

5.1. Prevalence and Incidence

Between the inception of national laboratory-based *Salmonella* surveillance in 1962 and 1976, the incidence of reported *Salmonella* isolations in humans increased slightly.

Table 1. Rates of Resistance to Specific Antimicrobials for *Salmonella* Isolates, 1979–1980 and 1984–1985 Sentinel County Surveys[a]

Antimicrobial	No. of isolates resistant		P
	1979–1980 (n=511)	1984–1985 (n=485)	
Ampicillin	42 (8%)	44 (9%)	NS
Cephalexin	7 (1.4)	4 (0.8)	NS
Chloramphenicol	4 (0.8)	10 (2)	NS
Colistin	0 (0)	2 (0.4)	NS
Gentamicin	0 (0)	3 (0.6)	NS
Kanamycin	18 (3.5)	17 (3.5)	NS
Nalidixic acid	0 (0)	6 (1.2)	<0.05
Nitrofurantoin	6 (1)	18 (3.7)	0.055
Streptomycin	63 (12)	59 (12.2)	NS
Sulfamethoxazole	41 (8)	34 (7.0)	NS
Tetracycline	44 (8.6)	64 (13)	0.05
Sulfamethoxazole and trimethoprim	1 (0.2)	3 (0.6)	NS

[a]Adapted from Macdonald *et al.*[51]

Between 1976 and 1986, the incidence rose by more than 60%, from 10.6/100,000 in 1976 to 17.4/100,000 in 1986 (Fig. 2). The actual incidence of infection is probably closer to 15/1000 (see Section 3.2). The increase has been relatively steady except for a marked peak in 1985 due to a massive outbreak of *S. typhimurium* from pasteurized milk. This increase in reported isolates was paralleled by an increase in clinical cases reported to the *Morbidity and Mortality Weekly Report* during the same period (Fig. 1). It is likely that the increasing number of isolates reflects a true increase in the incidence of *Salmonella* infections, rather than improved reporting, for the following reasons: During this time, the incidence of *Shigella* infections reported through a parallel laboratory-based system remained constant, no major changes occurred in the technology of *Salmonella* isolation and diagnosis, nor were any changes recognized in physicians' ordering of stool cultures. The isolation rate in a Washington health maintenance organization (HMO) in 1985 was 21/100,000, close to the national surveillance figure.[52]

The epidemiology of *Salmonella* infection varies considerably by serotype. *S. typhimurium* accounts for 25–30% of human isolates; the ten most common serotypes together account for over 70% of isolates. Six of these serotypes, *S. typhimurium, S. heidelberg, S. agona, S. montevideo, S. enteritidis,* and *S. newport,* are also among the top ten isolates reported from animals (Table 2). In the past 10 years, the isolation rates for *S. enteritidis* and *S. heidelberg* have more than tripled. *S. hadar,* first isolated in the United States in 1976, has become the fifth most common serotype

(1552 isolates reported in 1986), while the incidence of *S. saint-paul* and *S. infantis* have decreased slightly.

The increase in the incidence of salmonellosis in the United States is not well understood, but it parallels increases seen in many other industrialized nations. This increase probably represents the combination of many factors, including changes in production and slaughter of meat and poultry, use of *Salmonella*-contaminated animal feeds, and changes in the cooking and eating practices of the population. These changes may include a decline in what children learn about cooking at home and in school, increased use of precooked convenience foods, the increased popularity of restaurants, the use of microwave ovens that can result in inconsistent heating, and changes in the knowledge and practice of safe food-handling by food service workers and the public. A large portion of the increase in *S. enteritidis* infection may be due to a new route of contamination of shell eggs and egg-containing foods.[80]

The prevalence of *Salmonella* carriage among the general population is not known with accuracy in the United States, but it is estimated to be between 0.15 and 0.2%.[9,19]

5.2. Epidemic Behavior and Contagiousness

Most cases of human salmonellosis result from contaminated food, although infection has been transmitted by an enormous variety of other vehicles (see Section 6). Cases may occur as part of recognized outbreaks but the majority occur as sporadic cases.

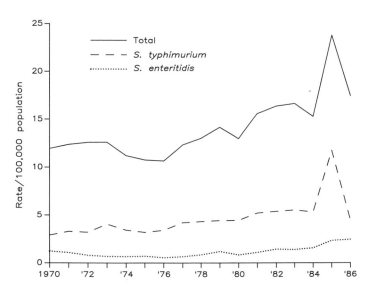

Figure 2. Isolation rates for *Salmonella* and for selected serotypes in the United States by year, 1970–1986. From Hargrett-Bean *et al.*[37]

Table 2.   Ten Most Frequently Reported Serotypes of *Salmonella* from Human and Nonhuman Sources[a]

Serotype	Human 1986		Serotype	Nonhuman 1985	
	Number	Percent		Number	Percent
S. typhimurium[b]	10,888	25.9	*S. typhimurium*[b]	1,956	26.4
S. enteritidis	5,967	14.2	*S. cholerae-suis*[c]	563	7.6
S. heidelberg	5,595	13.3	*S. heidelberg*	432	5.8
S. newport	2,431	5.8	*S. agona*	259	3.5
S. hadar	1,552	3.7	*S. montevideo*	258	3.5
S. infantis	1,104	2.6	*S. anatum*	244	3.3
S. agona	912	2.2	*S. saint-paul*	220	3.0
S. montevideo	775	1.8	*S. enteritidis*	197	2.7
S. muenchen	694	1.7	*S. sandiego*	186	2.5
S. braenderup	616	1.5	*S. newport*	165	2.2
Subtotal	30,534	72.7		4,480	60.4
Total	42,028			7,417	

[a]Data reported to CDC and USDA; from Ref. 37 and unpublished data.
[b]*S. typhimurium* includes var. Copenhagen.
[c]*S. cholerae-suis* includes var. Kunzendorf.

Recognized outbreaks of salmonellosis that are reported to CDC account for less than 10% of reported isolates in most years. In 1982, the mean size of reported *Salmonella* outbreaks was 37 persons, suggesting that only relatively large outbreaks were identified and reported.[17] In the 1979–1980 sentinel county survey, only 21% of reported isolates were associated with outbreaks or linked to other cases reported to local health departments. The remaining cases were not associated with other cases or recognized outbreaks and are considered "sporadic."[66] It is likely that sporadic cases come from the same sources as outbreak-associated cases, since when epidemiologic markers have been available, it has been possible to link many apparently "sporadic" cases to a known outbreak.[64]

Salmonella outbreaks often have distinctive patterns. Most distinctive is the explosive outbreak from a common source of exposure, dramatically exemplified by the massive milk-borne outbreak in Illinois in 1985 involving more than 16,000 reported cases.[71] A pattern more difficult to recognize is the prolonged epidemic curve associated with continued exposure to a contaminated food source or product, such as the outbreaks due to *S. newport*-contaminated roast beef in several northeastern states,[64] *S. eastborne* in contaminated chocolate,[28] *S. newbrunswick* in powdered milk,[27] or marijuana contaminated with *S. muenchen*.[83] These outbreaks are most easily recognized when they involve an unusual serotype. It is likely, though, that many small foodborne outbreaks occur in families, and this has

led to difficulty determining the relative importance of foodborne versus intrafamilial spread. In one study, 39% of cases of salmonellosis in infants were preceded by gastroenteritis in an adult family member, suggesting that intrafamilial spread to infants may follow salmonellosis in other family members.[93]

5.3. Geographic Distribution

Worldwide, the proportion of *Salmonella* infections due to nontyphoid serotypes of *Salmonella* appears to increase with the degree of economic development, while the proportion due to *S. typhi* declines (Fig. 3). Although *Salmonella* infections are universal, nontyphoidal salmonellosis appears to be predominantly a disease of industrialized nations and industrialized agriculture.

Isolation rates vary considerably across the United States. Differences in reported isolation rates between states must be interpreted with caution since it has been shown that isolation rates correlate with per capita state laboratory expenditure, and with the number of stool cultures submitted to the state laboratory.[73] Consistent regional differences exist, however, with the highest rates observed in the New England, Middle Atlantic, and Pacific states, and the lowest rates in the West and West–North Central states, suggesting that real variations may exist in *Salmonella* exposure.

Within the United States, considerable geographic

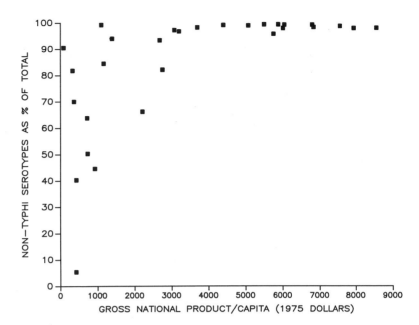

Figure 3. Nontyphoid serotypes as a percentage of all *Salmonella* isolates (including *S. typhi*) as a function of per capita gross national product, showing the increasing importance of nontyphoidal salmonellosis with increased economic development. Data from Rowe[70] and United Nations.[87]

variation exists among serotypes. For example, *S. enteritidis* is particularly common in the Northeast and Middle Atlantic states, almost equaling the number of *S. typhimurium* isolates. On the Pacific coast, *S. newport* is an important strain. *S. javiana* is associated with the Southeast and virtually all *S. weltevreden* isolates are reported from Hawaii.

5.4. Temporal Distribution

Salmonella isolation shows a consistent seasonal pattern, with a summer and fall peak (Fig. 4). This seasonal pattern is thought to result from seasonal variation in the contamination of raw foods of animal origin, and from the more rapid growth of the organism at higher ambient temperature. This pattern varies somewhat for specific serotypes and probably reflects differences in vehicles of transmission.

5.5. Age and Sex

The age- and sex-specific isolation rates for *Salmonella* is shown in Fig. 5. The isolation rate is highest in the first year of life, peaking at more than 180 cases per 100,000 population per year in the second month of life. The rate of infection declines rapidly among individuals 10 to 19 years old and then begins to rise among those older than 60. Some degree of detection bias probably exists, since infants and

the elderly may be more likely to have stool cultures performed when they are diagnosed with gastrointestinal infection. Nonetheless, this pattern probably reflects real age-specific differences in host susceptibility and in exposure rates.

The age-specific isolation rate for males is slightly higher than that for females between the age of 6 months and 4 years. The rate for females in most years slightly exceeds that for males in the age group 20 through 40, perhaps reflecting the greater likelihood that women will be involved in food preparation or maternal exposure to infected infants. The curious excess of isolates among male children is unexplained.

5.6. Race

Data on race are not routinely collected in national laboratory-based surveillance and no national data on the relative isolation rates by race have been reported.

5.7. Occupation

Few data are available to demonstrate that high-risk occupations for salmonellosis exist. Some studies have found higher rates of *Salmonella* carriage among food handlers, which may reflect their high level of contact with raw food and the frequency with which they are cultured.[29] In the past, sewage workers were considered to be at high risk

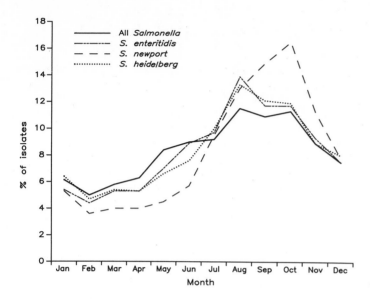

Figure 4. Monthly distribution of *Salmonella* isolates, United States 1975–1986, for all *Salmonella* isolates and selected serotypes. CDC (unpublished data).

of *Salmonella* infections, particularly typhoid fever, but existing evidence does not suggest that they are currently at increased risk.[72]

5.8. Occurrence in Different Settings

Salmonella outbreaks may create particular problems at institutions, including schools, prisons, nursing homes, hospitals, mental hospitals, and institutions for the retarded.

Between 1963 and 1972, 28% of all *Salmonella* outbreaks reported to CDC occurred in institutions; two thirds of these occurred in acute-care hospitals, pediatric wards, and newborn nurseries.[5] Institutional outbreaks tend to be more serious than those in other settings; the case-fatality rate for all institutional outbreaks between 1963 and 1972 was 2.3% and for those occurring in nursing homes, 8.7%. In the past, nosocomial outbreaks have occurred due to the use of contaminated medical and pharmaceutical products including

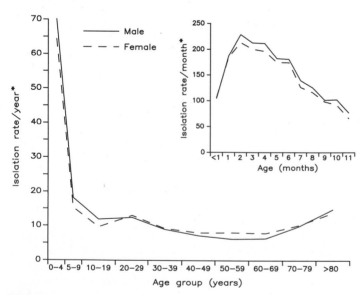

Figure 5. *Salmonella* isolation rates by age and sex, per 100,000 population, United States, 1984–1986. Adapted from Hargrett-Bean *et al.*[37]

carmine dye, pancreatic enzymes, platelets, and extracts of thyroid, adrenal cortex, pancreas, and pituitary.[5] Other important hospital outbreaks have been caused by contaminated foods, including powdered eggs, dried milk, and human breast milk.[90] The number of nosocomial *Salmonella* outbreaks reported to CDC has decreased in recent years, but several outbreaks due to *S. enteritidis* in shell eggs have occurred in nursing homes and hospitals in the northeastern United States, reflecting an increase in the role of eggs as the vehicle of *S. enteritidis*.[80]

Although person-to-person spread is frequently suspected in institutional outbreaks of *Salmonella*, it has been rigorously demonstrated in relatively few. Most recent institutional outbreaks are caused by food products of animal origin. The risk of secondary transmission within hospitals probably varies according to the patient population and setting. Transmission is particularly likely to occur in neonatal nurseries, where peripartum transmission may result in an infected infant, and the high level of nursing intervention and the susceptibility of neonates to *Salmonella* predispose to secondary transmission. On regular hospital wards the risk may be considerably less. No secondary transmission was documented in a recent hospital outbreak involving more than 200 nurses who developed salmonellosis after a "nurse appreciation day" meal.[81] Infection control measures included emphasis on hand-washing and exclusion of nurses with enterocolitis until symptoms resolved; negative stool cultures before returning to duty were only required for those working in the neonatal or adult intensive care unit, nursery, or renal dialysis unit.

5.9. *Salmonella* Infections in the Compromised Host

A variety of conditions have been associated with increased risk of *Salmonella* infections, including gastric surgery, decreased gastric acidity, sickle-cell anemia, lymphoma, Hodgkin's disease, metastatic cancer, and AIDS.[9,15,94] These are related to different mechanisms of defense against *Salmonella* infections (see Section 7). Patients with sickle-cell anemia and other diseases that compromise the reticuloendothelial system have an increased rate of *Salmonella* bacteremia and *Salmonella* osteomyelitis. The decreased ability to clear opsonized bacteria of these patients and perhaps the increased availability of iron may play a major role.[7] Patients with neoplastic disease are also at increased risk of salmonellosis, and lymphoproliferative disorders appear to be more strongly associated with salmonellosis than are solid tumors[94] (see Section 8).

5.10. *Salmonella* Infections and AIDS

Salmonella has emerged as an important pathogen among patients with AIDS. In a San Francisco study, the annual incidence of salmonellosis among patients with AIDS was almost 20 times higher than that in men in a similar age group who did not have AIDS.[15] The proportion of bacteremic *Salmonella* infections is also increased in patients with AIDS; *S. typhimurium* and *S. dublin* were more likely to cause bacteremia among these patients than among patients without HIV infection. *Salmonella* bacteremia in patients with AIDS often occurs in the absence of an identifiable episode of enterocolitis and frequently recurs after appropriate antimicrobial treatment.[40] Recurrent *Salmonella* bacteremia was made an indicator disease in the AIDS case definition in 1987. *Salmonella* bacteremia in HIV-infected individuals may precede and foreshadow the development of AIDS; in one third of the patients in the San Francisco study, salmonellosis occurred shortly before they were diagnosed to have AIDS.[15] It is not clear whether particular exposures, such as raw milk, health-food preparations, nontraditional medications, or undercooked meat and eggs, are important among AIDS patients, but *Salmonella* infections represent a large and potentially preventable source of mortality in this group. Patient education and the avoidance of high-risk foods have an important role in prevention.

6. Mechanisms and Routes of Transmission

Human infection can follow transmission of the organism via a variety of routes, including foodborne, waterborne, animal-to-person contact, person-to-person contact (either direct or indirect), and transfusion. However, up to 90% of infections with *Salmonella* in the United States are foodborne in origin.[24] Data on the sources of foodborne salmonellosis outbreaks indicate that foods of animal origin are the most common source (Table 3). The typical foodborne outbreak is the result of at least two food-handling errors: one that permits the contamination to occur, and another that permits sufficient bacterial growth to reach the infectious dose.

The epidemiologic complexity of tracing the sources of specific contaminated foods can be challenging. A few serotypes are associated with a specific vehicle. For instance, *S. dublin* infection is strongly associated with the consumption of raw milk and *S. enteritidis* with undercooked eggs.[80,82] When a convenient bacteriologic strain marker is available, however, it has been possible to retrace

Table 3. Foodborne Outbreaks of Salmonellosis Reported 1973–1982, by Implicated Vehicle[a]

Food vehicle	No. of outbreaks	Percent of outbreaks
Beef	57	13
Poultry	43	10
Pork/ham	20	5
Other meat	13	3
Fish and shellfish	4	1
Eggs, eggnog, ice cream	37	8
Milk, cheese, other dairy	17	4
Other foods	59	13
Multiple vehicles	42	10
Unknown	145	33
Total	437	100

[a]CDC (unpublished data).

the chain of transmission to farms of origin.[38,79] If the serotype is rare, it may be possible to trace it considerably further. For instance, the international epidemic of *S. agona* infections was traced to Peruvian fish meal, used in poultry feed, that introduced this formerly rare serotype to several continents simultaneously, where it has since persisted.[22] *Salmonella* can be introduced and perpetuated on a farm through contaminated feeds, the introduction of infected stock, or by wild animals. Foods may be contaminated in different ways: meat by feces during the slaughter process, or *in vivo* if the animal was bacteremic at the time of slaughter; milk by feces during the milking process, or by mastitis in the milked cow; prepared foods during processing by the use of contaminated ingredients, or by cross-contamination within the processing plant itself. In the kitchen, food may be cross-contaminated from raw foods or other sources. Although food handlers are often found to be infected in the course of investigating a foodborne outbreak investigation, they are most often infected because of their exposure to contaminated foods, and are rarely shown to be the source of the contamination themselves.[29]

In addition to foodborne transmission, large waterborne outbreaks of salmonellosis have occurred, when drinking water supplies have been contaminated in the absence of proper chlorination.[1]

Salmonella can reach an individual from animal reservoirs via a variety of other routes. Persons in direct contact with ill animals may become infected themselves. Pet turtles, which were almost universally colonized with *Salmonella*, emerged as an important source of the disease in the United States in the early 1970s.[46] Chameleons, aquarium

fish, chicks, snakes, and other potential pets may also be colonized with *Salmonella* and may occasionally be sources of infection.[21,86] Marijuana contaminated with *S. muenchen* was the source of an interstate outbreak probably due to the presence of animal feces.[83] A series of outbreaks of *S. cubana* infections was traced to carmine dye made from powdered insects and used as a marker of gastrointestinal motility.[47] An outbreak of *S. arizona* was traced to powdered rattlesnake capsules sold as a folk remedy.[63]

Salmonellosis can also be transmitted from one infected person to another (see Section 5.2.). Nosocomial outbreaks of salmonellosis that are not foodborne typically occur in the nursery, and transmission from one child to the next occurs on the unwashed hands of the health care worker. Many other routes of nosocomial transmission are possible. Infection can follow transfer of the organism via endoscope from one patient to the next.[8,38] *S. kottbus* has been transmitted through unpasteurized human milk, collected for infants at a human milk bank, from a woman with asymptomatic mammary carriage.[74] *S. cholerae-suis* was transmitted through platelet transfusions after the platelets were collected from a bacteremic donor.[62]

Although epidemiologic data from developing countries are limited, transmission of salmonellosis in those countries may include all of the above routes. Nosocomial reservoirs may be of greater importance than in industrialized countries, particularly for multiply resistant and invasive strains of *S. typhimurium,* such as those described in Brazil, Rwanda, and South Africa.[48,65,68]

7. Pathogenesis and Immunity

The incubation period after ingestion of *Salmonella* usually ranges from 6 to 48 h. The pathogenesis of *Salmonella* infections is incompletely understood. The multiplicity of serotypes and animal hosts involved introduces much complexity; a serotype that is nonpathogenic in one animal species may produce severe illness in another. Laboratory models need to be interpreted with caution. For instance, *S. typhimurium* infections in the mouse may be more analogous to *S. typhi* than to *S. typhimurium* infections in humans. The clinical expression of infection is affected by serotype and strain of the bacteria; the status of the underlying health and gut flora of the host; and the dose, vehicle, and route of transmission. Following ingestion, the organisms traverse the gastric acid barrier and multiply in the small intestine. The bacteria penetrate and damage the intestinal mucosa, are ingested by macrophages, and may multiply in a limited fashion in mesenteric lymphoid tissues. In severe invasive infection, bacteremia and focal infections in distant tissues occur.

The process includes several distinct steps, no single one of which explains the entire pathogenic spectrum: (1) Attachment and penetration. Adhesins facilitate the attachment of salmonellae to intestinal mucosal cells, and may be necessary for mucosal invasion.[41] Strains of *S. ty-phimurium* that are lethal for mice have a plasmid-dependent ability to adhere to and penetrate HeLa cells.[42] (2) Secretory response. The diarrhea of salmonellosis may reflect bacterial properties that cause fluid loss. Some invasive strains of *Salmonella* can cause fluid to accumulate in the rabbit ileal-loop model, and the characteristics of the fluid suggest active secretion, rather than just passive leaking through a damaged and permeable mucosa.[34,78] This fluid accumulation is attended by high levels of tissue cyclic AMP, is abolished by indomethacin, and may reflect the action of an enterotoxin.[6,33] (3) Inflammation and tissue destruction. The fever, bloody diarrhea, and evidence of colitis that often accompany salmonellosis may be the result of local inflammation, effects of bacterial endotoxin, or of specific cytotoxins that cause mucosal cell death.[32] A cytotoxin has been identified in *Salmonella* that inhibits protein synthesis in cultured vero cells, in a manner analogous to the cytotoxins present in *Shigella dysenteriae* 1 and verotoxigenic *Escherichia coli*.[45] (4) Intracellular multiplication in macrophages. Lethality in the mouse model is associated with the ability to multiply in macrophages, which may be a function of the presence of flagella, serum resistance, and undefined plasmid-associated factors.[20,36,91]

The outcome of infection is partly dependent on the number of ingested bacteria that reach the intestine. Small numbers of ingested *Salmonella* may cause transient asymptomatic intestinal colonization, while larger doses of the same strain may produce overwhelming or even fatal illness. The minimum dose necessary to cause illness varies with the serotype, the vehicle, and a variety of host factors. Although early volunteer studies indicated the infectious dose ranged from 10^5 to 10^{10} organisms, the minimal dose that causes illness may in some circumstances be substantially lower, even as low as 10 organisms.[11]

There are several major barriers in the host's defense against *Salmonella* infection. The first is gastric acidity, which can reduce the number of viable organisms by several logs within minutes. The degree of protection provided by gastric acid depends on the vehicle of infection; *Salmonella* may traverse the stomach more rapidly when consumed in liquids than in solid foods, and contaminated foods that buffer gastric acid well, such as chocolate, cheese, or milk,

may transmit infection more efficiently than foods that do not. Persons with high gastric pH, such as the elderly, those taking antacids or other antiulcer medications, and those who have had gastric surgery, are at increased risk for infection.[9,66]

The normal intestinal flora are a second major barrier to infection with salmonellosis. Disruption of the flora, particularly with antimicrobials that are active against the anaerobic flora such as penicillin or tetracycline, decreases the infectious dose needed to produce illness.[12,71] If the infecting strain is resistant to the antimicrobial used, therapy for an unrelated condition may convert a silent transient colonization to overt clinical infection, when the normal flora are suppressed.[38,66] Cellular immunity is the third major defense against bacteremia and invasive illness. This can be overcome in the normal host by certain highly invasive serotypes, such as *S. cholerae-suis,* or *S. paratyphi,* or by very large doses of other serotypes.[84] Hemolytic conditions, such as sickle-cell disease, bartonellosis, or malaria, predispose to invasive infection.[23] Persons with defective cellular immunity, such as those receiving immunosuppressive therapy, with advanced malignancies, or AIDS, are also at increased risk for invasive illness (see Sections 5.9 and 5.10).

Immunity to *Salmonella* infection is partial at best. In volunteer experiments, patients rechallenged with the homologous strain became ill a second time, although with somewhat milder symptoms than on initial exposure.[53] In animal models, experimental vaccines can prevent death, but not infection; more than 100 years after it was first isolated, *S. cholerae-suis* remains an economically important pathogen in swine, without a commercially useful and effective vaccine.

The humoral response of humans to experimental infection has been defined. Agglutinating antibodies develop against the somatic (O) and flagellar (H) antigens, even following asymptomatic infections.[35] These antibodies do not always appear, they wane after several months, and sufficient cross-reactions occur with other enteric bacteria that they have been of little diagnostic or epidemiologic utility. The nature of the cellular immune response to salmonellosis in humans has not been clearly defined.

8. Patterns of Host Response

The host response to *Salmonella* infection includes asymptomatic colonization, gastroenteritis, focal soft-tissue infection, meningitis, bacteremia, sepsis, and death. The pattern of host response may be dictated by the virulence of the specific strain, the size of the inoculum, and specific host factors including age, gastric acidity, immunologic competence, prior antimicrobial exposure, and specific illnesses. Disorders of the gastrointestinal tract (gastrectomy, achlorhydria, esophageal, gastric, or intestinal malignancies) may predispose to enterocolitis, and defects of cellular immunity (leukemia, lymphoma, HIV infection) or reticuloendothelial cell function (sickle-cell anemia, bartonellosis, malaria) may predispose to bacteremia and invasive disease.[9,94] Age is also an important determinant of host response. The incidence of salmonellosis is higher among infants and the elderly and the frequency of bacteremia is higher in both of these age groups.[39] The mortality of *Salmonella* infection is also considerably higher at the extremes of age, as demonstrated by outbreaks in nurseries and nursing homes.[5]

The most important determinant of host response may be the organism itself. Certain serotypes appear to be unusually virulent and are isolated more often from the blood and CSF relative to their overall isolation rate. *S. cholerae-suis, S. dublin, S. paratyphi* A, and *S. schottmuelleri* (formerly *S. paratyphi* B) are more commonly isolated from blood, and *S. panama, S. heidelberg,* and *S. saint-paul* are disproportionately common isolates from CSF.[10,92]

8.1. Clinical Features

The clinical manifestations of infection with nontyphoidal *Salmonella* can be grouped into several clinical syndromes with some overlap.

Acute enterocolitis, or gastroenteritis, is the most common syndrome of *Salmonella* infection. Initial symptoms often include nausea, vomiting, and headache, followed by abdominal cramps and diarrhea, which are the predominant manifestations. The stools are normally loose and of moderate volume; blood is occasionally seen. Voluminous, choleralike diarrhea has been reported, as have small-volume, dysenteric stools associated with tenesmus, but these are unusual manifestations. Fever, often accompanied by chills, is present in about 50% of patients. Diarrhea usually lasts 3 to 7 days, but may be prolonged.[9,77]

The enteric fever syndrome is classically associated with *S. typhi,* but may at times occur with other serotypes. This syndrome is characterized by a prolonged course with prominent fever, anorexia, abdominal pain, splenomegaly, and headache. Respiratory symptoms may be prominent and hepatomegaly, neurologic manifestations, and relative bradycardia may occur in nontyphoidal enteric fever. Complications include intestinal hemorrhage and perforation, myocarditis, seizures, and localized infections, but are less common than in enteric fever due to *S. typhi.*

Bacteremia without enteric fever may also occur due to nontyphoidal *Salmonella.* In children, "silent" bacteremia during enterocolitis may occur in 5–10% of patients,[85] but *Salmonella* bacteremia with high fever may occur without other signs of enterocolitis or enteric fever. Localized extraintestinal infections may result. Endarteritis, particularly infection of atherosclerotic aortic aneurysms, may occur in patients with preexisting atherosclerotic disease. Endocarditis is rare, and usually occurs on abnormal valves; infection of prosthetic heart valves has also been reported. *S. cholerae-suis* is responsible for a disproportionate number of endothelial infections. These infections can rarely be cured by antibiotics alone and surgical intervention is often necessary.[9] *Salmonella* meningitis occurs primarily in infants, and even with adequate antibiotic therapy, the mortality is high. Osteomyelitis and arthritis due to *Salmonella* may occur in normal hosts but are more common in immunocompromised persons, particularly those with hemolytic disorders. *Salmonella* is the most common cause of osteomyelitis in patients with sickle-cell anemia. Other complications of *Salmonella* bacteremia include pneumonia, empyema, endocarditis, intracranial abscess, urinary tract infections, and abscesses of the spleen, liver, and other soft tissue.[23] Another consequence of acute infection is chronic carriage. Although the median duration of excretion after infection is approximately 5 weeks and 90% of adults are culture-negative by 9 weeks, approximately 1% of patients continue to excrete *Salmonella* for more than 1 year. The duration of excretion tends to be longer in children less than 5 years old.[14]

8.2. Diagnosis

The diagnosis of *Salmonella* enterocolitis is made by stool culture. The diagnosis should be considered in any patient with moderate to severe gastroenteritis; the presence of headache or fever makes the possibility of this disease more likely. Fecal leukocytes may be present, but are not diagnostic. The differential diagnosis of *Salmonella* enterocolitis includes viral gastroenteritis and other bacterial enteric infections, including those caused by *Shigella,* enterotoxigenic, enterohemorrhagic, and enteropathogenic *E. coli, Campylobacter* species, *Vibrio* species, and *Yersinia enterocolitica.* The disorder must also be differentiated from toxin-mediated foodborne illnesses including those caused by *Staphylococcus aureus, Bacillus cereus,* and *Clostridium perfringens.* Compared to patients with these toxin-mediated disorders, persons with salmonellosis usually have less prominent vomiting and are more likely to have prolonged diarrhea and fever. The shorter incubation periods of toxin-mediated foodborne illness can be an important clue to distinguish them from salmonellosis. The presence of frequent, small-volume, bloody or mucus-streaked stools, tenesmus, and large numbers of fecal leukocytes makes campylobacterosis or shigellosis more likely than salmonellosis. A recent history of ingestion of raw milk, undercooked eggs or meat, or exposure to farm animals within the 48 h before onset of illness may suggest the diagnosis of salmonellosis. Ultimately, however, the diagnosis depends on cultures of stool, or in the case of high fever or invasive disease, blood, CSF, or other body fluids.

9. Control and Prevention

The control of salmonellosis depends on understanding the widespread and complex cycles of transmission well enough to interrupt them. Many control measures are implemented to prevent person-to-person transmission. The potential for this transmission makes it prudent to exclude from work food-handlers or health care workers with acute *Salmonella* enterocolitis, and convalescent persons in sensitive occupations who continue to shed the organism are often excluded until stool cultures no longer yield *Salmonella*. The risk posed by the entirely asymptomatic shedder is low and does not justify routine periodic stool cultures of food-handlers or health care providers. Nosocomial salmonellosis can be controlled by taking routine precautions to prevent transmission of enteric organisms from patients with acute salmonellosis, including strict hand-washing and other basic tenets of hospital infection control.[90] The ban on the sale of small pet turtles in 1975, following unsuccessful efforts to educate the turtle-owning public in methods to reduce risk, led to a dramatic decrease in the isolation rate of turtle-associated serotypes.[26]

The control of foodborne salmonellosis requires efforts at multiple levels, including those involving the cook, the processor, and the farm. Educating consumers in proper food-handling techniques to reduce their exposure to mishandled food is a constant effort of the public health community. The licensing and inspection of food-service establishments, particularly when coupled with food-handler education and certification, is an integral part of the effort to prevent foodborne illness of all sorts, including salmonellosis.

Many effective efforts to control foodborne salmonellosis focus on specific vehicles of transmission, after critical control points for intervention are identified. The single most successful such control measure has been the pasteurization of milk, which protects the consumer against many raw-milk-associated infections including *Salmonella*. The continued popularity of unpasteurized milk in some

parts of the country and the attendant risk of salmonellosis and campylobacteriosis led to the ban on interstate sale of raw milk in 1987. Irradiating other raw foods that are potentially contaminated is a theoretically effective, but thus far socially unacceptable way of controlling salmonellosis.[69] Changes in production practices within the food-processing industry can increase or decrease the risk of *Salmonella* contamination of the finished product. Following a series of *S. newport* outbreaks traced to precooked roast beef in the late 1970s, the cooking process was found to be inadequate to kill *Salmonella* entering the plant on raw beef. The series of outbreaks ended after the required times and temperatures of the cooking process were increased and measures were taken to prevent recontamination.[61] Modifications of techniques for producing dried powdered milk or eggs have reduced the contamination of those products. At slaughter plants, means to reduce the contamination of meat with feces at the time of slaughter have been proposed, but few have been widely studied or adopted.[59] The increasing concern over the need for microbiologic standards for raw foods means that reassessment of current practices of slaughter and inspection is likely.[57]

Animals entering the slaughter plant may be free of *Salmonella*, may have asymptomatic intestinal colonization, or may be ill or even moribund with systemic salmonellosis. The proportion of slaughtered animals that are moribund has been shown to be associated with the level of contamination of the carcass.[79] The carcass is condemned if evidence of bacteremia is found on simple visual inspection, and is sold for pet food or rendered into meal used to make animal feed. Rendering plants produce meat and bone meals that are frequently contaminated with *Salmonella*, despite the high temperatures used in the rendering process. These contaminated meals return the *Salmonella* to the farm animal. Many countries, but not the United States, require the pasteurization of animal feeds to interrupt this cycle.

Control of *Salmonella* contamination on the farm is also challenging. The larger farms and greater concentration of animals that characterize industrialized agriculture are conducive to the spread of salmonellosis. Many serotypes that are pathogenic in humans produce limited illness or asymptomatic colonization in the animal, and the direct cost of *Salmonella* contamination to the producer is often low. Nonetheless, significant advances have been made. In Scandinavia, the prevalence of salmonellosis in chicken flocks has been greatly reduced by exposing the chicks to normal fecal flora shortly after hatching, which increases their resistance to subsequent colonization with *Salmonella*.[58] In many countries, including the United States, two serotypes that are highly pathogenic for poultry, *S. pullorum* and *S. gallinarum*, have been virtually eradicated by a vigorous program of serologic testing and destruction of infected birds.[2]

10. Unresolved Problems

Salmonellosis will continue to be an important public health problem in the industrialized world and an increasing problem in developing countries for the foreseeable future. Although the pathogen has been well known for more than 100 years, many fundamental questions remain unanswered. Microbiologic issues in need of further study include clarifying the mechanisms of virulence, which may ultimately permit the successful development of vaccines. If programs of food safety that depend on bacteriologic monitoring are to be widely implemented, more rapid and sensitive means of detecting the organism in foods need to be developed.

Several important clinical issues are unresolved. The relationship between dose and incubation period has not been clearly defined. The risk factors for invasive infection in infants, particularly meningitis, are poorly defined, and the use of antimicrobials to treat *Salmonella* enterocolitis in infants to prevent invasive infections is presently unproven. The paradoxic and important ability of the organism to persist in the individual who is treated with antimicrobials, even when the organism is sensitive to those antimicrobials *in vitro*, needs to be explained. Developing new antimicrobial agents or other modes of treatment that would eliminate long-term carriage would be of benefit. The increasing antimicrobial resistance of strains isolated from humans in the United States will pose clinical challenges for the treatment of invasive infections, and increases the risk that resistant salmonellosis will complicate the therapy of other infections. The problem of increasing antimicrobial resistance would benefit greatly from a rational approach to defining the choice and indications for use of antimicrobials in animal husbandry and human medicine. Invasive infections are likely to be an increasing clinical problem, as the population ages and the prevalence of AIDS increases.

Unresolved epidemiologic issues include determining risk factors for salmonellosis in infants, and further assessing the risk of transmission associated with the human carrier. Reducing the contamination of our food supply without using radiation will require a continuing effort to identify specific critical control points at the farm, the rendering plant, the slaughterhouse, and the food-processing factory, and to implement cost-effective control measures.

11. References

1. Anon. A waterborne epidemic of salmonellosis in Riverside, California, 1965: Epidemiologic aspects, *Am. J. Epidemiol.* **93**:33–48 (1971).
2. Anon. The national poultry improvement plan and auxiliary provisions, Animal Science Research Division, Agriculture Research Service, U.S. Department of Agriculture, Beltsville, Md. (1982).
3. ASERKOFF, B., AND BENNETT, J. V., Effect of therapy in acute salmonellosis on *Salmonellae* in feces, *N. Engl. J. Med.* **281**:3–7 (1969).
4. ASERKOFF, B., SCHROEDER, S. A., AND BRACHMAN, P. S., Salmonellosis in the United States—A five-year review, *Am. J. Epidemiol.* **92**:13–24 (1970).
5. BAINE, W. B., GANGAROSA, E. J., BENNETT, J. V., AND BARKER, W. H., JR., Institutional salmonellosis, *J. Infect. Dis.* **128**:357–360 (1973).
6. BALODA, S. B., FARIS, A., KROVACEK, K., AND WADSTROM, T., Cytotonic enterotoxins and cytotoxic factors produced by *Salmonella enteritidis* and *Salmonella typhimurium*, *Toxicon* **21**:785–796 (1983).
7. BARRETT-CONNOR, E., Bacterial infection and sickle cell anemia: An analysis of 250 infections in 166 patients and a review of the literature, *Medicine* **50**:97–112 (1971).
8. BEECHAM, H. J., COHEN, M. L., AND PARKIN, W. E., *Salmonella typhimurium:* Transmission by fiberoptic upper gastrointestinal endoscopy, *J. Am. Med. Assoc.* **241**:1013–1015 (1979).
9. BLACK, P. H., KUNZ, L. J., AND SWARTZ, M. N., Salmonellosis—A review of some unusual aspects, *N. Engl. J. Med.* **262**:811–816, 846–870, 921–927 (1960).
10. BLASER, M. J., AND FELDMAN, R. A., *Salmonella* bacteremia: Reports to the Centers for Disease Control, 1968–1979, *J. Infect. Dis.* **143**:743–746 (1981).
11. BLASER, M. J., AND NEWMAN, L. S., A review of human salmonellosis: I. Infective dose, *Rev. Infect. Dis.* **4**:1096–1106 (1982).
12. BOHNHOFF, M., MILLER, C. P., AND MARTIN, W. R., Resistance of the mouse's intestinal tract to experimental *Salmonella* infection. II. Factors responsible for its loss following streptomycin treatment, *J. Exp. Med.* **120**:817–828 (1964).
13. BRYAN, F. L., What the sanitarian should know about *Staphylococci* and *Salmonellae* in non-dairy products: II. *Salmonellae*, *J. Milk Food Technol.* **31**:131–140 (1968).
14. BUCHWALD, D. S., AND BLASER, M. J., A review of human salmonellosis: II. Duration of excretion following infection with nontyphi *Salmonella*, *Rev. Infect. Dis.* **6**:345–356 (1984).
15. CELUM, C. L., CHAISSON, R. E., RUTHERFORD, G. W., BARNHART, J. L., ECHENBERG, D. F., Incidence of salmonellosis in patients with AIDS, *J. Infect. Dis.* **156**:998–1002 (1987).
16. Centers for Disease Control, Annual summary 1983: Reported morbidity and mortality in the United States, *Morbid. Mortal. Weekly Rep.* **32**(54) (1984).

17. Centers for Disease Control, *Foodborne Disease Outbreaks Annual Summary 1982,* CDC, Atlanta.

18. Centers for Disease Control, Summary of notifiable diseases, United States, 1986, *Morbid. Mortal. Weekly Rep.* **35**(55): 1986.

19. CHALKER, R. B., AND BLASER, M. J., A review of human salmonellosis: III. Magnitude of *Salmonella* infection in the United States, *Rev. Infect. Dis.* **9**:111–124 (1988).

20. CHIKAMI, G. K., FIERER, J., AND GUINEY, D. G., Plasmid-mediated virulence in *Salmonella dublin* demonstrated by use of a Tn5-oriT construct, *Infect. Immun.* **50**:420–424 (1985).

21. CHIODINI, R. J., AND SUNDBERG, J. P., Salmonellosis in reptiles: A review, *Am. J. Epidemiol.* **113**:494–499 (1981).

22. CLARK, G. M., KAUFMANN, A. F., GANGAROSA, E. J., AND THOMPSON, M. A., Epidemiology of an international outbreak of *Salmonella agona, Lancet* **2**:1–10 (1973).

23. COHEN, J. I., BARTLETT, J. A., AND COREY, G. R., Extraintestinal manifestations of *Salmonella* infections, *Medicine* **66**:349–388 (1987).

24. COHEN, M. L., AND TAUXE, R. V., Drug-resistant *Salmonella* in the United States: An epidemiologic perspective, *Science* **234**:964–969 (1986).

25. COHEN, M. L., FONTAINE, R. E., POLLARD, R. A., VON ALLMEN, S. D., VERNON, T. M., AND GANGAROSA, E. J., An assessment of patient-related economic costs in an outbreak of salmonellosis, *N. Engl. J. Med.* **299**:459–460 (1978).

26. COHEN, M. L., POTTER, M. E., POLLARD, R., AND FELDMAN, R. A., Turtle-associated salmonellosis in the United States: Effect of public health action. 1970–1976, *J. Am. Med. Assoc.* **243**:1247–1249 (1980).

27. COLLINS, R. N., TREGER, M. D., GOLDSBY, J. B., BORING, J. R., COOHAN, D. B., AND BARR, R. N., Interstate outbreak of *Salmonella new-brunswick* infection traced to powdered milk, *J. Am. Med. Assoc.* **203**:838–844 (1968).

28. CRAVEN, P. C., MACKEL, D. C., BAINE, W. B., BARKER, W. H., GANGAROSA, E. J., GOLDFIELD, M., DEWITT, W. E., FODO, T., FISH, S. M., DOUGHERTY, W. J., MURPHY, J. B., FELDMAN, J., AND VOGEL, H., International outbreak of *Salmonella eastbourne* infection traced to contaminated chocolate, *Lancet* **1**:788–793 (1975).

29. CRUICKSHANK, J. G., AND HUMPHREY, T. J., The carrier food-handler and non-typhoid salmonellosis, *Epidemiol. Infect.* **98**:223–230 (1987).

30. FARMER, J. J., III, MCWHORTER, A. C., BRENNER, D. J., AND MORRIS, G. K., The *Salmonella–Arizona* group of *Enterobacteriaceae:* Nomenclature, classification and reporting, *Clin. Microbiol. Newsl.* **6**:63–66 (1984).

31. FARMER, J. J., WELLS, J. G., GRIFFIN, P. M., AND WACHSMUTH, I. K., *Enterobacteriaceae* infections, in: *Diagnostic Procedures for Bacterial Infections,* 7th ed. (B. Wentworth, ed.), American Public Health Association, Baltimore, 1987.

32. GIANNELLA, R. A., Importance of intestinal inflammatory reaction in *Salmonella*-mediated intestinal secretion, *Infect. Immun.* **23**:140–145 (1979).

33. GIANNELLA, R. A., GOTS, R. E., CHARNEY, A. N., GREENOUGH, W. B., AND FORMAL, S. B., Pathogenesis of *Salmonella*-mediated intestinal fluid secretion. Activation of adenylate cyclase and inhibition by indomethacin, *Gastroenterology* **69**:1238–1245 (1975).

34. GIANNELLA, R. A., FORMAL, S. B., AND COLLINS, H., Role of plasma filtration in the intestinal fluid secretion mediated by infection with *Salmonella typhimurium, Infect. Immun.* **13**:470–474 (1976).

35. GOTOFF, S. P., LEPPER, M. K., AND FIEDLER, M. A., Immunologic studies in an epidemic of *Salmonella* infections, *Am. J. Med. Sci.* **251**:61–66 (1966).

36. GULIG, P. A., AND CURTISS, R., Plasmid-associated virulence of *Salmonella typhimurium, Infect. Immun.* **55**:2891–2901 (1987).

37. HARGRETT-BEAN, N.T., PAVIA, A. T., AND TAUXE, R. V., *Salmonella* isolates from humans—United States, 1984–1986, *Morbid. Mortal. Weekly Rep.* **37**(SS-2):25–31 (1988).

38. HOLMBERG, S. D., OSTERHOLM, M. T., SENGER, K. A., AND COHEN, M. L., Drug-resistant *Salmonella* from animals fed antimicrobials, *N. Engl. J. Med.* **311**:617–622 (1984).

39. HOOK, E. W., Salmonellosis: Certain factors influencing the interaction of *Salmonella* and the human host, *Bull. N.Y. Acad. Med.* **37**:499–512 (1961).

40. JACOBS, J. L., GOLD, J. W., MURRAY, H. W., ROBERTS, R. B., AND ARMSTRONG, O., *Salmonella* infections in patients with the acquired immunodeficiency syndrome, *Ann. Intern. Med.* **103**:186–88 (1985).

41. JONES, G. W., AND RICHARDSON, L. A., The attachment to, and invasion of HeLa cells by *Salmonella typhimurium:* The contribution of mannose-sensitive and mannose-resistant haemagglutinating activities, *J. Gen. Microbiol.* **127**:361–370 (1981).

42. JONES, G. W., ROBERT, D. K., SVINARICH, D. M., AND WHITFIELD, H. J., Association of adhesive, invasive and virulent phenotypes of *Salmonella typhimurium* with autonomous 60-megadalton plasmids, *Infect. Immun.* **38**:476–486 (1982).

43. KARLINSKI, J., Zur kenntnis des Bacillus enteritidis gaertner, *Zentralbl. Bakteriol. Parasitenkd.* **6**:289–292 (1889).

44. KAUFFMANN, F., *Die Bakteriologie der Salmonella-gruppe,* Munksgaard, Copenhagen, 1941.

45. KOO, F. C. W., PETERSON, J. W., HOUSTON, C. W., AND MOLINA, N. C., Pathogenesis of experimental salmonellosis: Inhibition of protein synthesis by cytotoxin, *Infect. Immun.* **43**:93–100 (1984).

46. LAMM, S. H., TAYLOR, A., GANGAROSA, E. J., ANDERSON, H. W., YOUNG, W., CLARK, M. H., AND BRUCE, A. R., Turtle-associated salmonellosis. 1. An estimation of the magnitude of the problem in the United States, 1970–1971, *Am. J. Epidemiol.* **95**:511–517 (1972).

47. LANG, D. J., KUNZ, L. J., MARTIN, A. R., SCHROEDER, S. A., AND THOMSON, L. A., Carmine as a source of nosocomial salmonellosis, *N. Engl. J. Med.* **276**:829–832 (1967).

48. LEPAGE, P., BOGAERTS, J., NSENGUMUREMYI, F., HITIMANA, D. G., VAN GOETHEM, C., VANDEPITTE, J., AND BUTZLER,

J. P., Severe multiresistant *Salmonella typhimurium* systemic infections in central Africa—Clinical features and treatment in a pediatric department, *J. Antimicrob. Chemother.* **14**(Suppl. B):153–159 (1984).

49. LOEFFLER, F., Ueber Epidemieen unter den im hygienischen Institute zu Greifswald gehaltenen maeusen und ueber die Bekaempfung der Feldmausplage, *Zentralbl. Bakteriol. Parasitenkd.* **12**:1–17 (1892).

50. MACCREADY, R. A., REARDON, J. P., AND SAPHRA, I., Salmonellosis in Massachusetts. A sixteen-year experience, *N. Engl. J. Med.* **256**:1121–1127 (1957).

51. MACDONALD, K. L., COHEN, M. L., HARGRETT-BEAN, N. T., WELLS, J. G., PUHR, N. D., COLLIN, S. F., AND BLAKE, P. A., Changes in antimicrobial resistance of *Salmonella* isolated from humans in the United States, *J. Am. Med. Assoc.* **258**:1496–1499 (1987).

52. MACDONALD, K. L., O'LEARY, M. J., NORRIS, P., COHEN, M. L., WELLS, J. G., KOBAYASHI, J. M., AND BLAKE, P. A., *Escherichia coli* O157:H7, an emerging gastrointestinal pathogen: Results of a one-year prospective population-based study, *J. Am. Med. Assoc.* **259**:3567–3570 (1988).

53. MCCULLOUGH, N. B., AND EISELE, C. W., Experimental human salmonellosis. II. Immunity studies following experimental illness with *Salmonella meleagridis* and *Salmonella anatum*, *J. Immunol.* **66**:595–608 (1951).

54. MCWHORTER, A. C., FIFE-ASBURY, M. A., HUNTLEY-CARTER, G. P., AND BRENNER, D. J., Modified Kauffman–White schema for *Salmonella* and *Arizona*, HEW Publ. (CDC) 78-8363 (1977).

55. MITSCHERLICH, E., AND MARTIN, E. H., *Microbial Survival in the Environment*, Springer-Verlag, Berlin, 1984.

56. MURRAY, M. J., *Salmonella:* Virulence factors and enteric salmonellosis, *J. Am. Med. Assoc.* **189**:145–147 (1986).

57. National Research Council, *Poultry Inspection: The Basis for a Risk-Assessment Approach*, National Academy Press, Washington, D.C., 1987.

58. NURMI, E., Use of competitive exclusion in prevention of *Salmonellae* and other enteropathogenic bacteria infections in poultry, in: Proceedings of the International Symposium on *Salmonella*, New Orleans, July 1984 (G. H. Snoeyenbos, ed.), pp. 64–73, University of Pennsylvania, Kennett Square, 1984.

59. OOSTEROM, J., AND NOTERMANS, S., Further research into the possibility of *Salmonella*-free fattening and slaughter of pigs, *J. Hyg.* **91**:59–69 (1983).

60. PACER, R. E., THURMOND, M. L., RYAN, C. P., SPIKA, J. J., AND POTTER, M. E., *Salmonella newport* in cattle: An animal and human health problem, in: Proceedings of the Nineteenth Annual Meeting of the U.S. Animal Health Association, pp. 374–380 (1986).

61. PARHAM, G. L., *Salmonellae* in cooked beef products, in: Proceedings of the International Symposium on *Salmonella*, New Orleans, July 1984 (G. H. Snoeyenbos, ed.), pp. 275–280, University of Pennsylvania, Kennett Square, 1984.

62. RHAME, F. S., RAAT, R. K., MACLOWRY, J. D., DADISMAN, T. A., AND BENNETT, J. V., *Salmonella* septicemia from platelet transfusions: Study of an outbreak traced to a hematogenous carrier of *Salmonella cholerae-suis*, *Ann. Intern. Med.* **78**:633–641 (1973).

63. RILEY, K. B., ANTONISKIS, D., MARIS, R., AND LEEDOM, J. M., Rattlesnake capsule-associated *Salmonella arizona* infections, *Arch. Intern. Med.* **148**:1207 (1988).

64. RILEY, L. W., DIFERDINANDO, G. T., DEMELFI, T. M., AND COHEN, M. L., Evaluation of isolated cases of salmonellosis by plasmid profile analysis: Introduction and transmission of a bacterial clone by precooked roast beef, *J. Infect. Dis.* **148**:12–14 (1983).

65. RILEY, L. W., CEBALLOS, B. S., TRABULSI, L. R., DE TOLEDO, M. R., AND BLAKE, P. A., The significance of hospitals as reservoirs for endemic multiresistant *Salmonella typhimurium* causing infection in urban Brazilian children, *J. Infect. Dis.* **150**:236–241 (1984).

66. RILEY, L. W., COHEN, M. L., SEALS, J. E., BLASER, M. J., BIRKNESS, K. A., HARGRETT, N. T., MARTIN, S. M., AND FELDMAN, R. A., Importance of host factors in human salmonellosis caused by multiresistant strains of *Salmonella*, *J. Infect. Dis.* **149**:878–883 (1984).

67. ROANTREE, R. J., *Salmonella* O antigens and virulence, *Annu. Rev. Microbiol.* **21**:443–466 (1967).

68. ROBBINS-BROWNE, R. M., ROWE, B., RAMSAROOP, R., NARAN, A. D., THRELFALL, E. J., WARD, L. R., LLOYD, D. A., AND MICKEL, R. E., A hospital outbreak of multiresistant *Salmonella typhimurium* belonging to phage type 193, *J. Infect. Dis.* **147**:210–216 (1983).

69. ROBERTS, T., Microbial pathogens in raw pork, chicken and beef: Benefit estimates for control using irradiation, *Am. J. Agric. Econ.* **67**:957–965 (1985).

70. ROWE, B., *Salmonella* surveillance: Reports received from centers participating with WHO Programme, 1981, Central Public Health Laboratory, London, 1984.

71. RYAN, C. A., NICKELS, M. K., HARGRETT-BEAN, N. T., POTTER, M. E., ENDO, T., MAYER, L., LANGKOP, C. W., GIBSON, C., MCDONALD, R. C., KENNEY, R. T., PUHR, N. D., MCDONNELL, P. J., MARTIN, R. J., COHEN, M. L., AND BLAKE, P. A., Massive outbreak of antimicrobial-resistant salmonellosis traced to pasteurized milk, *J. Am. Med. Assoc.* **258**:3269–3274 (1987).

72. RYAN, C. A., HARGRETT-BEAN, N. T., AND BLAKE, P. A., *Salmonella typhi* infections in the United States, 1975–1984: Increasing role of foreign travel, *Rev. Infect. Dis.* **11**:1–8, 1989.

73. RYDER, R. W., MERSON, M. H., POLLARD, R. A., JR., AND GANGAROSA, E. J., Salmonellosis in the United States, 1968–1974, *J. Infect. Dis.* **133**:483–486 (1976).

74. RYDER, R. W., CROSBIE-RITCHIE, A., MCDONOUGH, B., AND HALL, W. J., Human milk contaminated with *Salmonella kottbus*: A cause of nosocomial illness in infants, *J. Am. Med. Assoc.* **238**:1533–1534 (1977).

75. SACK, R. B., Serologic tests for the diagnosis of enterobacterial infections, in: *Manual of Clinical Laboratory Immunology* (N. ROSE, ed.), pp. 359–362, American Society for Microbiology, Washington, D. C., 1986.

76. SALMON, D. E., AND SMITH, T., Report on swine plague, U.S. Bureau of Animal Industry, 2nd Annual Report (1885).

77. SAPHRA, I., AND WINTER, J. W., Clinical manifestations of salmonellosis in man. An evaluation of 7779 human infections identified at the New York *Salmonella* Center, *N. Engl. J. Med.* **256:**1128–1134 (1957).

78. SEDLOCK, D. M., AND DEIBEL, R. H., Detection of *Salmonella* enterotoxin using rabbit ileal loops, *Can. J. Microbiol.* **24:**268–273 (1978).

79. SPIKA, J. S., WATERMAN, S. H., SOO HOO, G. W., ST. LOUIS, M. E., PACER, R. E., JAMES, S. M., BISSET, M. L., MAYER, I. W., CHIU, J. Y., HALL, B., GREENE, K., POTTER, M. E., COHEN, M. L., AND BLAKE, P. A., Chloramphenicol-resistant *Salmonella newport* traced through hamburger to dairy farms, *N. Engl. J. Med.* **316:**565–570 (1987).

80. ST. LOUIS, M. E., MORSE, D. L., POTTER, M. E., DeMELFI, T. M., GUZEWICH, J. J., TAUXE, R. V., AND BLAKE, P. A., The emergence of grade A eggs as a major source of *Salmonella enteritidis* infections. New implications for the control of salmonellosis, *J. Am. Med. Assoc.* **259:**2103–2107 (1988).

81. TAUXE, R. V., HASSAN, L. F., FINDEISEN, K. O., SHARRAR, R. G., AND BLAKE, P. A., Salmonellosis in nurses: Lack of transmission to patients, *J. Infect. Dis.* **157:**370–373 (1988).

82. TAYLOR, D. N., BIED, J. M., MUNRO, J. S., AND FELDMAN, R. A., *Salmonella dublin* infections in the United States, 1979–1980, *J. Infect. Dis.* **146:**322–327 (1982).

83. TAYLOR, D. N., WACHSMUTH, I. K., SCHANGKUAN, Y.-H., SCHMIDT, E. V., BARRETT, T. J., SCHRODER, J. S., SCHERACH, C. S., MCGEE, H. B., FELDMAN, R. A., AND BRENNER, D. J., Salmonellosis associated with marijuana: A multistate outbreak traced by plasmid finger-printing, *N. Engl. J. Med.* **306:**1249–1253 (1982).

84. TAYLOR, D. N., BOPP, C., BIRKNESS, K., AND COHEN, M. L., An outbreak of salmonellosis associated with a fatality in a healthy child: A large dose and severe illness, *Am. J. Epidemiol.* **119:**907–912 (1984).

85. TORREY, S., FLEISHER, G., AND JAFFE, D., Incidence of *Salmonella* bacteremia in infants with *Salmonella* gastroenteritis, *J. Pediatr.* **108:**718–721 (1986).

86. TRUST, T. J., AND BARTLETT, K. H., Aquarium pets as a source of antibiotic-resistant *Salmonellae, Can. J. Microbiol.* **25:**535–541 (1979).

87. United Nations, *Demographic Yearbook,* United Nations, New York, 1983.

88. U.S. National Office of Vital Statistics, Reported incidence of selected notifiable diseases, *Vital Statistics—Special Reports* **37**(9) (1953).

89. WACHSMUTH, K., Molecular epidemiology of bacterial infections: Examples of methodology and investigations of outbreaks, *Rev. Infect. Dis.* **8:**682–692 (1986).

90. WEICKEL, C. S., AND GUERRANT, R. L., Nosocomial salmonellosis, *Infect. Control* **6:**218–220 (1985).

91. WEINSTEIN, D. L., CARSIOTIS, M., LISSNER, C. R., AND O'BRIEN, A. D., Flagella help *Salmonella typhimurium* survive within murine macrophages, *Infect. Immun.* **46:**819–825 (1984).

92. WILSON, R., AND FELDMAN, R. A., Reported isolates of *Salmonella* from cerebrospinal fluid in the United States, 1968–1979, *J. Infect. Dis.* **143:**504–506 (1981).

93. WILSON, R., FELDMAN, R. A., DAVIS, J., AND LAVENTURE, M., Salmonellosis in infants: The importance of intrafamilial transmission, *Pediatrics* **69:**436–438 (1982).

94. WOLFE, M. S., ARMSTRONG, D., LOURIA, D. B., AND BLEVINS, A., Salmonellosis in patients with neoplastic disease. A review of 100 episodes at Memorial Cancer Center over a 13-year period, *Arch. Intern. Med.* **128:**546–554 (1971).

12. Suggested Reading

HARGRETT-BEAN, N., PAVIA, A. T., TAUXE, R.V., *Salmonella* isolates from humans in the United States, 1984–1986, in *COC Surveillance Summaries, June 1988, MMWR* **37**(No 55–2):25–31 (1988).

HOOK, E. W., *Salmonella* species (including typhoid fever), in: *Principles and Practice of Infectious Diseases,* 3rd ed. (G. L. Mandell, R. G. Douglas, and J. E. Bennett, eds.), Wiley, New York, 1989.

KELTERBORN, E., *Salmonella Species: First Isolations, Names, and Occurrence,* Junk, The Hague, 1967.

National Research Council, Poultry inspection: The basis for a risk-management approach, National Academy Press, Washington, D.C., 1987.

SCHWABE, C. W., Food safety, in: *Veterinary Medicine and Human Health,* 3rd ed., pp. 539–559, Williams & Wilkins, Baltimore, 1984.

CHAPTER 29

Shigellosis

Gerald T. Keusch and Michael L. Bennish

1. Introduction

Shigellosis, an acute infectious enteritis of humans and on occasion subhuman primates, is often referred to as bacillary dysentery. The reason is that dysentery, a syndrome manifested by frequent passage of small-volume, bloody mucoid stools, abdominal cramps, and tenesmus, is widely considered to be the principal clinical presentation of the infection.[87] However, watery diarrhea without blood or mucus is common in all forms of shigellosis and may be the only intestinal sign of infection.[2,55] In addition, there are a myriad of manifestations described in shigellosis, some common and some rare, that without doubt qualify the organism as a protean pathogen.[10,114] The objective of this chapter is to present the salient features of shigellosis in sufficient detail to understand the spectrum of the disease and its distinctive epidemiology.

2. Historical Background

Dysentery has long been clinically recognized.[1] The classic syndrome is depicted in the Old Testament, and mention of it appears in the descriptions of war, so common in our history, from Thucydides in the Levant to Montgomery at the battle of El Alamein.[80] According to Thomas Willis in 1684[235]:

> A dysentery is a distemper, so frequent in continual feavers, that some years it becomes epidemical and not more mild than the plague, kills many—the cause of it is wont to be not any humor produced within the viscera that corrodes the intestines with its acrimony, as some affirm, but a certain infection impressed on the blood.

There are two principal causes of this syndrome, *Shigella* species and *Entamoeba histolytica,* and a number of minor causes, including *Salmonella* and *Campylobacter.* Under circumstances of epidemic dysentery, *Shigella* is more likely to be the agent involved, while sporadic disease in adults associated with liver involvement is probably due to *E. histolytica.* However, in individual patients, the specific etiology of the syndrome can be determined only by laboratory investigation. This first became possible after Losch described *E. histolytica* and demonstrated its virulence in dogs in 1875[148] and Councilman and Lafleur[44] reported the anatomic criteria for the diagnosis in humans in 1891. The problem of assigning etiology to cases of dysentery in which neither the organism nor characteristic histology was present, however, remained. The loop was closed in 1898 by Dr. Kioshi Shiga,[210] who isolated the organism now known as *Shigella dysenteriae* 1 (Shiga's bacillus). The bacterium was found in the stools of patients with epidemic dysentery in Japan during a particularly widespread (almost 90,000 cases) and severe (25% mortality) outbreak. Shiga was able to demonstrate the presence of specific serum agglutinins in individuals convalescent from the disease,

Gerald T. Keusch · Department of Medicine, Division of Geographic Medicine and Infectious Diseases, New England Medical Center Hospitals, Boston, Massachusetts 02111. **Michael L. Bennish** · International Centre for Diarrhoeal Disease Research–Bangladesh, Ohaka Bangladesh; Departments of Pediatrics and Medicine, Division of Geographic Medicine and Infectious Diseases, New England Medical Center Hospitals, Boston, Massachusetts 02111.

but not in the healthy or in patients with other illnesses. In fact, the identical organism had been reported a decade earlier by Chantemesse and Widal[37] as the cause of non-amoebic dysentery, but the description was less complete and lacked the epidemiological proof of Shiga's study, and it is the Japanese microbiologist who is honored in the genus name. Two years later, Shiga's results were confirmed in the Philippines by Flexner and in Germany by Kruse.[15]

The following year, Kruse[132] isolated a similar but serologically distinct organism during an outbreak of "asylum dysentery," which he called *Bacillus pseudodysenteriae*. Identical organisms were soon described in the Philippines by Flexner and by Strong and Musgrave, and in Ceylon by Castellani, who suggested the name *B. paradysenteriae* instead. Somewhat later, Todd referred to this same strain as *B. dysenteriae* Flexner, and to clear the confusion, the name *Shigella flexneri* was ultimately adopted. A third species was defined by Duval, Castellani, and Kruse, who found a serologically distinct, late lactose-fermenting *Shigella,* which Kruse originally called *B. pseudodysenteriae* type E. To honor the subsequent extensive work of Sonne on Kruse's type E organism, the name was first modified to *B. dysenteriae* Sonne and then shortened to *Shigella sonnei.*

The final stage in classification on shigellae began in 1929 with Boyd's studies in Bangalore, India, of non-lactose-fermenting, mannitol-positive organisms resembling *S. flexneri* that were not agglutinated by *flexneri* antisera. Boyd[24] showed the presence of well-defined distinctive serological reactions with homologous antisera to the inagglutinable Flexner group, and on this basis such strains were classified together as *S. boydii*. By 1938, then, fully 40 years after the first complete description of the prototypic organism, *S. dysenteriae* 1, the four species of *Shigella* were defined [*dysenteriae* (10 serotypes), *flexneri* (6 serotypes), *boydii* (15 serotypes), and *sonnei* (1 serotype but multiple colicin types)].

At the beginning of this century, when it was commonly believed that pathogenic bacteria exerted their effects via toxins, Conradi[43] and Todd[224] separately described the animal toxicity of cell-free culture supernates of Shiga's bacillus, but not of the other related species. This toxic activity was known as Shiga neurotoxin because when injected parenterally into certain experimental animals, it caused a characteristic limb paralysis, terminating in death. The neurotoxic material was clearly shown to be distinct from lipopolysaccharide endotoxin by McCartney and Olitsky[163] in 1923, while van Heyningen and Gladstone[228] achieved significant purification of the protein toxin in 1953 and showed it to be one of the most potent known poisons.

From the time of its discovery, however, neurotoxin remained a biological activity in search of pathogenetic relevance until almost 70 years later, when Keusch and colleagues[121] found that neurotoxin-containing cell-free preparations from Shiga's bacillus were also enterotoxic, capable of inducing both fluid secretion by rabbit small intestine and an inflammatory enteritis resembling the colitis of human dysentery.[122] When *Shigella* species other than *S. dysenteriae* 1 were found to produce a similar toxin *in vitro*[119,181] and neutralizing serum antibody was demonstrated in human patients convalescent from infection due to *S. dysenteriae, S. flexneri,* and *S. sonnei,*[118] an *in vivo* role of toxin seemed plausible. That toxin is involved in pathogenesis of clinical shigellosis, however, remains a tempting, but unproven hypothesis.[125]

3. Methodology

3.1. Sources of Mortality and Morbidity Data

It is difficult to accurately determine morbidity or mortality rates due to shigellosis. There is first of all a "numerator problem." A clinical diagnosis of an isolated case is difficult to make due to the similarity of symptoms with other enteric infections. However, a clinical diagnosis can be made with greater confidence if the case occurs among a cluster of related cases, at least one of which is laboratory confirmed. The "laboratory" diagnosis of an individual case depends on good microbiological technique. Certain media used for isolation of enteric pathogens are inhibitory to the growth of shigellae[45,112,158] and multiple cultures may be needed to establish the diagnosis. In addition, shigellae do not survive well in media, such as Cary–Blair, that are commonly used to transport fecal specimens for culture.[171] Second, there is a "denominator problem," because the population to be considered in calculation of morbidity rates is less than the population at risk. *Shigella* infection is most often identified in patients, usually children, who either have the dysenteric form of the illness or have specific complications, such as seizures.[135] More mildly affected patients, particularly those without clinical dysentery, are usually treated symptomatically, and specific etiology is not determined. The problem of underdiagnosis is even more pronounced in many less developed countries, where access to health care facilities is limited and laboratory services are, as a general rule, not available.

Such data as are available generally come from three sources: (1) hospital-based reports; (2) etiological investigations of diarrhea in either the hospital or the community setting; (3) national surveillance. The first source will miss most of the disease in the community.[102] The third, such as the national surveillance system maintained by the United States Centers for Disease Control (CDC), depends on multiple uncontrolled reporting sources based on cultures submitted to local and state health departments.[21] Only community studies of the second sort can provide reliable estimates of morbidity or mortality.[18,86,154] These data are usually time and place specific; however, they are not universally applicable.

3.2. Surveys

Both bacteriological and serological methods have been used in prospective community-based surveys of the incidence and prevalence of *Shigella* infection.[18,154,216] Bacteriological surveys can underestimate the true disease incidence because the organisms die during transport of the specimen, or because patients are sampled either late in the course of their illness or after antibiotic therapy has been initiated.

A variety of serological methods have been employed for detecting both acute infection as well as evidence of past infection, but their usefulness is limited because there is cross-reactivity between different species and serotypes of *Shigella,* they have limited sensitivity, and titers wane rather quickly after infection.[9,185] Newer methods that detect antibodies directed at somatic antigens, Shiga toxin, outer-membrane proteins, or other plasmid-encoded surface antigens have been developed,[50,60,118,119,145,179] but their utility for diagnostic or epidemiological purposes has not been extensively evaluated.

3.3. Laboratory Diagnosis, Isolation, and Identification of the Organism

Shigellae are slender, gram-negative, nonmotile rods. They are members of the family Enterobacteriaceae and tribe Eschericheae, and are closely related to *Escherichia coli*. Routine isolation and identification of *Shigella* species involves the use of selective bacteriological media that spotlight certain biochemical properties of the genus and allow a presumptive microbiological diagnosis. Identity can be quickly confirmed by the use of serological agglutination reactions, employing group-specific anti-O-(somatic) antigen sera. Unfortunately, many of the commercially available typing sera are of poor quality, being too dilute or too cross-reactive to identify group- or type-specific antigens.[62] Even so, the grouping sera are reasonably good for

S. dysenteriae 1, *S. flexneri* (except *flexneri* 6), and *S. sonnei* bearing Form I antigen, which are the most important isolates to identify in the United States.

Because feces is the most frequently submitted specimen for isolation of *Shigella*, representing a complex ecosystem of many different organisms, differential bacteriological media are used with two purposes in mind: (1) to suppress the growth of the usual nonpathogenic normal flora that might numerically overwhelm and obscure the growth of *Shigella* and (2) to dramatically contrast the colonial appearance of the possible pathogen with that of the common commensal so that suspect colonies may be picked for further study. This is accomplished by inclusion in the media of either substances inhibitory to the growth of nonpathogens or a dye indicator system to detect rapid fermentation of lactose, since all shigellae are unable to perform this reaction, but commensals can. A variety of media have been developed for this purpose; the most successful and currently used are MacConkey's bile salt, xylose–lysine–deoxycholate (XLD), Hektoen enteric (HE), and tergitol-7-triphenyl tetrazolium chloride (TTC) agars. These media permit the growth of all *Shigella* species reasonably well, are inhibitory to normal flora, and clearly distinguish the lactose-negative organisms by color reactions. *Salmonella–Shigella* (SS) agar is far too inhibitory to shigellae, especially to *S. dysenteriae* 1,[158,171,191] to be recommended for general use, particularly if only one differential medium is to be used. Indeed, it is microbiologically sound to employ more than one screening medium to maximize the yield of positives.[171] When the number of organisms in the sample is small, isolation may be facilitated by brief enrichment in broth inhibitory to nonpathogens, such as Hajna's gram-negative (GN) broth. After 6–8 h of incubation of the sample in broth, the resulting growth is streaked onto the same differential media used in direct isolation as above.

Three technical details should be followed to minimize the number of false-negative cultures: (1) whenever possible, inoculate from a stool sample, rather than a swab, selecting blood-tinged mucus plugs as the source of culture; (2) if a swab is to be used, be certain that it passes beyond the anal sphincter; (3) if there is to be any appreciable delay in processing the sample, place it in buffered glycerol-saline holding medium.[233]

Lactose-negative colonies are picked to a medium such as triple sugar iron (TSI) agar, which allows confirmation of the lactose-negative phenotype and detects glucose fermentation and lack of motility, which are additional properties of shigellae. Both the agar surface (slant) and the butt are inoculated with the colony to be tested, to achieve aerobic and anaerobic conditions, respectively. In the butt, fermentation of glucose results in a pH change and a change in color of the phenol red indicator to yellow (acid), but without gas bubbles, while on the slant, the failure of the organism to use lactose (or sucrose, which is also contained in TSI) precludes sufficient drop in pH to change the pink (alkaline) color. In contrast to the non-lactose-fermenting enteric pathogens in the genus *Salmonella*, no black reaction product is deposited due to H_2S formation. The presumptive diagnosis based on TSI is then confirmed by serological agglutinations using group-specific antisera. Of course, more thorough biochemical study can be done, but this is rarely necessary, and the criteria enumerated above, included in standard schemata for the identification of Enterobacteriaceae, are sufficient for diagnostic purposes.

4. Biological Characteristics of the Organism

4.1. Invasiveness

Probably the single most important property of the shigellae in determining virulence is their ability to penetrate mammalian epithelial cells.[55,57,74,81,94,95,133] Invasion of intestinal epithelial cells confers on the organism a means to secure an ecological niche for multiplication wherein the bacteria are sequestered away from host antibacterial factors including antibody, complement, and phagocytic cells. It is presumably this property that permits establishment of infection with as few as 10–200 viable *S. dysenteriae* 1 organisms ingested by mouth.[139] The tiny infective dose, in turn, permits effective contact spread from host to host without the need for enrichment growth in some vehicle such as food or water.

In experimental studies in animals, the invasive process *per se* has been found to be surprisingly innocuous for the cell, at least early in the infection.[68,219] While such a mechanism might be expected to cause lysis of the cell, this does not happen, perhaps because the invading bacteria are at first contained within membrane-bound vesicles. In time, however, with escape of the organism from the vesicle and subsequent multiplication to produce an intracellular microcolony, cell damage and death do occur (see Section 7).

Invasion and intracellular survival of shigellae are determined by factors controlled by both chromosomal and plasmid genes.[94,161,202,203] Conjugal transfer or transduction of chromosomal DNA from *E. coli* to *Shigella* indicates that at least three regions are involved, including one bounded by the xylose and rhamnose loci, the histidine locus, and the purine E locus.[95] *Shigella–E. coli* hybrids

involving these regions are able to invade mammalian cells in culture but seem unable to survive within the host and are avirulent in animal models and volunteers. In *S. flexneri,* the xylose–rhamnose regions are known to code for the iron-binding protein, aerobactin, and for an iron-regulated outer-membrane protein (OMP) that may be important for bacterial iron metabolism.[89,175] The histidine region regulates expression of the specific carbohydrate side chains of lipopolysaccharide endotoxin, which probably serves to protect the organism from host defense mechanisms.[82]

However, conjugal transfer of these three regions (or for that matter, almost the entire bacterial chromosome) from *S. flexneri* to an avirulent *E. coli* K12 does not confer virulence in animal models,[203] suggesting that additional factors are needed. Such factors (at least four loci) have been identified on large 120- to 140-megadalton (MDa) plasmids present in all virulent shigellae (and in the biologically similar invasive *E. coli* serotypes).[200–202] These plasmids are both highly conserved and functionally equivalent. Several noncontiguous genes are present within a cloned smaller 22-MDa fragment of the 140-MDa plasmid from *S. flexneri* 5, which are necessary to confer the invasive phenotype. Two loci are included, the *ipa* gene (invasion plasmid antigen) coding for several polypeptides expressed on the outer membrane, where they may function to recognize ligands on the surface of mammalian cells and initiate the internalization of the organism,[28] and the *inv* (invasion) genes, which may serve to insert the OMPs into the outer membrane.[229]

The 140-MDa plasmid also contains virulence genes outside of the 22-MDa region,[205] including *virF* (which codes for Congo red binding, a marker of surface charge)[197] and *virG* (which codes for a hemolysin activity that correlates with the ability of the organism to rapidly escape from endocytic vesicles in which it is internalized, to diffuse throughout the infected cell, and to spread from cell to adjacent cell).[150,204] These latter properties are obviously critical for the bacterium to survive in the mammalian host.

Characteristics of the epithelial cell surface may also be important determinants of invasion. Rout *et al.* have shown that oral infection of rhesus monkeys with virulent *S. flexneri* 2a produces a noninvasive secretory diarrhea in proximal jejunum and an invasive bacterial colitis.[195] This difference in invasive capacity of one organism in two locations in the gut strongly suggests that the epithelial cell surface also determined invasion by shigellae. Studies by Hale *et al.*[93] employing eukaryotic cell-culture lines also demonstrate differences in susceptibility to invasion from cell type to cell type, as well as differences among HeLa cell isolates obtained from different sources.

Invasive qualities of *Shigella* isolates can be demonstrated by the Sereny test, in which a culture is inoculated into the conjunctival sac of an experimental animal such as a guinea pig.[208] Invasive organisms produce a visible purulent keratoconjunctivitis within 24–48 h. This property is encoded in a chromosomal locus called *kcp* that is cotransducible with *purE*.[72] Although patient isolates are invariably Sereny test positive, *Shigella–E. coli* hybrids incorporating the 140-MDa plasmid and *his* region may be invasive in HeLa cells but Sereny test negative, while Sereny-positive strains possessing the *kcp* locus do not necessarily cause fluid secretion in the ligated rabbit ileal-loop model.[95] However, it is hardly necessary to document the invasive ability of clinical isolates of *Shigella;* these organisms are invariably invasive.

4.2. Toxigenicity

It is now believed that a bacterial cytotoxin, present in the periplasmic space,[48] is a second key factor in virulence.[121,124,125] It has been known since 1903 that at least one *Shigella* species (*S. dysenteriae* 1 or Shiga's bacillus) produces a toxin designated Shiga neurotoxin[43] because it caused limb paralysis and death when inoculated parenterally into sensitive animal species such as the rabbit or mouse. The toxin could also elicit neutralizing antibodies in animals.[43,182,224] Although a role in pathogenesis was suggested initially, by the late 1960s it was concluded that Shiga toxin was produced only by one *Shigella* species and was not a virulence attribute of the genus.[124]

However, cytotoxins are produced by all *Shigella* species, albeit much less efficiently *in vitro* by non-*S. dysenteriae* 1 strains.[11,119,181] Quantitative studies suggest that *S. dysenteriae* 1 produces 1000- to 10,000-fold more toxin than does *S. flexneri* 2a under equivalent cultural conditions, but detailed comparative studies of many strains are still lacking. It is not yet clear whether a family of structurally related cytotoxins exists or if there are two or more distinct toxins.[180] Using a monoclonal antibody capture ELISA test, Shiga toxin has been found in stool of approximately 80% of patients in Bangladesh with *S. dysenteriae* 1 infection but in fewer than 20% of those with *S. flexneri* infection.[50] Clinical evidence also indicates that the highly toxigenic *S. dysenteriae* 1 strain produces a more virulent form of illness than does either *S. flexneri* or *S. sonnei*.[55,139,149,156,210] In volunteers with induced experimental shigellosis, the mean incubation period is shorter and the severity of clinical disease greater in individuals infected with a fully toxigenic *Shigella* strain compared to a derived hypotoxigenic mutant.[139] Similar findings have been obtained by assay of *in vitro* cytotoxicity in HeLa cells using the same bacterial strains.[93]

The toxin has two biological properties that may be relevant to virulence.[121,122] First, it causes secretion of isotonic fluid without histological damage in proximal intestine in rabbits, which resembles the jejunal response in monkeys infected with viable *S. flexneri* 2a.[195] Second, toxin is taken up by cells via receptor-mediated endocytosis,[106] resulting in damage to absorptive intestinal epithelial cells by a process of apoptosis, associated with crypt hyperplasia and mild inflammatory changes in the lamina propria.[113,172] If crude toxin preparations are employed, a marked inflammatory reaction is observed, with epithelial cell death, microulcer formation, and exudation of leukocytes into the bowel lumen along with blood and mucus, resembling the events in the colon during clinical dysentery.[122]

4.3. Antimicrobial Resistance

Resistance to antimicrobial agents commonly used in the treatment of shigellosis is a major problem both in developed and in developing countries.[34,35,91,98,152,209] Increasing resistance to ampicillin and sulfamethoxazole–trimethoprim (SXT), the drugs of choice for the treatment of shigellosis,[137] has in many situations forced practitioners to use alternative drugs, which are often more expensive (third-generation cephalosporins),[109] less effective (oral, nonabsorbable agents),[99] or newer drugs that have not yet been approved by the Federal Drug Administration for use in children (ciprofloxacin and norfloxacin).[4] At the Treatment Centre of the International Centre for Diarrhoeal Disease Research, Bangladesh (ICDDR,B), the percentage of isolates of *Shigella* that were resistant to both ampicillin and SXT increased from less than 5% in 1983 to 25% in 1986; among *S. dysenteriae* type 1 isolates, resistance increased from 5% to 70% during that period (Fig. 1). As a consequence, nalidixic acid is now the drug of choice for treating patients with presumed shigellosis at the ICDDR,B.[198]

Plasmid-mediated resistance to antimicrobial agents was originally described in *Shigella*[230] and transfer of resistance between *Shigella* and other Enterobacteriaceae inhabiting the gut may account in part for the rapidity with which shigellae have developed resistance to newly introduced antimicrobial agents. Resistance to ampicillin continues to be primarily plasmid mediated.[64,76,184] Resistance to SXT in an epidemic strain of *S. dysenteriae* type 1 from Africa[76] and three fourths of isolates of *S. flexneri* from Brazil,[222] were plasmid-mediated. In Thailand, SXT resistance in shigellae mediated by an alteration in di-

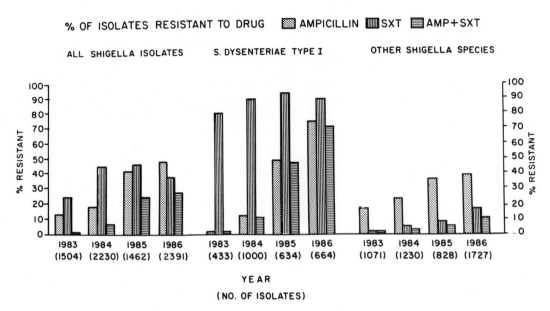

Figure 1. Prevalence of ampicillin and sulfamethoxazole–trimethoprim (SXT)-resistant *Shigella* isolated at the International Centre for Diarrhoeal Disease Research, Bangladesh (ICDDR,B), from 1983 to 1986.

hydrofolate reductase, was plasmid-borne in only 24% of 58 strains studied.[38] Although quinolone resistance is not believed to be plasmid-mediated, a recent report suggests that nalidixic acid resistance was transferable in some *S. dysenteriae* 1 strains in Bangladesh.[174] This has still to be confirmed, but if true, it signals that resistance to nalidixic acid will spread, perhaps limiting the utility of the newer 6-fluoroquinolones as well. This would be very unfortunate, as there is tremendous expectation for these drugs in treatment of multiresistant shigellosis,[117] since chromosomally mediated resistance among the Enterobacteriaceae has developed much more slowly to the new agents than to the original quinolone drug, nalidixic acid.[177]

Epidemic strains of *S. dysenteriae* 1 resistant to multiple antimicrobial agents in common use in the community have emerged in the past two decades in Central America, Africa, the Indian subcontinent and elsewhere in Asia.[38,76,78,91,109,152,155,158,174,184,209] Since the most obvious alteration in the epidemic strain, compared to the preepidemic strain, was the acquisition of a drug-resistance plasmid, the question has been raised as to whether the virulence of the strain is a consequence of genes associated with the drug-resistance factor.[79] Such an epidemic-associated virulence factor has never been identified, and an alternative explanation is that epidemic strains quickly acquire resistance as they spread through the community and come under intensive antimicrobial selective pressure.

5. Descriptive Epidemiology

5.1 Prevalence and Incidence

An estimated 140 million cases and 576,000 deaths occur annually due to *Shigella* infection in children under 5 years of age, even excluding data from China.[3] Because of the problems described in Section 3, such an estimate of worldwide prevalence and incidence is only a gross approximation of the actual number. For certain populations, however, good data do exist. In a study by Mata and colleagues of young Mayan Indian children in the village of Santa Maria Cauque, Gautemala, during 1964–1969, a cohort of 45 newborns was followed prospectively with intensive disease surveillance and regular and frequent culturing of stool samples to determine colonization by normal flora and infection by pathogens.[154] *Shigella* infections were common in these young children, accounting for 21% of the diarrheal episodes, and indeed this genus was the most frequently identified enteric bacterial pathogen. Age-specific prevalence rates in the routine cultures are shown in Table 1 and are ·compared with earlier data from India.[65] Prevalence was higher in the first 6 months of life than in the second 6 months in Guatemalan infants, reflecting a combination of a surprisingly high prevalence of 1.6% during the first week of life and the natural resistance of the breast-fed infant to *Shigella* infection thereafter. Prevalence rose dramatically

Table 1. Prevalence of *Shigella* Infections in Two Developing Countries

Age interval (months)	Routine cultures positive for *Shigella* species	
	Guatemala[154]	Vellore, India[65]
0–5	1.4%	0.7%
6–11	0.4	7.1
12–17	6.8	
18–23	15.8	} 8.5
24–29	19.1	
30–35	22.1	} 7.7

Table 2. *Shigella* Infections in Children in Santa Maria Cauque, Guatemala[a]

Age (weeks)	Incidence (per 100,000/year)
0–25	3,120
26–51	36,400
52–77	88,400
78–103	176,800
104–129	187,200
130–155	192,400

[a]From Mata.[154]

at the end of the second year, reaching about 20% in the third year of life because of circumstances favoring exposure and the effects of malnutrition in the weanling infant in that setting. Incidence rates can also be calculated from the data, if the assumption is made that repeat isolation of the same serotype following a culture-negative period of 2 weeks or more indicates a new infection (Table 2). Incidence increased progressively, reaching a level of 189,900/100,000 per year in the third year of life. These prevalence and incidence rates are enormous compared to those of well-nourished populations in the industrialized nations (see below).

Shigella infections in Santa Maria Cauque children were often prolonged (Table 3). *S. dysenteriae* 1 and *S. flexneri* produced the most chronic infections, while *S. sonnei* was the shortest in duration. Nearly 20% of all documented *Shigella* infections lasted more than 2 months. Observations in a group of young children recovering from acute infections in a convalescent home in Guatemala and followed for at least 8 weeks, and up to 20 weeks,[156] showed that nearly 33% of 110 children initially surveyed

were positive for *Shigella* compared to a prevalence of 7–8% in rural Guatemalan preschool populations. Of these children, 20, including 6 documented *Shigella*-infected subjects, were then followed with daily examinations and cultures. Of these 20, 8 remained negative for *Shigella*, while 12 harbored the agent at one time or another during the study. Of the latter, 8 were asymptomatic carriers, 1 was an acute case, and 3 had chronic recurrent diarrheal disease. There was a strong association between isolation of *Shigella* and the presence of malnutrition. In 2 patients, there was transition from carrier to acute case after 13 and 15 days of symptomless documented carriage. These 2 patients highlight the problem of differentiating the healthy carrier state from carriers who subsequently develop disease. It is generally believed that clinical illness occurs within a period of 5–6 days, or not at all, but this may not be correct. The chronic relapsing form of illness was characterized by continuous presence of organisms and periods of acute active diarrhea with intervals of low-grade or indefinite symptomatology. The organism was excreted during 75 of 154 person-weeks of observation (in 27 weeks of acute illness

Table 3. Duration of *Shigella* Infections in Children in Santa Maria Cauque, Guatemala[a]

Duration (weeks)	Percentage of total *Shigella* species				
	S. dysenteriae	*S. flexneri*	*S. boydii*	*S. sonnei*	All species
1	24	24	67	100	35
2–4	35	28	28	—	28
5–8	14	24	5	—	17
9–12	10	12	—	—	9
13–16	7	7	—	—	5
>16	10	5	—	—	5
	100	100	100	100	100

[a]From Mata.[154]

and 48 weeks of asymptomatic carriage). Following acute shigellosis, 17% of the children excreted organisms for at least 1 month and 11% for more than 2 months.

Earlier studies in 1954 in Sindbis village, Egypt, are in general confirmatory of the high incidence of *Shigella* infection in developing countries.[104] The incidence of symptomatic *Shigella* infections was 101,200/100,000 per year and an equal number of asymptomatic *Shigella* infections were detected so that the total incidence was 202,400 per 100,000 per year. Twenty-two percent of the children had two or more attacks during the year. As the bacteriological methods employed were not optimal for isolation of the organism, it is likely that these rates are minimum figures and underestimate the true incidence in this community.

Shigellosis is also a significant diarrheal disease problem in the United States and other industrial countries. In 1987, there were 16,567 isolations of *Shigella* reported to CDC through nationwide passive surveillance system [35]; 67.7% were *S. sonnei*, 22.2% *S. flexneri*, 2.1% *S. boydii*, 1.4% *S. dysenteriae,* and 6.6% unknown species. During the 12-year period, 1976 through 1987, a total of 167,915 isolates were reported.

However, there are groups in the United States that have incidence and prevalence rates that begin to resemble those seen in developing countries. One such group are Native Americans, with an incidence rate 3.6 times that of the general population,[21] predominantly *S. flexneri,* rather than *S. sonnei* as the rest of the American population. In Israel, a country with attributes of both a developed and a developing nation, the incidence of shigellosis is reported to be 150/100,000 per year, with a predominance (70%) of *S. sonnei.*[88] Another group in the United States with high incidence are the institutionalized mentally retarded, in whom "asylum dysentery" was an early recognized epidemiological entity.[63] In one study in the United States extending over 2 years, 541 of 5310 individuals (10.2%) living at one institution had *Shigella* isolated from at least one culture, and 247 of those (46%) were symptomatic at the time the first culture was obtained.[56] The incidence rate for clinical infections in persons newly admitted to the institution was nearly 37,000/100,000. In addition, 7% of the children excreted organisms intermittently for over a year, because of either establishment of a carrier state, or frequent reinfection. Prolonged carriage of shigellae is not the usual pattern for otherwise healthy individuals in developed nations.[55] In a study in England, for example, only 2.4% of patients excreted the organism for as long as 4 months and none beyond 7 months.[221] Thus, in both incidence and carriage, institutionalized populations in the United States epidemiologically resemble the children of Santa Maria Cauque.

Children in day-care centers are a third group with a high incidence of shigellosis.[187] With the increase in the number of children in day-care facilities in recent years, these centers are playing an increasingly important role in transmission of the disease in the United States.[232] In 1392 children enrolled in day-care centers in Houston, Texas, who were followed prospectively for up to 19 months, the incidence of culture-confirmed shigellosis was 6689/100,000 per year.[187,188] Secondary cases of shigellosis occurred in 24 (26%) of 91 families when a child in day-care developed shigellosis. During extended outbreaks of the illness in Louisville and Cleveland, infection was first introduced into the household by a child attending a day-care center in 25% of affected families investigated.[231]

5.2. Epidemic Behavior and Contagiousness

The first bacteriologically documented description of epidemic shigellosis was that of Shiga during the 1896 epidemic of *S. dysenteriae* 1 in Japan[210] involving some 90,000 clinical cases. For the first two decades of this century, this organism was the cause of numerous outbreaks of shigellosis throughout the world with high morbidity and mortality.[211] Inexplicably, the organism became less prevalent after 1920, and various serotypes of *S. flexneri* became dominant.[130] After World War II, *S. sonnei* gradually replaced *S. flexneri* in industrialized nations,[17,21,90,194,221] while *S. flexneri* persisted in developing countries.[19,65,66,86,131,216] For example, in the first decade of surveillance in the United States by the CDC,[194] the prevalence of *S. flexneri* went from 60.6% in 1964 to 15.5% in 1973, while the isolation of *S. sonnei* rose from 38.1% to 83.6%. The absolute number of *S. flexneri* decreased and that of *S. sonnei* increased, so that overall nearly two thirds of the isolates were *S. sonnei* and just over one third were *S. flexneri,* a complete reversal in the relative frequency of the two organisms over this 10-year period of time. This same pattern of change is also being observed in the more developed urban centers in developing countries, such as Bangkok, Thailand (P. Echeverria, personal communication).

Engrafted on this unexplained, changing world picture has been the reappearance of epidemic Shiga bacillus dysentery since 1969. After many years of playing a minor role in the etiology of shigellosis in Central America, *S. dysenteriae* 1 suddenly and dramatically became the dominant enteric pathogen in 1969–1970. It resulted in epidemic spread of infection, affecting adults as well as children, with an adult often being the index case, and it caused a degree of severity in the disease much beyond the accustomed level. For example, in 18 Guatemalan communities surveyed, the dysentery mortality increased from 39/100,000 in 1968 to 170/100,000 in 1969 when the outbreak occurred.[155] All age groups were affected, the youngest and the oldest most significantly. The death rate for the entire country was estimated to be 250/100,000, varying from 334/100,000 in the lowlands to 190/100,000 in the highlands. The case-fatality rate was also quite high in untreated patients, ranging from 8.4% of village patients to 10–15% of those hospitalized because of acute illness. This rate decreased later in the epidemic when better therapy was employed. These features are in contrast to endemic shigellosis principally due to *S. flexneri* and *S. sonnei*, primarily affecting young children in the under-5-year-old group, with the index case in families generally a preschool or school-age child and with mortality in adults an unusual event.[136,221,232]

5.3. Geographic Distribution

The shigellae are worldwide in distribution. The incidence of infection in different regions will vary, of course, with the level of sanitation and exposure. In the United States, the highest isolation rates are from the western states, and the ratio of *S. flexneri* to *S. sonnei* is higher than for the rest of the country. In Alaska, isolations of *S. flexneri* actually outnumber those of *S. sonnei*. In developed countries, infection with *S. dysenteriae* 1, and to a lesser extent *S. flexneri*, is often related to travel to developing countries.[90] Incidence rates also vary according to socioeconomic levels, including the standard of hygiene in the community and in the home, and especially the availability of water for washing.

5.4. Temporal Distribution

Different temporal patterns of shigellosis have been found. In the United States, peak incidence of both *S. sonnei* and *S. flexneri* infection is mid to late summer.[21] In both urban[216] and rural[18] Bangladesh, isolation of *Shigella* peaks in the postmonsoon season of December and January, and again in the hot dry premonsoon period of April and May. In southern India, the incidence of shigellosis is highest during the monsoon season itself. In Egypt, peak incidence is during the early summer months of June and July.[66,67] In Guatemala, the illness tends to peak just before and in the early weeks of the rainy season.[84–86] A variety of explanations, none entirely satisfactory, have been offered for the different temporal patterns observed, which must relate to specific epidemiological features in the various environments that lead to seasonal transmission.

Explanations for summertime peaks in temperate climates include increased social activity of children during this time, promoting person-to-person transmission, and perhaps longer survival of organisms in the environment. Summertime peaks during the hot dry season in tropical climates have been explained by decreased availability of water and the attendant decrease of water use for personal hygiene.[22] Lastly, peaks before or during the rainy season have been explained by increased contamination of water supplies, or seasonal worsening of nutritional status and increased susceptibility to infection.[84–86]

5.5. Age

Endemic shigellosis is a childhood disease in both developed and developing nation settings, whereas epidemic shigellosis can be expected to affect all age groups.[21,78,84,85,136,158,194,221] But, even where shigellosis is highly endemic, neonatal shigellosis is rare[67,154,157] and is usually traceable to infection in the mother. In the developed nations, this disease is severe and frequently complicated by gram-negative rod bacteremia.[12,97] In the developing nations, neonatal infection is generally transient and asymptomatic.[157] The pattern of acquisition of shigellosis in the remainder of the first year of life is one of increasing incidence in Dallas, Texas,[97] and decreasing incidence in Guatemala.[154] The most important determinant of this difference is the use of bottle-feeding in Dallas and breast-feeding in Santa Maria Cauque. An additional factor is the age at which table foods are introduced into the diet. Incidence rises at age 2–3 months in Dallas,[97] after 6 months in Egypt,[67] or later in Guatemala[154] as solid foods are introduced. There is a dramatic further increase in the period following weaning in children in the developing countries, as the combined effects of infection and nutritional inadequacy of the diet result in enhanced susceptibility of the child.[67,84,120,154] In Bangladesh, the highest incidence of *Shigella* bacteremia and death is in infants under the age of 1, and the associated risk factors are weaning and evidence of malnutrition.[218] During the recent epidemics of Shiga bacillus dysentery, the very young and the elderly have experienced the most severe illness, with clustering of mortality as well.[78,158,192] Beyond the first few years of life, increasing age is associated with lowered prevalence, diminished severity, and a relative increase in the proportion of mild and subclinical infections. With decreasing prevalence of infection in the community, there is an apparent shift in the age-specific peak to a somewhat older age group.[102,154,221]

5.6. Sex

Age-specific attack rates for *Shigella* infection show no sex differences except for an increase in females aged 10–29 and 60–79 in the United States, presumably reflecting the greater exposure of mothers and grandmothers to young children. In contrast, in areas with a large male homosexual population, there may be a preponderance of infection in young and middle-aged males due to venereal transmission.[52] Approximately one fourth of the *S. flexneri* isolates in the United States are now from young adult men, largely the result of venereal transmission. This appears to be the major explanation for the recent rise in the median age of males infected with *S. flexneri* from 5 to 24 years of age, with no change in median age in women and a decrease in children. This population may also account for the stabilization in the number of *S. flexneri* isolates reported to the CDC over the past decade, in contrast to the steady decrease in the two decades before.

5.7. Race

There is no evidence that race *per se* affects susceptibility to the disease. Genetic factors, such as HLA-B27 antigen, do predispose to joint involvement and postdysenteric Reiter's syndrome,[42,178,226] and this may explain the frequency of these complications in Scandinavians, who have a high prevalence of this histocompatibility antigen.

5.8. Occupation

Certain occupations may increase exposure to shigellae. Notable examples of the increased incidence of shigellosis in women caring for young children at home were cited in Section 5.6. Attendants in custodial institutions for the mentally retarded, teachers in day-care centers or in grade school, microbiology laboratory technicians, nurses, and physicians should also be at greater risk of contracting the disease than is the general population, but with the exception of anecdotal and isolated instances, convincing data are not available. The lack of a striking relationship may point to the protective value of good personal hygiene and ready access to clean water for washing.

5.9. Occurrence in Different Settings

Shigellosis can readily spread among individuals living in close quarters where personal hygiene and environmental sanitation are inadequate. Bacillary dysentery has been a classic problem of the army at war,[80] and it occurs in other similar settings such as closed populations in custodial institutions[56] or aboard ship.[167] Introduction of illness into the household often results in intrafamilial spread, and the family should therefore be considered an epidemiological entity in this instance.[8,221,222] The secondary attack rate is greater in children than in adults (Table 4) and infection is more likely to be symptomatic in the young as well. Although breast-fed neonates appear to be protected from symptomatic shigellosis when infected,[39,157] the same cannot be said for those being bottle-fed. Spread of shigellosis in a nursery can result in serious clinical manifestations, frequently terminating fatally.[97]

5.10. Socioeconomic Factors

Endemic shigellosis is associated with poverty, crowding, poor sanitation, water sources inadequate in quantity and quality, and malnutrition.[86] Both cross-sectional and longitudinal studies show the inverse relationship between socioeconomic status and *Shigella* infection (Table 5).[215,231] Each of the factors considered—water availability,[105] sanitary disposal of feces,[160] and control of flies[81]—can be demonstrated to affect the infection rate individually (Table 6). However, these factors usually occur together, which may exacerbate the problem. Effects of malnutrition have already been noted. Bottle-feeding young infants in such environments will considerably worsen the situation, whereas breast-feeding appears to be protective until the weaning age.[84]

6. Mechanisms and Routes of Transmission

The shigellae are, like the typhoid bacillus, highly host-adapted; the only natural hosts for *Shigella* are humans and a few nonhuman primates.[173] For this reason, more than 99% of all *Shigella* isolates in the United States are from human sources.[21,194] Thus, the route of transmission is inevitably traceable to an infected human (or, on rare

Table 4.   Secondary Attack Rates among Household Contacts of Shigellosis Patients

Age of exposed contact	Secondary attack rates	
	S. flexneri[102]	*S. sonnei*[222]
Child	42%	42%
Adult	14	20

Table 5. Incidence and Prevalence of *Shigella* Infection according to Socioeconomic Status

Fresno County, California, 1953[231]

Socioeconomic status	Water supply	No. studied	Prevalence of *Shigella* infection (per 100,000)
Low	Outside; >15 people per faucet	1051	9200
Low	Outside; <15 people per faucet	2182	5300
Low	In home	376	2100
Moderate	In home	278	400

Southwest Georgia, 1955[215]

Sanitation	Environmental features	Person-months of observation	Incidence of new *Shigella* infection (per 100,000)
Poor	Outside water, surface privy, no screens, high fly counts	2782	6200
Fair	Single inside faucet, pit privy, inadequate screens, high fly counts	5392	2200
Good	Complete inside plumbing, adequate screening	1279	600
Very good	Complete inside plumbing, adequate screening, not near fair or poor housing	1709	300

occasion, to a simian contact). The route can be further described as a circle from the stool to the mouth and back to the stool again, and indeed shigellosis is most frequently spread by person-to-person contact.[85,102,232] Large numbers of shigellae (10^5–10^8/g) are present in stools of clinical cases, and even healthy carriers have 10^2 organisms/g feces.[45] Even under epidemic conditions, such as the Shiga outbreak in Central America from 1969–1972, the epidemiological evidence may favor contact spread.[78] This is encouraged by conditions of poverty, crowding, and poor

Table 6. Relationship of Environmental Factors and Prevalence of *Shigella* Infections

Environmental factor	*Shigella* infections (prevalence/100,000) in relation to evaluation of factor		
	Poor	Fair	Moderate
Water availability[105]	7200	4800	700
Feces disposal[162]	4700	2800	—
Fly control[147]	3200	—	800

sanitation, which facilitate the transfer of the small inoculum needed to initiate the infection. The index case within households is most often a young child under the age of 10.[21,86,102,194,221]

Organisms can, of course, find their way to food or water sources and thereby initiate common-source epidemics.[17,50,52,166,167,214,234] These may occur in households, towns, or larger groupings of people or under special circumstances such as in hospitals, resort clubs, or aboard ship. Foodborne epidemics are generally traceable to infected food handlers,[214] and are especially associated with foods eaten raw or handled after preparation.[153] Resort clubs represent an ideal environment for widespread dissemination of foodborne disease, with large numbers of short-stay visitors who eat virtually all of their meals at the club, and who return home within the incubation period of shigellosis.[36] Waterborne transmission is not restricted to contamination of drinking water or use of ice. Even swimming or surfing in contaminated waters can lead to infection.[46,151]

In the developing countries, a combination of contact and waterborne spread can contribute to a prolonged, smoldering epidemic that lasts for months rather than weeks, until the population of susceptibles is exhausted.[84-86] In the Central American epidemic of 1969–1972, waterborne spread within some communities is suggested by the clustering of cases in place and time, the presence of multiple index cases in families, and the relationship between defective water distribution and illness.[78] However, the occurrence of the disease in widely separated places that do not share food or water supplies also indicates the likely role of the human carrier in spread. In the initial Bangladesh outbreak,[192] strong circumstantial evidence suggested waterborne transmission; the epidemic occurred during the monsoon, when the ground was saturated with rain water; there were poor sanitation and high coliform counts in drinking and wash water, indicative of extensive fecal contamination; and the epidemic terminated when chlorination of water was begun. The introduction of the organisms into this insular community was undoubtedly from an infected human, and the early slow spread of disease is probably explained by initial person-to-person contact. The later spread was likely caused by contamination of water sources from the excreta of the slowly increasing number of patients.

A variation on the mechanism, but not the route, of transmission has been clearly demonstrated in recent years among homosexual men engaging in anal–oral sex practices.[168] Recently, five cases of severe *Shigella* septicemia have been reported in patients with AIDS, associated with concomitant cryptosporidiosis in two and herpetic perirectal disease in three.[13] The presumptive route of transmission in these individuals is venereal, which is often associated with simultaneous transmission of other enteric pathogens, such as *Giardia lamblia*.[52,168]

7. Pathogenesis and Immunity

7.1. Pathogenesis

The incubation period for shigellosis can be estimated at approximately 2–5 days based on experimental human infections with *S. flexneri* 2a and *S. dysenteriae* 1.[54,139] Surprisingly, the more virulent *S. dysenteriae* 1 strain had a longer mean incubation period than the *S. flexneri* 2a isolate.

Following oral ingestion of the organisms, a sufficient inoculum must survive gastric acidity and other intestinal defense mechanisms to initiate infection. Human shigellosis is clearly a colonic process.[2,27,159,212] However, in experimental shigellosis in the rhesus monkey,[195] there is evidence of involvement of both the proximal small bowel and the colon. Whether this is true in humans as well remains uncertain.

It is now quite well established that the colonic disease involves the direct invasion of epithelial cells and the multiplication of bacilli in the cytoplasm.[69,139,159,195] Bacteria then invade adjacent cells, spreading the infection in a focal fashion. An inflammatory process develops in the lamina propria, with epithelial cell death and sloughing, leading to formation of microulcers and an inflammatory-cell exudate in the stool.[2,159] This lesion is the cause of the dysentery syndrome. It is, however, still unknown how the organism invades the epithelial cell and how it produces this basic colonic lesion.

In the course of investigating the microbial invasion genes carried on large (120–140 MDa) plasmids in the genus *Shigella*,[200-202] a number of other plasmid-mediated characteristics have been discovered that suggest that a series of events occurs during and after the invasion process.[40,41,161,197,204] There may be separate genes within a complex operating together as an operon,[160] since mutants defective in just one property can be obtained. Such genes may individually control initial bacterial–epithelial cell contact (? adhesin), rearrangement of the epithelial cell cytoskeleton leading to bacterial uptake within a phagocytic vesicle, rapid escape from the vesicle to the cytoplasm, distribution throughout the cell along actin filaments, and cell-to-cell invasion. What triggers epithelial cell death and the inflammatory response is not certain, although *Shigella* cytotoxins both damage and kill cells[113,121,122,124,172] *in vitro* and *in vivo* and this property could be central to the pathological processes observed in humans.

Small-bowel involvement has been best demonstrated in the rhesus monkey model.[195] In the monkey, organisms appear to proliferate first in the proximal small-bowel lumen and, without invading the bowel mucosa itself, cause a local secretory diarrhea with characteristics reminiscent of the watery diarrhea of cholera (see Chapter 10). Early colonization of the human small bowel occurs in some patients,[54] raising the speculation that a small-bowel secretory phase may occur in humans as well,[125] but this has yet to be substantiated and evidence to the contrary has been presented.[27] Later in the course of infection organisms reach the colon, initiating the invasive bacterial colitis characteristic of dysentery. This temporal sequence of watery diarrhea first followed by colonic involvement and dysentery is found in shigellosis due to all species of the genus.[2,55,158]

In vitro and *in vivo* experiments employing rabbits have provided insights into the mechanisms that may be involved in the small bowel of the monkey. In the rabbit,

Shiga toxin recognizes a glycolipid receptor in the microvillus membrane of the proximal small-bowel cell,[77] which has been identified as globotriaosylceramide, Gb3.[107] This globoseries glycolipid is a trisaccharide of Galα1→4Ga1β1→4Gluβ1-ceramide. The binding of toxin is specific for the terminal disaccharide[107,146] and is necessary for the fluid secretory response in the rabbit to occur.[169] The receptor is present only in villus cells and not in the crypt, and thus toxin targets the villus cell alone, inhibiting its protein synthesis.[110] This leads to depression of villus cell functions, including neutral and glucose- or alanine-facilitated sodium absorption, with no apparent effect on chloride secretion by the crypt cell. Net accumulation of fluid in the lumen is due to diminished sodium absorption, without change in unidirectional transport of chloride from the blood to the lumen. Attempts to detect a small-bowel "net secretory" phase of disease in humans have not provided clear-cut answers. Colonoscopy and colonic perfusion methods were employed in one complex study designed to measure fluid movement across the ileocecal valve as a marker of the small-bowel origin of secretion,[27] but by the time the patients were prepared and ready for study, all were in the dysenteric phase of illness. Thus, while this study did not find evidence of small-bowel involvement, it does not rule out this possibility in the watery disease phase of shigellosis.

In spite of its marked activity in gut tissue, the role of Shiga toxin in pathogenesis remains a subject in need of further clarification. In studies in Bangladesh, a monoclonal antibody-capture ELISA[50] has been used to detect toxin in stool of infected patients. High levels of toxin antigen were present in most individuals with *S. dysenteriae* 1 (over 80%), but in fewer than 20% of patients with *S. flexneri*. The low incidence of positives in *S. flexneri*-infected patients may be because this species produces less toxin than does *S. dysenteriae* 1. Alternatively, it could be related to the recent report that non-*S. dysenteriae* 1 species make cytotoxins that differ immunologically from Shiga toxin.[11] However, these non-cross-reactive toxins are not well characterized as yet, their properties are not fully defined, and their role in pathogenesis is as uncertain as that of Shiga toxin itself. The possible importance of these cytotoxins is suggested by the correlation between the clinical picture of bloody diarrhea and the production of toxin *in vitro* by the patient's own isolate.[189] This correlation is strengthened by the observation that certain *E. coli* strains that cause a characteristic bloody diarrhea, hemorrhagic colitis, are noninvasive and do not make the classical LT or ST toxins of *E. coli,* but produce large amounts of a cytotoxin that is identical to or very closely related to Shiga toxin.[30,61,180] These

toxins have been called Shiga-like toxins in the United States and Verotoxin by workers in the United Kingdom and in Canada. The former name is preferred, since the name Shiga toxin antedates Verotoxin, which is also physiologically incorrect, since the toxin is neither made by nor is specific for Vero cells.

A number of systemic complications occur in shigellosis as well, most with uncertain pathogenesis. Bacteremia, most commonly encountered in infection due to *S. dysenteriae* 1 or *S. flexneri,* may be a consequence of tissue damage and host defense defects.[170,218] In Bangladesh, bacteremia occurs primarily in children under 1 year of age and is significantly associated with malnutrition.[218] Leukemoid reactions occur most often in Shiga bacillus dysentery,[26] often associated with hemolytic–uremic syndrome (HUS).[129,193] The role of toxin in pathogenesis of HUS is suggested by the observation that HUS also occurs during infection with high Shiga-like toxin-producing *E. coli* causing hemorrhagic colitis.[111] Toxic megacolon is an uncommon but severe problem, reflecting extreme inflammatory colitis,[31] and may result in perforation of the gut.[7] What determines why this occurs in some patients is not known. Encephalopathy and seizures are present with a greater frequency in shigellosis than in any other diarrheal disease.[5,6,134,199] Seizures occur during infection with all *Shigella* species, and are associated with high fever. While it may be nothing more than a febrile seizure,[127] its pathogenesis is not known. Reactive arthritis appears to be associated with *S. flexneri* infection, but its pathogenesis is not clear.[32,178,226,227] Whereas the majority of patients with reactive arthritis are B27-positive, only a minority of B27-positive subjects develop joint disease after bacillary dysentery.[226] *S. flexneri* (and some other enterobacteriaceae) possess cell envelope components that resemble B27 antigens, but this cross-reactivity alone is insufficient to initiate the complication.[227]

7.2. Immunity

There is much epidemiological evidence suggesting acquired immunity to *Shigella* infections. While shigellosis is primarily a childhood disease,[21,84,86,136,194] introduction of an epidemic strain, not previously prevalent in the population (such as the spread of the Shiga bacillus in Central America in 1969–1972), involves all age groups.[78,155,158] This indicates that the widespread prevalence of certain serotypes of the organism in the community results in immunity to reinfection by that specific serotype. This idea is supported by live oral vaccination studies (see Section 9.3) that clearly indicate development of type-specific immunity following infection by attenuated avirulent vaccine strains.[138,142,165] Rechallenge of volunteers who previously had experimental dysentery with the same serotype also demonstrates serotype-specific protection.[53] These data suggest that the protection is probably antibacterial. However, the specific mechanism involved is not known at present, and in any event can be overcome by exposure to heavily contaminated environments.[140]

Among the likely microbial surface structures available for antibacterial immunity is the O-antigen of the lipopolysaccharide endotoxin. The structural basis of O-antigen specificity in the shigellae is now known to a considerable extent, and both unique and cross-reactive determinants exist, including many *Shigella* antigens identical to or cross-reactive with *E. coli* as well.[114] Compared to the older agglutination reactions such as passive hemagglutination using LPS-coated erythrocytes, new serological methods such as radioimmunoassay (RIA) and enzyme immunoassay (EIA) offer the advantages of greater sensitivity, reproducibility, and the ability to measure IgG as well as IgM antibody. Sera from Vietnamese patients have been analyzed with an EIA to *S. dysenteriae* 1 somatic antigen.[145] A specific IgA and IgM antibody response was present by day 10 and remained significantly elevated over Vietnamese control values for at least 45 and 180 days, respectively. IgG antibody was present on day 30, and remained detectable at least through 180 days. *S. flexneri* antigens represent a problem, since serotypes 1–5 possess a common tetrasaccharide repeating unit,[114] to which D-glucosyl and/or O-acetyl groups are added to produce serotype specificity. The immune response therefore produces antibodies to both common repeat unit epitopes and to type-specific epitopes. Rises in titer indicate a recent *S. flexneri* infection but cannot distinguish among types 1–5. The antigen for *S. flexneri* type 6 is distinct,[144] and could be used for a specific test. *S. sonnei* has a distinctive O-antigen containing polymerized disaccharide repeat units of two unusual sugars.[114] It is known to cross-react only with a *Pleisiomonas shigelloides* C27 antigen, and appears to result in specific antibodies in the majority of patients with documented *S. sonnei* infections.[60]

OMPs are also antigenic.[95,96,179] The major OMP is a chromosomally determined antigen, present in both virulent and avirulent *Shigella* strains.[179] Antibody responses to the plasmid-controlled OMPs believed to be involved in invasion develop as well, but the currently available data suggest that young children under the age of 3 respond poorly or not at all.[179]

Serum toxin-neutralizing antibodies develop in acute shigellosis due to all serotypes.[118] This antibody activity has been recovered in the IgM fraction of immunoglobulin, rises rapidly after infection, and disappears some time after 9 months.[119,123] Although this time course is similar to that of the antisomatic O-antigen response,[29,123] there is no relationship between the titers of the two antibodies in individual patients.[123] There is no apparent protection from serum antitoxin. Rhesus monkeys parenterally immunized with toxin and orally challenged with viable *S. dysenteriae* 1 develop high serum antitoxin levels, but infection proceeds as in unimmunized control animals.[164] The question of a role for antitoxin antibodies at the level of the mucosa itself has not been answered.

8. Patterns of Host Response

Most clinical shigellosis is gastrointestinal disease.[47,51,56,63] This spans a spectrum from mild to severe watery diarrhea,[2,55,189,216] with or without blood and mucus, to the bacillary dysentery syndrome.[55,139,216] A clear-cut dose–response curve can be seen in adult volunteers experimentally infected with known numbers of bacteria (Table 7). The prevalence of asymptomatic infection will depend on the presence of acquired resistance (especially in endemic regions) and the inoculum size (especially in virgin populations in nonendemic regions). However, first postweaning exposure to *Shigella*, wherever and whenever it occurs, will likely result in symptomatic disease.[56,136,154] In most recent common-source outbreaks in the United States, the attack rate in adults has varied from 10 to 85% with a mean of 40%.[17,47,194] In outbreaks involving children in day-care centers, attack rates have ranged from 26 to 48%.[34,187,188,220]

Under most circumstances, extraintestinal manifesta-

Table 7.   Relationship of Inoculum to Illness in Shigellosis

Bacterial challenge (no. of organisms)	Volunteers ill	
	S. flexneri 2a[55]	*S. dysenteriae* 1[139]
100,000	58%	—
10,000	59	83%
5,000	57	—
2,000	—	70
200	22	50
10	—	10

tions occur uncommonly. They may include involvement of the central nervous system. (usually seizures, but also nuchal rigidity, meningismus, and delirium), the blood (bacteremia with the infecting *Shigella* or another gram-negative rod, leukemoid reactions, thrombocytopenia, microangiopathic hemolysis), the kidney (hyponatremia, uremia), the eye (keratoconjunctivitis, iritis), and the joints (nonsuppurative arthritis).[5,6,10,13,16,26,193,218,223]

Postdysenteric Reiter's syndrome (iritis, urethritis, arthritis) is particularly likely to present in subjects who possess HLA-B27 antigen[226] and is usually associated with *S. flexneri* infection.[32,112,178] Joint manifestations in the genetically prone subjects are frequently chronic and destructive. Hematological manifestations, including bacteremia, occur primarily in subjects with Shiga bacillus dysentery.[26,129,193,218] Indeed, microangiopathic hemolytic anemia appears to occur exclusively in Shiga infections.[193] Rare patients may exhibit metastatic infection of skin, wounds, the lungs, the joints, the urinary tract, or the meninges.[10]

8.1. Clinical Features

The initial manifestations of acute shigellosis are usually fever, malaise, abdominal pain, and watery diarrhea.[54,115] There is nothing pathognomonic about this presentation, however, until the disease progresses with the appearance of blood and mucus in the stools. The entire colon may be involved, but the rectum and sigmoid area are the most severely affected.[212] The intense inflammation and ulceration result in tenesmus and frequent passage of small-volume stools that often consist of only blood and mucus (Fig. 2). In very severe cases, toxic megacolon[33] or colonic perforation[7,33] may ensue. The more virulent the organism (dysenteriae 1 > *flexneri* > *sonnei*), the more likely and the more rapid is the appearance of dysentery after onset of diarrhea[54,55,101,149,156]; in fact, the course may be so rapid in Shiga bacillus infection that it is hardly possible to distinguish the diarrheal phase at all.

In well-nourished subjects, the illness is generally self-limited in 7–10 days.[55,57,101,139] In the malnourished,

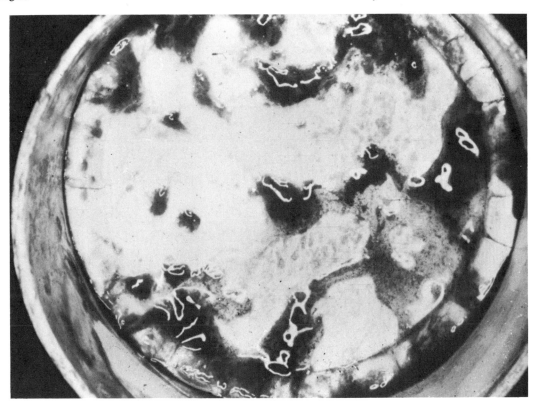

Figure 2. Classic "red currant jelly" stool of *Shigella* dysentery. Even in this black-and-white photograph, the bloody mucoid character of the dysentery stool is readily apparent, as is the scanty volume of the bowel movement. Courtesy of Myron M. Levine.

it may cause a chronic relapsing disease extending over months.[84,85,104,154,156] At the ICDDR, where the majority of patients admitted to the inpatient unit are malnourished (mean weight for age = 59% of the NCHS 50% standard),[25] the fatality rate in 4150 patients over a 5-year period was 9% (Table 8).[14] There was little difference in fatality rate with the four *Shigella* species, suggesting that debilitation of the host affects his/her ability to defend against even the least virulent *Shigella* species. Early deaths in shigellosis are generally due to septicemia, toxic megacolon with or without perforation, or renal failure. Later fatalities are the result of complex interactions of infection and nutritional status.[84,85,154,218] In these circumstances, kwashiorkor or marasmic kwashiorkor usually develops and the terminal event is often another infection.

8.2. Diagnosis

Shigellosis should be suspect when a febrile, bloody, mucoid diarrhea or the dysentery syndrome occurs. The definitive diagnosis of shigellosis depends on isolation of the organism from a stool specimen. However, because early treatment can markedly shorten the duration and intensity of symptoms in more severely ill patients, presumptive diagnosis on the basis of clinical symptoms can be useful. This is easiest for patients in endemic areas, or patients infected during outbreaks, who have the dysenteric form of the illness. In rural Bangladesh, recent prospective community-based studies show that bloody, mucoid diarrhea accounts for two-fifths of diarrhea episodes and two-thirds of fatalities, about half being associated with documented shigellosis. In Dallas, Texas, a correct presumptive diagnosis based on clinical features alone was possible in 34 of 47 (72%)

Shigella-infected patients who came to a general outpatient clinic.[176] However, the prevalence of *Shigella* infection in diarrhea patients attending this clinic was 33%, a rate much higher than in most outpatient settings in the United States.[92] In children with acute diarrhea and fever, the presence of gross blood and mucus in the stool or detection of large numbers of leukocytes by microscopic examination of stool stained with methylene blue is suggestive, but not diagnostic, of *Shigella* infection.[92,103,127,128,186,217] In patients who present with nonbloody watery diarrhea there is often little to differentiate *Shigella* infection from other, more common causes of watery diarrhea. While the presentation of fever, diarrhea, and seizures in children is most characteristic of shigellosis, the seizures occasionally can occur prior to the development of intestinal symptoms, prompting the initial diagnosis of acute meningitis. Examination of the CSF is completely normal in nearly all,[5,6,10] and the real diagnosis becomes apparent when the intestinal manifestations occur and the stool is cultured.

In the developing countries, where the vast majority of *Shigella* infections occur, laboratory facilities for isolation of the organism are often not available, and diagnosis is dependent on clinical evaluation, at times aided by stool microscopy for white blood cells. The major differential diagnosis, *E. histolytica*, is much less common a cause of dysentery in children,[18,154] and does not cause a purulent stool.[213] In practice, all children with clinical dysentery in endemic regions should be presumed to have *Shigella* and treated accordingly. Under optimal conditions, the stool should be examined for motile amoebic trophozoites containing ingested erythrocytes to rule out amoebiasis. In adults, the incidence of amoebic dysentery is higher than in children and a microscopic examination of stool is important to discriminate between the two illnesses.[213]

Table 8. Outcome of Patients Infected with *Shigella* Admitted to the ICDDR, B Inpatient Unit, 1983 through 1987

Species or serotype	Total admissions	Discharged alive	Left against advice	Transferred to other hospital	Died in hospital
S. flexneri	2319	1841 (79)	211 (9)	37 (2)	230 (10)
S. dysenteriae type 1	1251	976 (78)	136 (11)	40 (3)	99 (8)
S. dysenteriae types 2–10	132	112 (85)	5 (4)	2 (2)	13 (10)
S. boydii	303	245 (81)	24 (8)	3 (1)	31 (10)
S. sonnei	145	119 (82)	12 (8)	2 (1)	12 (8)
	4150	3293 (79)	388 (9)	84 (2)	385 (9)

9. Control and Prevention

9.1. General Concepts

Even though the infective inoculum for *Shigella* infection is small and person-to-person contact spread is common, it is surprising how effective simple hygiene measures can be in control and prevention of shigellosis.[105,146,162,215,231] Hand-washing and sanitary disposal of feces constitute the keystones of personal hygiene and will minimize the spread of infection within the household.[126,162] Within the community, the integrity of the water supply and its protection from fecal contamination is important; this is most obvious when breaks in the system permit waterborne disease. This is true whether the community is an institution, a town, or a ship at sea and its passengers and crew. Breast-fed infants are at lesser risk of symptomatic *Shigella* infection than are bottle-fed neonates, and good nutritional state may limit the chronicity of established illness.[39]

While vector spread may contribute to the transmission of shigellosis, it is certainly not necessary. None the less, vector control might be a useful measure, but is difficult to achieve in the developing countries. In Beirut, Lebanon, two families of flies were cultured for enteric bacteria, including Muscidae, which congregate around human feces, and Calliphoridae, which rest chiefly on decaying meat and fruit. Pathogens were recovered in 29 of 156 fly pools studied; 10/29 were shigellae, and these were entirely from Muscidae. This association is probably more useful as an indicator of exposure of the flies to human feces than it is a real risk for transmission. Therefore, fly cultures may be a surrogate measure for sanitary level of the community, analogous to coliform counts in water. A high level of association should suggest the need for attention to sanitary waste disposal.

It is wise for physicians making the diagnosis of acute shigellosis in one family member, usually a young child, to consider the whole family to be at risk.[8,102,221] Depending on the ability of the household to contain fecal spread, the physician may decide to either culture other family members or initiate antimicrobial therapy. Younger contacts of the index case are at greater risk of symptomatic secondary infection than are adults.[102,221]

9.2. Antibiotic and Chemotherapeutic Approaches to Prophylaxis

Bismuth subsalicylate (BSS) tablets have recently been shown to be effective, at least in travelers to Mexico.[58] Two 300-mg BSS tablets four times a day provide 35–40% protection during a 3-week exposure.[59] In a placebo-controlled trial of liquid BSS for prevention of diarrhea in North American students traveling to Mexico,[58] symptomatic *Shigella* infections occurred in 7/68 students receiving placebo, compared to 1/61 students who received BSS prophylaxis. Because of its salicylate content, BSS should not be used in children under 3, in those with aspirin sensitivity or gout, or in patients taking anticoagulants, probenecid, methotrexate, or aspirin-containing preparations. In addition, BSS contains 350 mg $CaCO_3$ per tablet, and could result in milk-alkali syndrome in susceptible subjects. However, the FDA considers the threshold dose to be 8 g/day, which is considerably higher than the amount contained in the recommended dose of BSS. BSS administration is associated with increased frequency of adverse side effects, most notably constipation and nausea. In addition, it should be noted that 60% of BSS is the bismuth component, which is converted to bismulth oxycholoride in the stomach. Excess bismuth salts, consumed over years, can result in encephalopathy, associated with plasma levels greater than 100 parts per billion (ppb). However, only one case due to BSS has been reported over the 80 years of the use of the drug. This patient was a 60-year-old diabetic with chronic diarrhea due to ulcerative colitis resulting in proctocolectomy and ileostomy. Blood bismuth levels measured in a small group of subjects given BSS four times daily never exceeded 34 ppb (mean 15 + 7.9 ppb).

There is little information on the utility of prophylactic antimicrobials for shigellosis. In endemic settings, exposure to infection occurs much too frequently to make prophylaxis a consideration.[23] In outbreak situations, the potential use of antimicrobial agents for prophylaxis is limited by the increasingly common resistance of *Shigella* to the drugs that might be used, and by the fear that prophylactic use of these agents would result in increased prevalence of resistant strains.[108,196,222]

9.3. Immunization

There is no vaccine for shigellosis at this time, but not because of a lack of effort to develop one. In fact, effective prototype vaccines have been prepared for oral use in humans,[53,140,142] but none to date is both effective and safe. The best tested of these is a trivalent live oral vaccine using streptomycin-dependent strains of *S. flexneri* 2a and 3 and *S. sonnei*.[165] This vaccine produces significant, but serotype-specific, protection, the duration of which is unclear. However, on a practical basis, multiple doses in bicarbonate are needed for protection, the incidence of gastrointestinal side effects produced by the vaccine equals the incidence of the disease it is designed to prevent in a moderate endemic area,[165] and reversion to virulence may occur.[141] The vaccine is therefore not acceptable for general use.

Parenteral immunization with killed organisms has never been shown to be protective. Instead, the approach has been to stimulate local intestinal mucosal immune defenses with live oral vaccines. Attenuated live vaccine strains of *S. flexneri* 2a have been prepared by hybridization to incorporate regions of the *E. coli* chromosome,[70] and these strains are protective in experimental studies.[53,70,71,140] Large-scale tests in humans have yet to be done. Another approach employed *E. coli* strains that express *Shigella* antigens on their surfaces.[143] To obtain these strains, the genes for type- and group-specific antigens were transferred from *S. flexneri* 2a to *E. coli*. The preparation is well tolerated and proliferates in the gastrointestinal tract, but does not appear to be protective.

A refinement of this general approach has employed the avirulent *Salmonella typhi* vaccine strain, Ty21a, a gal E mutant, defective in the enzyme UDP-Gal-4-epimerase.[83] This lesion allows the organism to be normally invasive and to make normal somatic antigens but it fails to survive in the host because of the accumulation of galactose-1-phosphate and UDP-galactose. When the 120-MDa plasmid from *S. sonnei* was conjugally transferred to Ty21a, the recipient strains produced both *S. sonnei* and *S. typhi* somatic antigens and mice were protected against intraperitoneal challenge with either organism.[73] The bivalent vaccine strain was shown to be safe and immunogenic in volunteers,[225] but only some vaccine preparations have produced protection from experimental challenge,[20] and the reason for this variability is not clear. A similar approach is being studied for *S. flexneri*, and a recombinant plasmid containing the chromosomal genes for the type and group antigens of *S. flexneri* 2a has been transferred to Ty21a.[9] Mice were shown to be protected against intraperitoneal challenge with the *Shigella*, but not the *Salmonella*, apparently because the synthesis of *Shigella* antigens interfered with the synthesis of *Salmonella* antigens. By combining the hybrid with unmodified Ty21a, immunity to both pathogens was induced in the mouse model.

Another prototype *S. flexneri* vaccine has been constructed by conjugally transferring the 140-MDa invasion plasmid into an *E. coli* K12 that also had the *his* and *pro* regions of the *S. flexneri* 2a chromosome inserted to express the somatic antigen.[75] The strain is safe and protec-

tive in monkeys, and human challenge studies are eagerly awaited. We may expect to see many new vaccine candidates constructed on the basis of new data on virulence factors.

Because of the possible role of Shiga toxin, attempts to develop a safe toxin immunogen have been initiated. Toxin is a complex protein consisting of one biologically active A subunit and five B subunits involved in binding to host cells.[49] Based on the amino acid sequence of the toxin B subunit and an analysis of its hydrophilicity and surface exposure (since hydrophilic and surface sequences can be predicted to be immunogenic),[207] a synthetic peptide vaccine has been prepared and used to immunize rabbits.[100] This induces serum antibodies that neutralize all of the toxin effects in experimental systems. Further work is certainly warranted, especially if immunity is inducible at the mucosal surface itself.

10. Unresolved Problems

10.1. Epidemiology

Because the shigellae are so host-adapted to humans and a few subhuman primates, there is an absolute need for constant passage of the organisms through these hosts. At first glance, it would seem improbable that the organism could survive this restriction when environmental sanitation and protected water supplies limit transmission by the water route. Under these conditions, frequent reintroduction of the organism would be necessary unless continual person-to-person or foodborne transmission were occurring. It is uncertain how, in fact, the organism does maintain itself, and for this reason it is difficult to plan for rational disease prevention or to consider eradication of the organism. In addition, the reasons for the major shifts in prevalence of *Shigella* species in different regions over time are not known.

10.2. Pathogenesis

The possible occurrence of small-intestinal colonization by shigellae, the mechanism of epithelial-cell invasion, and the role of toxin in both diarrhea and dysentery are not clear, although a start has been made in each of these areas. Elucidation of the specific mechanisms involved is essential for the planning of therapeutic and prophylactic measures. For example, vaccine development using attenuated noninvasive mutants or mutant-hybrids may not work well because the attenuation removes a critical virulence factor from the organism to which a protective response could be elicited. However, if this factor were a surface protein[95] or membrane glycolipid of the organism,[183] it might be possible to induce a protective immune response to the isolated material. Similarly, antitoxin immunity, which is ineffective when induced in serum, might prevent activation of the secretory process in *Shigella* diarrhea if present at the mucosal surface.

Manipulation of the host–pathogen and host cell–toxin interactions for therapeutic benefit based on the specific receptor-binding chemistry involved is obviously dependent on clarification of the processes occurring at the surface of the intestinal epithelial cell.[107] For example, neither the presence nor role of the Gb3 glycolipid villus cell receptor for toxin in the human gut has been defined; however, if this glycolipid is present and involved in pathogenesis, then use of Gb3 analogues or antibodies to inhibit toxin binding are possible strategies. Rational pharmacological manipulation of the secretory or inflammatory processes is equally dependent on such knowledge. These take on particular significance when the problems of epidemiology (see Section 10.1) and antimicrobial drug resistance (see Section 10.3) are considered.

10.3. R-Factor Antibiotic Resistance

Transferable multiple antimicrobial drug resistance mediated by plasmid DNA was first discovered in the shigellae.[230] This led to a spectacular rise in the prevalence of highly drug-resistant shigellae in Japan and elsewhere in the world as antibiotic pressures led to selection of the plasmid-bearing organisms. Resistance clearly restricts the antimicrobial therapy of acute shigellosis, which is effective when susceptible organisms are treated with the appropriate agent. Plasmid-mediated resistance is, of course, a problem with organisms other than shigellae and is a major impediment to successful chemotherapy. The principal strategy in dealing with this has been to develop new or modified drugs to which the organism is still sensitive.[117] This merely buys time—the ultimate solution is to learn how to control plasmids. It would be advantageous to clinically cure the plasmids and thus restore susceptibility to the drugs already available for safe use. This could have the added advantage of curing plasmids bearing essential virulence traits, rendering the survivors nonpathogenic. Because the rise in prevalence of resistant strains in a given area is often abrupt, rather than gradual, it has also been suggested that there may be some sort of threshold phenomenon in which a given degree of antibiotic usage for a certain period of time is necessary before widespread transmission of the plasmid occurs.[206] Perhaps this time is

necessary for the resistance transfer factor that modulates plasmid mobility to link up with the resistance genes, or perhaps influences other than antibiotic pressure orchestrate the emergence of drug-resistant strains. In either event, understanding the biology of plasmid movement in nature could lead to ecological measures to reduce their transfer from organism to organism and thus minimize the drug-resistance problem encountered clinically.

10.4. Clinical Complications

The pathogenesis of most of the clinical complications that occur in shigellosis is not well understood. Since certain of these complications, including microangiopathic hemolytic anemia, uremia, hyponatremia, and thrombocytopenia, occur almost exclusively in association with *S. dysenteriae* 1 infection, speculation has centered about the role of high levels of Shiga toxin with this organism. This suspicion is heightened by the recent discovery that HUS frequently occurs during infection by high-level Shiga toxin-producing strains of *E. coli*.[111] However, there are no specific data that provide any insights into the mechanisms of HUS.

Toxic megacolon is another complication associated with significant mortality. It is logical to assume that the extent of the inflammatory changes is the major determinant of toxic dilatation, but little is known in fact. Therapy is principally the use of appropriate antimicrobials and general support with fluids, with surgery reserved for those who do not respond or whose colon becomes perforated. There is no information about other possible options, and clearly oral rehydration is not the answer to these problems.

In the case of Reiter's arthritis, there is a clear genetic predilection for HLA-B27-positive subjects. The mechanisms underlying this particular host response to the infection need to be understood. Therapy, or even better, prevention could then be considered. This is clearly important because of the chronic destructive joint disease initiated by the organisms.

Shigella infection is associated with the most severe nutritional consequences of all the diarrheal diseases. In developing countries, this malnutrition is strongly associated with mortality,[120] and there is growing evidence that the mortality rate in patients discharged from the hospital after shigellosis is far greater than in those discharged after watery diarrhea due to *E. coli* , cholera, or rotavirus. Nutritional effects of the infection may account for this in large part. The relative importance of mucosal inflammation, systemic catabolic responses,[120] and protein-losing enteropathy[190] is uncertain, and there is no clear approach to treatment.

10.5. Vaccines

Because of unresolved questions of pathogenesis and the failure to develop acceptable vaccines, the whole question of prophylaxis is open to investigation. When success does not come easily with conventional approaches, it is time to stop and reason. In the present context, this means more studies to define the host's protective immune response, to define the protection-eliciting antigens of the organisms, and to find a way to present these to the host without toxicity or unacceptable side effects to achieve the protection desired.

11. References

1. ACKERKNECHT, E. H., *History and Geography of the Most Important Diseases*, Hafner, New York, 1965.
2. ANAND, B. S., MALHORTRA, V., BHATTACHARYA, S. K., DATTA, P., DATTA, D., SEN, D., BHATTACHARYA, M. K., MUKHERJEE, P. P., AND PAL, S. C., Rectal histology in acute bacillary dysentery, *Gastroenterology* **90**:654–660 (1986).
3. Anonymous, The prospects for immunizing against *Shigella* spp., in: *New Vaccine Development—Establishing Priorities, Volume II, Diseases of Importance in Developing Countries* (S. L. KATZ, ed.), pp. 329–337, National Academy Press, 1986.
4. Anonymous, Ciprofloxacin, *The Medical Letter* **30**:11–13 (1988).
5. ASKENAZI, S., DINARI, G., ZEVULUNOV, A., AND NITZAN, M., Convulsion in shigellosis: Evaluation of possible risk factors, *Am. J. Dis. Child.* **141**:208–210 (1987).
6. AVITAL, A., MAAYAN, C., AND GOITEIN, K. J., Incidence of convulsion and encephalopathy in childhood Shigella infection, *Clin. Pediatr.* **21**:645–648 (1982).
7. AZAD, M. A. K., ISLAM, M., AND BUTLER, T., Colonic perforation in *Shigella dysenteriae* type 1 infection, *Pediatr. Infect. Dis. J.* **5**:103–104 (1986).
8. BAINE, W. B., HERRON, C. A., BRIDSON, K., BARKER, W. H., JR., LINDELL, S., MALLISON, G. F., WELLS, J. G., MARTIN, W. T., KOSURI, M. R., CARR, F., AND VOELKER, E., SR., Waterborne shigellosis at a public school, *Am. J. Epidemiol.* **101**:323–332 (1975).
9. BARON, L. S., KOPECKO, D. J., FORMAL, S. B., SEID, R., GUERRY, P., AND POWELL, C., Introduction of *Shigella flexneri* 2a type and group antigen genes into oral typhoid vaccine strain *Salmonella typhi* Ty21a, *Infect. Immun.* **55**:2797–2801 (1987).
10. BARRETT-CONNOR, E., AND CONNOR, J. D., Extraintestinal manifestations of shigellosis, *Am. J. Gastroenterol.* **53**:234–245 (1970).
11. BARTLETT, A. V., III, PRADO, D., CLEARY, T. G., AND PICKERING, L. K., Production of Shiga toxin and other cytotoxins by serogroups of *Shigella*, *J. Infect. Dis.* **154**:996–1002 (1986).
12. BARTON, L. L., AND PICKERING, L. K., Shigellosis in the first week of life, *Pediatrics* **51**:437–438 (1973).
13. BASKIN, D. H., LAX, J. D., AND BARENBERG, D., *Shigella bacteremia* in patients with the acquired immune deficiency syndrome, *Am. J. Gastroenterol.* **82**:338–341 (1987).
14. BENNISH, M. L., CLEMENS, J., AND HARRIS, J., Risk factors for death among patients with shigellosis, Interscience Conference on Antimicrobial Agents and Chemotherapy, October 1984, American Society for Microbiology, Washington, D.C., 1984.
15. BENSTED, H. J., Dysentery bacilli-shigella: A brief historical review, *Can. J. Microbiol.* **2**:163–174 (1956).
16. BIEDNER, B., ROSENBLATT, I., DOGAN, R., AND YASSAI, Y., Corneal ulcer caused by *Shigella flexneri* in an infant, *Am. J. Ophthal Mol.* **104**:90 (1987).
17. BLACK, R. E., GRAUN, G. F., AND BLAKE, P. A., Epidemiology of common-source outbreaks of shigellosis in the United States 1961–1975, *Am. J. Epidemiol.* **108**:47–52 (1978).
18. BLACK, R. E., BROWN, K. H., BECKER, S., ALIM, A. R. M. A., AND HUQ, I., Longitudinal studies of infectious diseases and physical growth of children in rural Bangladesh, *Am. J. Epidemiol.* **115**:315–324 (1982).
19. BLACK, R. E., BROWN, K. H., AND BECKER, S., Effects of diarrhea associated with specific enteropathogens on the growth of children in rural Bangladesh, *Pediatrics* **73**:79–85 (1984).
20. BLACK, R. E., LEVINE, M. M., CLEMENTS, M. L., LOSONSKY, G., HERRINGTON, D., BERMAN, S., AND FORMAL, S. B., Prevention of shigellosis by a *Salmonella typhi–Shigella sonnei* bivalent vaccine, *J. Infect. Dis.* **155**:1260–1265 (1987).
21. BLASER, M. J., POLLARD, R. A., AND FELDMAN, R. A., *Shigella* infections in the United States, 1974–1980, *J. Infect. Dis.* **147**:771–775 (1983).
22. BLUM, D., The role of water supplies and sanitation in prevention of acute diarrhoeal diseases, in: *Diarrhoeal Disease and Malnutrition: A Clinical Update* (M. GRACEY, ed.), pp. 207–210, Churchill Livingstone, Edinburgh, 1985.
23. BOYCE, J. M., HUGHES, J. M., ALIM, A. M. R. A., KHAN, M., AZIZ, K. M. A., WELLS, J. G., AND CURLIN, G. T., Patterns of *Shigella* infection in families in Bangladesh, *Am. J. Trop. Med. Hyg.* **31**:1015–1020 (1982).
24. BOYD, J. S. K., The antigenic structure of the mannitol-fermenting group of dysentery bacilli, *J. Hyg.* **38**:477–499 (1938).
25. BRIEND, A., DYKEWICZ, C., GRAVEN, K., MAZUMDER, R. N., WOJTNYIAK, B., AND BENNISH, M., Usefulness of nutri-

tional indices and classifications in predicting death of malnourished children, *Br. Med. J.* **293**:373–375 (1986).

26. BUTLER, T., ISLAM, M. R., AND BARDHAN, P. K., The leukemoid reaction in shigellosis, *Am. J. Dis. Child.* **138**:162–165 (1984).

27. BUTLER, T., SPEELMAN, P., KABIR, I., AND BANWELL, J., Colonic dysfunction during shigellosis, *J. Infect. Dis.* **154**:817–824 (1986).

28. BUYSSE, J., STOVER, C. K., OAKS, E. V., VENKATESAN, M., AND KOPECKO, D. J., Molecular cloning of invasion plasmid antigen (*ipa*) genes from *Shigella flexneri*: Analysis of *ipa* gene products and genetic mapping, *J. Bacteriol.* **169**:2561–2569 (1987).

29. CACERES, A., AND MATA, L. J., Serologic response of patients with Shiga dysentery, *J. Infect. Dis.* **129**:439–443 (1974).

30. CALDERWOOD, S. B., AUCLAIR, F., DONOHUE-ROLFE, A., KEUSCH, G. T., AND MEKALANOS, J. J., Nucleotide sequence of the iron-regulated Shiga-like toxin genes of *Escherichia coli*, *Proc. Natl. Acad. Sci. USA* **84**:4364–4368 (1987).

31. CALDWELL, G. R., DE CARLE, D. J., REISS-LEVY, E., AND HUNT, D. R., *Shigella dysenteriae* type 1 enterocolitis, *Aust. N.Z. J. Med.* **16**:405–407 (1986).

32. CALIN, A., AND FRIES, J. F., An "experimental" epidemic of Reiter's syndrome revisited: Follow-up evaluation on genetic and environmental factors, *Ann. Intern. Med.* **84**:564–566 (1976).

33. CASTRO, F., ROSAL, J. E., AND SANCHEZ, E., Hallazgos anatomopatologicos en 173 casos de disenteria bacilar, Simposio sobre disenteria Shiga en Centroamerica, Organization Panamericana de la Salud, Publicacion Cientifica No. 283, pp. 17–26, 1974.

34. Centers for Disease Control, Multiply resistant shigellosis in a day-care center—Texas, *Morbid. Mortal. Weekly Rep.* **35**:753–55 (1986).

35. Centers for Disease Control, Nationwide dissemination of multiply resistant *Shigella sonnei* following a common-source outbreak, *Morbid. Mortal. Weekly Rep.* **36**:633–634 (1987).

36. Centers for Disease Control, Multistate outbreak of *Shigella sonnei* gastroenteritis—United States, *Morbid Mortal. Weekly Rep.* **36**:440–449 (1987).

37. CHANTEMESSE, A., AND WIDAL, F., Sur les microbes de la dysenteria epidemique, *Bull. Acad. Med. (Paris* **19**:522–529 (1888).

38. CHATKAEOMORAKOT, A., ECHEVERRIA, P., TAYLOR, D. N., SERIWATANA, J., AND LEKSOMBOON, U., Trimethoprim-resistant *Shigella* and enterotoxigenic *Escherichia coli* strains in children in Thailand, *Pediatr. Infect. Dis. J.* **6**:735–739 (1987).

39. CLEMENS, J. D., STANTON, B., STOLL, B., SHAHID, N. S., BANU, H., AND CHOWDHURY, A. K. A. M. A., Breast feeding as a determinant of severity in shigellosis, *Am. J. Epidemiol.* **123**:710–718 (1986).

40. CLERC, P. L., RYTER, A., MOUNIER, J., AND SANSONETTI, P. J., Plasmid-mediated early killing of eucaryotic cells by *Shigella flexneri* as studied by infection of J774 macrophages, *Infect. Immun.* **55**:521–527 (1987).

41. CLERC, P. L., AND SANSONETTI, P. J., Entry of *Shigella flexneri* into HeLa cells: Evidence for directed phagocytosis involving actin polymerization and myosin accumulation, *Infect. Immun.* **55**:2681–2688 (1987).

42. COLIN, A., AND FRIES, J. F., An "experimental" epidemic of Reiter's syndrome revisited: Follow-up evaluation of genetic and environmental factors, *Ann. Intern. Med.* **84**:564–566 (1976).

43. CONRADI, H., Uber losliche durch aseptische autolyse erhalten giftstoffe von ruhr and Typhusbazillen, *Dtsch. Med. Wochenschr.* **29**:26–28 (1903).

44. COUNCILMAN, W. T., AND LAFLEUR, H. A., Amoebic dysentery, *Johns Hopkins Hosp. Rep.* **2**:393–548 (1891).

45. DALE, D. C., AND MATA, L. J., Studies of diarrheal disease in Central America. XI. Intestinal bacterial flora in malnourished children with shigellosis, *Am. J. Trop. Med.* **17**:397–403 (1968).

46. DEWAILLY, E., POIRIER, C., AND MEYER, F. M., Health hazards associated with wind surfing on polluted water, *Am. J. Public Health* **76**:690–691 (1986).

47. DONADIO, J., AND GANGAROSA, E., Foodborne shigellosis, *J. Infect. Dis.* **119**:666–668 (1969).

48. DONOHUE-ROLFE, A., AND KEUSCH, G. T., *Shigella dysenteriae* 1 cytotoxin: Periplasmic protein releasable by polymyxin B and osmotic shock, *Infect. Immun.* **39**:270–274 (1983).

49. DONOHUE-ROLFE, A., KEUSCH, G. T., EDSON, C., THORLEY-LAWSON, D., AND JACEWICZ, M., Pathogenesis of Shigella diarrhea. IX. Simplified high yield purification of Shigella toxin and characterization of subunit composition and function by the use of subunit specific monoclonal and polyclonal antibodies, *J. Exp. Med.* **160**:1767–1781 (1984).

50. DONOHUE-ROLFE, A., KELLEY, M. A., BENNISH, M., AND KEUSCH, G. T., Enzyme-linked immunosorbent assay for Shigella toxin, *J. Clin. Microbiol.* **24**:65–68 (1986).

51. DRACHMAN, R. H., PAYNE, F. J., JENKINS, A. A., MACKEL, D. C., PETERSEN, N. J., BORING, J. R., GAREAU, F. E., FRASER, R. S., AND MYERS, G. G., An outbreak of water borne shigella gastroenteritis, *Am. J. Hyg.* **72**:321–324 (1960).

52. DRITZ, S. K., AINSWORTH, T. E., GARRARD, W. F., BACK, A., PALMER, R. D., BOUCHER, L. A., AND RIVER, E., Patterns of sexually transmitted enteric diseases in a city, *Lancet* **2**:3–4 (1977).

53. DUPONT, H. L., Enteropathogenic organisms: New etiologic organisms and concepts of disease, *Med. Clin. North Am.* **62**:945–960 (1978).

54. DUPONT, H. L., HORNICK, R. H., DAWKINS, A. T., SNYDER, M. J., AND FORMAL, S. B., The response of man to virulent *Shigella flexneri* 2a, *J. Infect. Dis.* **119**:296–299 (1969).

55. DuPont, H. L., Gangarosa, E. J., Reller, L. B., Wood-ward, W. E., Armstrong, R. W., Hammond, J., Glaser, K., and Morris, G. K., Shigellosis in custodial institutions, *Am. J. Epidemiol.* **92:**172–179 (1970).

56. DuPont, H. L., Hornick, R. B., Snyder, M. J., Li-bonati, J. P., Formal, S. B., and Gangarosa, E. J., Immunity in shigellosis. I. Response of man to attenuated shigella strains, *J. Infect. Dis.* **125:**5–11 (1972).

57. DuPont, H. L., Hornick, R. B., Snyder, M. J., Libonati, J. P., Formal, S. B., and Gangarosa, E. J., Immunity in shigellosis. II. Protection induced by oral live vaccine or primary infection, *J. Infect. Dis.* **125:**12–16 (1972).

58. DuPont, H. L., Sullivan, P., Evans, D. G., Pickering, L. K., Evans, D. J., Vollet, J. J., Ericsson, C. D., Ackerman, P. B., and Tjoa, W. S., Prevention of traveler's diarrhea (*Emporiatric enteritis*): Prophylactic administration of subsalicylate bismuth, *J. Am. Med. Assoc.* **243:**237–241 (1980).

59. DuPont, H. L., Ericsson, C. D., Johnson, P. C., Bit-sura, J. A., DuPont, M. M., and de la Calada, F. S., Prevention of travelers' diarrhea by the tablet formulation of bismuth subsalicylate, *J. Am. Med. Assoc.* **257:**1347–1350 (1987).

60. Ekwall, E., Haeggman, S., Kalin, M., Svenungsson, B., and Lindberg, A. A., Antibody response to *Shigella sonnei* infection determined by an enzyme-linked immu-nosorbent assay, *Eur. J. Clin. Microbiol.* **2:**200–205 (1983).

61. Endo, Y., Tsurugi, K., Yutsudo, T., Takeda, Y., Ogasawara, T., and Igarashi, K., Site of action of a Vero toxin (VT2) from *Escherichia coli* O157:H7 and of Shiga toxin on eukaryotic ribosomes. RNA N-glycosidase activity of the toxins, *Eur. J. Biochem.* **171:**45–50 (1988).

62. Evins, G. M., Gheesling, L. L., and Tauxe, R. V., Quali-ty of commercially produced *Shigella* serogrouping and serotyping antisera, *J. Clin. Microbiol.* **26:**438–442 (1988).

63. Eyre, J. W. H., Asylum dysentery in relation to *S. dysen-teriae*, *Br. Med. J.* **1:**1002–1004 (1904).

64. Farrar, W. E., and Ridson, M., Antibiotic resistance in *Shigella* mediated by R factors, *J. Infect. Dis.* **123:**477–484 (1971).

65. Feldman, R. A., Bhat, P., and Kamath, K. R., Infection and disease in a group of South Indian families. IV. Bac-teriologic methods and a report of the frequency of enteric bacterial infection in preschool children, *Am. J. Epidemiol.* **92:**367–375 (1970).

66. Floyd, T. M., The incidence of *Shigella* organisms in a group of Egyptian village children, *Am. J. Trop. Med. Hyg.* **3:**294–302 (1954).

67. Floyd, T. M., Higgins, A. R., and Kadar, M. A., Studies in shigellosis. V. The relationship of age to the incidence of shigella infections in Egyptian children, with special refer-ence to shigellosis in the newborn and in infants in the first six months of life, *Am. J. Trop. Med.* **5:**119–130 (1956).

68. Formal, S. B., Abrams, G. D., Schneider, H., and Sprinz, H., Experimental *Shigella* infections. VI. Role of

69. Formal, S. B., LaBrec, E. H., Kent, T. H., and Falkow, S., Abortive intestinal infection with an *Escherichia coli–Shigella flexneri* hybrid strain, *J. Bacteriol.* **89:**1374–1382 (1965).

70. Formal, S. B., Kent, T. H., May, H. C., Palmer, A., Falkow, S., and LaBrec, E. H., Protection of monkeys against experimental shigellosis with a living attenuated oral polyvalent dysentery vaccine, *J. Bacteriol.* **92:**17–22 (1966).

71. Formal, S. B., Kent, T. H., Austin, S., and LaBrec, E. H., Fluorescent-antibody and histological study of vaccinated and control monkeys challenged with *Shigella flexneri*, *J. Bacteriol.* **91:**2368–2376 (1966).

72. Formal, S. B., Gemski, P., Baron, L. S., and LaBrec, E. H., A chromosomal locus which controls the ability of *Shigella flexneri* to evoke keratoconjunctivitis, *Infect. Im-mun.* **3:**73–79 (1971).

73. Formal, S. B., Baron, L. S., Kopecko, D. J., Wash-ington, O., Powell, C., Life, C. A., Construction of a potential bivalent vaccine strain: Introduction of *Shigella son-nei* form I antigen genes into the galE-*Salmonella typhi* Ty21a typhoid vaccine strain, *Infect. Immun.* **34:**746–750 (1981).

74. Formal, S. B., Hale, T. L., and Sansonetti, P. J., Inva-sive enteric pathogens, *Rev. Infect. Dis.* **5:**S702–S707 (1983).

75. Formal, S. B., Hale, T. L., Kapfer, C., Cogan, J. P., Snoy, P. J., Chung, R., Wingfield, M. E., Elisberg, B. L., and Baron, L. S., Oral vaccination of monkeys with an invasive *Escherichia coli* K-12 hybrid expressing *Shigella flexneri* 2a somatic antigen, *Infect. Immun.* **46:**465–469 (1984).

76. Frost, J. A., Willshaw, G. A., Barclay, E. A., Rowe, B., Lemmens, P., and Vandepitte, J., Plasmid charac-terization of drug-resistant *Shigella dysenteriae* 1 from an epidemic in central Africa, *J. Hyg.* **94:**163–172 (1985).

77. Fuchs, G., Mobasaleh, M., Donohue-Rolfe, A., Montgomery, R. K., Grand, R. J., and Keusch, G. T., Pathogenesis of shigella diarrhea. XII. Rabbit intestinal cell microvillus membrane binding site for shigella toxin, *Infect. Immun.* **53:**372–377 (1986).

78. Gangarosa, E. J., Perera, D. R., Mata, L. J., Men-dizabal-Morris, C., Guzman, G., and Reller, L. B., Epi-demic Shiga bacillus dysentery in Central America. II. Epide-miologic studies in 1969, *J. Infect. Dis.* **122:**181–190 (1970).

79. Gangarosa, E. J., Bennett, J. V., Wyatt, C., Pierce, P. E., Olarte, J., Hernandes, P., Vasquez, V., and Bes-sudo, D., An epidemic associated episome? *J. Infect. Dis.* **126:**215–218 (1972).

80. Gear, H. S., Hygiene aspects of the El Alamein victory, 1942, *Br. Med. J.* **1:**383–387 (1944).

81. Gemski, P., Jr., and Formal, S. B., Shigellosis: An invas-ive infection of the gastrointestinal tract, in: *Microbiology 1975* (D. Schlessinger, ed.), pp. 165–169, American Soci-ety for Microbiology, Washington, D.C., 1975.

82. GEMSKI, P., SHEAHAN, D. G., WASHINGTON, O., AND FORMAL, S. B., Virulence of *Shigella flexneri* hybrids expressing *Escherichia coli* somatic antigens, *Infect. Immun.* **6**:104–111 (1972).

83. GERMANIER, R., AND FURER, E., Isolation and characterization of *galE* mutant Ty21A of *Salmonella typhi*: A candidate strain for a live, oral typhoid vaccine, *J. Infect. Dis.* **131**:553–558 (1975).

84. GORDON, J. E., Acute diarrheal disease, *Am. J. Med. Sci.* **248**:345–365 (1964).

85. GORDON, J. E., GUZMAN, M., ASCOLI, W., AND SCRIMSHAW, N. S., Acute diarrheal disease in less developed countries. 2. Patterns of epidemiological behavior in rural Guatemalan villages, *Bull. WHO* **31**:9–20 (1964).

86. GORDON, J. E., ASCOLI, W., PIERCE, V., GUZMAN, M., AND MATA, L. J., Studies of diarrheal disease in Central America. VI. An epidemic of diarrhea in a Guatemalan highland village, with a component due to *Shigella dysenteriae* type 1, *Am. J. Trop. Med. Hyg.* **14**:404–411 (1965).

87. GRADY, G. F., AND KEUSCH, G. T., Pathogenesis of bacterial diarrheas, *N. Engl. J. Med.* **285**:831–841, 891–900 (1971).

88. GREEN, M. S., COHEN, D., BLOCK, C., ROUACH, Z., AND DYCIAN, R., A prospective epidemiologic study of shigellosis in the Israel Defense Forces: Implications for the use of *Shigella* vaccines, *Isr. J. Med. Sci.* **23**:811–815 (1987).

89. GRIFFITHS, E., STEVENSON, P., HALE, T. L., AND FORMAL, S. B., Synthesis of aerobactin and a 76,000-dalton iron-regulated outer membrane protein by *Escherichia coli* K-12–*Shigella flexneri* hybrids and by enteroinvasive strains of *Escherichia coli, Infect. Immun.* **49**:67–71 (1985).

90. GROSS, R. J., THOMAS, L. V., AND ROWE, B., *Shigella dysenteriae*, *S. flexneri* and *S. boydii* infections in England and Wales: The importance of foreign travel, *Br. Med. J.* **2**:744 (1979).

91. GROSS, R. J., ROWE, B., CHEASTY, T., AND THOMAS, L. V., Increase in drug resistance among *Shigella dysenteriae*, *S. flexneri*, and *S. boydii*, *Br. Med. J.* **283**:575–576 (1981).

92. GUERRANT, R. L., SHIELDS, D. S., THORSON, S. M., SCHORLING, J. B., AND GROSCHEL, D. H. M., Evaluation and diagnosis of acute infectious diarrhea, *Am. J. Med.* **78**(Suppl. 6B):91–98 (1985).

93. HALE, L. H., AND FORMAL, S. B., Protein synthesis in HeLa or Henle 407 cells infected with *Shigella dysenteriae* 1, *Shigella flexneri* 2a, or *Salmonella typhimurium* W118, *Infect. Immun.* **32**:137–144 (1981).

94. HALE, L. H., AND FORMAL, S. B., Genetics of virulence in *Shigella, Microbial. Pathogenesis* **1**:511–518 (1986).

95. HALE, L. H., AND FORMAL, S. B., Pathogenesis of Shigella infections, *Pathol. Immunopathol. Res.* **6**:117–127 (1987).

96. HALE, L. H., OAKS, E. V., AND FORMAL, S. B., Identification and antigenic characterization of virulence-associated, plasmid-coded proteins of *Shigella* spp. and enteroinvasive *Escherichia coli, Infect. Immun.* **50**:620–629 (1985).

97. HALTALIN, K. C., Neonatal shigellosis: Report of 16 cases and a review of the literature, *Am. J. Dis. Child.* **114**:603–611 (1967).

98. HALTALIN, K. C., NELSON, J. D., RING, R., SLADJOE, M., AND HINTON, L. V., Double-blind treatment study of shigellosis comparing ampicillin, sulfadiazine, and placebo, *J. Pediatr.* **70**:970–981 (1967).

99. HALTALIN, K. C., NELSON, J. D., HINTON, L. V., KUSMIESZ, H. T., AND SLADOJE, M., Comparison of orally absorbable and nonabsorbable antibiotics in shigellosis. A double blind study with ampicillin and neomycin, *J. Pediatr.* **72**:708–720 (1968).

100. HARARI, I., DONOHUE-ROLFE, A., KEUSCH, G., AND ARNON, R., Synthetic peptides of Shiga toxin B-subunit induce antibodies which neutralize the biological activities of the toxin, *Infect. Immun.* **56**:1618–1624 (1988).

101. HARDY, A. V., AND WATT, J., Studies of the acute diarrheal diseases. XIV. Clinical observations, *Public Health Rep.* **60**:521–532 (1945).

102. HARDY, A. V., AND WATT, J., Studies of the acute diarrheal diseases. XVIII. Epidemiology, *Public Health Rep.* **63**:363–378 (1948).

103. HARRIS, J. C., DUPONT, H. L., AND HORNICK, R. B., Fecal leukocytes in diarrheal illness, *Ann. Intern. Med.* **76**:697–703 (1972).

104. HIGGINS, A. R., FLOYD, T. M., AND KADER, M. A., Studies in shigellosis. II. Observations on incidence and etiology of diarrheal disease in Egyptian village children, *Am. J. Trop. Med. Hyg.* **4**:271–278 (1955).

105. HOLLISTER, A. C., BECK, M. D., GITTELSOHN, A. M., AND HEMPHILL, E. C., Influence of water availability on shigella prevalence in children of farm labor families, *Am. J. Public Health* **45**:354–362 (1955).

106. JACEWICZ, M., AND KEUSCH, G. T., Pathogenesis of shigella diarrhea. VIII. Evidence for a translocation step in the cytotoxic action of Shiga toxin, *J. Infect. Dis.* **148**:844–854 (1983).

107. JACEWICZ, M., CLAUSEN, H., NUDELMAN, E., DONOHUE-ROLFE, A., AND KEUSCH, G. T., Pathogenesis of shigella diarrhea. XI. Isolation of a shigella toxin binding glycolipid from rabbit jejunum and HeLa cells and its identification as globotriaosylceramide, *J. Exp. Med.* **163**:1391–1404 (1986).

108. JOHNSON, P. C., ERICSSON, C. D., MORGAN, D. R., DUPONT, H. L., AND CABADA, F. J., Lack of emergence of resistant fecal flora during successful prophylaxis of traveler's diarrhea with norfloxacin, *Antimicrob. Agents Chemother.* **30**:671–674 (1986).

109. KABIR, I., BUTLER, T., AND KHANAM, A., Comparative efficacies of single intravenous dose of ceftriaxone and ampicillin for shigellosis in a placebo-controlled trial, *Antimicrob. Agents Chemother.* **29**:645–648 (1986).

110. KANDEL, G., DONOHUE-ROLFE, A., DONOWITZ, M., AND KEUSCH, G. T., Pathogenesis of *Shigella* diarrhea. XV. Selective targeting of shiga-toxin to villus cells explains the

effect of the toxin on intestinal electrolyte transport. *J. Clin. Invest.* **84:**1509–1517 (1989).

111. KARMALI, M. A., PETRIC, M., LIM, C., FLEMING, P. C., ARBUS, G. S., AND LIOR, H., The association between idiopathic hemolytic uremic syndrome and infection by verotoxin-producing *Escherichia coli, J. Infect. Dis.* **151:**775–782 (1985).

112. KASLOW, R. A., RYDER, R. W., AND CALIN, A., Search for Reiter's syndrome after an outbreak of *Shigella sonnei* dysentery, *J. Rheumatol.* **6:**562–566 (1979).

113. KEENAN, K. P., SHARPNACK, D. D., COLLINS, H., FORMAL, S. B., AND O'BRIEN, A. D., Morphologic evaluation of the effects of Shiga toxin and *E. coli* Shiga-like toxin on the rabbit intestine, *Am. J. Pathol.* **125:**69–80 (1986).

114. KENNE, L., AND LINDBERG, B., Bacterial polysaccharides, in: *The Polysaccharides* (G. O. Aspinall, ed.), pp. 287–363, Academic Press, New York, 1983.

115. KEUSCH, G. T., Shigella infections, *Clin. Gastroenterol.* **8:**645–662 (1979).

116. KEUSCH, G. T., Shigellosis, in: *Bacterial Infections of Humans* (A. S. EVANS AND H. A. FELDMAN, eds.), pp. 487–509, Plenum Medical, New York, 1982.

117. KEUSCH, G. T., Antimicrobial therapy for enteric infections and typhoid fever: State-of-the art, *Rev. Infect. Dis.* **10**(Suppl.):S199–S205 (1988).

118. KEUSCH, G. T., AND JACEWICZ, M., Serum enterotoxin-neutralizing antibody in human shigellosis, *Nature New Biol.* **241:**31–32 (1973).

119. KEUSCH, G. T., AND JACEWICZ, M., Pathogenesis of shigella diarrhea. VI. Toxin and antitoxin in *S. flexneri* and *S. sonnei* infections in humans, *J. Infect. Dis.* **135:**552–556 (1977).

120. KEUSCH, G. T., AND SCRIMSHAW, N. S., Selective primary health care. Strategies for control of disease in the developing world. XIV. The control of infection to reduce the prevalence of infantile and childhood malnutrition, *Rev. Infect. Dis.* **8:**273–287 (1986).

121. KEUSCH, G. T., GRADY, G. F., MATA, L. J., AND MCIVER, J. M., The pathogenesis of Shigella diarrhea. 1. Enterotoxin production by *Shigella dysenteriae* I, *J. Clin. Invest.* **51:**1212–1218 (1972).

122. KEUSCH, G. T., GRADY, G. F., TAKEUCHI, A., AND SPRINZ, H., The pathogenesis of Shigella diarrhea. II. Enterotoxin induced acute enteritis in rabbit ileum, *J. Infect. Dis.* **126:**92–95 (1972).

123. KEUSCH, G. T., JACEWICZ, M., LEVINE, M. M., HORNICK, R. B., AND KOCHWA, S., Pathogenesis of shigella diarrhea: Serum anticytotoxin antibody response produced by toxigenic and nontoxigenic *Shigella dysenteriae* 1, *J. Clin. Invest.* **57:**194–202 (1976).

124. KEUSCH, G. T., DONOHUE-ROLFE, A., AND JACEWICZ, M., Shigella toxin(s): A review, *Pharmacol. Thera.* **15:**403–438 (1982).

125. KEUSCH, G. T., DONOHUE-ROLFE, A., AND JACEWICZ, M., Shigella toxin and the pathogenesis of shigellosis, *Ciba Found. Symp.* **112:**193–214.

126. KHAN, W. W., Interruption of shigellosis by handwashing, *Trans. R. Soc. Trop. Med. Hyg.* **66:**164–168 (1982).

127. KNOWLESSAR, M., AND FORBES, G. B., The febrile convulsion in shigellosis, *N. Engl. J. Med.* **258:**520–526 (1958).

128. KORZENIOWSKI, D. M., BARADA, F. A., ROUSE, J. D., AND GUERRANT, R. L., Value of examination for fecal leukocytes in the early diagnosis of shigellosis, *Am. J. Trop. Med. Hyg.* **28:**1031–1035 (1979).

129. KOSTER, F., LEVIN, J., WALKER, L., TUNK, K. S. K., GILMAN, R. H., RAHAMAN, M. M., MAJID, M. A., ISLAM, S., AND WILLIAMS, R. C., Hemolytic–uremic syndrome after shigellosis: Relation to endotoxin and circulating immune complexes, *N. Engl. J. Med.* **298:**927–933 (1978).

130. KOSTREWSKI, J., AND STYPULKOWSKA-MISIUREWICZ, H., Changes in the epidemiology of dysentery in Poland and the situation in Europe, *Arch. Immunol. Ther. Exp.* **16:**429–451 (1968).

131. KOURANY, M., VASQUEZ, M. A., AND MATA, L. J., Prevalence of pathogenic enteric bacteria in children of 31 Panamanian communities, *Am. J. Trop. Med. Hyg.* **20:**608–615 (1971).

132. KRUSE, W., Weitere Untersuchungen uber die Ruhr und Ruhrbazillen, *Dtsch. Med. Wochenschr.* **27:**370–372 (1901).

133. LABREC, E. H., SCHNEIDER, H., MAGNANI, T. J., AND FORMAL, S. B., Epithelial cell penetration is an essential step in the pathogenesis of bacillary dysentery, *J. Bacteriol.* **88:**1503–1518 (1964).

134. LAHAT, E., ALADJEM, M., HEIPERT, J., AND MUNDEL, G., Shigellosis: Incidence of convulsions and resistance to antibiotics, *Helv. Paediatr. Acta* **39:**123–128 (1984).

135. LEIGHTON, P. M., An outbreak of shigellosis in the province of New Brunswick, *Can. J. Public Health* **68:**249–252 (1977).

136. LEVINE, M. M., Shigella and Salmonella diarrhoeal disease, *Trop. Doctor* **9:**4–9 (1979).

137. LEVINE, M. M., Antimicrobial therapy for infectious diarrhea, *Rev. Infect. Dis.* **8**(Suppl. 2):S207–S216 (1986).

138. LEVINE, M. M., DUPONT, H. L., GANGAROSA, E. J., HORNICK, R. B., SNYDER, M. J., LIBONATI, J. P., GLASER, K., AND FORMAL, S. B., Shigellosis in custodial institutions. II. Clinical, immunologic and bacteriologic response of institutionalized children to oral attenuated shigella vaccines, *Am. J. Epidemiol.* **96:**40–49 (1972).

139. LEVINE, M. M., DUPONT, H. L., FORMAL, S. B., HORNICK, R. B., TAKEUCHI, A., GANGAROSA, E. J., SNYDER, M. J., AND LIBONATI, J. P., Pathogenesis of *Shigella dysenteriae* (Shiga) dysentery, *J. Infect. Dis.* **127:**261–270 (1973).

140. LEVINE, M. M., GANGAROSA, E. J., WERNER, M., AND MORRIS, G. K., Shigellosis in custodial institutions. 3. Prospective clinical and bacteriologic surveillance of children vaccinated with oral attenuated shigella vaccines, *J. Pediatr.* **84:**803–806 (1974).

141. LEVINE, M. M., GANGAROSA, E. J., BARROW, W. B., MORRIS, G. K., WELLS, J. G., AND WEISS, C. G., Shigellosis in

custodial institutions. IV. *In vivo* stability and transmissibility of oral attenuated streptomycin-dependent shigella vaccines, *J. Infect. Dis.* **131:**704–707 (1975).

142. LEVINE, M. M., GANGAROSA, E. J., BARROW, W. B., AND WEISS, C. F., Shigellosis in custodial institutions. V. Effect of intervention with streptomycin-dependent *Shigella sonnei* vaccine in an institution with endemic disease, *Am. J. Epidemiol.* **104:**88–92 (1976).

143. LEVINE, M. M., WOODWARD, W. E., FORMAL, S. B., GEMSKI, P., JR., DUPONT, H. L., HORNICK, R. B., AND SNYDER, M. J., Studies with a new generation of oral attenuated shigella vaccine: *Escherichia coli* bearing surface antigens of *Shigella flexneri*, *J. Infect. Dis.* **136:**577–582 (1977).

144. LINDBERG, A. A., AND HOLME, T., Evaluation of some extraction methods for the preparation of bacterial lipopolysaccharides for structural analysis, *Acta Pathol. Microbiol. Scand. Sect. B* **80:**751–759 (1972).

145. LINDBERG, A. A., HAEGGMAN, S., KARLSSON, K., CAM, P. D., AND TRACH, D. D., The humoral antibody response to *Shigella dysenteriae* type 1 infection, as determined by ELISA, *Bull. WHO* **62:**597–606 (1984).

146. LINDBERG, A. A., BROWN, J. E., STROMBERG, N., WESTLING-RYD, M., SCHULTZ, J. E., AND KARLSSON, K.-A., Identification of the carbohydrate receptor for Shiga toxin produced by *Shigella dysenteriae* type 1, *J. Biol. Chem.* **262:**1779–1785 (1987).

147. LINDSAY, D. R., STEWART, W. H., AND WATT, J., Effect of fly control on diarrheal disease in an area of moderate morbidity, *Public Health Rep.* **68:**361–367 (1953).

148. LOSCH, F., Massenhafte entwickelung von aeroben in dickdarm, *Arch. Pathol. Anat. Physiol.* **65:**196–211 (1875).

149. MACOMBER, H. H., Acute bacillary dysentery: Clinicopathologic study of 263 consecutive cases, *Arch. Intern. Med.* **69:**624–635 (1942).

150. MAKINO, S., SASAKAWA, C., KAMATA, K., KURATA, T., AND YOSKIKAWA, M., A genetic determinant required for continuous reinfection of adjacent cells on a large plasmid in S. flexneri 2a, *Cell* **46:**551–555 (1986).

151. MAKINTUBEE, S., MALLONEE, J., AND ISTRE, G. R., Shigellosis outbreak associated with swimming, *Am. J. Public Health* **77:**166–168 (1987).

152. MALENGREAU, M., MOLIMA-KOBA, GILLIEAUX, M., DE-FEYTER, M., KYELE-DUIBONE, MUKOLO-NDJOLO, Outbreak of *Shigella* dysentery in eastern Zaire, 1980–1982, *Ann. Soc. Belge Med. Trop.* **63:**59–67 (1983).

153. MARTIN, D. L., GUSTAFSON, T. L., PELOSI, J. W., SUAREZ, L., AND PIERCE, G. V., Contaminated produce—A common source for two outbreaks of *Shigella* gastroenteritis, *Am. J. Public Health* **76:**299–305 (1986).

154. MATA, L. J., *The Children of Santa Maria Cauque: A Prospective Field Study of Health and Growth*, MIT Press, Cambridge, Mass., 1978.

155. MATA, L. J., AND CASTRO, F., Epidemiology, diagnosis and impact of Shiga dysentery in Central America, *Ind. Trop. Health* **8:**30–37 (1974).

156. MATA, L. J., CATALAN, M. A., AND GORDON, J. E., Studies of diarrheal disease in Central America. IX. Shigella carriers among young children of a heavily seeded Guatemalan convalescent home, *Am. J. Trop. Med. Hyg.* **15:**632–638 (1966).

157. MATA, L. J., URRUTIA, J. J., GARCIA, B., FERNANDEZ, R., AND BEHAR, M., *Shigella* infection in breast-fed Guatemalan Indian neonates, *Am. J. Dis. Child.* **117:**142–146 (1969).

158. MATA, L. J., GANGAROSA, E. J., CACERES, A., PERERA, D. R., AND MEJICANOS, M. L., Epidemic Shiga bacillus dysentery in Central America. I. Etiologic investigations in Guatemala, 1969, *J. Infect. Dis.* **122:**170–180 (1970).

159. MATHAN, M. M., AND MATHAN, V. I., Ultrastructural pathology of the rectal mucosa in *Shigella* dysentery, *Am. J. Pathol.* **123:**25–38 (1986).

160. MAURELLI, A. T., AND SANSONETTI, P. J., Identification of a chromosomal gene controlling temperature-regulated expression of *Shigella* virulence, *Proc. Natl. Acad. Sci. USA* **85:**2820–2824 (1988).

161. MAURELLI, A. T., BAUDRY, B., D'HAUTEVILLE, H., HALE, T. L., AND SANSONETTI, P. J., Cloning of plasmid DNA sequences involved in invasion of HeLa cells by *Shigella flexneri*, *Infect. Immun.* **49:**164–171 (1985).

162. MCCABE, C. J., AND HAINES, T. W., Diarrheal disease control by improved human excreta disposal, *Public Health Rep.* **72:**921–928 (1957).

163. MCCARTNEY, J. E., AND OLITSKY, P. K., Separation of the toxins of *Bacillus dysenteriae* Shiga, *J. Exp. Med.* **37:**767–779 (1923).

164. MCIVER, J., GRADY, G. F., AND FORMAL, S. B., Immunization with *Shigella dysenteriae* type 1: Evaluation of antitoxic immunity in prevention of experimental disease in rhesus monkeys (*Macaca mulatta*), *J. Infect. Dis.* **136:**416–421 (1977).

165. MEL, D. M., ARSIC, B. L., NIKOLIC, B. D., AND RADOVANOVIC, M. L., Studies on vaccination against bacillary dysentery. 4. Oral immunization with live monotypic and combined vaccines, *Bull. WHO* **39:**375–380 (1968).

166. MERSON, M. H., GOLDMANN, D. A., BOYER, K. M., PETERSEN, N. J., PATTON, C., EVERETT, L. G., DOWNS, H., STECKLER, A., AND BARKER, W. H., An outbreak of *Shigella sonnei* gastroenteritis on Colorado River raft trips, *Am. J. Epidemiol.* **100:**186–196 (1974).

167. MERSON, M. H., TENNEY, J. H., MEYERS, J. D., WOOD, B. T., WELLS, J. G., RIMZO, W., CLINE, B., DEWITT, W. E., SKALIY, P., AND MALLISON, G. F., Shigellosis at sea: An outbreak aboard a passenger cruise ship, *Am. J. Epidemiol.* **101:**165–175 (1975).

168. MILDVAN, D., GELB, A. M., AND WILLIAM, D., Venereal transmission of enteric pathogens in male homosexuals: Two case reports, *J. Am. Med. Assoc.* **238:**1387–1389 (1977).

169. MOBASSALEH, M., DONOHUE-ROLFE, A., JACEWICZ, M., GRAND, R. J., AND KEUSCH, G. T., Pathogenesis of shigella diarrhea. XIII. Evidence for a developmentally regulated glycolipid receptor for shigella toxin involved in the fluid

secretory response of rabbit small intestine, *J. Infect. Dis.* **157:**1023–1031 (1988).

170. MORDUCHOWICZ, G., HUMINER, D., SIEGMAN-IGRA, Y., DRUCKER, M., BLOCK, C. S., AND PITLIK, S. D., Shigella bacteremia in adults. A report of five cases and review of the literature, *Arch. Intern. Med.* **147:**2034–2037 (1987).

171. MORRIS, G. K., KOEHLER, J. A., GANGAROSA, E. J., AND SHARRAR, R. G., Comparison of media for direct isolation and transport of shigellae from fecal specimens, *Appl. Microbiol.* **19:**434–437 (1970).

172. MOYER, M. P., DIXON, P. S., ROTHMAN, S. W., AND BROWN, J. E., Cytotoxicity of Shiga toxin for primary cultures of human colonic and ileal epithelial cells, *Infect. Immun.* **55:**1533–1535 (1987).

173. MULDER, J. B., Shigellosis in nonhuman primates: A review, *Lab. Anim. Sci.* **21:**734–738 (1971).

174. MUNSHI, M. H., SACK, D. A., HAIDER, K., AHMED, Z. U., RAHAMAN, M. M., AND MORSHED, M. G., Plasmid mediated resistance to nalidixic acid in *Shigella dysenteriae* type 1, *Lancet* **2:**419–421 (1987).

175. NASSIF, X., MAZERT, M.-C., MOUNIER, J., AND SANSONETTI, P., Evaluation with an iuc::Tn10 mutant of the role of aerobactin production in the virulence of *Shigella flexneri,* *Infect. Immun.* **55:**1963–1969 (1987).

176. NELSON, J. D., AND HALTALIN, K. C., Accuracy of diagnosis of bacterial diarrheal disease by clinical features, *J. Pediatr.* **78:**519–522 (1971).

177. NEU, H. C., Bacterial resistance to fluoroquinolones, *Rev. Infect. Dis.* **10**(Suppl. 1):S57–S63 (1988).

178. NOER, H. R., An "experimental" epidemic of Reiter syndrome, *J. Am. Med. Assoc.* **198:**693–698 (1966).

179. OAKS, E. V., HALE, T. L., AND FORMAL, S. B., Serum immune response to Shigella protein antigens in rhesus monkeys and humans infected with *Shigella* spp., *Infect. Immun.* **53:**57–63 (1986).

180. O'BRIEN, A. D., AND HOLMES, R. K., Shiga and Shiga-like toxins, *Microbiol. Rev.* **51:**206–220 (1987).

181. O'BRIEN, A. D., THOMPSON, M. R., GEMSKI, P., DOCTOR, B. P., AND FORMAL, S. B., Biological properties of *Shigella flexneri* 2a toxin and its serological relationship to *Shigella dysenteriae* 1 toxin, *Infect. Immun.* **15:**796–798 (1977).

182. OLITSKY, P. K., AND KLIGLER, I. H., Toxins and anti-toxins of *Bacillus dysenteriae* Shiga, *J. Exp. Med.* **31:**19–33 (1920).

183. OSADA, Y., AND OGAWA, H., A possible role of glycolipids in epithelial cell penetration by virulent *Shigella flexneri* 2a, *Microbial Immunol.* **21:**405–410 (1977).

184. PALCHAUDHURI, S., KUMAR, R., SEN, D., PAL, R., GHOSH, S., SARKAR, B., BHATTACHARYA, S. K., AND PAL, S. C., Molecular epidemiology of plasmid patterns in *Shigella dysenteriae* type 1 obtained from an outbreak in west Bengal (India), *FEMS Microbiol. Lett.* **30:**187–191 (1985).

185. PATTON, C. M., GANGAROSA, E. J., WEISSMAN, J. B., MERSON, M. H., AND MORRIS, G. K., Diagnostic value of indirect hemagglutination in the seroepidemiology of shigella infections, *J. Clin. Microbiol.* **3:**143–148 (1976).

186. PICKERING, L. K., DUPONT, H. L., OLARTE, J., CONKLIN, R., AND ERICSSON, C. Fecal leukocytes in enteric infections, *Am. J. Clin. Pathol.* **68:**562–565 (1977).

187. PICKERING, L. K., EVANS, D. G., DUPONT, H. L., VOLLET, J. J., AND EVANS, D. J., Diarrhea caused by *Shigella,* rotavirus, and *Giardia* in day-care centers: Prospective study, *J. Pediatr.* **99:**51–56 (1981).

188. PICKERING, L. K., BARTLETT, A. V., AND WOODWARD, W. E., Acute infectious diarrhea among children in day care: Epidemiology and control, *Rev. Infect. Dis.* **8:**539–547 (1986).

189. PRADO, D., CLEARY, T. G., PICKERING, L. K., ERICSSON, C. D., BARTLETT, A. V., III, DUPONT, H. L., AND JOHNSON, P. C., The relation between production of cytotoxin and clinical features in shigellosis, *J. Infect. Dis.* **154:**149–155 (1986).

190. RAHAMAN, M. M., AND WAHED, M. A., Direct nutrient loss and diarrhea, in: *Diarrhea and Malnutrition: Interactions, Mechanisms, and Interventions* (L. C. Chen and N. S. Scrimshaw, eds.), pp. 268–286, Plenum Press, New York, 1983.

191. RAHAMAN, M. M., HUQ, I., AND DEY, C. R., Superiority of MacConkey's agar over *Salmonella–Shigella* agar for isolation of *Shigella dysenteriae* type 1, *J. Infect. Dis.* **131:**700–703 (1975).

192. RAHAMAN, M. M., KHAN, M. M., AZIZ, K. M. S., ISLAM, M. S., AND GOLAM KIBRIYA, A. K. M., An outbreak of dysentery caused by *Shigella dysenteriae* type 1 on a coral island in the Bay of Bengal, *J. Infect. Dis.* **132:**15–19 (1975).

193. RAHAMAN, M. M., ALAM, A. R. M. J., ISLAM, M. R., GREENOUGH, W. B., AND LINDENBAUM, J., Shiga bacillus dysentery associated with marked leukocytosis and erythrocyte fragmentation, *Johns Hopkins Med. J.* **135:**65–70 (1975).

194. ROSENBERG, M. L., WEISSMAN, J. B., GANGAROSA, E. J., RELLER, L. B., AND BEASLEY, R. P., Shigellosis in the United States: Ten year review of nationwide surveillance, *Am. J. Epidemiol.* **104:**543–551 (1976).

195. ROUT, W. R., FORMAL, S. B., GIANNELLA, R. A., AND DAMMIN, G. J., Pathophysiology of shigella diarrhea in the rhesus monkey: Intestinal transport, morphological and bacteriological studies, *Gastroenterology* **68:**270–278 (1975).

196. SACK, R. B., SANTOSHAM, M., FROELICH, J. L., MEDINA, C., ORSKOV, F., AND ORSKOV, I., Doxycycline prophylaxis of travelers' diarrhea in Honduras, an area where resistance is common among enterotoxigenic *Escherichia coli, Am. J. Trop. Med. Hyg.* **33:**460–466 (1984).

197. SAKAI, T., SASAKAWA, C., MAKINO, S., AND YOSHIKAWA, M., DNA sequence and product analysis of the virF locus responsible for Congo red binding and cell invasion in Shigella flexneri 2a, *Infect. Immun.* **54:**395–402 (1986).

198. SALAM, M. A., AND BENNISH, M. L., Randomized, double blind trial of nalidixic acid vs. ampicillin in the treatment of childhood shigellosis, IX International Congress of Infectious and Parasitic Diseases, Munich, July 1986.

199. SANDYK, R., AND BRENNAN, M. J. W., Fulminating enceph-alopathy associated with *Shigella flexneri* infection, *Arch. Dis. Child.* **58:**70–72 (1983).

200. SANSONETTI, P. J., KOPECKO, D. J., AND FORMAL, S. B., *Shigella sonnei* plasmids: Evidence that a large plasmid is necessary for virulence, *Infect. Immun.* **34:**75–83 (1981).

201. SANSONETTI, P. J., KOPECKO, D. J., AND FORMAL, S. B., Involvement of a plasmid in the invasive ability of *Shigella flexneri, Infect. Immun.* **35:**852–860 (1982).

202. SANSONETTI, P. J., D'HAUTEVILLE, H., ECOBICHON, C., AND POURCEL, C., Molecular expression of virulence plas-mids in *Shigella* and enteroinvasive *Escherichia coli, Ann. Microbiol. (Paris)* **134A:**295–318 (1983).

203. SANSONETTI, P. J., HALE, T. L., DAMMIN, G. I., KAPPER, C., COLLINS, H. H., AND FORMAL, S. B., Alterations in the pathogenicity of *Escherichia coli* K 12 after transfer of plas-mids and chromosomal genes from *Shigella flexneri, Infect. Immun.* **39:**1392–1402 (1983).

204. SANSONETTI, P. H., RYTER, A., CLERC, P., MAURELLI, A. T., AND MOUNIER, J., Multiplication of *Shigella flexneri* within HeLa cells: Lysis of the phagocytic vacuole and plas-mid-mediated contact hemolysis, *Infect. Immun.* **51:**461–469 (1986).

205. SASAKAWA, C., MAKINO, S., KAMATA, K., AND YOSHIKAWA, M., Isolation, characterization, and mapping of Tn5 insertions into the 140 megadalton invasion plasmid de-fective in mouse Sereny test in Shigella flexneri 2a, *Infect. Immun.* **54:**32–36 (1986).

206. SCHLOSSBERG, D., AND MCGOWAN, J. E., Shigella infection and antibiotic resistance, *Ann. Intern. Med.* **83:**120–121 (1975).

207. SEIDAH, N. G., DONOHUE-ROLFE, A., LAZURE, C., AUCLAIR, F., KEUSCH, G. T., AND CHRETIEN, M., Complete amino acid sequence of *Shigella* toxin B-chain. A novel poly-peptide containing 69 amino acids and one disulfide bridge, *J. Biol. Chem.* **261:**13928–13931 (1986).

208. SERENY, B., Experimental *Shigella* conjunctivitis, *Acta Mi-crobiol. Acad. Sci. Hung.* **2:**293–296 (1955).

209. SHAHID, N. S., RAHAMAN, M. M., HAIDER, K., BANU, H., AND RAHMAN, N., Changing pattern of resistant Shiga bacillus (*Shigella dysenteriae* type 1) and *Shigella flexneri* in Bangladesh, *J. Infect. Dis.* **152:**1114–1119 (1985).

210. SHIGA, K., Ueber den Dysenterie-bacillus (*Bacillus dysen-teriae*), *Zentralbl. Bakteriol. Orign.* **24:**913–918 (1898).

211. SHIGA, K., The trend of prevention, therapy and epidemiolo-gy of dysentery since the discovery of its causative organism, *N. Engl. Med.* **26:**1205–1211 (1936).

212. SPEELMAN, P., KABIR, I., AND ISLAM, M., Distribution and spread of colonic lesions in shigellosis: A colonoscopic study, *J. Infect. Dis.* **150:**899–903 (1984).

213. SPEELMAN, P., MCGLAUGHLIN, R., KABIR, I., AND BUTLER, T., Differential clinical features and stool findings in shigellosis and amoebic dysentery, *Trans. R. Soc. Trop. Med. Hyg.* **81:**549–551 (1987).

214. SPIKA, J. S., DABIS, F., HARGRETT-BEAN, N., SALCEDO, J., VEILLARD, S., AND BLAKE, P. A., Shigellosis at a Caribbean

resort. Hamburger and North American origin as risk factors, *Am. J. Epidemiol.* **126:**1173–1180 (1987).

215. STEWARD, W. H., MCCABE, L., JR., HEMPHILL, E. C., DE-CAPITO, T., Diarrheal disease control studies. IV. The rela-tionship of certain environmental factors to the prevalence of Shigella infection, *Am. J. Trop. Med. Hyg.* **4:**718–724 (1955).

216. STOLL, B. J., GLASS, R. I., HUQ, M. I., KHAN, M. U., BANU, H., AND HOLT, J., Epidemiologic and clinical fea-tures of patients infected with *Shigella* who attended a diar-rheal disease hospital in Bangladesh, *J. Infect. Dis.* **146:**177–183 (1982).

217. STOLL, B. J., GLASS, R. I., BANU, H., HUQ, M. I., KHAN, M. U., AND AHMED, M., Value of stool examination in pa-tients with diarrhoea, *Br. Med. J.* **285:**2037–2040 (1983).

218. STRUELENS, M. J., PATTE, D., KABIR, I., SALAM, A., NATH, S. N., AND BUTLER, T., *Shigella septicemia:* Preva-lence, presentation, risk factors, and outcome, *J. Infect. Dis.* **152:**784–790 (1985).

219. TAKEUCHI, A., SPRINZ, H., LABREC, E. H., AND FORMAL, S. B., Experimental bacillary dysentery: An electron micro-scopic study of the response of the intestinal mucosa to bacte-rial invasion, *Am. J. Pathol.* **47:**1011–1044 (1965).

220. TAUXE, R. V., JOHNSON, K. E., BOASE, J. C., HELGERSON, S. D., AND BLAKE, P. A., Control of day-care shigellosis: A trial of convalescent day care in isolation, *Am. J. Public Health* **76:**627–630 (1986).

221. THOMAS, M. E. M., AND TILLET, H. E., Dysentery in gener-al practice: A study of cases and their contacts in Enfield and an epidemiological comparison with salmonellosis, *J. Hyg.* **71:**373–389 (1973).

222. TIEMENS, E. M., SHIPLEY, P. L., CORREIA, R. A., SHIELDS, D. S., AND GUERRANT, R. L., Sulfamethoxazole–tri-methoprim-resistant *Shigella flexneri* in northeastern Brazil, *Antimicrob. Agents Chemother.* **25:**653–654 (1985).

223. TOBIAS, J. D., STARKE, J. R., AND TOSI, M. F., Shigella keratitis: A report of two cases and a review of the literature, *Pediatr. Infect. Dis. J.* **6:**79–81 (1987).

224. TODD, C., On a dysentery toxin and anti-toxin, *J. Hyg.* **4:**480–494 (1904).

225. TRAMONT, E. C., CHUNG, R., BERMAN, S., KEREN, D., KAPFER, C., AND FORMAL, S. B., Safety and antigenicity of typhoid–*Shigella sonnei* vaccine (strain 5076-1C), *J. Infect. Dis.* **149:**133–136 (1984).

226. VAN BOHEMEN, C. G., LIONARONS, R. J., VAN BODEGOM, P., DINANT, H. J., LANDHEER, J. E., NABBE, A. J., GRUMET, F. C., AND ZANEN, H. C., Susceptibility and HLA-B27 in post-dysenteric arthropathies, *Immunology* **56:**377–379 (1985).

227. VAN BOHEMEN, C. G., NABBE, A. J. J. M., GRUMET, F. C., LANDHEER, J. E., DINANT, H. J., AND ZANEN, H. C., Lack of correlation between HLA-B27-like antigenic epitopes on *Shigella flexneri* and the occurrence of reactive arthritis, *Clin. Exp. Immunol.* **65:**679–682 (1986).

228. VAN HEYNINGEN, W. E., AND GLADSTONE, G. P., The neu-rotoxin of *Shigella shiga.* 1. Production, purification and

properties of the toxin, *Br. J. Exp. Pathol.* **34:**202–216 (1953).

229. WATANABE, H., AND NAKAMURA, A., Identification of *Shigella sonnei* form I plasmid genes necessary for cell invasion and their conservation among *Shigella* species and enteroinvasive *Escherichia coli, Infect. Immun.* **53:**352–358 (1986).

230. WATANABE, T., Infective heredity of multiple drug resistance in bacteria, *Bacteriol. Rev.* **27:**87–115 (1963).

231. WATT, J., HOLLISTER, A. C., JR., BECK, M. D., AND HEMPHILL, E. C., Diarrheal diseases in Fresno County, California, *Am. J. Public Health* **43:**728–741 (1953).

232. WEISSMANN, J. B., SCHMERLER, A., WEILER, P., FILICE, G., GODBEY, N., AND HANSEN, I., The role of preschool children and day-care centers in the spread of shigellosis in urban communities, *J. Pediatr.* **84:**797–802 (1974).

233. WELLS, J. G., AND MORRIS, G. K., Evaluation of transport methods for isolating *Shigella, J. Clin. Microbiol.* **13:**789–790 (1981).

234. WHITE, F. M. M., AND PEDERSEN, A. T., Epidemic shigellosis on a worktrain in Labrador, *Can. Med. Assoc. J.* **115:**647–649 (1976).

235. WILLIS, T., *Practice of Physick,* T. Dring, C. Harper, & J. Leigh, London, 1684.

12. Suggested Reading

ANONYMOUS, The prospects for immunizing against *Shigella* spp., in: *New Vaccine Development—Establishing Priorities,* Volume II, *Diseases of Importance in Developing Countries* (S. L. KATZ, ed.), pp. 329–337, National Academy Press, 1986.

BLACK, R. E., GRAUN, G. F., AND BLAKE, P. A., Epidemiology of common-source outbreaks of shigellosis in the United States 1961–1975, *Am. J. Epidemiol.* **108:**47–52 (1978).

BLASER, M. J., POLLARD, R. A., AND FELDMAN, R. A., *Shigella* infections in the United States, 1974–1980, *J. Infect. Dis.* **147:**771–775 (1983).

KEUSCH, G. T., Shigella infections, *Clin. Gastroenterol.* **8:**645–662 (1979).

PICKERING, L. K., BARTLETT, A. V., AND WOODWARD, W. E., Acute infectious diarrhea among children in day care: Epidemiology and control, *Rev. Infect. Dis.* **8:**539–547 (1986).

CHAPTER 30

Staphylococcal Infections

Frederick L. Ruben and Carl William Norden

1. Introduction

Although staphylococci, as a cause of sporadic infection, produce severe morbidity and mortality for the individual, the public-health importance of infections with this organism is its potential to cause epidemics. Major public-health problems resulting from infection with staphylococci include spread of the organism in newborn nurseries and outbreaks of postoperative wound infections. Also of importance is staphylococcal food poisoning, caused by the ingestion of food containing enterotoxin produced by coagulase-positive strains of *Staphylococcus aureus*.

A definitive diagnosis of staphylococcal disease is made when *S. aureus,* coagulase-positive, is isolated from a purulent lesion or from the blood, urine, peritoneal fluid, or cerebrospinal fluid (CSF) of a patient with clinical signs of infection. The diagnosis of *S. epidermidis,* coagulase-negative, as the causative agent of infection depends upon repeated isolation of this organism in appropriate clinical circumstances such as endocarditis involving a prosthetic heart valve, infected peritoneal fluid in a patient undergoing dialysis, urinary tract infection in a young woman, infection of CSF from a ventriculoatrial or a ventriculoperitoneal shunt, or bacteremia in an immunocompromised host or a patient with an intravenous catheter.

2. Historical Background

Approximately 100 years ago, von Recklinghausen[34] applied the term "micrococci" to gram-positive cocci observed in disease tissue and in pus from human abscesses. In 1881, Sir Alexander Ogston[111] published extensive observations showing that a cluster-forming coccus was the cause of certain pyogenic abscesses in man. He subsequently named the organisms *Staphylococcus,* derived from the Greek nouns *staphyle* (grapes) and *coccus* (grain or berry). He distinguished staphylococci from streptococci and produced disease in mice by subcutaneous inoculation of staphylococci recovered from pus.

In 1884, Rosenbach[127] observed that isolates of staphylococci formed two types of colonies, distinguishable from each other by color; he named the orange colonies *S. aureus* and the white *S. albus.*

From the time of Job, staphylococcal infections have plagued man. The advent of penicillin initially checked the spread of staphylococci, but in the 1950s, penicillinase-producing staphylococci were the cause of widespread hospital and nursery epidemics. The development of new penicillinase-resistant penicillins appeared to reverse this tide, and for a period staphylococcal infections have been less important as causes of nosocomial disease than infections caused by gram-negative bacilli. Methicillin-resistant staph-

Frederick L. Ruben and Carl William Norden · Infectious Diseases Unit, Department of Medicine, Montefiore Hospital, University of Pittsburgh School of Medicine, Pittsburgh, Pennsylvania 15213.

ylococci have emerged, however, as a cause of disease and are particularly prevalent in Europe. Thus, it appears that the cycle of resistant bacteria and antibiotics designed to check such organisms will continue for the staphylococcus.

3. Methodology

3.1. Sources of Mortality Data

Most staphylococcal disease is localized to the skin and is not fatal. Once infection becomes generalized and bacteremia occurs, mortality is great despite appropriate antibiotic therapy. Data on mortality from bacteremic staphylococcal infections have come from national surveillance[59] and from hospital studies[23,109] with comparable findings.

3.2. Sources of Morbidity Data

The incidence of all staphylococcal disease in the community can be assessed only indirectly, since minor disease may never come to medical attention.[108] The incidence of more serious disease including bacteremia can be estimated.[59,94] Surveillance has provided reliable data on hospital-acquired staphylococcal disease.[18,94,95,130,131]

3.3. Surveys

Household- and population-based surveys have provided the only data on community-acquired morbidity from staphylococci.[108] Hospital-based surveillance for staphylococcal disease, community- and nosocomially acquired, allows for ongoing assessment of serious staphylococcal disease.[95,118,128,130] Hospital surveillance begins from laboratory cultures reporting staphylococci; hence, it may underestimate the incidence of disease when cultures are not taken. Typing of staphylococci in the laboratory permits identification of strains responsible for outbreaks or epidemics.[11]

3.4. Laboratory Diagnosis

Staphylococci can be recognized quickly and reliably on Gram strains of exudates from most clinical specimens. Their lack of fastidiousness permits their growth on ordinary laboratory media.[104] Selective media such as that containing mannitol have expedited recognition of staphylococci grown from swabs of throat, nose, or other contaminated areas and have permitted rapid evaluation of staphylococcal carriage by individuals. Once grown, *S. aureus* is identified by a positive coagulase test, which permits differentiation from coagulase-negative *S. epidermidis*. Antibiotic sensitivity of staphylococci as measured by a Kirby–Bauer disk technique is widely used,[30] although in selected instances tube-dilution techniques permitting the determination of minimal inhibitory and bactericidal concentrations are more valuable.[5] Phage typing of staphylococci has permitted identification of specific strains and allowed for the recognition of prevalent and epidemic strains. Such typing is currently less widely available, and the routinely available antibiotic-sensitivity pattern has become more used for strain identification, although it is neither as sensitive nor as reliable as phage typing.

Serological studies have not proved useful, since the normal human adult possesses antibodies to several staphylococcal antigens.[76] Staphylococci contain a variety of antigens, each of which might be important, so that the question of which antigen(s) may be useful for serological studies remains controversial.[101] Antibodies to *S. aureus* teichoic acid have been demonstrated in human sera[93]; studies suggest that their presence in bacteremic patients might indicate a more serious form of the disease[56,104,146] including endocarditis,[103] osteomyelitis,[57,157] and metastatic abscesses.[149]

4. Biological Characteristics of the Organism

The two species of staphylococci are *S. aureus* and *S. epidermidis* (sometimes called *S. albus*). Pigment production is only a minor criterion for identification; the coagulase reaction is the major test used to distinguish the two species. The following enzymes and toxins that are produced by staphylococci are often considered of importance in human virulence:

1. Coagulase: *S. aureus* produces two antigenically distinct enzymes, bound and free coagulase, both capable of coagulating human serum. Their role in infection is unclear, but the presence of this enzyme serves to distinguish the more virulent species, *S. aureus*, from *S. epidermidis*.
2. Leukocidin: This extracellular protein acts on human polymorphonuclear leukocytes *in vitro*. It causes death of white blood cells, but its role in infection is unclear.
3. Enterotoxin: Most *S. aureus* strains produce enterotoxin, which is responsible for the syndrome of staphylococcal food poisoning. A smaller percentage of *S. epidermidis* strains produce enterotoxin; these have rarely been implicated in food poisoning.[13]
4. Exfoliative toxin: Staphylococci of phage group II produce

a toxin responsible for the dermatological manifestations of infection, which go under the general heading of "scalded-skin syndrome."

5. Toxic shock syndrome toxins: This syndrome is caused by a toxin or toxins produced by *S. aureus.* Toxic shock syndrome toxin 1 (TSST-1) is a specific toxin identified to date, but other exotoxins and enterotoxins may also be responsible for the syndrome.[12,126] It seems unlikely that TSST-1 can be produced by *S. epidermidis.*[114]

Susceptible staphylococci may be lysed by viruses that infect bacteria (phages). The patterns formed by lysis and lack of lysis permit classification of staphylococci into several major groups.[156] The technique of phage typing has been a useful guide in identifying staphylococci for epidemiological study. Phage type, however, is not an absolute criterion of identity, since lysis of *S. aureus* can be altered through lysogenization with wild phages, loss of prophage, or transduction.

Clinical isolates of coagulase-negative staphylococcus, from patients with clinical infections, appear to produce an extracellular polysaccharide ("slime factor") that enhances adherence to plastic or metal surfaces.[7,22] This slime layer also inhibits diffusion of antibiotics, impairing their ability to reach organisms.[136] In addition, the slime material interferes with the lymphoproliferative response to mitogens[49] and also alters polymorphonuclear functions such as decreasing responsiveness to chemotactic stimuli[60] and inhibiting phagocytosis of coagulase-negative staphylococci.[60] Coagulase-negative staphylococci have the ability to erode into polyethylene catheters and prosthetic devices, which may also allow increased adherence of the organisms.[20,115] Catheter-adherent coagulase-negative staphylococci appear to possess survival mechanisms under adverse conditions (absence of conventional nutrients), which may be important in the genesis of occult foreign-body-associated infections.[46]

5. Descriptive Epidemiology

5.1. Prevalence and Incidence

S. aureus may be carried by normal people in a variety of body sites without disease being present. The nose is the principal site of carriage; cross-sectional studies reveal rates of 30–50% in persons outside hospitals and higher rates in hospital nursing personnel.[158] Longitudinal studies have shown persons to be intermittent carriers, persistent noncarriers, or persistent carriers. The latter are more common

among children, only 10–20% of normal adults being chronic carriers.[158] Skin carriage has been demonstrated in 85% of persons with atopic dermatitis, suggesting a strong predisposition to carriage.[9] In newborn nurseries, colonization of the umbilical stump precedes nasal carriage, and up to 75% of infants become carriers at one or more body sites by the 5th day.[39]

Carriage may precede or, indeed, lead to disease in susceptible individuals.[158] Conversely, not all carriers develop *S. aureus* lesions or any other form of staphylococcal disease. General practitioners in England have reported the annual incidence for *S. aureus* disease in their practice populations at 1.5–5.0%,[52,96] certainly lower than population carriage rates. The nasal carrier in the hospital has been shown to have a higher rate of staphylococcal postoperative sepsis (7.0%) than the noncarrier (2.0%).[160] Insulin-using diabetics have increased carriage rates.[148] The true rate of minor disease in nasal carriers postoperatively and in the newborn with umbilical carriage is not known, since these patients may be discharged from the hospital before disease becomes manifest.[105]

Serious staphylococcal disease including sepsis may be acquired outside the hospital. One report from a community-type hospital noted that 14% of all community-acquired episodes of sepsis were caused by staphylococci, while the rate of sepsis for all bacterial types was 340/100,000 admissions.[130] Other more recent reports found that 7 to 14% of community-acquired episodes were caused by *S. aureus.*[14,36]

5.2. Epidemic Behavior and Contagiousness

S. aureus can be highly contagious through direct contact with the large numbers of organisms present in lesions. The condition of the host clearly influences the frequency and severity of disease produced by staphylococci. Within a household, any strain of *S. aureus* can colonize family members and cause disease sporadically, or it may cause continuous and repeated episodes of infection.[108]

Community and worldwide epidemics of *S. aureus* disease have been recognized. Finland[41] has conceptualized these epidemic features of *S. aureus:* First are local and short-term epidemics of staphylococcal disease exemplified by outbreaks of antibiotic-related staphylococcal diarrhea noted in the late 1950s and early 1960s, by outbreaks in burn units, and by excess staphylococcal pneumonia complicating the influenza type A outbreaks of 1941 and 1957. To this, one can add more recent outbreaks of methicillin-resistant staphylococcal disease.[69,73,78,112] Second, there have been worldwide and long-term epidemics of *S. aureus* disease noted in nurseries and hospitals throughout the world, coincident with the appearance and spread of new bacteriophages 80, then 81, and then 80/81 in the late 1950s. Following this occurrence, S. aureus disease has shown a cyclical character with periods of increased cases followed by periods of declining incidence. The phage-type patterns of S. aureus have also changed during these cycles, with different phage groups predominating.

Several factors may have contributed to the epidemic of phage type 80/81 staphylococci.[106] Its arrival was associated with the widespread availability of penicillin and use of broad-spectrum antibiotics that allowed selection of penicillin-resistant strains.[40] The number of susceptible persons increased as a result of medical advances. Finally, the transmission of S. aureus was enhanced by the reliance on antibiotics instead of aseptic techniques in caring for hospitalized persons. The demise of the 80/81 strain may have resulted from vigorous control efforts, the advent of semisynthetic penicillinase-resistant penicillins, and also unknown factors.

Finland[41] and others[59,78] suggest that the epidemic character of S. aureus may relate in part to genetic properties of the organism. The changing susceptibility and resistance of S. aureus to bacteriophages or properties of the phages themselves may create within S. aureus the changes required for enhanced virulence. The changing antigenic character and epidemic properties of S. aureus may thus be analogous to the changing influenza A viruses and their epidemiological virulence.

S. epidermidis is among the most common causes of sepsis in newborns requiring umbilical vein catheters and in patients with cancer who require long-term vascular catheterization. Two outbreaks of catheter-related S. epidermidis sepsis in intensive-care units have been reported; the bacteremia was correlated with the duration of catheterization and the use of parenteral hyperalimentation.[21,45] In one outbreak, 13 episodes of S. epidermidis sepsis occurred over a 20-month period; these episodes were characterized by fever, toxicity, multiple positive blood cultures, and uniformly colonized intravascular catheters.[21] An additional 16 patients had possible sepsis. Four associated deaths occurred; in the three autopsies, all patients had multiple pulmonary abscesses in which gram-positive cocci were profusely present.[21] A prominent feature of the S. epidermidis isolates was resistance to many commonly used antimicrobial agents.[21] Most of the patients were hospitalized in the intensive-care unit; nose and hand cultures taken from personnel showed frequent carriage of multiply resistant S. epidermidis strains.[21]

5.3. Geographic Distribution

Infections with S. aureus are worldwide in distribution.[41] While the penicillin-resistant phage type 80/81 caused infections worldwide, the more recent methicillin-resistant strains have been of several phage types[69] or were nontypable,[73] and have been more prevalent in Europe than elsewhere.[68,73]

Penicillin-resistant forms of S. aureus do occur in nature,[137] and penicillinase-producing strains from the preantibiotic era have been reported.[113] In contrast, there is no clear documentation of resistance to other antistaphylococcal drugs prior to their clinical use.[119]

5.4. Temporal Distribution

Annual rates for S. aureus bacteremia have varied in both the United States[41] and Europe.[17] S. aureus pneumonia with bacteremia has shown a peak incidence in winter and summer months,[22] whereas postoperative wound rates have peaked in winter months.[142]

Bullous impetigo from S. aureus has a seasonal peak in late summer and early fall.[26] Pyomyositis caused by S. aureus is a common condition in tropical areas such as eastern Africa,[53] whereas it occurs rarely in temperate-climate areas such as the United States.[31,83]

5.5. Age

As noted in Section 5.1, children have higher rates of carriage and persist as carriers more commonly than do adults.[3] Rates for bacteremia are higher in the age groups 5–15 years[51,59] and 50–80 years[59] whether the bacteremia was acquired inside or outside the hospital. Mortality from bacteremia is age-related, with higher rates in the very young and older age groups.[59,109]

5.6. Sex

Males and females carry S. aureus at a similar rate.[3] Males have an increased rate of disease during the first month of life[141] and have more disseminated infections in childhood.[51] In adults, results are conflicting for sex differences in rates of disease.[38,44,59,66,70,122] Males are reported to have more S. aureus pneumonia[44] and to have more fatal infections.[122] A problem with all the reports showing sex differences is actually assessing the population at risk.[141]

5.7. Race

No racial predisposition for *S. aureus* disease has been noted.

5.8. Occupation

Persons such as physicians and nurses in hospitals who may come in contact with patients with *S. aureus* lesions have higher rates of nasal carriage than persons not in such contact[139,158] and may develop diseases from such carriage.[105]

5.9. Occurrence in Different Settings

Staphylococci have been long recognized as a hospital problem, and the policy of routine ongoing surveillance for hospital-acquired staphylococcal disease is well justified.[38,39,105] Nationwide surveillance[18] for nosocomial *S. aureus* bacteremia, in hospitals of multiple types, showed a rate of 21/100,000 discharges and an overall disease rate of 458, placing *S. aureus* in a virtual tie with *Escherichia coli* as a pathogen in surgical wounds. The bulk of *S. aureus* illness came from surgical wounds, where the rate was 189. Intermediate rates were reported for lower-respiratory, urinary, and cutaneous infections. *S. aureus* ranks second to *E. coli* in proclivity for causing hospital-acquired infections.[18] Altemeier[1] noted that prior to 1956, *S. aureus* and other gram-positive cocci accounted for approximately 65% of all surgical wound infections.

Because of the rate of colonization with *S. aureus* of newborn infants in nurseries, there have been serious outbreaks of *S. aureus* sepsis in nursery populations.[39] Staphylococci in nurseries are spread via personnel handling the infants,[161] suggesting an important role for hand-washing in the control of nursery colonization. Reduced handling and segregation of colonized cohorts have reduced colonization and disease rates within nurseries,[39] as has umbilical-cord care using bacitracin ointment.[61]

Heroin addicts who take their drugs by injection are at considerable risk for developing *S. aureus* endocarditis.[89] While neither the injection paraphernalia nor the drugs[147] have contained *S. aureus,* it has been shown that addicts actively using heroin have significantly higher carriage rates than addicts not on drugs.[144] The organisms recovered from the blood of heroin addicts with endocarditis are usually of the same phage type as those carried on the skin and in the nose.[145]

5.10. Socioeconomic Factors

There is little to suggest that socioeconomic factors influence the occurrence of staphylococcal disease. Overcrowding, poor skin hygiene, or a minor skin trauma may play a role in predisposing to *S. aureus* bullous impetigo, but the association is greater for streptococcal pyoderma.[27]

5.11. Other Factors

Certain persons with altered host resistance are particularly prone to *S. aureus* infections.[3,76,102,107] Very old and very young individuals were mentioned in Section 5.5. To these we add persons with influenza A, exfoliative skin disorders, starvation, neoplasms, diabetes mellitus, chronic granulomatous disease, agammaglobulinemia, liver disease, and renal failure, as well as persons undergoing cardiovascular surgery with prosthesis insertion and those receiving cancer chemotherapy or steroids. Recognized sources for staphylococcal infections include arteriovenous fistulas or shunts in patients undergoing hemodialysis[88,110] and intravenous cannulas used to administer fluid.[91]

The use of antibiotics has clearly influenced the epidemiology of *S. aureus* infections. Following the widespread use of penicillin and broad-spectrum antibiotics, diarrhea associated with overgrowth of *S. aureus* in the stools became a recognized complication.[41] In addition, changing antibiotic-susceptibility patterns have been dictated by the antibiotics being used.[42,50,128] Resistance to penicillin has increased progressively over the years whereas with the declining indiscriminate use of other broad-spectrum antibiotics, *S. aureus* strains have regained sensitivity to these drugs. Methicillin-resistant *S. aureus,* while rare in U.S. hospitals until the mid-1970s, is now widespread in hospitals of all sizes, in rehabilitation facilities, and in nursing homes.[63] The mechanisms for this spread are not known.[87,129]

Quite possibly, the virulence of the organism itself has influenced the occurrence of infection. Phage types such as the 52, 52A, and 80/81 complex[107] of the 1950s that were resistant to penicillin have been called "epidemiologically virulent."[39,105] Whether disease incidence alone was the result of intense exposure to these strains or whether they were inherently more virulent is unresolved.

An association has been shown between the use of vaginal tampons by younger women during their menses[100] and the entity called toxic shock syndrome.[143] *S.*

aureus has been cultured from the vagina in over 90% of patients with this syndrome,[100] whereas a much lower prevalence of colonization, 2–15%, of the cervix and vagina with *S. aureus* was found in healthy women.[6,100] Toxic shock syndrome not associated with menstruation has also been described[125] in conjunction with *S. aureus* infections such as surgical wound infections or with childbirth by vaginal delivery and cesarean section. Toxic shock syndrome has also been a complication of influenza.[90]

Coagulase-negative staphylococci are part of the normal skin flora and are uncommon pathogens except in the presence of foreign bodies (prosthetic valves, CSF shunts, prosthetic joints, and intravascular catheters). Immunocompromised hosts and neutropenic patients appear to have an increased susceptibility to severe infections, such as bacteremia, with these organisms. It is sometimes hard to separate the roles of foreign bodies versus immunocompromised status. For example, intravascular catheters are an important portal of entry in immunocompromised hosts; however, overgrowth at respiratory and gastrointestinal sites may also serve as sites of entry in such hosts, even without a foreign body.

6. Mechanisms and Routes of Transmission

Transmission of *S. aureus* outside the hospital consists of person-to-person spread within families or intimate contacts.[108] Studies within the hospital show that the nasal carrier is predisposed to postoperative infection with the same strain.[160] Also within hospitals, other vectors for infection exist with infected patients,[39] health-care personnel[105] who are infected or are carriers, and fomite contamination.[51,138] Airborne spread of *S. aureus* can be demonstrated[29,85,158,159]; however, it has been difficult to correlate counts of staphylococci in air with infection rates.[158] Patients on broad-spectrum antibiotics have been shown to have increased shedding of resistant staphylococci.[158] The infected lesion sheds heavy concentrations of organisms and is potentially the greatest hazard for spreading infection.[39] In nurseries, the nurse carrier usually conveys *S. aureus* to infants by handling them.[161] Other potential vectors for spreading *S. aureus* are the "cloud baby"[32] and the adult carrier who has chronic dermatological disease or who becomes an effective disseminator for unknown reasons.[39]

Too little is currently known of animal staphylococci and human *S. aureus* interrelationships to determine their importance in human disease.[24]

Humans are the natural reservoir for *S. epidermidis;*

these bacteria are part of the normal skin flora and are the commonest staphylococcal species isolated from cutaneous sites. The organism is easily shed from skin and can contaminate inanimate environmental surfaces, other people, and the air. The resistance of the organism to drying and temperature changes produces a long viability.[74] *S. epidermidis* infections result from contamination of a site (usually surgical) by organisms from the patient's skin or nasopharynx or from exogenous sources. One study reported the recovery of organisms, primarily *S. epidermidis* and diptheroids, in about 55% of cultures taken from the site of the valvular prosthesis during open-heart surgery.[75]

7. Pathogenesis and Immunity

7.1. Pathogenesis

Foreign bodies enhance the likelihood that staphylococcal infection will develop by reducing the number of organisms needed to initiate infection. Healthy persons require more than 10^6 virulent staphylococci to initiate a minor infection, whereas 10^2 organisms can infect when a foreign body is present.[35] Sutures, intravascular catheters, or needles left in place,[91] prosthetic joint devices,[19] artificial heart valves,[28] and tracheostomy tubes[37] are examples of commonly used foreign bodies that may become infected. Bacteremia may arise from the local site and can lead to *S. aureus* infection and abscess formation in any organ of the body.[109] Sequelae include such entities as meningitis,[155] osteomyelitis,[152] and endocarditis.[154]

Damaged tissues, e.g., the skin in burns and the airways in influenza, are predisposed to colonization and then proliferation of *S. aureus*. A consequence in burn patients is septicemia[4] and in influenza patients, *S. aureus* pneumonia.[43]

Other abnormalities of host defense such as neutropenia,[71,77] chronic granulomatous disease,[123] immunosuppression,[23] and renal failure[99] predispose to more frequent occurrence and greater severity of *S. aureus* disease.

The factors responsible for virulence of different strains of staphylococci are unknown. *S. aureus* organisms shed from fresh tissues are more virulent than desiccated organisms in air or on fomites.[92] Some strains such as the epidemic 80/81 complex are epidemiologically more virulent.[41,105,107] *S. aureus* is a complex organism with a variety of bacterial products with the potential for promoting disease.[102] Two extracellular products—enterotoxin, which produces food poisoning, and exfoliatin, which causes the scalded-skin syndrome—clearly produce disease. In toxic shock syndrome, an extracellular toxin (now known as TSST-1) of *S. aureus* related to phage group I is believed to mediate the multiple clinical manifestations seen.[143]

As with *S. aureus*, the presence of foreign bodies markedly enhances the likelihood of infection with coagulase-negative staphylococci. Indeed, *S. epidermidis* is generally not a pathogen except in the presence of a foreign body, in an immunocompromised host, or in patients with neutropenia. As described earlier, the ability of a coagulase-negative strain of staphylococcus to secrete a slime layer appears to offer it advantages in terms of colonization, persistence, and infection. In one study, 81% of 59 infectious episodes in patients with a prosthetic device were due to a slime-positive coagulase-negative staphylococcus.[25] In contrast, 22 noninfectious episodes (in which the organisms were considered contaminants) were equally distributed between episodes due to slime-positive or slime-negative isolates.[25] Slime-positive organisms producing infection were significantly harder to eradicate than slime-negative organisms.[25]

7.2. Immunity

Man enjoys a high degree of natural resistance to *S. aureus*. The exact nature of this natural immunity is not clear and may be nonspecific.[33] While man shows little resistance to superficial colonization with *S. aureus*, there is great resistance to progressive forms of disease.[33] Spread of staphylococcal infections is limited by reticuloendothelial system clearance[98] and polymorphonuclear leukocyte chemotaxis and ingestion of bacteria.[77,124] Although IgG antibodies to specific components of *S. aureus* have been demonstrated,[93] and components of the classic and alternative complement systems have been shown to be at times necessary for efficient phagocytosis of staphylococci,[150] the overall significance of opsonization in immunity to *S. aureus* is unclear.[77,102] IgE antibodies to *S. aureus*, demonstrated in patients with recurrent "cold" abscesses, may represent an abnormal immunological response to *S. aureus*[133] and more specifically to the cell walls of the bacteria.[134]

The role of cell-mediated immunity to *S. aureus* remains to be defined.[82,102] Filtrates from strains of *S. aureus* contain mitogens for human lymphocytes.[140] Delayed hypersensitivity reactions to *S. aureus* have been demonstrated in animals, but are not associated with increased resistance.[82] Indeed, repeated skin infections in a rabbit model produced increased susceptibility to *S. aureus*

skin and joint infections, suggesting that delayed hypersensitivity may have a pathogenetic role in staphylococcal disease.[62]

8. Patterns of Host Response

Staphylococci may infect and cause disease in virtually every organ system of the body. The organism is highly virulent for man and, with the exception of the anterior nares, the pharynx, and skin, rarely lives in symbiosis with the host. Within the nose and pharynx and on the skin, staphylococci may exist as part of the "carrier" state; their importance in such locations is the capacity to be spread to other sites within the host or to other susceptible individuals. The manifestations of staphylococcal infection vary depending on site involved and will be described separately. Table 1 summarizes some of the features of selected forms of *S. aureus* infections.

8.1. Clinical Features

8.1.1. Boils, Furuncles, and Carbuncles. A boil or furuncle is an acute abscess of the skin and subcutaneous tissues. Such lesions occur most commonly on the face, neck, buttocks, thighs, perineum, or axillae. Exquisite tenderness is the hallmark of these lesions, which swell with pus and eventually drain spontaneously. Carbuncles are collections of interconnected furuncles that are less likely to drain externally. Carbuncles become larger, are more painful, and are associated with systemic signs and bacteremia; they appear more commonly in diabetics.

8.1.2. Wound Infections. The bulk of wound infections are caused by *S. aureus*.[1,16] Factors that have been associated with an increased incidence of wound infection are age, diabetes, steroid administration, obesity, malnutrition, increased duration of time in the operating room, and presence of other infected sites. Wound infections are usually associated with frank purulent drainage, breakdown of the wound, fever, and lack of well-being of the patient.

8.1.3. Breast Infections. Mastitis due to staphylococci generally occurs in newborns and in women (frequently in the puerperium). In neonates, the breast shows marked redness with induration resembling a furuncle. In adults, infection can be superficial, presenting only with pain and a lump, but more extensive involvement may occur, with marked tenderness, fever, and leukocytosis.

8.1.4. Pneumonia. Staphylococcal pneumonia may present in one of three ways: (1) lobar pneumonia; (2) dif-

Table 1.   Clinical Forms of Staphylococcal Infections

Category	Age most often afflicted	Special risk factors
Boils, furuncles, carbuncles	All ages	Diabetes mellitus
Wound infections	All ages	Diabetes mellitus, steroid therapy, obesity, malnutrition, prolonged surgery, foreign body (e.g., prosthesis)
Breast infections	Newborn, women in puerperium	None
Pneumonia	All ages	Drug addiction, influenza outbreaks
Endocarditis	All ages	Heroin addiction, prosthetic heart valve
Skin infections		
Bullous impetigo	Childhood	None
Scalded-skin syndrome	Childhood	Compromised host
Thrombophlebitis	All ages	Intravenous catheters
Bacteremia	All ages	Diabetes mellitus, leukemia, lymphoma
Osteomyelitis	Children	None
Septic arthritis	All ages	None
Food poisoning	All ages	None
Parotitis	Elderly	Dehydration
Toxic shock syndrome	Younger women	Use of vaginal tampons during menses, after childbirth, surgical wounds, influenza
Peritonitis	All ages	Continuous peritoneal dialysis
Urinary tract infection	Young women	None or urinary tract abnormality
Cerebrospinal fluid shunt infection	All ages	Presence of shunt
Pyomyositis	Young men and boys	Tropical climate
Meningitis	Newborn infants, all ages	Prematurity, endocarditis, CNS disorders

fuse interstitial pneumonia; (3) localized areas of pneumonia secondary to septic emboli with infarction. In lobar pneumonia, the patients are usually acutely ill with high fever, tachypnea, and cough productive of yellow bloody sputum; on smear of the sputum, large numbers of neutrophils and staphylococci are seen. Empyema is a frequent occurrence, and in infants, the development of pneumatoceles is a hallmark of staphylococcal pneumonia. Diffuse interstitial pneumonia usually occurs after or coincident with influenza. The most prominent clinical feature is tachypnea and cyanosis with refractory hypoxia. Localized areas of pneumonia secondary to septic emboli can occur with bacteremia alone or in the presence of endocarditis, particularly involving the tricuspid valve. Pleuritic chest pain, dyspnea, fever, and chills are prominent, whereas cough and purulent sputum are less likely. Roentgenographic examination frequently reveals multiple small densities at the periphery of the lung that frequently increase in size and cavitate.

8.1.5. Endocarditis. Endocarditis caused by *S. aureus* usually presents as an acute fulminant illness with high fever and metastatic abscesses and has the potential for lethal damage to heart valves. Staphylococcal endocarditis should be suspected in any patient with staphylococcal bacteremia and particularly in heroin addicts. Many of the classic features of endocarditis may be absent, and staphylococcal disease frequently involves normal heart valves.[67]

Only 5% of all cases of infective endocarditis on native cardiac valves are caused by coagulase-negative staphylococci.[66] The disease is subacute and resembles that caused by viridans streptococci. In contrast to the low frequency of coagulase-negative infections of native cardiac valves, these organisms are the single most common etiological agent in infection of prosthetic valves.[2] Coagulase-negative staphylococci were implicated as the cause of approximately 40% of the cases of prosthetic valve endocarditis at two large medical centers.[2] Generally, *S. epidermidis* is the species most frequently implicated.[65] The infections are usually serious with evidence of prosthetic valve dysfunction. It is presumed that cases caused by coagulase-negative staphylococci occurring in the year following surgery are probably the result of inoculation of organisms at the time of surgery. Diagnosis of coagulase-negative prosthetic valve endocarditis requires a high level of suspicion and the findings of fever and blood cultures positive for these organisms.

8.1.6. Skin Infections. Staphylococci of phage group II have been associated with several manifestations of infection in the skin.[97] These include bullous impetigo, a nonstreptococcal scarlatiniform rash, and toxic epidermal necrolysis (the scalded-skin syndrome). Infected individuals show an abrupt onset with diffuse erythema over most of the body. The skin is exquisitely sensitive to touch and within 1–2 days begins to peel off after light stroking (Nikolsky's sign). Large bullae filled with clear sterile fluid appear in the epidermis, which separates in sheets. Secondary desquamation continues 7–10 days after the onset of redness; recovery is complete.

8.1.7. Thrombophlebitis. *S. aureus* is the most common pathogen isolated from the tips of intravenous catheters and from bacteremias related to venous catheterization.[91] The area around the catheter may show signs of phlebitis, but it may also appear innocuous in a patient with high spiking fevers. Blood cultures will generally be positive, and on occasion pus may be found in the lumen of the vein. The risk of infection of the catheter increases with the duration of catheterization, and prevention by frequent changes of the catheter is mandatory.

Studies evaluating central hyperalimentation catheters, peripheral intravenous lines, subclavian catheters, and Hickman or Broviac central lines in immunocompromised patients have all reported *S. epidermidis* to be the most common infecting organism. Risk factors include the long periods of time that intravenous lines now stay in place, the pressure of multiple antibiotic usages in sick patients enhancing the likelihood of colonization with multiply resistant coagulase-negative staphylococci, the ability of the organism to produce a slime layer, the presence of neutropenia, and the administration of other drugs that produce immunosuppression. Distinguishing significant catheter-acquired bacteremia from contaminated blood cultures may be difficult and there is often a lack of any local sign of infection in these patients. It seems wise to regard as significant repeatedly positive blood cultures that grow *S. epidermidis* and that are obtained from patients who have indwelling catheters or are immunocompromised or neutropenic.

8.1.8. Bacteremia. Staphylococcal bacteremia may arise from any site where staphylococci produce infection. Hospital procedures such as surgery with subsequent wound infection or parenteral infusion via intravenous catheters are a frequent source. Patients who develop staphylococcal bacteremia frequently have underlying diseases such as di-

abetes, leukemia, and lymphoma.[79] The clinical picture of staphylococcal bacteremia is generally a fulminant illness with high fever, tachycardia, and frequently shock. Disseminated intravascular coagulation may also occur.

There have been many reports suggesting an increase in the rate of coagulase-negative staphylococcal bacteremia in hospitalized patients.[120] Part of this increase is clearly attributable to the increased number of immunocompromised patients who are living longer and spending more time in hospitals. Investigators at the Baltimore Cancer Research Center identified *S. epidermidis* as the single most common cause of bacteremia in their patients between 1977 and 1979.[151] The majority of patients were neutropenic; they were also heavily colonized with the organism in their rectum. Both the gastrointestinal tract and intravenous catheters appeared to be important portals of entry or sources for the bacteremia. The infections were clinically significant with a substantial mortality rate (34% in one series), which is similar to that reported for bacteremia with coagulase-positive staphylococci.[120]

8.1.9. Osteomyelitis. *S. aureus* is the most common cause of acute osteomyelitis. It occurs most frequently in children under 12 years of age, but may also be seen in adults. The clinical picture begins abruptly with fever, chills, and pain at the site of involvement. The skin overlying the bone is often warm, red, and swollen. Cultures of bone or pus will generally reveal staphylococci; bacteremia is present in about half of the patients. Long bones are most commonly afflicted in children, while vertebrae are a more common site in adults. The clinical picture of vertebral osteomyelitis may be only that of malaise and vague back pain; an elevated erythrocyte sedimentation rate may be the only laboratory abnormality. With progression, painful muscle spasms, limitation of motion of the spine, and low-grade fever will usually develop. Chronic staphylococcal osteomyelitis may occur if therapy of the acute disease is delayed or even in some instances following proper treatment. The characteristic clinical course is an indolent one in which sinuses drain purulent material for many years.

8.1.10. Septic Arthritis. Septic arthritis, in all age groups, is frequently caused by staphylococcus. The typical presentation occurs with fever, pain and chills; the diagnosis rests on aspiration, Gram stain, and culture of the joint fluid.

S. epidermidis is the second most common cause (*S. aureus* is first) of infections of prosthetic hips and knees.[55] It is presumed that infections with coagulase-negative staphylococci are a result of operative contamination; however, there may be a prolonged latent period before clinical infection occurs and it is not possible to exclude hematogenous dissemination as a mechanism. The symptoms of infection may be mild, consisting only of pain in the area of the prosthesis and fever. The diagnosis must be made by culture of the joint space. Although such infections are not common, they are devastating complications because removal of the prosthesis is usually required.

8.1.11. Food Poisoning. Staphylococcal food poisoning is produced by the ingestion of food containing enterotoxin produced by *S. aureus*. The usual interval between ingestion of food containing the toxin and the onset of symptoms is relatively short, ranging from 30 min to 7 h. Onset is usually abrupt with severe nausea and cramps followed by vomiting, diarrhea, and prostration. Fever is usually absent, and the duration of illness is generally less than 24 h. The short incubation period, brief duration of illness, and absence of fever help distinguish staphylococcal food poisoning from other forms of food poisoning. (See Chapter 4 for more details.)

8.1.12. Parotitis. *S. aureus* has been recognized to cause severe and fatal parotitis.[116] Patients were elderly, severely debilitated from chronic disease, and dehydrated. The parotid gland was erythematous and tender. Fever and markedly elevated white-cell counts were typical. Suppurative parotitis has also been reported in neonates[80] and children[81] with *S. aureus* isolated from parotid pus.

8.1.13. Toxic Shock Syndrome. This entity[143] has been described, predominantly in young women who are actively menstruating but also following all types of surgery, after childbirth, with wounds, or after influenza. These individuals develop fever, an erythematous macular rash that subsequently desquamates, falling blood pressure, and then multisystem involvement. The latter has included gastrointestinal, renal, hepatic, hematological, central nervous, and cardiopulmonary systems. *S. aureus* has been found in the vaginal cultures of nearly all menstrual cases and has been recovered from wounds in other cases. A significantly higher proportion of menstruating women with this syndrome used vaginal tampons when compared with controls.[100] Other diseases must be excluded, such as meningococcemia, Rocky Mountain spotted fever, or bacteremia.

Toxic shock has been reported to be caused by strains of coagulase-negative staphylococci that produce TSST-1.[64] In such cases, coagulase-negative staphylococci that produce this toxin were isolated from the vagina and no coagulase-positive staphylococci were recovered.

8.1.14. Peritonitis. Chronic ambulatory peritoneal dialysis is an attractive alternative to hemodialysis for patients with chronic renal failure. One complication, however, is the development of peritonitis and the organism

most frequently isolated from such patients is *S. epidermidis* (17 to 40% of episodes).[117] Because the number of organisms in the peritoneum may be small, inoculation of larger volumes of peritoneal fluid, filtration of large volumes of fluid followed by culture of the filter, etc. have been tried to enhance the likelihood of diagnosis. Treatment of these infections is generally successful without catheter removal, either with systemic therapy or with intraperitoneal administration of antibiotics.[117]

8.1.15. Urinary Tract Infection. Although not commonly thought of as a urinary tract pathogen, coagulase-negative staphylococcus (*S. saprophyticus*) is the second most common cause of acute urinary tract infections in young women.[54] The organism is cultured infrequently from the genitourinary tract of young women, but there is a high correlation between colonization and subsequent development of urinary tract infection.[54] Identification of the organism is facilitated in the clinical microbiology laboratory because of its resistance to novobiocin. The organism causes both upper and lower urinary tract disease and the signs, symptoms, and examination of the urine of women infected with this organism are indistinguishable from those of patients infected with gram-negative enteric organisms. Other coagulase-negative staphylococci do not generally infect the urine, but do account for some infections in older patients who are usually hospitalized and have underlying urinary tract complications (e.g., indwelling urinary catheter, recent urinary surgery, bladder dysfunction, obstruction).[84] These latter infections with coagulase-negative staphylococci account for less than 5% of all episodes of significant bacteriuria in hospitalized patients.

8.1.16. CSF Shunt Infection. The most common organism causing infection of CSF shunts is coagulase-negative staphylococcus.[153] In one series, close to 50% of the infections were caused by *S. epidermidis*.[153] The diagnosis often depends on the type of shunt; patients with ventriculoatrial shunts usually have bacteremia while those with ventriculoperitoneal shunts most often have peritonitis. The signs and symptoms may be only low-grade temperature and shunt malfunction. Examination of the spinal fluid is important, but pleocytosis is usually mild. In general, shunt removal is required to cure infection.

8.1.17. Pyomyositis. *S. aureus* can infect a single muscle or less commonly several muscles in healthy young men or boys in tropical climates. Fever, muscle pain and swelling, and leukocytosis are common. Bacteremia can occur. Drainage and antibiotic therapy are usually effective.[15]

8.1.18. Meningitis. Approximately 1–9% of bacterial meningitis is caused by *S. aureus* in published studies.[132] Newborn infants, either premature or low birth weight, and CNS disorders, as well as endocarditis (in predominantly intravenous drug abusers) appear to predispose to staphylococcal meningitis.[132]

8.2. Diagnosis

Because of the multiplicity of manifestations, there are no pathognomonic features that allow one to establish a diagnosis of staphylococcal infection immediately. There are, however, certain epidemiological, clinical, and laboratory features that help to establish the diagnosis or to raise suspicion. Outbreaks of nursery infections or postoperative surgical wound infections generally are caused by staphylococci; recovery of the causative organism and identification of an individual who may be responsible for shedding the organism should be considered promptly. Heroin addicts appear particularly prone to staphylococcal infections, and this organism should be considered when such patients present with fever. Other groups of patients such as diabetics, patients with hematological malignancies, and patients with granulocytopenia appear particularly prone to staphylococcal infections. Skin manifestations of the scalded-skin syndrome may be sufficient to establish a diagnosis of staphylococcal infection. Ultimately, however, with rare exceptions, the definitive diagnosis of staphylococcal infection depends on isolating the organism (or visualizing it by Gram stain) from pus or other body tissues and fluids. Measurement of antibodies to teichoic acid[103] may be helpful in the diagnosis of severe staphylococcal infections when organisms cannot be recovered; however, this is not helpful in rapid diagnosis, since time must be allowed for antibody formation in the host.

9. Control and Prevention

The basic concept in control and prevention of staphylococcal infection is to minimize contact with persons with active lesions.[76] In the hospital setting, isolation of the patient with a lesion best serves this purpose. Strict enforcement of hand-washing for anyone coming in contact with the patient or dressings from the patient is necessary. Hospital personnel with active lesions should be removed from patient contact. Other measures that are effective and necessary include avoiding the use of unnecessary antibiotics, minimizing intravenous therapy and tracheotomy use when possible, and judicious use of therapeutic agents that alter host resistance.

Control measures based on routine surveillance are of demonstrated value in the hospital. Patients with disease must first have cultures made from infected sites to determine the presence of *S. aureus*. Thus, the laboratory serves as the point from which surveillance begins.[39] After the nosocomial infection rate is determined, increases from this baseline rate need close investigation to determine whether a problem exists and whether action need be taken.

In the nursery, where the umbilical cord serves[58] as a reservoir for *S. aureus,* attempts to reduce colonization have evolved over time. Initially, prophylactic antibiotics were tried, but their use fostered selection of resistant staphylococci.[39] Hexachlorophene skin care, while effective,[48] was deemed unsafe for extensive routine use.[61] Attempts to use the staphylococcal strain 502A to colonize the infants and thereby "block" colonization with virulent strains of staphylococci were successful,[86] except that the 502A strain itself was subsequently shown to be a cause of disease in some patients.[8,10] Bacitracin ointment has been used to abort outbreaks and has been tried routinely with success,[61,72] as has the application of triple dye (brilliant green, proflavin hemisulfate, and crystal violet) to the umbilicus.[47]

Prophylactic antibiotics used in certain surgical procedures may prevent *S. aureus* infection. Their use is justified only in circumstances where *S. aureus* infection rates are unacceptably high or where infection may not be cured once present. Examples of such circumstances are cardiac surgery with prosthetic valve insertion, CSF shunt insertion, and prosthetic joint placement. Narrow-spectrum agents such as a semisynthetic penicillin during the intraoperative period and for a short time following surgery seem reasonable in such circumstances, although the effectiveness of this practice has not been shown in controlled trials.

Surveillance of intravenous catheter-related infection and septicemia is worthwhile for infections with both coagulase-positive and -negative staphylococci. Several studies with indwelling catheters in immunocompromised patients or patients with malignancy indicate that Hickman or Broviac catheters should have infection rates of less than 0.15/100 catheter days.[121] Review of procedures, when catheter rates exceed this desired goal or if a single infecting strain appears to be increasing in frequency, is indicated.

Prevention of infection due to coagulase-negative staphylococcus at sites other than intravenous catheters involves adherence to basic principles of infection control. Reducing the occurrence of bacterial contamination during surgery by precise and gentle technique is of critical import in lowering the incidence of endocarditis and septic joints in which foreign bodies are in place. The role of antimicrobial prophylaxis is not clear and deserves further study in controlled prospective trials.

10. Unresolved Problems

Despite many years of intensive work toward control of *S. aureus,* there are numerous areas for continued investigation. Factors related to the host or organism itself that make for chronic as opposed to transient carriage remain undefined. We still do not know the rates of endogenous infection among transient compared with persistent carriers outside the hospital setting. Studies of well-defined populations are needed to assess whether sex differences exist for rates of *S. aureus* disease. With new ways to treat formerly fatal diseases, we need ongoing studies to define additional populations at high risk for serious *S. aureus* disease.

Our understanding of natural and acquired immunity to *S. aureus* is sorely lacking when compared to our understanding of other bacterial pathogens. What is lacking in the "normal" child that allows for disseminated *S. aureus* infection? Conversely, in the "normal" adult, why is disseminated disease so infrequent? If mortality from *S. aureus* is to be reduced in the high-risk population already defined, further means need to be identified that could either reduce exposure to *S. aureus* or immunize against this pathogen. The use of autogenous vaccines and toxoids has not been proven to be effective. Immunization will probably remain only a prospect until determination of the specific fraction(s) of the organism needed to immunize for protection is achieved.

As more is learned about the toxins causing toxic shock syndrome, the development of a toxoid vaccine would seem worthwhile.

A major problem with *S. epidermidis* is determining whether the organism, when isolated from blood, is a true pathogen or a contaminant. If one looks at all patients in hospitals, only about 5 to 10% of individuals having one or more blood cultures positive for coagulase-negative staphylococci have a "true" clinically significant episode of bacteremia.[135] In contrast, in patients who are immunocompromised or have malignancies with indwelling intravenous catheters, the likelihood that a blood culture growing *S. epidermidis* represents significant clinical infection is substantially higher. The availability of sensitive, specific, inexpensive, and easily performed typing systems for coagulase-negative staphylococci could be of help to the clinical microbiology laboratory, to clinicians, and to infec-

tion control personnel trying to contain the spread of nosocomial infection caused by these organisms.

A second major problem with *S. epidermidis* is determining optimal antimicrobial therapy. Many of these organisms are resistant to multiple different antibiotics and often the clinician is left with only vancomycin to use as treatment. The precise role of the addition of rifampin is not clear and further controlled studies are needed to determine whether addition of this agent truly improves the outcome of infection with *S. epidermidis.*

11. References

1. ALTEMIER, W., Current infection problems in surgery, in: *Proceedings of the International Conference on Nosocomial Infections* (P. S. BRACHMAN AND T. C. EICKHOFF, eds.), pp. 82–87, Waverly Press, Baltimore, 1971.
2. ARCHER, G. L., Staphylococcus epidermidis and other coagulase-negative staphylococci, in: *Principles and Practices of Infectious Diseases* (G. L. MANDELL, R. G. DOUGLAS, AND J. E. BENNETT, eds.), pp. 1117–1123, Wiley, New York, 1985.
3. ARMSTRONG-ESTHER, C. A., AND SMITH, J. E., Carriage patterns of *Staphylococus aureus* in a healthy non-hospital population of adults and children, *Ann. Hum. Biol.* **3**(3):221–227 (1976).
4. ARTZ, C. P., AND MONCRIEF, J. A., *The Treatment of Burns,* Saunders, Philadelphia, 1969.
5. BARRY, A. L., AND BADAL, R. E., Reliability of the microdilution technic for detection of methicillin-resistant strains of *Staphylococus aureus, Am. J. Clin. Pathol.* **67**:489–495 (1977).
6. BARTLETT, J. G., ONDERDONK, A. B., DRUDE, E., GOLDSTEIN, C., ALPERT, S., AND McCORMACK, W. M., Quantitative bacteriology of the vaginal flora, *J. Infect. Dis.* **136**:271–277 (1977).
7. BAYSTON, R., AND PENNY, S., Excessive production of mucoid substance in staphylococcus SIIA, a possible factor in colonization of Holter shunts, *Dev. Med. Child. Neurol.* **14**:25–28 (1972).
8. BENNETT, J. V., SHULMAN, J. A., ROSENSTEIN, B. J., TREMBATH, B. J., EICKHOFF, T. C., AND BORING, J. R., Staphylococcal interference studies, *Am. J. Epidemiol.* **88**:410–421 (1968).
9. BIBEL, D. J., GREENBERG, J. H., AND COOK, J. L., *Staphylococcus aureus* and the microbial ecology of atopic dermatitis, *Can. J. Microbiol.* **23**:1062–1068 (1977).
10. BLAIR, E. B., AND TULL, A. H., Multiple infections among newborns resulting from colonization with *Staphylococcus aureus* 502A, *Am. J. Clin. Pathol.* **52**:42–49 (1969).
11. BLAIR, J. E., AND WILLIAMS, R. E. O., Phage typing of staphylococci, *Bull. WHO* **24**:771–784 (1961).

12. Bonventre, P. F., Weckbach, L., Staneck, J., Schlievert, P. M., and Thompson, M., Production of staphylococcal enterotoxin F and pyrogenic exotoxin C by *Staphylococcus aureus* isolates from toxic shock syndrome-associated sources, *Infect. Immun.* **40**:1023–1029 (1983).

13. Breckenridge, J., and Bergdoll, M., Outbreak of food-borne gastroenteritis due to coagulase-negative entero-toxin producing staphylococcus, *N. Engl. J. Med.* **284**:541–543 (1971).

14. Brenner, E. R., and Bryan, C. S., Nosocomial bacteremia in perspective: A community-wide study, *Infect. Control* **2**:219–226 (1981).

15. Brown, J. D., and Wheeler, B., Pyomyositis, report of 18 cases in Hawaii, *Arch. Intern. Med.* **144**:1749–1751 (1984).

16. Burke, J. F., Identification of the sources of staphylococci contaminating the surgical wound during operation, *Ann. Surg.* **158**:898–904 (1963).

17. Caswell, H. T., Groschel, D., Rogers, F. B., Learner, N., Schreck, K. M., and Schuman, C. R., A ten year study of staphylococcal disease: Surveillance, control, and prevention of hospital infections, 1956 to 1965, *Arch. Environ. Health* **17**:221–224 (1968).

18. Centers for Disease Control, *National Nosocomial Infections Study Report,* No. 78-8257, February, 1978.

19. Charnley, J., and Eftehkar, N., Postop infection in total prosthetic replacement of hip joint, *Br. J. Surg.* **56**:641–649 (1969).

20. Christensen, G. D., Simpson, W. A., Bisno, A. L., and Beachey, E. H., Adherence of slime-producing strains of *Staphylococcus epidermidis* to smooth surfaces, *Infect. Immun.* **37**:318–326 (1982).

21. Christensen, G. D., Bisno, A. L., Parisi, J. T., McLaughlin, G., Hester, M. G., and Luther, R. W., Nosocomial septicemia due to multiple antibiotic-resistant *Staphylococcus epidermidis*, *Ann. Intern. Med.* **96**:1–10 (1982).

22. Cluff, L. E., Reynolds, R. C., Page, D. L., and Breckenridge, J. L., Staphylococcal bacteremia: Demographic, clinical and microbiological features of 185 cases, *Trans. Am. Clin. Climatol. Assoc.* **79**:205–213 (1967).

23. Cluff, L. E., Reynolds, R. C., Page, D. L., and Breckenridge, J. L., Staphylococcal bacteremia and altered host resistance, *Ann. Intern. Med.* **69**:859–873 (1968).

24. Courter, R. D., and Galton, M. M., Animal staphylococcal infections and their public health significance, *Am. J. Public Health* **52**:1818–1827 (1962).

25. Davenport, D. S., Massanari, R. M., Pfaller, M. A., Bale, M. J., Streed, S. A., and Hierholzer, W. J., Jr., Usefulness of a test for slime production as a marker for clinically significant infections with coagulase-negative staphylococci, *J. Infect. Dis.* **153**:332–339 (1986).

26. Dillon, H. C., Impetigo contagiosa: Suppurative and non-suppurative complications. I. Clinical, bacteriologic and epidemiologic characteristics of impetigo, *Am. J. Dis. Child.* **115**:530–541 (1968).

27. Dillon, H. C., Impetigo, in: *Communicable and Infectious Diseases* (F. H. Top, Sr., and P. F. Wehrle, eds.), pp. 362–368, Mosby, St. Louis, 1976.

28. Dismukes, W. E., Karchmer, A. W., Buckley, M. J., Austen, W. G., and Swartz, M. N., Prosthetic valve endocarditis: Analysis of 38 cases, *Circulation* **48**:365–377 (1973).

29. Drake, C. T., Goldman, E., Nichols, R. L., Piatruszka, K., and Nyhus, L. M., Environmental air and airborne infections, *Ann. Surg.* **185**:219–223 (1977).

30. Drew, W. L., Barry, A. L., O'Toole, R., and Sherris, J. C., Reliability of the Kirby–Bauer disc diffusion method for detecting methicillin-resistant strains of *Staphylococcus aureus*, *Appl. Microbiol.* **24**:240–247 (1972).

31. Echeverria, P., and Vaughn, M. C., "Tropical pyomyositis," a diagnostic problem in temporate climates, *Am. J. Dis. Child.* **129**:856–857 (1975).

32. Eichenwald, H. F., Kotsevalov, O., and Fasso, L. A., The "cloud baby"—An example of bacterial–viral synergism, *Am. J. Dis. Child.* **100**:161–173 (1960).

33. Ekstedt, R. D., Immunity to the staphylococci, in: *The Staphylococci* (J. O. Cohen, ed.), pp. 385–418, Wiley, New York, 1972.

34. Elek, S. D., *Staphylococcus pyogenes,* Livingstone, London, 1959.

35. Elek, S. D., and Conen, P. E., The virulence of *Staphylococcus pyogenes* for man: A study of the problems of wound infection, *Br. J. Exp. Pathol.* **38**:573–586 (1957).

36. Elhag, K. M., Mustafa, A. K., and Sethi, S. K., Septicemia in a teaching hospital in Kuwait. 1. Incidence and aetiology, *J. Infect.* **10**:17–24 (1985).

37. Espinosa, H., Palmer, D. L., Kisch, A. L., Ulrich, J., Eberle, B., and Reed, W. P., Clinical and immunologic response to bacteria isolated from tracheal secretions following tracheostomy, *J. Thorac. Cardiovasc. Surg.* **68**:432–439 (1974).

38. Farrer, S., and MacLeod, C. M., Staphylococcal infections in a general hospital, *Am. J. Hyg.* **72**:38–58 (1960).

39. Fekety, F. F., The epidemiology and prevention of staphylococcal infection, *Medicine* **43**:593–613 (1964).

40. Finland, M., Changing ecology of bacterial infections as related to antibacterial therapy, *J. Infect. Dis.* **122**:419-431 (1970).

41. Finland, M., Changing patterns of susceptibility of common bacterial pathogens to antimicrobial agents, *Ann. Intern. Med.* **76**:1009–1036 (1972).

42. Finland, M., Excursions into epidemiology: Selected studies during the past four decades at Boston City Hospital, *J. Infect. Dis.* **128**:76–124 (1973).

43. Finland, M., Peterson, O. L., and Strauss, E., Staphylococcal pneumonia occurring during an epidemic of influenza, *Arch. Intern. Med.* **70**:183–205 (1942).

44. Fisher, A. M., Trever, R. W., Curtin, J. A., Schulze, G., and Miller, D. F., Staphylococcal pneumonia: A review of 21 cases in adults, *N. Engl. J. Med.* **258**:919–928 (1958).

45. FORSE, R. A., DIXON, C., BERNARD, N., MARTINEZ, L., MCLEAN, A. P., AND MEAKINS, J. L., *Staphylococcus epidermidis:* An important pathogen, *Surgery* **86:**507–514 (1979).

46. FRANSON, T. R., SHETH, N. U., MENON, L., AND SOHNLE, P. G., Persistent in vitro survival of coagulase-negative staphylococci adherent to intravascular catheters in the absence of conventional nutrients, *J. Clin. Microbiol.* **24:**559–561 (1986).

47. GLASGOW, L. A., AND OVERALL, J. C., Infections of the newborn, in: *Nelson Textbook of Pediatrics* (V. C. VAUGHAN, R. J. MCKAY, R. E. BEHRMAN, AND W. E. NELSON, eds.), pp. 468–475, Saunders, Philadelphia, 1979.

48. GLUCK, L., AND WOOD, H. F., Staphylococcal colonization in newborn infants with and without antiseptic skin care, *N. Engl. J. Med.* **268:**1265–1268 (1963).

49. GRAY, E. D., PETERS, G., VERSTEGEN, M., AND REGELMANN, W. E., Effect of extracellular slime substance from *Staphylococcus epidermidis* on the human cellular immune response, *Lancet* **1:**365–367 (1984).

50. HASSAM, Z. A., SHAW, E. J., SHOOTER, R. A., AND CARO, D. B., Changes in antibiotic sensitivity in strains of *Staphylococcus aureus,* 1952–78, *Br. Med. J.* **2:**536–537 (1978).

51. HIEBER, J. P., NELSON, A. J., AND MCCRACKEN, G. H., Acute disseminated staphylococcal disease in childhood, *Am. J. Dis. Child.* **131:**181–185 (1977).

52. HORDER, J., AND HORDER, E., Illness in general practice, *Practitioner* **173:**177–187 (1954).

53. HORN, C. V., AND MASTER, S., Pyomyositis tropicans in Uganda, *East. Afr. Med. J.* **45:**463–471 (1968).

54. HOVELIUS, B., AND MARDH, P., *Staphylococcus saprophyticus* as a common cause of urinary tract infections, *Rev. Infect. Dis.* **6:**328–337 (1984).

55. HUNTER, G., AND DANDY, D., The natural history of the patient with an infected total hip replacement, *J. Bone Jt. Surg.* **59B:**293–297 (1977).

56. JACKSON, L. J., SOTTILE, M. I., AGUILAR-TORRES, F. G., DEE, T. H., AND RYTEL, M. W., Correlation of antistaphylococcal antibody titers with severity of staphylococcal disease, *Am. J. Med.* **64:**629–633 (1978).

57. JACOB, E., DURHAM, L. C., FALK, M. C., WILLIAMS, T. J., AND WHEAT, L. J., Antibody response to teichoic acid and peptidoglycan in *Staphylococcus aureus* osteomyelitis, *J. Clin. Microbiol.* **25:**122–127 (1987).

58. JELLARD, J., Umbilical cord as a reservoir of infection in a maternity hospital, *Br. Med. J.* **1:**925–928 (1957).

59. JESSEN, O., ROSENDAL, K., BULOW, P., FABER, V., AND ERIKSEN, K. R., Changing staphylococci and staphylococcal infections: A ten-year study of bacteria and cases of bacteremia, *N. Engl. J. Med.* **281:**627–635 (1969).

60. JOHNSON, G. M., LEE, D. A., REGELMANN, W. E., GRAY, E. D., PETERS, G., AND QUIE, P. G., Interference with granulocyte function by *Staphylococcus epidermidis* slime, *Infect. Immun.* **54:**13–20 (1986).

61. JOHNSON, J. D., MALACHOWSKI, N. C., VOSTI, K. L., AND

SUNSHINE, P., A sequential study of various modes of skin and umbilical care and the incidence of staphylococcal colonization and infection in the neonate, *Pediatrics* **58:**354–361 (1976).

62. JOHNSON, J. E., CLUFF, L. E., AND GOSHI, K., Studies on the pathogenesis of staphylococcal infection. I. The effect of repeated skin infections, *J. Exp. Med.* **113:**235–270 (1961).

63. JORGENSEN, J. H., Laboratory and epidemiologic experience with methicillin-resistant *Staphylococcus aureus* in the USA, *Eur. J. Clin. Microbiol.* **5:**693–696 (1986).

64. KAHLER, R. C., BOYCE, J. M., BERGDOLL, M. S., LOCKWOOD, W. R., AND TAYLOR, M. R., Case report: Toxic shock syndrome associated with TSST-1 producing coagulase-negative staphylococci, *Am. J. Med. Sci.* **292:**310–312 (1986).

65. KARCHMER, A. W., ARCHER, G. L., AND DISMUKES, W. E., *Staphylococcus epidermidis* prosthetic valve endocarditis: Microbiological and clinical observations as guides to therapy, *Ann. Intern. Med.* **98:**447–455 (1987).

66. KAY, C. R., Sepsis in the home, *Br. Med. J.* **1:**1048–1052 (1962).

67. KAYE, D., Infecting microorganisms, in: *Infective Endocarditis* (D. KAYE, ed.), p. 43, University Park Press, Baltimore, 1976.

68. KAYSER, F. H., Methicillin-resistant staphylococci 1965–75, *Lancet* **2:**650–652 (1975).

69. KAYSER, F. H., AND MAK, T. M., Methicillin-resistant staphylococci, *Am. J. Med. Sci.* **264:**197–205 (1972).

70. KEENE, W. R., MINCHEW, B. H., AND CLUFF, L. E., Studies of the epidemiology of staphylococcal infection. III. Clinical factors in susceptibility to staphylococcal disease, *N. Engl. J. Med.* **269:**332–337 (1963).

71. KILTON, L. J., FOSSIECK, B. E., COHEN, M. H., AND PARKER, R. H., Bacteremia due to gram-positive cocci in patients with neoplastic disease, *Am. J. Med.* **66:**596–602 (1979).

72. KLAINER, L. M., AGRAWAL, H. S., MORTIMER, E. A., AND WOLINSKY, E., Bacitracin ointment and neonatal staphylococci, *Am. J. Dis. Child.* **103:**546–568 (1962).

73. KLIMEK, J. J., MARSIK, F. J., BARTLETT, R. C., WEIR, B., SHEA, P., AND QUINTILIANI, R., Clinical epidemiologic and bacteriologic observations of an outbreak of methicillin-resistant *Staphylococcus aureus* at a large community hospital, *Am. J. Med.* **61:**340–345 (1976).

74. KLOOS, W. E., AND SMITH, P. B., Staphylococci, in: *Manual of Clinical Microbiology* (E. H. LENNETT, W. J. HAUSLER, JR., AND J. P. TRUANT, eds.), pp. 83–87, American Society for Microbiology, Washington, D.C., 1980.

75. KLUGE, R. M., CALIA, F. M., MCLAUGHLIN, J. S., AND HORNICK, R. B., Sources of contamination in open heart surgery, *J. Am. Med. Assoc.* **230:**1415–1418 (1974).

76. KOENIG, M. G., Staphylococcal infections—Treatment and control, *Dis. Mon.* pp. 2–36 (April 1968).

77. KOENIG, M. G., The phagocytosis of staphylococci, in: *The Staphylococci* (J. O. COHEN, ed.), pp. 365–383, Wiley, New York, 1972.

78. LACEY, R. W., Genetic basis, epidemiology, and future sig-

nificance of antibiotic resistance in *Staphylococcus aureus, J. Clin. Pathol.* **26:**899–913 (1973).

79. LADISCH, S., AND PIZZO, P. A., *Staphylococcus aureus* sepsis in children with cancer, *Pediatrics* **61:**231–234 (1978).
80. LEAKE, D., AND LEAKE, R., Neonatal suppurative parotitis, *Pediatrics* **46:**203–207 (1970).
81. LEAKE, D. L., KRAKOWIAK, F. J., AND LEAKE, R. C., Suppurative parotitis in children, *Oral Surg.* **31:**174–179 (1971).
82. LENHART, N., AND MUDD, S., Staphylococcidal capability of rabbit peritoneal macrophages in relation to infection and elicitation: Delayed-type hypersensitivity without increased resistance, *Infect. Immun.* **5:**757–762 (1971).
83. LEVIN, M. J., GARDNER, P., AND WOLDVOGEL, F. A., "Tropical" pyomyositis: An unusual infection due to *Staphylococcus aureus, N. Engl. J. Med.* **284:**196–198 (1971).
84. LEWIS, J. F., BRAKE, S. R., ANDERSON, D. J., AND VREDEVELD, G. N., Urinary tract infection due to coagulase-negative staphylococcus, *Am. J. Clin. Pathol.* **77:**736–739 (1982).
85. LIDWELL, O. M., BROCK, B., SHOOTER, R. A., COOKE, E. M., AND THOMAS, G. E., Airborne infection in a fully air-conditioned hospital. IV. Airborne dispersal of *Staphylococcus aureus* and its nasal acquisition by patients, *J. Hyg.* **75:**445–474 (1975).
86. LIGHT, I. J., WALTON, R. L., SUTHERLAND, J. M., SHINEFIELD, H. R., AND BRACKVOGEL, V., Use of bacterial interference to control a staphylococcal nursery outbreak, *Am. J. Dis. Child.* **113:**291–300 (1967).
87. LINNEMANN, C. C., MASON, M., MOORE, P., KORFHAGEN, T. R., AND STANECK, J. L., Methicillin-resistant *Staphylococcus aureus:* Experience in a general hospital over four years, *Am. J. Epidemiol.* **115:**941–950 (1982).
88. LINNEMANN, C. C., MCKEE, E., AND LAVER, M. C., Staphylococcal infections in a hemodialysis unit, *Am. J. Med. Sci.* **276:**67–75 (1978).
89. LOURIA, D. B., Infectious complications of nonalcoholic drug abuse, *Annu. Rev. Med.* **25:**219–232 (1974).
90. MACDONALD, K. L., OSTERHOLM, M. T., HEDBERG, C. W., SCHROCH, C. G., PETERSON, G. F., JENTZEN, J. M., LEONARD, S. A., AND SCHLIEVERT, P. M., Toxic shock syndrome: a newly recognized complication of influenza and influenzalike illness, *J. Am. Med. Assoc.* **257:**1053–1058 (1987).
91. MAKI, D., GOLDMAN, D., AND RHAME, F., Infection control in intravenous therapy, *Ann. Intern. Med.* **79:**867–887 (1973).
92. MALTMAN, J. R., ORR, J. H., AND HINTON, N. A., The effect of desiccation on *Staphylococcus pyogenes* with special reference to implications concerning virulence, *Am. J. Hyg.* **72:**335–342 (1960).
93. MARTIN, R. R., DAUGHARTY, H., AND WHITE, A., Staphylococcal antibodies and hypersensitivity to teichoic acids in man, in: *Antimicrobial Agents and Chemotherapy—1965* (G. L. HOBBY, ed.), pp. 91–96, American Society for Microbiology, Washington, D.C., 1966.
94. MCGOWEN, J. E., BARNES, M. W., AND FINLAND, M., Bacteremia at Boston City Hospital: Occurrence and mortality during 12 selected years (1953–1972), with special reference to hospital acquired cases, *J. Infect. Dis.* **132:**316–335 (1975).
95. MCGOWEN, J. E., PARROTT, P. L., AND DUTY, V. P., Nosocomial bacteremia: Potential for prevention of procedure-related cases, *J. Am. Med. Assoc.* **237:**2727–2729 (1977).
96. MCGREGOR, R. M., The work of a family doctor, *Edinburgh Med. J.* **57:**433–453 (1950).
97. MELISH, M., AND GLASGOW, L., Staphylococcal scalded skin syndrome: The expanded clinical syndrome, *J. Pediatr.* **78:**958–967 (1971).
98. MILES, A. A., Non-specific defense reactions in bacterial infections, *Ann. N.Y. Acad. Sci.* **66:**356–369 (1956).
99. MONTGOMERIE, J. Z., KALMANSON, G. M., AND GUSE, L. B., Renal failure and infection, *Medicine* **47:**1–32 (1968).
100. *Morbidity and Mortality Weekly Report,* **29:**229–230, 297–299, 441–445, 495–496 (1980).
101. MORSE, S. I., Pathogenesis of staphylococcal infections, in: *Symposium on New Approaches for Inducing Natural Immunity to Pyogenic Organisms* (J. B. ROBBINS, R. E. HORTON, AND R. M. KRAUSE, eds.), pp. 131–136, DHEW Publ. 74-553, Washington, D.C., 1973.
102. MUSHER, D. M., AND MCKENZIE, S. O., Infections due to *Staphylococcus aureus, Medicine* **56:**383–409 (1977).
103. NAGEL, J. G., TUAZON, C. U., CARDELLA, T. A., AND SHEAGREN, J. N., Teichoic acid serologic diagnosis of staphylococcal endocarditis: Use of gel diffusion and counterimmunoelectrophoretic methods, *Ann. Intern. Med.* **82:**13–17 (1975).
104. NAGEL, J. G., SHEAGREN, J. N., TUAZON, C. U., AND CARDELLA, T. A., Teichoic acids in pathogenic *Staphylococcus aureus, J. Clin. Microbiol.* **6:**233–237 (1977).
105. NAHMIAS, A. J., AND EICKHOFF, T. C., Staphylococcal infections in hospitals: Recent developments in epidemiologic and laboratory investigation, *N. Engl. J. Med.* **265:**74–81, 120–128, 177–182 (1961).
106. NAHMIAS, A. J., AND SCHULMAN, J. A., Epidemiologic aspects and control methods, in: *The Staphylococci* (J. O. COHEN, ed.), pp. 483–502, Wiley, New York, 1972.
107. NAHMIAS A., SAKURAI, N., BLUMBERG, R., DOEGE, A., AND SULZER, C., The staphylococcus "80/81 complex": Epidemiological and laboratory observations, *J. Infect. Dis.* **109:**211–222 (1961).
108. NAHMIAS, A. J., LEPPER, M. H., HURST, V., AND MUDD, S., Epidemiology and treatment of chronic staphylococcal infections in the household, *Am. J. Public Health* **52:**1828–1843 (1962).
109. NOLAN, C. M., AND BEATY, H. N., *Staphylococcus aureus* bacteremia: Current clinical patterns, *Am. J. Med.* **60:**495–500 (1976).
110. NSOULI, K. A., LAZARUS, J. M., SCHOENBAUM, S. C., GOTTLIEB, M. N., LOWRIE, E. G., AND SCHOCAIR, M., Bac-

teremic infection in hemodialysis, *Arch. Intern. Med.* **139:**1255–1258 (1979).

111. OGSTON, A., Report upon microorganisms in surgical diseases, *Br. Med. J.* **1:**369–375 (1881).

112. O'TOOLE, R. D., DREW, L. D., DAHLGREN, B. J., AND BEATY, H. N., An outbreak of methicillin-resistant *Staphylococcus aureus* infection: Observations in hospital and nursing home, *J. Am. Med. Assoc.* **213:**257–263 (1970).

113. PARKER, M. T., AND LAPAGE, S. P., Penicillinase production by *Staphylococcus aureus* strains from outbreaks of food poisoning, *J. Clin. Pathol.* **10:**313–317 (1957).

114. PARSONNET, J., HARRISON, A. E., SPENCER, S. E., READING, A., PARSONNET, K. C., AND KASS, E. H., Nonproduction of toxic shock syndrome toxin 1 by coagulase-negative staphylococci, *J. Clin. Microbiol.* **25:**1370–1372 (1987).

115. PETERS, G., LOCCI, R., AND PULVERER, G., Adherence and growth of coagulase-negative staphylococci on surfaces of intravenous catheters, *J. Infect. Dis.* **146:**479–482 (1982).

116. PETERSDORF, R. G., FORSYTH, B. R., AND BERNANKI, D., Staphylococcal parotitis, *N. Engl. J. Med.* **259:**1250–1254 (1958).

117. PETERSON, P. K., MATZKE, G., AND KEANE, W. F., Current concepts in the management of peritonitis in patients undergoing continuous ambulatory peritoneal dialysis, *Rev. Infect. Dis.* **9:**604–612 (1987).

118. PHAIR, J. P., WATANAKUNAKORN, C., GOLDBERG, L., AND CARLETON, J., Ecology of staphylococci in a general medical service, *Appl. Microbiol.* **24:**967–971 (1973).

119. PLORDE, J. J., AND SHERRIS, J. C., Staphylococcal resistance to antibiotics: Origin, measurement, and epidemiology, *Ann. N.Y. Acad. Sci.* **236:**413–434 (1974).

120. PONCE DE LEON, S., AND WENZEL, R. P., Hospital acquired bloodstream infections with *Staphylococcus epidermidis*. Review of 100 cases, *Am. J. Med.* **77:**639–644 (1984).

121. PRESS, O. W., RAMSEY, P. G., LARSON, E. B., FEFER, A., AND HICKMAN, R. O., Hickman catheter infections in patients with malignancies, *Medicine* **63:**189–200 (1984).

122. PURSER, B. N., Fatal staphylococcal infections, *Med. J. Aust.* **2:**441–443 (1958).

123. QUIE, P. G., Infections due to neutrophil malfunction, *Medicine* **52:**411–417 (1973).

124. QUIE, P. G., HILL, H. R., AND DAVIS, A. T., Defective phagocytosis of staphylococci, *Ann. N.Y. Acad. Sci.* **236:**233–243 (1974).

125. REINGOLD, A. L., DAN, B. B., SHANDS, K. N., AND BROOME, C. V., Toxic-shock syndrome not associated with menstruation, *Lancet* **1:**1–4 (1982).

126. ROBBINS, R. N., REISIER, R. F., HEHL, G. L., AND BERGDOLL, M. S., Production of toxic shock syndrome toxin 1 by *Staphylococcus aureus* as determined by tampon disk–membrane–agar method, *J. Clin. Microbiol.* **25:**1446–1449 (1987).

127. ROSENBACH, F. J., *Mikroorganismen bei den Wundinfections-krankheiten des Menschen*, Bergmann, Wiesbaden, 1884.

128. ROSENDAL, K., BULOW, P., BENTZON, M. W., AND ERIKSON, K. R., *Staphylococcus aureus* strains isolated in Danish hospitals from January 1st, 1966, to December 31st, 1974, *Acta Pathol. Microbiol. Scand. Sect. B* **84:**359–368 (1976).

129. SCHAEFLER, S., JONES, D., PERRY, W., BARADET, T., MAYR, E., AND RAMPERSAD, C., Methicillin-resistant *Staphylococcus aureus* strains in New York City hospitals: Interhospital spread of resistant strains of type 88, *J. Clin. Microbiol.* **20:**536–538 (1984).

130. SCHECKLER, W. E., Septicemia in a community hospital 1970 through 1973, *J. Am. Med. Assoc.* **237:**1938–1941 (1977).

131. SCHECKLER, W. E., Nosocomial infections in a community hospital, 1972 through 1976, *Arch. Intern. Med.* **138:**1792–1794 (1978).

132. SCHLESINGER, L. S., ROSS, S. C., AND SCHABERG, D. R., *Staphylococcus aureus* meningitis: A broad-based epidemiologic study, *Medicine* **66:**148–156 (1987).

133. SCHOPFER K., BAERLOCHER, K., PRICE, P., KRECH, U., QUIE, P. G., AND DOUGLAS, S. D., Staphylococcal IgE antibodies, hyperglobulinemia E and *Staphylococcus aureus* infections, *N. Engl. J. Med.* **300:**835–838 (1979).

134. SCHOPFER, K., DOUGLAS, S. D., AND WILKINSON, B. J., Immunoglobulin E antibodies against *Staphylococcus aureus* cell walls in the sera of patients with hyperimmunoglobulin E and recurrent staphylococcal infection, *Infect. Immun.* **27:**563–568 (1980).

135. SHEAGREN, J. N., Significance of blood culture isolates of *Staphylococcus epidermidis*, *Arch. Intern. Med.* **147:**635 (1987).

136. SHETH, N. K., FRANSON, T. R., AND SOHNLE, P. G., Influence of bacterial adherence to intravascular catheters on in vitro antibiotic susceptibility, *Lancet* **2:**1266–1268 (1985).

137. SMITH, J. M. B., AND MARPLES, M. J., A natural reservoir of penicillin-resistant strains of *Staphylococcus aureus*, *Nature* **201:**844 (1964).

138. SPERS, R., SHOOTER, R. A., GAYA, H., PATEL, N., AND HEWITT, J. H., Contamination of nurses' uniforms with *Staphylococcus aureus*, *Lancet* **2:**233–235 (1969).

139. STOKES, E. J., BRADLEY, J. M., THOMPSON, R. E. M., HITCHCOCK, N. M., PARKER, M. J., AND WALKER, J. S., Hospital staphylococci in three London teaching hospitals, *Lancet* **1:**84–88 (1972).

140. TARANTA, A., Lymphocyte mitogens of staphylococcal origin, *Ann. N.Y. Acad. Sci.* **236:**362–375 (1974).

141. THOMPSON, D. J., GEZON, H. M., RODGERS, K. D., YEE, R. B., AND HATCH, T. F., Excess risk of staphylococcal infection and disease in newborn males, *Am. J. Epidemiol.* **84:**314–328 (1966).

142. THORNTON, G. F., FEKETY, F. R., AND CLUFF, L. E., Studies of the epidemiology of staphylococcal infection. VIII. Seasonal variation, *N. Engl. J. Med.* **271:**1333–1337 (1964).

143. TODD, J., AND FISHAUT, M., Toxic-shock syndrome associated with phage-group-I staphylococci, *Lancet* **1:**1116–1118 (1978).

144. TUAZON, C. U., AND SHEAGREN, J. N., Increased rate of carriage of *S. aureus* among narcotic addicts, *J. Infect. Dis.* **129:**725–727 (1974).

145. TUAZON, C. U., AND SHEAGREN, J. N., Staphylococcal endocarditis in parenteral drug abusers: Source of the organism, *Ann. Intern. Med.* **82:**788–791 (1975).

146. TUAZON, C. U., AND SHEAGREN, J. N., Teichoic acid antibodies in the diagnosis of serious infections with *Staphylococcus aureus, Ann. Intern. Med.* **84:**543–546 (1976).

147. TUAZON, C. U., HILL, R., AND SHEAGREN, J. N., The microbiologic study of street heroin and injection paraphernalia, *J. Infect. Dis.* **129:**327–329 (1974).

148. TUAZON, C. U., PEREZ, A., KISHABA, T., AND SHEAGREN, J. N., Increased carrier rate of *Staphylococcus aureus* in insulin-injecting diabetics, *J. Am. Med. Assoc.* **231:**1272 (1975).

149. TUAZON, C. U., SHEAGREN, J. N., CHOA, M. S., MARCUS, D., AND CURTIN, J. A., *Staphylococcus aureus* bacteremia: Relationship between formation of antibodies to teichoic acid and development of metastatic abscess, *J. Infect. Dis.* **137:**57–62 (1978).

150. VERHOEF, J., PETERSON, P. K., KIM, Y., SABATH, L. D., AND QUIE, P. G., Opsonic requirements for staphylococcal phagocytosis: Heterogeneity among strains, *Immunology* **33:**191–197 (1977).

151. WADE, J. C., SCHIMPFF, S. C., NEWMAN, K. A., AND WIERNER, P. H., *Staphylococcus epidermidis:* An increasing cause of infection in patients with granulocytopenia, *Ann. Intern. Med.* **97:**503–508 (1982).

152. WALDVOGEL, F. A., MEDOFF, G., AND SWARTZ, M. N., Osteomyelitis: A review of clinical features, therapeutic considerations and unusual aspects, *N. Engl. J. Med.* **282:**198–206 (1970).

153. WALTERS, B. C., HOFFMAN, H. J., HENDRICK, E. B., AND HUMPHREYS, R. P., Cerebrospinal fluid shunt infection. Influences on initial management and subsequent outcome, *J. Neurosurg.* **60:**1014–1021 (1984).

154. WATANAKUNAKORN, C., AND BAIRD, I. M., *Staphylococcus aureus* bacteremia and endocarditis associated with a removable infected intravenous device, *Am. J. Med.* **63:**253–256 (1977).

155. WELLMAN, W. E., AND SENFT, R. A., Bacterial meningitis. III. Infections caused by *Staphylococcus aureus, Mayo Clin. Proc.* **39:**263–269 (1964).

156. WENTWORTH, B., Bacteriophage typing of the staphylococcus, *Bacteriol. Rev.* **27:**253–272 (1963).

157. WHEAT, L. J., WHITE, A. C., AND NRODEN, C., Serological diagnosis of *Staphylococcus aureus* osteomyelitis, *J. Clin. Microbiol.* **21:**764–767 (1985).

158. WILLIAMS, R. E. O., Healthy carriage of *Staphylococcus aureus:* Its prevalence and importance, *Bacteriol. Rev.* **27:**56–71 (1963).

159. WILLIAMS, R. E. O., Epidemiology of airborne staphylococcal infection, *Bacteriol. Rev.* **30:**660–672 (1966).

160. WILLIAMS, R. E. O., JEVONS, M. P., SHOOTER, R. A., HUNTER, C. J. W., GIRLING, J. A., GRIFFITHS, J. D., AND TAYLOR, G. W., Nasal staphylococci and sepsis in hospital patients, *Br. Med. J.* **2:**658–662 (1959).

161. WOLINSKY, E., LIPSITZ, P. J., MORTIMER, E. A., AND RAMMELKAMP, C. H., Acquisition of staphylococci by newborns: Direct versus indirect transmission, *Lancet* **2:**620–622 (1960).

12. Suggested Reading

ELEK, S. D., *Staphylococcus pyogenes,* Livingstone, London, 1959.

MUSHER, D. M., AND McKENZIE, S. O., Infections due to *Staphylococcus aureus, Medicine* **56:**383–409 (1977).

NOLAN, C. M., AND BEATY, H. N., *Staphylococcus aureus* bacteremia: Current clinical patterns, *Am. J. Med.* **60:**495–500 (1976).

PLORDE, J. J., AND SHERRIS, J. C., Staphylococcal resistance to antibiotics: Origin, measurement, and epidemiology, *Ann. N.Y. Acad. Sci.* **235:**413–434 (1974).

SHEAGREN, J. N., *Staphylococcus aureus,* the persistent pathogen, *N. Engl. J. Med.* **310:**1368–1373, 1437–1442 (1984).

CHAPTER 31

Streptococcal Infections

Barry M. Gray

1. Introduction

The streptococci are a large heterogeneous group of gram-positive spherically shaped bacteria found widely distributed in nature. They include some of the most important agents of human disease, as well as members of the normal human flora. Some streptococci have been associated mainly with disease in animals, while others have been domesticated and used for the culture of buttermilk, yogurt, and certain cheeses. Those known to cause human disease can be thought of as comprising two broad categories: First are the pyogenic streptococci, including the familiar β-hemolytic streptococci and the pneumococcus. These organisms are not generally part of the normal flora but cause acute, often severe, infections in normal hosts. Second are the more diverse enteric and oral streptococci, which are nearly always part of the normal flora and which are more frequently associated with opportunistic infections.

Measured in terms of mortality, morbidity, and economic costs, five streptococcal species are of major importance in human disease. (1) The group A streptococcus, *Streptococcus pyogenes*, produces a wide range of infections, from pharyngitis and impetigo to puerperal sepsis and erysipelas. Their nonsuppurative sequelae include acute rheumatic fever and acute glomerulonephritis. (2) The group B streptococcus, *S. agalactiae,* is currently a leading cause of sepsis in newborn infants and a frequent cause of postpartum infections in mothers. (3) The pneumococcus, *S. pneumoniae,* remains the most frequent cause of bacterial pneumonia in all age groups and is a common agent in otitis media, bacteremia, and meningitis. (4) The enterococcus, now considered to form a separate genus of the same name, is part of the normal bowel flora but has been increasingly isolated as an opportunistic invader. (5) Among the oral streptococci, *S. mutans* is by far the most important as the principal agent of dental caries. This chapter will focus mainly on infections caused by group A and B streptococci and will include current information on pneumococci and other streptococci associated with human disease. Further details on *S. pneumoniae* may be found in Chapter 25 on pneumococcal infections.

2. Historical Background

Streptococcal infections were recognized by Greek physicians by the 3rd century B.C. A description of erysipelas is recorded in *Epidemicus* and attributed to Hippocrates. In the Middle Ages, scarlet fever, or "scarlatina," as it was called in Italy, was an eye-catching and notable disease. Sydenham's description in 1676 clearly differentiated this disease from measles and other rashes, but it was not until 1924 that G.F. and G.H. Dick showed conclusively that streptococci were the causative agents. Until the advent of penicillin, childbed fever, or puerperal sepsis, remained one of the most frequent causes of death among

Barry M. Gray · Department of Pediatrics, University of Alabama School of Medicine, Birmingham, Alabama 35294.

otherwise healthy young women. The classic works of
Holmes, in 1858, and Semmelweiss, in 1861, described the
transmission of this disease and provided guidelines for
effective preventive measures that are still applicable today.
Rheumatic fever was first described by Wells in 1812, and
Bouillaud described the association of acute rheumatism
and heart disease in 1835. In 1836 Bright published his
account of "renal disease accompanied with secretion of
albuminous urine." Thus, the most severe forms of streptococcal disease and their nonsuppurative sequelae were
well known long before the discovery of the bacterium
itself.[159]

In the late 19th century, many investigators contributed
to the understanding of streptococci and their relation to
human disease. By the 1880s many species had been given
names such as *S. epidemicus, S. erysipelatus, S. scar-
latinae,* and *S. rheumaticus,* which reflected different manifestations of streptococcal infection. The name *S. pyogenes*
dates from this period but is probably of less descriptive
value than the term "*S. haemolyticus,*" which was commonly used through the early part of this century. The formal classification of streptococci began when blood agar
came into use and the hemolytic properties of various organisms were noted. In 1919 Brown used the term "beta" to
describe streptococci that produced a 2- to 4-mm zone of
clear hemolysis around colonies grown on blood agar. "Alpha" streptococci were those producing incomplete, green-
ish, hemolysis. Most of the isolates from severe human
disease were β-hemolytic. It was not until 1928, when
Lancefield introduced methods of serotyping streptococci
based upon immunologic reactions with cellular components, that groups and types within groups could be clearly
distinguished. The group antigens were eventually shown to
be specific cell-wall carbohydrates. The group A streptococci were further differentiated by the M and T protein
antigens. The β-hemolytic streptococci from most human
infections proved to be those of group A. Armed with these
new epidemiologic tools, Lancefield and Hare investigated
cases of puerperal sepsis at Queen Charlotte's Hospital in
London, beginning in the early 1930s.[116] Of 46 cases of
postpartum sepsis, all but one isolate was group A, and the
exception was identified as the prototype of a new serologic
group, designated group G. A year earlier, Hare and Cole-
brook observed that hemolytic streptococci resembling
those associated with sepsis were never found in vaginal
cultures of healthy women, but that some women carried
streptococci that resembled those isolated in bovine mastitis. The latter organisms proved to be members of streptococcus group B.[116]

By the late 1930s the group B streptococci were recog-

nized as important, if occasional, pathogens causing postpartum sepsis, amnionitis, endocarditis, and septic abortion.[53,78] The advent of antibiotics, along with better
methods for preventing nosocomial spread, resulted in a
dramatic decline in streptococcal infections on obstetrical
services. At Queen Charlotte's Hospital there were very few
maternal deaths due to either group A or group B streptococci
from 1940 through the mid-1960s.[69] In this same period
there were few cases of neonatal sepsis or meningitis attributed to streptococci of any kind in large series published
in the pediatric literature. It appears unlikely that group B
streptococci went simply unrecognized as perinatal pathogens for over 20 years. Rather, there seems to have been a
real increase in group B disease, beginning in the United
States and Europe during the 1960s.[32,58,94] In New Zealand, Becroft *et al.* examined all neonatal deaths and stillbirths from 1966 to 1974.[16] They reported about a fourfold
increase in group B-related deaths beginning in 1970 and
noted especially the high frequency of congenital pneumonia. By the mid-1970s, numerous reports of group B
disease appeared in the literature, and the group B streptococcus was said to have come of age.[53]

The pneumococcus has an interesting and important
history,[7,125] and the reader is referred to Section 2 of
Chapter 25.

The enterococci, as they were called by Thiercelin in
1899, were noted as a major aerobic component of feces.
Extremely hardy, they grow in bile, at high or low temperatures, in salt, and at high pH. Because of these biologic
characteristics, as well as genetic differences, *S. faecalis*
and *S. faecium* have recently been accorded a separate
genus, *Enterococcus.*[162] These and several new *Enterococcus* species are clearly distinct from the "nonenterococ-
cal" group D streptococci. Enterococci have long been
known as an occasional cause of bacteremia and endocarditis, but in the early 1970s they began to appear with
increasing frequency in reports of bacteremia in obstetric,
trauma, and surgical patients.[89,119] Frequently found in
mixed infections, they were difficult to eradicate and resistant to many conventional antibiotics.

The history of *S. mutans* began in 1924, when Clark
first isolated the organism from human dental caries. It was
another 50 years, however, before the role of *S. mutans* was
established, first in animal models and later in human subjects.[122] Since dental caries are chronic rather than acute
infections and are not directly life-threatening, the global
significance of *S. mutans* has only recently been appreciated. Dental caries, a complex but diagnosable and treatable
infection, is perhaps the most common bacterial infection in
humans.

3. Methodology

3.1. Sources of Mortality Data

There are no reliable sources of mortality data for any of the streptococcal diseases. Cause-of-death coding classifications have been revised about every decade, usually without sufficient details regarding a particular etiologic agent. For example, patients may die of heart failure without rheumatic heart disease being specified; puerperal sepsis may be due to group A or group B streptococci as well as other organisms; pneumococcal pneumonia deaths are frequently counted with those attributed to influenza virus.

3.2. Sources of Morbidity Data

There are likewise no accurate data on morbidity from streptococcal infections. Streptococcal sore throat, scarlet fever, and acute rheumatic fever have been reported only optionally since 1971, with the result that data were deemed so unreliable that the Centers for Disease Control (CDC) no longer tabulates or publishes the data it does receive. Monitoring of recent outbreaks of rheumatic fever by the CDC has been incomplete, and no mechanism for systematic nationwide reporting has yet been adopted. Group B streptococcal disease is also reported on an optional basis. Although CDC workers have tried to estimate the national incidence of early onset neonatal group B streptococcal infections, using birthweight stratification and local incidence rates, their estimate of 7000 cases per year[42] is probably low. The National Academy of Science Institute of Medicine has issued two volumes of reports on new vaccine development, with estimates of disease burden (a combined morbidity and mortality estimate) of major infectious diseases in the United States[43] and in developing countries.[44] Although these sources are helpful and also offer estimates of the economic cost of some of the diseases discussed here, they rely mainly on survey data.

3.3. Surveys

A considerable number of surveys have been published on diseases caused by various streptococcal species. The most informative have been prospective epidemiologic studies, certain family studies, and surveys of defined populations. These will be reviewed in the description of epidemiologic features of specific diseases in Section 5.1.

3.4. Laboratory Diagnosis

The major streptococcal species associated with human disease are listed in Tables 1 and 2, along with selected biologic and clinical features. Our grouping of species is more for convenience than for taxonomic purposes, and various bacteriology textbooks will have different schemes, as well as more detailed information on laboratory methods. The laboratory procedures and the particular approach to identification will of course depend upon whether isolation is for clinical or research purposes and the degree of specificity required.

3.4.1. Isolation and Identification

a. Media and Growth Conditions. Most streptococci grow poorly on ordinary nutrient media but grow quite well on media enriched with blood, brain or heart infusion, serum, or glucose.[60,145] Todd–Hewitt broth is an enriched buffered medium that has become a standard liquid medium for most streptococci. A recently described chemically defined medium gives better growth and is more suitable for use in biochemical studies where extraneous proteins may be a problem.[173] In the United States most laboratories use 5–7% sheep blood agar, whereas in Britain horse blood is generally used. Both give good hemolysis, although with sheep blood it may be necessary to "stab" the agar in the area of inoculation to ensure subsurface growth for the action of oxygen-sensitive hemolysins. While most streptococci grow well in a normal atmosphere, some species, particularly the milleri group and the peptostreptococci, do not show good growth or hemolysis without a reduced oxygen atmosphere. Pneumococci prefer to grow in 5% CO_2 or in a candle jar. Most streptococci grow best at 35 to 37°C, although the enterococci will also grow at 10 and at 45°C.

Selective media are not generally employed for routine isolation of group A streptococci but have been used for some epidemiologic studies. For colonization studies of group B streptococci a selective medium is required to minimize overgrowth of gram-negative organisms and staphylococci in cultures from the lower gastrointestinal and genital tracts. Although some workers have used gentamicin plus nalidixic acid, we have found that the gentamicin inhibits some group B strains and have preferred a medium containing nalidixic acid, polymyxin, and crystal violet.[83] A fairly satisfactory commercially available medium is Columbia CNA agar, which contains colistin and nalidixic acid. For isolation of pneumococci from nasopharyngeal carriers a selective medium is also essential; we have favored blood agar containing 4 mg/liter of gentamicin sulfate.[47] Mouse inoculation, the standard of an earlier era, is seldom used today. The enterococci grow on nearly all con-

Table 1. The Major Streptococcal Species Causing Disease in Humans: The Pyogenic Streptococci

	Species designation	Lancefield group	Hemolysis	Presumptive identification	Definitive identification	Ecologic niche	Normal flora	Association with disease
Group A streptococci	S. pyogenes	A	β	Bacitracin sensitive	M proteins, T proteins, Opacity factor	Oropharynx	No	Pharyngitis, impetigo, erysipelas, bacteremia
Group B streptococci	S. agalactiae	B	β	CAMP test positive	Capsular polysaccharides, c-protein, Bacteriophage	Lower bowel, genital tract	High carrier rate in normal population	Neonatal sepsis, meningitis, postpartum infections, endocarditis, cellulitis
Group C streptococci	S. equisimilis	C	β	"Not A or B"	Bacteriocin	(Swine, humans)	Occasional	Pharyngitis, bacteremia, wound infections, cellulitis often veterinary-related
	S. zooepidemicus	C	β	"Not A or B"	Bacteriophage	(Horses, cattle, other animals)	No	
	S. equi	C	β	"Not A or B"	DNA fingerprint		No	
Group G streptococci	"Large colony" group G	G	β	"Not A or B"	Some with M-12 protein	Pharynx, bowel	Occasional	Pharyngitis, cellulitis, bacteremia
Pneumococci	S. pneumoniae	None (has pneumococcal C-polysaccharide)	α	Optochin sensitive, Bile soluble	Capsular polysaccharides, Surface protein	Nasopharynx	High carrier rate in normal population	Lobar pneumonia, otitis media, bacteremia, meningitis

Table 2. The Major Streptococcal Species Causing Disease in Humans: Enteric and Oral Streptococci

Group	Species designation	Lancefield group	Hemolysis	Presumptive identification	Definitive identification	Ecologic niche	Normal flora	Association with disease
Enterococci (now classified as genus *Enterococcus*)	*E. faecalis*	D	None, β	Growth in bile–esculin, 6.5% NaCl	Biochemical	Bowel	Yes	Bacteremia, endocarditis, opportunistic infections
	E. faecium	D	α, β, none		Biochemical	Bowel	Yes	Bacteremia, endocarditis, opportunistic infections
Nonenterococcal group D	*S. bovis*	D	α	—	Biochemical	Bowel	Yes	Bacteremia, endocarditis, opportunistic infections
	S. equinus	D	α	—	Biochemical	Bowel	Yes	Endocarditis
Dental/oral streptococci	Viridans group	Various	α, none	—	Biochemical	Oral cavity	Yes	Endocarditis
	S. mutans	None, E	None	—	Cell wall carbohydrate DNA hybridization	Tooth surface, dental plaque	Yes	Dental caries, endocarditis
	S. sanguis	None, H	α, β, none	—	Biochemical	Dental plaque	Yes	Endocarditis, brain abscesses, bacteremia
	S. mitis	None, O, K, M	α, β, none	—	Biochemical	Oral cavity	Yes	
	S. salivarius	None, K	None	—	Biochemical	Tongue	Yes	
Milleri group	*S. anginosis* (*S. "milleri"*)	None, A, C, F, G	α, β, none	—	Biochemical	Oral cavity	Yes	Endocarditis, dental abscesses,
	S. anginosis	F	β	—	Biochemical	Oral cavity	Yes	brain abscesses, liver abscesses
	Minute colony group A	A	β	—	Biochemical	Oral cavity	Yes	
	Minute colony group C	C	β	—	Biochemical	Oral cavity	Yes	
	Minute colony group G	G	β	—	Biochemical	Oral cavity	Yes	
Nutritionally deficient streptococci	*S. mitis* (mutant)	Various	α, β, none	Require pyridoxal	Biochemical	Oral cavity	Yes	Endocarditis
	S. sanguis (mutant)	Various	α, β, none		Biochemical	Oral cavity	Yes	Endocarditis
	S. salivarius (mutant)	Various	α, none	Require pyridoxal	Biochemical	Oral cavity	Yes	Endocarditis
Microaerophilic and anaerobic streptococci	*Peptostreptococcus* (five species)	Some D	None	—	Biochemical	Oral cavity, bowel	Yes	Abscesses, otitis media, pelvic inflammatory disease

ventional media, including EMB (eosin–methylene blue) used for gram-negative enteric organisms. The dental streptococci are best isolated on MSB medium, made with mitis–salivarius agar (M), sucrose (S), and bacitracin (B).[122]

   b. Colony Morphology and Hemolysis. The first step in identifying a streptococcus is examining colonies grown on blood agar for characteristic morphology and hemolysis. A throat culture, for example, will have much extraneous growth, but the bacteriologist will be looking for group A streptococci that have small (0.5–1 mm) opaque white colonies surrounded by a wide zone of clear β-hemolysis. Stabs made into the medium in the area of inoculation will usually clear first because the streptolysin O is more active in the absence of air. Streptolysin S, which is active on the surface, does not always produce complete hemolysis in young cultures. Group A, C, and G streptococci are similar in appearance, but group B streptococci are usually larger, more mucoid, and have a narrower zone of hemolysis that is often less distinct. About 1% of wild group B strains are nonhemolytic, but this depends to some degree on the media used. Streptococci of the milleri group have very tiny colonies but usually have comparatively large zones of β hemolysis; these include group F and the "minute colony" group A, C, and G streptococci. Enterococci have larger, rather buttery colonies, compared to other streptococci, and usually produce no hemolysis or may be β hemolytic on horse blood and α hemolytic on sheep blood. The α-hemolytic streptococci are quite heterogeneous and are difficult to distinguish even to the practiced eye. The pneumococci, however, are usually smooth and glossy with central craters formed by autolysis as the colonies grow beyond 18–24 h. Colonies of type 3 pneumococci are often very large and have a distinctive mucoid appearance.

   c. Presumptive Identification. For practical purposes, group A streptococci can be identified presumptively by the bacitracin sensitivity test of Maxted in which a 0.04-unit bacitracin (TAXO[R]) disk is placed on a pure subculture of a β-hemolytic streptococcus. Group A streptococci are extremely sensitive and uniformly show a zone of inhibition, whereas only 5–10% of group C or G strains may give a false-positive result. The simplest of several tests for group B streptococci is the CAMP test, described by Christie, Atkins, and Munch-Petersen in 1944.[37] The test is performed by inoculating a streak of the streptococcus perpendicular to a streak of *Staphylococcus aureus* on a sheep blood agar plate; an arrowhead-shaped area of complete hemolysis indicates the presence of CAMP factor, which enhances the effect of the staphylococcal β lysin. Streptococci reported simply as "not A or B" on the basis of

presumptive tests usually prove to be group C or G. Pneumococci are distinguished from other α-hemolytic streptococci by sensitivity to optochin in a manner similar to that of the bacitracin test for group A streptococci. In addition, the bile solubility test of Neufeld remains useful for separating pneumococci from the occasional optochin-sensitive viridans streptococcus. Enterococci are identified by growth on bile–esculin media and in 6.5% NaCl. Further identification of these and the viridans streptococci is done with various panels of biochemical tests.

   d. Definitive Identification. Streptococci are classified into Lancefield groups on the basis of their cell wall carbohydrate antigens, except for the enterococci in which the group D antigen is a glycerol teichoic acid. The classical methods of grouping employ an extraction step, usually hot acid (Lancefield method) or nitrous acid, followed by detection of liberated antigens with specific rabbit antisera. More recently, latex and similar particle agglutination kits make it possible for any laboratory to provide rapid and accurate group identification without having to maintain serologic supplies.

   Typing of group A streptococci is done by precipitation of M and T proteins with specific antisera. The T proteins are trypsin-resistant antigens that are useful as markers for certain M types and for strains having no detectable M protein. Over 60 M types have been described, but up to a quarter of isolates are not typable with existing antisera. Because group A typing is not readily available, the opacity factor (OF) neutralization test described by Fraser and Maxted in 1979 has recently been reevaluated and modified by Johnson and Kaplan.[103] This test is relatively simple and correlates well with M typing. The epidemiologic importance of group A typing is obvious when it is noted that certain M types are commonly associated with specific kinds of infection or sequelae. Table 3 lists the most common types associated with nephritis[52] and with recent outbreaks of rheumatic fever in Utah and Ohio.[109]

   The typing of group B streptococci is based upon the detection of capsular polysaccharides, as outlined in Table 4. There are four major types: Ia, Ib, II, and III, and two newly recognized provisional types: IV and V. In her original description of the type polysaccharides, Lancefield noted that, finding no antigens analogous to the M proteins of group A streptococci, she was looking for capsular materials like those found in the capsules of pneumococci. The group B polysaccharides are all similar in structure, composed of glucose, galactose, and glucosamine, with side chains containing terminal sialic acid residues that are major antigenic determinants.[157,182] Type Ib strains and some type II and type III strains also carry the c protein, formerly

Table 3. Group A Streptococcal Serotypes Commonly Associated with Acute Glomerulonephritis and Acute Rheumatic Fever

	M serotypes	T antigens	Usual infection site
Nephritis[a]	2	8/25/Imp. 19	Skin
	49	T-14/'49'	Skin
	55	8/25/Imp. 19	Skin
	57	8/25/Imp. 19	Skin
	60	T-4/'60'	Skin
	1	T-1	Throat
	12	T-12	Throat
Rheumatic fever[b]	1	T-1	Throat
	18	T-18	Throat
	3	T-3	Throat
	5	T-5/27/44	Throat
	6	T-6	Throat

[a]Data on nephritis serotypes from Dillon *et al.*[52]
[b]Data on rheumatic fever serotypes from Kaplan *et al.*[109]

called the "Ibc protein." The R antigen occurs on some type II and III strains but is not seen frequently among human isolates. The X antigen is found almost exclusively in veterinary strains, particularly those from bovine mastitis. To distinguish among strains of the same capsular type, a bacteriophage typing scheme has been employed.[22]

The pneumococci are divided into serologic types, according to capsular polysaccharides. The Danish typing system currently in use recognizes 48 types, many of which have several closely related subtypes that correspond to individual types of the American system. The subtypes are denoted by the Arabic type number plus a letter to indicate the subtype. For example, types 1–5 each contain only one distinct type; type 6 (sometimes called "group" 6) includes type 6A (America type 6) and type 6B (American type 26); type 9 includes four subtypes, of which only type 9N (American type 9) and 9V (American type 68) are at all common among clinical isolates. Knowledge of the distribution of types in human infections led directly to the selection of the most important types in the formulation of pneumococcal vaccines.[161] Type-specific "M protein" antigens of pneumococci were described by Austrian 40 years ago but were not found to be of biologic importance or useful for taxonomic purposes. More recently, Waltman *et al.* have developed a protein typing scheme using monoclonal antibodies against a pneumococcal surface protein that permits the differentiation of many strains within capsular serotypes.[179]

Group D and viridans streptococci are usually speciated by their pattern of biochemical reactions, carried out as individual tests or as panels of tests, such as the API 20 Strep system. Various test kits and automated equipment are in general use in most clinical laboratories and give basically similar results. Two major identification schemes are

Table 4. Type-Specific Antigens of Group B Streptococci[a]

	Ia	Ib	II	III	(IV)	(V)
Capsular polysaccharides						
c protein	−	+	(+)	(+)	?	?

[a]Serologic classification is determined according to the capsular polysaccharide. The c protein was formerly called the "Ibc protein" because of its association with Ib and Ic strains. Ib strains (which always have this protein) are now designated Ib/c, and Ic strains (which have the Ia capsule) are designated Ia/c. About one-third of type II strains have the c protein and are noted as II/c; the frequency of c protein in provisional types IV and V is unknown. The R antigen occurs occasionally in type II and III strains, but like the X antigen is more common in veterinary than in human isolates.

currently in use, one from Great Britain, the other from the CDC in the United States.[60,145] They differ mainly in the classification of group F and the milleri group. However, the entire viridans group is presently being reevaluated and a new classification should be expected in a few years. *S. mutans* is further divided into eight serologic types based on cell wall carbohydrates, and into four genetic groups based on the guanine-plus-cytosine content of DNA.[122] Nutritionally deficient streptococci causing endocarditis are thought to be mostly mutant subspecies of *S. mitis* that require pyridoxal for growth.[167]

e. Rapid Diagnostic Tests. A number of rapid antigen detection systems for group A streptococcus have been developed and made commercially available over the past 10 years.[108] Most of these methods are based upon the extraction of cell wall antigens from throat swabs and their detection by agglutination of particles coated with antibody against the group A polysaccharide. These "rapid strep tests" yield results in 10 to 60 min and permit the physician to appropriately treat streptococcal pharyngitis without the delay of conventional cultures. In general, the specificity of these tests is excellent: 90–95%. The sensitivity, however, varies from 60 to 85%. Those patients with strong positive cultures are nearly always detected, but up to half of those with "1+" cultures (one to ten colonies per plate) may go undetected. The clinical significance of this shortcoming is not entirely clear. The latter group may include some patients who are "carriers" and not at risk in terms of the acute infection or sequelae. However, 35–45% of those with false-negative rapid tests (but 1+ positive cultures) have evidence of true infection as determined by a rise in streptococcal antibody titers. Left untreated, some of these patients could be at risk for developing acute rheumatic fever. For this reason it is recommended that a throat culture be done when the rapid test is negative. Two other problems limit the usefulness of rapid strep tests. One is that they detect only group A streptococci, whereas acute pharyngitis is sometimes caused by group C or G streptococci and may require antibiotic therapy. The other is cost, which may be considerably more than that of a conventional throat culture.

The same methodology has also been employed for rapid diagnostic methods for detecting specific antigens in CSF or urine samples. False-positive reactions may be eliminated by heating samples for 2 min in a boiling water bath. Reagents for group B streptococci are usually based upon detection of the group antigen. They are fairly reliable in detecting antigen from infants infected with group B streptococci, but are not sensitive enough to determine maternal colonization directly from vaginal swabs. The sensitivity of antigen tests for pneumococci is rather low, because antibodies of multiple capsular serotypes must be fixed to the reagent particles and the sensitivity varies enormously for antigens of different serotypes. A possible solution is the use of reagents made with antibodies against phosphocholine or teichoic acid antigens common to all pneumococcal strains.[178]

3.4.2. Serologic and Immunologic Diagnostic Methods. Antibody tests have been developed as clinical and epidemiologic tools in the study of group A, group B, and pneumococcal infections. In general, antibodies are markers of past experience with the organisms and do not indicate when an infection took place. For this reason they are most useful when acute and convalescent antibody levels are compared in relation to an episode of presumed infection.

Assays for the group A streptococcus are based upon the development of antibodies either to cellular antigens or to extracellular enzymes. These are listed in Table 5 and further described in Section 4. Tests for antibody to M proteins, which confer immunity, and to the group A carbohydrate have been used primarily for research purposes. Of the assays used clinically, the antistreptolysin O (ASO) is the most widely employed for confirming recent respiratory infection. A rise in titer is usually seen 3–6 weeks after infection, and a rise, even if modest, is more helpful than a single determination. Responses after skin infections are usually feeble, compared to those after pharyngitis, but only about 80% of patients with rheumatic fever or acute glomerulonephritis following respiratory infection will mount a significant ASO response. Test kits give a titer of >166 Todd units as elevated for adults, but there is considerable variation in the "normal" values among populations and laboratories. In general, single ASO titers above 250 in adults and above 300 in school-aged children are considered elevated. The anti-DNase B titer usually peaks 6–8 weeks after either skin or throat infections. The antihyaluronidase is less frequently used but probably comparable. The Streptozyme-hemagglutination test is a crude screening test based on reactions with an unspecified mixture of streptococcal enzymes. It is not considered sufficiently reliable by many authorities and cannot be recommended in its present form. When used, antibody responses appear earlier (1–2 weeks), but results should be confirmed with one or more of the standardized assays whenever rheumatic fever or acute glomerulonephritis is suspected.

Assays for antibody to pneumococcal and group B streptococcal capsular polysaccharides have employed radioimmunoassay (RIA) for total antibody and enzyme-linked immunosorbent assays (ELISA) for total and class-specific

Table 5. Group A Streptococcal Antigens and Antibodies[a]

	Antibody	Clinical interpretation
Cellular antigens		
M protein	(M protein)	Type-specific, confers immunity. Some antigens cross-reactive with sarcolemma of heart muscle
Group A carbohydrate	(Group A CHO)	Slow response following infection
Hyaluronic acid capsule	None	Not antigenic
Extracellular enzymes		
Streptolysin O	Antistreptolysin O (ASO)	Increases after most group A infections, more reliable for throat than skin infections
Deoxyribonuclease A, B, C, D	Anti-DNase B	Most useful test for skin infections, also reliable for throat infections; anti-DNase A and C inconsistent
Hyaluronidase	Antihyaluronidase	Increases after most group A infections
Streptokinase	Antistreptokinase (ASK)	Increases after most group A infections. Streptokinase A more common than B
Nicotinamide adenine dinucleotidase	Anti-NADase (anti-DPNase)	Response better after throat than skin infections. Common to group A, C, and G streptococci
Proteinase	Antiproteinase	Antibodies appear in small amounts following infection with group A
Erythrogenic toxins A, B, and C	Antierythrogenic toxin	Toxin produces rash of scarlet fever; Dick skin test for immunity or susceptibility

[a]Adapted from Quinn.[159]

antibody determinations. Since both pneumococci and group B streptococci have multiple capsular types, antibody to specific types must be considered. Although it has proved impossible to establish an absolute or minimal protective antibody level, infection appears to be more common in subjects with low antibody levels against the specific capsular antigen of the type causing infection. Assays for pneumococcal antibodies have been important in the development of the pneumococcal vaccines and in evaluating vaccine failures. Assays for several common types are now commercially available and are also useful in screening selected patients for immunoglobulin deficiencies, especially when a generalized unresponsiveness to polysaccharide antigens is suspected.

4. Biological Characteristics of the Organisms

The various streptococcal species have many biologic similarities and differences. The genus name suggests a "twisted chain," which describes the microscopic appearance of many species. The pneumococci are commonly described (and were formerly named) as diplococci because of their propensity to occur in pairs, but they are often indistinguishable from other streptococci when grown in

blood cultures. All the streptococci have a tough cell wall composed of cross-linked peptidoglycans. Most have a polysaccharide group antigen associated with the cell wall, and some have teichoic acids as major or additional components. The pneumococci and the group B streptococci have polysaccharide capsules as their major surface antigens. The group A streptococci, in contrast, have the M proteins, but these appear to play a similar role in helping the organisms resist phagocytosis. Other streptococci, especially the oral and enteric species, have little or no protective outer layer. With few exceptions, streptococci are aerobic and facultatively anaerobic. They are cytochrome-negative, catalase-negative, and ferment sugars mainly to lactic acid but not to gas. All streptococci secrete enzymes extracellularly, but those of group A have been studied most extensively.

4.1. Cellular Antigens and Enzymes

4.1.1. Group A Streptococcal Cellular Antigens and Enzymes. The major components of group A streptococci are the cellular antigens and the extracellular enzymes listed in Table 5.

M proteins, noted above, are the major virulence factors of group A streptococci, contributing to the organism's resistance to phagocytosis in the absence of type-specific antibody. M proteins bind host proteins, especially fibrinogen, as a ploy to evade host defense mechanisms. [36,155] Although immunity appears to be life-long, most humans are usually infected by only a few different types and remain susceptible to the other types. Thus, repeated episodes of streptococcal infection may be due to different types rather than to a failure of host response. Evidence for the cross-reactivity of certain M proteins with heart tissue suggests a mechanism for the etiology of acute rheumatic fever, but direct evidence is incomplete. [49]

Group A carbohydrate, also noted above, is a polymer of rhamnose with N-acetylglucosamine side chains. [98] Humans normally make antibodies to this antigen but antibodies play no role in protection. There is no conclusive evidence that this antigen plays a role in sequelae of streptococcal infections.

Hyaluronic acid capsules are also produced by some strains, giving colonies a highly mucoid appearance. This material is indistinguishable from the ground substance of mammalian connective tissue and is not immunogenic. Its effect on virulence in mice is small, although similar capsules may occur on group C streptococci and have greater virulence than unencapsulated strains. [110] Nevertheless, mucoid group A strains have been associated with severe disease in humans and with rheumatic fever. [109]

Lipoteichoic acids are composed of polyglycerophosphate attached to lipids. These surface molecules are directly involved in attachment of organisms to host epithelia and are of importance in the initiation of infection. [15]

Other cellular components are less well defined in terms of their role in disease. As in other gram-positive bacteria, there is a rigid cell wall structure made from polymers of alternating glucosamine and muramic acid units cross-linked by peptide side chains. This serves to stabilize the organisms against outside osmotic changes. The peptidoglycan components are highly inflammatory and may play a role in inciting nonspecific host responses. The T proteins, noted above, occur in families that may be shared by a number of M types. The serum opacity factor proteins are coexpressed with specific M types and are not shared among M types. [103] The R antigen is an antigenic surface protein that occurs in strains of various types but appears to play no role in virulence or protection. Like group C and G streptococci, group A and other streptococci also have antibody binding proteins that bind antibodies nonspecifically via the Fc fragment, presumably to help the organism avoid specific, complement-fixing, antibody binding. [186]

Extracellular substances are released by group A streptococci into the surrounding milieu and may contribute to the pathogenic process. [180] There are two well-described

hemolysins capable of lysing red blood cells and injuring other cell membranes and subcellular organelles. Streptolysin O is the antigenic, oxygen-labile hemolysin used in the ASO test. Streptolysin S is nonantigenic, oxygen-stable, and is responsible for hemolysis at the surface of cultures grown on blood agar under aerobic conditions.

Deoxyribonucleases (DNases) are elaborated by group A, B, C, and G streptococci. [71] DNase B is the most common and most immunogenic of the group A DNases and is the basis of the antibody test of the same name. While a pathogenic role is not established, it is thought that these enzymes along with hyaluronidase and streptokinase combine to produce the thin pus seen in streptococcal infections, in contrast to the thick pus often associated with infections due to other pyogenic bacteria. [159]

Streptococcal hyaluronidase (produced by groups A and C) is capable of hydrolyzing the hyaluronic acid of group A capsules and of mammalian connective tissue. Although formerly called "spreading factor," its biologic role remains uncertain with regard either to cell metabolism or to the production of disease. [71]

The streptokinases are antigenic proteins that convert plasminogen to plasmin, which in turn lyses fibrin clots. Group A streptococci produce either streptokinase A, the most common, or streptokinase B. An antibody test based on the former antigen is often employed in the clinical assessment of group A disease. The group C streptococci produce an enzyme similar to streptokinase A that has been used clinically in attempts to lyse pleural adhesions in patients with lung infections and clots in patients with coronary artery occlusions. A distinctive low-molecular-weight streptokinase, called "nephritis strain-associated protein," has also been identified from group A streptococci recovered from patients with acute nephritis. [104]

Nicotinamide adenine dinucleotidase (NADase; also called diphosphopyridine nucleotidase, DPNase) is produced by streptococci of groups A, C, and G. [71] Anti-NADase antibodies are produced by the majority of patients recovering from group A streptococcal pharyngitis, but responses are poor following skin infections. NADase is toxic to leukocytes, but the role of this enzyme in human infection is not certain, since some serotypes, such as M type 1, 5, and 19, do not produce NADase and yet are fully capable of causing disease.

Streptococcal proteinases have been carefully studied and shown to exert pathologic effects *in vitro* and *in vivo*. Their role in human disease has yet to be directly established. [71] A specialized peptidase has recently been described that diminishes chemotactic activity by inactivation of the C5a complement component. [141]

Erythrogenic toxins, also known as pyrogenic exotoxins, are responsible for the characteristic rash of scarlet fever.[180] There are three antigenically distinct toxins, A, B, and C, thus making it possible to have scarlet fever more than once, due to different toxins. Not all group A streptococci carry an erythrogenic toxin, but only those strains infected by certain lysogenic bacteriophages coding for the toxin. The Dick test, seldom used today, is based upon the observation that patients with antibody to the toxin show no response to a small intradermal injection of toxin (negative Dick test). Susceptible individuals, who have no antibody to neutralize the toxin, develop inflammation at the injection site within 24 h (positive Dick test). Pyrogenic exotoxin A has been implicated in a toxic shock syndrome similar to that produced by staphylococcal enterotoxins[46] (see Chapter 35). Both are thought to be mediated by inducing the production of tumor necrosis factor by monocytes.[61]

4.1.2. Group B Streptococcal Cellular Antigens and Enzymes.

The group B streptococci differ from group A in that their virulence may be accounted principally by capsular polysaccharides rather than proteins. The capsular types, noted in Section 3.4.1 and in Table 4, are antigenically distinct by virtue of variations in linkages of the same essential sugars. A key feature is that all have terminal *N*-acetylneuraminic acid (sialic acid) residues that are major immunodeterminants. The capsules are antiphagocytic and require specific antibody for efficient opsonization. An exception may be the prototype strain of type Ia, which may be opsonized by direct antibody-independent activation of the C1 complement component.[57] The quantity of sialic acid-containing antigen appears to be directly related to size and density of the capsule and to virulence in animal models.[90,187] The capsular material itself appears to inhibit the activation and chemotactic functions of neutrophils.[134] Many group B strains are also capable of binding fibrinogen to their surface in a manner that competes with the nonspecific binding of C3 complement.[36]

The group B antigen is a complex glucitol-containing polysaccharide associated with the peptidoglycan cell wall. Antibodies to the group B antigen are generally not protective, presumably because it is covered by capsular material.[157] Recently, a human monoclonal antibody to the group B antigen has been described that opsonizes strains of all serotypes and has been proposed as an adjunctive therapeutic agent.[160]

The major protein antigen of group B streptococci is the c protein, which occurs on all type Ib and some type II and III strains. Antibodies to this antigen are protective,[117] but common variants of the protein apparently confer resistance to intracellular killing by neutrophils.[147] An important property of the c protein may be its ability to nonspecifically bind human IgA.[41] The R and X antigens are rarely seen in human isolates and probably play no role in protection or disease. Also present are lipoteichoic acids that are involved with adherence of organisms to host epithelial cells.

The group B streptococci elaborate a number of extracellular enzymes, including CAMP factor, DNases, and neuraminidase.[71,145] The neuraminidase is thought to have a possible role in virulence.[137] The CAMP factor potentiates the activity of sphingomyelinase and may have effects on cell membranes. Purified CAMP factor appears to enhance the lethality of live organisms injected into mice.[106]

4.1.3. Pneumococcal Cellular Antigens and Enzymes.

S. pneumoniae is the paradigm of encapsulated bacteria.[145] Its polysaccharide capsules are essential to virulence, and antibodies against the capsule are the major specific defense against infection, and the development of antibody is important in convalescence from disease. The 82 recognized type-specific polysaccharides vary in composition, including linear polymers, branched chains, and teichoic acid-like antigens. The most frequently occurring types have been selected for inclusion in the presently licensed vaccines.[161]

The C-polysaccharide corresponds to the group carbohydrates of other streptococci but differs significantly in structure. Its major antigenic determinant is phosphocholine, linked to ribitol phosphate, galactosamine, and other sugars. Antibodies to the phosphocholine moiety protect mice from experimental infection. Although humans make natural antibodies to this antigen, its role in human infection is not clear.[27] The phophocholine determinant is also the site of binding for C-reactive protein (CRP), an acute-phase reactant elevated in acute disease. The Forssman antigen is a membrane teichoic acid with a similar composition but linked to a lipid, forming what is essentially the lipoteichoic acid of the pneumococcus.

Cell surface proteins, notably a newly described antigen designated pneumococcal surface protein A (PspA), may also play a role in virulence.[133] Mutant type 2 strains lacking PspA were less virulent in infected mice than their otherwise identical parent strain with intact PspA. Antibodies to PspA were protective against various encapsulated strains that carried the protein. The importance of these proteins in human disease has not yet been determined. Nevertheless, the concept of a protein antigen that can elicit protective responses is especially attractive, since infants under 2 years of age are known to have poor responses to the conventional polysaccharide vaccines.

Enzymes produced by pneumococci include pneumolysin, amidase (the autolytic enzyme that breaks down cell wall material), neuraminidase, and IgA proteases. Although none of these has been conclusively shown to be associated with virulence, all have at least theoretical implications. The pneumolysin gene bears extensive amino acid sequence homology to streptolysin O and to the theta-toxin of *Clostridium perfringens*.[172] Pneumolysin is an intracellular enzyme and is released only by cell lysis. The neuraminidase is directly toxic to mice and may play a role either in modifying epithelial cells during invasion or in damaging sialylated cell surfaces in meningitis. IgA proteases cleave the Fc fragment from IgA, making it incapable of preventing adhesion to epithelial cells and possibly also preventing the recognition of IgA by tissue macrophages.[71]

4.1.4. Components of Other Streptococci. Other streptococci share many characteristics noted above. All have rigid peptidoglycan cell walls, with various distinctive or group antigens, and usually with some form of lipoteichoic acid. Group C streptococci may have hyaluronic acid capsules like those of group A. Group G streptococci may have the type 12 M protein of group A or similar surface proteins, as well as antibody binding proteins. Group C and G streptococci also produce streptokinases. We have recently described a patient with nephritis following infection with a group G strain that had a low-molecular-weight enzyme similar to the nephritis strain-associated protein of group A.[73]

The enteric and oral streptococci are usually unencapsulated. Streptococci of the milleri group appear to require at least 50% of cells to have capsules in order to produce abscesses in experimental animals. Capsule production can be induced in some species, but capsular materials from this group have not been defined.[76] Few toxins or noxious enzymes have been described among the enteric and oral streptococci. The inflammatory response to infection probably relates largely to the properties of the cell wall breakdown products. Characteristics that enable them to cause disease often relate to their ability to adhere to host tissues, such as tooth enamel, heart valves or prostheses, or to intravascular catheters. *S. mutans,* for example, adheres to the pellicle coating the tooth surface and is further aided by the presence of sucrose. Caries occur when the secretion of acids demineralizes the tooth surface.[122] Enterococci and milleri group streptococci are frequently found in mixed infections, especially in association with anaerobic bacteria, suggesting that additional factors are required for them to cause disease. Serious enterococcal disease also occurs as superinfection in patients receiving broad-spectrum antibi-

otics that may disturb the normal ecology of this unusually benign organism.

4.2. Antibiotic Susceptibility

The streptococci are generally quite susceptible to penicillin, as indicated by the usual range of minimal inhibitory concentrations (MIC) listed in Table 6. The exceptions are group D, particularly the enterococcus, and certain strains of pneumococcus. Although streptococci are generally resistant to aminoglycosides, gentamicin is sometimes used for its synergistic effect in combination with a penicillin. Chloramphenicol has occasionally been substituted in penicillin-allergic patients with pneumococcal infections, although other drugs are considered to be superior.

Group A and B streptococci have never developed resistance to penicillins. They are somewhat less sensitive to vancomycin and the cephalosporins but are resistant to aminoglycosides and moderately resistant to chloramphenicol. Group B strains have shown some tolerance to penicillin, but the clinical significance of such observations is unknown. Tolerance to penicillin has been suggested as one mechanism by which group A streptococci persist after treatment of pharyngitis, allowing either relapses or asymptomatic carriage to follow.[113] Another mechanism is thought to be the protection of susceptible streptococci by the production of β-lactamases by other bacteria in the pharynx or tonsils.[29] Resistance to erythromycin occurs in 1–5% of group A strains in most parts of the world, but resistance rates as high as 60% have been reported in Japan.

Penicillin resistance in pneumococci was first reported in 1967 from Australia and New Guinea. Since then, strains with intermediate susceptibility (MIC 0.1–1.0 μg/ml) have been identified throughout the world, and highly resistant strains (MIC > 1.0 μg/ml) have been reported from South Africa and Spain.[4] Strains resistant to multiple antibiotics have been especially frequent in the latter two countries, with some isolates resistant to all common antibiotics except vancomycin, rifampin, bacitracin, novobiocin, and fusidic acid. In South Africa, Spain, and other European countries, intermediate and resistant strains account for up to 50% of all pneumococcal isolates. Few highly resistant strains have been reported from the United States, but intermediately resistant strains now occur at rates of 1–15%.[4,184] The National Committee for Clinical Laboratory Standards recommends screening of pneumococci by disk diffusion on Mueller–Hinton/5% sheep blood agar using 1-μg oxacillin disks. The criterion for susceptible strains is an inhibition zone diameter ≥ 20 mm. About half

Table 6.   Antibiotic Susceptibility of Various Streptococcal Species: Range of Minimal Inhibitory Concentrations (MIC) in μg/ml

| | Group A streptococci | Group B streptococci | Pneumococci | | Group D/ enterococci |
			Penicillin-susceptible	Penicillin-resistant	
Penicillin G	<0.01	<0.03	<0.06	1–16	0.5–2
Ampicillin	<0.01	<0.03	<0.12	1–16	0.5–2
Vancomycin	<0.1	<0.1	0.25–0.5	0.25–0.5	2–6
Cephalothin	0.01–0.4	<0.03	0.03–0.2	2–32	16–64
Cefotaxime	<0.1	<0.1	<0.5	0.25–2	>256
Ceftriaxone	<0.1	<0.1	<0.06	<0.1	1–>64
Gentamicin	>4	>4	>4	>4	5–64
Chloramphenicol	2–4	2–4	2–8	2–8	50

of strains with zones <20 mm may prove borderline susceptible when retested for MIC by the agar dilution method.[184]

The basis for resistance among pneumococci are the alterations in penicillin-binding proteins in combination with changes in the peptidyl chains on the muramic acid units of the cell wall matrix.[100] There is no evidence for β-lactamase coding plasmids in pneumococci. Penicillin acts as a false substrate in the cross-linking of cell wall precursors, preventing the formation of normal peptidoglycan chains and rendering the organisms susceptible to damage by osmotic forces. It is thought that resistant strains have arisen in response to the environmental pressures of widespread use of penicillins. Stable chromosomal changes have led to penicillin-binding proteins with lower binding affinities for penicillin, while at the same time, the predominant cell wall peptides have shifted from straight- to branched-chain peptide moieties. The resulting organisms no longer bind penicillin in preference to the new cell wall precursors, and intact peptidoglycan chains are formed. At least three genetically related groups of resistant strains have been identified and show clear indications of clonal origin.

Group D enterococci are moderately resistant to penicillins alone, because of the intrinsic properties of their penicillin-binding proteins. Infections are usually treated with penicillin or ampicillin plus an aminoglycoside, which exert a synergistic effect against the organisms. Some enterococci have developed high-level resistance (MIC > 500 μg/ml) to gentamicin, but the extent of this problem is not known because most isolates are not routinely tested for susceptibility to gentamicin.

5. Descriptive Epidemiology

5.1. Prevalence and Incidence

Group A streptococcal pharyngitis is one of the most common acute bacterial infections, especially in children, accounting for up to 10% of patient visits in a private pediatric practice.[25] While current data are incomplete, Fig. 1 clearly shows that scarlet fever, a major recognizable form of group A disease, has declined dramatically since the beginning of this century.[159] The severity of the disease, reflected by mortality rates, declined concomitantly. This trend began long before the advent of antibiotics, suggesting a decrease in virulence or an increase in host resistance, or both. In the 1940s penicillin became widely available, and deaths attributed to scarlet fever and puerperal sepsis, the two most common lethal forms of group A streptococcal disease, became a rarity. The number of reported cases of streptococcal sore throat increased during the 1950s and 1960s, probably because of increased physician awareness of its relation to rheumatic fever, greater use of throat cultures, and the availability of antibiotics for treatment and prevention.

Figure 2 shows the number of positive throat cultures and number of cases of acute rheumatic fever and acute glomerulonephritis in private pediatric practices participating in surveillance studies in Rochester, New York, 1967–1988. These data were compiled and kindly supplied by Caroline Breese Hall, University of Rochester. Of approximately 23,000 throat cultures done annually, 18–25% were positive for group A streptococci in this relatively stable population. Meanwhile, the number of cases of acute

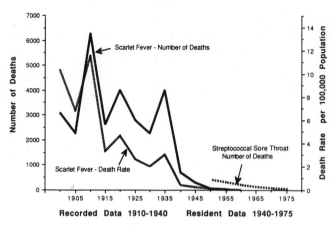

Figure 1. The number of deaths (left-hand scale) from scarlet fever (1900–1960) and from all streptococcal sore throat (1950–1975), with death rates (right-hand scale) per 100,000 population in the United States. Appropriate comparability ratios were applied beginning in 1940, and recorded data compiled according to the geographic locale where the event occurred without regard to residence (1900–1940); resident data were compiled according to the usual place of residence without regard to locale where the event occurred (1940–1975). The population used for determining rates was that of the registration area. Data were not available for streptococcal sore throat for 1900–1950. The number of states reporting for 1900–1905 was 10, gradually increasing to 48 in 1935 and to 50 states in 1960. After 1975, reporting was optional, and no accurate data are available. Sources of data: U.S. Bureau of the Census, *Historical Statistics of the United States: Colonial Times to 1970,* Bicentennial ed., Part I, p. 77, 1975; National Office of Vital Statistics, *Vital Statistics Reports,* Vol. 37, No. 9 (1920–1950); Centers for Disease Control, *Morbidity and Mortality Weekly Report,* Annual Supplement, 1960 and 1970. Figure redrawn from Quinn.[159]

glomerulonephritis declined from nearly 40 in 1967 to an average of 1 case per year from 1981 to 1988. Confirmed cases of acute rheumatic fever dropped from 20–28 per year to a very few from 1975 through 1985 but have since begun to rise. A similar pattern has been observed elsewhere.[130] In Baltimore, between 1960 and 1964, the incidence of rheumatic fever was 26 per 100,000 among 5- to 19-year-olds. By 1980 the rates had fallen to 0.2–0.8 per 100,000 nationwide among whites, with rates several times higher among other races. Beginning in 1985, an increase in new cases was seen in Utah, Pennsylvania, Ohio, New York,

and other areas.[96,130,174,177] Disease incidence in Utah was 18 per 100,000 population age-adjusted for 5- to 17-year-olds. Of particular interest was the observation that throughout this period incidence rates went essentially unchanged in Hawaii, where the disease is especially prevalent among Polynesian children.[39] Contemporary data from Kuwait suggest similar rates for a developing country, with about 20 cases per 100,000 childhood population.[127] Deaths from acute rheumatic fever are rare at the present time, but deaths associated with chronic rheumatic heart disease continue to occur in persons who had acute rheu-

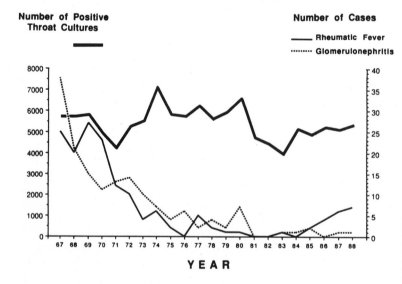

Figure 2. The number of positive throat cultures (left-hand scale) and number of confirmed cases of rheumatic fever and acute glomerulonephritis (right-hand scale) seen in private pediatric practices participating in streptococcal surveillance studies in Rochester, New York, 1967–1988. The data were kindly provided by Caroline Breese Hall, University of Rochester.

matic fever in childhood. In 1975, for example, 9255 of 12,775 deaths attributed to rheumatic heart disease were in patients over 50 years of age.[159]

Acute poststreptococcal glomerulonephritis occurs with about the same frequency as rheumatic fever in Kuwait (18 per 100,000 childhood population)[127] but no data are available on current rates for skin infection or associated nephritis in the United States. Prospective studies in Alabama (1966–1969) revealed 91 cases of nephritis relative to 1149 cases of uncomplicated streptococcal pyoderma treated in a clinical setting—an 8% attack rate.[52] Acute glomerulonephritis has declined markedly in subsequent years, along with the frequency of nephritigenic serotypes (Table 3) isolated from children with impetigo. As typified by data from Rochester, New York, in Fig. 2, nephritis is now relatively uncommon.

Another change in group A streptococcal disease in recent years has been the reappearance of serious acute infections, especially bacteremia and streptococcal "toxic shock."[37,46,67,99,168] Since 1980, the number of septicemic deaths has increased in the United Kingdom out of proportion with other streptococcal infections, but precise incidence figures are not available.[67] A hospital survey in Nottingham found that group A streptococci accounted for 2% of all bacteremias over a 7-year period. The mortality rate was 35% and was particularly high in males over 60 years of age.[99]

Group B streptococcal infections continue to be common in neonates, with attack rates of early onset disease of 2 per 1000 live births in defined populations from Chicago, Illinois, and from Birmingham, Alabama.[22,54] Late-onset disease (usually occurring after hospital discharge up to about 3 months of age) adds another 2 infections per 1000 births, for a total of about 4 neonatal group B infections per 1000 live births.[54] Exact incidence data are very difficult to obtain and interpret, and few accurate data are available outside of Europe and North America. Rates appear to be much lower (about 0.5 per 1000 live births) in Scandinavia and the United Kingdom than in the United States and parts of western Europe.[132] Maternal and infant colonization rates are similar in Hong Kong, but the neonatal disease rate is 0.6 per 1000 live births.[120] Maternal sepsis due to group B streptococci occurs in 0.5–2 per 1000 deliveries in Alabama, depending upon the population studied.[78] Lowest rates were seen when particular attention was paid to aggressive antibiotic use in mothers undergoing cesarean section delivery.

The incidence of pneumococcal disease[33,63,114,163,169] is summarized in Section 5.1 of Chapter 25.

Enterococcal infections now account for nearly 10% of nosocomial infections, and for 5–6% of all bacteremias in hospitalized patients.[101,181] Rates of bacteremic infection are often twice as high on trauma, surgical, and obstetric–gynecologic services.[30,89,119] Three-fourths of enterococcal bacteremias are nosocomial, but endocarditis is more frequently community-acquired.[128] Case-fatality rates are in the range of 40%, and many of these patients are debilitated, immunocompromised, or have serious predisposing conditions.[30,56,89,128]

In terms of sheer numbers, *S. mutans,* the principal organism in dental caries, probably infects more persons than all other streptococci combined. Of the 40 to 50% of the population of developed countries who regularly visit a dentist, most receive treatment related to restoration of teeth or decayed tooth substance. Treatment of dental infections in the United States cost an estimated $24 billion in 1984.[122] Inasmuch as dental caries is a chronic disease that varies within and among populations, several measures of morbidity have been developed. Prevalence, defined as the percentage of a population showing any evidence of caries, may be so widespread as to have little epidemiologic significance. The most commonly used index is that counting the number of *decayed, filled,* and *missing teeth* (DFM or DFMT). Because of the difficulty of examining representative groups of subjects beyond school age, population surveys are often standardized at an index age of 12 years.[118] By this measure the World Health Organization can monitor trends from the more than 1000 surveys submitted to the WHO Global Oral Data Bank, set up in 1970. The WHO goal of 3 DFM teeth per person has been realized in 84 of 148 countries for which data are currently available. Dental health in industrialized countries, most of which had moderate to high DFMT rates in 1969, has improved greatly over the past two decades. Meanwhile, developing countries have seen a rise in DFMT thought to be associated with changes in diet and other factors associated with urbanization. Since the populations of developing countries are skewed toward the younger age groups, who have fewer caries relative to the older populations in the developed world, a population-weighted mean DFMT at age 12 is used for global comparisons. From 1980 to 1986 DFMT rates have increased from 1.63 to 2.16 in developing countries and have decreased from 4.53 to 3.82 in developed countries.[118] Rates also vary within countries. In the United States highest DFMT rates have always been found in northeastern states, with lowest rates in south-central states. This has been attributed in part to differences in natural fluoridation.

The incidence of dental caries may be estimated from DFMT data, but a more sensitive method makes use of individual counts of new *decayed* and *filled surfaces* (DFS) observed over a defined period of time. These counts may be further adjusted to calculate annual mean DFS rates per 100 surfaces at risk. Using this approach, Glass *et al.* observed American males 35 to 80 years of age in a 10-year longitudinal study.[72] The mean annual incidence of new DFS per 100 surfaces at risk was 1.36 and was similar in each of three age cohorts. Within the mouth the rate was highest for molars (mean = 2.69), followed by premolars (1.93) and anterior teeth (0.91), and was higher for upper than lower teeth. The conventional DFMT rate was 23 for these patients at the beginning of the study. The DFS incidence rates, however, were similar to those reported from children aged 7 to 12 years.

5.2. Epidemiology and Contagiousness

Of all the streptococcal infections only scarlet fever has been feared as an epidemic disease in the same sense as cholera and plague. In most areas of the world, group A streptococcal disease is endemic, with fluctuations exceeding the normal prevalence levels occurring seasonally or sometimes over an extended period. Occasional localized epidemics of streptococcal pharyngitis or skin infections are reported from newborn nurseries, military installations, closed communities, or institutions.[10,35,140]

The epidemiology of streptococcal infections reflects the ecologic features peculiar to the species in question. Streptococci associated primarily with the respiratory tract, such as group A and the pneumococcus, cause infections that are initially related to that portal of entry. Of course, some group A strains prefer to colonize the skin and cause impetigo, while others affect either skin or throat. The group B streptococci, in contrast, are gut organisms. Asymptomatic gastrointestinal, and to a lesser extent genitourinary, colonization is common. Their infections relate to the aberrations induced by pregnancy, labor, and delivery, and to the unique conditions of infants in the newborn period. The enterococci are also normal gut organisms, but their infections are more generally opportunistic in nature.

Group A streptococci are not considered part of the normal flora of the respiratory tract. Their presence is generally associated with overt infection. Transmission to other persons is greatest from an infected individual, and communicability appears to be dose-related. Nevertheless, a large reservoir of asymptomatic carriers exists with endemic rather than epidemic characteristics. These individuals carry relatively small numbers of organisms. They are at little risk for acute disease or sequelae and are probably an uncom-

mon source of new infection. However, the identification of the carrier state, usually defined by the absence of a serologic response, is fraught with difficulties that continue to cloud the relationship between colonization and disease.[68,107]

Group B streptococci cause serious disease in the perinatal period, but only a small number of infections occur among colonized mothers and infants exposed *in utero,* during, or after delivery. Maternal group B infections may be initially subclinical and possibly contribute to premature labor or septic abortion.[78] Amnionitis may be present before the onset of fever or other symptoms. After delivery, a previously asymptomatic mother may develop endometritis usually without bacteremia. Classical puerperal sepsis due to group A streptococci, in contrast, was often transmitted via obstetric personnel and occurred as a fulminant infection after delivery, sparing the infant. With group B streptococci, infected infants are usually exposed *in utero* to the serotype carried by the mother. Infants with this "early onset" form of infection are usually bacteremic at delivery and become symptomatic within a few hours of birth.[158] Infection is directly related to the size of the inoculum to which the infant is exposed, by swallowing or aspirating infected amniotic fluid. Most infants are lightly colonized and at little risk for infection, whereas those who are infected are almost invariably heavily colonized at birth.[54] Some infants may acquire organisms via the respiratory tract during transit through the birth canal, or from persons other than the mother, and become symptomatic at a later time. Development of the late-onset form of disease may be delayed for days or weeks, and only about half of these infants will be infected by an organism acquired at birth or from the mother.[54]

Pneumococci are often thought of as normal respiratory flora, but pneumococcal infections are not opportunistic in the sense that they are caused by any pneumococcus that happens to reside in the nasopharynx. In a classical investigation, Hodges and MacLeod reported extensive epidemiologic studies at a United States Air Force training facility in 1946.[93] Upon arrival at the base, recruits frequently carried pneumococci of serotypes common to the population at large. Within about 6 weeks they acquired one of a small number of "epidemic" types prevalent at the base—types 1, 2, 4, 5, 7, and 12. The peak incidence of pneumonia due to these types occurred 4–6 weeks after the entry of a new contingent of trainees. Although the rate of carriage of the epidemic types was relatively low, the "infectivity factor" (measured by the ratio of infections to the number of carriers) was much higher than that of other common types, such as 3, 6, 14, 19, and 23. In our epidemiologic studies in infants, we also observed a relationship between acquisition and infection.[81,84] Infants frequently carried types 6, 14, 19, and 23 for prolonged periods, but neither carriage *per se* nor overall rates correlated with disease. Most infections, which were due to these same common types, occurred within a month of acquiring a new type never before carried by a particular child. The infecting type was often isolated together with a former carriage type from the nasopharynx, but only the new type was recovered from middle ear fluid or other infected sites. In terms of exposure to new strains, 15% of acquisitions resulted in disease.

5.3. Geographic Distribution

Streptococcal diseases are of worldwide importance. Group A streptococci appear to be well adapted to humans living in temperate or tropical climates, although differences in the temporal distribution and perhaps the characteristics of disease may vary.[91] In some tropical areas, group C and G streptococci are more frequently isolated in cases of pharyngitis than are group A strains. Pneumococci are the leading cause of bacterial respiratory infection in all parts of the world. In some areas, such as sub-Saharan Africa where seasonal epidemics of meningococcal disease are common, pneumococcal disease remains endemic and accounts for many cases of meningitis throughout the course of the year. As noted above, group B streptococcal carriage is widespread, but infection rates are highest in North America and western Europe, with lowest rates reported from the United Kingdom, northern Europe, and parts of Asia.[132]

Dental caries occur worldwide, but are more common in industrialized areas than in developing countries, as noted above. This has been attributed in part to the higher use of sucrose, prepared and refined foodstuffs, and other dietary and social changes associated with urbanization; it is mitigated to some extent by the availability of artificial fluoridation in dentifrices and water supplies, and of dental care. Caries have always been less common in areas with natural fluoridation.

5.4. Temporal Distribution

Group A streptococcal infections follow characteristic seasonal patterns.[91] In northern parts of the United States streptococcal pharyngitis is typically seen over the winter months, peaking in February or March, while skin infections occur mainly in the summer. Figure 3 illustrates this pattern in surveillence data from private pediatric practices

in Rochester, New York, for the 12 years 1977–1988. In the southeastern states there is both a late fall and a late winter peak of respiratory infection, coinciding with the beginning of school in the fall and with increased indoor activity or crowding during colder months. Seasonal variation is less evident in tropical or subtropical areas, although gathering of children at school or other institutions appears to increase the incidence of disease at certain times of the year. Streptococcal skin infections are most common in the rainy season in tropical areas. Such conditions favor the exposure of unprotected skin to the assault of minor trauma and the bites of mosquitoes and other insects. Organisms present on the skin surface, or rarely from the respiratory tract, may be inoculated into damaged skin by itching or scratching.

Pneumococcal infections tend to peak in winter months.[82] The disease incidence is not related to the carriage rate, which varies only slightly over the year, but parallels the markedly seasonal rate of acquisition of new strains.[84,85,93] In the study of Hodges and MacLeod there was also a strong correlation of pneumococcal lobar pneumonia with the seasonal peaks of influenza virus infection, with about one case of pneumonia for every ten recruits admitted to the infirmary with nonbacterial respiratory disease.[93]

5.5. Age

Group A streptococcal pharyngitis is uncommon in children under 4 years of age. It increases in frequency as children enter school, peaking at 9 to 12 years of age. These children are the primary source of respiratory infections that occur among families and are thus a source of exposure for parents and other adults in the household. Streptococcal impetigo, in contrast, is chiefly a disease of younger children. It is frequently seen in toddlers and children under 4 and typically reaches a peak incidence at about 6 years of age. Adolescents tend to be subject to milder and often self-limited disease.

Group B streptococcal sepsis or meningitis is essentially limited to neonates and infants under 3 months of age and to their mothers around the time of delivery. Group B streptococci are a common though sometimes disregarded cause of urinary tract infection among adult women, especially during pregnancy. This has been associated with late abortions and problems of the perinatal period.[51,185] Rarely does an older child or adult develop a serious infection in the absence of some compromise of normal host defenses. Among older adults, especially diabetics, group B streptococci are frequently isolated from cellulitis and bed sores.[32,58,95,143]

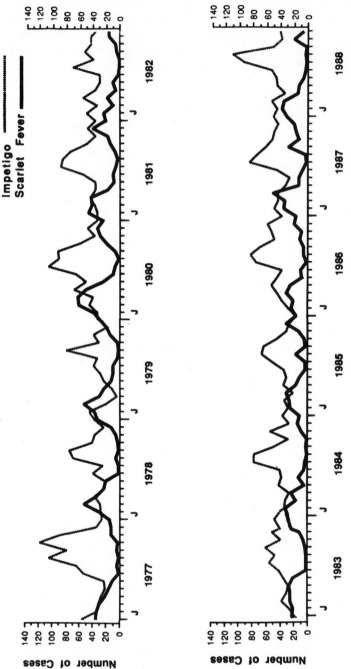

Figure 3. The number of cases of scarlet fever (solid lines) and streptococcal impetigo (dotted lines) seen monthly in private pediatric practices participating in streptococcal surveillance studies in Rochester, New York, 1977–1988. The data were kindly provided by Caroline Breese Hall, University of Rochester.

Pneumococcal disease is seen in all age groups, but principally affects the very young and the very old. Among children, 70% of meningitis and bacteremia occurs in those under 24 months of age, peaking at 8 to 12 months of age.[79] Deaths are also most frequent in this age group, with an overall fatality rate of 6%. Pneumococcal infections are least common among adolescents but increase in frequency with advancing age. The incidence of bacteremic infections reaches 25 per 100,000 among those over 55 years of age, and the case-fatality rate in this group is over 80%.[138]

Serious infections by enteric and oral streptococci are less subject to the effects of age than to the natural defenses of the host. Low-birthweight babies, however, are increasingly infected by group D and viridans streptococci, perhaps because of the kinds of interventions required for the management of very premature infants or changes in patterns of antibiotic use.[124,166]

Dental caries (*S. mutans*) is a chronic disease that continues throughout life. Longitudinal studies from the United States and from Africa show that rates of development of new caries are about the same in adults as they are in children, despite considerable differences in overall caries incidence for the two localities.[72,129]

5.6. Sex

Sex is not a factor in the development of streptococcal disease, except as it relates to pregnancy and to specific genitourinary infections. The peptostreptococci are recognized in pelvic inflammatory disease but are rarely encountered (or looked for) elsewhere. Group B streptococci may be transmitted by sexual contact, but genital colonization is not associated with symptoms in either sex. Colonization may be higher in women during the first half of the menstrual cycle, perhaps because of greater adherence to vaginal epithelial cells at this time.[189]

5.7. Race and Genetic Factors

No one is spared from susceptibility to streptococcal infections. Much of the association between race and susceptibility can probably be accounted for extrinsic factors, such as poverty, crowding, and lack of medical care. Nevertheless, there is growing evidence that certain persons within racial groups may have some genetic host predisposition. Studies of histocompatibility leukocyte antigen (HLA) distributions point to increased risk of rheumatic fever for blacks expressing the DR2 phenotype and for whites with the DR4 phenotype.[9] Agammaglobulinemia and IgG sub-

class deficiencies are associated with recurrent pneumococcal infection.[23,131] Various complement deficiencies, especially that of the second component (C2), should also be considered in children with repeated pneumococcal disease.[19] Down's syndrome and cleft palate are associated with increased frequency of otitis media due to pneumococci and other organisms.

5.8. Occupation

Occupation is rarely a factor in the development of group A streptococcal infections. Physicians, nurses, and laboratory workers in close contact with infected patients or their cultures seldom develop disease. Epidemics of skin infections have occasionally appeared in meat packers in the United States and Britain.[34] Group B streptococci are a major cause of mastitis in cattle. Spread is thought to occur mainly via the hands of dairy workers from human or bovine sources. Consumers of raw infected milk may become colonized with group B streptococci but do not appear to be at risk for disease.[102] Group A and C streptococcal diseases have occasionally been associated with milk-borne transmission. Group C infections have also been associated with exposure to horses and other animals.[5] Workers in the pork industry occasionally develop meningitis due to *S. suis,* at a rate in the Netherlands of about 3 per 100,000, or 1500-fold higher than in the population at large.[6]

5.9. Other Settings and Predisposing Factors

Family studies of respiratory bacteria have indicated that the group A streptococcus and the pneumococcus enter a family unit most commonly via the school-aged children.[28,92] These organisms spread rather slowly to other family members, some becoming colonized and very few developing overt infection. Spread is often facilitated by concomitant viral respiratory infections. Socioeconomic factors, crowding, and substandard housing have frequently been cited as contributing to the spread of these organisms and to the development of acute rheumatic fever and bronchopneumonia. Schools and day-care centers may experience periodic problems with group A streptococci. In a recent day-care outbreak of streptococcal pharyngitis, the overall rate of positive cultures was 49% for 187 children and 33% for 27 adult staff.[165] Spread of pneumococci occurs slowly in day-care centers and seldom leads to serious disease.[121]

The military has been associated for over a century with increased risk for developing streptococcal disease, especially acute rheumatic fever and pneumococcal pneumonia. Our present understanding of the epidemiology of rheumatic fever and methods for antibiotic prophylaxis date from important studies done in the U.S. Armed Forces during and after World War II.[171] Rates of streptococcal pharyngitis are much lower in recruit camps where penicillin prophylaxis is routinely used, and rheumatic fever cases have recently appeared at installations that discontinued the practice.[35,171] There may be an incidental effect of prophylactic penicillin on rates of pneumococcal pneumonia, but this has not been studied. Pneumococcal vaccines, however, have been a priority. Nearly 30 years before the current generation of vaccines was licensed in the United States, several purified polysaccharide vaccines were developed for the military and proven efficacious.[125]

Nosocomial spread of group A, B, and C streptococci continues to be reported occasionally, especially from obstetric and surgical services and newborn nurseries.[21,74,140] Sources of infection may be other patients or personnel who carry organisms in the nose, throat, skin, vagina, or anus. Enterococcal infections in neonates and surgical patients usually originate from the patient's own flora, under the influence of physical interventions and antibiotic therapy.[89,124] Intraabdominal wounds, burns, intravascular catheters, and the urinary tract are the most frequent sites associated with nosocomial enterococcal bacteremia.[128] Epidemic group A streptococcal puerperal sepsis such as described by Holmes and Semmelweiss has largely been eliminated by infection control measures and antibiotics.[53,69]

Predisposing host factors may be genetic or acquired, such as sickle-cell disease, immunodeficiency, or splenectomy. Splenectomized patients have a 50- to 200-fold greater risk of serious bacteremic infection. The spleen is injured most commonly by external abdominal trauma and incidentally during abdominal operations not directly involving the spleen. Surgical repair, rather than removal, of a traumatized spleen is frequently possible and should always be preferred.[31] Overall, about a fourth of children with pneumococcal bacteremia or meningitis have some underlying condition or host defense abnormality, and risk for these children persists well beyond 24 months of age.[79] Patients with human immunodeficiency virus (HIV) infection or acquired immunodeficiency syndrome (AIDS) have a higher incidence of bacteremic pneumococcal infection compared to patients in population-based studies done before the AIDS epidemic. In San Francisco the rate in AIDS patients is 9.4 per 1000 patient-years, or almost 1% per annum.[161] Intravenous drug abuse, also a known AIDS risk factor, is associated with an increase in group G streptococcal infection.[48]

6. Mechanisms and Routes of Transmission

The transmission of streptococci, introduced in Section 5.2, depends on such factors as the usual ecologic niche of the species, its occurrence as part of the normal flora, and the ease with which it may be carried by hands, in secretions, or possibly in droplets. The group A streptococci are transmitted principally by direct contact. Contagiousness is greatest during acute respiratory infection, whereas the chronic carrier is a relatively low risk as an infectious source. This probably reflects the fact that development of infection requires a fairly large inoculum. About 10^5 organisms are required to infect adult volunteers by directly inoculating the tonsils and pharynx with organisms on a cotton swab.[50] Although streptococci may occur in droplets and survive in dust, an individual is unlikely to acquire a large enough inoculum to become infected from these sources. Streptococci recovered from contaminated blankets and dust may also be less infective.[149,150] Direct transmission of respiratory secretions may occur via hands, person-to-person contact such as kissing, or projection of large droplets during coughing or sneezing. Treatment of infected persons eliminates the risk of spread within 24–48 h, permitting resumption of work or school activities as soon as constitutional symptoms have abated.

Pneumococci are thought to be transmitted by similar routes. Coughing is a more regular feature of pneumonia than it is of other pneumococcal infections or of streptococcal pharyngitis. Transmission appears to be favored by symptoms of cold and coryza.[28] Dust particles may harbor pneumococci but do not play a significant role in transmission.[93] Direct spread of secretions containing viable organisms is the most likely source. Covering one's mouth with a hand may deflect a cough or sneeze, but the hand may then transmit fresh secretions.

Common-source outbreaks of streptococcal disease are rarely observed, but group A and C infections have been associated with contaminated foods, such as egg salad, or with improperly pasteurized milk from cows with mastitis. Despite the prevalence of group B streptococci in bovine mastitis, milk-borne group B infections have not been reported.[102]

Skin infections due to group A streptococci are usually caused by serotypes different from those associated with throat infections (see Table 3). Streptococci may occur on normal skin but do not cause infection unless there is a break in the cutaneous epithelium. Minor injuries such as scratches, abrasions, cuts, or insect bites may become points of entry.[126] Mosquito bites are an especially common site of inoculation, where organisms are rubbed into the wound during itching. In Trinidad, streptococcal impetigo may be transmitted by flies of the genus *Hippelates,* which feed on open skin sores.[14] Streptococci from the nasopharynx may be transmitted to skin sites, but it is more common for the skin to be colonized first and the throat later. Classical erysipelas, in contrast, is thought to be transmitted via the respiratory tract, either from the patient or from a caretaker. Erysipelas is occasionally seen following superinfection of chicken pox lesions.

The group B streptococci causing early onset perinatal infections are those carried by the mother in the lower gastrointestinal and genitourinary tracts. Organisms may enter the amniotic cavity following rupture of amniotic membranes, but the fetus may become infected with membranes intact.[58,111] Although rupture of membranes for greater than 12 h is a recognized risk factor for ascending infection,[22] the duration of labor is also important, perhaps because of the entry of organisms via microscopic defects in the membranes.[16] Among twins, who have a higher rate of infection than singletons, it is usually the first twin who is closer to the source of infection and at greater risk.[146] Once the streptococci have entered the amniotic fluid, they proliferate rapidly and are aspirated or swallowed by the fetus. Late-onset infections may have a maternal source in about half of cases, with colonization occurring at delivery.[54] Other infants may acquire streptococci later from persons outside the immediate family, presumably via the oral or respiratory route.

Enteric and oral streptococci are part of the normal flora, acquired early in life from the mother and family members. They generally cause opportunistic infection only after perturbations of normal defenses. Nosocomial infections are usually due to a patient's own flora. Transient bacteremia may occur with dental manipulation, transurethral prostate resection, or gynecologic and gastrointestinal surgery. Patients with known history of rheumatic heart disease, mitral valve prolapse, or artificial heart valves are at higher risk for developing endocarditis due to otherwise "benign" streptococcal species. In such cases a prophylactic antibiotic, usually penicillin, is administered just prior to the dental or surgical treatment (see Section 9.2).

7. Pathogenesis and Immunity

7.1. Pathogenesis

The development of infection involves a multitude of interrelated bacterial and host factors that vary enormously

among streptococcal species. The biologic characteristics associated with virulence among various streptococci are summarized in Section 4; certain host factors and modes of transmission are noted in Sections 5.9 and 6. The pathogenic process is not clearly understood for any streptococcal disease, but it may be useful to consider three general stages. First, organisms are acquired by the host and either succeed in colonizing their preferred sites or are eliminated by host defenses at the epithelial surface. For many streptococcal species the specific mechanisms of adherence are known.[2,15,122] Adherence may be important in the establishment of colonization but is not necessarily a property that distinguishes virulent from commensal species or strains. To ward off bacterial invasion the host has epithelial barriers, mucus layers, and secretions containing enzymes and antibodies. The second stage begins when organisms succeed in breaching local defenses and enter the epithelial and subepithelial tissues, or in the case of *S. mutans* get into and through the tooth enamel.[122] Most of the acute pathologic effects of group A streptococci occur at this stage by causing pharyngitis or skin infection, frequently accompanied by lymphadenitis but rarely progressing to bacteremia. In pneumococcal pneumonia and in otitis media the initial insult is not a direct breach of epithelium but rather the invasion of a normally sterile compartment; symptoms of disease ensue as organisms multiply and induce inflammation in surrounding tissue. The host responds with nonspecific secretory and serum forces, including the release of vasoactive and chemotactic mediators, activation of the alternative complement pathway, and with the mobilization of neutrophils and tissue macrophages. Eventually, specific secretory and serum antibodies develop and contribute to resolution of the disease. The third stage is systemic infection, in which organisms multiply in blood and tissues. Further alterations in host physiology occur by direct and indirect effects on hemodynamics, metabolism, and the function of individual organs.

Some of the mechanisms thought to be involved in acute group B streptococcal sepsis have been studied *in vitro* and in animal models. The infusion of a cell-free extract of group B streptococci was shown to reduce neutrophil counts and induce neutrophil infiltration in the lungs of newborn lambs.[142] This may be mediated by activation of C5a. A similar picture of pneumonia/sepsis may be seen in some human neonates, but in others there is a minimal inflammatory response despite the presence of bacteria in the lung or other tissue.[148] The type III capsular polysaccharide may act directly to diminish inflammation and adherence of neutrophils to vascular endothelia.[134] Group B streptococci also appear to produce an enzyme that inactivates C5a, similar to that described in group A streptococci. The immediate effect of intravenous infusions of washed heat-killed type III group B streptococci in chronically instrumented piglets is a marked increase in pulmonary artery pressure,[151] as also observed in septic neonates. The pulmonary hypertension could be blocked with indomethacin, a cyclooxygenase inhibitor, and dazmagrel, an inhibitor of thromboxane synthesis. Similar drugs could be useful clinically but remain experimental at present. Other streptococci, including group A, and pneumococci, also induce hemodynamic aberrations that could contribute to severe forms of systemic disease.

The pathogenesis of the nonsuppurative sequelae of group A infections has yet to be elucidated. The cross-reactivity of certain M proteins and components of heart tissue has long been considered to play an important role in the development of rheumatic fever. Recent studies have identified M protein epitopes that cross-react with myosin and DNA, and α-helically coiled proteins such as tropomyosin, actin, and keratin.[49] The diverse manifestations of acute rheumatic fever might be explained in part by the specificity and titer of antibodies cross-reactive with different tissue components. In a similar fashion, acute glomerulonephritis may involve the development of antibodies that cross-react with basement membrane collagen and laminin.[112,188] The cationic charge of the antigens may also influence their affinity for the glomerular basement membrane and the nature of immune complexes formed.[175] Another feature of nephritogenic streptococci is the presence of a nephritis strain-associated protein.[104] This distinctive low-molecular-weight streptokinase is a plasminogen activator and could induce proliferation of cells, release of inflammatory products, and activate complement, thus contributing to known pathologic features of the disease.

7.2. Immunity

Specific immunity to streptococcal infections is thought to depend on the development of antibodies to capsular and other surface determinants. Antibody assays for various streptococcal antigens have been noted in Section 3.4.2, and current developments in streptococcal vaccines are further discussed in Section 9.6. Although most of our knowledge of the immune response relates to the occurrence of antibodies in the serum, recent studies of mucosal immunity suggest that the first line of host defenses are at the local level. The precise role of secretory antibodies in preventing, modifying, or eradicating bacterial colonization is not presently understood. Conversely, the effects of bacterial antigens at respiratory and gastrointestinal sites are poorly understood in regard to the systemic antibody response and the development of autoantibodies. In some cases it is likely that the organisms have developed a form of mimicry to confuse or evade the immune response of the host. Many streptococci have antigens that cross-react with other organisms, common foodstuffs, or components of the host's own tissue. Antibodies undoubtedly have functions other than protection against disease. They are known to be important in the recovery from established infection and probably function in the removal of antigens from local and systemic sites.

Assays for group A streptococcal antibodies (Table 5) are used clinically to determine if a patient has had a recent infection. Although humans normally make antibodies to streptolysin O and other extracellular components, only antibodies to M proteins are associated with protection against subsequent disease. Serum IgG antibodies to M proteins arise in response to infection or immunization and can initiate bactericidal activity in whole blood opsonophagocytic assays. These antibodies, however, are not as efficient as secretory IgA antibodies in protecting mice against infection via the intranasal route.[17] Intranasal immunization of volunteers with purified M protein resulted in greater resistance to colonization with live streptococci than did subcutaneous immunization, and serum antibody response was not a reliable predictor of resistance to pharyngitis.[50] At present, group A vaccines remain experimental, but it appears that local immune mechanisms may be more efficiently utilized and less likely to result in systemic side effects (see Section 9.6).

Antibodies to the capsular polysaccharides of group B streptococci are thought to mediate protection against systemic invasion. This concept is based upon the finding that few infants with group B streptococcal disease have antibodies to the offending type, and that antibodies are protective against bacterial challenge in animal models.[12,77] Naturally occurring antibodies in mothers are often of the IgM class and do not readily cross the placenta,[3] and less IgG antibody is transferred to the premature than to the term fetus. Despite the presumed importance of antibodies, it should be pointed out that the prevalence of group B streptococcal antibodies is generally low, with about 6% of cord sera having > 2 μg/ml against types II and III in a defined population.[86,88] Thus, the vast majority of infants, including most of those colonized, are "antibody deficient," yet a very small number become infected. The presence of mucosal antibodies may modify colonization, but so far a clearly defined role for secretory immunity is not apparent.[87]

Most of our knowledge of pneumococcal immunity comes from studies of purified polysaccharide vaccines.[161] Adults respond well to most of the antigens, but infants respond poorly. Children over 2 years of age have more consistent responses but still respond poorly to types common in childhood illnesses, especially types 6 and 14.[55,115] Although repeated doses of vaccine produce little or not booster effect, systemic tolerance does not appear to develop in humans.[115] Efforts to improve the immunogenicity of vaccines have been directed toward the use of proteins coupled to the polysaccharides in order to elicit T-helper cell cooperation.[1] Theoretically, this approach should also increase the proportion of IgG antibodies. The B-cell response can be monitored by enumerating the peripheral blood leukocytes that secrete specific antibodies at about 7 days after systemic immunization.[123] The majority of cells secreted IgA antibodies, although the later serum response was predominantly IgG and IgM. The secretory antibody response was relatively modest. There is no consensus as to what constitutes a protective serum antibody level, whether IgG is required in preference to IgM antibodies, or what role secretory antibodies play in vaccine-induced immunity.[123,139,161]

The poor response of infants to vaccines should not be interpreted to mean that they lack antibody to pneumococci. Antibodies to pneumococcal polysaccharides occur naturally and in response to infection or asymptomatic nasopharyngeal colonization.[80] The response to polysaccharide antigens is commonly regarded as "T-cell independent," but animal studies suggest that this independence relates only to the participation of the T-helper cell system. The direction and magnitude of response is apparently de-

termined by T-amplifier and T-suppressor cells and possibly other components. Oral tolerance has been described in humans ingesting a vaccine containing *H. influenzae* type b[40] and in animals fed gum arabic, a complex carbohydrate food additive that cross-reacts with pneumococcus type 23.[170] In human infants serum antibody levels were highest at the time of acute otitis media, presumably in response to prior colonization, but levels frequently declined over succeeding months despite the continued carriage of the organism.[80] This suggests that specific antibodies in serum were not associated with protection against otitis media and that some form of oral tolerance may be involved in the response to natural exposure. The role of secretory immunity in natural infections remains entirely unexplored.

8. Patterns of Host Response

8.1. Clinical Features

The manifestations of streptococcal diseases are remarkably diverse. Their clinical presentation, diagnosis, and therapy are discussed in detail in many of the medical, pediatric, and infectious disease textbooks. The most common and most important diseases caused by the major streptococcal group are listed in Table 7. Diseases associated with other streptococci are noted in Tables 1 and 2.

The typical form of group A streptococcal respiratory disease in children and adults is acute exudative phar-

Table 7. Diseases Associated with Major Streptococcal Groups

Group A streptococci	Group B streptococci	Pneumococci	Enterococci
Most common	Early onset neonatal disease	Infants and children	Nosocomial
Pharyngitis/tonsillitis	Undifferentiated sepsis	Otitis media	Bacteremia
Scarlet fever	Meningitis	Conjunctivitis	Intraabdominal infection
Impetigo/pyoderma	Pneumonia	Pneumonia	Surgical wounds
Cellulitis	Maternal infections	Bacteremia	Burn wounds
Less common	Amnionitis	Meningitis	Vascular catheter
Peritonsillar abscess	Endometritis	Adults	Urinary tract infection
Otitis media	Urinary tract infection	Sinusitis	Postpartum infections
Mastoiditis	Bacteremia/sepsis	Pneumonia	Community acquired
Sinusitis	Septic abortion	Pleural empyema	Urinary tract infection
Erysipelas	Late-onset neonatal disease	Bacteremia	Endocarditis
Pneumonia/empyema	Meningitis	Meningitis	Biliary infection
Puerperal sepsis	Bacteremia/sepsis	Endocarditis	Pelvic infection
Meningitis	Bone and joint infection		
Endocarditis	Skin and soft tissue infection		
Nonsuppurative sequelae	Otitis media		
Acute rheumatic fever	Omphalitis		
Acute glomerulonephritis			

yngitis. The onset is abrupt, with fever, chills, a sore throat with pain on swallowing, malaise, headache, often with abdominal pain, nausea, or vomiting. On physical examination, the pharyngeal mucosae are erythematous, edematous, and streaked with a purulent nonadherent exudate over the tonsils or posterior pharynx; petechiae may be present. The anterior cervical lymph nodes may be enlarged and are usually acutely tender. In young children the findings may be less specific, often with fever and lymphadenitis but relatively little inflammation of the upper respiratory mucosae. Mild or subclinical infection may occur at any age and may be missed. This is of concern because up to half of patients developing rheumatic fever do not give a clear history of an antecedent sore throat. With scarlet fever the pharyngitis is accompanied within 24 to 28 h by a fine red exanthem beginning on the trunk and intertriginous areas, later spreading to the extremities. The face is usually spared, but the tongue may be inflamed with a "strawberry" appearance. Streptococcal impetigo may appear as single lesions of the epidermis, frequently on the lower extremities,

spreading to other areas as new insect bites or breaks in the skin become infected. Early lesions are pustular and rapidly develop into mature lesions about 1 cm in diameter with a characteristic honeylike crust. Lesions may become concomitantly infected by staphylococci, which may be resistant to penicillin therapy. Erysipelas is a serious fulminant form of cellulitis that appears as an elevated erythematous lesion with a rapidly advancing well-demarcated border. Erysipelas often involves the face, a surgical wound, an umbilical stump, or a chicken pox lesion. The patient is febrile, toxic, and may be bacteremic. Group A streptococci are also associated with many of the same clinical entities as the pneumococcus and other pyogenic organisms.

The nonsuppurative sequelae of group A infections may present acutely, or less often insidiously. Acute rheumatic fever varies greatly in its manifestations, the diagnosis being made with the guidance of the Jones Criteria (revised in 1984),[105] described in Table 8. The onset is typically abrupt, with fever and polyarthritis. Myocarditis

Table 8.   Jones Criteria (Revised) for Guidance in the Diagnosis of Acute Rheumatic Fever, as Recommended by the American Heart Association[105]

Major manifestations	Minor manifestations
Carditis	*Clinical*
Polyarthritis	Fever
Chorea	Arthralgia
Erythema marginatum	Previous rheumatic fever or
Subcutaneous nodules	rheumatic heart disease
	Laboratory
	Acute-phase reactions
	Abnormal erythrocyte sedimentation
	rate, C-reactive protein, or leukocytosis
	Prolonged P-R interval

Supporting evidence of streptococcal infection
  Increased antistreptolysin O or other streptococcal antibody
  Positive throat culture for group A streptococcus
  Recent scarlet fever

The presence of two major, or one major and two minor, manifestations *plus* evidence of a preceding streptococcal infection indicates a high probability of rheumatic fever.
Manifestations with a long latent period, such as chorea and late-onset carditis, are exempt from the latter requirement.
The WHO Study Group recommends that the following groups be considered separately and exempted from the Jones criteria: "pure" chorea, insidious or late-onset carditis, and rheumatic recurrence.[183]

or valvulitis, most commonly involving the mitral valve, occurs in about half of patients suffering their first attack. Carditis may be the only major manifestation in some patients and may develop insidiously, presenting as heart failure without any clear history of prior rheumatic fever or obvious streptococcal infection.[174,183] Because of difficulties in making the diagnosis, other conditions, such as collagen–vascular diseases and infective endocarditis, must be considered whenever acute rheumatic fever is suspected. Acute glomerulonephritis presents fewer diagnostic problems. A recent skin or throat infection is usually evident by examination, history, culture, or antibody tests. The urine is dark, containing many red blood cells and casts. The patient usually has edema and elevated blood pressure; the blood urea nitrogen and creatinine are usually elevated and the C3 complement level is low. With appropriate acute care, nearly all patients have a complete recovery.[156]

Group B streptococcal disease in the neonate usually begins *in utero* with nonspecific symptoms appearing within the first few hours of birth.[54,148] Unexplained apnea, respiratory distress, temperature instability, or poor feeding may be the only clues to early onset disease. Infection usually takes the form of undifferentiated sepsis with, or more often without, meningitis. The disease is well advanced by the time hypoxia, cyanosis, acidosis, or vascular collapse becomes obvious. Lung involvement is frequent but the chest X-ray is typical of hyaline membrane disease more often than of discrete pneumonia. Similarly, there is rarely a CSF pleocytosis even when bacteria are recovered from the spinal fluid. In general, the inflammatory response parallels the maturity of the infant, the specificity of clinical signs and symptoms, and to some extent the prognosis. Late-onset infections, occurring beyond the immediate newborn period, often tend to be more localized and have a better outcome. Meningitis is common, but sepsis without meningitis is frequently seen.[54] Bacteremia or meningitis may be associated with an infective focus, such as omphalitis, otitis media, or osteomyelitis. The long-term outcome of infants who survive group B streptococcal meningitis is generally good.[176] Very occasionally, neonates develop similar disease due to group G streptococci or pneumococci. Maternal group B streptococcal disease may occur during gestation, notably urinary tract infections and septic abortion.[51,185] Infection around the time of delivery, especially amnionitis, is a threat to both fetus and mother.[78] Endometritis and bacteremia are the most frequent postpartum infections. Endocarditis is an unusual complication of perinatal infection or septic abortion and is more often seen in older individuals with some underlying heart disease or other predisposing condition.[66]

The clinical features of pneumococcal disease vary with the site of infection and the age of the patient. Meningitis in young infants does not commonly present with neck stiffness and headache, as it does in adults, but more often with nonspecific symptoms, such as fever, irritability or inconsolable crying, poor feeding, or vomiting. Patients presenting with a second episode of meningitis must be suspected of having a CSF leak, skull fracture, or immunologic deficiency. Pneumonia in children is similar to that seen in adults, but classic features of chills, hacking cough, pleuritic pain, and rusty sputum may be subdued or absent. Bacteremia in children is associated with pneumonia in about a third of cases, with otitis media in another third, and the remainder with no focus of infection.[79] While most infants with bacteremia present with fever, leukocytosis, and a clinically apparent focus of infection, some have "occult" bacteremia with few physical findings and a marginal leukocytosis.[24]

8.2. Diagnosis

The isolation and identification of streptococci from properly cultured infected sites provides the definitive means of establishing the diagnosis. A careful evaluation of the patient is essential in forming an accurate clinical diagnosis, after which the physician must decide what sites are to be cultured and what ancillary tests are appropriate. Streptococcal pharyngitis cannot reliably be diagnosed without a throat culture, because many other agents may cause acute pharyngitis. Conversely, an asymptomatic carrier may have a positive throat culture coincidental with a viral pharyngitis. It is in the best interest of the patient and the community to avoid prescribing antibiotics without a specific indication; it is also preferable to treat a positive throat culture rather than risk untoward sequelae. In some cases, however, it is valuable to confirm the diagnosis by antibody tests and follow-up cultures. The efficacy of treatment regimens depends upon accurate etiologic diagnoses; patients with recurrent infection may actually prove to be chronic carriers or have multiple disease episodes due to different streptococcal serotypes; a definitive diagnosis is needed for the clinical management of patients with nephritis or symptoms suggesting rheumatic fever.

The microbiologic diagnosis of other forms of streptococcal disease is no less important, inasmuch as it directs both the clinical approach and the choice of antibiotics. Blood cultures may be indicated when infection is suspected in the absence of an obvious infected site, especially for those at risk for nosocomial disease and infants who may have occult bacteremias. Cultures of blood, spinal fluid, skin, lung or empyema, sinus or middle ear fluid, may be required to confirm the appropriateness of antibiotics selected empirically upon suspicion of infection. While most streptococci remain susceptible to the penicillins, some pneumococci are intermediate or resistant, as are many oral and enteric species. With the exception of streptococcal pharyngitis, cultures of normal carriage sites, including the nasopharynx and lower bowel, are rarely useful in making an etiologic diagnosis of clinically diagnosed infection. Otitis media, for example, is frequently caused by the pneumococcus, but pneumococci are frequently isolated from the nasopharynx of children with otitis media due to *Haemophilus influenzae*. Similarly, many infants are colonized by group B streptococci at delivery but relatively few are infected. In some instances, however, it may not be possible to obtain a definitive culture, as is often the case in pneumonia. A sputum culture growing pneumococci, in a patient with an alveolar consolidation on chest X-ray and a typical clinical course, supports the diagnosis of "putative" pneumococcal pneumonia.

9. Control and Prevention

9.1. General Preventive Measures

Personal hygiene, adequate nutrition and housing, health education, and access to medical care are all important factors in prevention of streptococcal diseases. Inspection of food and milk production, and proper pasteurization of dairy products are taken for granted in most developed countries but remain problems in certain areas. Strict asepsis is required in surgical and obstetric procedures. Simple infection control measures, especially hand-washing, must be continually encouraged, and attention must be paid to the health of hospital employees working in patient areas.

9.2. Antibiotics in Prevention of Group A Streptococcal Disease

Primary prevention of acute rheumatic fever consists of identifying and treating persons with acute streptococcal pharyngitis. Antibiotic therapy is aimed at eradicating streptococci from the respiratory tract. Penicillin is the drug of choice, given as a single intramuscular injection of ("long-acting") benzathine benzylpenicillin or as a 10-day course of oral phenoxymethyl penicillin. Other oral penicillins, such as amoxicillin and dicloxacillin, are also effective but are more expensive and offer no particular advantage. Alternative drugs include erythromycin (except in some areas of

eastern Asia or eastern Europe where resistance may be a problem) and oral cephalosporins (cephalexin, cefaclor, cephradine, cefadroxil). Clindamycin is effective but is costly and has a small potential risk of pseudomembranous enterocolitis. Tetracyclines, sulfonamides, and chloramphenicol are not effective. Mass penicillin prophylaxis has been used in some epidemic situations but is now chiefly confined to certain military populations.[171]

Secondary prevention consists of the regular administration of antibiotic to persons who have had rheumatic fever in order to prevent subsequent group A infections that could trigger recurrent attacks or exacerbate existing rheumatic heart disease.[183] Secondary prophylaxis is cost-effective, reduces the risk of recurrence, and in many patients allows for healing of valvular damage occurring in the initial attack. Long-acting intramuscular penicillin is usually given at monthly intervals, but may be required every 3 weeks in high-risk situations. Alternatively, oral penicillin may be given daily, but lack of compliance is a major problem. Patients unable to take penicillin may be given sulfadiazine or erythromycin. The duration of secondary prophylaxis is not certain but must be tailored to the individual. Patients with valvular rheumatic heart disease are given prolonged, even life-long, prophylaxis. Those without cardiac involvement should have prophylaxis for at least 5 years and at least through age 18. Patients with carditis as part of their initial attack are usually given prophylaxis until age 25.[183]

Patients with rheumatic heart disease, as well as others with prosthetic valves, other valvular lesions, and probably mitral valve prolapse, are at risk for developing infective endocarditis when undergoing dental or surgical manipulations. Prophylaxis is required for dental procedures that cause bleeding, especially when gingival disease is present; for respiratory procedures including tonsillectomy, adenoidectomy, bronchoscopy, or mucosal biopsy; for genitourinary or gastrointestinal procedures, such as prostate resection or intestinal biopsy. Recommended antibiotic regimens vary and are subject to change.[45,183] High-risk patients, who have prosthetic valves, severely damaged native valves, or history of previous endocarditis, are usually given penicillin or ampicillin plus gentamicin, to cover oral or enteric streptococci, as well as other organisms. Antibiotic doses are given 1 h prior and 6 h after the procedure. "Standard risk" patients are usually given only a penicillin for dental manipulations, but an aminoglycoside is added for genitourinary or gastrointestinal procedures. Patients allergic to penicillin or who are on long-term penicillin prophylaxis are given erythromycin or vancomycin.

The prevention of acute glomerulonephritis by antibiotic therapy has not been convincingly demonstrated, and prophylaxis may not be practical in most patient populations. Prompt treatment of minor skin trauma and insect bites with topical antibiotic ointment has been shown to reduce the occurrence of streptococcal skin infections and could reduce the risk of subsequent nephritis.[126]

9.3. Surgical Approaches to Recurrent Group A Streptococcal Disease

Tonsillectomy or tonsillectomy with adenoidectomy are frequently performed because of recurrent throat infections. Although children who have surgery experience fewer throat infections over the subsequent 2 years, the difference in rates compared to controls is not impressive. These findings were confirmed by Paradise *et al.* in a carefully controlled study with stringent entry criteria.[144] Surgical intervention was beneficial for severely affected children over at least the 2 years following surgery. Nevertheless, a substantial proportion of those managed nonsurgically had relatively little throat infection during the period of study, and the actual reduction in group A streptococcal infection rates was small. Their results appeared to "justify but by no means to mandate the performance of tonsillectomy" in carefully selected children. Treatment should be individualized, and should be considered only for severely affected children. More clearly defined indications for surgical intervention include patients with peritonsillar abscess or severe obstructive symptoms.

9.4. Intrapartum Chemoprophylaxis against Group B Streptococcal Disease

Most efforts to prevent group B streptococcal infections have focused on the early onset disease of neonates. Because most of these infections begin *in utero,* a dose of "prophylactic" penicillin given at delivery does little to stem the progress of established disease.[158] A more effective approach, reported by Boyer and Gotoff, is based upon the use of ampicillin given during labor to selected women whose infants are at high risk for group B streptococcal disease.[20] Mothers were cultured for group B colonization during gestation. Colonized mothers presenting in labor were selected for assignment to treatment or control groups if they had premature labor (< 37 weeks of gestation) or prolonged rupture of amniotic membranes (> 12 h). Patients in the treatment group received 2 g of ampicillin intravenously, followed by 1 g every 4 h until delivery. [Mothers in either group who developed intrapartum fever (> 37.5°C) were excluded form the study and were treated

with ampicillin.] Infants of study mothers receiving ampicillin were given four doses of ampicillin at 12 h intervals until their initial culture results were available. There were no cases of group B streptococcal disease among 83 mothers given intrapartum ampicillin, while bacteremic infections occurred in 5 of 79 infants in the control group. In addition to efficacy, an advantage of selective intrapartum prophylaxis is that it limits the use of antibiotic to a small proportion of patients at greatest risk. It requires prenatal cultures for colonization and the cooperation of obstetric and pediatric care providers. It could be easier to implement if rapid diagnostic methods (Section 3.4.1) for detection of group B streptococcal colonization proved to be feasible. Estimates indicate that this should be a cost-effective as well as practical approach to preventing perinatal group B streptococcal disease.

9.5. Passive Immune Prophylaxis against Streptococcal Infections

The administration of gamma globulin has been employed for prevention of various bacterial infections in immunodeficient patients. The spectrum of host defense abnormalities that may benefit from this approach now includes patients with hypogammaglobulinemias, IgG subclass deficiencies, malignancy and immunosuppression, severe burns, bone marrow transplantation, and HIV infection.[75] Immunoglobulin preparations suitable for intravenous administration (IVIG) are also under investigation for prevention and adjunctive therapy of group B streptococcal disease in neonates.[65,160] Specialized IVIG preparations have been made from serum donors immunized with group B streptococcal vaccines to increase the concentrations of relevant antibodies. Similar preparations have been developed for studies of prevention of pneumococcal infections in certain high-risk populations. It is too early to tell how effective these approaches will be, but it should be noted that passive immunotherapy was used with some success in the treatment of pneumococcal pneumonia prior to the advent of penicillin.[64]

9.6. Immunization against Streptococcal Infections

A vaccine against rheumatic fever has been the goal of many investigators over the years. The difficulties involved are considerable and as yet only partially solved. The multitude of M protein types makes a simple vaccine impossible. Although a single broadly protective M protein epitope does not appear to exist,[136] certain conserved epitopes have been found to be common among different M types.[17] This feature has been used to make oral synthetic peptide vaccines (coupled to a cholera toxin subunit adjuvant) that induce mucosal immunity in mice and reduce the effects of nasopharyngeal challenge of streptococci.[17] Another approach uses cloned M protein expressed in live attenuated strains of *Salmonella* given orally to mice.[154] The possibility of inducing antibodies that cross-react with human tissue is of obvious concern but could be minimized by the oral route of administration and by the identification and selection of vaccine epitopes that have no homology with host proteins.

Group B polysaccharide vaccines have been under investigation for nearly a decade.[11,59] The goal of the vaccine approach is to immunize women in order to induce antibody that will later be capable of protecting the fetus against early onset disease and perhaps afford protection for several months against late-onset disease. Ideally, a vaccine should induce antibodies of the IgG class and be effective against all four major serotypes; it should be safe for administration to pregnant women or induce long-lived immunity if administered prior to pregnancy. One candidate type III vaccine has been tested in a small number of women at about 30 weeks of gestation.[13] The results indicated that antibody could be induced in about 60% of mothers, and that this antibody was predominantly IgG with functional activity demonstrated in the infant's cord serum. Given the feasibility of a vaccine, several problems remain to be solved: Vaccines against other types need to be developed and tested; the immunogenicity of the vaccine needs to be improved; the target population needs to be defined. Since only a minimal amount of maternally derived antibody is able to cross the placenta before the last trimester, the prospect of protecting the more premature fetus is uncertain. Nevertheless, it would be reasonable to suggest that any degree of protection afforded the mother would indirectly affect the fetus. Here a better understanding of the determinants of colonization and the mechanisms of mucosal immunity is clearly needed.

Pneumococcal vaccines have been studied for nearly 80 years. Their history and current recommendations[1,18,62,70,138,164] for use are summarized in Section 9.2 of Chapter 25.

Vaccines against dental caries, based upon antigens derived from *S. mutans*, have been under investigation for a number of years.[135] Several candidate vaccines have been successful in preventing caries in experimental animals. Limited human studies have shown that oral vaccines induce salivary IgA antibody responses, but long-term evaluations of efficacy have not been supported to date. One reason is that caries is not a life-threatening disease. Another is the concern that the antigens of *S. mutans*, like those of group A streptococci, could induce antibodies cross-reactive with human tissues. The latter problem has not been substantiated and may be minimized by the oral route, but further study is obviously needed.

10. Unresolved Problems

Despite the availability of antibiotics, the diagnosis and treatment of group A streptococcal pharyngitis continue to pose problems for the clinician.[26] The distinction between infection and carrier state is frequently blurred.[68] The new rapid diagnostic tests make it possible to treat promptly and reduce clinical symptoms, but the price paid may be a higher rate of symptomatic disease recurrence.[152] This has led some pediatricians to return to the old way of blood agar plates, postponing therapy for 48 h.[153] It is unlikely that changes in clinical practice have influenced the resurgence of acute rheumatic fever in recent years. The reasons for its reappearance remain unknown.

Group B streptococci are the most common cause of serious bacterial disease in newborn infants in many Western countries. Despite similar maternal colonization rates and presumably similar risk of exposure, the disease is infrequent in some areas of Europe and Asia.[132] The reasons for this are not clear but could be of considerable practical importance. Methods for intrapartum antibiotic prophylaxis have been established but remain to be implemented on a wide scale.[21] Meanwhile, we still have little understanding of the local and systemic defense mechanisms required to prevent infection by this usually benign organism. Other streptococci, particularly oral and enteric species, are constant companions that cause disease only under specialized circumstances. It is not clear whether some of these organisms are in fact "virulent" in certain settings, or whether the disease is due mainly to predisposing conditions in the host. The question may be moot, but answers would help us direct attention to better ways of preventing nosocomial and opportunistic infections.

Few bacteria have been studied as intensely as the pneumococci, yet our knowledge of their virulence and pathogenesis is extremely limited. It is especially curious that certain serotypes are most frequently associated with children and childhood infections. These are among the least immunogenic types but are uncommon in adults.[79] Virulent pneumococcal serotypes appear to differ in the binding and degradative processing of the C3b complement component in ways that may affect both phagocytosis and the ability to stimulate antibody production.[97] The regulation of the immune response to pneumococcal polysaccharides is not at all understood, and the role of systemic and secretory antibodies has yet to be fully explored.

The unanswered questions apparent from the discussions in this chapter remain: how do streptococci cause disease, and why do some individuals become infected while others do not? Major virulence factors, such as M proteins and polysaccharide capsules, have been identified, but the pathophysiologic mechanisms by which they interact with the host remain uncertain and do not completely explain the disease process. The determinants of colonization, the defenses of the host at the mucosal level, and the development of local and systemic immunity are not well understood. Much has to be learned before the development of effective vaccines or other preventive measures becomes a reality.

ACKNOWLEDGMENTS

The author thanks Marilyn J. Crain, Department of Pediatrics, University of Alabama at Birmingham, and Edward L. Kaplan, Department of Pediatrics, University of Minnesota, for review and suggestions for this chapter. Data for Figs. 2 and 3 were kindly supplied by Caroline Breese Hall, University of Rochester, New York. Supported in part by Program Project Grant P01-17812 from the National Institute of Child Health and Human Development.

11. References

1. ANDERSON, P., AND BETTS, R., Human adult immunogenicity of protein-coupled pneumococcal capsular antigens of serotypes prevalent in otitis media, *Pediatr. Infect. Dis. J.* **8**:S50–S53 (1989).
2. ANDERSSON, B., GRAY, B. M., DILLON, H. C., JR., BAHRMAND, A., AND SVANBORG-EDEN, C., Role of adherence of *Streptococcus pneumoniae* in acute otitis media, *Pediatr. Infect. Dis. J.* **7**:476–480 (1988).
3. ANTHONY, B. F., CONCEPCION, N. F., WASS, C. A., AND HEINER, D. C., Immunoglobin G and M composition of naturally occurring antibody to type III group B streptococci, *Infect. Immun.* **46**:98–104 (1984).
4. APPELBAUM, P. C., World-wide development of antibiotic resistance in pneumococci, *Eur. J. Clin. Microbiol.* **6**:367–377 (1987).
5. ARDITI, M., SHULMAN, S. T., DAVIS, T., AND YOGEV, R., Group C β-hemolytic streptococcal infections in children: Nine pediatric cases and review, *Rev. Infect. Dis.* **11**:34–45 (1989).
6. ARENDS, J. P., AND ZANEN, H. C., Meningitis caused by

7. AUSTRIAN, R., Pneumococcus: The first one hundred years, *Rev. Infect. Dis.* **3**:183–189 (1981).
8. AVERY, O. T., MacLEOD, C. M., AND McCARTY, M., Studies on the chemical nature of the substance inducing transformation of pneumococcal types: Induction of transformation by a desoxyribonucleic acid, *J. Exp. Med.* **79**:137–158 (1944).
9. AYOUB, E. M., BARRETT, D. J., MACLAREN, N. K., AND KRISCHER, J. P., Association of class II human histocompatibility leukocyte antigens with rheumatic fever, *J. Clin. Invest.* **77**:2019–2026 (1986).
10. BACKHOUSE, C. I., AND CARTWRIGHT, R. Y., An outbreak of streptococcal skin sepsis in a closed community, *Br. Med. J.* **3**:497–499 (1974).
11. BAKER, C. J., AND KASPER, D. L., Group B streptococcal vaccines, *Rev. Infect. Dis.* **7**:458–467 (1985).
12. BAKER, C. J., EDWARDS, M. S., AND KASPER, D. L., Role of antibody to native type III polysaccharide of group B streptococcus in infant infections, *Pediatrics* **68**:544–549 (1981).
13. BAKER, C. J., RENCH, M. A., EDWARDS, M. S., CARPENTER, R. J., HAYS, B. M., AND KASPER, D. L., Immunization of pregnant women with a polysaccharide vaccine of group B streptococcus, *N. Engl. J. Med.* **319**:1180–1185 (1988).
14. BASSETT, D. C. J., Hippelates flies and acute nephritis, *Lancet* **1**:503 (1967).
15. BEACHEY, E. H., AND COURTNEY, H. S., Bacterial adherence: The attachment of group A streptococci to mucosal surfaces, *Rev. Infect. Dis.* **9**(Suppl.):S475–S481 (1987).
16. BECROFT, D. M. O., FARMER, J., MASON, J. H., AND MORRIS, M. C., Perinatal infections by group B β-hemolytic streptococci, *Br. J. Obstet. Gynaecol.* **83**:960–966 (1976).
17. BESSEN, D., AND FISCHETTI, V. A., Influence of intranasal immunization with synthetic peptides corresponding to conserved epitopes of M protein on mucosal colonization by group A streptococci, *Infect. Immun.* **56**:2666–2672 (1988).
18. BOLAN, G., BROOME, C. V., FACKLAM, R. R., PLIKAYTIS, B. D., FRASER, D. W., AND SCHLECH, W. F., III, Pneumococcal vaccine efficacy in selected populations in the United States, *Ann. Intern. Med.* **104**:1–6 (1986).
19. BORZY, M. S., WOLFF, L., GEWURZ, A., BUIST, N. R., AND LOVRIEN, E., Recurrent sepsis with deficiencies of C2 and galactosidase, *Am. J. Dis. Child.* **138**:186–191 (1984).
20. BOYER, K. M., AND GOTOFF, S. P., Prevention of neonatal group B streptococcal disease with selective intrapartum chemoprophylaxis, *N. Engl. J. Med.* **314**:1665–1669 (1986).
21. BOYER, K. M., VOGEL, L. C., GOTOFF, S. P., GADZALA, C. A., STRINGER, J., AND MAXTED, W. R., Nosocomial transmission of bacteriophage type 7/11/12 group B streptococci in a special care nursery, *Am. J. Dis. Child.* **134**:964–966 (1980).
22. BOYER, K. M., GADZALA, C. A., BURD, L. I., FISHER, D. E., PATON, J. B., AND GOTOFF, S. P., Selective intrapartum

Streptococcus suis in humans, *Rev. Infect. Dis.* **10**:131–137 (1988).

chemoprophylaxis of neonatal group B streptococcal early-onset disease. I. Epidemiologic rationale, *J. Infect. Dis.* **148:**795–801 (1983).

23. BRACONIER, J. H., NILSSON, B., OXELIUS, V. A., AND KARUP-PEDERSEN, F., Recurrent pneumococcal infections in a patient with lack of specific IgG and IgM pneumococcal antibodies and deficiency of serum IgA, IgG$_2$ and IgG$_4$, *Scand. J. Infect. Dis.* **16:**407–410 (1984).

24. BRATTON, L., TEELE, D. W., AND KLEIN, J. O., Outcome of unsuspected pneumococcemia in children not initially admitted to the hospital, *J. Pediatr.* **90:**703–706 (1977).

25. BREESE, B. B., DISNEY, F. A., AND TALPEY, W., The nature of a small pediatric group practice. II. The incidence of beta streptococcal illness in a private pediatric practice, *Pediatrics* **38:**277–285 (1966).

26. BREESE, B. B., DENNY, F. W., DILLON, H. C., JR., STILLERMAN, M., NELSON, J. D., AND MCCRACKEN, G. H., Consensus: Difficult management problems in children with streptococcal pharyngitis, *Pediatr. Infect. Dis. J.* **4:**10–13 (1985).

27. BRILES, D. E., SCOTT, G., GRAY, B. M., CRAIN, M. J., BLAESE, M., NAHM, M., SCOTT, V., AND HABER, P., Naturally occurring antibodies to phosphocholine as a potential index of antibody responsiveness to polysaccharides, *J. Infect. Dis.* **155:**1307–1314 (1987).

28. BRIMBLECOMBE, F. S. W., CRUICKSHANK, R., MASTERS, P. L., AND REID, D. D., Family studies of respiratory infections, *Br. Med. J.* **1:**119–128 (1958).

29. BROOK, I., Role of beta-lactamase-producing bacteria in the failure of penicillin to eradicate group A streptococci, *Pediatr. Infect. Dis. J.* **4:**491–495 (1985).

30. BRYAN, C. S., REYNOLDS, K. L., AND BROWN, J. S., Mortality associated with enterococcal bacteremia, *Surg. Gynecol. Obstet.* **160:**557–561 (1985).

31. BUNTAIN, W. L., AND LYNN, H. B., Splenorrhaphy: Changing concepts for the traumatized spleen, *Surgery* **86:**748–760 (1979).

32. BUTTER, M. N., AND deMOOR, C. E., *Streptococcus agalactiae* as a cause of meningitis in the newborn, and of bacteraemia in adults, *Antonie van Leeuwenhoek J. Microbiol. Serol.* **33:**439–450 (1967).

33. Centers for Disease Control, Update: Pneumococcal polysaccharide vaccine usage—United States, *Morbid. Mortal. Weekly Rep.* **33:**273–281 (1984).

34. Centers for Disease Control, Group A, β hemolytic *Streptococcus* skin infections in a meat-packing plant—Oregon, *Morbid. Mortal. Weekly Rep.* **35:**629–630 (1986).

35. Centers for Disease Control, Acute rheumatic fever at a Navy training center, San Diego, California, *Morbid. Mortal. Weekly Rep.* **37:**101–104 (1988).

36. CHHATWAL, G. S., DUTRA, I. S., AND BLOBEL, H., Fibrinogen binding inhibits the fixation of the third component of human complement on surface of group A, B, C, and G streptococci, *Microbiol. Immunol.* **29:**973–980 (1985).

37. CHRISTIE, C. D. C., HAVENS, P. L., AND SHAPIRO, E. D.,

Bacteremia with group A streptococci in childhood, *Am. J. Dis. Child.* **142:**559–561 (1988).

38. CHRISTIE, R., ATKINS, N. E., AND MUNCH-PETERSEN, E., A note on a lytic phenomenon shown by group B streptococci, *Aust. J. Exp. Biol. Med. Sci.* **22:**197–200 (1944).

39. CHUN, L. T., REDDY, D. V., AND YAMAMOTO, L. G., Rheumatic fever in children and adolescents in Hawaii, *Pediatrics* **79:**549–552 (1987).

40. CLANCY, R. L., CRIPPS, A. W., HUSBAND, A. J., AND BUCKLEY, D., Specific immune response in the respiratory tract after administration of an oral polyvalent bacterial vaccine, *Infect. Immun.* **39:**491–496 (1983).

41. CLEAT, P. H., AND TIMMS, K. N., Cloning and expression in *Escherichia coli* of the Ibc protein genes of group B streptococci: Binding of human immunoglobin A to the beta antigen, *Infect. Immun.* **55:**1151–1155 (1987).

42. COCHI, S., AND FELDMAN, R., Estimating national incidence of group B streptococcal disease: The effect of adjusting for birth weight, *Pediatr. Infect. Dis. J.* **2:**414–415 (1983).

43. Committee on Issues and Priorities for New Vaccine Development, National Academy of Science Institute of Medicine, *New Vaccine Development: Establishing Priorities,* Volume I, *Diseases of Importance in the United States,* National Academy Press, Washington, D.C., 1985.

44. Committee on Issues and Priorities for New Vaccine Development, National Academy of Science Institute of Medicine, *New Vaccine Development: Establishing Priorities,* Volume II, *Diseases of Importance in Developing Countries,* National Academy Press, Washington, D.C., 1986.

45. Committee on Prevention of Rheumatic Fever and Bacterial Endocarditis of the American Heart Association, Prevention of bacterial endocarditis, *Circulation* **70:**1123A (1984).

46. CONE, L. A., WOODWARD, D. R., SCHLIEVERT, P. M., AND TOMORY, G. S., Clinical and bacteriologic observations of a toxic shock-like syndrome due to *Streptococcus pyogenes,* *N. Engl. J. Med.* **317:**146–149 (1987).

47. CONVERSE, G. M., III, AND DILLON, H. C., JR., Epidemiological studies of *Streptococcus pneumoniae* in infants: Methods of isolating pneumococci, *J. Clin. Microbiol.* **5:**293–296 (1977).

48. CRAVEN, D. E., RIXINGER, A. I., BISNO, A. L., GOULARTE, T. A., AND MCCABE, W. R., Bacteremia caused by group G streptococci in parenteral drug abusers: Epidemiological and clinical aspects, *J. Infect. Dis.* **153:**988–992 (1986).

49. CUNNINGHAM, M. W., MCCORMACK, J. M., TALABER, L. R., HARLEY, J. B., AYOUB, E. M., MUNEER, R. S., CHUN, L. T., AND REDDY, D. V., Human monoclonal antibodies reactive with antigens of the group A streptococcus and human heart, *J. Immunol.* **141:**2760–2766 (1988).

50. D'ALESSANDRI, R., PLOTKIN, G., KLUGE, R. M., AND WALDMAN, R. H., Protective studies with group A streptococcal M protein vaccine. III. Challenge of volunteers after systemic or intranasal immunization with type 3 or type 12 group A streptococcus, *J. Infect. Dis.* **138:**712–718 (1978).

51. DAUGAARD, H. O., THOMSEN, A. C., HENRIQUES, U., AND

OSTERGAARD, A., Group B streptococci in the lower urogenital tract and late abortions, *Am. J. Obstet. Gynecol.* **158:**28–31 (1988).

52. DILLON, H. C., DERRICK, C. W., AND DILLON, M. S., M-antigens common to pyoderma and acute glomerulonephritis, *J. Infect. Dis.* **103:**257–267 (1974).

53. DILLON, H. C., JR., GBS: The childhood and adolescent years, *Antibiot. Chemother.* **35:**1–9 (1985).

54. DILLON, H. C., JR., KHARE, S., AND GRAY, B. M., Group B streptococcal carriage and disease: A 6 year prospective study, *J. Pediatr.* **110:**31–36 (1987).

55. DOUGLAS, R. M., PATON, J. C., DUNCAN, S. J., AND HANSMAN, D. J., Antibody response to pneumococcal vaccination in children younger than five years of age, *J. Infect. Dis.* **148:**131–137 (1983).

56. DUMA, R. J., WEINBERG, A. N., MEDREK, T. F., AND KUNTZ, L. G., Streptococcal infections, *Medicine* **48:**87–127 (1969).

57. EADS, M. E., LEVY, N. J., KASPER, D. L., BAKER, C. J., AND NICHOLSON-WEBER, A., Antibody-independent activation of C1 by type Ia group B streptococci, *J. Infect. Dis.* **146:**665–671 (1982).

58. EICKHOFF, T. C., KLEIN, J. O., DALY, A. K., INGAL, P., AND FINLAND, M., Neonatal sepsis and other infections due to group B beta-hemolytic streptococci, *N. Engl. J. Med.* **271:**1221–1228 (1964).

59. EISENSTEIN, T. K., DE CUENINCK, B. J., RESAVY, D., SHOCKMAN, G. D., CAREY, R. B., AND SWENSON, R. M., Quantitative determination in human sera of vaccine induced antibody to type-specific polysaccharides of group B streptococci using an enzyme-linked immunosorbant assay, *J. Infect. Dis.* **147:**847–856 (1983).

60. FACKLAM, R. R., AND CAREY, R. B., Streptococci and aerococci, in: *Manual of Clinical Microbiology,* 4th ed. (E. H. LANNETTE, ed.), pp. 154–175, American Society for Microbiology, Washington, D.C., 1985.

61. FAST, D. J., SCHLIEVERT, P. M., AND NELSON, R. D., Toxic shock syndrome-associated staphylococcal and streptococcal pyrogenic toxins are potent inducers of tumor necrosis factor production, *Infect. Immun.* **57:**291–294 (1989).

62. FEDSON, D. S., Improving the use of pneumococcal vaccine through a strategy of hospital-based immunization, *J. Am. Geriatr. Soc.* **33:**142–150 (1985).

63. FINCH, R., Is pneumococcal infection a preventable disease? *J. Infect.* **17:**95–98 (1988).

64. FINLAND, M., SPRING, W. C., AND LOWELL, F. C., Specific treatment of the pneumococcic pneumonias: An analysis of the results of serum therapy and chemotherapy at the Boston City Hospital from July 1938 through June 1939, *Ann. Intern. Med.* **13:**1567–1593 (1940).

65. FISCHER, G. W., Immunoglobin therapy of neonatal group B streptococcal infections: An overview, *Pediatr. Infect. Dis. J.* **7**(Suppl.):S13–S16 (1988).

66. GALLAGHER, P. G., AND WATANAKUNAKORN, C., Group B streptococcal endocarditis: Report of seven cases and review of the literature, 1962–1985, *Rev. Infect. Dis.* **8:**175–188 (1986).

67. GAWORZEWSKA, E., AND COLMAN, G., Changes in the pattern of infection caused by *Streptococcus pyogenes, Epidemiol. Infect.* **100:**257–269 (1988).

68. GERBER, M. A., RANDOLPH, M. F., AND MAYO, D. R., The group A streptococcal carrier state: A reexamination, *Am. J. Dis. Child.* **142:**562–565 (1988).

69. GIBBERD, G. F., Puerperal sepsis 1930–1965, *J. Obstet. Gynaecol. Br. Commonw.* **73:**1–10 (1966).

70. GIEBINK, G. S., Preventing pneumococcal disease in children: Recommendations for using pneumococcal vaccine, *Pediatr. Infect. Dis. J.* **4:**343–348 (1985).

71. GINSBURG, I., Streptococcal enzymes and virulence, in: *Bacterial Enzymes and Virulence* (I. A. HOLDER, ed.), pp. 122–144, CRC Press, Boca Raton, 1985.

72. GLASS, R. L., ALMAN, J. E., AND CHAUNCY, H. H., A 10-year longitudinal study of caries incidence rates in a sample of male adults in the USA, *Caries Res.* **21:**360–367 (1987).

73. GNANN, J. W., JR., GRAY, B. M., GRIFFIN, F. M., JR., AND DISMUKES, W. E., Acute glomerulonephritis following group G streptococcal infection. *J. Infect. Dis.* **156:**411–412 (1987).

74. GOLDMANN, D. A., AND BRETON, S. J., Group C streptococcal surgical wound infections transmitted by an anorectal and nasal carrier, *Pediatrics* **61:**235–237 (1978).

75. GOOD, R. A., AND PAHWA, R. N. (eds.), The recognition and management of immunodeficient disorders, *Pediatr. Infect. Dis. J.* **7**(Suppl.):S2–S125 (1988).

76. GOSLING, J., Occurrence and pathogenicity of the *Streptococcus milleri* group, *Rev. Infect. Dis.* **10:**257–285 (1988).

77. GOTOFF, S. P., ODELL, C., PAPIERNIAK, C. P., KLEGERMAN, M. E., AND BOYER, K. M., Human IgG antibody to group B *Streptococcus* type III: Comparison of protective levels in a murine model with levels in infected human neonates, *J. Infect. Dis.* **153:**511–519 (1986).

78. GRAY, B. M., AND DILLON, H. C., JR., GBS infections in mothers and their infants, *Antibiot. Chemother.* **35:**225–236 (1985).

79. GRAY, B. M., AND DILLON, H. C., JR., Clinical and epidemiologic studies of pneumococcal infections in children, *Pediatr. Infect. Dis. J.* **5:**201–207 (1986).

80. GRAY, B. M., AND DILLON, H. C., JR., Epidemiologic studies of *Streptococcus pneumoniae* in infants: Antibody to types 3, 6, 14, and 23 in the first two years of life, *J. Infect. Dis.* **158:**948–955 (1988).

81. GRAY, B. M., AND DILLON, H. C., JR., Natural history of pneumococcal infections, *Pediatr. Infect. Dis. J.* **8**(Suppl.): S23–S25 (1989).

82. GRAY, B. M., CONVERSE, G. M., III, AND DILLON, H. C., JR., Serotypes of *Streptococcus pneumoniae* causing disease, *J. Infect. Dis.* **140:**979–983 (1979).

83. GRAY, B. M., PASS, M. A., AND DILLON, H. C., JR., Laboratory and field evaluation of selective media for isolation of group B streptococci, *J. Clin. Microbiol.* **9:**466–470 (1979).

84. GRAY, B. M., CONVERSE, G. M., III, AND DILLON, H. C., JR., Epidemiologic studies of *Streptococcus pneumoniae* in infants: Acquisition, carriage and infection during the first 24 months of life, *J. Infect. Dis.* **146**:923–933 (1980).

85. GRAY, B. M., TURNER, M. E., AND DILLON, H. C., JR., Epidemiologic studies of *Streptococcus pneumoniae* in infants: The effects of season and age on pneumococcal acquisition and carriage in the first 24 months of life, *Am. J. Epidemiol.* **116**:692–703 (1982).

86. GRAY, B. M., PRITCHARD, D. G., AND DILLON, H. C., JR., Seroepidemiological studies of group B *Streptococcus* type II, *J. Infect. Dis.* **151**:1073–1080 (1985).

87. GRAY, B. M., DILLON, H. C., JR., PRITCHARD, D. G., FEINSTEIN, R. A., OH, K., AND MICHALEK, S. M., Type-specific antibodies against group B streptococci in human serum, saliva and vaginal secretions, *Adv. Exp. Med. Biol.* **216**:995–1003 (1987).

88. GRAY, B. M., PRITCHARD, D. G., AND DILLON, H. C., JR., Seroepidemiology of group B *Streptococcus* type III at delivery, *J. Infect. Dis.* **159**:1139–1142 (1989).

89. GULLBERG, R. M., The enterococcus, *Infect. Control* **7**:600–606 (1986).

90. HÅKANSSON, S., HOLM, S. E., AND WAGNER, M., Density profile of group B streptococci, type III, and its possible relation to enhanced virulence, *J. Clin. Microbiol.* **25**:714–718 (1987).

91. HAVERKORN, M. J. (ed.), *Streptococcal Disease and the Community*, American Elsevier, New York, and Excerpta Medica, Amsterdam, 1974.

92. HENDLEY, J. O., SANDE, M. A., STEWART, P. M., AND GWALTNEY, J. M., JR., Spread of *Streptococcus pneumoniae* in families. I. Carriage rates and distribution of types, *J. Infect. Dist.* **132**:55–61 (1975).

93. HODGES, R. G., AND MACLEOD, C. M., Epidemic pneumococcal pneumonia, *Am. J. Hyg.* **44**:183–213 (1946).

94. HOOD, J., AND JANNEY, A., Beta hemolytic streptococcus group B associated with problems of the perinatal period, *Am. J. Obstet. Gynecol.* **82**:809–818 (1961).

95. HOOK, E. W., HOOTON, T. M., HORTON, C. A., COYLE, M. B., RAMSEY, P. G., AND TURCK, M., Microbiologic evaluation of cutaneous cellulitis in adults, *Arch. Intern. Med.* **146**:295–297 (1986).

96. HOSIER, D. M., CRAEMEN, J. M., TESKE, D. W., AND WHELLER, J. J., Resurgence of acute rheumatic fever, *Am. J. Dis. Child.* **141**:730–732 (1987).

97. HOSTETTER, M. K., Serotypic variations among virulent pneumococci in deposition and degradation of covalently bound C3b: Implications for phagocytosis and antibody production, *J. Infect. Dis.* **153**:682–693 (1986).

98. HUANG, D. H., KRISHNA, N. R., AND PRITCHARD, D. G., Characterization of the group A streptococcal polysaccharide by two-dimensional ^{1}H-nuclear-resonance spectroscopy, *Carbohydr. Res.* **155**:193–199 (1986).

99. ISPAHANI, P., DONALD, F. E., AND AVELINE, A. J. D., *Streptococcus pyogenes* bacteremia: An old enemy subdued but not defeated, *J. Infect.* **16**:37–46 (1988).

100. JABES, D., NACHMAN, S., AND TOMASZ, A., Penicillin-binding protein families: Evidence for the clonal nature of penicillin resistance in clinical isolates of pneumococci, *J. Infect. Dis.* **159**:16–25 (1989).

101. JARVIS, W. R., WHITE, J. W., MANN, P. W., MOSSER, J. L., EMORI, T. G., CULVER, D. H., THORNSBERRY, C., AND HUGHES, J. M., Nosocomial infection surveillance, 1983, *Morbid. Mortal. Weekly Rep.* **33**:9SS–21SS (1984).

102. JENSEN, N. E., Epidemiological aspects of human/animal interrelationships in GBS, *Antibiot. Chemother.* **35**:40–48 (1985).

103. JOHNSON, D. R., AND KAPLAN, E., Microtechnique for serum opacity factor for characterization of group A streptococci adaptable to the use of human sera, *J. Clin. Microbiol.* **26**:2025–2030 (1988).

104. JOHNSTON, K. H., AND ZABRISKIE, J. B., Purification and partial characterization of the nephritis strain-associated protein from *Streptococcus pyogenes*, group A, *J. Exp. Med.* **163**:697–712 (1986).

105. Jones Criteria (Revised) for Guidance in Diagnosis of Rheumatic Fever, *Circulation* **69**:203A–208A (1984).

106. JURGENS, D., STERZIK, B., AND FEHRENBACH, F. J., Unspecific binding of group B streptococcal cocytolysin (CAMP factor) to immunoglobins and its possible role in pathogenicity, *J. Exp. Med.* **165**:720–732 (1987).

107. KAPLAN, E. L., The group A streptococcal upper respiratory tract carrier state: An enigma, *J. Pediatr.* **97**:337–345 (1980).

108. KAPLAN, E. L., The rapid identification of group A beta-hemolytic streptococci in the upper respiratory tract, *Pediatr. Clin North Am.* **35**:535–543 (1988).

109. KAPLAN, E. L., JOHNSON, D. R., AND CLEARY, P. P., Group A streptococcal serotypes isolated from patients and sibling contacts during the resurgence of rheumatic fever in the United States in the mid-1980s, *J. Infect. Dis.* **159**:101–103 (1989).

110. KASS, E. H., AND SEASTONE, C. V., The role of the mucoid polysaccharide (hyaluronic acid) in the virulence of group A streptococci, *J. Exp. Med.* **79**:319–330 (1944).

111. KATZ, V., AND BOWES, W. A., Perinatal group B streptococcal infections across intact amniotic membranes, *J. Reprod. Med.* **33**:445–449 (1988).

112. KEFALIDES, N. A., PEGG, M. T., OHNO, N., POON-KING, T., ZABRISKIE, J., AND FILLIT, H., Antibodies to basement membrane collagen and to laminin are present in sera from patients with poststreptococcal glomerulonephritis, *J. Exp. Med.* **163**:588–602 (1986).

113. KIM, K. S., AND KAPLAN, E. L., Association of penicillin tolerance with failure to eradicate group A streptococci from patients with pharyngitis, *J. Pediatr.* **107**:681–684 (1985).

114. KLEIN, J. O., FEIGIN, R. D., AND MCCRACKEN, G. H., JR., Report of the task force on diagnosis and management of meningitis, *Pediatrics* **78**(Suppl.):959–982 (1986).

115. KOSKELA, M., LEINONEN, M., HAIVA, V., AND MAKALA, P. H., First and second dose antibody responses to pneumococ-

cal polysaccharide vaccine in infants, *Pediatr. Infect. Dis. J.* **5:**45–50 (1986).

116. LANCEFIELD, R. C., AND HARE, R., The serological differentiation of pathogenic and nonpathogenic strains of hemolytic streptococci from parturient women, *J. Exp. Med.* **61:**335–349 (1935).

117. LANCEFIELD, R. C., MCCARTY, M., AND EVERLY, W. N., Multiple mouse-protective antibodies directed against group B streptococci, *J. Exp. Med.* **142:**165–179 (1975).

118. LECLERCQ, M. H., BARMES, D. E., AND SARDO INFIRRI, J., Oral health: Global trends and projections, *World Health Stat. Q.* **40:**116–128 (1987).

119. LEDGER, W., NORMAN, M., GEE, C., AND LEWIS, W., Bacteremia on an obstetric-gynecologic service, *Am. J. Obstet. Gynecol.* **121:**205–212 (1975).

120. LIANG, S. T., LAU, S. P., CHAN, S. H., FOK, T. F., MURAI, T., AND KANEKO, Y., Perinatal colonization of group B streptococcus—An epidemiological study in a Chinese population, *Aust. N.Z. Obstet. Gynaecol.* **26:**138–141 (1986).

121. LODA, F. A., COLLIER, A. M., GLEZEN, W. P., STRANGERT, K., CLYDE, W. A., AND DENNY, F. W., Occurrence of *Diplococcus pneumoniae* in the upper respiratory tract of children, *J. Pediatr.* **87:**1087–1093 (1975).

122. LOESCHE, W. J., Role of *Streptococcus mutans* in human dental decay, *Microbiol. Rev.* **50:**353–380 (1986).

123. LUE, C., TARKOWSKI, A., AND MESTECKY, J., Systemic immunization with pneumococcal polysaccharide vaccine induces a predominant IgA2 response of peripheral blood leukocytes and increases of both serum and secretory antipneumococcal antibodies, *J. Immunol.* **140:**3793–3800 (1988).

124. LUGINBUHL, L. M., ROTBART, H. A., FACKLAM, R. R., ROE, M. H., AND ELLIOT, J. A., Neonatal enterococcal sepsis: Case–control study and description of an outbreak, *Pediatr. Infect. Dis. J.* **6:**1022–1026 (1987).

125. MACLEOD, C. M., HODGES, R. G., HEIDELBERGER, M., AND BERNHARD, W. G., Prevention of pneumococcal pneumonia by immunization with specific capsular polysaccharides, *J. Exp. Med.* **82:**445–465 (1945).

126. MADDOX, J. S., WARE, J. C., AND DILLON, H. C., JR., The natural history of streptococcal skin infection: Prevention with topical antibiotics, *Am. J. Acad. Dermatol.* **13:**207–212 (1985).

127. MAJEED, H. A., KHUFFASH, F. A., SHARDA, D. C., FARWANA, S. S., EL-SHERBINY, A., AND GHAROUR, S. Y., Children with acute rheumatic fever and acute poststreptococcal glomerulonephritis and their families in a subtropical zone: A three-zone prospective comparative epidemiological study, *Int. J. Epidemiol.* **16:**561–586 (1987).

128. MAKI, D. G., AND AGGER, W. A., Enterococcal bacteremia: Clinical features, the risk of endocarditis, and management, *Medicine* **67:**248–269 (1988).

129. MANJI, F., FEJERSKOV, O., AND BAELUM, V., Pattern of dental caries in an adult rural population, *Caries Res.* **23:**55–62 (1989).

130. MARKOWITZ, M., AND GERBER, M. D., Rheumatic fever: Recent outbreaks of an old disease, *Conn. Med.* **51:**229–233 (1987).

131. MATTER, L., WILHELM, J. A., ANGEHRN, W., SKVARIL, F., AND SCHOPFER, K., Selective antibody deficiency and recurrent pneumococcal bacteremia in a patient with Sjogren's syndrome, hyperimmunoglobulinemia G, and deficiencies of IgG$_2$ and IgG$_4$, *N. Engl. J. Med.* **312:**1039–1042 (1985).

132. MAYON-WHITE, R. T., The incidence of GBS disease in neonates in different countries, *Antibiot. Chemother.* **35:**17–27 (1985).

133. MCDANIEL, L. S., YOTHER, J., VIJAYAKUMAR, M., MCGARRY, L., GUILD, W. R., AND BRILES, D. E., Use of insertional inactivation to facilitate studies of biological properties of pneumococcal surface protein A (PspA), *J. Exp. Med.* **165:**381–394 (1987).

134. MCFALL, T. L., ZIMMERMAN, G. A., AUGUSTINE, N. H., AND HILL, H. R., Effect of group B streptococcal type-specific antigen on polymorphonuclear leukocyte function and polymorphonuclear leukocyte–endothelial cell interaction, *Pediatr. Res.* **21:**517–523 (1987).

135. MICHALEK, S. M., AND CHILDERS, N. K., Development and outlook for a caries vaccine, *Crit. Rev. Oral Biol. Med.* **1:**37–54 (1990).

136. MILLER, L., BURDETT, V., POIRIER, T. P., GRAY, L. D., BEACHEY, E. H., AND KEHOE, M. A., Conservation of protective and nonprotective epitopes in M proteins of group A streptococci, *Infect. Immun.* **56:**2198–2204 (1988).

137. MILLIGAN, T. W., BAKER, C. J., STRAUS, D. C., AND MATTINGLY, S. J., Association of elevated levels of extracellular neuraminidase with clinical isolates of type III group B streptococci, *Infect. Immun.* **21:**738–746 (1978).

138. MUFSON, M. A., OLEY, G., AND HUGHEY, D., Pneumococcal disease in a medium-sized community in the United States, *Am. Med. Assoc.* **248:**1486–1489 (1982).

139. MUSHER, D. M., CHAPMAN, A. J., GOREE, A., JONSSON, S., BRILES, D., AND BAUGHN, R. E., Natural and vaccine-related immunity to *Streptococcus pneumoniae*, *J. Infect. Dis.* **154:**245–256 (1986).

140. NELSON, J. D., DILLON, H. C., JR., AND HOWARD, J. B., A prolonged nursery epidemic associated with a newly recognized type of group A streptococcus, *J. Pediatr.* **89:**792–796 (1976).

141. O'CONNOR, S. P., AND CLEARY, P. P., In vivo *Streptococcus pyogenes* C5a peptidase activity: Analysis using transposon- and nitrosoguanidine-induced mutants, *J. Infect. Dis.* **156:**495–504 (1987).

142. OLSON, T. A., FISCHER, G. W., HEMMING, V. G., O'BRIAN, W. F., GOLDEN, S. M., AND MAYBEE, D. A., A group B streptococcal extract reduces neutrophil counts and induces neutrophil aggregation, *Pediatr. Res.* **21:**326–330 (1988).

143. OPAL, S. M., CROSS, A., PALMER, M., AND ALMAZAN, R., Group B streptococcal sepsis in adults and children: Contrasts and comparisons, *Arch. Intern. Med.* **148:**641–645 (1988).

144. PARADISE, J. L., BLUESTONE, C. D., BACHMAN, R. Z., COLBORN, D. K., BERNARD, B. S., TAYLOR, F. H., ROGERS, K. D., SCHWARZBACH, R. H., STOOL, S. E., FRIDAY, G. A.,

SMITH, I. H., AND SAEZ, C. A., Efficacy of tonsillectomy for recurrent throat infection in severely affected children, *N. Engl. J. Med.* **310:**674–683 (1984).

145. PARKER, M. T., Streptococcus and lactobacillus, in: *Topley and Wilson's Principles of Bacteriology, Virology and Immunity,* Volume 2 (M. T. PARKER, ed.), pp. 173–217, Williams & Wilkins, Baltimore, 1983.

146. PASS, M. A., KHARE, S., AND DILLON, H. C., JR., Twin pregnancies: Incidence of group B streptococcal colonization and disease, *J. Pediatr.* **94:**635–637 (1980).

147. PAYNE, N. R., KIM, Y., AND FERRIERI, P., Effect of differences in antibody and complement requirements on phagocytic uptake and intracellular killing of "c" protein-positive and -negative strains of type II group B streptococci, *Infect. Immun.* **55:**1243–1251 (1987).

148. PAYNE, N. R., BURKE, B. A., DAY, D. L., CHRISTENSON, P. D., THOMPSON, T. R., AND FERRIERI, P., Correlation of clinical and pathologic findings in early onset neonatal group B streptococcal infection with disease severity and prediction of outcome, *Pediatr. Infect. Dis. J.* **7:**836–847 (1988).

149. PERRY, W. D., SIEGEL, A. C., AND RAMMELKAMP, C. J., JR., Transmission of group A streptococci. II. The role of contaminated dust, *Am. J. Hyg.* **66:**96–101 (1957).

150. PERRY, W. D., SIEGEL, A. C., RAMMELKAMP, C. J., JR., WANNAMAKER, L. W., AND MARPLE, C. E., Transmission of group A streptococci. I. The role of contaminated bedding, *Am. J. Hyg.* **66:**85–95 (1957).

151. PHILIPS, J. B., III, LYRENE, R. K., GODOY, G., GRAYBAR, G., BAREFIELD, E., SAMS, J. E. P., AND GRAY, B. M., Hemodynamic responses of chronically instrumented piglets to bolus injections of group B streptococci, *Pediatr. Res.* **23:**81–85 (1988).

152. PICHICHERO, M. E., DISNEY, F. A., TALPEY, W. B., GREEN, J. L., FRANCIS, A. B., ROGHMANN, K., AND HOEKELMAN, R. A., Adverse and beneficial effects of immediate treatment of group A beta-hemolytic streptococcal pharyngitis with penicillin, *Pediatr. Infect. Dis. J.* **6:**635–643 (1987).

153. PICHICHERO, M. E,. DISNEY, F. A., TALPEY, W. B., GREEN, J. L., FRANCIS, A. B., ROGHMANN, K., AND HOEKELMAN, R. A., Delayed treatment for strep throat (reply), *Pediatr. Infect. Dis. J.* **6:**1140 (1987).

154. POIRIER, T. P., KEHOE, M. A., AND BEACHEY, E. H., Protective immunity evoked by oral administration of attenuated *aroA Salmonella typhimurium* expressing cloned streptococcal M protein, *J. Exp. Med.* **168:**25–32 (1988).

155. POIRIER, T. P., KEHOE, M. A., WHITNACK, E., DOKTER, M. E., AND BEACHEY, E. H., Fibrinogen binding and resistance to phagocytosis of *Streptococcus sanguis* expressing cloned M protein of *Streptococcus pyogenes, Infect. Immun.* **57:**29–35 (1989).

156. POTTER, E. V., LIPSCHULTZ, S. A., ABIDH, S., POON-KING, T., AND EARLE, D. P., Twelve to seventeen-year follow-up of patients with poststreptococcal acute glomerulonephritis in Trinidad, *N. Engl. J. Med.* **307:**725–729 (1982).

157. PRITCHARD, D. G., EGAN, M. E., GRAY, B. M., AND DIL-

LON, H. C., JR., Immunochemical characterization of the polysaccharide antigens of group B streptococci, *Rev. Infect. Dis.* **10**(Suppl. 2):S367–S371 (1988).

158. PYATI, S. P., PILDES, R. S., JACOBS, N. M., RAMAMURTHY, R. S., YEH, T. F., RAVAL, D. S., LILLIEN, L. D., AMMA, P., AND METZGER, W. I., Penicillin in infants weighing two kilograms or less with early-onset group B streptococcal disease, *N. Engl. J. Med.* **308:**1383–1389 (1983).

159. QUINN, R. W., Streptococcal infections, in: *Bacterial Infections of Humans* (A. S. Evans and H. A. Feldman, eds.), pp. 525–552, Plenum Medical, New York, 1982.

160. RAFF, H. V., SISCOE, P. J., WOLFF, E. A., MALONEY, G., AND SHUFORD, W., Human monoclonal antibodies to group B streptococcus, *J. Exp. Med.* **168:**905–917 (1988).

161. ROBBINS, J. B., AUSTRIAN, R., LEE, C., RASTOGI, S. C., SCHIFFMAN, G., HENRICHSEN, J., MAKALA, P. H., BROOME, C. V., FACKLAM, R. R., TIESJEMA, R. H., AND PARK, J. C., JR., Considerations for formulating the second-generation pneumococcal capsular polysaccharide vaccine with emphasis on the cross-reactive type within groups, *J. Infect. Dis.* **148:**1136–1159 (1983).

162. SCHLEIFER, K. H., AND KILPPER-BALZ, R., Transfer of *Streptococcus faecalis* and *Streptococcus faecium* to the genus *Enterococcus* nom. rev. as *Enterococcus faecalis* comb. nov. and *Enterococcus faecium* comb. nov., *Int. J. Syst. Bacteriol.* **34:**31–34 (1984).

163. SHANN, F., Etiology of severe pneumonia in children in developing countries, *Pediatr. Infect. Dis. J.* **5:**247–252 (1986).

164. SHAPIRO, E. D., AND CLEMENS, J. D., A controlled evaluation of the protective efficacy of pneumococcal vaccine for patients at high risk for serious pneumococcal infections, *Ann. Intern. Med.* **101:**325–330 (1984).

165. SMITH, T. D., WILKINSON, V., AND KAPLAN, E. L., Group A *Streptococcus*-associated upper respiratory tract infections in a day-care center, *Pediatrics* **83:**380–384 (1989).

166. SPIGELBLATT, L., SAINTONGE, J., AND CHICOINE, R., Changing pattern of neonatal streptococcal septicemia, *Pediatr. Infect. Dis. J.* **4:**56–58 (1985).

167. STEIN, D. S., AND NELSON, K. E., Endocarditis due to nutritionally deficient streptococci, *Rev. Infect. Dis.* **9:**908–916 (1987).

168. STOLLERMAN, G. H., Changing group A streptococci: The reappearance of streptococcal "toxic shock," *Arch. Intern. Med.* **148:**1268–1270 (1988).

169. STOOL, S. E., AND FIELD, M. J., The impact of otitis media, *Pediatr. Infect. Dis. J.* **8**(Suppl):S11–S14 (1989).

170. STROBEL, S., AND FERGUSON, A., Induction of oral tolerance, in mice, to gum arabic, *Food Addit. Contam.* **3:**43–46 (1986).

171. THOMAS, R. J., CONWELL, D. E., MORTON, D. E., BROOKS, T. J., HOLMES, C. K., AND MAHAFFEY, W. B., Penicillin prophylaxis for streptococcal infections in United States Navy and Marine Corps recruit camps, 1951–1985, *Rev. Infect. Dis.* **10:**125–130 (1988).

172. TWETEN, R., Nucleotide sequence of the gene for perfingolysin O (theta-toxin) from *Clostridium perfringens:* Significant homology with genes for streptolysin O and pneumolysin, *Infect. Immun.* **56:**3235–3240 (1988).

173. VAN DER RIJN, I., AND KESSLER, R. E., Growth characteristics of group A streptococci in a new chemically defined medium, *Infect. Immun.* **27:**444–448 (1980).

174. VEASY, L. G., WIEDMEIER, S. E., ORSMOND, G. S., RUTTENBERG, H. D., BOUCEK, M. M., ROTH, S. J., TAIT, V. F., THOMPSON, J. A., DALY, J. A., KAPLAN, E., AND HILL, H. R., Resurgence of acute rheumatic fever in the intermountain area of the Untied States, *N. Engl. J. Med.* **316:**421–427 (1987).

175. VOGT, A., BATSFORD, S., RODRIGUEZ-ITURBE, B., AND GARCIA, R., Cationic antigens in poststreptococcal glomerulonephritis, *Clin. Nephrol.* **20:**271–279 (1983).

176. WALD, E. R., BERGMAN, I., TAYLOR, H. G., CHIPONIS, D., PORTER, C., AND KUBEK, K., Long-term outcome of group B streptococcal meningitis, *Pediatrics* **77:**217–221 (1986).

177. WALD, E. R., DASHEFSKY, B., FEIDT, C., CHIPONIS, D., AND BYERS, C., Acute rheumatic fever in western Pennsylvania and the tristate area, *Pediatrics* **80:**371–374 (1987).

178. WALTMAN, W. D., GRAY, B., MCDANIEL, L. S., AND BRILES, D. E., Cross-reactive monoclonal antibodies for diagnosis of pneumococcal meningitis, *J. Clin. Microbiol.* **26:**1635–1640 (1988).

179. WALTMAN, W. D. I., MCDANIEL, L. S., ANDERSSON, B., BLAND, L., GRAY, B. M., EDEN, C. S., AND BRILES, D. E., Protein serotyping of *Streptococcus pneumoniae* based on reactivity to six monoclonal antibodies, *Microb. Pathogenesis* **5:**159–167 (1988).

180. WANNAMAKER, L. W., Streptococcal toxins, *Rev. Infect. Dis.* **5**(Suppl.)**:**S723–S732 (1983).

181. WEINSTEIN, M. P., RELLER, L., MURPHY, J. R., AND LICHTENSTEIN, K. A., The clinical significance of positive blood cultures. A comprehensive analysis of 500 episodes of bacteremia and fungemia in adults—I. Laboratory and epidemiologic observations, *Rev. Infect. Dis.* **5:**35–53 (1983).

182. WESSELS, M. R., POZSGAY, V., KASPER, D. L., AND JENNINGS, H. J., Structure and immunochemistry of an oligosaccharide repeating unit of the capsular polysaccharide of type III group B *Streptococcus, J. Biol. Chem.* **262:**8262–8267 (1987).

183. WHO Study Group, Rheumatic fever and rheumatic heart disease, *WHO Tech. Rep. Ser.* **764:**1–58 (1988).

184. WILLETT, L. D., DILLON, H. C., JR., AND GRAY, B. M., Penicillin-intermediate pneumococci in a children's hospital, *Am. J. Dis. Child.* **139:**1054–1057 (1985).

185. WOOD, E. G., AND DILLON, H. C., JR., A prospective study of group B streptococcal bacteriuria in pregnancy, *Am. J. Obstet. Gynecol.* **140:**515–520 (1981).

186. YARNALL, M., AND BOYLE, M. D. P., Isolation and characterization of type IIa and type IIb Fc receptors from group A streptococcus, *Scand. J. Immunol.* **24:**549–557 (1986).

187. YEUNG, M. K., AND MATTINGLY, S. J., Biosynthetic capacity for type-specific antigen synthesis determines the virulence of serotype III strains of group B streptococci, *Infect. Immun.* **44:**217–221 (1984).

188. YOSHIMOTO, M., HOSOI, S., FUJISAWA, S., SUDO, M., AND OKUDA, R., High levels of antibodies to streptococcal cell membrane antigens specifically bound to monoclonal antibodies in acute poststreptococcal glomerulonephritis, *J. Clin. Microbiol.* **25:**680–684 (1987).

189. ZAWANEH, S. M., AYOUB, E. M., BAER, H., CRUZ, A. C., AND SPELLACY, W. N., Factors influencing the adherence of group B streptococci to human vagina epithelial cells, *Infect. Immun.* **26:**441–447 (1979).

12. Suggested Reading

CHRISTENSEN, K. K., CHRISTENSEN, P., AND FERRIERI, P. (eds.), Neonatal Group B Streptococcal Infections, *Antibiot. Chemother.* **35:**1–347 (1985).

DUNNING, J. M., *Principles of Dental Public Health,* Harvard University Press, Cambridge, Mass., 1986.

HEFFRON, R., *Pneumonia with Special Reference to Pneumococcus Lobar Pneumonia,* Commonwealth Fund, New York, 1939; reprinted by Harvard University Press, Cambridge, Mass., 1979.

KIMURA, Y., KOTAMI, S., AND SHIOKAWA, Y. (eds.), *Recent Advances in Streptococci and Streptococcal Diseases,* Reedbooks, Brackness, Birkshire, U.K., 1985.

MAKI, D. G., AND AGGER, W. A., Enterococcal bacteremia: Clinical features, the risk of endocarditis, and management, *Medicine* **67:**248–269 (1988).

MARKOWITZ, M., AND GORDIS, L. *Rheumatic Fever,* 2nd ed., Saunders, Philadelphia, 1972.

Third International Conference on Rheumatic Fever and Rheumatic Heart Disease, Rotorua 16–18 April 1987, *N.Z. Med. J.* **101:**387–411 (1987).

WANNAMAKER, L. W., AND MATSEN, J. M. (eds.), *Streptococci and Streptococcal Diseases,* Academic Press, New York, 1972.

WHITE, B. (with the collaboration of ROBINSON, E. S., AND BARNES, L. A.), *The Biology of the Pneumococcus: The Bacteriological, Biochemical and Immunological Characters and Activities of Diplococcus pneumoniae,* Commonwealth Fund, New York, 1938; reprinted by Harvard University Press, Cambridge, Mass., 1979.

WHO Study Group, Rheumatic fever and rheumatic heart disease, *WHO Tech. Rep. Ser.* **764:**1–58 (1988).

CHAPTER 32

Syphilis

Joseph G. Lossick and Stephen J. Kraus

1. Introduction

Since its appearance in Europe over four centuries ago, syphilis has had a major impact on society. Its history is characterized by myth and superstition, and it has come to represent the prototype of venereal diseases that has been as associated with character weaknesses or debauchery as it has as a communicable disease.

Although the organism remains highly susceptible to a variety of inexpensive antibiotics, the disease has managed to survive and flourish in many populations. Its very survival speaks to the lack of concerted commitment to its eradication and the frailties of human personal behavior. Contemporary approaches to the control of syphilis have been impacted by an era of cost consciousness and an awareness of competing health expenditure needs. Recent circumstances surrounding the epidemic of the human immunodeficiency virus (HIV) resemble many of the historical events that were typical of syphilis in the past. These include public fear and prejudice against infected patients, calls for widespread quarantine, controversy regarding widespread testing, concerns about confidentiality, debate about laws dealing with contact tracing and public health reporting, conflict between public health science and moral views, individual versus public rights, and a broad-based movement in society for a reappraisal of personal behavior and educational and religious approaches to same. HIV disease with its associated immune dysfunction provokes a

need to reassess the diagnostic, therapeutic, and control strategies of syphilis. Limited public health resources are being strained to deal with an expanding panorama of sexually transmitted diseases (STDs) and the additional burden of the HIV problem. Many tough challenges lie ahead for those public health officials responsible for the containment of these diseases.

2. Historical Background

It is not possible to determine precisely the origin of syphilis or to be sure whether syphilis is a disease of antiquity (pre-Columbian theory) or one imported from the New World by sailors of Columbus's expedition. Whether these sailors introduced syphilis to the European continent (Columbian theory) or the outbreak of disease was simply coincidental with their return, there is general agreement among historians that syphilis epidemics of unprecedented intensity swept through Europe during the late 15th and 16th centuries. The disease was highly virulent for about 50 years and many thousands died during the secondary stage of the disease. Authorities resorted to banishment or quarantine of infected individuals in an effort to contain the disease. Between 1496 and 1569, the disease spread in epidemic proportions to the rest of the world. It acquired its present name in 1530 from a poem about an afflicted shepherd named Syphilis (Syphilis Sive Morbus Gallicus) written by the physician-poet, Hieronymi Fracastorii. The importance of sexual intercourse in the transmission of syphilis was recognized early and nongenital transmission associated with poor hygienic conditions was postulated. During the 16th century the severity of the disease lessened significantly and

Joseph G. Lossick and Stephen J. Kraus · Clinical Research Branch, Division of Sexually Transmitted Disease, Center for Prevention Services, Centers for Disease Control, Atlanta, Georgia 30333.

although epidemic disease continued, death was uncommon and the disease assumed a clinical course similar to what it is today. In fact, the disease became somewhat romanticized and became known as a disease of the aristocrats with a variety of famous individuals succumbing to this malady. Its victims included the popes, Alexander VI, Julius II, and Leo X; Peter the Great (the First), Ivan the Terrible (IV), Catherine the Great, the kings, Charles VIII, Henry VIII of England, Louis XIV of France, and the authors, John Keats, Oscar Wilde, and Guy de Maupassant. From the 16th to the 19th century, syphilis and gonorrhea were presumed to be different clinical manifestations of the same infection. In 1837 the French venereologist, Phillipe Ricord, characterized the three stages of syphilis and differentiated it from gonorrhea by a series of inoculations with syphilitic chancres.[36] Two of his students, Paul Diday and Alfred Fournier, identified and described the clinical syndrome of congenital syphilis (1854) and the familial impact of this disease (1880). This introduced the competing notions of confidentiality and the physician's responsibility to the patient versus public disclosure for the good of society. Although it was known to be a sexually communicable disease, medical prejudice abounded and many clinics and hospitals refused to care for patients with syphilis.

In the United States, courts increasingly recognized the introduction of venereal disease into marriage as grounds for divorce. In 1899, Michigan was the first U.S. state to make venereal disease a bar to matrimony and soon thereafter several other states passed similar laws. These laws generally required men to swear to being free from a venereal disease. Women were exempt from such laws since they were an affront to their dignity. The 1891 Immigration Act barred entrance to the United States based on the presence of a venereal disease. The next few years were characterized by the association of syphilis and other venereal diseases with lower social groups and immigrants, and raised the specter of segregation of social classes to minimize the risks of transmission. Calls for education about these diseases abounded, generating significant controversy, particularly from religious groups. The need to improve morals versus that of safer sex was a common debate.

In 1901, it was estimated that 5–18% of New York men were afflicted with syphilis.[32] Early 20th century society increasingly began to view syphilis as a threat to the family unit of innocent women and children. Again, controversy occurred about the rights of society and the loss of patient confidentiality through reporting of venereal disease cases or notification of potentially exposed individuals.[22, 33,35,42] In 1905 Fritz Schaudin and Eric Hoffman identified the etiological agent of syphilis, *Spirochaeta pallida*. A

year later, August Wassermann, Albert Neisser, and Carl Bruck introduced a new blood test for syphilis. In 1909, Paul Erlich introduced a new treatment for syphilis, Salvarsan.

These developments stimulated increasing interest in the public health implications of this disease, and in 1911 California was the first state to require the reporting of the number of syphilis cases for morbidity purposes. These laws were viewed by many as possible impediments to the control of disease. Many physicians contended that mandatory reporting would drive the infected patients underground forcing them to avoid testing and to seek care by quacks and cultists,[43] but ultimately all states adopted similar laws. The reticence of the private medical sector to treat syphilis cases and their reluctance to involve themselves in breaking the transmission chains of infection prompted the development of public health clinics for the diagnosis and treatment of syphilis. These facilities initiated and refined contact tracing activities as a means of disrupting chains of infection. By the mid-1920s, prenatal serologic screening to prevent congenital syphilis was common.

The public health sector was often criticized for concentrating on the scientific aspects of the venereal diseases and ignoring the moral issues. The American Social Health Association (ASHA) was formed to integrate both the hygienic and moral issues surrounding sexually transmitted infections. Scare tactics used by the public health sector and others resulted in considerable syphilophobia in the U.S. population.

During World War I, control efforts were focused on safe sex education and personal prophylaxis. Morality issues and concerns regarding the contribution of alcohol to sexual promiscuity were emphasized and prostitution became the target of organized groups, as well as the local and federal governments. Congress amended the Selective Service Act to establish "moral zones" around military bases that were free of alcohol and prostitution. Voluntary organizations rallied to provide canteens and clubs where servicemen could safely socialize. By 1918, 32 states passed laws requiring involuntary compulsory testing of prostitutes for venereal diseases. The federal government supported the constitutional right of communities to quarantine individuals with venereal disease. Forceful detention of prostitutes became the rule and many red-light districts throughout the United States were closed. In 1918, President Wilson allocated $250,000 from the National Security and Defense Fund for the establishment of detention–treatment centers. Congress also passed the Chamberlain–Kahn bill, which provided additional monies for civilian quarantine and isolation. Between 1918 and 1920, 18,000 women were committed to these institutions for an average of 10 weeks until they were considered noninfectious. In spite of these efforts, venereal disease in the military remained high and it was ultimately recognized that much of the disease transmission was not prostitute-related.

In 1935, Connecticut was the first state to require premarital syphilis serology testing and examination. In 1938, New York and Rhode Island were the first to mandate prenatal screening for syphilis. In 1936, Dr. Thomas Parran, the surgeon general of the United States Public Health Service (USPHS), advocated widespread screening and contact tracing activities to control syphilis. The following year he published a book, *Shadow on the Land,* which detailed the main thrust of his campaign against syphilis. In 1938, The National Venereal Disease Control Act provided $15 million over a 3-year period for assistance to the states for screening and updating clinical facilities for the diagnosis and treatment of STDs. Serologic screening became widespread throughout the United States.

In 1941, Congress passed the May Act, which made vice activities near a military establishment a federal crime. As a result, 700 cities closed their red-light districts and thousands of prostitutes were detained and tested. Because of the overflowing jails, "civilian conservation camps" were established. Although highly visible and apparently productive, this campaign had little impact on syphilis rates and it was subsequently determined that prostitutes accounted for only 10–15% of the venereal disease cases. The advent of World War II brought a return to emphasis on prophylaxis and venereal disease education and U.S. servicemen were exposed to innumerable safe sex educational films. In contrast to World War I, little emphasis was placed on the moral aspects of venereal disease. During the war, 50 million condoms were sold or given away yearly. Some expressed concerns that this emphasis on safe sex would only encourage promiscuity and diminish the morals of the servicemen.

In 1943, Dr. John Mahoney of the USPHS began his experiments on penicillin treatment for syphilis and the Office of Scientific Research and Development expended $2 million on the production and testing of the drug. Within the first year, over 10,000 patients were treated with a cure rate of 90–97% and a new era in the treatment of syphilis began.

3. Methodology

3.1. Sources of Mortality Data

Statistics on syphilis mortality rates are derived from death certificates. The accuracy of these data over time is significantly influenced by changes in coding methods, diagnostic methods, physician reporting candor, and the autopsy percentages. The validity of case definitions may vary significantly over time, place, and patient population. Because of this, these data must be considered "soft" and observations, especially those relating to comparisons over time, must be viewed very conservatively. Each revision of the International Statistical Classification of Diseases, Injuries, and Causes of Death (ISC) (which occurs about every decade) has influenced these data. This is especially true of the Sixth Revision in 1949, which significantly affected death certificates by requiring listing of multiple causes of death. This revision used the first disease listed as the underlying cause of death for tabulation rather than using a fixed set of priority tables such as was used prior to 1949. This artifactually reduced the number of syphilis deaths by 28%.[2] Because of the stigma associated with syphilis, it is probable that many physicians do not list it on death certificates and that the frequency of this would vary over time and by socioeconomic class and locale. Because late syphilis, especially cardiovascular involvement, may be difficult to diagnose premortem, documentation of this cause of death is highly dependent on the autopsy rate, which has varied significantly over time and between patient subpopulations.

3.2. Sources of Morbidity Data

The national syphilis morbidity data base is collected by the Centers for Disease Control (CDC) by formal case reporting from the states. Data may vary in accuracy, dependent upon the quality and quantity of the STD control programs. These morbidity data tend to be more accurate in states that have laws requiring reporting of positive serologic tests for syphilis. Because private physicians are less reliable sources of morbidity data, public health syphilis morbidity data are overrepresentative of patients seen in the public sector and thus tend to underestimate disease in the more affluent and older patient populations. The case mix of early versus late disease is significantly related to the quantity of serologic screening, which tends to detect latent rather than early infectious disease cases. Trend data, particularly those relating to latent disease, may be less accurate than those related to early infectious syphilis because of a progressive trend over time to concentrate investigational efforts on early disease detection (duration < 1 year). Low-titer reactive serologies, especially in older patients, which may represent latent (possibly untreated) cases, are often not investigated. Thus, there are no accurate national or local data on the frequency of late or latent syphilis cases in the United States. The latent syphilis cases currently documented in the morbidity base represent only a portion of the real prevalence of disease, a proportion that varies markedly by regional and STD control program priorities and staffing. Data relating to the incidence of congenital syphilis are particularly confounded by diagnostic errors. Because public health investigational activities are directed at interrupting infectious syphilis, early syphilis morbidity data tend to be more accurate, especially those relating to the primary and secondary phases, which are associated with signs of disease. In tropical settings endemic for yaws, positive tests for syphilis may occur that are indistinguishable from those due to *Treponema pallidum*.

Data on private-sector case rates and disease sequelae in the United States are derived from three major sources: (1) hospital data are provided by the National Center for Health Statistics (NCHS), which surveys 7500 randomly selected U.S. hospitals to provide the Hospital Discharge Survey; (2) the National Ambulatory Medical Care Survey (NAMCS), which is a probability sampling of the diagnoses of 1900 physicians conducted by the NCHS; and (3) the National Disease and Therapeutic Index (NDTI), which is a random sample survey of office visit data derived from U.S. physicians in office-based practices. The major shortcoming of these data bases is small numbers with subsequent wide confidence intervals in specific areas and patient subpopulations. The data are best viewed in aggregate and are thus characterized by the ecologic fallacy associated with these types of analyses.

3.3. Serologic Surveys

Serologic testing for syphilis provides a method of case finding and disease surveillance. Contemporary syphilis serology may represent the ideal in seroepidemiologic tools. The disease characteristically mimics a variety of maladies and thus often presents diagnostic difficulties or may be latent and inapparent to both patient and examiner. The available serologic tests are inexpensive, simple to do, sensitive, specific, and readily available. Positive tests are run in tandem with readily available and affordable confirmatory tests to substantiate the diagnosis. The infection is easily and inexpensively treated and the sequelae averted are serious and life-threatening. Because syphilis tends to be clustered within the population, random or routine serologic testing of the general population may be a rather insensitive measure of disease trends. Serologic screening for syphilis primarily identifies inapparent latent disease cases for which treatment is needed to prevent sequelae. Its moderate sensitivity in very early infectious syphilis limits its use as

an early case-finding tool. Unless selectivity is applied to high-risk patient populations, widespread serologic testing is expensive, but appropriately applied, may be a good method for disease surveillance and is the only way to identify latent syphilis before the development of irreversible sequelae.

It has been estimated that about 45 million serologic tests are run in the United States annually and about 1.4 million (3.1%) are reactive.[41] About one-third of these positive reactors prove to be newly identified cases of syphilis. Of these, about 25% have clinically evident primary or secondary syphilis while the remainder have latent inapparent infection. It is estimated that serologic screening has generally accounted for the identification of about 25% of primary and secondary syphilis morbidity, about 40% of the early latent cases, and most of the late latent cases in the United States.

Routine serologic screening has generally been done by hospitals, blood banks, the military, preemployment physicians, prenatal facilities, and as a requirement for marriage in the United States. Although early syphilis case rates have been increasing in the last few years, there has been an increasing trend to discontinue serologic screening in hospitals and many states have repealed their premarital testing laws because of their apparent low yields.

There are few published data on contemporary seroprevalence estimates in the United States. Hospital screening provides some measure of disease frequency in community patient populations. One study of hospital admission screening[6] found that the test identified 19 of 20 patients with early syphilis and that routine testing of hospital admissions identified a new case in need of treatment about every third day. Another study yielded a positivity rate of 2.6% with 75% of those positive identified as having had syphilis.[45] A study conducted in a community medical practice[20] found an infection prevalence of 1.1% in 8100 tests of which about one-half of the positive patients were in need of treatment. A recent study of sera collected for the second National Health and Nutritional Survey (NHANES-II), which is a national probability survey done between 1976 and 1980 that studied 13,000 sera, revealed a syphilis prevalence of 1.3% with 8.5% of those positive (or 1/1000) in need of treatment.[14] If this sample were representative of the U.S. population, this translates into a projection of about 200,000 unidentified syphilis cases in the United States who are in need of treatment.

Premarital syphilis screening was originally instituted as a syphilis testing dragnet designed to test a broad segment of the population who were usually in the peak age group for syphilis infection. It was also designed to serve as an adjunct to prenatal screening to diminish the frequency of congenital syphilis. The cost of this activity is borne by the patients rather than the public health sector and the benefits accrued are usually for the individual (cases brought to treatment to avert sequelae) rather than the population (new cases averted). Most of the cases detected by this method are latent rather than early infectious cases. As the frequency of syphilis in the United States declined, so did the cost benefit of this testing. Also, the emphasis of syphilis control has changed from interdiction of disease sequelae to case finding of early infectious syphilis. There is a general feeling among public health workers and the medical community that many of the undetected latent cases of syphilis would often be ultimately cured with treatment with antibiotics for other medical conditions. Concerns have been expressed in the medical literature about the lack of value and cost-effectiveness of premarital syphilis testing.[8,9,15,16,18] Since no state had collected data on the discrete clinical situations of individual premarital screening tests, these studies used proxy rate data. Numerator data were derived from the reported number of early syphilis cases brought to treatment from premarital syphilis testing. Denominator data were derived from the number of marriages in the state. Unfortunately, since public health data collection processes are tailored for early infectious syphilis, latent cases beyond 1 year are often not documented. Our own experience and that of others suggests that the current reporting system in most states underestimates syphilis cases brought to treatment by serologic testing such as premarital screening by as much as 5- to 60-fold. In response to some of these articles, public health experts at CDC expressed concerns about premature decisions about premarital syphilis testing based on incomplete data and oversimplified cost-effectiveness analyses based only on an early infectious syphilis perspective.[26,38] In spite of this, and an increasing frequency of early infectious syphilis nationwide, the trend has been to discontinue premarital syphilis screening. In 1964, 45 states required premarital syphilis screening; in 1986, only 19 states still retained the practice. The private resources previously used for syphilis screening have not been reallocated to more productive control activities.

State and federal public health officials have not used mandated syphilis screening programs such as premarital and prenatal testing as surveillance tools to identify high-risk patient populations. Data collection of this type would permit better trend estimates of disease morbidity and permit more appropriate targeting of public health resources.

Serologic screening programs could be made more cost-effective if targeted to populations at high risk for in-

fection. In the United States, this may be of only theoretical importance, since it may not be politically expedient to apply mandated screening to only selected populations, especially if these populations are minority groups. With the proper resources and public health resolve, it may be possible to promote widespread voluntary testing of high-risk populations.

3.4. Laboratory Diagnosis

3.4.1. Identification of the Organism.
Claims have been made regarding successful *in vitro* culture of *Treponema pallidum,* but the techniques have been difficult to reproduce and have no current place in syphilis diagnosis. Dark-field microscopy identification of the motile *T. pallidum* in secretions from primary, secondary, and early congenital lesions constitutes a rapid, reliable, sensitive, and specific test during these syphilis stages. The organism can also be identified in the aqueous humor of late ocular syphilis. *T. pallidum* can be differentiated from genital saprophytic spirochetes by its length, number and symmetry of its concentric spirals, and smooth rotating motility along its long axis. Dark-field microscopy is less helpful with mouth chancre and mucous patch specimens because *T. pallidum* and oral *T. denticola* are morphologically similar. A positive dark-field finding in an oral lesion should be confirmed by a direct fluorescent antibody procedure.

T. pallidum can also be identified from lesions and in biopsy material by direct fluorescent-antibody techniques, which are commercially available. This procedure is more expensive than dark-field microscopy and the test results may not be available before the patient leaves the doctor's office or clinic. The advantages of direct fluorescent-antibody testing for *T. pallidum* are that the specimen does not need to be examined immediately and can be transported to a laboratory where an experienced microscopist can make the proper identification. This procedure is ideally suited for testing oral and anorectal lesion secretions because it will differentiate *T. pallidum* from *T. denticola* and other spirochete strains.

Specimens for either dark-field or fluorescent-antibody microscopy tests are best obtained from the moist lesions of primary and secondary syphilis because these contain the greatest numbers of *T. pallidum.* Genital lesions can be secondarily infected with pyogenic bacteria and leukocytes in clinical specimens can make it difficult to detect *T. pallidum.* Chancre exudate should therefore be wiped away prior to specimen collection. The clean lesion is then grasped between the thumb and index finger and compressed to yield enough clear secretion such that a bead of fluid will collect when a microscope slide coverslip is touched to the lesion. If enough secretion is not produced with the first try, compression for a longer period or re-grasping the lesion from another angle will usually produce an adequate specimen. The relatively painless nature of syphilitic lesions facilitates their vigorous compression with minimal patient complaints. Healing chancres become dry and specimen collection may require abrasion with cotton gauze prior to compression. *T. pallidum* can also be found in the dry macular and papular lesions of secondary syphilis and in the enlarged nodes that drain the chancre of primary syphilis, but the numbers of *T. pallidum* are considerably fewer. Dark-field examination under these circumstances is therefore more difficult and, in addition, patients resist the invasive procedures needed to obtain specimens from dry lesions or lymph nodes.

Falsely negative dark-field and direct fluorescent-antibody tests may occur even with adequate clinical specimens. Patient self-treatment with even a single penicillin tablet, for instance, can render a chancre dark-field-negative within hours. The same occurs when antiseptic ointments are locally applied to syphilis lesions.

3.4.2. Serology. Serologic tests are valuable in syphilis diagnosis when moist lesions are not available for dark-field examination. They should not replace dark-field tests in primary syphilis because in this stage of syphilis all serologic tests are less sensitive than direct visualization of *T. pallidum*. Cases of primary syphilis will be missed if clinicians rely only on serologic tests. When syphilis has reached the secondary stage, antibody levels have risen and nearly all serologic tests are reactive. The rare exception, referred to as the prozone phenomena, is a falsely negative nontreponemal test in secondary syphilis due to excess antibody interfering with the test. The phenomena can be eliminated and a positive test obtained by diluting the serum specimen before rerunning the test. Clinicians suspicious of secondary syphilis, but confronted with a negative nontreponemal syphilis serology, should request that the test be repeated with diluted serum.

Based on the character of the test antigen, two major categories of syphilis serologic tests exist (Table 1). The first syphilis serologic test, the Wassermann test, used an antigen that has subsequently been called cardiolipin. The test has been refined by the use of more purified versions of cardiolipin antigen. The current antigen is a defined combination of cardiolipin, cholesterol, and lecithin. Wassermann extracted his antigen from a congenital syphilis liver that contained many *T. pallidum*. Sometime thereafter, it was unexpectedly shown that a similar extract from a nonsyphilitic liver worked equally well as test antigen. Car-

Table 1. Antibody Tests for Syphilis

Nontreponemal
  Rapid plasma reagin (RPR)
  Venereal disease research laboratory (VDRL)
  Unheated serum reagin (USR)
  Reagin screen test (RST)
Treponemal
  Fluorescent treponemal antibody absorption (FTA-ABS)
  Fluorescent treponemal antibody absorption double staining (FTA-ABS DS)
  Microhemagglutination assay for antibody to *Treponema pallidum* (MHA-TP)
  Hemagglutination treponemal test for syphilis (HATTS)
  Bio-enzaBead test (ELISA)

diolipin is now known to be a component of many normal animal tissues. At the present time, cardiolipin is extracted from beef hearts. For this reason, syphilis serologies using cardiolipin antigen are referred to as nontreponemal tests. This terminology may not be completely correct because *T. pallidum* itself contains a cardiolipin antigen. Current cardiolipin tests have similar sensitivities and specificities and include the venereal disease research laboratory (VDRL) and the rapid plasma reagin (RPR) tests (Table 2).

The other major category of syphilis serologic tests comprises the treponemal tests. Intact *T. pallidum* organisms are the antigens used in the *T. pallidum* immobilization (TPI) and fluorescent treponemal antibody absorption (FTA-ABS) tests. The TPI test was very labor-intensive and is now used only in research laboratories. The newest treponemal tests employ *T. pallidum* extracts fixed to erythrocytes and involve hemagglutination procedures. Sheep erythrocytes are used in the microhemagglutination test for *T. pallidum* (MHA-TP) and turkey erythrocytes carry the

Table 2. Comparative Sensitivities of Serologic Tests for Syphilis[a,b]

Syphilis stage	Sensitivity of test			
	VDRL	RPR	FTA-ABS	MHA-TP
Primary	80	82	98	85
Secondary	/100	/100	/100	/100
Latent	90	90	100	100
Late	80	80	98	96

[a]The specificity of all the test procedures is approximately 99%.
[b]/ = Approximately.

antigen in the hemagglutination treponemal test for syphilis (HATTS). The hemagglutination tests may be slightly more specific than the FTA-ABS, but are less sensitive in primary syphilis.

Falsely positive nontreponemal tests were described shortly after it was realized that the tests' antigen was not specific for *T. pallidum*. These false-positive tests are usually of low titer ($\leq 1:4$), although some of the highest titers ($> 1:30,000$) have occurred in nonsyphilitic patients who have a lymphoma. False-positive nontreponemal tests are divided into acute and chronic (Table 3), based on the fact that acute reactions revert to negative in less than 6 months, whereas others (chronic) remain positive for more than 6 months. It was initially felt that the treponemal tests would be specific for syphilis and the other treponemal infections such as yaws, pinta, and bejel. Now it is realized that some false-positive treponemal tests may be associated with lupus erythematosus, pregnancy, and intravenous drug abuse.

4. Biological Characteristics of the Organism

T. pallidum is classified in the order Spirochaetales, genus *Treponema*. The latter includes both human pathogens and nonpathogenic organisms. The pathogens and the diseases they cause are *T. pallidum* (syphilis), *T. pertenue* (yaws), *T. carateum* (pinta), and *T. pallidum* variant (endemic syphilis). Morphologically, these four treponemes are identical and their antigenic and biochemical differences remain to be described. DNA homology has demonstrated a close similarity between *T. pallidum* and some of the other pathogens and marked differences between the pathogens and the nonpathogenic treponemes.[11] Cross-resistance between *T. pallidum* infection and the other treponemal infections suggests immunologic similarities. Syphilis nontreponemal and treponemal tests are reactive in patients with yaws, pinta, and endemic syphilis. Syphilis incidence is low in areas where yaws is endemic, but has increased following active yaws eradication programs. The pathogenic treponemes can be differentiated by the host response in various animal models.

T. pallidum, like other treponemes, is a gram-negative bacterium. It is best identified, however, by finding it in fresh, moist, unstained specimens. Here, dark-field microscopy is advantageous because the organism is very thin, 0.1 μm to 0.2 μm, which is beyond the usual resolution of conventional light microscopy. Its length varies from 6 μm to 15 μm, possibly because its reproductive cycle consists of growth in length followed by division halfway along its axis. *T. pallidum*'s forward and backward motility is associated with screwlike rotation along its long axis. It can also bend to form "C" and "O" configurations or flex to produce "V" forms. Concentric spirals, in contrast to asymmetric bends, and smooth motility, in contrast to jerking movements, are the morphologic differences between *T. pallidum* and many of the nonpathogenic treponemes. One saprophytic organism that can be morphologically confused with *T. pallidum* is *T. denticola* (*T. microdentium*), which is found in the mouth.

Special staining techniques suggest that *T. pallidum* is surrounded by an amorphous capsulelike layer.[47] The outermost structure, as seen by conventional electron microscopy, is an outer envelope or membrane that covers the axial filaments (periplastic flagella). Three of these filaments originate at each end of the treponeme, wrap around the organism's surface, and extend about halfway down its length. An outer peptidoglycan and an inner cytoplasmic membrane enclose the cytoplasm and its contents. Six to eight cytoplasmic tubules attach to each end of the treponeme and wind around the organism just inside the cytoplasmic membrane. A nuclear region, ribosomes, and mesosomes are present in the cytoplasm.

T. pallidum is a fragile organism very susceptible to osmolarity and temperature fluctuations. It does not survive in dried secretions and it is readily destroyed by disinfectants commonly used in laboratories and clinics. Within a heavy concentration of *T. pallidum,* as occurs in a laboratory extraction of a rabbit syphilitic orchitis, some organisms will still be viable after several days of refrigeration. *T. pallidum* utilizes oxygen and is microaerophilic. None of the human pathogenic treponemes have been grown in broth

Table 3. Causes of False-Positive Nontreponemal Syphilis Serologic Tests[a]

Acute (remain positive < 6 months)
  Pregnancy
  Infections
  Immunizations
  Narcotic addiction[b]
Chronic (remain positive > 6 months)
  Autoimmune diseases
  Malignancies
  Elderly
  Narcotic addiction[b]
  Yaws

[a] Table derived from best estimates compiled from available published information.
[b] May be acute or chronic.

or on bacteriologic media. Limited replication is said to occur in certain cell culture systems.[23]

5. Descriptive Epidemiology

Because syphilis passes through both clinical and subclinical phases, case definition presents a dilemma for morbidity analysts. Since the disease passes into a latent phase if untreated and accumulates in the population, incidence and prevalence rates may be significantly different. Primary and secondary syphilis, due to their symptomatic clinical presentations and relatively short duration, provide us with a measure of disease incidence. This is especially true in men, where the signs of primary disease most often occur on the external genitalia. In contrast, primary infections of women are uncommonly identified. Latent disease rates, on the other hand, are highly dependent on the level of screening and contact tracing activities. In many ways, trends in latent disease rates may reflect the levels of program resources devoted to syphilis control and serologic screening activities. Thus, changes in the descriptive epidemiologic features of syphilis may vary artifactually, by sex and the level and quality of program activities in any geographic area.

5.1. Prevalence and Incidence

After the advent and widespread use of penicillin treatment, syphilis cases dropped dramatically. Sixteen years after the introduction of penicillin (1958), the reported number of syphilis cases had dropped 75% (Fig. 1). Between 1962 and 1978 the total number dropped another 48%. Since then, total syphilis cases have increased. Congenital syphilis cases followed a similar trend (Fig. 2). In 1987, 34,008 cases of primary and secondary syphilis were reported in the United States. This represented a 25% increase over the 1986 cases, the largest single-year increase since 1960. The case rates increased by 23.5%, from 11.5/100,000 in 1986 to 14.2/100,000 in 1987. Except for a brief period between 1976 through 1978, primary and secondary syphilis rates in U.S. men increased greatly between 1969 and 1982 (Fig. 3). During this period the number of cases more than doubled. Beginning in 1983 the number of primary and secondary cases in men dropped 24%, but again increased 20% between 1986 and 1987. In women, the incidence of primary and secondary cases showed a different trend. It remained relatively stable between 1969 and 1973, and after a decrease of 36% between 1973 and 1979, the number of cases began to increase. Since 1979 there has been a progressive 64% increase in

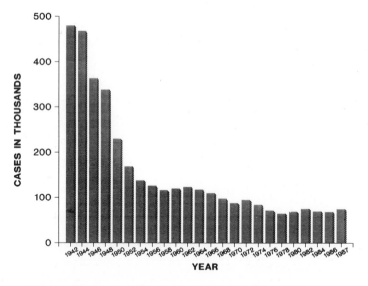

Figure 1. Total cases of syphilis, all stages, United States, 1942–87.

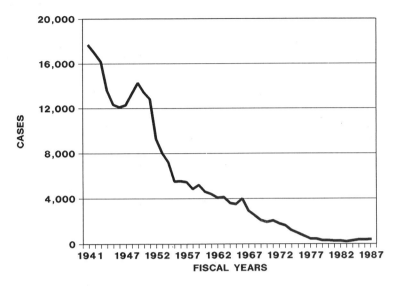

Figure 2. Total congenital syphilis cases (all ages), United States, 1941–1987.

cases and between 1986 and 1987 the number of cases sharply increased by 34%. In aggregate, between 1978 and 1987 the number of primary and secondary syphilis cases in women has more than doubled. Congenital syphilis cases have paralleled the trends in female primary and secondary disease (Fig. 3). Between 1983 and 1987 the number of congenital syphilis cases has increased by almost threefold.

5.2. Epidemic Behavior and Contagiousness

Except for intrauterine infection, syphilis is transmitted by sexual activity that provides intimate contact between infected epithelial surfaces and mucosa or abraded skin. The attack rate is high, especially after repeated exposures, and is inversely proportional to the stage of the disease. One

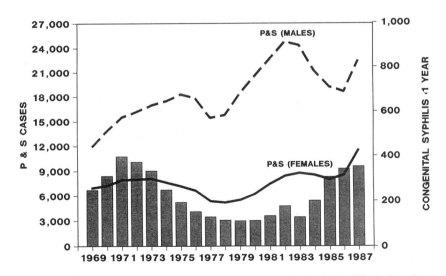

Figure 3. Primary and secondary syphilis cases by sex, and congenital syphilis (< 1 year) cases

study of married couples found an attack rate of 81% when one partner was exposed to infectious lesions and also found that no disease transmission occurred when exposed to a person infected for more than 4 years.[27] Another study of married partners found an attack rate of 77% for infectious syphilis cases and 69% for early latent cases.[4] In a study of untreated nonconjugal sexual contacts to patients with primary and secondary syphilis, 30% acquired infection.[40]

The infectious dose for the transmission of *T. pallidum* infection may be very low. The ID_{50} of the rabbit-acclimated Nichols strain for the production of intracutaneous infection in human volunteers has been found to be about 50 organisms.[30]

Perinatal transmission of syphilis has been shown to occur as early as week 9 of gestation.[17] The risk of intrauterine transmission of infection in maternal syphilis is high and it varies with the stage of maternal disease. One analysis identified the risk of congenital syphilis acquisition to be 50% in maternal primary and secondary infection, 40% in

early latent infection, and only 10% in late latent infection.[12] Healthy term infants were born to 20% of mothers with early latent maternal infections and to 70% of those with late latent disease.

5.3. Geographic Distribution

Syphilis morbidity is characterized by a geographic clustering of infections. This clustering may not be as tight as that seen with gonorrhea.[39] In 1983, 63 cities with populations of 200,000 or more accounted for 60% of the reported cases of primary and secondary syphilis although only accounting for 26% of the population.[44] In the United States, infectious syphilis is clustered in the South and Southeast, with heavy concentrations also in California and New York (Fig. 4). Five states—Florida, California, Georgia, New York, and Texas—accounted for 70% of all the primary and secondary syphilis cases reported in the United States in 1987. The primary and secondary case

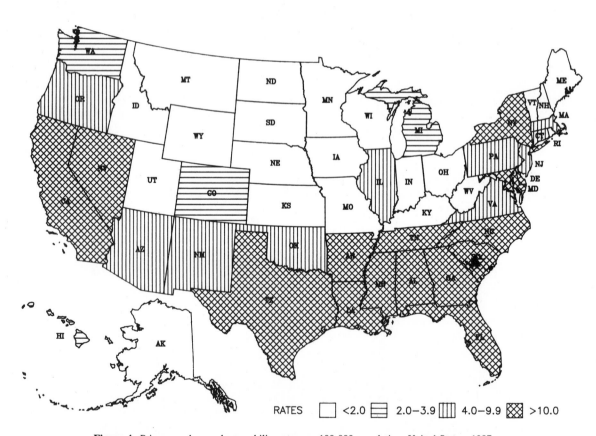

Figure 4. Primary and secondary syphilis, rates per 100,000 population, United States, 1987.

rate/100,000 in the United States in 1987 was 14.2 and ranged by state from 0.3 (North Dakota) to 59.6 (Florida), a difference of almost 200-fold. The median primary and secondary case rate for this period was 4.6 and the mean was 8.7. The states with the highest primary and secondary syphilis morbidity during 1987 were Florida (59.6), California (27.9), Georgia (27), Mississippi (25.1), and New York (25). The states with the lowest primary and secondary syphilis rates were North Dakota (0.3), Minnesota (0.5), Kentucky (0.6), Nebraska (0.6), Vermont (0.6), and West Virginia (0.6). Only nine states had rates greater than 16/100,000 whereas 25 states had rates less than 4/100,000. A similar pattern is seen in congenital syphilis cases. In 1985, three states (Texas, Florida, California) and one city (New York) accounted for 80% of the reported congenital syphilis cases in the United States.[5] In 1986, the cities with the highest primary and secondary syphilis rates were Atlanta (118), Miami (68), Dallas (64), Newark (57), Memphis (56), the District of Columbia (49), and San Francisco (49). The lowest case rates were seen in Minneapolis (1.0), Wichita (1.0), Des Moines (1.3), Tucson (1.4), Akron (1.8), and St. Paul (1.9). The range between cities was between 1.0 and 118, with a median of 12 and a U.S. metropolitan city rate of 24.5.

Because of major differences in surveillance activities and record-keeping practices worldwide, it is not possible to reliably compare case rates by country. In general, the trend of syphilis in Europe and Canada usually parallels that in the United States with a lag of about 2 years. The disease appears to be hyperendemic in Africa where congenital syphilis continues to regularly occur. The transmission of syphilis in some developing countries is associated with prostitution, which, in some areas, is more socially accepted as a sexual outlet for men.

5.4. Temporal Distribution

A seasonal trend has not been demonstrated for syphilis. The secular trend of syphilis incidence by geographic region has been similar over the last decade.

5.5. Age and Sex

The highest incidence of syphilis occurs in the age group 20–24 years old and it varies by sex. Table 4 shows the distribution of primary and secondary case rates by age group and sex. In women, the highest case rates are seen in those 15–30 years old. The highest incidence in men are seen in a somewhat older age group, 20–39. The case rates for men are 2.5-fold those of women and this ratio increased

Table 4. 1985 Primary and Secondary Syphilis Case Rates/100,000 by Age Group and Sex

Age group	Men	Women	M/F ratio
0–9	0	0.1	0.0
10–14	0.5	1.4	0.4
15–19	16.3	17.7	0.9
20–24	50.5	25.9	1.9
25–29	45.3	16.4	2.8
30–34	32.8	9.3	3.5
35–39	21.7	5.4	4.0
40–44	16.5	3.4	4.9
45+	4.3	0.6	7.2
Total	16.6	6.7	2.5

with age. Part of this sex difference is undoubtedly due to the difficulty in identifying primary infections in women, but the comparative case ratio differences suggest that other factors are operative. It is likely that at least a part of this difference, if not the major part, relates to homosexual practices in men. Part of it may be associated with the decreasing accuracy of the ratios as the case numbers get smaller as they do with ascending age. The secular trend in the male/female primary and secondary syphilis case ratios is shown in Fig. 5. From a low point in 1966, this ratio more than doubled by 1980. This coincides with the data indicating that the proportion of early syphilis that occurred in homosexual and bisexual males increased from 25% in 1969 to 52% in 1979. These data support the observation of an epidemic of syphilis in male homosexuals beginning in the late 1960s and continuing into the 1980s. Between 1980 and 1986, the male/female ratio for primary and secondary syphilis cases declined by 32% and between 1980 and 1983 (the last year these data were kept) the proportion of early syphilis in men with same-sex sexual partners declined by 19%.

5.6. Race

Most studies have found higher syphilis case rates in blacks compared to whites. These data are often biased by the higher utilization by the black population of public clinics, which disproportionately report cases for morbidity purposes. Military draft screening in the 1940s revealed that the syphilis rates in black males were 272/1000, compared with 23.5/1000, almost a 12-fold difference.[46] A U.S. probability sample, the National Health Examination Sur-

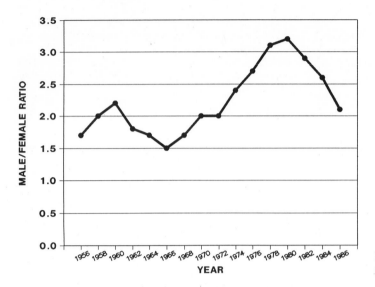

Figure 5. Male/female primary and secondary syphilis case ratios, United States, 1956–1986.

vey (NHES-I) taken in 1960–1962, found serologic evidence of syphilis in ten times as many black men and eight times as many black women as white.[34] A similar study conducted between 1976 and 1980 examined about 13,000 sera from throughout the United States (NHANES-II). Controlling for the effects of age, marital status, residence, education, income, and gender, serologic evidence of syphilis was found to be 4.7 times more prevalent in blacks than whites (Dr. Robert Hahn, personal communication). These data and another study that evaluated the race-specific trends of syphilis between 1967 and 1979[10] indicate that the race-specific syphilis rates and the black versus white case ratios have gone down between 1940 and 1980.

The reasons for the higher syphilis rates in blacks are currently unknown. It is probable that racial social segregation, which somewhat confines sexual activity within a population with a previously elevated prevalence of disease, contributes to it.

5.7. Occupation

Except for prostitution, occupation bears no specific relationship to the risk of acquisition of syphilis. Occupations that employ predominantly younger, sexually active individuals, especially from syphilis endemic areas, would likely yield higher infection rates.

5.8. Occurrence in Different Settings

As mentioned previously, higher syphilis case rates are often seen in urban centers, especially in the southern and

southeastern United States. Like many other STDs, the spread of syphilis is favored in highly promiscuous socially disadvantaged populations, and has been associated with prostitution, alcoholism, and drug abuse.

5.9. Socioeconomic Factors

Although syphilis has been more frequent in lower socioeconomic groups, all social strata are at risk for sexually transmitted infections such as syphilis. Factors such as educational and income level, which are directly related to the frequency of use of prophylactic and therapeutic measures to circumvent disease, are often important determinants of the frequency of disease and the rate of disease transmission.

5.10. Other Factors

There is an increasing body of circumstantial evidence that the level of promiscuity in the United States has increased during the prior two decades. This appears to apply to both heterosexuals and homosexuals. This, combined with decreased condom use (for pregnancy and disease prophylaxis) has surely influenced the epidemic of STDs seen in the past two decades. Recently, the proportion of syphilis in gay men has decreased significantly, probably as a reflection of safer sex practices brought about by concern about AIDS. Preliminary evidence suggests that the recent increase in heterosexual syphilis are predominantly occurring in minority populations and are increasingly associated with prostitution and drug abuse, especially the cocaine product "crack." It is possible that given an introduction of syphilis within the drug-abusing population, the social–sexual preferences that favor sex with members of the same social environment and the lack of good health-seeking habits may tend to favor rapid transmission of syphilis in these populations.

Several factors influence the occurrence of congenital syphilis.[5] In a study of 437 infants with congenital syphilis, it was found that about half of the maternal cases did not have prenatal care. One fourth of the cases acquired their infections after the initial serologic test for syphilis was found to be negative and 14% of the cases were the result of failure to treat mothers with positive serologies.

6. Mechanisms and Routes of Transmission

T. pallidum is usually transmitted during sexual contact between an infectious individual and a susceptible recipient. Infection of a sexual partner occurs in about one third of such exposures. Initial infection fails to occur unless adequate numbers of treponemes are transferred to the partner's mucosae or abraded skin. Normal serum has some antitreponemal activity, but it is weak and probably of little clinical relevance because no natural resistance has been found in experimental infection of volunteers not previously exposed to *T. pallidum*.[30]

Infected individuals are not continually infectious to others. Patients may remain infected with *T. pallidum* from the time of inoculation until their death, but they are infectious to others only during the several weeks of the primary and secondary stage of syphilis and early latent disease when clinical lesions may recur; late latent and late syphilis are not infectious stages.

For syphilis infection to be transmitted, there must be adequate numbers of *T. pallidum* on the surface of the organ that contacts the recipient's skin or mucosae. The exact number needed to infect is unknown, but experimental intracutaneous injection of *T. pallidum* required only 57 organisms.[30] *T. pallidum* can penetrate mucosal surfaces but penetration is resisted by intact skin. *T. pallidum* can penetrate through the skin abrasions that occur in sexual activity. Rabbits resist syphilis when *T. pallidum* is placed on normal skin, but the minimal trauma associated with shaving the animal allows the same skin to be infected. A similar situation may occur in childbirth, when *T. pallidum* from a mother's genital chancre is transmitted to the child as it passes through the vagina. Under this circumstance, the chancre(s) in the newborn develops several weeks postpartum in the site(s) of birth trauma, such as where extraction

forceps were applied to the head. The more common mode of congenital syphilis transmission is via a maternal septicemia with passage of *T. pallidum* through the placenta and into the developing fetus. Such a septicemia is most likely when the pregnant mother has an early stage of syphilis. Treatment of an infectious mother in the first trimester may prevent congenital syphilis because placental passage usually occurs during the second and third trimesters.

Hematogenous spread of *T. pallidum* has been described with blood transfusions, but is quite rare. Treponemes are present in blood for only the short duration of the primary and secondary phases. In addition, blood is screened with a syphilis serologic test before it is transfused into a recipient. Intravenous illicit drug use probably transmits infection but there are no good supporting data for this.

Fomite transmission of syphilis is very rare or may not occur because *T. pallidum* is rapidly killed by drying. *T. pallidum* has not been found in urine, milk, or sweat. Syphilis transmission has anecdotally been reported to occur by sharing razors, drinking from the same container, and chewing the same gum.[25]

7. Pathogenesis and Immunity

The interval between infection with *T. pallidum* and development of the first clinical sign of syphilis varies from 10 to 90 days with the typical case developing an ulcer (the primary chancre) in 3 weeks. The incubation period's upper limit is important because failure of a syphilis sexual contact to develop a chancre or a positive cardiolipin serology within 90 days is strong evidence that syphilis infection did not occur.

T. pallidum infection evokes both humoral and cellular immune responses. The first evidence of a cellular immune response in syphilis was a delayed type of reaction following the intracutaneous injection of killed *T. pallidum*. More recently, *in vitro* culture of syphilis patients' lymphocytes with *T. pallidum* antigens produced lymphocyte blast transformation.

Treponemal (anti-*T. pallidum*) and nontreponemal (anticardiolipin) antibodies begin developing in primary syphilis and, in the secondary stage, all patients have high titers of both antibodies. Titers of anticardiolipin antibodies then start to decline slowly and spontaneously revert to negative in about one-third of untreated patients. Anti-*T. pallidum* antibodies remain detectable for the life of the patient. Cell-mediated immunity also develops in primary syphilis, appears to be suppressed during the secondary stage, and is again detected in the latent and late stages.[28]

The roles of antibodies and cellular immunity in resistance to infection are not completely understood. Human inoculation experiments have shown that some syphilis infections confer a degree of resistance to reinfection.[30] Patients treated previously for primary and secondary syphilis were easily reinfected with *T. pallidum* despite the fact that they showed an anamnestic antibody response to both cardiolipin and *T. pallidum* antigens. Patients with untreated late latent syphilis were most resistant; many patients with this stage of syphilis resisted an intracutaneous challenge of 100,000 *T. pallidum*. This compares with an infectious dose of about 50 organisms for an initial syphilis infection. Resistance to reinfection correlated better with cellular immunity than with antibodies. It is not known how coinfection with HIV influences the immunologic and clinical course of syphilis.

Resistance to reinfection is to be differentiated from chancre immunity. The latter is failure of *T. pallidum* to produce a second chancre while the primary chancre is still present. Chancre immunity may be secondary to cellular immunosuppression in early syphilis.

8. Patterns of Host Response

8.1. Clinical Features

The clinical features of syphilis as it passes through the various phases resemble, and must be differentiated from, a variety of other diseases. Because of this, it has become known as "the great imitator."

8.1.1. Primary Stage.
When infection occurs, the first sign of syphilis develops at the site of inoculation and consists of a pink to red macule. This flat lesion rapidly becomes a palpable nodule and within several days its surface erodes to produce the characteristic chancre. Chancres are usually single, without pain, and accompanied by painless regional lymphadenopathy. The asymptomatic character of such a large genital ulcer contrasts markedly with the pain of smaller genital herpes and chancroid ulcers. Lack of pain not only alerts the clinician to the possibility of syphilis but also allows compression of the ulcer to produce adequate specimens for diagnostic dark-field microscopy. Multiple chancres can occur, as with the "kissing" lesions on opposing surfaces of a skin of mucosal fold. Chancres can be painful if secondarily infected by pyogenic bacteria. Such secondary infection can also cause a painless adenopathy to become painful. Syphilis chancres are so often different in appearance from textbook presentations that clinicians should do dark-field microscopy on all acute genital ulcers in sexually active patients to avoid missing cases of early syphilis.

A primary syphilis chancre heals spontaneously, usually within 2 to 3 weeks, even without treatment, but occasionally may persist for up to 8 weeks. A residual scar in the area of the chancre is rare unless the lesion was secondarily infected. The regional adenopathy requires a longer time to resolve spontaneously.

8.1.2. Secondary Stage.
Several weeks after the chancre has healed, or in rare instances while it is still present, the manifestations of secondary syphilis emerge and are the manifestations of hematogenous spread of the spirochete to various organs. Nonspecific symptoms of this stage include low-grade fever, headache, sore throat, malaise, anorexia, and arthralgias. Somewhat more specific manifestations include mild hepatitis in about 10% of patients and, rarely, the nephrotic syndrome. The most characteristic signs of secondary syphilis, although not pathognomonic, are changes in the skin, hair, and mucous membranes. Skin lesions are discrete and may be macular (flat) or papular (small palpable elevations). The macular lesions on the trunk most closely mimic pityriasis rosea. Macular lesions on the palms and soles are frequently hyperpigmented and somewhat characteristic but must be differentiated from hereditary macular palmar–plantar hyperpigmentation. Psoriasis and lichen planus can look very much like the papular lesions of secondary syphilis. Hair loss may occur in secondary syphilis. Patches of scalp hair are thinned rather than completely denuded and the result is a moth-eaten appearance to the scalp. Glistening, grayish superficial plaques of secondary syphilis may appear in the mouth and, to a lesser extent, on the genital mucosae. These are mucous patches and must be differentiated from precancerous leukoplakia. Secondary syphilis in intertriginous sites presents as nodules or plaques with eroded surfaces. These lesions are referred to as condylomata lata and may appear similar to venereal warts (condylomata acuminata).

A patient with secondary syphilis may have one, several, or all signs of the secondary stage. Since each of the signs includes a differential diagnosis, none is specific to syphilis. However, when more of these signs are present, the diagnosis of syphilis is more likely to be accurate. The diagnosis of secondary syphilis is confirmed by the identification of *T. pallidum* in mucosal lesions or by the conversion of a syphilis serologic test from negative to positive. Almost all treponemal and nontreponemal syphilis serologies are reactive in this stage of syphilis.

The manifestations of secondary syphilis last 2 to 8 weeks and then, as with primary syphilis, heal spontaneously without residual scarring. When healing is complete, the patient enters into a latent phase where there are no clinical signs or symptoms of syphilis. The serologic tests for syphilis, however, remain positive.

8.1.3. Clinical (Infectious) Secondary Relapse. About 25% of untreated patients in the Oslo study done in 1890 to 1910[13] relapsed from latency back into secondary syphilis. This occurred during the first 5 years of latency, although most relapses took place in the first year. Such relapses are now infrequent, possibly related to inadvertent syphilis treatment by systemic antibiotics used to treat another infection.

8.1.4. Late Benign Syphilis. Late or tertiary syphilis occurs much less often than was reported in the Oslo study of untreated syphilis.[3] As with the reduction in secondary syphilis relapses, this is probably related to inadvertent syphilis treatment when systemic antibiotics are used to treat a variety of other infectious diseases. This trend, however, may be reversing. A recent report suggests that concurrent HIV infection may facilitate early syphilis progression to symptomatic neurosyphilis.[24] This occurred in both untreated and treated syphilis patients.

One third of untreated syphilis patients in the Oslo study progressed from the latent stage to one or more of the tertiary stages of syphilis. The remaining two thirds of syphilis patients remained asymptomatic during the remainder of their lives. The sera of some of these asymptomatic patients also become nonreactive in the cardiolipin syphilis serologic tests. Such serologic conversion suggested a spontaneous cure, but an occasional patient with late syphilis can be seronegative in the cardiolipin tests.

There are three types of tertiary syphilis: gummas, cardiovascular syphilis, and central nervous system syphilis. Gummatous lesions developed in about 15% of the Oslo study patients. These lesions have their onset 2 to 40 years after primary syphilis. Seventy percent of gummas involve the skin, 10% are found in bone, and a similar percentage are present on mucosal surfaces. Gummas can involve any organ. Skin and bone gummas are disfiguring, but involvement of a vital organ such as the heart or liver could be fatal. Skin gummas frequently have an annular configuration; the surface of early lesions is elevated above surrounding normal skin. These lesions slowly progress, creating a depression below adjacent skin. Such atrophic skin easily erodes, producing chronic ulcerations.

8.1.5. Cardiovascular Syphilis. Cardiovascular tertiary syphilis develops 10 to 30 years after primary syphilis and was clinically evident in about 10% of the Oslo study's untreated syphilis patients. Another 20 to 30% of untreated patients have cardiovascular changes that do not produce signs or symptoms. The microscopic pathology of cardiovascular syphilis is similar to that of neurosyphilis: blood vessel inflammation that progresses to vessel occlusion. The vessels clinically involved in cardiovascular syphilis are those that provide metabolites and oxygen to the cells and tissues of the aorta and of the heart's coronary vessels. Loss of this blood supply results in blood vessel wall death and scar formation. Scar tissue within the aorta weakens its walls such that the aorta either balloons outwards and into adjacent structures, or ruptures, causing hypovolemic shock and death. Aorta dilation just outside the heart spreads the aortic valve ring and separates the valve's leaflets. This allows blood to leak back into the heart through the damaged aortic valve. Progression of syphilitic aortic valve damage results in congestive heart failure and possible death. Incomplete syphilitic occlusion of the coronary vessels causes intermittent anginal cardiac chest pain. Myocardial infarction can occur when the coronary vessel occlusion is complete.

8.1.6. Neurosyphilis. Neurosyphilis develops 1 to 30 years after primary syphilis and involved 5 to 10% of Oslo's untreated patients. The earliest form of symptomatic neurosyphilis, syphilitic meningitis, is also the least common (10% of neurosyphilis patients). It occurs no more than several years after primary syphilis and is manifest by typical meningitis symptoms: fever, headache, photophobia, and stiff neck. The spinal fluid findings are those of aseptic meningitis—normal sugar and elevated lymphocytes and protein. It is differentiated from other types of aseptic meningitis by having a positive cerebrospinal fluid (CSF) cardiolipin test.

Later manifestations of neurosyphilis are due to blood vessel changes consisting of vascular inflammation leading to vessel occlusion. Some of the brain's blood vessels are affected more than others. Vessel occlusion results in the death of brain tissue served by that vessel. The clinical manifestations of vascular neurosyphilis, as with other neurologic diseases, depend upon which areas of the brain are damaged. Strokes and seizures are early presentations of vascular neurosyphilis. Progression of vascular neurosyphilis consists of the involvement of more and more blood vessels with the subsequent loss of more brain tissue. This loss can be so extensive that at autopsy it can be appreciated grossly as a shrunken brain. The associated clinical state is referred to as paresis and is a combination of neurologic and psychiatric changes. The latter is primarily a dementing process with loss of intellectual function, although some patients experience grandiose delusions. Common paresis neurologic changes are eye pupil abnormalities (Argyll–Robertson pupils), slurred speech, and tremors.

Spinal cord neurosyphilis consists of degeneration of

the posterior columns. Nerve fibers in these columns transmit deep pain and proprioception sensations. Early clinical manifestations include transient (lasting minutes) sharp pains that radiate into the legs or abdomen. Loss of deep pain sensation in the legs results in repeated painless trauma to the knees and feet. The knees enlarge (Charcot's joints) and ulcers develop on the bottom of the feet (mal perforant).

8.2. Diagnosis

The clinical diagnosis of syphilis is based on its signs and symptoms and, to a lesser extent, on epidemiology and demography. The laboratory diagnosis of syphilis is based on demonstration of *T. pallidum* or antibody to this pathogen or cardiolipin antigen. Occasionally, the gross and microscopic pathology may be available and aid in the diagnosis.

No single finding or test is absolutely diagnostic of syphilis. The most accurate single diagnostic test is the dark-field or direct fluorescent-antibody demonstration of *T. pallidum*. The accuracy of these two tests, however, depends on how and where the clinical specimen was obtained, how it was transported to the laboratory, and who did the test.

The diagnosis of primary syphilis would not be questioned in a patient who presents to an STD clinic because a steady sexual partner has recently been diagnosed as having secondary syphilis, with a single, indurated, nontender, dark-field-positive penile ulcer, and respective RPR and FTA-ABS tests, and whose genital sore heals within a week of receiving 2.4 million units of benzathine penicillin G. However, imagine another patient who presents to a private gynecologist because she develops a tongue ulcer 10 days after having oral–genital sexual contact with a man who had an undiagnosed penile ulcer. Her physician orders a stat RPR serologic test and dark-field examination of the tongue lesion; both tests are positive. The woman is diagnosed as having primary syphilis and her tongue heals within 1 week of receiving benzathine penicillin G therapy. This woman may have syphilis, but her presentation may be more consistent with the diagnosis of herpes simplex. Among the various causes of sexually transmitted ulcerative diseases seen by private physicians, herpes simplex is much more common than syphilis. Herpes simplex infection is also a cause of some false-positive cardiolipin tests. In addition, mouth *T. denticola* can be confused with *T. pallidum*. Herpes simplex lesions heal spontaneously, unrelated to penicillin or other concurrent antibiotic therapy. The diagnosis of primary syphilis in the woman with the tongue ulcer could have been better confirmed by a positive FTA-

ABS or MHA-TP serology or a positive direct fluorescent-antibody test on secretions from her tongue lesion.

The typical diagnostic findings associated with secondary syphilis include a high serologic titer (usually > 8 dils), body rash, the presence of condyloma lata, regional adenopathy, often accompanied by systemic symptoms such as mild fever, cephalgia, and malaise.

The diagnosis of latent syphilis requires a spinal tap to differentiate it from asymptomatic neurosyphilis. The differential is important because neurosyphilis requires more prolonged therapy and posttherapy spinal taps to document therapeutic success.

Treatment of syphilis is often much easier than diagnosis. This infection was one of the first treated with penicillin when this antibiotic became available in the mid-1940s. Unlike many other bacteria, *T. pallidum* has not developed resistance to this antibiotic although it has been the syphilis treatment-of-choice for over 30 years. A single dose of 2.4 million units of benzathine penicillin G is the treatment for primary, secondary, and latent syphilis of less than 1 year duration. The same penicillin preparation and dose is the treatment for latent syphilis of more than 1 year duration but here it is given on each of 3 days 1 week apart for a total of 7.2 million units. Patients with neurosyphilis may not respond adequately to this benzathine penicillin regimen and require hospitalization for 10 days for treatment with intravenous aqueous crystalline penicillin G. It is not clear whether patients with CNS involvement during secondary syphilis require treatment for neurosyphilis. Syphilis occurring in pregnancy is treated with the same penicillin regimens. Nonpregnant patients allergic to penicillin can be treated with tetracycline or erythromycin. Pregnant patients with a history of penicillin allergy present a therapeutic dilemma and should have the allergy confirmed by skin tests. Tetracycline treatment is contraindicated during pregnancy and erythromycin's low transplacental activity makes it a poor choice for treatment of the infected pregnant patient. Those found not allergic can be carefully treated with penicillin and those with positive skin tests could receive oral desensitization, followed by treatment with standard penicillin doses. The role of cephalosporins in the treatment of syphilis is still not clear and potential cross-reactivity in those allergic to penicillin mitigates against simple substitution therapy.

Syphilis treatment, like that of many other infectious diseases, requires follow-up to assure cure. Besides observing the resolution of the signs and symptoms of early syphilis, the cardiolipin serologic tests should be repeated 3, 6, and 12 months after treatment. A decline of at least two dilutions in test titers should occur after treatment and most tests will revert to negative in cases of primary and secondary syphilis. The anatomic damage occurring in late syphilis cannot be reversed, but treatment will prevent progression of the disease. Management of syphilis patients, as with other STDs, requires evaluation and treatment of sexual partners.

The treatment of syphilis is still clouded by continuing controversies. The documentation of central nervous involement in some cases of early syphilis continues to stir debate about the adequacy of the sole use of long-acting penicillin for this infection. Predictably effective alternative treatment for pregnant patients with penicillin allergy has still not been well defined. The association of immunodeficiency with decreased treatment efficacy has served as a new impetus for increased investigational efforts in the area of syphilis treatment. For a more comprehensive review of current syphilis therapy the reader is referred to the CDC 1989 Sexually Transmitted Diseases Treatment Guidelines in the Suggested Reading Section.

9. Control and Prevention

9.1. General Concepts

The only known vector for the transmission of *T. pallidum* infection is man. Thus, primary prevention of syphilis and other STDs involves the self-control of personal behavior. This involves careful selection of sexual partners, accepting sexual promiscuity as a socially unacceptable behavior, and knowledge of safe sexual practices, including the proper use of condoms. Education on these concepts needs to be started early and clearly directed at target populations and in a manner consistent with the population-specific hierarchy of social and personal values. These same measures would also help limit the spread of HIV and other sexually transmissible infections.

Because of human nature and the frequent failure of the above efforts to be uniformly successful, secondary prevention strategies by the medical and public health sector are important. The federal government, primarily through the CDC, provides grant funds, personnel, program and quality assurance guidelines, and data analysis to the states to assist in the control of the STD. The current public health syphilis control programs in the United States consist of the provision of clinic facilities, serologic reactor follow-up, sexual partner contact tracing, epidemiologic treatment of exposed individuals, and selective serologic screening.

Disease control occurs at the local level and the available resources that are committed to control activities

strongly depend on the state and local government commitment to supplement the federal disease control funding.

Almost all major cities in the United States have at least one or more public STD clinics that provide low-cost (usually on a sliding scale) or no-cost diagnosis and treatment of a variety of STDs, including syphilis. They are often the only source for dark-field testing in the community. The quality and efficiency of these clinics vary markedly and are highly dependent on local public health awareness of the extent of the STD problem and the degree of commitment to the provision of quality clinical services. These clinics serve as a hub around which most of the other control strategies work.

The serology reactor program, which was officially started in 1962, consists of a formalized attempt to follow-up the positive serologic tests reported through a variety of reporting mechanisms. This program provides a morbidity reporting device aimed at the identification of early infectious syphilis cases. It is necessary because of the incomplete reporting of syphilis cases by the private medical sector and because patients often ignore symptoms and signs of early infectious syphilis and do not seek medical care. Most, but not all, states have laws requiring laboratories and physicians to report positive serologic reactions for syphilis to the health department. In the reactor program, the public health workers attempt to investigate the clinical and treatment status of the positive patients and initiate contact tracing efforts to locate potentially infected sexual partners. A central file of these patients is kept (reactor file) and the first step in the reactor follow-up process is to check this file to determine if the patient is an old case with persistent seroreactivity. Because of limited staff and numerous reactors, the degree of follow-up will usually be ranked into high- and low-priority reactors with the low-titered blood (< 4 dils) in older patients (> 35 years) often placed in the low-priority categories. These may not get any further follow-up and be closed out by administrative closure if time does not permit additional action. As a consequence, substantial numbers of late latent disease may not be identified and counted. In 1983, serologic follow-up identified about 23% of the 55,797 early infectious syphilis cases reported. Unfortunately, because the reactor program concentrates solely on numerator data, it has not been a reliable surveillance tool. Further refinement of this program that would permit better estimates of rates in specific programs such as prenatal screening or others would provide a measure of surveillance not currently available.

Contact tracing consists of interviewing early syphilis patients for the identification of all sexual partners who may have been exposed to infectious lesions during a critical period. It has been the backbone of syphilis control activities. For primary syphilis cases the critical period is 90 days, for secondary disease it is 6 months, and for early latent disease, it is 1 year. The major goal of these activities is to identify the source of infection in the index as well as other cases that have spread out from the original source or index case. This is accomplished by examination and interviewing of all contacts elicited. Contact-tracing activities generate several indices that are helpful from an administrative and public health perspective. The contact index refers to the number of sexual partners elicited per case interviewed. This averaged out to about two contacts elicited per early infectious case interviewed in the United States in 1983. The brought-to-treatment index is the number of infected contacts brought to treatment per infected patient interviewed and in 1983 this was 0.18. The epidemiologic index is the total number of infected cases identified (including previously treated cases) per index case interviewed. The lesion-to-lesion index is the number of contacts identified with primary or secondary syphilis per case of primary or secondary syphilis interviewed. This is often a better measure of the speed and efficiency of the contact-tracing process. Cluster contact tracing involves interviewing and examining high-risk patients known to the index case (cluster suspect) or to the examined contacts (cluster associate). This method of contact tracing is usually implemented during epidemic outbreaks of infections where it is usually more productive. Of the approximately 20,000 cluster contacts initiated in the United States in 1983, 7% were found to be untreated cases of syphilis. In the same year, public health workers interviewed 92% of the early infectious syphilis cases and contact-tracing efforts identified 24% of the early syphilis cases reported. The source of infection for the index cases was identified 32% of the time. This source identification yield is lower than the usual 60% seen in primary and secondary cases since the source yield for early latent syphilis cases is considerably lower.

About 10% of serologically negative contacts who were exposed to infectious syphilis lesions are incubating the disease.[31] Because of this, it is the policy in the United States to provide "epidemiologic treatment" of exposed contacts regardless of the clinical or laboratory findings.

9.2. Prophylaxis

Standard penicillin treatment for gonorrhea is probably effective in aborting incubating syphilis infection.[40] Other antibiotics in therapeutic dosages, except for spectinomycin, may also be effective in aborting infection but clinical studies are lacking. Condom usage is probably at least moderately effective in preventing infection, dependent on the location of the lesion. It is also probable that vaginal creams containing nonoxynol-9 reduce the risk of infection.

9.3. Immunization

There is no vaccine available for the prevention of syphilis. It is unlikely that one will be available soon.

10. Unresolved Problems

Although the etiologic agent of syphilis is well defined and treatment is inexpensive, effective, and readily available, congenital infection continues to occur and the disease remains endemic in some areas of the United States. Also, minority groups continue to have a disproportionate share of both congenital disease and early infectious syphilis. In spite of recent emphasis in the United States on the epidemic of AIDS and the need for personal sexual responsibility and safe sex practices, the largest increase in early syphilis cases in 27 years occurred in 1987. This has occurred despite the fact that the incidence of syphilis in homosexual males has been dropping dramatically. The recent upsurge in syphilis cases appears clustered in a few states with known high rates of endemic disease and is predominantly a problem of heterosexual minority populations and appears to have links to prostitution and drug-abusing activities. Innovative strategies will be needed to reach these difficult high-risk populations. It is time to reappraise the role of prostitution in the spread of syphilis and it may be appropriate to formalize screening programs in definable prostitute populations that appear epidemiologically linked to high-frequency disease transmission. The best strategy to prevent congenital syphilis is to decrease the frequency of syphilis. Innovative approaches to getting high-risk patient populations to prenatal care facilities are needed. In some endemic areas, repeat serologic testing during pregnancy may need to be routine. An incentive for minorities is needed for improved syphilis control in high-risk communities.

More research is needed into the population-specific factors associated with personal behavior that is relevant to sexual promiscuity and risk-taking behavior associated with continued unsafe sexual practices in areas of endemic disease. STD control managers must take advantage of the recent trend prompted by the AIDS epidemic to promote educational efforts in modifying sexual behavior. Confidentiality statutes should be strengthened and should include syphilis and the other STDs, as well as AIDS.

The recent outbreak of HIV infections in the United States may be portending a new era of syphilis control and treatment strategies. Data identifying problems in the reliability of serologic diagnosis have been reported for AIDS patients with coccidioidomycosis,[37] toxoplasmosis,[29] and cytomegalovirus infection[7] and suggest the possibility of diagnostic problems for syphilis in significantly immunocompromised patients. This has recently been substantiated in a secondary syphilis case that displayed aberrant serologic reactivity.[19] On the positive side, a recent study has shown that HIV-positive men were able to develop appropriate antibody responses to both influenza and pneumococcal vaccines although the responses were mildly impaired.[21] The very fact that the vast majority of patients with HIV infection develop an antibody response to their infection suggests functioning immunoreactivity in a substantial proportion of patients. It is not known what effect HIV infection could have on the duration of antibody response. It is probable that the ability of patients to respond with antibodies to syphilis infection depends on the degree of immunodeficiency present. For the vast majority of HIV-infected individuals, this will probably not present diagnostic problems in the use of serologic tests for syphilis. For patients with AIDS and other forms of immunodeficiency, we should stay cognizant of the potential fallibilities of sole dependence upon serologic markers for clinical disease diagnosis. It is not yet clear what effect HIV infections will have on the clinical course of syphilis and the treatment efficacy of currently recommended treatment regimens. A recent case report raises concerns in this area.[1] Recent case reports have suggested that HIV infection may alter the clinical course of early syphilis so that it becomes a more severe disease or is associated with early sequelae. It is probable that antimicrobial cure of syphilis infections also requires humoral and cell-mediated responses. It is theoretically probable that treatment outcomes with currently recommended treatment will depend to a great extent on the quantitative degree of immunodeficiency present and that in some patients, larger and longer treatment regimens will be needed. Further collection of data and prospective studies are needed to determine the extent to which HIV infections contribute to both diagnostic and therapeutic problems in syphilis infections. It is evident that the advent of the AIDS infection era has introduced new challenges to the control of syphilis and possibly to other epidemic infections as well. On the other hand, it may also provide new incentives for the study of innovative educational and case-finding approaches to infection control.

11. References

1. BERRY, C. D., HOOTEN, T. M., COLLIER, A. C., AND LUKEHART, S. A., Neurologic relapse after benzathine penicillin therapy for secondary syphilis in a patient with HIV infection, *N. Engl. J. Med.* **316:**1587–1589 (1987).
2. BROWN, W. J., DONOHUE, J. F., AXNICK, N. W., BLOUNT, J. H., EWEN, N. H., AND JONES, O. G., Mortality caused by syphilis and its sequelae and other late manifestations of untreated venereal disease, in: *Syphilis and Other Venereal Diseases,* pp. 98–134, Harvard University Press, Cambridge, Mass., 1970.
3. Centers for Disease Control, *Sexually Transmitted Disease Statistics 1985,* Issue No. 135, U.S. Department of Health and Human Services.
4. CLARKE, E. G., Studies in the epidemiology of syphilis. I. Material on which epidemiological studies are based; II. Contact investigation, *Vener. Dis. Inf.* **21:**349–369 (1941).
5. Congenital syphilis—United States, 1983–1985, *Morbid. Mortal. Weekly Rep.* **35:**625–628 (1986).
6. DRUSIN, L. M., TOPF-OLSTEIN, B., AND LEVY-ZOMBEK, E., Epidemiology of infectious syphilis in a tertiary hospital, *Arch. Intern. Med.* **139:**901–904 (1979).
7. DYLEWSKI, J., CHOU, S., AND MERIGAN, T. C., Absence of detectable IgM antibody during cytomegalovirus disease in patients with AIDS [Letter], *N. Engl. J. Med.* **309:**493 (1983).
8. FELDMAN, Y. M., Should premarital syphilis serologies continue to be mandated by law? *Am. Med. Assoc.* **240:**459–460 (1978).
9. FELDMAN, Y. M., Repeal of mandated premarital tests for syphilis: A survey of state health officers, *Am. J. Public Health* **71:**155–159 (1981).
10. FICHTNER, R. R., ARAL, S. O., BLOUNT, J. H., ZAIDI, A. A., REYNOLDS, G. H., AND DARROW, W. W., Syphilis in the United States: 1967–1979, *Sex. Transm. Dis.* **10:**77–80 (1983).
11. FIELDSTEEL, A. H., AND MIAO, R. H., Genetics of treponema, in: *Pathogenesis and Immunology of Treponemal Infection* (R. F. SCHELL AND D. M. MISHER, eds.), Dekker, New York, 1982.
12. FIUMARA, N., FLEMING, W. L., DOWNING, J. G., AND GOOD, F. L., The incidence of prenatal syphilis at the Boston City Hospital, *N. Engl. J. Med.* **247:**48–52 (1952).
13. GJESTLAND, T., The Oslo study of untreated syphilis: An epidemiologic investigation of the natural course of the syphilitic infection based on a re-study of the Boeck–Bruusgaard material, *Acta Derm. Venereol.* **35**(Suppl. 34) (1955).
14. HAHN, R. A., JOHNSON, R. E., MAGDER, L. S., AND LARSEN, S. A., Follow-up study of syphilis infections detected in a 1978 U.S. survey, Presented at the 1987 Epidemic Intelligence Service Conference, p. 59, CDC, Atlanta, April 1987.
15. HALPIN, T. J., Costly and unnecessary syphilis serology, *Ohio State Med. J.* **7:**536–537 (1980).
16. HART, G., Screening to control infectious diseases: Evaluation

of control programs for gonorrhea and syphilis, *Rev. Infect. Dis.* **2:**701–712 (1980).

17. HARTER, C. A., AND BENIRSCHKE, K., Fetal syphilis in the first trimester, *Am. J. Obstet. Gynecol.* **124:**705–711 (1976).

18. HASKELL, R. J., A cost–benefit analysis of California's mandatory premarital screening program for syphilis, *West. J. Med.* **141:**538–541 (1984).

19. HICKS, C. B., BENSEN, P. M., LUPTON, G. P., AND TRAMONT, E. C., Seronegative secondary syphilis in a patient infected with the human immunodeficiency virus (HIV) with Kaposi sarcoma, *Ann. Intern. Med.* **107:**492–495 (1987).

20. HO, P. W., PIEN, F. D., AND PRUETT, K. A., Routine serological testing for syphilis in a community medical practice, *West. J. Med.* **132:**485–487 (1980).

21. HUANG, K. L., RUBEN, F. L., RINALDO, C. R., KINGSLEY, L., LYTER, D. W., AND HO, M., Antibody responses after influenza and pneumococcal immunization in HIV-infected homosexual men, *Am. Med. Assoc.* **257:**2047–2050 (1987).

22. HUBERICH, C. H., Venereal disease in the law of marriage and divorce, *Am. Law Rev.* **37:**226–236 (1903).

23. JENKINS, H., Cultivation of treponemes, in: *Pathogenesis and Immunology of Treponemal Infections* (R. F. Schell and D. M. Musher, eds.), Dekker, New York, 1982.

24. JOHNS, D. R., TIERNEY, M., AND FELSENSTEIN, D., Alteration in the natural history of neurosyphilis by concurrent infection with the human immunodeficiency virus, *N. Engl. J. Med.* **316:**1569–1572 (1987).

25. KAMPMEIER, R. H., Syphilis, in: *Bacterial Infections of Humans* (A. S. EVANS AND H. A. FELDMAN, eds.), pp. 553–577, Plenum Medical, New York, 1982.

26. KINGON, R. J., AND WIESNER, P. J., Premarital syphilis screening: Weighing the benefits, *Am. J. Public Health* **71:** 160–162 (1981).

27. KLINGBEIL, L. J., AND CLARK, E. G., Studies in the epidemiology of syphilis. III. Conjugal syphilis, *Vener. Dis. Inf.* **22:**1–6 (1941).

28. LEVENE, G. M., TURK, J. L., WRIGHT, D. M. J., AND GRIMBLE, A. G. S., Reduced lymphocyte transformation due to a plasma factor in patients with active syphilis, *Lancet* **2:**246–247 (1969).

29. LUFT, D. J., CONLEY, F., REMINGTON, J. S., LAVERDIERE, M., WAGNER, K. F., LEVINE, J. F., CRAVEN, P. C., STRANDBERG, D. A., FILE, T. M., RICE, N., AND MEUNIER-CARPENTIER, F. Outbreak of central-nervous system toxoplasmosis in western Europe and North America, *Lancet* **1:**781–784 (1983).

30. MAGNUSON, H. J., THOMAS, E. W., ORLANSKY, S., KAPLAN, B. I., DE MELLO, L., AND CUTLER, J. C., Inoculation syphilis in human volunteers, *Medicine* **35:**33–82 (1956).

31. MOORE, M. D., PRICE, E. V., KNOX, J. M., AND ELGIN, L. W., Epidemiological treatment of contacts to infectious syphilis, *Public Health Rep.* **78:**966–970 (1963).

32. MORROW, P. A., Report of the Committee of Seven of the Medical Society of the County of New York on the prophylaxis

of venereal disease in New York City, *N.Y. Med. J.* **74:**1146 (1901).

33. MORROW, P. A., The relations of social diseases to the family, *Am. J. Soc.* **14:**635 (1909).

34. National Center for Health Statistics, Findings on the serologic test for syphilis in adults: United States—1960–1962, *Vital Health Stat.* **11:**1031 (1965).

35. PURRINGTON, W. A., Professional secrecy and the obligatory notification of venereal diseases, *N.Y. Med. J.* **85:**1207 (1907).

36. PUSEY, W. A., *The History and Epidemiology of Syphilis,* pp. 53–61, Thomas, Springfield, Ill., 1933.

37. ROBERTS, C. J., Coccidioidomycosis in acquired immune deficiency syndrome. Depressed humoral as well as cellular immunity, *Am. J. Med.* **76:**734–736 (1984).

38. ROTHENBERG, R., Premarital syphilis serologies [Letter], *J. Am. Med Assoc.* **241:**2007 (1979).

39. ROTHENBERG, R., The geography of syphilis: A demonstration of epidemiologic diversity, in: *Advances in Sexually Transmitted Diseases* (MORISSET, R. AND KURSTAK, E., eds.), pp. 125–133, Academic Press, New York, 1984.

40. SCHROETER, A. L., TURNER, R. H., LUCAS, J. B., AND BROWN, W. J., Therapy for incubating syphilis: Effectiveness of gonorrhea treatment, *J. Am. Med. Assoc.* **218:**711–713 (1971).

41. STD Fact Sheet, Edition 35, Centers for Disease Control, Atlanta, 1979.

42. STEVENARD, L., The professional secret in syphilis and marriage, *Am. J. Urol.* **12:**33–37 (1916).

43. STRONG, S. L., A symposium on the reportability and control of venereal diseases, *Boston Med. Surg. J.* **169:**903–907 (1913).

44. Syphilis—United States, 1983, *Morbid. Mortal. Weekly Rep.* **33**(30):433–436 (1984).

45. TOMECKI, K. J., AND TOMECKI, E. C., Neglect of syphilis in hospitalized patients, *South. Med. J.* **77:**1118–1120 (1984).

46. VONDERLEHR, R. A., AND USILTON, L. J., Syphilis among men of draft age in the United States, *J. Am. Med. Assoc.* **120:**1369–1372 (1942).

47. ZIEGLER, J. A., JONES, A. M., AND KUBICA, K. M., Demonstration of extracellular material at the surface of pathogenic *T. pallidum* cells, *Br. J. Vener. Dis.* **52:**1–8 (1976).

12. Suggested Reading

BRANDT, A. M., *No Magic Bullet: A Social History of Venereal Diseases in the United States Since 1880,* Oxford University Press, London, 1985.

BROWN, W. J., DONOHUE, J. F., AXNICK, N. W., BLOUNT, J. H., EWEN, N. H., AND JONES, O. G., *Syphilis and Other Venereal Diseases,* Harvard University Press, Cambridge, Mass., 1970.

Centers for Disease Control, *Morbid. Mortal. Weekly Rep.* STD Treatment Guidelines **34**(4S):21–23 (1985).

Centers for Disease Control, Guidelines for the Prevention and Control of Congenital Syphilis, *Morbid. Mortal. Weekly Rep.* **37**(5–1): 1–13 (1988).

Centers for Disease Control, 1989 Sexually Transmitted Disease Treatment Guidelines. *Morbid. Mortal. Weekly Rep.* **38**:1–43 (1989).

CLARK, E. G., AND DANBOLT, N., The Oslo study of the natural history of untreated syphilis, *J. Chron. Dis.* **2**:311–344 (1955).

GJESTLAND, T., The Oslo study of untreated syphilis: An epidemiologic investigation of the natural course of the syphilitic infection based on a re-study of the Boeck–Bruusgaard material, *Acta Derm. Venereol.* **35**(Suppl. 34) (1955).

HOLMES, K. K., MARDH, P. A., SPARLING, P. F., WEISNER, P. J., CATAS, W., LEMON, S. M., AND STAMM, W. E., *Sexually Transmitted Diseases,* McGraw–Hill, New York, 1990.

WHO Expert Committee on Venereal Diseases and Treponematoses, Sixth Report, World Health Organization Technical Report Series 736, World Health Organization, Geneva, 1986.

CHAPTER 33

Nonvenereal Treponematoses

Peter L. Perine

1. Introduction

The endemic treponematoses are a group of chronic diseases affecting primarily the skin of children and young adults who live in remote, impoverished areas between the tropics of Cancer and Capricorn. They are considered as a group because they have many clinical, pathologic, and epidemiologic features in common (Table 1). They are also caused by spirochetes that are closely related to one another and to *Treponema pallidum* of venereal syphilis.[11] These diseases with their etiologic treponeme in order of their worldwide prevalence are: yaws (*T. pallidum* ssp. *pertenue*), endemic syphilis (*T. pallidum* ssp. *endemicum*), and pinta (*T. carateum*).[18] Other related treponemes cause venereal syphilis in rabbits (*T. cuniculi*) and asymptomatic infections in African baboons (*T. freiborg-blanc)* but they have no epidemiologic significance as far as human infections are concerned.

2. Historical Background

There are two theories about the origin of the treponematoses. The unitarian theory suggests that they are all caused by a single treponeme that has been modified by the environment, and the Columbian theory states that these diseases are caused by distinct species of treponemes.[7,8] The unitarian theory seems to be the more tenable in light of recent DNA hybridization and other studies that indicate almost complete homology between the *T. pallidum* of venereal and nonvenereal syphilis and *T. pertenue*.[4,11] The controversy about the origins of the treponematoses is focused on venereal syphilis, which appeared in Europe in the late 15th century as a highly contagious and fatal disease. Its appearance in Europe coincided with the return of Columbus from the New World and historians ascribed its origin to the New World.[6,25] A more plausible explanation is that endemic syphilis, long prevalent in west Africa, became venerally transmitted among Europeans after its importation into Europe by sailors and African slaves.[21]

Yaws was one of the most prevalent infectious diseases of the tropics before the penicillin era (Fig. 1). The development of long-acting penicillin preparations, producing a treponemicidal blood level for 3 to 4 weeks after a single injection, made mass treatment of treponemal infections feasible.[2] In 1949, the World Health Organization (WHO) agreed to conduct coordinated mass treatment campaigns against yaws, endemic syphilis, and pinta. Demonstration projects in yaws endemic areas confirmed the efficacy of single injections of penicillin aluminum monostearate in mass treatment campaigns, the need to examine at least 90% of the target population during the initial survey, and to conduct resurveys of treated populations to treat new cases and reinfections.[2] From 1952 to 1968, an estimated 160 million persons were examined during yaws campaigns worldwide and 50 million persons with clinical or latent

Peter L. Perine · Division of Tropical Public Health, Department of Preventive Medicine, F. Edward Hébert School of Medicine, Uniformed Services University of the Health Sciences, Bethesda, Maryland 20814.

Table 1.   Major Features of the Treponematoses

	Venereal syphilis	Endemic syphilis	Yaws	Pinta
	T. pallidum ssp. *pallidum*	*T pallidum* ssp. *endemicum*	*T. pallidum* ssp. *pertenue*	*T. carateum*
Age of infection	15–40	2–10	5–15	10–30
Occurrence	Worldwide	Africa, Middle East	Africa, South America, Oceania, Asia	Central and South America
Climate	All	Dry, arid	Warm, humid	Warm
Transmission				
Direct				
Venereal	Common	Rare	No	No
Nonvenereal	Rare	Common	Common	Probable
Congenital	Yes	Unproven	No	No
Indirect				
Contaminated utensils	Rare	Common	Rare	No
Insects	No	No	Possible	No
Reservoir of infection	Adults	Infectious and latent cases	Infectious and latent cases	Infectious cases
Ratio of infectious to latent cases	1:3	1:2	1:3–5	?
Late complications	+	+	+	+
Skin, bone, cartilage	+	+	+	No
Neurologic	+	Unproven	No	No
Cardiovascular	+	Unproven	No	No

infections and their contacts were treated with penicillin.[2,5] At the end of these campaigns, the endemic treponematoses appeared to be on their way to extinction, especially in view of the improvements in living standards that occurred in many of the endemic areas.

3. Methodology

The endemic treponematoses are reportable diseases in most countries where reservoirs of active disease persist. The best sources for these data are the regional offices of WHO and its *Weekly Epidemiological Record*[26] and the proceedings of recent yaws symposia.[9,15,27]

3.1. Sources of Mortality Data

There is little pathologic or epidemiologic evidence that the endemic treponematoses acquired in childhood subsequently cause fatal late cardiovascular or CNS complica-

tions usually associated with venereal syphilis. Where venereal syphilis is prevalent together with yaws or endemic syphilis, however, it is impossible to differentiate visceral, ocular, and neurologic lesions caused by venereal syphilis from those that might result from yaws or endemic syphilis.[16,23]

3.2. Sources of Morbidity Data

The WHO through its regional offices periodically reports on the prevalence of active and latent cases of the endemic treponematoses in its *Weekly Epidemiological Record*.

3.3. Surveys

Clinical and seroprevalence surveys for yaws and endemic syphilis have been conducted by many African and Asian countries since 1980 as part of a WHO initiative to

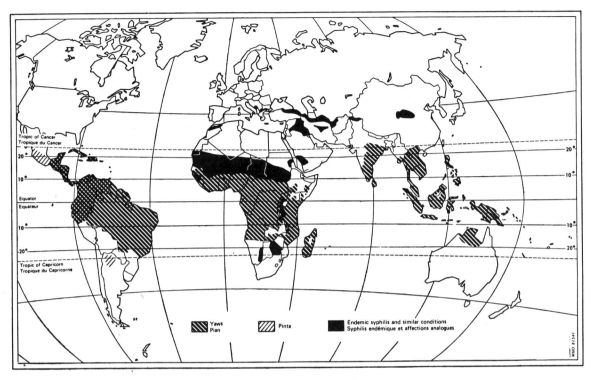

Figure 1. Geographic distribution of the endemic treponematoses in the early 1950s.

control the resurgence of these diseases. The results of these surveys are usually reported to the WHO.

3.4. Laboratory Diagnosis

3.4.1. Isolation and Identification of the Organism. The pathogenic treponemes cannot be cultured *in vitro* and their identification by dark-field microscopy of lesion exudate is the standard diagostic test.[13] Lesion exudate can also be collected in heparinized blood capillary tubes and sent to a reference laboratory to be examined by specific fluorescein-tagged antibodies.[14]

3.4.2. Serologic and Diagnostic Methods. Serologic tests routinely employed in seroprevalence surveys are the venereal disease research laboratory (VDRL) and rapid plasma reagin (RPR) tests.[13] These tests are not specific but their reactivity and titer in an appropriate clinical setting give a good idea of the prevalence of latent treponemal infection.

4. Biological Characteristics of the Organism

T. pallidum and its subspecies are obligate anaerobes. The lack of a cell-free *in vitro* culture method has limited comparative studies of their genetic and antigenic structure. Prototype strains of yaws and endemic syphilis treponemes produce lesions in only a few experimental animals. The lesions produced in these animals are similar to those occurring during the early stages of infection in man. Subtle differences in virulence and lesion morphology exist between subspecies and strains of *T. pallidum endemicum* and *pertenue* and variable degrees of immunity are produced to superinfection by the other pathogenic treponemes.[22] Similar subspecies and strain differences exist in most species of pathogenic bacteria.

The pathogenic treponemes are exquisitely sensitive to penicillin. Their multiplication by binary fission takes an estimated 32 h to complete[10] and is the reason why long-acting penicillin preparations that produce low but persistent penicillin blood concentrations for 3 to 4 weeks are recommended for therapy. Despite the widespread use of penicillins in medical practice, there is no evidence that the pathogenic treponemes have developed resistance to the drugs.

T. carateum is pathogenic only in man.[22] Persons infected with this treponeme produce antibodies that react in standard treponemal and nontreponemal antigen tests for syphilis. These antibodies react against the full spectrum of antigenic molecules of *T. pallidum* ssp. *pallidum,* indicating a close genetic relationship.[4]

5. Descriptive Epidemiology

5.1. Prevalence and Incidence

In 1950, an estimated 70 to 100 million people living in large areas of Africa and Southeast Asia, the western Pacific islands, and parts of the Americas had yaws, another 1 million living in the Middle East, the Balkans, and north and west Africa had endemic syphilis, and 700,000 mostly American Indians of Central and South America had pinta (Fig. 1).[5] The ratio of infectious to latent yaws was 1 : 3 or more and most infections occurred in children under 15 years of age. Improved living conditions and penicillin treatment campaigns from 1950 to 1970 dramatically reduced the prevalence of the endemic treponematoses. However, reservoirs of untreated disease persisted in many remote impoverished areas because surveillance was prematurely curtailed or discontinued.[2]

The Third International Symposium on yaws and the endemic treponematoses, held in Washington, D.C., in 1984, assessed the current extent of these diseases and the feasibility of their global eradication and/or control. Resurgence of both yaws and endemic syphilis was noted to have occurred in many formerly endemic areas of the world, especially among impoverished rural children and young adults born after penicillin treatment campaigns were completed. Several countries had taken recent steps to control these diseases, including mass penicillin treatment of selected affected populations. This meeting and others held in Indonesia, the Congo, and Jordan concluded that new control initiatives, integrated into primary health care activities wherever possible, were needed to interrupt transmission and spread of yaws and endemic syphilis in Africa.

Since 1980, cases of yaws have been reported from more than two dozen African nations and there are at present an estimated 1 million children infected with yaws in Ghana, Benin, Logo, and Ivory Coast and perhaps 200,000 cases of endemic syphilis in Niger, Mali, and Burkina Faso. Foci of yaws also persist in some areas of the southern Pacific, particularly in Papua New Guinea and Indonesia. India, Thailand, and Malaysia have also experienced small epidemics of yaws in the past decade. Africa is the major reservoir of yaws and endemic syphilis.

5.2. Epidemic Behavior and Contagiousness

Yaws is highly contagious and can spread rapidly in susceptible populations when environmental conditions favor development of cutaneous lesions teeming with spirochetes. Endemic syphilis tends to affect isolated, nomadic populations, and its epidemic potential is less than that of yaws. Pinta is very difficult to transmit by person-to-person contact and has little epidemic potential.

5.3. Geographic Distribution

The worldwide distribution of the endemic treponematoses in the mid-1980s is shown in Fig. 2.

5.4. Temporal Distribution

There is no seasonality in occurrence of the endemic treponematoses, but the number, morphology, and infectiousness of cutaneous yaws lesions change during the wet and dry seasons in Africa and Asia. The high humidity associated with seasonal rains promotes an exuberant growth of papillomas and the survival of treponemes in their serous exudate, thus increasing infectiousness and the probability of person-to-person transmission. The skin is also softened by high humidity and is more susceptible to abrasions and lacerations, which are a portal of entry for treponemes. This contrasts with a paucity of infectious yaws lesions during dry seasons.

5.5. Age

In endemic areas yaws is usually acquired before age 15 from infected siblings or playmates, and active early lesions are found almost exclusively in this age group. Endemic syphilis tends to occur in family groups, the infection being acquired first by children who spread it to susceptible adults. Pinta usually first appears in young adults.

5.6. Sex

Pinta tends to occur more frequently in men but there is no sexual predilection for yaws or endemic syphilis.

5.7. Race

Race is not a factor.

5.8. Occupation

The diseases have no relationship to occupation *per se,* but the vast majority of those affected live in communities that survive by subsistence farming.

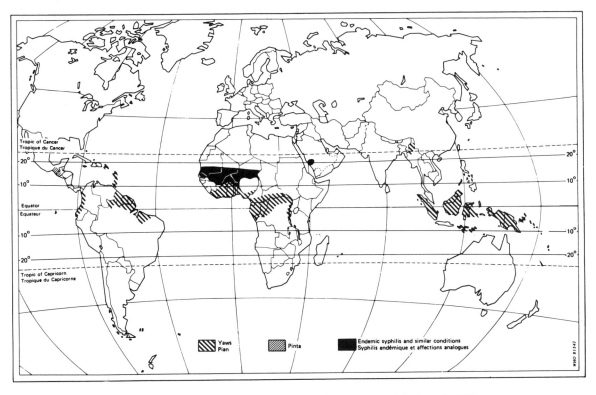

Figure 2. Geographic distribution of the endemic treponematoses in the early 1980s.

5.9. Occurrence in Different Settings

These treponematoses are usually found within families and among playmates.

5.10. Socioeconomic Factors

The endemic treponematoses are prevalent today in impoverished, remote, rural populations lacking adequate clothing, water, sanitation, and medical care.

6. Mechanisms and Routes of Transmission

Transmission of yaws and endemic syphilis occurs by person-to-person contact, probably more often than not by fingers contaminated with fresh lesion exudate. Papillomas are pruritic and scratching removes loosely adherent, crusty eschars, contaminating the fingers with serous exudate

loaded with viable treponemes. Various species of flies are attracted to such lesions and it is possible that they mechanically transmit viable treponemes to the abraded or lacerated skin of nearby susceptible individuals.[17] The efficiency of such transmission by flies is probably epidemiologically insignificant.

Endemic syphilis is transmitted by person-to-person contact or by sharing of drinking cups contaminated with treponemes present in the serous exudate from lesions on the oral mucous membranes or at the corners of the mouth. Congenital transmission of yaws or endemic syphilis has not been convincingly documented.

Transmission of yaws or endemic syphilis can occur during sexual intercourse providing one partner has infectious lesions in the genital area and the other is susceptible to infection.

The transmission of pinta requires prolonged intimate contact with an adult with active disease as takes place in a household. Infection rates are low, even between marital couples.[10]

7. Pathogenesis and Immunity

The endemic treponematoses manifest histopathologic changes and serologic responses that closely resemble those of venereal syphilis. The only practical means of comparing their pathogenicity is by experimental animal infections. *T. pallidum* ssp. *pallidum* is more invasive and pathogenic than is *T. pallidum* ssp. *pertenue*. *T. carateum* is pathogenic only for man and higher primates.

The prototype pathologic lesion of yaws and endemic syphilis is a granuloma. This reflects a strong delayed-hypersensitivity response to the presence of treponemes in skin and bone. Normal skin and bone are replaced by scar tissue, causing disfigurement and occasional disability. Although treponemes enter the circulation early in the course of yaws and endemic syphilis, the cardiovascular, neurologic, and visceral lesions characteristic of late venereal syphilis seldom occur.[16] Indeed, infection by yaws or endemic syphilis appears to protect against venereal syphilis, which is very uncommon where these diseases are endemic.

Immunity waxes and wanes during the course of untreated yaws and endemic syphilis, especially during the 5 years following initial infection. This is manifested by the reappearance of infectious cutaneous lesions, and is the reason why penicillin must be given to asymptomatic persons living in highly endemic communities who are very likely to have latent infections. Persons with yaws or endemic syphilis are probably immune to reinfection if they have untreated infections of more than 1 year's duration.

8. Patterns of Host Response

The manifestations of yaws and endemic syphilis are usually mild and lesions are restricted to the skin and mucous membranes, heal spontaneously after several months, and leave few scars. About 10% of those infected experience more aggressive disease with destruction of skin and bone. Those who suffer severe disease may be genetically predisposed.

In populations where the endemic treponematoses are prevalent, serologic surveys invariably detect more persons who have latent infections than have clinically manifest disease. Many of these patients have no recollection of early disease manifestations, suggesting that asymptomatic infection is frequent or that their earlier lesions were inconsequential or mistakenly interpreted as something else.

8.1. Clinical Features

The incubation periods of yaws, endemic syphilis, and pinta are directly related to the number of treponemes in the inoculum. The initial lesion(s) appears at the portal of entry after an incubation period of 9 to 90 days.

Pinta, yaws, endemic and venereal syphilis are chronic infections with early and late clinical manifestations. Early lesions are infectious and usually are not destructive, whereas late lesions are not infectious but are destructive.

8.1.1. Pinta. The painless initial papular lesion on an arm or leg spreads to form an irregular, reddish or bluish patch 5 to 10 cm in diameter with raised borders. Several weeks or months later, disseminated lesions ("pintides") with a morphology similar to that of the initial lesion appear on different parts of the body. Hyperkeratosis with desquamation, itching, and formation of fissures within the borders of lesions is common and may be accompanied by lymph node enlargement. The skin is the only organ pathologically affected.

In the late stage the involved skin becomes atrophic, and the bluish coloration of the initial lesion caused by accumulation of melanin pigment in the dermis fades. This leaves the patient disfigured by red, blue, and white spots on the face, neck, arms, hands, legs, and feet. Eventually the lesions cause sclerosis of the dermis and depigmentation, leaving scars that resemble vitiligo. The evolution from the time of the appearance of the initial lesion to its late depigmented scarring may be several years.

8.1.2. Yaws. The initial lesion of yaws is usually a papule. This painless, pruritic, elevated lesion appears at the site of treponemal invasion after an incubation period of 9–90 days. The site of entry is often a preexisting abrasion, laceration, or insect bite. The treponemes multiply at the infection site, invade subcutaneous lymphatics, cause local lymph node enlargement, and spread systemically through the bloodstream.

The yaws papule enlarges to become a papilloma (frambesioma) that lasts 3–6 months. It may ulcerate and become secondarily infected with bacteria or heal spontaneously, thereby creating a brief period of latency. Secondary yaws lesions then appear in crops on the skin near the initial lesion or elsewhere on the body, including bone and cartilage, as a result of systemic spread and autoinoculation. Constitutional symptoms are rare but nocturnal pain of the long bones of the leg due to periostitis and papillomas on the soles of the feet preventing weight-bearing are common.

Secondary papillomas are prominent during wet seasons and involute to form micropapules and macules during dry seasons. The lesions heal spontaneously and do not leave permanent scars unless they ulcerate and become secondarily infected by pyogenic bacteria. The disease then enters a noninfectious latent period that may last the lifetime of the patient.

During the first 5 years after infection, the state of latency may be interrupted at any time by the reappearance of infectious yaws lesions. Destructive gummatous lesions appear in the skin or osseous tissue in about 10% of those infected, usually several years after the initial infection. These late lesions mutilate and cripple.

8.1.3. Endemic Syphilis. A primary lesion is rarely seen in endemic syphilis. The first lesions to appear are painless ulcerations on the oropharyngeal mucosa. These are followed by a variety of skin, bone, and joint lesions that are indistinguishable from those of yaws. Skin lesions prefer the moist body surfaces such as the axillary and genital areas. Angular stomatitis or split papules at the corners of the mouth are more common than in yaws and are ideally situated to contaminate drinking vessels.

Osteoperiostitis of the long bones occurs more frequently in endemic syphilis than in yaws. It usually involves the long bones of the lower extremities, causing nocturnal leg pains. Gummas of the nasopharynx, skin, and bone are common in late endemic syphilis and may progress to destructive ulcers. Such ulceration may destroy nasal tissue, producing a terrible disfiguring lesion known as gangosa. Chronic osteoperiostitis and gangosa are still frequently encountered among adult nomadic Bedouins of the Arabian peninsula[12] and occasionally in children and adults suffering from late yaws in west Africa.[13]

8.2. Diagnosis

A presumptive diagnoses of yaws, pinta, or endemic syphilis can usually be made by careful assessment of the clinical features that characterized each infection in appropriate epidemiologic settings. Pinta is easily differentiated clinically from yaws, endemic and venereal syphilis. The differentiation between sporadic cases of yaws and endemic syphilis may not be possible because they may coexist in the same geographic area and their clinical and serologic manifestations are indistinguishable.

The most sensitive and specific diagnostic test for treponemes is dark-field microscopic examination of freshly isolated lesion exudate. With this technique, motile treponemes appear as brilliant coiled threads on a dark background. Lesion exudate can also be collected and fixed on microscope slides and sent to a reference laboratory for microscopic examination using *T. pallidum*-specific monoclonal antibodies.[14]

A number of different serologic tests are used to detect antibodies produced in response to treponemal infections. These tests were originally designed for use in venereal syphilis and none are specific for a given treponematosis. The most commonly used serologic tests are the VDRL and RPR tests, which are highly sensitive in the early stages of disease. They are widely used in screening programs to detect latent yaws or endemic syphilis. Other tests employ treponemal antigens to detect "specific" antibodies. These tests are best performed in reference laboratories; serum specimens for this purpose can be collected on filter paper and sent by mail.

Following adequate penicillin treatment, the titer of VDRL and RPR serologic tests declines but, depending upon the duration of the infection, may remain positive for several years or a lifetime. Such is often the case in persons who immigrate from yaws or endemic syphilis endemic areas to parts of the world where only venereal syphilis is encountered. Based on reactive serologic tests for syphilis, many of these patients are diagnosed and treated inappropriately for active latent venereal syphilis.

9. Control and Prevention

The provision of adequate clothing and soap and water would greatly reduce the transmission of pinta, yaws, and endemic syphilis. Marginal improvements in standards of living together with occasional access to medical care may partly explain why the mutilating complications of yaws and endemic syphilis are seen much less frequently today compared to the preantibiotic era.

The experience gained from pilot programs of the 1950s established a set of principles and procedures that is still valid today and should be used to control yaws and endemic syphilis.[13] The most important principle is to conduct periodic assessments of communities or nomadic groups where one or more members have infectious lesions resulting from recently acquired or relapse infections. The population of a village or family group should be seen and evaluated at an initial treatment survey and those with active disease should be treated with a single intramuscular injection of 2.4 million units of benzathine penicillin (half-doses for children under 12) as should all of their household members and playmates. Control activities should be expanded in such a way that an ever-enlarging disease-free area is established, so that reintroduction of yaws or endemic syphilis by persons from untreated areas is minimized. Because penicillin is inexpensive compared to other costs associated with surveys, many authorities recommend that treatment be given to entire communities that have one or more infectious cases.[2] Treated populations should be reexamined for active yaws within 6 months and at intervals thereafter so that missed cases and their contacts can be treated. The price of freedom from yaws and endemic syphilis is eternal vigilance.

9.1. Antibiotic and Chemotherapeutic Approaches to Prophylaxis

Prophylaxis other than penicillin treatment of contacts of infectious cases of yaws and endemic syphilis is not indicated.

9.2. Immunization

Although theoretically possible, a treponemal vaccine does not exist and the prospects for one are remote.

10. Unresolved Problems

The lack of a cell-free *in vitro* culture system has limited studies of the genetic structure and the immunopathogenesis of the pathogenic treponemes. Control of the endemic treponematoses may result in increased transmission of venereal syphilis with congenital transmission and the serious and potentially fatal cardiovascular and neurologic complications. The perennial problem posed by the endemic treponematoses is the low priority they are given by most health authorities when faced with limited resources and more serious disease problems.

11. References

1. ALEMAENA, O., Yaws situation in the Solomon Islands, *Southeast Asian J. Trop. Med. Public Health* **17**(Suppl.):14–18 (1986).
2. ANTAL, G. M., AND CAUSSE, G., The control of endemic treponematoses, *Rev. Infect. Dis.* **7**(Suppl. 2):S220–S226 (1985).
3. CSONKA, G., AND PACE, J., Endemic nonvenereal treponematosis (Bejel) in Saudi Arabia, *Rev. Infect. Dis.* **8**(Suppl. 2): S260–S265 (1985).
4. FOHN, M. J., WIGNALL, F. S., BAKER-ZANDER, S. A., AND LUKEHART, S. A., Specificity of antibodies from patients with pinta for antigens of *Treponema pallidum* subspecies *pallidum*, *J. Infect. Dis.* **157**:32–37 (1988).
5. GUTHE, T., AND LUGER, A., The control of endemic syphilis of childhood, *Dermatol. Int.* **5**:179–199 (1966).
6. HACKETT, C. J., On the origin of the human treponematoses, *Bull. WHO* **29**:7–41 (1963).
7. HOLLANDER, D. H., Treponematosis from pinta to venereal syphilis revisited: Hypothesis for temperature determination of disease patterns, *Sex. Transm. Dis.* **8**:34–37 (1981).
8. HUDSON, E. H., *Non-venereal Syphilis, a Sociologic and Medical Study of Bejel*, Livingstone, Edinburgh, 1958.
9. International symposium on yaws and other endemic treponematoses, Washington, D.C., *Rev. Infect. Dis.* **7**(Suppl.): S217–S351 (1985).
10. MAGNUSON, H. J., EAGLE, H., AND FLEISCHMAN, R., The minimal infectious inoculum of *Spirocheaeta pallidum* (Nichols strain) and a consideration of its rate of multiplication *in vivo*, *Am. J. Syph.* **32**:1–18 (1948).
11. MIAO, R. M., AND FIELDSTEEL, A. H., Genetic relationship between *Treponema pallidum* and *Treponema pertenue*, two noncultivable human pathogens, *J. Bacteriol.* **144**:427–429 (1980).
12. PACE, J. L., AND CSONKA, G. W., Endemic non-venereal syphilis (bejel) in Saudi Arabia, *Br. J. Vener. Dis.* **60**:293–297 (1984).
13. PERINE, P. L., HOPKINS, D. R., NIEMEL, P. L. A., ST. JOHN, R. K., CAUSSE, G., AND ANTAL, G. M., *Handbook of Endemic Treponematoses*, World Health Organization, Geneva, 1984.
14. PERINE, P. L., NELSON, J. W., LEWIS, J. O., LISKA, S., HUNTER, E. F., LARSEN, S. A., AGADZI, V. K., KOFI, F., OFORI, J. A. K., TAM, M. R., AND LOVETT, M. A., New technologies for use in the surveillance and control of yaws, *Rev. Infect. Dis.* **8**(Suppl. 2):S295–S299 (1985).
15. Proceedings of the inter-regional meeting on yaws and other endemic treponematoses, Cipanas, Indonesia, *Southeast Asian J. Trop. Med. Public Health* **17**(Suppl.):1–96 (1986).
16. ROMAN, G. C., AND ROMAN, L. N., Occurrence of congenital, cardiovascular, visceral, neurologic, and neuro-ophthalmologic complications in late yaws; a theme for future research, *Rev. Infect. Dis.* **8**:760–770 (1986).
17. SATCHELL, G. H., AND HARRISON, R. A., Experimental observations on the possibility of transmission of yaws by wound-feeding diptera in western Samoa, *Trans. R. Soc. Trop. Med. Hyg.* **47**:148–153 (1953).
18. SMIBERT, R. M., *Treponema*, in: *Bergey's Manual of Systematic Bacteriology* (N. R. KREIG AND J. C. HOLT, eds.), pp. 50–52, Williams & Wilkins, Baltimore, 1984.
19. SOSA-MARTINEZ, J., AND PERALTA, S., An epidemiologic study of pinta in Mexico, *Am. J. Trop. Med. Hyg.* **10**:556–565 (1961).
20. SOSROAMIDJOJO, S., RAI, K., AND SUESEN, N., Yaws in Indonesia, *Southeast Asian J. Trop. Med. Public Health* **17**(Suppl.): 19–34 (1986).
21. SYDENHAM, T., Epistle II: Venereal disease, in: *The Works of Thomas Sydenham, M.D.*, Volume 2, pp. 29–50, The Sydenham Society, London, 1848–1850.
22. TURNER, T. B., AND HOLLANDER, D. H., *Biology of the Treponematoses*, pp. 193–213, World Health Organization, Geneva, 1957.
23. WELLER, C. V., The visceral pathology in Haitian treponematoses, *Am. J. Syph. Gonorrhea Vener. Dis.* **21**:357–369 (1937).
24. WIDEY-WIRSKI, R., Surveillance and control of resurgent yaws in the African region, *Rev. Infect. Dis.* **7**(Suppl. 2): S227–S232 (1985).

25. WILLCOX, R. R., Evolutionary cycle of the treponematoses, *Br. J. Vener. Dis.* **36:**78–90 (1960).
26. World Health Organization, Endemic treponematoses, *Weekly Epidemiol. Rec.* **61:**198–202 (1986).
27. World Health Organization, Report on a regional meeting on yaws and other endemic treponematoses, Brazzaville, 1986.

12. Suggested Reading

BURKE, J. P., HOPKINS, D. R., HUME, J. C., PERINE, P. L., AND ST. JOHN, R. (eds.), International syposium on yaws and other endemic treponematoses, Washington, D.C., 1984, *Rev. Infect. Dis.* **8**(Suppl. 2):S217–S351 (1985).

GUTHE, T., RIDET, J., VORST, F., D'COSTA, J., AND GRAB, B., Methods for the surveillance of endemic treponematoses and sero-immunological investigations of "disappearing" diseases, *Bull. WHO* **46:**1–14 (1972).
HACKETT, C. J., *An International Nomenclature of Yaws Lesions,* World Health Organization, Geneva, 1957 (Monograph Series No. 36).
HILL, K. R., KODIJAT, R., AND SARDADI, M., Atlas of framboesia: A nomenclature and clinical study of the skin lesions, *Bull. WHO* **4:**201–246 (1954).
PERINE, P. L., HOPKINS, D. R., NIEMEL, P. L. A., ST. JOHN, R. K., CAUSSE, G., AND ANTAL, G. M., *Handbook of Endemic Treponematoses,* World Health Organization, Geneva, 1984.

CHAPTER 34

Tetanus

Walter A. Orenstein and Steven G. F. Wassilak

1. Introduction

Tetanus is a noncommunicable infectious disease of humans and certain animal species, acquired through environmental exposure. *Clostridium tetani* is an anaerobic, spore-forming resident of the soil as well as the intestinal tracts of a large proportion of animals and humans. The ubiquitous spores germinate to vegetative bacilli when introduced into the soft tissues of the host under conditions in which the partial pressure of molecular oxygen is low. The vegetative organisms produce a potent neurotoxin that acts on the central nervous system leading to the muscular contractions characteristic of the illness. Although a significant proportion of tetanus cases occur in wounded adults and children, the major burden of tetanus in the world is borne by neonates, who are both (1) contaminated at or soon after birth and (2) born to mothers who are not adequately immunized. Prevention of tetanus can be achieved by passive immunization following wounds in which presumptive contamination with spores occurred; however, a more efficient means of prevention is by active immunization with tetanus toxoid, which is chemically inactivated toxin.

Tetanus toxoid, which protects by inducing production of neutralizing antibodies, is both highly immunogenic and safe. Nearly 100% of recipients of a primary immunization series are protected.

2. Historical Background

The clinical characteristics of tetanus are described in the writings of Hippocrates. Until 1884, however, the etiol-

Walter A. Orenstein and Steven G. F. Wassilak · Division of Immunization, Center for Prevention Services, Centers for Disease Control, Atlanta, Georgia 30333.

ogy of tetanus remained unknown. In that year, Carle and Rattone demonstrated artificial transmission in animals.[42] The contents of a pustule from a fatal human case led to typical symptoms in rabbits when injected into the sciatic nerve; the disease could subsequently be passed to other rabbits from infected nervous tissue. Also in 1884, Nicolaier induced tetanus in experimental animals after injection of soil samples; he observed gram-positive bacilli in the exudate at the inoculation site but not in nervous tissue, leading him to hypothesize that a locally produced poison led to the neurologic symptoms.[133] In 1886, Rosenbach observed spore-forming bacilli in the exudate obtained from a case in a human.[150] In 1889, Kitasato demonstrated that *C. tetani* spores survived heating and germinated under anaerobic conditions; injection of pure cultures reproducibly caused disease in animals.[110] After Behring and Kitasato identified and purified the toxin in 1890, they showed that repeated inoculation of animals with small quantities of toxin led to the production of antibodies in survivors.[16] Preparations of antitoxin from animal sera, particularly horses, became the first means of preventing and treating tetanus. In 1924, Descombey prepared toxoid, chemically altered toxin, which induced neutralizing antibodies without causing illness.[57] This paved the way for large-scale tetanus prophylaxis.

3. Methodology

3.1. Sources of Mortality Data

In the United States and most developed countries, data on tetanus deaths come from national compilations of death certificates listing tetanus as the underlying cause of death.[108] In such countries, death data probably are a reasonable estimate of the total deaths from diagnosed tetanus.

However, in developing countries where the great majority of deaths occur in the neonatal period often outside the hospital, death certificate information may not be reliable. In those settings, community-based surveys have been used to obtain accurate estimates of mortality from neonatal tetanus.[168,169] The National Center for Health Statistics (NCHS) compiles death certificate information from all deaths occurring in the United States.

3.2. Sources of Morbidity Data

In many developed countries, tetanus is a reportable disease. In the United States, tetanus became notifiable in 1947. Most notification systems do not have a specific case definition and rely on physician diagnoses. Case notification is passive, depending on physician initiative, which makes reporting efficiency highly variable. It is likely that only a proportion of the cases actually occurring are reported to national health authorities. In the United States, additional available information reported to the Centers for Disease Control (CDC) includes a patient's immunization status, wound history, postexposure prophylaxis and outcome. Between 1980 and 1984, 123 tetanus deaths were reported to NCHS compared to 110 deaths reported via the passive surveillance system maintained by the CDC. Also, during this period, the reported death-to-case ratio (using CDC reports only) varied from 28 to 36%. Case series from other developed countries have reported death-to-case ratios as low as 10–20%.[63,79,95,174,175] It is likely that there is a bias toward reporting the most severe cases in passive surveillance systems. By matching demographic information for individuals with death following tetanus from both NCHS mortality data and tetanus morbidity reporting, the efficiency of the reporting of tetanus deaths to CDC has been estimated at 40%[171]; therefore, the efficiency of morbidity reporting is likely also not to be optimal.

3.3. Serologic Surveys

Serologic tests measure the level of circulating antitoxin, which correlates directly with protection from disease.[65,121,126,159,193] In general, detectable antitoxin is induced almost exclusively through immunization. Tetanus disease generally does not result in production of circulating antitoxin.[22,41,167,177] Therefore, serologic surveys, particularly in developed countries, serve an important purpose to measure the impact of immunization but cannot measure the impact and epidemiologic characteristics of disease.

Toxin neutralization assays, usually in mice, correlate best with clinical protection since they assess prevention of disease in a living host.[121,126] Injecting the animals with various dilutions of serum and a lethal dose of tetanus toxin allows detection of levels as low as 0.001 IU/ml when compared to a reference serum.[9,46,88,123,128] However, because the test is time-consuming and expensive, a variety of other tests have been employed. These include passive hemagglutination, enzyme immunoassays (EIA), radioimmunoassays (RIA), immunofluorescent tests (IFA), latex agglutination, and a variety of methods using agar gel precipitation.[19,54,88,90,113,123,128,135,136,140,143,156,184,191] The sensitivity and specificity vary with the technique. Agar gel and IFA tests tend to have low sensitivities. Specificity is usually good provided the test is standardized to toxin neutralization. Most population studies have employed the passive hemagglutination technique.[84,85,88,90,123,140,143,184,191] This assay is both sensitive and specific although false-positive results may occur at low levels. Use of turkey erythrocytes is helpful in enhancing specificity, reproducibility, and speed of the assay.[123,143] The passive hemagglutination assay measures both IgG and IgM.[85,90] Neutralization results primarily from IgG antitoxin.[65,135] Thus, measurement of antitoxin by PHA shortly after the first or second dose of toxoid may give falsely high antibody levels secondary to IgM. This should not be a problem for serosurveys, however, when only IgG antibody would be expected. EIA, RIA, and IFA assays measure specific immunoglobulins and avoid this problem. Serologic tests for tetanus have been recently reviewed.[123]

3.4. Laboratory Diagnosis

Tetanus is primarily a clinical diagnosis and the laboratory usually plays little role. Anaerobic culture of wounds is frequently negative although the yield can be improved by inoculating part of the specimen in cooked-meat medium and heating to 80°C for 5 to 20 min to destroy nonsporulating competing microorganisms.[6,161] Even isolation of the organism does not necessarily confirm tetanus. The organism has been grown from wounds in the absence of clinical symptoms or signs. Serologic tests also are of little use since most tetanus patients do not mount a serologic response against the toxin.[177] Levels of circulating antitoxin less than 0.01 IU/ml at the time of onset of illness suggest susceptibility to the agent and are compatible with the diagnosis. However, several recent reports have documented higher levels of circulating antitoxin in some patients at the time of presentation suggesting that even higher levels of antitoxin are needed to prevent disease in some instances.[17,137] Although such instances are probably rare, tetanus should still be considered in the differential diagnosis as long as the illness is clinically compatible even when circulating antitoxin is greater than 0.01 IU/ml.

4. Biological Characteristics of the Organism

C. tetani is a gram-positive, spore-forming, anaerobic bacillus.[24,38,190] Flagella attached bilaterally on nonsporulating bacteria add motility. The organism typically measures 0.3 to 0.5 μm in diameter and 2 to 2.5 μm in length although long filamentous forms may be seen in culture. Spores typically form in the terminal position and give the organism its characteristic drumsticklike appearance.

While there may be some tolerance for oxygen when the oxidation–reduction potential is low, for the most part *C. tetani* can be considered an obligate anaerobe. It grows optimally at 33–37°C although, depending on the strain, growth can occur from 14 to 43°C. The organism can be grown on a variety of anaerobic media such as cooked meat, casein hydrolysate, and thioglycolate. Growth is usually characterized by production of gas with a fetid odor. Compact colonies formed in a meshwork of fine filaments are usually seen on blood agar. Addition of reducing substances at neutral to alkaline pH enhances growth.

Formation of spores can be promoted or inhibited by a variety of factors including media composition, temperature, and pH.[24,38] Sporulation is enhanced in aging cultures and by physiologic temperatures (i.e., 37°C), and in the presence of oleic acid, phosphates, 1–2% NaCl, and manganese. In contrast, low pH, extremes of temperature (> 41 or < 25°C), glucose, assorted saturated fatty acids, antibiotics, and potassium can inhibit sporulation.

Spores are highly resistant to environmental agents and may persist in soil for months to years, if not exposed to sunlight.[24,185,190] Spores can be destroyed by a variety of disinfectants and heat although susceptibility varies by agent. Aqueous iodine or 2% glutaraldehyde at pH 7.5 to 8.5 kills spores within 3 h. In contrast, phenol (5%), formalin (3%), chloramine (1%), and hydrogen hyperoxidates (6%) require 15 to 24 h to destroy spores. Spores are resistant to boiling but heating to 120°C for 15 to 20 min will inactivate them.

C. tetani produces two exotoxins, tetanolysin and tetanospasmin.[24] Tetanolysin is an oxygen-sensitive hemolysin that may play a role in establishing infection but does not cause disease.[160] It appears to be related to streptolysin and the theta toxin of *C. perfringens*. Tetanospasmin, the cause of the clinical signs and symptoms of tetanus, is a highly potent neurotoxin that accumulates intracellularly during the logarithmic growth phase and is released into the medium upon autolysis. Toxin production appears to be under the control of a plasmid.[74,112] The molecule of approximately 150,000 daltons is synthesized as a single polypeptide chain that may be cleaved into light and heavy chains bound by two disulfide bonds when released into the medium.[25,124,148]

The toxin is one of the most potent poisons on a weight basis although species sensitivities vary considerably.[81] Guinea pigs are exquisitely sensitive with doses of 0.3 ng/kg usually fatal. About 1 ng/kg will kill a mouse while the estimated minimum human lethal dose is < 2.5 ng/kg. Monkeys, sheep, goats, and horses also are extremely susceptible to the effects of the toxin while cats, dogs, and particularly birds and poikilotherms are relatively resistant.[195] The differences in species susceptibility cannot be explained by differences in circulating antitoxin.[161]

5. Descriptive Epidemiology

5.1. Prevalence and Incidence

In spite of the availability of a highly effective immunizing agent, tetanus exerts a substantial health impact throughout the world. In 1973, there were an estimated 1 million tetanus deaths worldwide, with 60–90% of that mortality due to tetanus neonatorum (tetanus during the first month of life).[40] An estimate in 1987 was that annually there are approximately 1 million cases of neonatal tetanus with 800,000 deaths[77] and up to 680,000 cases of nonneonatal tetanus with up to 230,000 deaths.[147] Improved hygiene and childbirth practices, improvements in wound care, reduction in exposure to tetanus spores, and active immunization have led to major declines in tetanus incidence since the 1950s in most developed countries. Similar improvements and especially increasing immunization of pregnant women have led to a reduction of occurrence in many developing countries.[77]

In the United States, death certificate data from 1920 onwards indicate a decline in annual tetanus death rates, which may have accelerated with the use of equine antitoxin in prophylaxis and treatment beginning in the mid-1920s (Fig. 1). Cases of tetanus have been monitored nationally since 1947, when the incidence was 0.39/100,000 total population; secular trends in tetanus occurrence since that time reflect changes in wound management and the use of

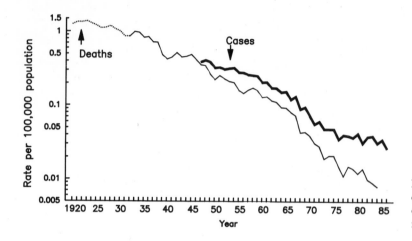

Figure 1. Reported tetanus mortality and incidence rates, United States 1920–1986. Incomplete reporting for 1920–1932; national reporting began in 1947.

toxoid. A continual decline in reported cases occurred until 1976 to about 0.040/100,000. Since then, a less pronounced decline in incidence rates has led to a rate of 0.020/100,000 in 1987, with an all-time low of 48 reported cases; provisionally, six deaths have been reported.

5.2. Epidemic Behavior

C. tetani spreads from the environment to humans generally through contamination of wounds. The organism does not spread person to person and so tetanus cannot be considered a contagious disease. Therefore, tetanus lacks epidemic potential.

5.3. Geographic Distribution

C. tetani organisms are distributed across the globe. However, the greatest concentrations are in warm climates with moist, fertile soil.[37] The highest rates of tetanus occur in the developing world, particularly in countries near the equator.[40] In the United States, tetanus has been and remains predominantly a disease of the Southeast; however, all states report cases. The occurrence of tetanus in regions at high altitude may be lower than in low-lying areas.[5]

5.4. Temporal Distribution

Tetanus is generally distinctly seasonal with a midsummer or "wet" season peak. This is consistent with multiplication of the organisms in the soil and sporulation. This likely also reflects more frequent host behaviors associated with injury during the warmer months.[26,37]

5.5. Age

As noted earlier, tetanus in developing countries occurs most frequently in neonates. Even in the United States in the 1950s, over one third of tetanus deaths were in children under 1 year of age.[89] Aside from neonatal tetanus, the major proportion of victims in developing nations are older children and young adults. Wherever immunization programs are in place, tetanus occurrence declines.[37] In the face of immunization programs, age (and sex) distributions shift to reflect the underimmunized. In the United States since 1965, average annual age-specific tetanus incidence rates reflect declines in all age groups. However, only slight declines were registered in the elderly while drastic declines were reported for younger age groups. Thus, in recent years, the elderly have become the group at highest risk for tetanus (Fig. 2). In 1975–1986, persons ≥ 60 years of age were at a sixfold greater risk of acquiring tetanus than those of all younger ages (incidence of 0.13 versus 0.02/100,000). Limited serosurveys in the United States have supported a high susceptibility in adults ≥ 60—up to 59% of males and up to 71% of females.[55,186] Susceptibility in younger age groups is substantially lower.[110a]

5.6. Sex

In much of the world, reported tetanus appears to be more common in males than in females at all ages.[37] In the neonatal period, particularly in developing countries, this may in part be due to a greater likelihood that parents of males may seek medical attention more frequently than do parents of females.[168] Among children and adults, males generally appear to have a somewhat higher reported inci-

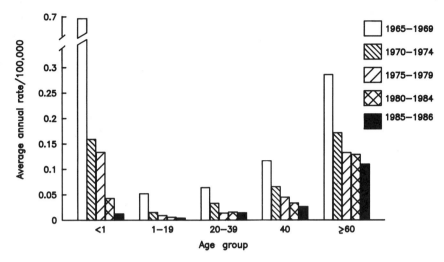

Figure 2. Reported age-group-specific tetanus incidence rates, by selected intervals, United States, 1965–1986.

dence, which could also be due to surveillance artifact and/or perhaps due to exposure factors, such as injury-incurring behaviors outdoors.

In the United States for the period 1975–1986, two-thirds of the 21 neonatal tetanus cases were in males. Outside of the neonatal period, the pattern by sex seen in the United States is different from that seen in developing countries; tetanus age-specific incidence rates were equal in both sexes until age 50. Above age 50, female incidence rates were higher; this sex discrepancy probably represents lower immunization levels among females of this age group since males entering military service during World War II were routinely vaccinated.

5.7. Race

In the 1950s in the United States, nonwhite individuals had an incidence more than five times that in whites, and rates of neonatal tetanus were ten times higher.[89] In the United States in 1975–1986, extrapolating from the patients of known race, the estimated average annual incidence rate was 0.034/100,000 for whites, 0.065/100,000 for blacks, and 0.038/100,000 for all other races. These differences are felt to be attributable primarily to lower levels of tetanus toxoid immunization in the nonwhite populations but could also reflect differences in health care following injury. Case-fatality ratios also differed by race—31% for whites, 43% for blacks, and 34% for all other races—and probably reflect differences both in access to health care and in immune

status. In the 1975–1986 case series, having two or more prior doses of tetanus toxoid put one at lower risk of death with tetanus.

5.8. Occupation and Location

Although the differentiation of the type of surroundings under which tetanus-associated wounds are acquired in the United States has not been collected on cases occurring recently, earlier data suggested that the vast majority occurred indoors in the home, and that wounds were incurred in decreasing frequency in farm, gardening, hospital and factory settings.[26]

5.9. Occurrence in Different Settings

Because of the field and wound conditions, war injuries frequently were associated with tetanus; it has been estimated that, prior to the availability of toxoid, 1 out of 100 serious wounds in battle conditions was complicated by tetanus.[39] As a result of routine tetanus toxoid prophylaxis and vigorous prophylaxis in wound management, only 12 cases of tetanus occurred among 2.73 million wounded U.S. Army personnel on all fronts in World War II (0.44/100,000) versus 70 out of 520,000 wounded in World War I (13.4/100,000).[117]

Parenteral drug abuse, both intravenous and subcutaneous, is known to place individuals at higher risk compared to the general population. Indeed, quinine used to "cut" the concentration of opiates may decrease local redox potential, favoring spore germination; in addition, contaminating organisms other than *C. tetani* may contribute to a hypoaerobic environment.[45,116]

Operative procedures, particularly bowel surgery, infrequently can put some individuals at risk, as can dental procedures, puerperal sepsis, and septic abortion[4,118]; these conditions accounted for 23 of the 977 nonneonatal cases (2%) of tetanus reported in 1975–1986.

5.10. Socioeconomic Factors

The incidence and complications of tetanus are inversely related to access to (1) routine prophylactic immunization, (2) immunization with appropriate wound care following wounds, and (3) care following onset of symptoms. Availability and use of these services probably correlate directly with socioeconomic status. The differences in racial incidence and the characteristics of mothers of patients with neonatal tetanus are strongly felt to reflect poorer immunization levels associated with lower socioeconomic status.

6. Mechanisms and Routes of Transmission

Tetanus is caused by the *in vivo* elaboration of tetanospasmin. Spores of *C. tetani* are usually introduced through breaks in the epithelium. Activation of the spores with production of toxin leads to disease. Since neonatal tetanus is the most common form of tetanus in the world, accounting for approximately 80%–90% of the deaths, the usual site of entry is the umbilical cord stump.[21,47,87, 91,99,153,168] Outside the neonatal period, a variety of conditions have been associated with tetanus. In the United States, information is available for 896 of the 977 nonneonatal cases reported between 1975 through 1986. Acute injuries were the predisposing event in 686 (77%) while chronic wounds or other medical conditions were associated with 135 cases (15%). Parenteral drug abuse was the only predisposing condition in 2% and was present in an additional 1%. For 6% of patients, no acute injury, chronic wound, or associated medical condition was known.

Of the patients reporting acute injuries, puncture wounds were most common (40%) followed by lacerations (30%). The circumstances of the wound were known for 77% of these cases. Injuries in outdoor settings (e.g., yard, garden, or farm settings) accounted for 27% of cases with acute wounds, injuries incurred indoors accounted for 34%

of cases, and 12% were incurred under special circumstances. These included animal bites and/or scratches in 4%, major trauma (burns, bullet wounds, and compound fractures) in 4%, and surgical wounds, many of which were contaminated (e.g., bowel wounds), in 4%.

Chronic medical conditions associated with tetanus included decubitus ulcers, gangrene, and frostbite, as well as dental and other abscesses and parental drug abuse. Cases without known wounds or portals of entry have been described for many years.[37] In some instances, these are thought to arise from minor wounds not recalled by those patients or from intraintestinal toxin production. There are some reports indicating that up to 40% of human intestines are colonized with *C. tetani*.[7,15,48,105,119,172, 173,176]

Other conditions associated with tetanus include contaminated injections, e.g., vaccinations, earlobe infections, foreign bodies, and the practice of tattooing.

7. Pathogenesis and Immunity

7.1. Pathogenesis

Tetanus results when spores inoculated through the epithelium germinate, leading to the production of tetanospasmin and its transport to the central nervous system (CNS). The period of time between an identified acute injury and onset of tetanus signs and symptoms is 3 days to 3 weeks for the majority of cases. In the United States in 1975–1986, the median incubation period in reported cases was 7 days.

Germination is enhanced by anaerobic conditions associated with significant tissue injury and accumulation of lactic acid.[161] Calcium may increase the likelihood that injected spores germinate because it can increase local necrosis.[36] The presence of calcium in soil along with tetanus spores may be one reason why wounds contaminated by soil are predisposed to tetanus.

The means by which tetanospasmin reaches the CNS has been debated for years. Toxin injected or produced in the subcutaneous tissue appears to enter muscle first. Tetanus can be prevented by treating the muscle with antitoxin prior to subcutaneous administration of toxin.[111] Once in the muscle, toxin can reach the bloodstream via the lymphatics and reach the CNS through hematogenous transport, or toxin can get to the CNS directly through retrograde transport via neurons.

Hematogenous transport was supported by a variety of studies showing that most of the toxin produced or injected reached the bloodstream and from there arrived in a variety of tissues.[1,111] However, because the toxin does not appear to cross the blood–brain barrier, neuronal transport is now believed to be the predominant means by which toxin gains access to the CNS.[23,75,83,1111,155] Experimental data indicate that toxin is found at motor end plates of muscle nerves.[73,196] From there, it gains entry to the nerve by binding to gangliosides or other receptors and is transported to the ventral horns of the spinal cord or motor nuclei of cranial nerves. Transmission within nerves can result from either intraaxonal transport, travel through perineural spaces between fibers, or by spreading via lymphatics associated with nerves. Radiolabeled toxin studies suggest that intraaxonal transport is most likely.[145]

Tetanospasmin acts by causing disinhibition of spinal cord reflex arcs, allowing excitatory reflexes to multiply unchecked resulting in the classical tetanic spasms.[27,30,31,111] Disinhibition appears to be caused by interfering with release of the neurotransmitters glycine and γ-aminobutyric acid from presynaptic inhibitory fibers.[111] In addition, the toxin can impede release of a variety of other neurotransmitters including acetylcholine in autonomic and peripheral somatic nerves.[187] The toxin can affect peripheral motor end plates, the spinal cord, the brain, and the sympathetic nervous system.[35,94,103,104,111] More detail on the toxin and its effects can be found in reviews by van Heyningen, Wellhoner, and Bizzini.[25,179,187]

7.2. Immunity

Immunity to tetanus does not generally follow disease since the quantity of toxin that causes illness is usually less than the quantity needed to induce an immune response.[177] Second cases of tetanus have been reported.[22,41,167]

Most serosurveys in unimmunized populations fail to find much evidence for natural immunity. However, a few recent reports of serosurveys in unimmunized populations of developed and particularly of developing countries suggest that some persons may develop such immunity.[56,125,146,181,183] These latter studies have been criticized because documentation of no prior immunizations may be lacking and because the assays used may have measured cross-reacting (nonneutralizing) antibodies at low levels. Nonetheless, these data suggest that at least in some developing countries, asymptomatic infection/colonization, presumably of the intestine, does occur resulting in the production of antitoxin. Nevertheless, natural immunization cannot be relied upon to control tetanus. Further study is needed in developed countries before the concept of natural immunity in those populations can be accepted.

It is generally agreed that a circulating level of antitoxin of 0.01 IU/ml is the level needed to guarantee protection against tetanus.[65,121,126,159] This comes from experiments both with humans and with animals. A review by McComb in 1964 reported that clinical tetanus could be prevented in horses by administration of 1500 IU/ml of antitoxin after acute injury, which corresponded to a serum level of 0.01 IU/ml.[126] Following immunization with tetanus toxoid, Wolters and Dehmel were able to resist challenge in themselves with "2–3 fatal doses" of tetanus toxin. They had achieved serum levels of 0.007 to 0.01 antitoxin unit (AU)/ml (prior to international standardization of the assay).[193] Further evidence that 0.01 IU/ml was protective came from trials to prevent neonatal tetanus. Induction of antitoxin levels of 0.01 IU/ml or higher in mothers resulted in protection of infants from neonatal tetanus.[121]

The protective level of circulating tetanus antitoxin has recently been challenged by reports of 12 patients who had serum levels greater than 0.01 IU/ml at the time they presented with clinical tetanus.[17,137] The highest level noted was 0.16 IU/ml. In some instances, large-scale production of toxin may overcome this barrier (i.e., 0.01 IU/ml) or perhaps rapid uptake through nerve endings may prevent neutralization of toxin. Whatever the explanation, these data suggest that the 0.01 level cannot be considered absolute. Nevertheless, the fact that tetanus is rare in adequately immunized persons, and with all the experimental animal and human data noted above, it seems reasonable to conclude that 0.01 IU/ml is protective in all but the rarest situations.

8. Patterns of Host Response

8.1. Clinical Features in Children and Adults

The reported incubation period for tetanus ranges from 1 day to several months. However, the majority of cases occur within 3 days to 3 weeks after an injury. In the United States, the median incubation period for cases with injury-associated wounds reported between 1975 and 1986 was 7 days. The incubation period varies with distance between the wound and the CNS. The longest periods are reported for injuries farthest away from the CNS while injuries to the head and trunk have the shortest incubation periods.[111,185] Historically, shorter incubation periods have been associated with more severe disease although this has not been the case in patients recently reported in the United States.[2,26,33,35,78,138]

Clinical tetanus can take one of three forms: (1) localized, (2) generalized, and (3) cephalic.[185] Local tetanus, which is rare in humans, consists of painful spasms in a confined area around the site of the original injury.[129,149] The spasms may persist for weeks to months. The prognosis of tetanus that remains localized is excellent; however, localized tetanus often will progress to generalized tetanus, which carries a more ominous prognosis. Over 80% of cases of tetanus fit this category. Patients most often present with trismus or lockjaw, i.e., spasm of the muscles of mastication.[3,144,185] Risus sardonicus, the characteristic facial expression, occurs with trismus and spasm of the facial muscles. It consists of raised eyebrows, tight closure of the eyelids, wrinkling of the forehead, and extension of the corners of the mouth laterally. Initial signs may be followed by involvement of multiple other muscle groups, hyperreflexia, and generalized hypertonicity. Tetanospasms, generalized tetanic seizure activity, consist of sudden painful contraction of all muscle groups resulting in opisthotonos, abduction and flexion at the shoulders, flexion of the elbows and wrists, and extension of the legs. Spasm of the glottis can cause immediate death. Autonomic nervous system abnormalities consisting of hyper- or hypotension, tachycardia, and arrhythmias among other manifestations are frequently reported in severe cases.[34,94,103,104] Complications can result directly from the actions of the toxin, from spasms, or from chronic debility. Reported death-to-case ratios for generalized tetanus have varied from 10 to 75%.[26,35,63,79,95,174,175] With good intensive care, mortality should be less than 20%. The greatest mortality occurs at the extremes of age.

Cephalic tetanus occurs with injuries or lesions of the head and face.[182,185] It is characterized by short incubation periods, 1 to 2 days, and by atonic cranial nerve palsies particularly involving nerves III, IV, VII, IX, X, and XII, singly or in combination. Trismus may be present. Cephalic tetanus may progress to generalized tetanus.

8.2. Neonatal Tetanus

Tetanus occurring within the first month of life is a form of generalized tetanus. It occurs in newborn infants following infection by *C. tetani* (most commonly at the umbilical cord stump). Symptoms of neonatal tetanus generally begin 3–14 days after birth but can occur from 1 to 28 days of age. The illness starts with poor sucking and excessive crying. This is followed by variable degrees of trismus, difficulty swallowing, opisthotonos, and other tetanic spasms. Cases are often associated with unsterile conditions of childbirth, delivery personnel untrained in sterile care of the umbilical cord and stump, and particularly with births followed by

unhygienic cultural rituals involving the umbilical stump—such as application of herbs, clarified butter, or animal dung.[47,87,99,173a] The disease can be prevented through transplacental passage of circulating antitoxin from mother to infant, most of which is in the IgG1 subclass.[67,121] However, most newborns in the world are susceptible because their mothers have not received two or more doses of tetanus toxoid; it was estimated that from 1986–1989 only 15%–25% of pregnant women in developing countries have received at least two recent doses of tetanus toxoid.[69,70] The case-fatality ratio of neonatal tetanus is 25–90% with therapy, depending on the intensity of supportive care. Overall, the Expanded Programme on Immunization (EPI) of the World Health Organization estimates that 80% of affected infants die.[77]

The incidence of tetanus neonatorum in developing nations had been estimated in the 1960s to be under 50,000 cases annually, or approximately 0.5/1000 live births overall.[37] A better estimate of the general incidence of neonatal tetanus has recently been made with the use of community-based, house-to-house surveys of neonatal deaths, which have suggested that the reported incidence is less than 5% of the actual incidence. These surveys have shown the incidence rates of neonatal tetanus deaths to be over 50/1000 live births in some areas of developing countries, and above 5/1000 in most, i.e., a crude incidence of neonatal tetanus deaths of more than 25/100,000 total population.[168]

As indicated by death rates, the occurrence of neonatal tetanus in the United States was already on the decline prior to widespread tetanus toxoid use in women due to an increasing number of births in hospitals and improvements in postpartum hygiene. Deaths due to tetanus in those less than 1 year old, generally reflecting neonatal disease, declined from 0.64/1000 live births in 1900 to 0.07 in 1930 to 0.01 by the 1960s. Using age-specific reporting beginning in 1961, tetanus incidence could be directly monitored in those less than 1 year old and showed the same downward trend. From 1967 to 1968, the incidence rates of reported cases and of reported tetanus deaths in those less than 1 year old declined abruptly.[91] This abrupt decline occurred primarily because of a decrease of reported cases in Texas for uncertain reasons. Part of the decline may be attributable to an increase in the cohort of women of child-bearing age who had received tetanus toxoid in childhood.

Of the 21 cases reported in the first 4 weeks of life in the United States during 1975–1986, 19 were in infants born outside of a hospital. Fourteen of the cases (66%) occurred in Texas, which had only 6% of U.S. births. Only three mothers had a history of ever having received tetanus toxoid, and none were known to have received more than one dose. Seventeen of nineteen with known outcome survived.

Given its substantial impact in developing countries, the control of neonatal and nonneonatal tetanus is the subject of a major effort of EPI by routine immunization in infancy with DTP and by immunization of women of reproductive age with tetanus toxoid.

8.3. Diagnosis

The diagnosis of tetanus is made primarily on clinical grounds.[182,185] Generalized stiffness, hyperreflexia, trismus, and the characteristic generalized tetanic spasms strongly support the diagnosis. Absence of changes in the state of consciousness or sensory involvement add further support. The epidemiologic history can also be helpful. A preceding history of a wound, particularly if contaminated by soil, is suggestive although not all cases will have such histories. Lack of a history/record of adequate immunization or wound care is typical. Given the high efficacy of a course of tetanus toxoid, a clinically compatible case who presents with a complete primary series of toxoid with maintenance boosters should not be considered tetanus unless an exhaustive workup fails to reveal other potential causes. Significant rises in circulating antitoxin are not reliably seen in tetanus and cannot be used to make the diagnosis unless demonstrated.[177] Testing for antitoxin using ELISA or passive hemagglutination can be performed on a rapid basis to assist in assessment of immune status. Isolation of the organism from a wound as well as the absence of circulating antitoxin at 0.01 IU/ml or greater when the patient is first seen also support the diagnosis.

The differential diagnosis will depend on the clinical signs and symptoms.[182,185] Trismus may be caused by dental caries, tonsillitis, peritonsillar abscesses, parotitis, temporomandibular joint dysfunction, and CNS disturbances other than tetanus. Hyperreflexia may be seen in rabies; however, rabies is more often associated with changes in the state of consciousness and the seizures of rabies are more often clonic in contrast to the tonic seizures of tetanus. The history of an animal bite is generally present with rabies but could be present in tetanus. Encephalitis also can result in spasms but, like rabies, is much more likely to be associated with changes in the state of consciousness. In addition to infections, a variety of poisonings and metabolic conditions can simulate tetanus. Hypocalcemic tetany can cause generalized muscle spasms but is not usually associated with trismus.[165] Strychnine poisoning can resemble generalized tetanus both in mechanism, disinhibition of spi-

nal cord reflex arcs, and clinically.[28] However, strychnine poisoning is usually not associated with muscle rigidity between spasms and is rarely associated with temperature elevations, which are frequent in severe tetanus. Dystonias caused by phenothiazines should also be considered in the differential diagnosis. Finally, hysteria can mimic tetanus although such patients tend to relax on prolonged observation and their seizurelike activity tends to be clonic rather than tonic.

9. Control and Prevention

Tetanus is a totally preventable disease.[64] Prevention begins with universal, routine immunization and with appropriate attention toward averting wounds and injuries. A routine immunization program should ensure that the entire population has received a primary series (at least three doses) of tetanus toxoid with booster doses as needed. Substantial health benefits are derived from combined immunization with diphtheria and tetanus toxoids and pertussis vaccine (DTP) in childhood. It was estimated that in 1986 more than 40% of target children in the world excluding the United States and Canada had received three doses of DTP.[69]

Once injuries occur, efforts should be made to prevent contamination with spores and to eliminate those conditions that predispose to germination of spores. Wounds should be carefully cleaned and surgically debrided when necessary to remove devitalized tissue, which can serve as a nidus for infection, followed by tetanus toxoid and tetanus immune globulin, when needed. Since neonatal tetanus is the major worldwide cause of tetanus morbidity and mortality, greater attention must be paid to covering umbilical cord stumps with sterile or uncontaminated dressings. Training of midwives in proper sterile techniques has been demonstrated to reduce the incidence of neonatal tetanus substantially (although not as effectively as immunization) as well as result in declines in neonatal mortality due to causes other than tetanus.[18,87,106,132]

Only 45 (5%) of the 896 cases of nonneonatal tetanus reported in the United States from 1975 through 1986 reported receiving three or more doses of tetanus toxoid. Of these, 8 had received the third dose as part of wound management and 23 had not received a dose within the preceding 5 years. Of 209 patients with acute injuries who were known to have sought medical care, 92% did not receive the recommended tetanus toxoid with or without tetanus immune globulin. Thus, almost all cases of tetanus could be prevented with routine immunization and appropriate wound management.

9.1. Passive Immunization

Although animal models suggest that prompt passive immunization is protective against the development of tetanus following injury, there is limited information in humans; appropriately controlled trials have not been performed. Passive immunization with equine antitoxin for treatment and for prophylaxis following wounds became common practice in World War I, with a decrease in wound-associated tetanus at the same time that other improvements in wound care were becoming common practice.[33] Passive immunity conferred by equine antitoxin is of limited duration. The half-life of refined equine antitoxin in humans is less than 2 weeks and may be shorter in some individuals.[170] A major disadvantage is that persons receiving large doses of equine antitoxin can experience immediate hypersensitivity reactions or serum sickness.[130]

Tetanus immune globulin (TIG) is a human antibody preparation prepared by cold-ethanol fractionation of the plasma of hyperimmunized adults. TIG was introduced in the early 1960s and was found to have a fairly constant half-life of 28 days in humans.[126] The frequency of allergic and serum sickness reactions to equine antitoxin, along with its shorter half-life, made TIG more attractive for passive immunization. TIG has been shown not to pose a risk of hepatitis transmission. Additionally, TIG and other purified immune globulins pose no risk of human immunodeficiency virus (HIV) transmission since donors are screened to be at low risk, serum is screened for antibody to HIV prior to serum pooling, and, most importantly, cold-ethanol fractionation inactivates HIV.[43] It is distributed at a concentration of 250 IU/ml in 1-ml vials. Even in the developing world, TIG is beginning to supplant equine antitoxin as it becomes more widely available. Tetanus toxoid is always given with TIG to induce persistence of immunity beyond 28 days in those with any past exposure to toxoid and to initiate active immunization in those without any prior exposure.[115] In contrast to equine antitoxin, TIG should never be administered intravenously, because of aggregates. It is intended solely for intramuscular use. The cost in 1989 of a 250-IU vial of TIG is $4.67 in the United States; that of a 1500-IU vial of equine antitoxin is $5.00.

9.2. Active Immunization

Tetanus toxoid is one of the best immunogens available today. A primary series will induce protective levels of circulating antitoxin in virtually 100% of recipients.[10–14,20,32,52,59–62,76,86,134,141,142] Protective levels usually last at least 10 years and in the majority will be present even up to 25 years after the last dose.[82,139,154,157]

9.2.1. Production and Testing of Tetanus Toxoid.
To produce toxoid, *C. tetani* is cultured in large-capacity fermentors in liquid medium free of allergenic substances. The culture filtrate is precipitated with methanol or ammonium sulfate to purify partially extracellular toxin. Toxin is further purified and detoxified with 40% formaldehyde at 37°C. By WHO standards, the final product should contain 0.5% formaldehyde or less. In the United States, minimum requirements stipulate a residual formaldehyde content of 0.02% or less. A single dose of adsorbed toxoid must contain less than 1.25 mg of aluminum. All toxoid preparations in the United States have thimerosal as a bacteriostatic agent added to a final concentration of 0.1%.

Potency is determined by animal bioassays: for the fluid preparation, immunized guinea pigs are tested for survival after a toxin challenge; for precipitated toxoid, a serum pool from immunized guinea pigs must exceed 2 IU/ml of tetanus antitoxin. The toxoid content of commercial products is assessed by flocculation; this measure of toxoid protein content (Lf) does not equate directly with immunogenicity as measured by potency in guinea pigs. Adsorbed products available in the United States have a content of 4–10 Lf per dose; fluid products contain 4–5 Lf.

Tetanus toxoid is available in several preparations: Diphtheria and Tetanus Toxoids and Pertussis Vaccine Adsorbed (DTP; also referred to as DPT, particularly outside the United States) and Diphtheria and Tetanus Toxoids Adsorbed (For Pediatric Use) (DT) used in infants and children under 7 years of age. Universal use of DTP in infancy and childhood is recommended unless there are contraindications to pertussis vaccine. Tetanus and Diphtheria Toxoids Adsorbed (For Adult Use) (Td) is for use in persons 7 years of age and older; it contains less diphtheria toxoid (2 Lf or less) than the pediatric preparation (over 10 Lf). Td is the preferred preparation for tetanus prophylaxis in adults under all circumstances because the vast majority of adults in need of tetanus toxoid are likely to be susceptible to diphtheria. Single-antigen Tetanus Toxoid (fluid) and Tetanus Toxoid Adsorbed are also available in the United States for use in persons 7 years of age and older.

In the United States, aluminum hydroxide or aluminum phosphate is used as an adjuvant. These salts allow an adequate immune response after fewer doses of toxoid than with the fluid preparation.[101] Since fluid and adsorbed preparations do not differ substantially with regard to adverse events, adsorbed toxoid is preferred because it confers protective levels of antitoxin for a longer period of time.[49,92,100,101] Response to either form of toxoid as a booster dose is equally brisk. In combined active–passive immunization, TIG does not substantially alter the response to adsorbed toxoid as it does with fluid toxoid.[115,122] In some countries other than the United States, a calcium phosphate adsorbed product is also available.[107,180] The adsorbed toxoid is administered intramuscularly; fluid preparations can be given subcutaneously. Either can be given by jet-injector.

Preparations should be stored at 2–10°C and generally have a 2-year expiration date. Higher ambient temperatures for 3 days or under do not reduce the potency of the toxoid. Freezing reduces potency, particularly when the toxoid is a component of DTP.[24]

9.2.2. Use of Tetanus Toxoid. Most immunization schedules in developed countries call for two or three doses in the first year of life followed by a reinforcing dose 6 months to 1 year afterwards.[50,96,194] The routine schedule for tetanus immunization in the United States is given in Table 1. In children less than 7 years old, tetanus toxoid is usually combined with diphtheria toxoid and pertussis vaccine as DTP. When given as DTP, three doses starting at 6 weeks to 2 months of age are indicated 1 to 2 months apart followed by a fourth dose approximately 6 to 12 months after the third dose. If pertussis vaccine is contraindicated, a pediatric preparation of diphtheria and tetanus toxoids (DT)

is indicated. In the first year of life, the schedule is identical to the DTP schedule. However, beginning in the second year, only three doses are required for primary immunization, two doses 1 to 2 months apart followed by a third dose 6 to 12 months after the second. For developing countries, the EPI, with its emphasis on infants, recommends a total of three doses early in the first year of life without reinforcing or booster doses.[68]

Protective levels of antitoxin can be achieved with schedules starting in the newborn period.[14,52,59,61,62,76,86] However, in most countries immunization rarely starts before 2 months of age. In the past, it was thought that passively transferred maternal antitoxin would not interfere with the immune response of the infant.[12,14,59,60,141] However, most of these studies were done before women had been routinely immunized either as children or as adults.[86] More recent studies in the United States demonstrate that substantial proportions of infants have levels of circulating antitoxin at the time of initiating the DTP series, suggesting that the issue of interference should be reconsidered. The need for a full three doses in the first year of life was supported by a recent report by Barkin *et al.*,[11] who demonstrated that substantially higher levels of antitoxin are achieved after three doses in the first year of life compared to two doses. The height of the antitoxin response is directly related to the age at completion of the third dose.[32] There is no good evidence that intervals of 2

Table 1. Recommendations for Primary Immunization with Tetanus Toxoid by Age at Beginning Immunization[a]

	Age group		
	< 1 year	1–6 years	≥ 7 years
Vaccine	DTP or DT[b,c]	DTP[a]	DT[b,e]	Td[f]
Interval before				
Dose 1	First visit	First visit	First visit	First visit
Dose 2	1–2 months	1–2 months	1–2 months	1–2 months
Dose 3	1–2 months	1–2 months	6–12 months	6–12 months
Dose 4	~ 1 year[g]	~ 1 year		

[a]DTP, diphtheria and tetanus toxoids and pertussis vaccine; DT, diphtheria and tetanus toxoids for pediatric use; Td, tetanus and diphtheria toxoids for adult use.

[b]DT for those with contraindications to pertussis vaccine.

[c]Boosters with DT or DTP (dose 5) indicated at 4–6 years of age. Boosters with Td indicated every 10 years thereafter. First visit generally at 2 months of age.

[d]Dose 5 of DTP indicated at 4–6 years of age unless dose 4 administered at ≥ 4 years of age. In this instance, dose 5 not needed. Boosters with Td indicated every 10 years after dose 4 or 5.

[e]Dose 4 of DT indicated at 4–6 years of age unless dose 3 administered at ≥ 4 years of age. In this instance, dose 4 not needed. Boosters with Td indicated every 10 years after dose 3 or 4.

[f]Boosters with Td indicated every 10 years.

[g]Generally given at 15 months with measles, mumps, and rubella vaccine (MMR) and trivalent oral polio vaccine (OPV) or with OPV alone at 18 months of age.

months for the first three doses offer any advantage over 1 month. All achieve protective levels regardless of schedule although antitoxin levels are higher after the 2-month interval probably because these children are older at the time they complete their three-dose schedule. Nevertheless, by the time the fourth dose is indicated (approximately 1 year after the third dose), antitoxin levels are comparable in both groups. Preterm infants appear to respond similarly at a given chronologic age as term infants.[20,61]

Unimmunized children 7 years of age or older and adults require a three-dose primary series with two doses 1 to 2 months apart followed by a third dose 6 to 12 months after the second. In the United States, an adult preparation of combined tetanus and diphtheria toxoids (Td) that contains a decreased amount of diphtheria toxoid is used. The immune response to tetanus toxoid tends to decrease with increasing age. In comparative studies, children tend to achieve higher levels of antitoxin than do adults.[131] The elderly tend to make a poorer response to toxoid than do younger adults.[109,166] Nevertheless, almost all children and adults will achieve protective titers after a three-dose primary series.

In developing countries, immunization of adults is intended primarily for pregnant women or women of childbearing age to effect prevention of tetanus neonatorum. Induction of protective levels in mothers is associated with protection from neonatal tetanus by transfer of antitoxin across the placenta.[44,58,121,132] A minimum of two doses at least 1 month apart has been recommended by the EPI for pregnant women with the last dose at least 2 weeks prior to the estimated date of delivery. However, difficulties in finding and vaccinating pregnant women have led to efforts to vaccinate all women of childbearing age. In addition, vaccination with only two doses is less effective and does not provide long-term protection. The schedule listed in Table 2, which recommends a total of five tetanus toxoid doses

Table 2.   Recommendations of the Expanded Programme on Immunization for Immunization of Women of Childbearing Age[a]

Dose 1—First contact or as early in pregnancy as possible
Dose 2—4 weeks later
Dose 3—6–12 months later or during subsequent pregnancy
Dose 4—1–5 years after dose 3 or during subsequent pregnancy
Dose 5—1–10 years after dose 4 or during subsequent
        pregnancy; no further doses indicated

[a]See Ref. 71.

with the third at least 6 months after the first, has recently been adopted by the EPI in hopes of inducing sustained levels of circulating antitoxin in all women.[71]

After a three-dose primary series, circulating antitoxin remains at protective levels for years. Studies in Denmark demonstrate that 96 and 72% had levels ≥ 0.01 IU/ml at 13–14 and ≥ 25 years, respectively, after the third dose of a product containing 7–12 Lf.[154,157] Based on these studies and others, immunization advisory bodies in the United States have recommended routine boosters of a tetanus toxoid-containing preparation every 10 years.[50,96] The booster response is not impaired even with intervals of 20 or more years since the last dose.[102,157] There is no need to restart a primary series if the schedule has not been followed or booster doses have been missed. Instead, prior doses should be counted and the remaining doses given to finish the three-dose primary series. Missed boosters can be ignored. In the United States, a preschool booster of DTP is recommended at 4–6 years of age primarily to ensure immunity to pertussis in young school-aged children. Thereafter, doses of Td are recommended every 10 years.

9.2.3. Adverse Events. Reports of local reactions following tetanus toxoid vary greatly. In general, 50–85% of recipients of booster doses of adsorbed toxoid experience pain or tenderness at the injection site. While 20–30% experience edema and erythema,[49,100,120] marked swelling occurs in less than 2%. Controlled studies suggest that minor swelling or pain may occur more frequently in individuals receiving Td than among those receiving tetanus toxoid; however, substantial differences in marked swelling have not been demonstrated.[120,178,189] Several studies have found that the greater the preexisting antitoxin level, the higher is the incidence of local reactions, which generally begin within 2–8 h of an injection.[49,100,127,188] There have been several reports of massive local swelling, particularly in persons with a history of multiple booster doses of toxoid. Such persons are typically found to have high serum antitoxin levels, likely leading to the formation of immune complexes with the deposited toxoid (Arthus reaction).[66,114,127] Thus, frequent boosters of tetanus toxoid in wound management are currently discouraged.

Fever can accompany a local response, particularly a marked local reaction.[114] Overall, booster doses of Td are associated with fever in 0.5–7% with temperature over 39°C being rare.[158,188] Headache and malaise are unusual.

There have been several anecdotal reports of peripheral neuropathy hours to weeks following tetanus toxoid at an estimated incidence of 0.4 per million doses of toxoid.[93,152]

Table 3. Summary Guide to Tetanus Prophylaxis in Routine Wound Management[a]

History of adsorbed tetanus toxoid (doses)	Clean, minor wounds		All other wounds[b]	
	Td[c]	TIG	Td[c]	TIG
Unknown or < three	Yes	No	Yes	Yes
≥ three[d]	No[e]	No	No[f]	No

[a] From ACIP, 1985.[96]
[b] Such as, but not limited to, wounds contaminated with with dirt, feces, soil, saliva, etc.; puncture wounds; avulsions; and wounds resulting from missiles, crushing, burns, and frostbite.
[c] For children less than 7 years old; DTP (DT, if pertussis vaccine is contraindicated) is preferred to tetanus toxoid alone. For persons 7 years old and older, Td is preferred to tetanus toxoid alone.
[d] If only three doses of *fluid* toxoid have been received, then a fourth dose of toxoid, preferably an adsorbed toxoid, should be given.
[e] Yes, if more than 10 years since last dose.
[f] Yes, if more than 5 years since last dose. (More frequent boosters are not needed and can accentuate side effects.)

Anaphylactic reactions to purified tetanus toxoid appear to be rare.[164] In the United States, passive surveillance for the years 1985–1986 revealed 6.4 serious allergic reactions (stridor, bronchospasm, and anaphylaxis) reported per million doses of publicly distributed Td. Skin testing has been urged in management of patients with a history suggestive of such a reaction.[98] Interpretation of some skin test results should take into account some expected nonspecificity of skin test reactions.[72]

9.2.4. Wound Management. An individual who presents for medical care with any type of wound should be evaluated for tetanus prophylaxis. Removal of foreign bodies and debridement of devitalized tissue in a timely fashion is imperative; if necessary, drainage and irrigation should be performed.[163] Recommendations for the use of tetanus toxoid and TIG in the United States for tetanus prophylaxis in the management of wounds have been made by the Immunization Practices Advisory Committee (ACIP) and agree with those of the American Academy of Pediatrics (AAP) and the Committee on Trauma of the American College of Surgeons (ACS).[50,51,96] The recommendations of the ACIP are given in Table 3.

Although any wound can potentially give rise to tetanus infection, uncomplicated wounds are considered to have a low likelihood both of contamination by tetanus spores and of leading to an environment that would support germination of spores. For persons with this category of wounds, Td is recommended if the patient has received less than three doses of adsorbed toxoid in the past or it has been

more than 10 years since the previous toxoid dose; TIG administration is not necessary. Such individuals respond briskly to subsequent doses of tetanus toxoid within 7 days and generally within 4 days.[8,102]

Most patients who had received fluid toxoid in the past, and rarely individuals who received adsorbed toxoid, may have circulating antitoxin levels less than 0.01 IU/ml after 5 years.[9,139] Therefore, it is recommended that persons with wounds that are of higher risk of contamination receive a dose of toxoid if more than 5 years has elapsed since the last dose. Individuals with such wounds are also potential candidates for simultaneous passive immunization with TIG if the immunization history indicates fewer than three toxoid doses. When administered at a separate site, TIG does not interfere with the immune response to adsorbed tetanus toxoid; an intramuscular dose of 250 units (1cm3) is recommended by the ACIP.[96]

Almost all of the tetanus cases with wounds in the United States might have been prevented with appropriate wound management. Of the 686 patients in the United States in 1975–1986 with acute wounds, tetanus toxoid was given as prophylaxis in wound management to only 25%; of these, 74% had received toxoid within 3 days of injury. Tetanus toxoid alone is not sufficient in patients who have never received at least a three-dose primary series. Most of these individuals were also potential candidates for, but did not receive, TIG. Thirty percent of the 686 patients with acute wounds reportedly underwent debridement after injury and before onset of tetanus symptoms. Of these 209 patients, 92 percent did not receive the recommended Td with or without TIG based on their individual immunization histories.

However, underadministration of tetanus prophylaxis following wounds appears to be the exception rather than the rule; two studies suggest that when patients with wounds seek care in the United States, 1–6% receive less than the recommended prophylactic measures of Td with or without TIG indicated by their wound and immunization history, and 12–17% receive more than recommended.[29,80]

9.3. Antimicrobials

As a substitute for or adjunct to equine antitoxin prior to wide availability of TIG, antibiotics were once frequently used for tetanus prophylaxis in wound management.[162] Antimicrobials may sensitize patients and have been known to fail. Antimicrobials have not been proven to have superior or equal efficacy to antitoxin and are not currently recommended for tetanus prophylaxis.[119,163]

9.4. Summary

Tetanus is an infectious but noncommunicable disease caused by a toxin. The spores of *C. tetani* are ubiquitous in nature and when injected under the epithelium of the skin can germinate given anaerobic conditions leading to the production of tetanospasmin. The toxin travels to the CNS along peripheral nerves and causes disease by presynaptic interference with release of neurotransmitters leading to disinhibition of spinal cord reflex arcs and accumulation of excitatory stimulation. This results in the tetanospasm, a generalized muscular spasm. Death-to-case ratios vary from 10 to 75%.

The disease can be prevented by appropriate attention to routine immunization and wound management. Tetanus toxoid is one of the most effective immunogens known with essentially all recipients of a primary series protected for at least 10 years. Since wounds are probably the most frequent predisposing cause of tetanus, special attention should be paid to (1) wound cleansing and debridement to remove both spores and devitalized tissue and (2) providing protective levels of circulating antitoxin including both passive immunization to achieve protection rapidly and active immunization to increase levels rapidly in previously primed persons. Completion of a primary series will lead to sustained protection and would prevent cases not associated with acute injuries and circumvent the need for special procedures following wounds.

10. Unresolved Problems

The major problem in tetanus prevention today is the difficulty in delivering routine immunization to those in need. This is particularly a problem in developing countries where an estimated 800,000 infants die of neonatal tetanus annually.[71,77] Since most women do not have access to prenatal care and most children are born outside of a hospital, there needs to be greater emphasis on vaccination of women of childbearing age if the incidence of neonatal tetanus is to be reduced. Every contact of a susceptible female of childbearing age with the health care system should be taken as an opportunity to update her tetanus immunization status. More research is needed on one-dose delivery systems. While preliminary results with high-potency toxoids have been encouraging, there is concern about maintenance of protective levels of antibody. At the present time, at least two doses in pregnancy are recommended but a vigorous attempt to provide five doses early in the reproductive years will lead to a higher likelihood of protection against neonatal tetanus. New systems used to release drugs slowly over time offer promise for immunizations such as tetanus.[192]

Universal immunization of children with later boosting will also go a long way toward preventing tetanus in the children themselves as well as their offspring because protective levels appear to persist in the majority for over 25 years. In hopes of raising immunization levels in the United States, the ACIP recently simplified the immunization schedule to allow DTP together with oral polio vaccine (OPV) and measles, mumps, and rubella (MMR) vaccine at 15 months of age.[97] Previously, separate visits were recommended at 15 months for MMR and 18 months for the fourth dose of DTP. Combination of DTP with *Haemophilus influenzae* type b polysaccharide conjugated with various proteins has been considered for the future. In many developing countries, simultaneous administration of multiple other antigens with DTP could result in improved immunity levels against several diseases; one potential combination that has been evaluated preliminarily is DTP with inactivated polio vaccine (IPV) and hepatitis B vaccine (HBV).[53]

In the United States, the remaining morbidity and mortality from tetanus are in the elderly. Serologic surveys suggest that substantial majorities of these populations lack protection.[55,151,186] Greater efforts are needed by practitioners to review the immunization status of their elderly patients and offer Td as needed.

Finally, universal proper wound management would prevent a significant proportion of tetanus cases. All persons in emergency rooms as well as other health care providers need to become familiar with current recommendations for wound care, including administration of passive immunization to persons who are unimmunized or whose immunization status is unknown.

11. References

1. ABEL, J. J., FIROR W. M., AND CHALAIN, W., Researches on tetanus. IX. Further evidence to show that tetanus toxin is not carried to central nervous system by way of the axis cylinders of motor nerves, *Bull. Johns Hopkins Hosp.* **63:**373–402 (1938).
2. ADAMS, E. B., The prognosis and prevention of tetanus, *S. Afr. Med. J.* **42:**739–743 (1968).
3. ALFERY, D. D., AND RAUSCHER, L. A., Tetanus: A review, *Crit. Care Med.* **7:**176–181 (1979).
4. ANONYMOUS, Postoperative tetanus [editorial], *Lancet* **2:**964–965 (1984).

5. BALL, K., ELFORD, J., AND SEAMAN, J., Tetanus and altitude [letter], *Lancet* **1**:801–802 (1987).

6. BAND, J. D., AND BENNETT, J. V., Tetanus, in: *Infectious Diseases: A Modern treatise of Infectious Processes,* 3rd ed. (P. D. Hoeprich, ed.), pp. 1107–1114, Harper & Row, New York, 1983.

7. BANDMANN, F., Zum nachweis von tetanusbaccilen im darm von ulcus- und carcinomträgern, *Z. Hyg.* **136**:559–567 (1953).

8. BANTON, H. J., AND MILLER, P. A., An observation of antitoxin titers after booster doses of tetanus toxoid, *N. Engl. J. Med.* **240**:13–14 (1949).

9. BARILE, M. F., HARDEGREE, M. C., AND PITTMAN, M., Immunization against neonatal tetanus in New Guinea. 3. The toxin-neutralization test and the response of guinea-pigs to the toxoids as used in the immunization schedules in New Guinea, *Bull. WHO* **43**:453–459 (1970).

10. BARKIN, R. M., SAMUELSON, J. S., AND GOTLIN, L. P., DTP reactions and serologic response with a reduced dose schedule, *J. Pediatr.* **105**:189–194 (1984).

11. BARKIN, R. M., PICHICHERO, M. E., SAMUELSON, J. S., AND BARKIN, S. Z., Pediatric diphtheria and tetanus toxoids vaccine: Clinical and immunologic response when administered as the primary series, *J. Pediatr.* **106**:779–781 (1985).

12. BARR, M., GLENNY, A. T., AND BUTLER, N. R., Immunization of babies with diphtheria–tetanus–pertussis prophylactic, *Br. Med. J.* **2**:635–639 (1955).

13. BARRETT, C. D., TIMM, E. A., MOLNER, J. G., TIMM, E. A., AND WEISS, C. F., Multiple antigen immunization of infants against poliomyelitis, diphtheria, pertussis and tetanus. II. Response of infants and young children to primary immunization and eighteen-month booster, *Am. J. Public Health* **49**:644–655 (1959).

14. BARRETT, C. D., MCLEON, I. W., MOLNER, J. G., TIMM, E. A., AND WEISS, C. F., Multiple antigen immunization of infants against poliomyelitis, diphtheria, pertussis and tetanus. An evaluation of antibody responses of infants one day old to seven months of age at start of inoculations, *Pediatrics* **30**:720–736 (1962).

15. BAUER, J. H., AND MEYER, K. F., Human intestinal carriers of tetanus spores in California, *J. Infect. Dis.* **38**:295–305 (1926).

16. BEHRING, E. VON, AND KITASATO, S., Ueber das Zustandekommen der Diphtherie-Immunität und Tetanus-Immunität bie Thieren, *Dtsch. Med. Wochenschr.* **16**:1113–1114 (1890).

17. BERGER, S. A., CHERUBIN, L. E., NELSON, S., AND LEVINE, L., Tetanus despite preexisting antitetanus antibody, *J. Am. Med. Assoc.* **240**:769–770 (1978).

18. BERGGREN, G. G., BERGGREN, W., VERLY, A., GARNIER, N., PETERSON, W., EWBANK, O., AND DIEVDONNE, W., Traditional midwives, tetanus immunization, and infant mortality in rural Haiti, *Trop. Doct.* **13**:79–87 (1983).

19. BERNATH, S., AND HABERMANN, E., Solid-phase radioimmunoassay in antibody coated tubes for the quantitative determination of tetanus antibodies, *Med. Microbiol. Immunol.* **160**:47–51 (1974).

20. BERNBAUM, J. C., DAFT, A., ANOLIK, R., SAMUELSON, J., BARKIN, R., DOUGLAS, S., AND POLIN, R., Response of preterm infants to diphtheria–tetanus–pertussis immunizations, *J. Pediatr.* **107**:184–188 (1985).

21. BHAT, G. J., JOSHI, M. K., AND KANDOTH, P. W., Neonatal tetanus: A clinical study of 100 cases, *Indian Pediatr.* **16**:159–166 (1979).

22. BHATT, A. D., AND DASTUR, F. D., Relapsing tetanus: A case report, *J. Postgrad. Med.* **27**:184–186 (1981).

23. BIZZINI, B., Tetanus toxin, *Microbiol. Rev.* **43**:224–240 (1979).

24. BIZZINI, B., Tetanus, in: *Bacterial Vaccines* (R. Germanier, ed.), pp. 38–68, Academic Press, New York, 1984.

25. BIZZINI, B., The chemistry of tetanus toxin as a basis for understanding its immunological and biological activities, in: *Seventh International Conference on Tetanus* (G. Nistico, P. Mastroeni, and M. Pitzurra, eds.), pp. 11–28, Gangeni, Rome, 1985.

26. BLAKE, P. A., AND FELDMAN, R. A., Tetanus in the United States 1970–1971, *J. Infect. Dis.* **131**:745–748 (1975).

27. BLECK, T. P., Pharmacology of tetanus, *Clin. Neuropharmacol.* **9**:103–120 (1986).

28. BOYD, R. E., BRENNAN, P. T., DENJ, J.-F., ROCHESTER, D. F., AND SPYKER, D. A., Strychnine poisoning, *Am. J. Med.* **74**:507–512 (1983).

29. BRAND, D. A., ACAMPORA, D., GOTTLIEG, L., GLANCY, K. E., AND FRAZIER, W. H., Adequacy of antitetanus prophylaxis in six hospital emergency rooms, *N. Engl. J. Med.* **309**:636–640 (1983).

30. BROOKS, V. B., AND ASANUMA, H., Action of tetanus toxin in the cerebral cortex, *Science* **137**:674–676 (1962).

31. BROOKS, V. B., CURTIS, D. R., AND ECCLES, J. C., Mode of action of tetanus toxin, *Nature* **175**:120–121 (1955).

32. BROWN, G. C., VOLK, V. K., GOTTSHALL, R. Y., KENDRICK, P. L., AND ANDERSON, H. D., Responses of infants to DTP-P vaccine used in nine injection schedules, *Public Health Rep.* **79**:585–602 (1964).

33. BRUCE, D., Tetanus, *J. Hyg.* **19**:1–32 (1920).

34. BUCHANAN, N., CANE, G. W., AND DEANDRADE, M., Autonomic dysfunction in tetanus: The effects of a variety of therapeutic agents, with special reference to morphine, *Intensive Care Med.* **5**:65–68 (1979).

35. BUCHANAN, T. M., BROOKS, G. F., MARTIN, S., AND BENNETT, J. V., Tetanus in the United States, 1968 and 1969, *J. Infect. Dis.* **122**:564–567 (1970).

36. BULLOCH, W. E., AND CRAMER, W., On a new factor in the mechanism of bacterial infection, *Proc. R. Soc. London Ser. B* **90**:513–528 (1919).

37. BYTCHENKO, B., Geographical distribution of tetanus in the world, 1951–60, *Bull. WHO* **34**:71–104 (1966).

38. BYTCHENKO, B., Microbiology of tetanus, in: *Tetanus: Important New Concepts* (R. VERONESI, ed.), pp. 28–39, Excerpta Medica, Amsterdam, 1981.

39. BYTCHENKO, B., Current status of tetanus in the European region in: *Eighth International Conference on Tetanus* (G. NISTICO, B. BIZZINI, B. BYTCHENKO, AND R. TRIAU, eds.), Pythagora Press, Rome (in press).

40. BYTCHENKO, B. D., CAUSSE, G., GRAB, B., AND KERESELIDZE, T. S., Tetanus: Recent trends of world distribution, in: *Sixth International Conference on Tetanus* (C. Merieux, ed.), pp. 97–111, Collection Foundation Merieux, Lyon, 1981.

41. CAIN, H. D., AND FALCO, F. G., Recurrent tetanus, *Calif. Med.* **97**:31–33 (1962).

42. CARLE, AND RATTONE, Studio spetrimentale sull' etiologia del tetano, G. *Accad. Med. Torino* 32:174 (1884).

43. Centers for Disease Control, Safety of theraputic immune globulin preparations with respect to transmission of human T-lymphocytic virus type III/lymphadenopathy-associated virus infection, *Morbid. Mortal. Weekly Rep.* **35**:231–233 (1986).

44. CHEN, S. T., EDSALL, G., PEEL, M. M., AND SINNATHURAY, T. A., Timing of antenatal tetanus immunization for effective protection of the neonate, *Bull. WHO* **61**:159–163 (1983).

45. CHERUBIN, C. E., Epidemiology of tetanus in narcotic addicts, *N.Y. State J. Med.* **70**:267–271 (1970).

46. CHRISTIANSEN, G., Quantification of tetanus antitoxin by toxin neutralization test in mice. A comparison between lethal and paralytic techniques, *J. Biol. Stand.* **9**:453–460 (1981).

47. CLIFF, J., Neonatal tetanus in Maputo, Mozambique. Part I: Hospital incidence and childbirth practices, *Cent. Afr. J. Med.* **31**:9–12 (1985).

48. COLEMAN, G. E., AND MEYER, K. F., Study of tetanus agglutinins and antitoxin in human serums, *J. Infect. Dis.* **39**:332–336 (1926).

49. COLLIER, L. H., POLAKOFF, S., AND MORTIMER, J., Reactions and antibody responses to reinforcing doses of adsorbed and plain tetanus vaccines, *Lancet* **1**:1364–1368 (1979).

50. Committee on Infectious Diseases, American Academy of Pediatrics, *Report of the Committee on Infectious Diseases* (G. PETER, C. B. HALL, M. L. LEPOW, AND C. F. PHILLIPS, eds.), American Academy of Pediatrics, Elk Grove Village, Ill. 1988.

51. Committee on Trauma, American College of Surgeons, Prophylaxis against tetanus in wound management, *Am. Coll. Surg. Bull.* **69**:22–23 (1984).

52. COOKE, J. V., HOLOWACH, J., ATKINS, J. E., AND POWENS, J. R., Antibody formation in early infancy against diphtheria and tetanus toxoids, *J. Pediatr.* **33**:141–146 (1948).

53. COURSAGET, P., YVONNET, B., RELYVELD, E. H., AND BARNES, J. L., Simultaneous administration of diphtheria/tetanus/pertussis/polio vaccine and hepatitis B vaccine in a simplified immunization programme, *Dev. Biol. Stand.* **65**:169–175 (1986).

54. COX, J. C., PERMIER, R. R., FINGER, W., AND HURRELL, J. G., A comparison of enzyme immunoassay and bioassay for the quantitative determination of antibodies to tetanus toxin, *J. Biol. Stand.* **11**:123–128 (1983).

55. CROSSLEY, K., IRVINE, P., WARREN, B., LEE, B. K., AND MEAD, K., Tetanus and diphtheria immunity in urban Minnesota adults, *J. Am. Med. Assoc.* **242**:2298–2300 (1979).

56. DASTUR, D. D., AWATRAMANI, V. P., AND DIXIT, S. K., Response to single dose of tetanus vaccine in subjects with naturally acquired tetanus antitoxin, *Lancet* **2**:219–222 (1981).

57. DESCOMBEY, P., L'anatoxine tetanique, *Can. R. Soc. Biol.* **91**:239–241 (1924).

58. DHILLON, H., AND MENON, P. S., Active immunization of women in pregnancy with two injections of absorbed tetanus toxoid for prevention of tetanus neonaturum in Punjab, India, *Indian J. Med. Res.* **63**:583–589 (1975). 589 (1975).

59. DI SANT AGNESE, P. A., Combined immunization against diphtheria, tetanus, and pertussis in newborn infants. I. Production of antibodies in early infancy, *Pediatrics* **3**:20–33 (1949).

60. DI SANT AGNESE, P. A., Combined immunization against diphtheria, tetanus, and pertussis in newborn infants. II. Duration of antibody levels. Antibody titers after booster dose. Effect of passive immunity to diphtheria on active immunization with diphtheria toxoid, *Pediatrics* **3**:181–194 (1949).

61. DI SANT AGNESE, P. A., Combined immunization against diphtheria, tetanus, and pertussis in newborn infants. III. Relationship of age to antibody production, *Pediatrics* **3**:333–344 (1949).

62. DI SANT AGNESE, P. A., Simultaneous immunization of newborn infants against diphtheria, tetanus, and pertussis. Production of antibodies and duration of antibody levels in an eastern metropolitan area, *Am. J. Public Health* **40**:674–680 (1950).

63. EDMONDSON, R. S., AND FLOWERS, M. W., Intensive care in tetanus: Management, complications and mortality in 100 cases, *Br. Med. J.* **1**:1401–1404 (1979).

64. EDSALL, G., The inexcusable disease, *J. Am. Med. Assoc.* **235**:62–63 (1976).

65. EDSALL, G., Problems in the immunology and control of tetanus, *Med. J. Aust.* **2**:216–220 (1976).

66. EDSALL, G., ELLIOT, M. W., PEEBLES, T. C., AND ELONED, M. C., Excessive use of tetanus toxoid boosters, *J. Am. Med. Assoc.* **202**:17–19 (1967).

67. EINHORN, M. S., GRANOFF, D. M., NAHM, M. H., QUINN, A., AND SHACKELFORD, P. G., Concentrations of antibodies in paired maternal and infant sera: Relationship to IgG subclass, *J. Pediatr.* **111**:783–788 (1987).

68. Expanded Programme on Immunization, Global Advisory Group, *Weekly Epidemiol. Rec.* **60**:13–16 (1985).

69. Expanded Programme on Immunization, Information System, WHO/EPI/GEN/89.2, July 1989, p. 1.

70. Expanded Programme on Immunization, EPI Update. Neonatal Tetanus: The Invisible Killer, WHO, September 1986.

71. Expanded Programme on Immunization, Issues in Neonatal Tetanus Control, EPI/GAG/87/WP. 11, WHO, 1987.

72. FACKTOR, M. A., BERNSTEIN, R. A., AND FIREMAN, P., Hypersensitivity to tetanus toxoid, *J. Allergy Clin. Immunol.* **52**:1–12 (1973).

73. FEDINEC, A. A., Current studies on pathogenesis of tetanus, in: *Seventh International Conference on Tetanus* (G. Nistico, P. Mastroeni, and M. Pitzurra, eds.), pp. 61–68, Rome, 1985.

74. FINN, L. W., JR., SILVER, R. P., HABIG, W. H., AND HANDEGNEE, M. C., The structural gene for tetanus neurotoxin is on a plasmid, *Science* **224**:881–884 (1984).

75. FRIEDEMANN, U., ZUGER, B., AND HOLLANDER, A., Investigations on the pathogenesis of tetanus, *J. Immunol.* **36**:473–488 (1939).

76. GAISFORD, W. FELOMAN, G. V., AND PENKINS, F. T., Current immunization problems, *J. Pediatr.* **56**:319–330 (1960).

77. GALAZKA, A., GASSE, F., AND HENDERSON, R. H., Neonatal tetanus in the world and the global Expanded Programme on Immunization, in: *Eighth International Conference on Tetanus* (G. NISTICO, B. BIZZINI, B. BYTCHENKO, AND R. TRIAU, eds.), Pythagora Press, Rome (in press).

78. GARCIA-PALMIERI, M. R., AND RAMIREZ, R., Generalized tetanus: Analysis of 202 cases, *Ann. Intern. Med.* **47**:721–730 (1957).

79. GARNIER, M. J., Tetanus in patients 3 years of age and up, *Am. J. Surg.* **129**:459–463 (1975).

80. GIANGROSSO, J., AND SMITH, R. K., Misuse of tetanus immunoprophylaxis in wound care, *Ann. Emerg. Med.* **14**:573–579 (1985).

81. GILL, D. M., Bacterial toxins: A table of lethal amount, *Microbiol. Rev.* **46**:86–94 (1982).

82. GOTTLIEB, S., McLAUGHLIN, F. X., LEVINE, L., LATHAM, W. C., AND EDSALL, G., Long-term immunity to tetanus: A statistical evaluation and its clinical implications, *Am. J. Public Health* **54**:961–971 (1964).

83. GREEN, J., ERDMANN, J. G., AND WELLHOVER, H. H., Is there retrograde axonal transport of tetanus toxin in both alpha and gamma fibres? *Nature* **265**:370 (1977).

84. GUPTA, R. K., MAHESHWARI, S. C., AND SINGH, H., The titration of tetanus antitoxin. I. Factors affecting the sensitivity of the indirect haemagglutination test, *J. Biol. Stand* **12**:11–17 (1984).

85. GUPTA, R. K., MAHESHWARI, S. C., AND SINGH, H., The titration of tetanus antitoxin. II. A comparative evaluation of the indirect haemagglutination and toxin neutralization tests, *J. Biol. Stand.* **12**:137–143 (1984).

86. HALSEY, N. A., AND GALAZKA, A., The efficacy of DPT and oral poliomyelitis immunization schedules initiated from birth to 12 weeks of age, *Bull. WHO* **63**:1151–1169 (1985).

87. HAMID, E. D., DAULAY, A. P., LUBIS, C. P., RUSDIDJAS, AND SIREGAR, H., Tetanus neonatorum in babies delivered by traditional birth attendants in Medan, Indonesia, *Pediatr. Indones.* **25**:167–174 (1985).

88. HARDEGREE, M. C., BARILE, M. F., PITTMAN, M., MAL-

ONEY, C. J., SCHOFIELD, F., AND MacLENNAN, R., Immunization against neonatal tetanus in New Guinea. 4. Comparison of tetanus antitoxin titers obtained by haemagglutination and toxin neutralization in mice, *Bull. WHO* **43**:461–468 (1970).

89. HEATH, C. W., ZUSMAN, J., AND SHERMAN, I. L., Tetanus in the United States, 1950–1960, *Am. J. Public Health* **54**:769–779 (1964).

90. HERNANDEZ, R., JUST, M., AND BURGIN-WOLF, A., Immunoglobulin classes of human antitoxin after tetanus vaccination studies by immunofluorescence with agarose bound tetanus toxoid, *Z. Immunol. Forsch.* **145**:376–384 (1973).

91. HINMAN, A. R., FOSTER, S. O., AND WASSILAK, S. G. F., Neonatal tetanus: Potential for elimination in the USA and the world, *Pediatr. Infect. Dis. J.* **6**:813–816 (1987).

92. HOLDEN, J. M., AND STRANG, D. U., Reactions to tetanus toxoid: Comparison of fluid and adsorbed toxoids, *N. Z. Med. J.* **64**:574–577 (1965).

93. HOLLIDAY, P. L., AND BAUER, R. B., Polyradiculoneuritis secondary to immunization with tetanus and diphtheria toxoids, *Arch. Neurol.* **40**:56–57 (1983).

94. HOLLOW, V. M., AND CLARKE, G. M., Autonomic manifestations of tetanus, *Anaesth. Intensive Care* **3**:142–147 (1975).

95. HUMBERT, G., FILLASTRE, J. P., DORDAIN, M., LEROY, J., ROBERT, M., AND DeLAUNAY, P., One hundred cases of tetanus, *Scand. J. Infect. Dis.* **4**:129–131 (1972).

96. Immunization Practices Advisory Committee (ACIP), Diphtheria, tetanus and pertussis. Guidelines for vaccine prophylaxis and other preventive measures, *Morbid. Mortal. Weekly Rep.* **34**:405–414, 419–426 (1985).

97. Immunization Practices Advisory Committee (ACIP), New recommended schedule for active immunization of normal infants and children, *Morbid. Mortal. Weekly Rep.* **35**:577–579 (1986).

98. JACOBS, R. L., LOWE, R. S., AND LANIER, B. Q., Adverse reactions to tetanus toxoid, *J. Am. Med. Assoc.* **247**:40–42 (1982).

99. JAGETIYA, P., AND BHANDARI, B., Analysis of tetanus neonatorum cases admitted in a hospital during 1976–1977, *Indian J. Public Health* **23**:103–105 (1979).

100. JONES, A. E., MELVILLE-SMITH, M., WATKINS, J., SEAGROATT, V., RICE, L., AND SHEFFIELD, F., Adverse reactions in adolescents to reinforcing doses of plain and adsorbed tetanus vaccines, *Community Med.* **7**:99–106 (1985).

101. JONES, F. G., AND MOSS, J., Studies on tetanus toxoid. I: The antitoxic titer of human subject following immunization with tetanus toxoid and tetanus alum precipitated toxoid, *J. Immunol.* **30**:115–125 (1936).

102. KAISER, G. C., KING, R. D., LEMPE, R. E., AND RUSTER, M. H., Delayed recall of active tetanus immunization, *J. Am. Med. Assoc.* **178**:914–916 (1961).

103. KANAREK, D. J., KAUFMAN, B., AND ZWI, S., Severe sympathetic hyperactivity associated with tetanus, *Arch. Intern. Med.* **132**:602–604 (1973).

104. KERR, J. H., CORBETT, J. L., PRYS-ROBERTS, C., SMITH, A. C., AND SPALDING, J. M., Involvement of the sympathetic nervous system in tetanus: Studies on 82 cases, *Lancet* **2:**236–241 (1968).

105. KERRIN, J. C., The incidence of *B. tetani* in human feces, *Br. J. Pathol.* **9:**69–71 (1928).

106. KESSEL, E., Strategies for the control of neonatal tetanus, *J. Trop. Pediatr.* **30:**145–149 (1984).

107. KIELMAM, A. A., AND VOHRA, S. R., Control of tetanus neonatorum in rural communities—Immunization effects of high-dose calcium phosphate-adsorbed tetanus toxoid, *Indian J. Med. Res.* **66:**906–916 (1977).

108. KIRCHER, T., AND ANDERSON, R. E., Cause of death: Proper completion of the death certificate, *J. Am. Med. Assoc.* **77:**137–139 (1987).

109. KISHIMOTO, S., TOMINO, S., MITSUYA, H., FUJIWARA, H., AND TSUDA, H., Age-related decline in the in vitro and in vivo syntheses of anti-tetanus toxoid antibody in humans, *J. Immunol.* **125:**2347–2352 (1980).

110. KITASATO, S., Ueber den tetanusbacillus, *Z. Hyg.* **7:**225–234 (1889).

110a. KOBLIN, B. A., AND TOWNSEND, T. R., Immunity to diphtheria and tetanus in inner-city women of childbearing age, *Am. J. Public Health* **79:**1297–1298 (1989).

111. KRYZHANOVSKY, G. N., Pathophysiology, in: *Tetanus: Important New Concepts* (R. VERONESI, ed.), pp. 109–182, Excerpta Medica, Amsterdam, 1981.

112. LAIRD, W. J., AARONSON, W., SILVER, R. P., HABIG, W. H., AND HARDEGREE, M. C., Plasmid-associated toxigenicity in *Clostridium tetani, J. Infect. Dis.* **142:**623 (1980).

113. LAYTON, G. T., A micro-enzyme-linked immunosorbent assay (ELISA) and radioimmunosorbent technique (RIST) for the detection of immunity to clinical tetanus, *Med. Lab. Sci.* **37:**323–329 (1980).

114. LEVINE, L., AND EDSALL, G., Tetanus toxoid: What determines reaction proneness? *J. Infect. Dis.* **144:**376 (1981).

115. LEVINE, L., MCCOMB, J. A., DWYER, R. C., AND LATHAM, W. C. Active–passive tetanus immunization, *N. Engl. J. Med.* **274:**186–190 (1966).

116. LEVINSON, A. K., MARSKE, R. L., AND SHEIN, M. K., Tetanus in heroin addicts, *J. Am. Med. Assoc.* **157:**658–660 (1955).

117. LONG, A. P., AND SARTWELL, P. E., Tetanus in the U.S. Army in World War II, *Bull. U.S. Army Med. Dep.* **7:**371–385 (1947).

118. LOWBURY, E. J. L., AND LILLY, H. A., Contamination of operating-theatre air with *Cl. tetani, Br. Med. J.* **2:**1334–1336 (1958).

119. LOWBURY, E. J. L., KIDSON, A., LILLY, H. A., WILKINS, M. D., AND JACKSON, O. M., Prophylaxis against tetanus in non-immune patients with wounds: The role of antibiotics and of human antitetanus globulin, *J. Hyg.* **80:**267–274. (1978).

120. MACKO, M. B., Comparison of the morbidity of tetanus toxoid boosters with tetanus–diphtheria toxoid boosters, *Ann. Emerg. Med.* **14:**33–35 (1985).

121. MACLENNAN, R., SCHOFIELD, F. D., PITTMAN, M., HARDEGREE, M. C., AND BANILE, M. F., Immunization against neonatal tetanus in New Guinea: Antitoxin response of pregnant women to adjuvant and plain toxoids, *Bull. WHO* **32:**683–697 (1965).

122. MAHONEY, L. J., APRILE, M. A., AND MOLONEY, P. J., Combined active–passive immunization against tetanus in man, *Can. Med. Assoc. J.* **96:**1401–1404 (1967).

123. MARCONI, P., PITZURRA, M., AND BISTONI, F., Passive hemagglutination as the reference method for evaluation of tetanus immunity, in: *Seventh International Conference on Tetanus* (G. Nistico, P. Mastroeni, and M. Pitzurra, eds.), pp. 259–273, Gangeni, Rome, 1985.

124. MATSUDA, M., AND YONEDA, M., Isolation and purification of two antigenically active, "complementary" polypeptide fragments of tetanus neurotoxin, *Infect. Immun.* **12:**1147–1153 (1975).

125. MATZKIN, H., AND REGEV, S., Naturally acquired immunity to tetanus toxin in an isolated community, *Infect. Immun.* **48:**267–268 (1985).

126. McCOMB, J. A., The prophylactic dose of homologous tetanus antitoxin, *N. Engl. J. Med.* **270:**175–178 (1964).

127. McComb, J. A., and Levine, L., Adult immunization. II. Dosage reduction as a solution to increasing reactions to tetanus toxoid, *N. Engl. J. Med.* **265:**1152–1153 (1961).

128. MELVILLE-SMITH, M. E., SEAGROATT, V. A., AND WATKINS, J. T., A comparison of enzyme-linked immunosorbent assay (ELISA) with the toxin neutralization test in mice as a method for the estimation of tetanus antitoxin in human sera, *J. Biol. Stand.* **11:** 137–144 (1983).

129. MILLARD, A. H., Local tetanus, *Lancet* **2:**844–846 (1954).

130. MOYNIHAN, N. H., Serum sickness and local reactions in tetanus prophylaxis: A study of 400 cases, *Br. Med. J.* **2:**264–266 (1955).

131. MYERS, M. G., BECKMAN, C. W., VOSDINGH, R. A., AND HANKIN, S., Primary immunization with tetanus and diphtheria toxoids. Reaction rate and immunogenicity in older children and adults, *J. Am. Med. Assoc.* **248:**2478–2480 (1982).

132. NEWELL, K. W., DUENAS LEHMAN, A., LeBLANC, D. R., AND GARCES OSORIO, N., The use of toxoid for the prevention of tetanus neonatorum. Final report of a double-blind controlled field trial, *Bull. WHO* **35:**863–871 (1966).

133. NICOLAIER, A., Ueber infectiosen tetanus, *Dtsch. Med. Wochenschr.* **10:**842–844 (1884).

134. ORENSTEIN, W. A., WEISFELD, J. S., AND HALSEY, N. A., Diphtheria and tetanus toxoids and pertussis vaccine, combined, in: *Recent Advances in Immunization: A Bibliographic Review*, PAHO Scientific Publ. 451, 1983, pp. 30–51.

135. OURTH, D. D., AND MacDONALD, A. B., Neutralization of tetanus toxin by human and rabbit immunoglobulin classes and subunits, *Immunology* **3:**807–815 (1977).

136. OURTH, D. D., MURRAY, E. S., MacDONALD, A. B., AND SPIELMAN, J. M., An indirect immunofluorescent test for human antibodies to tetanus toxoid using an insoluble toxoid as antigen, *J. Clin. Exp. Immunol.* **19:**571–577 (1975).

137. PASSEN, E. L., AND ANDERSEN, B. R., Clinical tetanus de-

spite a 'protective' level of toxin-neutralizing antibody, *J. Am. Med. Assoc.* **255:**1171–1173 (1986).

138. PATEL, J. C., MEHTA, B. C., AND MODI, K. N., Prognosis in tetanus, in: *Proceedings of the International Conference on Tetanus, 1963* (J. C. PATEL, ed.), p. 181, PH Ramans, Bombay, 1965.

139. PEEBLES, T. C., LEVINE, L., ELDRED, M. L., EDSALL, G., Tetanus-toxoid emergency boosters: A reappraisal, *N. Engl. J. Med.* **280:**575–581 (1969).

140. PEEL, M. M., Measurement of tetanus antitoxin. I. Indirect haemagglutination, *J. Biol. Stand.* **8:**177–189 (1980).

141. PETERSON, J. C., AND CHRISTIE, A., Immunization in the young infant: Response to combined vaccines. VI. Tetanus, *Am. J. Dis. Child.* **81:**518–529 (1951).

142. PICHICHERO, M. E., BARKIN, R. M., AND SAMUELSON, J. S., Pediatric diphtheria and tetanus toxoids—adsorbed vaccine: Immune response to the first booster following the diphtheria and tetanus toxoids primary series, *Pediatr. Infect. Dis. J.* **5:**428–430 (1986).

143. PITZURRA, L. F., BISTONI, M., PITZURRA, L., BASTIANINI, L., PIENTO, S., VECCHIARELLI, A., AND MARCONI, P., Comparison of passive haemagglutination with turkey erythrocyte assay, enzyme-linked immunosorbent assay and counter immunoelectrophoresis assay for serological evaluation of tetanus immunity, *J. Clin. Microbiol.* **17:**432–435 (1983).

144. PRATT, E. L., Clinical tetanus: A study of fifty-six cases with special reference to methods of prevention and a plan for evaluating treatment, *J. Am. Med. Assoc.* **129:**1243–1247 (1945).

145. PRICE, D. L., GRIFFIN, J. W., YOUNG, A., PECK, K., AND STOCK, A., Tetanus toxin: Direct evidence for retrograde axonal transport, *Science* **188:**945–957 (1975).

146. RAY, S. N., RAY, K., AND GROVER, S. S., Sero-survey of diphtheria and tetanus antitoxin, *Indian J. Med. Res.* **68:**901–904 (1978).

147. REY, M., AND THIKHOMIROV, E., Non-neonatal tetanus over the world, in: *Eighth International Conference on Tetanus* (G. NISTICO, B. BIZZINI, B. BYTCHENKO, AND R. TRIAU, eds.), Pythagora Press, Rome (in press).

148. ROBINSON, J. P., AND HASH, J. H., A review of the molecular structure of tetanus toxin, *Mol. Cell. Biochem.* **48:**33–44 (1982).

149. ROISTACHER, K., AND GRIFFIN, J. W., Local tetanus, *Johns Hopkins Med. J.* **149:**84–88 (1981).

150. ROSENBACH, Zur aetiologie des wundstarrkrampfes beim menschen, *Arch. Klin. Chir.* **34:**306–317 (1886).

151. RUBEN, F. L., NAGEL, J., AND FIREMAN, P., Antitoxin responses in the elderly to tetanus–diphtheria (Td) immunization, *Am. J. Epidemiol.* **108:**145–149 (1978).

152. RUTLEDGE, S. L., AND SNEAD, O. C., Neurologic complications of immunizations, *J. Pediatr.* **109:**917–923 (1986).

153. SALIMPOUR, R., Cause of death in tetanus neonatorum: Study of 233 cases with 54 necropsies, *Arch. Dis. Child.* **52:**587–594 (1977).

154. SCHEIBEL, I., BENTZON, M. W., CHRISTENSEN, P. E., AND BIERING, A., Duration of immunity to diphtheria and tetanus after active immunization, *Acta Pathol. Microbiol. Scand.* **67:**380–392 (1966).

155. SCHWAB, M. E., AND THOENEN, H., Selective binding, uptake and retrograde transport of tetanus toxin by nerve terminals in the rat iris, *J. Cell Biol.* **77:**1–13 (1978).

156. SEDGWICK, A. K., BALLOW, M., SPARKS, K., AND TILTON, R. C., Rapid quantitative micro-enzyme-linked immunosorbent assay for tetanus antibodies, *J. Clin. Microbiol.* **18:**104–109 (1983).

157. SIMONSEN, O., KJELDSEN, K., AND HERON, I., Immunity against tetanus and effect of revaccination 25–30 years after primary vaccination, *Lancet* **2:**1240–1242 (1984).

158. SISK, C. W., AND LEWIS, C. E., Reactions to tetanus–diphtheria toxoid (adult), *Arch. Environ. Health* **11:**34–36 (1965).

159. SMITH, J. W. G., Diphtheria and tetanus toxoids, *Br. Med. Bull* **25:**177–182 (1969).

160. SMITH, J. W. G., Tetanus and its prevention, *Prog. Drug Res.* **19:**391–401 (1975).

161. SMITH, J. W. G., Tetanus, in: *Topley and Wilson's Principles of Bacteriology, Virology and Immunity*, Volume 3 (G. WILSON, A. MILES, AND M. T. PARKER, eds.), pp. 345–368, Williams & Wilkins, Baltimore, 1984.

162. SMITH, J. W. G., AND MacIVER, A. G., Studies in experimental tetanus infection, *J. Med. Microbiol.* **2:**385–393 (1969).

163. SMITH, J. W. G., LAURENCE, D. R., AND EVANS, D. G., Prevention of tetanus in the wounded, *Br. Med. J.* **3:**453–455 (1975).

164. SMITH, R. E., AND WOLNISTY, C., Allergic reactions to tetanus, diphtheria, influenza and poliomyelitis immunization, *Ann. Allergy* **20:**809–813 (1962).

165. SMITH, W. D., AND TOBIAS, M. A., Tetany, tetanus or drug reaction? *Br. J. Anaesth.* **48:**703–705 (1976).

166. SOLOMONOVA, K., AND VIZEV, S., Secondary response to boostering by purified aluminum-hydroxide-adsorbed tetanus antitoxin in aging and in aged adults, *Immunobiology* **158:**312–319 (1981).

167. SPENNEY, J. G., LAMB, R. N., AND COBBS, C. G., Recurrent tetanus, *South. Med. J.* **64:**859–862 (1971).

168. STANFIELD, J. P., AND GALAZKA, A., Neonatal tetanus in the world today, *Bull. WHO* **62:**647–669 (1984).

169. SULEMAN, O., Mortality from tetanus neonatorum in Punjab (Pakistan), *Pak. Pediatr. J.* **6:**152–183 (1982).

170. SURI, J. C., AND RUBBO, S. D., Immunization against tetanus, *J. Hyg.* **59:**29–48 (1961).

171. SUTTER, R. W., COCHI, S. L., BRINK, E. W., AND SIROTKIN, B. I., Assessment of vital statistics and surveillance data for monitoring tetanus mortality, 1979–1984 *Am. J. Epidemiol.* **131:**132–142 (1990).

172. TENBROECK, C., AND BAUER, J. H., The tetanus bacillus as an intestinal saprophyte in man, *J. Exp. Med.* **36:**261–271 (1922).

173. TENBROECK, C., AND BAUER, J. H., Studies on the relation of tetanus bacilli in the digestive tract to tetanus antitoxin in the blood, *J. Exp. Med.* **37:**479–489 (1923).

173a. TRAVERSO, H. D., BENNET, J. V., KAHN, A. J., AGHAN, S. B., RAHIM, H., KAMIL, S., AND LANG, M. H., Ghee application to the umbilical cord: A risk factor for tetanus, *Lancet* **1**:486–488 (1989).

174. TRUJILLO, M. J., CASTILLO, A., ESPANA, J. V., GUEVANA, P., AND EGANEZ, H., Tetanus in the adult: Intensive care and management experience with 233 cases, *Crit. Care Med.* **8**:419–423 (1980).

175. TRUJILLO, M. H., CASTILLO, A., ESPANA, J., MANZO, A., AND ZERPA, R., Impact of intensive care management on the prognosis of tetanus. Analysis of 641 cases, *Chest* **92**:63–65 (1987).

176. TULLOCH, W. J., Report of bacteriological investigation of tetanus carried out on behalf of the war office committee for the study of tetanus, *J. Hyg.* **18**:103–202 (1919).

177. TURNER, T. B., VELASCO-JOVEN, E. A., AND PRUDOVSKY, S., Studies on the prophylaxis and treatment of tetanus. II. Studies pertaining to treatment, *Bull. Johns Hopkins Hosp.* **102**:71–84 (1958).

178. ULLBERG-OLSSON, K., Vaccinationsreaktioner efter injektion: av tetanustoxoid med och utan tillsats av difteritoxoid, *Lakartidningen* **76**:2976 (1979).

179. VAN HEYNINGEN, S., Tetanus toxin, *Pharmacol. Ther.* **11**:141–157 (1980).

180. VASSILEV, T. L., Aluminum phosphate but not calcium phosphate stimulates the specific IgE response in guinea-pigs to tetanus toxoid, *Allergy* **33**:155–159 (1978).

181. VERONESI, R., Naturally acquired tetanus immunity: Still a controversial theme? in: *Seventh International Conference on Tetanus* (G. NISTICO, P. MASTROENI, AND M. PITZURRA, eds.), Gangeni, Rome, 1985, pp 365–372.

182. VERONESI, R., AND FOCACCIA, R., The clinical picture, in: *Tetanus: Important New Concepts* (R. Veronesi, ed.), pp. 459–463, Excerpta Medica, Amsterdam, 1981.

183. VERONESI, R., BIZZINI, B., FOCACCIA, R., COSCINA, A. L., MAZZA, C. C., FOCACCIA, M. T., CARRARO, F., AND HONNINGMAN, M. N., Naturally acquired antibodies to tetanus toxin in humans and animals from the Galapagos Islands, *J. Infect. Dis.* **147**:308–311 1983).

184. WANG, A. S., BURNS, G. F., KRONBORG, I. J., AND MACKEY, I. R., Detection of antibodies to tetanus toxoid: Comparison of a direct haemagglutination method with a radioimmunoassay, *J. Clin. Pathol.* **35**:1138–1141 (1982).

185. WEINSTEIN, L., Tetanus, *N. Engl. J. Med.* **289**:1293–1296. (1973).

186. WEISS, B. P., STRASSBURG, M. A., AND FEELEY, J. C., Tetanus and diphtheria immunity in an elderly population in Los Angeles County, *Am. J. Public Health* **73**:802–804 (1983).

187. WELLHONER, J. J., Tetanus neurotoxin, *Rev. Physiol. Biochem. Pharmacol.* **93**:1–68 (1982).

188. WHITE, W. G., BARNES, G. M., BARKER, E., GALL, D., KNIGHT, P., GRIFFITH, A.H., MORRIS-OWEN, R. M., AND SMITH, J. W., Reactions to tetanus toxoid, *J. Hyg.* **71**:283–297 (1973).

189. WILLIAMS, J. J., AND ELLINGSON, H. V., Field trial of commercially-prepared diphtheria–tetanus toxoid: Immunization reactions among recruits, Unpublished report to the Armed Forces Epidemiologic Board, 1954.

190. WILLIS, A. T., Clostridium: The spore-bearing anaerobes, in: *Topley and Wilson's Principles of Bacteriology, Virology and Immunity,* Volume 2 (G. WILSON, A. MILES, AND M. T. PARKER, eds.), pp. 442–475, Williams & Wilkins, Baltimore, 1983.

191. WINSNES, R., AND CHRISTIANSEN, G., Quantification of tetanus antitoxin in human sera. II. Comparison of counterimmunoelectrophoresis and passive haemagglutination with toxin neutralization in mice, *Acta Pathol. Microbiol. Scand. Sec. B* **87**:197–200 (1979).

192. WISE, D. L., TRANTOLO, J., MARINO, R. T., AND KITCHELL, J. P., Opportunities and challenges in the design of implantable biodegradable polymeric systems for the delivery of antimicrobial agents and vaccines, *Adv. Drug Delivery Rev.* **1**:19–30 (1987).

193. WOLTERS, K. L., AND DEHMEL, H., Abschliessende untersuchungen über die tetanus prophylaxe durch active immunisierung, *Z. Hyg.* **124**:326–332 (1942).

194. World Health Organization, Immunization Policies in Europe, Report on a WHO meeting, Karlovy Vary, Czechoslovakia, World Health Organization ICP/EPI 001 m01, 1430G, 1986 PS4.

195. WRIGHT, G. P., The neurotoxins of *Clostridium botulinum* and *Clostridium tetani, Pharmacol. Rev.* **7**:413–456 (1955).

196. ZACKS, S. I., AND SHEF, M. F., Tetanus toxin: Fine structure, localization of binding sites in striated muscle, *Science* **159**:643–644 (1968).

CHAPTER 35

Toxic Shock Syndrome

Arthur L. Reingold

1. Introduction

Toxic shock syndrome (TSS) is an acute, multisystem febrile illness caused by *Staphylococcus aureus*. The currently accepted criteria for confirming a case of TSS include fever, hypotension, a diffuse erythematous macular rash, subsequent desquamation, evidence of multisystem involvement, and lack of evidence of another likely cause of the illness (Table 1).

2. Historical Background

TSS was first described as such in 1978 by Todd *et al.*[91] However, cases of what we now believe to have been TSS have been reported in the medical literature since at least 1927 as "staphylococcal scarlet fever" or "staphylococcal scarlatina."[3,86] In addition, a number of patients reported more recently in the medical literature as having adult Kawasaki disease probably had TSS.[22] The association between illness and focal infection with *S. aureus* was, by definition, apparent in early reports of "staphylococcal scarlet fever," but was reinforced by the findings of Todd *et al.*[91] and later by the findings of other investigators.[20,83]

TSS achieved notoriety in 1980 when numerous cases

Arthur L. Reingold   Department of Biomedical and Environmental Health Sciences, University of California, Berkeley, California 94720.

were recognized and an association between illness (in women), menstruation, and tampon use was demonstrated.[14,15] While the early case reports of "staphylococcal scarlet fever" and the report by Todd *et al.*[91] clearly showed that TSS occurred in small children, men, and women who were not menstruating, most (but by no means all) of the cases initially recognized and reported in late 1979 and early 1980 were in menstruating women,[15,65,69] leading to the frequent misperception among the general public and many physicians that TSS occurred only in association with tampon use (hence, "the tampon disease"). This misperception undoubtedly led to subsequent biases in the diagnosing (and probably reporting) of TSS cases. However, later studies designed to eliminate such biases have shown that TSS does, in fact, occur disproportionately in menstruating women,[60,93] while case–control studies demonstrating an association between the risk of developing TSS during menstruation and tampon use preceded (indeed led to) the introduction of bias concerning the relationship between tampon use and menstrual TSS.[20,83]

Follow-up studies demonstrated that the risk of developing tampon-related menstrual TSS varies with the absorbency and/or chemical composition of the tampon,[9,56,72] although the relative importance of these and other tampon characteristics in determining that risk remains uncertain. As a result of both epidemiologic and *in vitro* laboratory studies, the formulation of available tampons has changed dramatically since 1980, such that absorbencies are substantially lower, and chemical composition is less varied across brands and styles. Recent studies have demonstrated that

Table 1. Case Definition of Toxic Shock Syndrome

Fever: temperature ≥ 38.9°C (102°F)
Rash: diffuse macular erythroderma
Desquamation: 1 to 3 weeks after onset of illness
Hypotension: systolic blood pressure ≤ 90 mm Hg for adults or below fifth percentile by age for children under 16 years of age,
    orthostatic drop in diastolic blood pressure ≥ 15 mm Hg from lying to sitting, orthostatic syncope, or orthostatic dizziness
Multisystem involvement: three or more of the following:
  Gastrointestinal: vomiting or diarrhea at onset of illness
  Muscular: severe myalgia or creatine phosphokinase level at least twice the upper limit of normal for laboratory
  Renal: blood urea nitrogen or creatinine at least twice the upper limit of normal for laboratory or urinary sediment with pyuria (≥ 5
    leukocytes per high-power field) in the absence of urinary-tract infection
  Hepatic: total bilirubin, serum aspartate transaminase, or serum alanine transaminase at least twice the upper limit of normal for
    laboratory
  Hematologic: platelets < 100,000
  Central nervous system: disorientation or alterations in consciousness without focal neurologic signs when fever and hypotension
    are absent
Negative results on the following tests, if obtained:
  Blood, throat, or cerebrospinal fluid cultures (cultures may be positive for *Staphylococcus aureus*)
  Rise in titer to Rocky Mountain spotted fever, leptospirosis, or rubeola

the incidence of TSS, particularly menstrual TSS, has risen and fallen in parallel with the absorbency of tampons,[60a] but that the risk of developing menstrual TSS continues to vary directly with tampon absorbency, despite the recent changes in tampon formulation.[66a]

3. Methodology

3.1. Sources of Mortality Data

Mortality rates for TSS have not been reported directly, but can be estimated from reported incidence rates and case-fatality rates.

3.2. Sources of Morbidity Data

Surveillance for TSS began in a few states in late 1979 and in other states and nationally in early 1980. Since that time, TSS has been made a reportable disease in most states. However, the level of intensity of surveillance activities has varied markedly between and within states. Thus, a few states have established active surveillance for TSS for brief periods of time, while others have done little to stimulate the diagnosis and reporting of cases. As a result, the completeness of diagnosing and reporting TSS cases undoubtedly has been inconsistent between states and over time. However, data from a national hospital discharge survey indicate that reporting of cases, while incomplete

and variable by region, has not been biased dramatically insofar as the age, race, sex, or menstrual status of the patients is concerned.[49] Hospital record review studies, in which both diagnosed and previously undiagnosed cases of TSS were ascertained in a consistent fashion, so as to minimize or eliminate both diagnostic and reporting biases, also have been conducted.[46,60,93] These studies demonstrate that, by and large, the patient characteristics and temporal trends observed in data collected through the largely passive network of TSS surveillance reflected true variation in the incidence of TSS by age, sex, race, and menstrual status. These same studies, taken together, demonstrate that at least some of the apparent geographic variation in the incidence of TSS in the United States is real.

3.3. Surveys

Numerous small surveys have demonstrated that many asymptomatic individuals carry in the nasopharynx and/or vagina strains of *S. aureus* that produce TSS toxin-1 (TSST-1), the toxin believed to be responsible for most TSS cases.[36,44,50,71,79] Similarly, large serosurveys have shown that antibodies to TSST-1 or to a cross-reacting antigen are extremely common.[12,36,71,98]

3.4. Laboratory Diagnosis

3.4.1. Isolation and Identification of the Organism. While recovery of *S. aureus* from the vagina or another site of infection is not one of the criteria of the TSS case definition, it is possible in most TSS cases if appropriate specimens are obtained before antimicrobial therapy is initiated.[20,67,68,83] *S. aureus* grows readily on most standard culture media and is readily identifiable by any clinical microbiology laboratory within 2 or 3 days. Testing of *S. aureus* strains for production of TSST-1, however, is performed in only a few research laboratories. Hence, the results of such testing are not readily available during the acute illness and are not of value in treating patients suspected of having TSS. Furthermore, because both *S. aureus* in general and TSST-1-producing strains of *S. aureus* in particular can be recovered from many patients without the clinical features of TSS and from asymptomatic individuals, microbiologic results cannot and do not prove that a given patient has TSS.

3.4.2. Serologic and Immunologic Diagnostic Methods. A variety of serologic and immunologic techniques have been used to test *S. aureus* strains for production of TSST-1. As noted above, these tests are not available outside a few research laboratories. Attempts to detect TSST-1 in clinical specimens have been unsuccessful in all but a few instances,[97] so antigen detection is not currently a diagnostic tool for TSS. Antibodies to TSST-1 can be measured using solid-phase radioimmunoassay and other techniques. However, most healthy individuals have detectable anti-TSST-1 antibodies.[12,36,71,98] Furthermore, some patients with TSS have demonstrable anti-TSST-1 antibodies at the time of onset, and many patients without such antibodies at the time of onset do not demonstrate an antibody rise in response to their illness.[12,87] Thus, testing for anti-TSST-1 antibodies (which is not available except in one or two research laboratories in any event) is of limited value in confirming the diagnosis of TSS, although it has been argued that the absence of detectable antibodies at the time of onset supports the diagnosis of TSS.

4. Biological Characteristics of the Organism

As noted above, there is convincing evidence that *S. aureus* is the cause of TSS. In patients with menstrual TSS, *S. aureus* can be recovered from the vagina and/or cervix in 95–100% of cases (usually as a heavy growth), but in only 5–15% of healthy control women.[19,20,29,47,50,53,54,83,84] In patients with nonmenstrual TSS associated with a focal wound, *S. aureus* is typically the only organism found in the lesion.[67,68] Furthermore, experimental studies demonstrate that TSS-associated *S. aureus* strains can cause a similar illness in rabbits (see below).

Similarly, there is strong evidence that the ability to make TSST-1, previously known as pyrogenic exotoxin C,[78] staphylococcal enterotoxin F,[8] and several other names, is characteristic of, although not universal among, TSS-associated *S. aureus* strains. Thus, 90–100% of *S. aureus* isolates recovered from the vagina, cervix, or used tampon in menstrual TSS cases produce TSST-1, compared with only 10–20% of vaginal or nasopharyngeal isolates from healthy controls.[1,2,8,78,79] On the other hand, only 60–70% of *S. aureus* strains recovered from normally sterile sites in patients with nonmenstrual TSS produce TSST-1,[27,76] suggesting that other staphylococcal toxins may be capable of inducing a clinically indistinguishable syndrome. Two studies of historical strains of *S. aureus* have demonstrated that the proportion of strains capable of making TSST-1 has changed over time and was generally higher in the mid to late 1970s than in earlier time periods.[1,31] Interestingly, that proportion appears to have declined somewhat in the early 1980s, when the incidence of TSS was peaking.

TSS-associated *S. aureus* strains also have been characterized phenotypically with respect to a number of other properties, including phage type, antimicrobial susceptibility, resistance to heavy metals, production or activity of various enzymes, and presence of plasmids and bacteriophages. The picture that emerges with regard to these characteristics, while consistent, is by no means invariable or unique. A higher proportion of TSS-related *S. aureus* strains are lysed by phage types 29 and/or 52 (58–82%), as compared to only 12–28% of control strains.[1,2] Similarly, TSS-associated strains generally are resistant to penicillin (and ampicillin), arsenate, and cadmium, while being susceptible to β-lactamase-resistant antimicrobial agents, most other commonly tested antimicrobial agents, bacteriocins, and mercury.[6,42,83] Other characteristics that appear to distinguish these strains from other *S. aureus* strains include decreased production of hemolysin, lipase, and nuclease[6,17]; tryptophan auxotypy[18]; decreased lethality in chick embryos[6]; increased pigment production[92]; and increased casein proteolysis.[92] TSS-associated strains also have been reported to be less likely to carry plasmids and more likely to carry lysogenic bacteriophage than are control strains. There is controversy over whether or not the gene coding for TSST-1 can be transferred by lysogeny.[41,64]

It should be noted that most of the strains examined in the above studies were recovered from the genital tract in menstrual TSS cases. Thus, the results are not necessarily applicable to *S. aureus* strains associated with nonmenstrual TSS, and there is some evidence to suggest that such strains, recovered from normally sterile sites in patients with nonmenstrual TSS, are less likely to be lysed by phage types 29 and/or 52 than are strains from menstrual TSS cases.[27] At the same time, as noted above, they also are less likely to make TSST-1.

5. Descriptive Epidemiology

5.1. Prevalence and Incidence

Carriage of *S. aureus* on the skin and in the nasopharynx and vagina is very common. Numerous cross-sectional studies have demonstrated that 30–40% of individuals carry *S. aureus* in the nasopharynx and 5–15% of women carry *S. aureus* in the vagina.[19,29,36,44,47,50,53,54,84] The corresponding figures for TSST-1-producing *S. aureus* are 5–15% (nasopharynx) and 1–5% (vagina). Thus, carriage of *S. aureus* strains believed to be capable of causing TSS is also very common.

In contrast, TSS is a rare disease. Since it became a notifiable disease in 1983, the number of cases reported annually in the United States has been in the range of 400–500. The most reliable estimates of incidence rates come from hospital-based record review studies. In these studies, both diagnosed and previously undiagnosed cases of TSS were ascertained in an unbiased way by reviewing thousands of medical records of hospitalized patients with one of a long list of discharge diagnoses likely to be indicative of misdiagnosed cases of TSS. In one such study in Colorado, the annual incidence of TSS in women between the ages of 10 and 30 was 15.8/100,000 in 1980.[93] In a similar study in California, the incidence rate in women between the ages of 15 and 34 was only 2.4/100,000 in 1980.[60] The incidence rate in men of the same age group in the latter study was consistently less than 0.5/100,000 in all of the years studied.

Estimates of the incidence of diagnosed TSS derive from statewide surveillance systems established in late 1979 or early 1980. The states with the most aggressive case-finding methods reported annual incidence rates at that time of 6.2/100,000 menstruating women (Wisconsin),[20] 8.9/100,000 menstruating women (Minnesota),[55] and 14.4/100,000 females 10–49 years of age (Utah).[38] An overall estimate of 0.8/100,000 total population of hospitalized, diagnosed TSS in the United States in 1981 and 1982 was derived from a national hospital discharge survey.[49] While TSS has been documented in numerous other countries, no estimates of incidence rates for other countries are available.

The discrepancy between the frequency of colonization and/or infection with TSST-1-producing *S. aureus* and the rarity of TSS is thought to be due to the fact that most individuals have detectable anti-TSST-1 antibodies. By age 30, more than 95% of men and women have such antibodies.[98] The origin of these antibodies is unknown.

5.2. Epidemic Behavior and Contagiousness

Because TSS increased dramatically in incidence in the United States beginning in 1979 in comparison with previous years,[46,60,93] it would be correct to say that an epidemic of TSS occurred at that time. TSS does not, however, occur in explosive epidemics in the same way that dengue and meningococcal disease do, although strains of *S. aureus* that produce TSST-1 are, like other *S. aureus* strains, transmitted readily by person-to-person spread (see below).

5.3. Geographic Distribution

5.3.1. United States. Cases of TSS have been reported in all 50 states and the District of Columbia, but the incidence of reported cases has varied substantially between states and regions.[65,69] Variation in the completeness of diagnosis and reporting of cases undoubtedly accounts for some of the observed differences, but there is substantial evidence that at least some of the observed differences are real. For example, a study of hospital discharge data in which differences in the reporting of cases could not have been a factor showed that the overall annual incidence of hospitalized cases varied by region between 0.24 and 1.43/100,000 in 1981–1982.[49] In this study, however, potentially large differences in the completeness with which TSS cases were diagnosed and different standards for hospitalizing patients suspected of having TSS could not be ruled out. More convincing evidence for true geographic differences in incidence rates comes from the virtually identical hospital record review studies conducted in Colorado and northern California, in which variation in the diagnosing and reporting of cases was largely or completely eliminated.[60,93] As noted above, the incidence of TSS in 1980 in females 10 to 30 years of age was 15.8/100,000 in Colorado, but only 2.4/100,000 females 15 to 34 years of age in northern California. A prospective study employing a similar chart review has recently been completed in five states (Missouri, New Jersey, Oklahoma, Tennessee, and Washington) and one large county (Los Angeles) and has yielded additional information on the geographic distribution of TSS.

Studies of *S. aureus* strains from the United States show no geographic differences in what proportion make TSST-1.[31] Similarly, anti-TSST-1 antibodies are found in similar proportions of healthy individuals in different parts of the United States.

5.3.2. Other Countries. Documented cases of TSS have been reported from Canada, most of western Europe, Australia, New Zealand, Japan, Israel, South Africa, and elsewhere. No information concerning incidence rates of TSS outside of the United States is available. However, the proportion of cases in other countries associated with menstruation and tampon use appears to be substantially lower than in the United States, in keeping with the fact that tampon use in general is less frequent in other countries and superabsorbent tampons are less widely available.

5.4. Temporal Distribution

Substantial controversy has surrounded the interpretation of observed changes over time in the diagnosis and reporting of TSS cases. Data from the passive national surveillance system suggested that the number of cases began to rise in 1978, peaked in 1980, and then declined and leveled off, with all of the observed differences being due to changes in the number of menstrual TSS cases reported[65,69] (Fig. 1). While this pattern also was observed in some individual states employing vigorous case-finding

methods (e.g., Utah and Wisconsin), a different pattern was seen in Minnesota, where no decline in the number of cases was observed in 1981.[16] Because of the documented impact of publicity on reporting of TSS cases and the undoubted fluctuations over time in the likelihood that cases would be diagnosed and/or reported, the results of studies that eliminate or minimize these influences are important in interpreting temporal trends.

While the three published hospital record review studies all suffer from having a relatively small number of cases of TSS to analyze statistically, the results of all three studies are consistent. In the California study, the incidence of TSS in women increased consistently through 1980, fell somewhat in 1981 and 1982, and then increased again in 1983, while the incidence in men remained consistently low (Fig. 2). In the Colorado study, the results were similar except that the decrease in 1981 compared with 1980 was sharper (Fig. 3). The similarity of the pattern in Colorado is even more apparent if cases meeting only the authors' proposed screening definition for TSS and not the more rigorous collaborative case definition are removed.[66] Similar trends are seen in the study from Cincinnati, although incidence rates cannot be estimated in this study.[46]

Thus, there is convincing evidence that hospitalized cases of TSS in females of menstrual age increased in the late 1970s, irrespective of any changes in the recognition and reporting of the disease. A similar increase was not

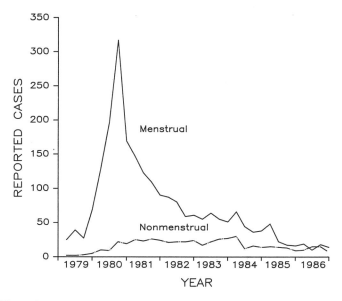

Figure 1. Reported cases of toxic shock syndrome, United States, 1979–1986.

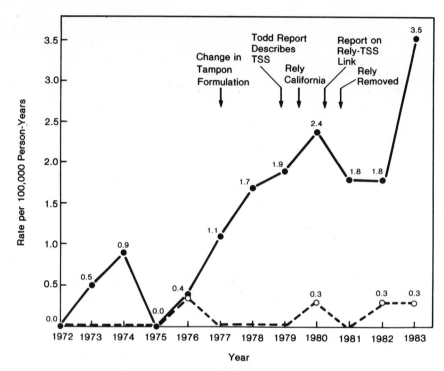

Figure 2. Incidence of hospitalized toxic shock syndrome cases in males (dashed line) and females (solid line), aged 15 through 34 years, northern California Kaiser-Permanente Medical Care Program, 1972 through 1983. Reproduced from Petitti *et al.* (60) with permission.

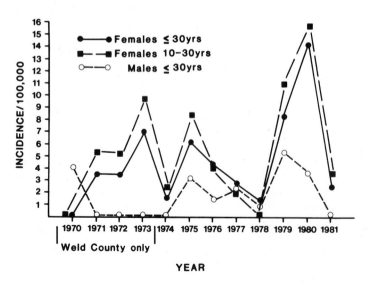

Figure 3. Annual incidence per 100,000 population of toxic shock syndrome in hospitalized patients ≤ 30 years of age meeting either the strict or the screening case definition in two Colorado counties, 1970–1981. Reproduced from Todd *et al.* (93) with permission.

apparent among men. There is also some evidence that this upward trend in the incidence of TSS through 1980 was reversed in several geographic areas, at least temporarily, in 1981. Studies currently in progress will shed more light on more recent temporal trends.

5.5. Age

TSS can occur in individuals of all ages and has been documented in a newborn baby and in patients up to 80 years of age. However, data from both passive and active surveillance systems and from the California record review study indicate that younger women are at greater risk of developing TSS than are older women. Of cases associated with menstruation reported nationally, almost 60% have been in women 15 to 24 years of age, compared with only 25% in women 25 to 34 years of age.[65,69] Cases in women 35 to 44 years of age are even less common. Furthermore, the highest age-specific incidence rates consistently have been observed in women 15–19 or 15–24 years of age. Thus, in the California record review study, the annual incidence rate was 2.6/100,000 women 15–19 years of age, compared with rates of 0.8 to 1.4/100,000 among women 20–24, 25–29, and 30–34 years of age.[60] Similarly, in Minnesota the annual incidence of menstrual TSS among women 15–24 years of age was 13.7/100,000, compared with rates of 2.3 in those < 15 years of age and 6.6 in those ≥ 25 years of age.[55] The age distribution of TSS cases unassociated with menstruation is more uniform, especially if cases in postpartum women are excluded.[68]

5.6. Sex

All available evidence clearly indicates that TSS is much more common among women of menstrual age than among men of the same age. Of U.S. cases reported through passive surveillance, 95% have been in women and 5% in men.[65,69] In the California record review study, the overall incidence of TSS in women 15 to 34 years of age during the time period 1972–1983 was 15 times that in men of the same age (1.5 versus 0.1/100,000 person-years).[60] This marked difference in incidence rates between men and women undoubtedly relates primarily to the fact that most cases of TSS are associated with menstruation and tampon use. What appears to be an increased risk of TSS during the postpartum interval and the apparent association between TSS and the use of barrier contraception probably contribute further to this pattern.[23,67,68] The incidence of TSS associated with other types of staphylococcal infections (e.g., surgical wound infections, cutaneous and subcutaneous lesions) appears to be similar in men and women.[67,68]

5.7. Race

Although it has been apparent since at least 1980 that TSS occurs in individuals of all racial groups,[15] the overwhelming majority (93–97%) of reported cases have been in whites, who make up only 80–85% of the U.S. population.[65,69] Likely explanations for this discrepancy fall into two categories—biases in the diagnosis and reporting of cases on the one hand, and true racial differences in either susceptibility to TSS or exposure to risk factors on the other. It has been postulated that increased difficulty in recognizing the rash on dark-skinned individuals, poorer access of minority groups to medical care, and the relative paucity of individuals of races other than white in areas with active TSS research efforts have all contributed to the observed racial distribution of cases. However, data from the California record review study indicate that in the 15–34 age group, TSS does, indeed, disproportionately affect whites.[60] All of the 54 definite cases (most of which are related to menstruation) found in that study were in whites, while only 81% of the population at risk was white ($p <$ 0.05; Fisher's exact test, two-tailed).

It has been noted that the racial distribution of patients with nonmenstrual TSS (87% white) more closely resembles the racial distribution of the U.S. population than does the racial distribution of patients with menstrual TSS (98% white).[69] Taken together with studies demonstrating that young white women use tampons far more often than do comparably aged women of other racial groups,[30,34,35] these results suggest that observed race-specific differences in incidence rates are due, at least in part, to different levels of exposure to an important risk factor for developing TSS during menstruation.

5.8. Occupation

There is no evidence to suggest that any given occupational group, including health care providers, is at increased risk of developing TSS.

5.9. Occurrence in Different Settings

As noted below, transmission of strains of *S. aureus* capable of causing TSS has been demonstrated in the hospital setting.[5,7,40] There is also evidence of spread of these strains and occasional clustering of cases in households and in military installations (CDC, unpublished observations).

5.10. Socioeconomic Factors

It is unclear to what extent the marked racial variation in tampon use, especially among adolescents, reflects socioeconomic rather than racial differences. Other socioeconomic factors have not been noted to play a role in TSS.

5.11. Other Factors

5.11.1. Menstrual TSS. Numerous case–control studies conducted in 1980–1981 examined risk factors for developing TSS during menstruation (Table 2). These studies consistently found that tampon use increased the risk of

menstrual TSS (the Oregon study, with its small number of cases, while not finding an association between menstrual TSS and tampon use in general, did find an association with a particular brand of tampon).[20,32,38,56,72,83] Included among these studies are two performed before any information concerning this association had appeared in the medical literature or lay press.[20,83] More recently, a study comparing tampon use among women with menstrual TSS in 1983 and 1984 with tampon usage patterns ascertained via a national survey found evidence of a continuing increased risk of menstrual TSS among tampon users.[9] Furthermore, a recently concluded multistate case–control study of menstrual TSS cases with onset in 1986–1987 documents that this association persists.[66a]

Two early case–control studies demonstrated that the risk of menstrual TSS varied with tampon brand and/or style (i.e., absorbency), suggesting that risk was a function of tampon absorbency and/or chemical composition.[56,72]

Table 2. Risk Factors for Menstrual TSS

Case onset dates	Date of study	Geographic area	Source of controls	No. cases	No. controls	Tampons			
						% cases	% controls	Relative risk[a]	p value
9/75–6/80	1980	Wisconsin	Clinic	35	105	97	76	10.6*	<0.01
12/76–6/80	6/80	USA (CDC)	Friend	52	52	100	85	20.1*	<0.05
7/80–8/80	9/80	USA (CDC)	Friend	50	150	100	83	20.5*	<0.01
1/76–8/80	5/80–8/80	Utah	Neighbor	29	91	100	77	18.0*	0.012
10/79–9/80	10/80–11/80	Minnesota, Wisconsin, Iowa	Neighbor	76	152	99	81	18.0	<0.001
12/79–11/80	1/81–3/81	Oregon	Friend	18	18	100	78	11.5*	NS[b]
			Clinic		18		89	5.6*	NS

Rely brand tampons				Absorbency		Oral contraceptives				
% cases	% controls	Relative risk	p value	Relative risk in multivariate model	p value	% cases	% controls	Relative risk	p value	Ref.
	NA[c]		NS	NA		17	36	0.36*	NS	20
33	27	NA	NS	NA		4	7	0.48*	NS	83
71	26	7.7	<0.0001	1.0	NS	NA	NA	NA		72
63	24	6.1	<0.0005	NA		3	11	0.29*	NS	38
53	29	2.5	0.005	3.2–10.4	0.01	12	20	0.55*	0.05	55
67	17	10.0*	<0.05	NA						32
	6	34.0*	<0.05							

[a]If relative risk not reported in reference, crude odds ratio estimated disregarding matching; 0.5 added to all cells in tables with a 0 value; estimated values indicated with an asterisk.
[b]NS, not significant.
[c]NA, data not available.

The two more recent studies document clearly that risk of menstrual TSS is directly correlated with measured *in vitro* tampon absorbency[9,66a] independent of chemical composition, but that chemical composition is also a factor.[9] It is interesting to note that the correlation with tampon absorbency has persisted, despite the major alterations in chemical composition and marked decreases in the absorbencies of available tampons that have occurred since 1980.

The early case–control studies also examined the role of a number of other factors in determining the risk of developing TSS during menstruation. Four of the studies found that women with TSS were less likely to use oral contraceptives than were controls, although the differences in individual studies were not statistically significant.[20,38,56,83] One study found that continuous use of tampons during the menstrual period was associated with an increased risk of TSS,[83] while in another study a similar association, present on univariate analysis, did not remain significant in a multivariate analysis.[56] Of four studies looking at the relationship between a history of a recent vaginal infection and the risk of TSS, only one found such an association. Factors found not to be related to the risk of developing menstrual TSS in one of more studies included marital status, income, parity, sexual activity, bathing, frequency of exercise, alcohol use, smoking, history of vaginal herpes infections, and frequency of changing tampons.

5.11.2. Postpartum TSS. Although numerous cases of TSS occurring during the postpartum interval have been reported, the lack of precise information concerning the incidence of TSS in various settings makes it difficult to be certain that the incidence in postpartum women is elevated. Those cases of postpartum TSS not related to infection of a cesarean section incision or an infection of the breast (i.e., mastitis and breast abscess) have occurred predominantly in association with the use of tampons to control the flow of lochia or the use of barrier contraception (i.e., diaphragms and contraceptive sponges).[68]

5.11.3. Postoperative TSS. TSS has been associated with *S. aureus* surgical wound infections following a wide array of surgical procedures.[7] It has been suggested, however, that patients undergoing nasal surgery are at particularly high risk, presumably due to the frequency of *S. aureus* carriage in the nasopharynx and the difficulty of eradiating such carriage.[36] The common use of "nasal tampons" and other packing material following nasal surgery also may play a role.

5.11.4. Other Nonmenstrual TSS. TSS can result from *S. aureus* infection at any body site. However, many nonmenstrual TSS cases are the result of cutaneous and subcutaneous *S. aureus* infections. Risk factors for the de-

velopment of such infections and/or associated TSS have not been studied. A relatively small proportion of nonmenstrual, nonpostpartum TSS cases are associated with vaginal *S. aureus* infections. One risk factor that has been identified in such cases is the use of contraceptive sponges.[23] It remains uncertain whether or not diaphragm use is similarly associated with an increased risk of nonmenstrual TSS.

6. Mechanisms and Routes of Transmission

Like all *S. aureus* strains, those capable of causing TSS appear to be transmitted readily by person-to-person spread, both within the hospital and in the community. There is convincing evidence that a nurse transmitted a TSS-associated strain of *S. aureus* to hospitalized burn patients[5] and suggestive evidence that some cases of postoperative TSS are due to nosocomial spread of the causative organism by hospital personnel.[7,40] In addition, vertical transmission from mother to newborn, with the development of TSS in both, has been reported.[28] Outside the hospital setting, transmission between husband and wife has been suggested by the almost simultaneous appearance of TSS in both, as has transmission between mother–daughter pairs (unpublished reports to the CDC). It is assumed, but not proven, that transmission in all these instances was by direct person-to-person spread. Nevertheless, it should be emphasized that in many TSS cases, particularly those associated with a focus of infection in the vagina, it may well be that disease is due to the introduction and/or multiplication of an endogenous *S. aureus* strain rather than to an exogenous source of infection.

7. Pathogenesis and Immunity

TSS results from an infection with an appropriate strain of *S. aureus* in a susceptible host. Once a nidus of infection is established, onset of symptoms typically occurs 1 to 3 days later. The best evidence concerning incubation period comes from patients with postoperative TSS due to surgical wound infections. In these patients, the date when the infection became established is usually the day of surgery and thus can be determined unequivocally. The median incubation period in such patients is 2 days.[7] When TSS is caused by *S. aureus* infection of the vagina during menstruation, onset of symptoms is typically on the third or fourth day of menstruation, although it can be earlier or later.

In most cases of TSS, the toxin TSST-1 is the bacterial product most likely to be responsible for many of the observed signs, symptoms, and abnormalities of laboratory values. There is, however, circumstantial evidence that one or more other staphylococcal products must be capable of causing an indistinguishable illness.[27,76] Furthermore, bacterial products other than TSST-1 that are made more commonly by *S. aureus* strains recovered from patients with TSS than by other strains have been described (see Section 4). For these reasons, it is likely that other staphylococcal products play a role in the pathogenesis of TSS. Furthermore, there is evidence that some of the multisystem derangements frequently observed in patients with TSS are due to the profound hypotension or shock that can occur, and only indirectly to any staphylococcal products. For example, renal failure in TSS is probably secondary to hypotension-induced acute tubular necrosis, which in turn is the result of multiple factors, including: hypovolemia due to vomiting, diarrhea, increased insensible losses associated with a high fever, and inability to ingest or retain fluids; and "third-spacing" of fluids. Uptake of "endogenous" endotoxin from gram-negative intestinal flora also has been proposed as playing a role in the pathogenesis of TSS.[73]

The biologic properties of TSST-1 have been studied *in vitro* and *in vivo*, and attempts have been made to develop an animal model of TSS. *In vitro*, purified TSST-1 has been shown to stimulate the proliferation of T lymphocytes,[61] to inhibit immunoglobulin synthesis,[62] and to be a potent stimulator of interleukin-1 production by macrophages and monocytes.[33,58] TSST-1 also has been shown to bind to and be internalized by epithelial cells,[43] suggesting that it can be absorbed from focal sites of infection. *In vivo*, TSST-1 has been shown to be pyrogenic,[78] to induce lymphopenia,[74] to decrease the clearance of endotoxin,[26] and to increase susceptibility to endotoxin-induced shock.[73] While initially reported to be an enterotoxin (as evidenced by induction of vomiting in monkeys), preparations of TSST-1 not contaminated with other staphylococcal enterotoxins do not appear to induce vomiting.[70]

Attempts to reproduce TSS in animals have included using mice, rabbits, goats, baboons, chimpanzees, and rhesus monkeys.[4,10,11,21,59,63,64,81,82,90,96] In these studies, investigators either have attempted to infect the animals with TSS-associated *S. aureus* strains at one of a variety of sites (previously implanted subcutaneous chambers, vagina, uterus, and muscle) or have injected purified TSST-1 as a bolus or continuous infusion. The animal models that come closest to reproducing the syndrome observed in humans have been those using rabbits. Live TSS-associated *S. aureus* organisms inside a previously implanted subcutaneous chamber and continuous infusion of purified TSST-1 both result in fever, hyperemia of mucous membranes, hypocalcemia, elevated CPK and hepatic enzymes, renal failure, and death in a high proportion of rabbits.[4,59] Also, the pathologic changes observed postmortem in these animals are similar to those reported in patients dying of TSS.[45,57]

These rabbit models have been used to study the host factors in susceptibility to TSS suggested as important by clinical and epidemiologic data or by *in vitro* results. It has been found that the age, sex, hormonal status, and strain of rabbits used all have a substantial impact on susceptibility to "rabbit TSS."[10,11] Thus, older rabbits have been reported to be more susceptible than are younger rabbits. Similarly, male rabbits appear to be more susceptible than are female rabbits, although castration abolishes this difference and estrogens protect male rabbits. Experiments concerning the contribution of endogenous endotoxin (i.e., endotoxin released by gut flora) to the pathogenesis of TSS have yielded conflicting results, although it appears that blocking the effect of endotoxin by giving polymyxin B does not consistently prevent "rabbit TSS."[59] Preexisting anti-TSST-1 antibody, however, does appear to protect against TSS in the rabbit,[82] and corticosteroids in high doses also decrease mortality.[59]

Because of the observed association between menstrual TSS and tampon use, many investigators have looked at the effect of tampons and their constituents on the growth of *S. aureus* and the production of TSST-1 in vitro. At the same time, the effect of environmental conditions such as pH, Po_2, Pco_2, and cation concentration on the production of TSST-1 has been investigated. In general, studies have shown that tampons and their individual components inhibit the growth of *S. aureus in vitro*, regardless of the growth medium.[13,80] Although some studies have suggested that *S. aureus* can use various tampon constituents as an energy source, these results have been challenged and their relevance to human disease questioned.[39,88,89] Also controversial is the effect of tampons on the production of TSST-1 *in vitro*, with some studies showing that certain tampons and tampon constituents increase TSST-1 production, and other studies showing no effect or inhibition of toxin production.[80,88] It has been suggested that the effect of tampons on TSST-1 production (and possibly on the risk of menstrual TSS) is mediated by changes in the availability of magnesium, which is bound by certain tampon components.[52]

Growth conditions appear to be important in determining the amount of TSST-1 produced. Thus, an aerobic environment, neutral pH, and low levels of glucose, magnesium, and tryptophan all increase TSST-1 production, although some controversy has arisen about the effect of magnesium concentration on TSST-1 levels.[37,51,52,75,77,94] It has been shown that in patients with TSS related to focal sites of *S. aureus* infection, growth conditions within the infected focus are well suited to TSST-1 production.[94] Also, while the vagina generally has been considered to be anaerobic, studies have shown that a substantial amount of oxygen is introduced when a tampon is inserted, leading to speculation that the amount of oxygen introduced with a tampon may be an important factor in explaining the increased risk of menstrual TSS among tampon users.[99] A role for proteases of either bacterial or human origin in the pathogenesis of TSS also has been suggested.[94] An earlier theory that the association between menstrual TSS and tampon use was mediated by the demonstrated induction of vaginal ulcerations by tampons[25] has received less attention ever since similar vaginal ulcerations were reported in at least one patient with menstrual TSS who did not use tampons.[45]

8. Patterns of Host Response

8.1. Clinical Features

An illness meeting all the criteria of the established TSS case definition is, by the very nature of the criteria, severe, and the vast majority of such patients are hospitalized for treatment. Some patients experience the relatively gradual onset of sore throat, fever, fatigue, headache, and myalgias over 24–48 h, followed by vomiting and/or diarrhea, signs of hypotension, and the appearance of the characteristic diffuse "sunburnlike" macular skin rash. Other patients appear to have a much more dramatic onset over the course of several hours, with some reporting that they can remember the exact moment when they suddenly felt overwhelmingly ill.

Because an established set of strict criteria is used to define someone as having or not having TSS, all of the cases so defined are, not surprisingly, alike, regardless of the site of infection with *S. aureus*. There is, however, some variation. The temperature elevation in patients with TSS, while sometimes modest, can be extreme, with temperatures in the range of 104–106°F being fairly common. The evidence of hypotension in an individual case can range from mild orthostatic dizziness to profound shock. The characteristic macular skin rash can be dramatic and obvious, with the patient appearing bright red throughout; it can be subtle and difficult to appreciate, particularly in

dark-skinned individuals; or it can be localized. Similarly, the desquamation that occurs during convalescence (usually 5–15 days after the acute illness) can be a subtle flaking and peeling of skin on the face and/or trunk or can involve the loss of full-thickness sheets of skin, particularly on the fingers, hands, and feet. Depending on which systems are affected most prominently in an individual case, the multisystem involvement in TSS can produce rather different clinical pictures. In some patients the involvement of the mucous membranes (e.g., sore throat, conjunctival and oropharyngeal injection) is severe and most prominent, while in other patients the gastrointestinal symptoms (vomiting and/or diarrhea) are predominant. Similarly, myalgias, thrombocytopenia, and involvement of the hepatic and renal systems can range from nil to severe.

Patients who receive aggressive supportive therapy (e.g., fluids), appropriate antimicrobial agents, and drainage of any focal *S. aureus* infection usually respond rapidly and improve over the course of several days. However, patients in whom therapy is either delayed or in whom a focal *S. aureus* infection is not eradicated can have a stormy, life-threatening course. In cases meeting all the established criteria, the case-fatality rate is currently 1–3% overall, although it increases with increasing age.[49]

The spectrum of illness of TSS has not been defined adequately due to the lack of a specific diagnostic laboratory test. It is evident that some illnesses not meeting all the criteria of the strict case definition, which was devised for use in epidemiologic studies, represent milder forms of TSS. For example, few would question that an individual whose highest recorded temperature was 101.8°F, but who otherwise met all of the established criteria, had TSS. A number of authors have described patients of this kind,[24,95] and some have attempted to fashion simplified and/or less rigorous case definitions for TSS.[100] It is apparent that less rigorous case definitions are likely to be more sensitive but less specific in identifying TSS cases. Ultimately, however, it is not possible, in the absence of a specific diagnostic test, to determine where along a spectrum of increasingly milder and/or more atypical cases illnesses cease to be TSS and start to be something else. Thus, it is unclear whether a tampon-using menstruating woman with *S. aureus* in the vagina (or anyone else) who experiences headache, fatigue, and nausea could represent a very mild form of TSS. Such distinctions are made all the more difficult because of the relative frequency with which completely asymptomatic individuals are colonized with TSST-1-producing *S. aureus* in the nasopharynx, vagina, and probably other sites that are not normally sterile (see above).

8.2. Diagnosis

As noted above, TSS can occur in individuals of any age, sex, and race. However, most recognized cases occur in a limited number of clinical settings. In women of reproductive age, TSS is most commonly seen during the menstrual period and the postpartum interval, although it can occur at other times as well, in association with focal *S. aureus* infections and in users of barrier contraception. TSS during pregnancy, however, is quite uncommon. Although patients undergoing nasal surgery may be at elevated risk, TSS related to a surgical wound infection is a possibility in any postoperative patient, particularly during the first 24–72 h. In many such instances, there will be few or no local signs that the operative site is infected.[7] As noted above, the median interval between surgery and onset of TSS in such cases is 2 days, but the range is 12 h to many weeks. TSS is an infrequent but serious consequence of focal *S. aureus* infections at every conceivable body site, although cutaneous and subcutaneous abscesses and other similar infections appear to predominate. In addition, TSS has been reported to be a life-threatening complication of postinfluenza *S. aureus* infections of the respiratory tract.[48,85]

The differential diagnosis for a patient suspected of having TSS depends, in part, on which features of the illness are most prominent. For example, patients in whom sore throat and fever predominate early are frequently suspected initially of having streptococcal or viral pharyngitis. In cases in which diarrhea and vomiting are more prominent, viral gastroenteritis is often considered. When the rash becomes apparent, scarlet fever and drug reactions are often suspected.

The differential diagnosis also can be influenced by the patient's age and sex, and the clinical setting in which the illness occurs. For example, cases in infants and very young children must be distinguished from Kawasaki syndrome and staphylococcal scalded skin syndrome. Similarly, in postpartum or postabortion women, other causes of fever and hypotension must be considered, such as endometritis and septic abortion. In individuals with appropriate exposure histories, leptospirosis, measles, and Rocky Mountain spotted fever should be included in the differential diagnosis. In summary, TSS can be confused fairly readily with a wide range of other conditions (Table 3).

9. Control and Prevention

9.1. General Concepts

9.1.1. Menstrual TSS. Most strategies for decreasing the incidence of TSS have focused on menstrual TSS and its relationship to tampon use. In light of the demonstrated association between tampon use and risk of developing menstrual TSS, women were advised in 1980 that they could minimize their risk of developing menstrual TSS by not using tampons. In response, many women stopped using tampons, at least temporarily. The proportion of menstruating women who used tampons fell from approximately 70% in 1980 to less than 50% in 1981, but has rebounded to approximately 65% since that time.

In response to epidemiologic and *in vitro* laboratory evidence concerning the possible roles of tampon absorbency and chemical composition in determining risk of menstrual TSS, most tampon manufacturers have dramatically altered both the absorbency and chemical composition of their products. After increasing markedly in the late 1970s, the measured *in vitro* absorbency of tampons has dropped sharply since 1979–1980, and one component, polyacrylate, has been eliminated from tampon formulations. In addition, one brand of tampons found to be associated with a high risk of menstrual TSS was withdrawn from the market altogether in 1980.

All tampons currently carry a label explaining the association between tampon use and menstrual TSS and describing the signs and symptoms of the illness. Tampon packages also carry a statement that women should use the lowest absorbency tampon consistent with their needs. However, until recently labeling standards have not required a uniform system of characterizing tampon absorbency, so it has been difficult for a woman to judge the relative absorbency of a given brand and style of tampon, and a tampon that

**Table 3. Differential Diagnosis
in Patients with Suspected TSS**

Kawasaki syndrome
Scarlet fever
Meningococcemia
Leptospirosis
Measles (especially "atypical")
Rocky Mountain spotted fever
Viral gastroenteritis
Viral syndromes with exanthems
Appendicitis
Pelvic inflammatory disease
Tubo-ovarian abscess
Staphylococcal scalded skin syndrome
Drug reactions/Stevens–Johnson syndrome

one company labeled "regular" might, in fact, have been more absorbent than tampons of another brand labeled "super." Uniform absorbency labeling of tampons was finally required by the Food and Drug Administration in 1989.

Although frequent changing of tampons has been recommended as a way of decreasing the risk of menstrual TSS, there is no evidence to suggest that changing tampons more often reduces risk. Evidence from one study suggests that alternating tampons and napkins during a menstrual cycle may decrease the risk of TSS.[83]

9.1.2. Postpartum TSS. Because women may be at increased risk of TSS during the postpartum period, they should avoid the use of tampons and barrier contraception during that interval.

9.1.3. Hospital-Acquired TSS. Other than those measures designed to minimize nosocomial infections in general (e.g., good hand-washing practices) and those recommended specifically for patients with other types of staphylococcal infections, there are no proven methods for decreasing the risk of TSS associated with infected surgical wounds and other nosocomial *S. aureus* infections.

9.2. Antibiotic and Chemotherapeutic Approaches to Prophylaxis

Appropriate antimicrobial therapy of an initial episode of menstrual TSS, combined with discontinuing tampon use, has been shown to reduce the risk of recurrent episodes during subsequent menstrual periods.[20] The value of follow-up cultures and prophylactic antimicrobial agents in women with a history of menstrual TSS is unproven, although such measures may be justified in women who have had recurrent episodes of TSS. Because carriage of *S. aureus* at various body sites is so common and cases of TSS are relatively rare, there is no role for obtaining cultures from or giving chemoprophylaxis to individuals without a prior history of TSS.

9.3. Immunization

Although some consideration was given to attempting to develop a toxoid vaccine from TSST-1 soon after its discovery, no concrete steps in this direction have been taken. Given the high proportion of the population with naturally occurring anti-TSST-1 antibodies and the relative rarity of TSS, it would be prohibitively expensive and impractical to demonstrate that such a vaccine yielded clinical protection.

10. Unresolved Problems

Unresolved problems in our understanding of TSS relate primarily to its pathophysiology. While a clear link between tampon use and risk of menstrual TSS has been established, what it is about tampons and their use that results in an increased risk is unknown. The relative importance of absorbency, chemical composition, oxygen content, and perhaps other tampon characteristics in determining risk is uncertain. Similarly, while a direct correlation between measured tampon absorbency and risk of menstrual TSS has been demonstrated, it remains unclear whether or not users of the lowest absorbency tampons are at greater risk than nontampon users. At the same time, the role of tampon chemical composition in determining risk is ill-defined. The importance of magnesium and its binding by tampon constituents in the pathophysiology of menstrual TSS is controversial. As a result of all these uncertainties, it is unknown whether or not the "perfect tampon" (i.e., one that offers menstrual protection and has no associated increased risk of menstrual TSS) currently exists or can be developed.

The roles of toxins other than TSST-1 and other bacterial or host products such as proteases in TSS remain to be elucidated. While there is convincing evidence that *S. aureus* strains that do not make TSST-1 can cause an illness clinically indistinguishable from that caused by TSST-1-producing strains, the responsible toxin(s) is (are) unidentified, although staphylococcal enterotoxin B is one likely candidate. Similarly, while it has been proposed that extracellular proteases may play a key role in the pathogenesis of TSS, evidence on this point is largely absent.

In the area of epidemiology, it remains uncertain to what extent observed geographic variation in the incidence of TSS in the United States is real, as opposed to artifactual. While there is convincing evidence that at least some of the geographic variation is real, explanations for such variation are lacking. In addition, controversy continues over the observed temporal trends in the incidence of TSS and to what extent these trends accurately reflect real variation over time. Again, while several studies have demonstrated that much of the variation over time is real, the small size of these studies leaves certain questions unanswered.

11. References

1. ALTEMEIER, W. A., LEWIS, S. A., SCHLIEVERT, P. M., BERGDOLL, M. S., BJORNSON, H. S., STANECK, J. L., AND CRASS, B. A., *Staphylococcus aureus* associated with toxic

shock syndrome: Phage typing and toxin capability testing, *Ann. Intern. Med.* **96**(Part 2)::978–982 (1982).

2. ALTEMEIER, W. A., LEWIS, S. A., SCHLIEVERT, P. M., AND BJORNSON, H. S., Studies of the staphylococcal causation of toxic shock syndrome, *Surg. Gynecol. Obstet.* **153**:481–485 (1981).

3. ARANOW, H., JR., AND WOOD, W. B., Staphylococcal infection simulating scarlet fever, *J. Am. Med. Assoc.* **119**:1491–1495 (1942).

4. ARKO, R. J., RASHEED, J. K., BROOME, C. V., CHANDLER, F. W., AND PARIS, A. L., A rabbit model of toxic shock syndrome: Clinicopathological features, *J. Infect.* **8**:205–211 (1984).

5. ARNOW, P. M., CHOU, T., WEIL, D., CRASS, B. A., AND BERGDOLL, M. S., Spread of a toxic-shock syndrome-associated strain of *Staphylococcus aureus* and measurement of antibodies to staphylococcal enterotoxin F, *J. Infect. Dis.* **149**:103–107 (1984).

6. BARBOUR, A. G., Vaginal isolates of *Staphylococcus aureus* associated with toxic shock syndrome, *Infect. Immun.* **33**:442–449 (1981).

7. BARTLETT, P., REINGOLD, A. L., GRAHAM, D. R., DAN, B. B., SELINGER, D. S., TANK, G. W., AND WICHTERMAN, K. A., Toxic shock syndrome associated with surgical wound infections, *J. Am. Med. Assoc.* **247**:1448–1450 (1982).

8. BERGDOLL, M. S., CRASS, B. A., REISER, R. F., ROBBINS, R. N., AND DAVIS, J. P., A new staphylococcal enterotoxin, enterotoxin F, associated with toxic-shock syndrome *Staphylococcus aureus* isolates, *Lancet* **1**:1017–1021 (1981).

9. BERKLEY, S. F., HIGHTOWER, A. W., BROOME, C. V., AND REINGOLD, A. L., The relationship of tampon characteristics to menstrual toxic shock syndrome, *J. Am. Med. Assoc.* **258**:917–920 (1987).

10. BEST, G. K., ABNEY, T. O., KLING, J. M., KIRKLAND, J. J., AND SCOTT, D. F., Hormonal influence on experimental infections by a toxic shock strain of *Staphylococcus aureus*, *Infect. Immun.* **52**:331–333 (1986).

11. BEST, G. K., SCOTT, D. F., KLING, J. M., CROWELL, W. F., AND KIRKLAND, J. J., Enhanced susceptibility of male rabbits to infection with a toxic shock strain of *Staphylococcus aureus*, *Infect. Immun.* **46**:727–732 (1984).

12. BONVENTRE, P. F., LINNEMANN, C., WECKBACH, L. S., STANECK, J. L., BUNCHER, C. R., VIGDORTH, E., RITZ, H., ARCHER, D., AND SMITH, B., Antibody responses to toxic-shock-syndrome (TSS) toxin by patients with TSS and by healthy staphylococcal carriers, *J. Infect. Dis.* **150**:662–666 (1984).

13. BROOME, C. V., HAYES, P. S., AJELLO, G. W., FEELEY, J. C., GIBSON, R. J., GRAVES, L. M., HANCOCK, G. A., ANDERSON, R. L., HIGHSMITH, A. K., MACKEL, D. C., HARGRETT, N. T., AND REINGOLD, A. L., In-vitro studies of interactions between tampons and *Staphylococcus aureus*, *Ann. Intern. Med.* **96**(Part 2):959–962 (1982).

14. Centers for Disease Control, Follow-up on toxic-shock syndrome—United States, *Morbid. Mortal. Weekly Rep.* **29**:297–299 (1980).

15. Centers for Disease Control, Toxic-shock syndrome—United States, *Morbid. Mortal. Weekly Rep.* **29**:229–230 (1980).

16. Centers for Disease Control, Toxic-shock syndrome—United States, 1970–1982, *Morbid. Mortal. Weekly Rep.* **31**:201–204 (1982).

17. CHOW, A. W., GRIBBLE, M. J., AND BARTLETT, K. H., Characterization of the hemolytic activity of *Staphylococcus aureus* strains associated with toxic shock syndrome, *J. Clin. Microbiol.* **17**:524–528 (1983).

18. CHU, M. C., MELISH, M. E., AND JAMES, J. F., Tryptophan auxotypy associated with *Staphylococcus aureus* that produce toxic-shock-syndrome toxin, *J. Infect. Dis.* **151**:1157–1158 (1985).

19. CORBISHLEY, C. M., Microbial flora of the vagina and cervix, *J. Clin. Pathol.* **30**:745–748 (1977).

20. DAVIS, J. P., CHESNEY, P. J., WAND, P. J., LAVENTURE, M., AND the Investigation and Laboratory Team, Toxic-shock syndrome: Epidemiologic features, recurrence, risk factors, and prevention, *N. Engl. J. Med.* **303**:1429–1435 (1980).

21. DE AZAVEDO, J. C. S., AND ARBUTHNOTT, J. P., Toxicity of staphylococcal toxic shock syndrome toxin-1 in rabbits, *Infect. Immun.* **46**:314–317 (1984).

22. EVERETT, E. D., Mucocutaneous lymph node syndrome (Kawasaki disease) in adults, *J. Am. Med. Assoc.* **242**:542–543 (1979).

23. FAICH, G., PEARSON, K., FLEMING, D., SOBEL, S., AND ANELLO, C., Toxic shock syndrome and the vaginal contraceptive sponge, *J. Am. Med. Assoc.* **255**:216–218 (1986).

24. FISHER, C. J., JR., HOROWITZ, B. Z., AND NOLAN, S. M., The clinical spectrum of toxic-shock syndrome, *West. J. Med.* **135**:175–182 (1981).

25. FRIEDRICH, E. G., AND SIEGESMUND, K. A., Tampon-associated vaginal ulcerations, *Obstet. Gynecol.* **55**:149–156 (1980).

26. FUJIKAWA, H., IGARASHI, H., USAMI, H., TANAKA, S., AND TAMURA, H., Clearance of endotoxin from blood of rabbits injected with staphylococcal toxic shock syndrome toxin-1, *Infect. Immun.* **52**:134–137 (1986).

27. GARBE, P. L., ARKO, R. J., REINGOLD, A. L., GRAVES, L. M., HAYES, P. S., HIGHTOWER, A. W., CHANDLER, F. W., AND BROOME, C. V., *Staphylococcus aureus* isolates from patients with nonmenstrual toxic shock syndrome, *J. Am. Med. Assoc.* **253**:2538–2542 (1985).

28. GREEN, S. L., AND LAPETER, K. S., Evidence for postpartum toxic-shock syndrome in a mother–infant pair, *Am. J. Med.* **72**:169–172 (1982).

29. GUINAN, M. E., DAN, B. B., GUIDOTTI, R. J., REINGOLD, A. L., SCHMID, G. P., BETTOLI, E. J., LOSSICK, J. G., SHANDS, K. N., KRAMER, M. A., HARGRETT, N. T., ANDERSON, R. L., AND BROOME, C. V., Vaginal colonization with *Staphylococcus aureus* in healthy women: A review of four studies, *Ann. Intern. Med.* **96**(Part 2):944–947 (1982).

30. GUSTAFSON, T. L., SWINGER, G. L., BOOTH, A. L., HUTCHESON, R. H., JR., AND SCHAFFNER, W., Survey of tampon use and toxic shock syndrome, Tennessee, 1979 to 1981, *Am. J. Obstet. Gynecol.* **143:**369–374 (1982).

31. HAYES, P. S., GRAVES, L. M., FEELEY, J. C., HANCOCK, G. A., COHEN, M. L., REINGOLD, A. L., BROOME, C. V., AND HIGHTOWER, A. W., Production of toxic-shock-associated protein(s) in *Staphylococcus aureus* strains isolated from 1956 through 1982, *J. Clin. Microbiol.* **20:**43–46 (1984).

32. HELGERSON, S. D., AND FOSTER, L. R., Toxic shock syndrome in Oregon: Epidemiologic findings, *Ann. Intern. Med.* **96**(Part 2):909–911 (1982).

33. IKEJIMA, T., DINARELLO, C. A., GILL, D. M., AND WOLFF, S. M., Induction of human interleukin-1 by a product of *Staphylococcus aureus* associated with toxic shock syndrome, *J. Clin. Invest.* **73:**1312–1320 (1984).

34. IRWIN, C. E., AND MILLSTEIN, S. G., Emerging patterns of tampon use in the adolescent female: The impact of toxic shock syndrome, *Am. J. Public Health* **72:**464–467 (1982).

35. IRWIN, C. E., AND MILLSTEIN, S. G., Predictors of tampon use in adolescents after media coverage of toxic shock syndrome, *Ann. Intern. Med.* **96**(Part 2):966–968 (1982).

36. JACOBSON, J. A., KASWORM, E. M., CRASS, B. A., AND BERGDOLL, M. S., Nasal carriage of toxigenic *Staphylococcus aureus* and prevalence of serum antibody to toxic-shock-syndrome toxin 1 in Utah, *J. Infect. Dis.* **153:**356–359 (1986).

37. KASS, E. H., KENDRICK, M. I., TSAI, Y.-C., AND PARSONNET, J., Interaction of magnesium ion, oxygen tension, and temperature in the production of toxic-shock-syndrome toxin-1 by *Staphylococcus aureus, J. Infect. Dis.* **155:**812–815 (1987).

38. KEHRBERG, M. W., LATHAM, R. H., HASLAM, B. R., HIGHTOWER, A., TANNER, M., JACOBSON, J. A., BARBOUR, A. G., NOBEL, V., AND SMITH, C. B., Risk factors for staphylococcal toxic-shock syndrome, *Am. J. Epidemiol.* **114:**873–879 (1981).

39. KIRKLAND, J. J., AND WIDDER, J. S., Hydrolysis of carboxymethylcellulose tampon material [letter], *Lancet* **1:**1041–1042 (1983).

40. KREISWIRTH, B. N., KRAVITZ, G. R., SCHLIEVERT, P. M., AND NOVICK, R. P., Nosocomial transmission of a strain of *Staphylococcus aureus* causing toxic shock syndrome, *Ann. Intern. Med.* **105:**704–707 (1986).

41. KREISWIRTH, B. N., LOFDAHL, S., BETLEY, M. J., O'REILLY, M., SCHLIEVERT, P. M., BERGDOLL, M. S., AND NOVICK, R. P., The toxic shock syndrome exotoxin structural gene is not detectably transmitted by a prophage [letter], *Nature* **305:**709–712 (1983).

42. KREISWIRTH, B. N., NOVICK, R. P., SCHLIEVERT, P. M., AND BERGDOLL, M., Genetic studies on staphylococcal strains from patients with toxic shock syndrome, *Ann. Intern. Med.* **96**(Part 2):974–977 (1982).

43. KUSHNARYOV, V. M., MACDONALD, H. S., REISER, R., AND BERGDOLL, M. S., Staphylococcal toxic shock toxin specifically binds to cultured human epithelial cells and is rapidly internalized, *Infect. Immun.* **45:**566–571 (1984).

44. LANSDELL, L. W., TAPLIN, D., AND ALDRICH, T. E., Recovery of *Staphylococcus aureus* from multiple body sites in menstruating women, *J. Clin. Microbiol.* **20:**307–310 (1984).

45. LARKIN, S. M., WILLIAMS, D. N., OSTERHOLM, M. T., TOFTE, R. W., AND POSALAKY, Z., Toxic shock syndrome: Clinical, laboratory, and pathologic findings in nine fatal cases, *Ann. Intern. Med.* **96**(Part 2):858–864 (1982).

46. LINNEMANN, C. C., JR., AND KNARR, D., Increasing incidence of toxic shock syndrome in the 1970s, *Am. J. Public Health* **76:**566–567 (1986).

47. LINNEMANN, C. C., STANECK, J. L., HORNSTEIN, S., BARDEN, T. P., RAUH, J. L., BONVENTRE, P. F., BUNCHER, C. R., AND BEITING, A., The epidemiology of genital colonization with *Staphylococcus aureus, Ann. Intern. Med.* **96**(Part 2):940–944 (1982).

48. MACDONALD, K. L., OSTERHOLM, M. T., HEDBERG, C. W., SCHROCK, C. G., PETERSON, G. F., JENTZEN, J. M., LEONARD, S. A., AND SCHLIEVERT, P. M., Toxic shock syndrome. A newly recognized complication of influenza and influenzalike illness, *J. Am. Med. Assoc.* **257:**1053–1058 (1987).

49. MARKOWITZ, L. E., HIGHTOWER, A. W., BROOME, C. V., AND REINGOLD, A. L., Toxic shock syndrome. Evaluation of national surveillance data using a hospital discharge survey, *J. Am. Med. Assoc.* **258:**75–78 (1987).

50. MARTIN, R. R., BUTTRAM, V., BESCH, P., KIRKLAND, J. J., AND PETTY, G. P., Nasal and vaginal *Staphylococcus aureus* in young women: Quantitative studies, *Ann. Intern. Med.* **96**(Part 2):951–953 (1982).

51. MILLS, J. T., PARSONNET, J., AND KASS, E. H., Production of toxic-shock-syndrome toxin-1: Effect of magnesium ion, *J. Infect. Dis.* **153:**993–994 (1986).

52. MILLS, J. T., PARSONNET, J., TSAI, Y.-C., KENDRICK, M., HICKMAN, R. K., AND KASS, E. H., Control of production of toxic-shock-syndrome toxin-1 (TSST-1) by magnesium ion, *J. Infect. Dis.* **151:**1158–1161 (1985).

53. NOBLE, V. S., JACOBSON, J. A., AND SMITH, C. B., The effect of menses and use of catamenial products on cervical carriage of *Staphylococcus aureus, Am. J. Obstet. Gynecol.* **144:**186–189 (1982).

54. ONDERDONK, A. B., ZAMARCHI, G. R., WALSH, J. A., MELLOR, R. D., MUNOZ, A., AND KASS, E. H., Methods for quantitative and qualitative evaluation of vaginal microflora during menstruation, *Appl. Environ. Microbiol.* **51:**333–339 (1986).

55. OSTERHOLM, M. T., AND FORFANG, J. C., Toxic-shock syndrome in Minnesota: Results of an active–passive surveillance system, *J. Infect. Dis.* **145:**458–464 (1982).

56. OSTERHOLM, M. T., DAVIS, J. P., AND GIBSON, R. W., Tri-state toxic-shock syndrome study. I. Epidemiologic findings, *J. Infect. Dis.* **145:**431–440 (1982).

57. PARIS, A. L., HERWALDT, L. A., BLUM, D., SCHMID, G. P., SHANDS, K. N., AND BROOME, C. V., Pathologic findings in twelve fatal cases of toxic shock syndrome, *Ann. Intern. Med.* **96**(Part 2):852–857 (1982).

58. PARSONNET, J., HICKMAN, R. K., EARDLEY, D. D., AND PIER, G. B., Induction of human interleukin-1 by toxic shock syndrome toxin-1, *J. Infect. Dis.* **151**:514–522 (1985).

59. PARSONNET, J., GILLIS, Z. A., RICHTER, A. G., AND PIER, G. B., A rabbit model of toxic shock syndrome that uses a constant, subcutaneous infusion of toxic shock syndrome toxin 1, *Infect. Immun.* **55**:1070–1076 (1987).

60. PETITTI, D. B., REINGOLD, A. L., AND CHIN, J., The incidence of toxic shock syndrome in northern California, 1972 through 1983, *J. Am. Med. Assoc.* **255**:368–372 (1986).

60a. PETITTI, D. B., AND REINGOLD, A. L., Update through 1985 on the incidence of toxic shock syndrome among members of a prepaid health plan, *Rev. Infect. Dis.* **11**(Suppl. 1):22–27 (1989).

61. POINDEXTER, N. J., AND SCHLIEVERT, P. M., Toxic-shock-syndrome toxin 1-induced proliferation of lymphocytes: Comparison of the mitogenic response of human, murine, and rabbit lymphocytes, *J. Infect. Dis.* **151**:65–72 (1985).

62. POINDEXTER, N. J., AND SCHLIEVERT, P. M., Suppression of immunoglobulin-screening cells from human peripheral blood by toxic-shock-syndrome toxin-1, *J. Infect. Dis.* **153**:772–779 (1986).

63. POLLACK, M., WEINBERG, W. G., HOSKINS, W. J., O'BRIEN, W. F., IANNINI, P. B., ANDERSON, S. E., AND SCHLIEVERT, P. M., Toxinogenic vaginal infections due to *Staphylococcus aureus* in menstruating rhesus monkeys without toxic-shock syndrome, *J. Infect. Dis.* **147**:963–964 (1983).

64. RASHEED, J. K., ARKO, R. J., FEELEY, J. C., CHANDLER, F. W., THORNSBERRY, C., GIBSON, R. J., COHEN, M. L., JEFFRIES, C. D., AND BROOME, C. V., Acquired ability of *Staphylococcus aureus* to produce toxic shock-associated protein and resulting illness in a rabbit model, *Infect. Immun.* **47**:598–604 (1985).

65. REINGOLD, A. L., Epidemiology of toxic-shock syndrome, United States, 1960–1984, Centers for Disease Control, *CDC Surveillance Summaries* **33**(3SS):19SS–22SS (1984).

66. REINGOLD, A. L., On the proposed screening definition for toxic shock syndrome by Todd et al. [letter], *Am. J. Epidemiol.* **122**:918–919 (1985).

66a. REINGOLD, A. L., BROOME, C. V., GAVENTA, S., HIGHTOWER, A. W., AND the TSS Study Group, Risk factors for menstrual toxic shock syndrome: Results of a multistate case-control study, *Rev. Infect. Dis.* **11**(Suppl. 1):35–42 (1989).

67. REINGOLD, A. L., DAN, B. B., SHANDS, K. N., AND BROOME, C. V., Toxic-shock syndrome not associated with menstruation: A review of 54 cases, *Lancet* **1**:1–4 (1982).

68. REINGOLD, A. L., HARGRETT, N. T., DAN, B. B., SHANDS, K. N., STRICKLAND, B. Y., AND BROOME, C. V., Non-

menstrual toxic shock syndrome: A review of 130 cases, *Ann. Intern. Med.* **96**(Part 2):871–874 (1982).

69. REINGOLD, A. L., HARGRETT, N. T., SHANDS, K. N., DAN, B. B., SCHMID, G. P., STRICKLAND, B. Y., AND BROOME, C. V., Toxic shock syndrome surveillance in the United States, 1980 to 1981, *Ann. Intern. Med.* **92**(Part 2):875–880 (1982).

70. REISER, R. F., ROBBINS, R. N., KHOE, G. P., AND BERGDOLL, M. S., Purification and some physicochemical properties of toxic-shock toxin, *Biochemistry* **22**:3907–3912 (1983).

71. RITZ, H. L., KIRKLAND, J. J., BOND, G. G., WARNER, E. K., AND PETTY, G. P., Association of high levels of serum antibody to staphylococcal toxic shock antigen with nasal carriage of toxic shock antigen-producing strains of *Staphylococcus aureus*, *Infect. Immun.* **43**:954–958 (1984).

72. SCHLECH, W. F., SHANDS, K. N., REINGOLD, A. L., DAN, B. B., SCHMID, G. P., HARGRETT, N. T., HIGHTOWER, A., HERWALDT, L. A., NEILL, M. A., BAND, J. D., AND BENNETT, J. V., Risk factors for the development of toxic shock syndrome: Association with a tampon brand, *J. Am. Med. Assoc.* **248**:835–839 (1982).

73. SCHLIEVERT, P. M., Enhancement of host susceptibility to lethal endotoxin shock by staphylococcal pyrogenic exotoxin type C, *Infect. Immun.* **36**:123–128 (1982).

74. SCHLIEVERT, P. M., Alteration of immune function by staphylococcal pyrogenic exotoxin type C: Possible role in toxic-shock syndrome, *J. Infect. Dis.* **147**:391–398 (1983).

75. SCHLIEVERT, P. M., Effect of magnesium on production of toxic-shock-syndrome toxin-1 by *Staphylococcus aureus*, *J. Infect. Dis.* **152**:618–620 (1985).

76. SCHLIEVERT, P. M., Staphylococcal enterotoxin B and toxic-shock syndrome toxin-1 are significantly associated with nonmenstrual TSS [letter], *Lancet* **1**:1149–1150 (1986).

77. SCHLIEVERT, P. M., AND BLOMSTER, D. A., Production of staphylococcal pyrogenic exotoxin type C: Influence of physical and chemical factors, *J. Infect. Dis.* **147**:236–242 (1983).

78. SCHLIEVERT, P. M., SHANDS, K. N., DAN, B. B., SCHMID, G. P., AND NISHIMURA, R. D., Identification and characterization of an exotoxin from *Staphylococcus aureus* associated with toxic-shock syndrome, *J. Infect. Dis.* **143**:509–516 (1981).

79. SCHLIEVERT, P. M., OSTERHOLM, M. T., KELLY, J. A., AND NISHIMURA, R. D., Toxin and enzyme characterization of *Staphylococcus aureus* isolates from patients with and without toxic shock syndrome, *Ann. Intern. Med.* **96**(Part 2):937–940 (1982).

80. SCHLIEVERT, P. M., BLOMSTER, D. A., AND KELLY, J. A., Toxic shock syndrome *Staphylococcus aureus:* Effect of tampons on toxic shock syndrome toxin 1 production, *Obstet. Gynecol.* **64**:666–670 (1984).

81. SCOTT, D. F., KLING, J. M., KIRKLAND, J. J., AND BEST, G. K., Characterization of *Staphylococcus aureus* isolates from patients with toxic shock syndrome, using polyethylene in-

fection chambers in rabbits, *Infect. Immun.* **39**:383–387 (1983).

82. SCOTT, D. F., KLING, J. M., AND BEST, G. K., Immunological protection of rabbits infected with *Staphylococcus aureus* isolates from patients with toxic shock syndrome, *Infect. Immun.* **53**:441–444 (1986).

83. SHANDS, K. N., SCHMID, G. P., DAN, B. B., BLUM, D., GUIDOTTI, R. J., HARGRETT, N. T., ANDERSON, R. L., HILL, D. L., BROOME, C. V., BAND, J. D., AND FRASER, D. W., Toxic-shock syndrome in menstruating women: Its association with tampon use and *Staphylococcus aureus* and the clinical features in 52 cases, *N. Engl. J. Med.* **303**:1436–1442 (1980).

84. SMITH, C. B., NOBLE, V., BENSCH, R., AHLIN, P. A., JACOBSON, J. A., AND LATHAM, R. H., Bacterial flora of the vagina during the menstrual cycle: Findings in users of tampons, napkins, and sea sponges, *Ann. Intern. Med.* **96**(Part 2):948–951 (1982).

85. SPERBER, S. J., AND FRANCIS, J. B., Toxic shock syndrome during an influenza outbreak, *J. Am. Med. Assoc.* **257**:1086–1087 (1987).

86. STEVENS, F. A., The occurrence of *Staphylococcus aureus* infection with a scarlatiniform rash, *J. Am. Med. Assoc.* **88**:1957–1958 (1927).

87. STOLZ, S. J., DAVIS, J. P., VERGERONT, J. M., CRASS, B. A., CHESNEY, P. J., WAND, P. J., AND BERGDOLL, M. S., Development of serum antibody to toxic shock toxin among individuals with toxic shock syndrome in Wisconsin, *J. Infect. Dis.* **151**:883–889 (1985).

88. TIERNO, P. M., JR., AND HANNA, B. A., *In vitro* amplification of toxic shock syndrome toxin-1 by intravaginal devices, *Contraception* **31**:185–194 (1985).

89. TIERNO, P. M., JR., HANNA, B. A., AND DAVIES, M. B., Growth of toxic-shock-syndrome strain of *Staphylococcus aureus* after enzymic degradation of 'Rely' tampon component, *Lancet* **1**:615–618 (1983).

90. TIERNO, P. M., JR., MALLOY, V., MATIAS, J. R., AND HANNA, B. A., Effects of toxic shock syndrome *Staphylococcus aureus,* endotoxin and tampons in a mouse model, *Clin. Invest. Med.* **10**:64–70 (1987).

91. TODD, J. K., FISHAUT, M., KAPRAL, F., AND WELCH, T., Toxic-shock syndrome associated with phage-group-I staphylococci, *Lancet* **2**:1116–1118 (1978).

92. TODD, J. K., FRANCO-BUFF, A., LAWELLIN, D. W., AND VASIL, M. L., Phenotypic distinctiveness of *Staphylococcus aureus* strains associated with toxic shock syndrome, *Infect. Immun.* **45**:339–344 (1984).

93. TODD, J. K., WIESENTHAL, A. M., RESSMAN, M., CASTAN, S. A., AND HOPKINS, R. S., Toxic shock syndrome. II. Estimated occurrence in Colorado as influenced by case ascertainment methods, *Am. J. Epidemiol.* **122**:857–867 (1985).

94. TODD, J. K., TODD, B. H., FRANCO-BUFF, A., SMITH, C. M., AND LAWELLIN, D., Influence of focal growth conditions on the pathogenesis of toxic shock syndrome, *J. Infect. Dis.* **155**:673–681 (1987).

95. TOFTE, R. W., AND WILLIAMS, D. N., Toxic-shock syndrome: Evidence of a broad clinical spectrum, *J. Am. Med. Assoc.* **246**:2163–2167 (1981).

96. VAN MIERT, A. S. J. P. A. M., VAN DUIN, C. T. M., AND SCHOTMAN, A. J. H., Comparative observations of fever and associated clinical hematological and blood biochemical changes after intravenous administration of staphylococcal enterotoxins B and F (toxic shock syndrome toxin-1) in goats, *Infect. Immun.* **46**:354–360 (1984).

97. VERGERONT, J. M., EVENSON, M. L., CRASS, B. A., DAVIS, J. P. BERGDOLL, M. S., WAND, P. J., NOBLE, J. H., AND PETERSEN, G. K., Recovery of staphylococcal enterotoxin F from the breast milk of a woman with toxic-shock syndrome, *J. Infect. Dis.* **146**:456–459 (1982).

98. VERGERONT, J. M., STOLZ, S. J., CRASS, B. A., NELSON, D. B., DAVIS, J. P., AND BERGDOLL, M. S., Prevalence of serum antibody to staphylococcal enterotoxin F among Wisconsin residents: Implications for toxic-shock syndrome, *J. Infect. Dis.* **148**:692–698 (1983).

99. WAGNER, G., BOHR, L., WAGNER, P., AND PETERSEN, L., Tampon-induced changes in vaginal oxygen and carbon dioxide tensions, *Am. J. Obstet. Gynecol.* **148**:147–150 (1984).

100. WIESENTHAL, A. M., RESSMAN, M., CASTON, S. A., AND TODD, J. K., Toxic shock syndrome. I. Clinical exclusion of other syndromes by strict and screening definitions, *Am. J. Epidemiol.* **122**:847–856 (1985).

12. Suggested Reading

CHESNEY, P. J., DAVIS, J. P., PURDY, W. K., WAND, P. J., AND CHESNEY, K. W., Clinical manifestations of the toxic shock syndrome, *J. Am. Med. Assoc.* **246**:741–748 (1981).

Division of Health Sciences Policy, Division of Health Promotion and Disease Prevention, Institute of Medicine, Toxic shock syndrome. Assessment of current information and future research needs, National Academy Press (1982).

FISHER, R. F., GOODPASTURE, H. C., PETERIE, J. D., AND VOTH, D. W., Toxic shock syndrome in menstruating women, *Ann. Intern. Med.* **94**:156–163 (1981).

Proceedings of the First International Symposium on Toxic Shock Syndrome, *Rev. Infect. Dis.* **11**: (1989).

STALLONES, R. A., A review of the epidemiologic studies of toxic shock syndrome, *Ann. Intern. Med.* **96**(Part 2):917–920 (1982).

CHAPTER 36

Tuberculosis

George W. Comstock and Richard J. O'Brien

1. Introduction

The term "tuberculosis" is used primarily to signify an infectious disease of the lungs caused by *Mycobacterium tuberculosis*. Many other organs may be involved, however, and similar illnesses caused by *M. bovis* are also called tuberculosis. The disease has long been a major killer of mankind. In 17th century England, John Bunyan referred to consumption, now recognized as one of the forms of pulmonary tuberculosis, as "the captain of all of these men of death." Tuberculosis is still a major cause of disability and premature death throughout most of the world today. Only among the economically favored nations has it become a relatively minor problem, concentrated among disadvantaged segments of the population.

Almost all human tuberculosis is caused by *M. tuberculosis*. Human disease due to *M. bovis* is rare except in areas where milk is not pasteurized. *M. africanum*, an organism with characteristics intermediate between *M. tuberculosis* and *M. bovis*, causes similar disease and is mostly confined to Africa. BCG (bacillus Calmette–Guérin), derived from an attenuated strain of *M. bovis*, is used as a vaccine but can cause disease in immunocompromised persons.

George W. Comstock · School of Hygiene and Public Health, The Johns Hopkins University, Baltimore, Maryland 21205. Richard J. O'Brien · Clinical Research Branch, Division of Tuberculosis Control, Center for Prevention Services, Centers for Disease Control, Atlanta, Georgia 30333.

2. Historical Background[36,65]

Descriptions of tuberculosis can be recognized in many older medical writings, usually as "phthisis" or "consumption," a chronic wasting illness associated with "ulcerations" of the lungs; as "galloping consumption," the pneumonic form of the disease; or as "scrofula," an involvement of the cervical lymph nodes. The term "tuberculosis" (literally "a condition of little knots or swellings") has only recently come into general use for all the many manifestations of this disease, although three centuries ago Franciscus Sylvius recognized in cases of phthisis little nodules that he called tubercula. That the various forms of tuberculosis had a common and infectious etiology was first established by Villemin in 1865. He showed that inoculation of material from the various forms of tuberculous lesions caused a similar disease in rabbits, as did the inoculation of sputum from patients with pulmonary lesions. Even more important in establishing the infectious nature of tuberculosis was the discovery of the tubercle bacillus by Koch in 1882. Only then did it become possible to make definitive diagnoses of tuberculosis and to identify disseminators of the organisms.

Koch made another fundamental contribution to the epidemiological armamentarium by discovering tuberculin in 1890. Although his claim for the therapeutic use of tuberculin was discredited, it was soon recognized that infected persons could be identified by the local reaction that followed the injection of a small amount of tuberculin into the skin.

The third major diagnostic procedure resulted from the discovery of X rays by Roentgen in 1895. Roentgenograms of the chest made it possible to demonstrate pulmonary disease that had developed in infected persons before it could be recognized clinically and often before it had become communicable.

Refinements of these fundamental diagnostic procedures occurred for the most part during the 1940s and 1950s and added greatly to their usefulness. Development of artificial culture media made it possible to detect much smaller numbers of tubercle bacilli than could be demonstrated by microscopic examination of stained specimens; furthermore, cultures were less expensive and more widely applicable than were guinea pig inoculations, which were originally used to confirm microscopic examinations. Photofluorography brought chest roentgenography to the general population in mass surveys designed to detect early asymptomatic cases of pulmonary tuberculosis. And improvements in the standardization, administration, and interpretation of the tuberculin test made it possible to identify, with minimal misclassification, persons who had been infected with *M. tuberculosis*.

The history of tuberculosis control is closely entwined with the sanatorium movement, which espoused healthful living, with particular emphasis on rest, good food, and fresh air. In addition, the concomitant isolation of patients during their treatment undoubtedly reduced the risk of transmission of their disease to others. Although the basic precepts of the sanatorium movement can be traced back to the temples of Asclepius in Greek and Roman civilizations, they did not receive wide public acceptance for treatment of tuberculosis until the successful establishment of sanatoriums by Brehmer in the mountains of Silesia in 1854 and by Trudeau in the Adirondack Mountains of the United States in 1882. Sanatorium treatment became the major tuberculosis-control activity for decades, diminishing in importance only with the introduction of effective antibiotics, notably streptomycin in 1946 and isoniazid in 1952. Successful treatment on an outpatient basis then became possible, and the days of the sanatoriums were over. Further advances in the treatment of tuberculosis and discovery of other antimycobacterial drugs have led to shortening of therapy to 6 months and supervised twice-weekly administration of medications.

Specific preventive measures began with the development of an attenuated strain of *M. bovis* by Calmette and Guérin between 1908 and 1922. A vaccine prepared from this strain came to be called bacillus Calmette–Guérin (BCG). Accepted at first with reluctance, vaccination with one of the many substrains descended from this organism has become a mainstay of tuberculosis-control programs in many parts of the world. The only other specific preventive

procedure is chemoprophylaxis, which provides the most recent landmark in the history of tuberculosis control. During the 1960s, large-scale controlled trials demonstrated that persons who had been infected with tubercle bacilli could be protected from the subsequent development of disease by the oral administration of isoniazid.

The impact of our increasing ability to detect, treat, and prevent tuberculosis on the course of the tuberculosis epidemic is uncertain. Skeptics note that the decline of tuberculosis mortality appears to have started prior to the present century, long before tuberculosis-control measures could have had any general effect. Some suspect that tuberculosis and other infectious diseases may have long-term cycles of waxing and waning and that much of the recent decline in tuberculosis may have resulted from this natural tendency. It is not necessary, however, to call upon arcane mechanisms. Dubos and Dubos[36] point out that in countries where the decline could be documented by death records, the sanitary and social reform movements in the early 19th century brought about many improvements in living conditions, notably in the field of housing with better ventilation, more illumination, and less crowding, all of which would tend to operate against the tubercle bacillus. Fortunately, unlike the fresh-air movement, sanatoriums, and mass chest X-ray surveys, more recent tuberculosis-control measures such as the use of drugs for treatment and prevention rest on secure ground, having had their effectiveness documented by large-scale controlled trials under actual field conditions.

3. Methodology

3.1. Sources of Mortality Data

Tuberculosis deaths and death rates are tabulated in the *World Health Statistics Annual*, published by the World Health Organization (WHO) in Geneva, and in various national vital statistics publications, such as *Vital Statistics of the United States*, published annually by the National Center for Health Statistics, Centers for Disease Control (CDC), U.S. Department of Health and Human Services. Annual reports on tuberculosis are also published by the Division of Tuberculosis Control, CDC.[8,9] Useful compendiums of official statistics are also available.[64,65]

Prior to the introduction of effective antibiotic therapy, tuberculosis mortality rates were relied on as indices of the magnitude of the tuberculosis problem. Because there appeared to be only moderate variation in case-fatality rates temporally or geographically, mortality rates correlated fairly well with morbidity rates. While mortality data have thus provided useful guidelines to problem areas and to progress in tuberculosis control, their use has to be tempered with a recognition of their deficiencies. Only in a few countries have mortality records been complete and reliable for many decades. In the United States, for example, the death-registration area did not include all states until 1933. With the introduction of antibiotic therapy in 1946 and the gradual but marked increase in its potential effectiveness, mortality statistics have come more and more to reflect the lack of access to or compliance with good medical treatment, rather than the incidence of the disease.

3.2. Sources of Morbidity Data

Tuberculosis cases and case rates are tabulated and summarized in the publications from the WHO and CDC mentioned in Section 3.1. In addition, the *Morbidity and Mortality Weekly Report* from the CDC and the monthly reports from state health departments give up-to-date accounts of reported cases. The disease is reportable in all states, and reporting is thought to be reasonably complete, particularly in areas that require laboratories to report bacteriological examinations that are positive for *M. tuberculosis*.

Changes in the definition of a reportable case have also influenced time trends. Although international advisory bodies have urged that only bacteriologically positive cases be reported, this recommendation has not been widely accepted. In 1961, the U.S. Public Health Service (PHS) recommended that new active cases for reporting purposes be defined as diagnosed cases of any site with positive bacteriology or with consistent X-ray or histological evidence, or cases of unexplained pleurisy with effusion.[65] In 1975, the definition was broadened to include previously reported cases whose disease had reactivated. In addition, in many jurisdictions, persons being treated with two or more antituberculosis drugs became reportable even in the absence of other criteria.

3.3. Surveys

Surveys for tuberculosis have been conducted by means of physical examinations, bacteriological examinations of sputum, chest photofluorography, and tuberculin testing. In 1917, an extensive antituberculosis campaign was carried out in Framingham, Massachusetts, in the course of which approximately 11,000 persons, two thirds of the population, were given physical examinations for

tuberculosis.[5] The findings of this survey resulted in the estimate that there were ten prevalent active cases for every annual tuberculosis death, a ratio used for the next three decades in the United States to estimate the size of the tuberculosis problem.

Sputum surveys are limited as a general rule to persons with abnormal findings on chest X-ray surveys either to identify cases that are most meaningful from the public health point of view or as a means of surveillance for drug-resistant organisms. Occasionally, in areas where mass radiography is impractical, sputum surveys of general populations have been done to estimate the prevalence of tuberculosis or to detect tuberculosis cases among persons with chronic cough.

With the demonstration in Brazil by de Abreu and de Paula[33] in 1936 of the practicability of mass photofluorography, it became feasible to examine the lungs of large numbers of apparently normal persons for tuberculosis. In the decade following World War II, millions of persons were examined in mass chest X-ray surveys. While it seems reasonable to believe that the detection of thousands of cases of tuberculosis before their disease became clinically manifest was beneficial, this belief has never been adequately tested. In only a few areas did the coverage approach completeness, and even there, careful follow-up of the examined population gave little evidence of an appreciable subsequent drop in the case rate.[13] Comparison of the results of tuberculin surveys in the two communities in Wales, one with nearly complete coverage by a mass X-ray campaign designed to identify and treat prevalent infectious cases, and the other community left unexamined, did indicate a decreased risk of new tuberculous infections among children in the examined community.[58]

In an evaluation of mass X-ray screening, survey films were reread 5 years after the initial survey. Two groups of persons with minimal roentgenographic evidence of disease were identified: those detected only by the initial reading and those detected only by the second reading 5 years later. The first group had been referred for medical advice and follow-up; the second group had not. Because the two groups were similar, differences in their fate since the initial survey could be attributed to the follow-up advice given the first group. At that time, such advice was likely to consist of suggestions for healthful living: adequate rest, good food, cutting down on tobacco and alcohol, and the like. Although mortality among the first group was lower than among the second during the 5 years after the survey, there was no difference in tuberculosis mortality among the two groups. The excess deaths among the second group were due to cardiovascular causes.[41]

There is no longer much place for mass radiography in tuberculosis control. Where it can be afforded, the yield is too low to justify the cost; where the prevalence of active disease is high enough to warrant this method of case-finding, funds are usually limited and must be spent on items of higher priority, such as providing adequate treatment for clinically manifest cases.

In the populations who have not been vaccinated with BCG, use of the tuberculin skin test can contribute a great deal to epidemiological knowledge. The applications of tuberculin testing to the delineation of the risks of having been infected with tubercle bacilli by time, place, and person are epitomized by the work of Palmer and Edwards and their colleagues.[37–39,65,67,87] By careful attention to the selection of study populations, to the techniques of administering and reading tuberculin tests, and to the interpretation of frequency distributions of reaction sizes, it has been possible to learn a great deal about the prevalence of infected persons under varied circumstances and the implications of these findings for temporal, geographic, and personal differences in the risk of becoming infected. Because classification of a given person as a positive tuberculin reactor or nonreactor may depend to a considerable extent on technical factors that can and usually do change with time, estimates of the rate of acquiring new infections derived from age-specific prevalence curves are likely to be more accurate than estimates derived from tests of the same persons at two points in time.[72]

3.4. Laboratory Diagnosis

3.4.1. Isolation and Identification of the Organism. Tubercle bacilli are commonly looked for in biological fluids and tissues by microscopic examination of preparations stained by the Ziehl–Neelson acid-fast technique. Staining of the organisms in fixed preparations with basic fuchsin is accomplished by the use of heat or detergents. Ethanol acidified with hydrochloric acid will decolorize most cells and other material promptly, but mycobacteria resist decolorization for many hours, thereby having acquired the name "acid-fast bacilli." Identification of the fuchsin-stained mycobacteria, which are rods 1–4 μm long, is facilitated by staining the preparation with a contrasting dye. Microscopic examination of stained specimens is relatively quick and inexpensive, but its sensitivity is low. It has been estimated that approximately 100,000 organisms/ml are needed to make their recognition by microscopy reasonably certain. With proper laboratory techniques in areas where tuberculosis is common, specificity is fairly high since acid-fast rods seen on microscopy are usu-

ally tubercle bacilli, which are readily distinguishable from most acid-fast artifacts. Nontuberculous mycobacteria, however, have a similar appearance and can occur as pathogens, as normal inhabitants in oral or genitourinary secretions, or even in water used to wash the slides.

Staining with fluorescent dyes has important advantages over the standard Ziehl–Neelson technique.[105] The times required for staining and for examination are considerably reduced, as is examiner fatigue. Both sensitivity and specificity of microscopy appear to be increased somewhat by the use of fluorescent staining.[83]

A much greater increase in sensitivity and specificity is obtained by culturing specimens, albeit at the cost of up to 8 weeks' delay. The most common culture media contain egg yolk and potato extract, although agar-based media may also be used. With a generation time of nearly 24 h, tubercle bacilli grow slowly, usually requiring 3–8 weeks to form identifiable colonies. Although they are aerobic, growth is stimulated by the presence of 5–10% carbon dioxide. Presumptive identification of the various mycobacteria is based on growth rate, colony characteristics, and pigment formation.[32] Tubercle bacilli (*M. tuberculosis* and *M. bovis*) are not pigmented. *M. tuberculosis* grows more readily than does *M. bovis,* especially on media that contain glycerol. The colonies of *M. tuberculosis* tend to be rough, dry, and friable; those of *M. bovis,* smaller and pyramidal. However, definitive speciation requires biochemical tests for the identification of *M. tuberculosis.* Niacin production, nitrate reduction, and quantitative catalase activity are commonly used. *M. tuberculosis* is niacin positive, reduces nitrate, and produces less than 45 mm of bubbles on catalase testing.[32]

A means of rapidly differentiating infectious tuberculosis from nontuberculous mycobacterial and other diseases is badly needed to replace time-consuming cultural identification. A method of considerable promise is based on the detection of radioactive carbon dioxide released by the growth of mycobacteria on a radiolabeled substrate. This radiometric method (BACTEC) can accurately detect the presence of mycobacteria within 1–2 weeks and distinguish *M. tuberculosis* complex from nontuberculous mycobacteria.[92]

3.4.2. Serological and Immunological Diagnostic Methods. A variety of serological tests for the diagnosis of tuberculosis have been evaluated.[30] At present, the only immunological test that can be applied widely enough to be useful for epidemiological purposes is the tuberculin skin test.

The standard tuberculin test is administered by the Mantoux technique, whereby 0.1 ml of test material is injected into the skin of the forearm by needle and syringe.[2] The test material is a purified protein derivative of old tuberculin (PPD or RT), which should come from a large, well-standardized batch of tuberculin and be protected against adsorption to vial or syringe by the addition of a detergent.[89] Injection at the proper depth produces a discrete pale elevation of the skin approximately 6–10 mm in diameter. The test is usually read 40–80 h after injection. Erythema is ignored except as a guide to the reaction site. Induration of the skin is detected by palpation and by visual inspection of the site, preferably under light that is indirect and oblique. The diameter of the visible (or palpable) induration transverse to the long axis of the arm is carefully measured and recorded in millimeters. The use of a caliper for measuring reactions reduces terminal digit preference if the scale cannot be seen until the caliper jaws have been set at the borders of the induration.

The definition of a positive reaction is best derived from a frequency distribution of reaction sizes in a population similar to the one under study.[2] The optimal dividing line between positive and negative will vary with the proportion of persons in the population who have been infected with tubercle bacilli, the frequency of cross-reactions caused by infections with nontuberculous mycobacteria, and technical factors related to administration and reading of the test. In many parts of the United States, an appropriate definition of a positive reaction is considered to be an area of induration 10 mm or more in diameter produced by the infection of 5 tuberculin units (TU) of PPD. If the likelihood of tuberculous infection is increased, as it is among persons with abnormal chest shadows or with a history of household exposure to an active case, reactions of 5 mm or more in diameter are considered to be positive and to indicate the occurrence of tuberculous infection at some time in the past. In persons at low risk of tuberculous infection and at increased risk of immunological cross-reactions (e.g., history of BCG vaccination or residence in an area endemic for nontuberculous mycobacteria), 15 mm of induration may be a more appropriate cutoff point.

Tuberculin testing may also be done by means of one of the multiple-puncture devices. These methods have the advantage of avoiding the fear induced by sight of a needle. Several of the multiple-puncture devices are both convenient and simple to use but the dose of tuberculin delivered by any of these devices cannot be predicted. Generally, the multiple-puncture devices with their highly concentrated tuberculin tend to classify some persons as positive who have negative reactions to the standard test. It is necessary, therefore, to retest positive reactors to a multiple-puncture test by the standard Mantoux technique. Some devices using dried

tuberculin have also been reported to fail to detect positive reactors.[35] Whether or not the advantages of administering tuberculin tests by multiple puncture outweigh the disadvantages depends a great deal on the proposed application. Multiple-puncture devices seem to be useful in clinical pediatric practice or in school surveys, where few positive reactors will need to be retested.

Although the accuracy of the tuberculin test in detecting past or present infection with tubercle bacilli compares favorably with that of many medical screening tests, there are important sources of error in addition to those associated with administration of the test by multiple-puncture devices. Errors in dosage, depth of injection, and measurement of reactions can result in misclassification. Many nontuberculous mycobacteria cause tuberculin hypersensitivity, which often results in reactions large enough to be classified as positive. False-negative reactions may occur up to weeks after infection while hypersensitivity is developing, in seriously ill tuberculosis patients, during and shortly after viral infections and vaccinations (notably measles), and with natural and induced immunosuppression (e.g., Hodgkin's disease, AIDS, therapy with large doses of corticosteroids).

Identifying recently infected persons by means of repeated tuberculin tests of initially negative reactors is simple in theory but difficult in practice. Even with fastidious technique, the results of two tests can vary by 6 mm or more in some instances.[71] Consequently, only persons whose reactions change from negative to positive and increase by at least 10 mm are considered to have had a true change in tuberculin sensitivity that may have been caused by a recent infection.

A further complication in the detection of newly infected persons results from the "booster effect," the analogue of the anamnestic reaction in serology. Many persons, especially those over 50 years of age, may have had a gradual decline in tuberculin sensitivity to the point where an initial test causes no detectable induration. Some of these previously positive persons may still have enough sensitivity left, however, that the stimulus of the initial test causes a "boost" of their sensitivity back to its original level. Boosting occurs within 1 week and appears to last for at least 2 years. If these persons are given a second test 6 or 12 months later, their positive reactions at that time may have resulted from either the booster effect or a new infection. To minimize the possibility of attributing a boosted reaction to a new infection, persons who are to be tested periodically and who have a low risk of becoming infected (i.e., those who are not household contacts) should have a second test given a week after the initial test if that initial test was negative. Persons still negative to the second test should then be included in the periodic testing program with reasonable assurance that any subsequent change to a positive reaction (with an increase of at least 10 mm) will have resulted from a recent infection. Persons who are positive to the second test of the initial series should be classified as initially positive reactors.[94]

Considerable work has been done in developing an enzyme-linked immunosorbent assay (ELISA) as a diagnostic test. Using a variety of purified antigens, sensitivities in 13 studies ranged from 49 to 94% and specificities from 88 to 100%.[30] The ELISA test appears to be most suitable among groups with a high prevalence of tuberculosis, such as tuberculosis suspects, and in detecting acute disease. Unfortunately, there is no good diagnostic test for tuberculous meningitis, a condition where delayed diagnosis can have catastrophic consequences. Recent development of several biochemical and immunological tests that can be applied to cerebrospinal fluid give reason to hope that this situation can soon be remedied.[29]

4. Biological Characteristics of the Organism

Tubercle bacilli are very resistant to drying and to most ordinary germicides, especially in the presence of organic material such as sputum. They are susceptible to moist heat, being killed in about 30 min by exposure to 60°C and in less than a minute by temperatures greater than 70°C. They are highly sensitive to sunlight or artificial ultraviolet light.

Their slow rate of growth, nearly 24 h from one generation to the next, undoubtedly contributes to the relatively slow development of disease in infected susceptible hosts. A factor that operates against the survival of tubercle bacilli in human populations is their proclivity to become buried within tissues. Only in the infrequent instances when pulmonary cavitation or airway ulceration occurs do the bacilli become surface dwellers and thus available for widespread dissemination to others.[47]

Whether or not *M. tuberculosis* varies in its virulence for man is uncertain. There is, however, considerable variation in virulence for guinea pigs. A significant fraction of wild strains from India, Southeast Asia, and Hong Kong show a low degree of virulence when injected into guinea pigs,[34] as do isoniazid-resistant tubercle bacilli. A study in India failed to show a significant difference between the acquisition of new infection by household contacts of patients with isoniazid-sensitive tubercle bacilli and that by

contacts of patients with resistant organisms.[82] This finding suggests that isoniazid resistance may not be related to the ability of the organisms to initiate infections in humans. Whether resistant organisms produce human disease following infection as readily as do sensitive organisms is not known.

5. Descriptive Epidemiology

In thinking epidemiologically about the development of tuberculosis in populations, it is important to look at each of the two stages of this disease—the acquisition of infection, as identified by an appropriate tuberculin test, and the subsequent development of significant disease, as diagnosed by radiological or bacteriological techniques. While all communicable diseases must go through these two stages, their separation is particularly important in tuberculosis, the reason being that tuberculosis differs from most other communicable diseases in a very important respect, namely, that the resistance that develops after successful recovery from the primary infection is often not sufficient to rid the body of invading organisms. As a consequence, an unknown but significant proportion of tuberculin reactors continue to harbor living organisms and are at risk of reactivation for the rest of their lives. In epidemiological terms, this means that the incubation period of tuberculosis is highly variable, ranging from a few weeks to a lifetime. For almost all other communicable diseases, the incubation period is fixed within a relatively short and discrete interval after infection. Once this interval is past, the individual has nothing to fear from that particular infection, and indeed is usually better off as a result of the immunity that follows, even though for some diseases this immunity may be transient. Not so for the person infected with tuberculosis: even those who pass through the highest-risk period shortly after infection still have a subsequent lifetime risk that may actually exceed the initial risk because of the cumulative effect of a low risk operating over many years.

It is useful to consider the development of tuberculosis as a two-stage process not only because the acquisition of infection is often far removed from the development of disease, but also because the known risk factors for infection are so different from the risk factors for the development of disease after infection. Despite the voluminous literature on tuberculosis, very little of the work has been done in such a way that these two risks can be disentangled. Even in determining the frequency of infection, there are serious problems because of insufficient attention to the tuberculin used, to the technique of administration and measurement, and to the detailed reporting of results.

5.1. Prevalence and Incidence

Information on the prevalence or incidence of tuberculous infections is rarely available on a communitywide basis, especially for recent years. Data have been selected for this section with an eye primarily toward their representativeness and comparability, using the most recent reports that meet these criteria. Estimating the frequency of tuberculous infections is also made difficult by the fact that positive reactions to the tuberculin skin test can result not only from infections with tubercle bacilli but also from BCG vaccination and from infections with a variety of nontuberculous mycobacteria as well. Frequency of cross-reactions from nontuberculous mycobacterial infections varies markedly by geography, being almost nonexistent in the Arctic and almost universal in some tropical and subtropical areas. Because disease caused by nontuberculous mycobacteria is uncommon, their presence has little effect on estimates of the frequency of tuberculous disease, which, however, can be seriously affected by the degree of access to adequate medical care, completeness of ascertainment and reporting, and variations in definition of cases.

The prevalence of tuberculous infections rises with age, tending to level off at about 40 to 50 years. In 1971, the overall prevalence in the United States was estimated at about 8%[54]; for white male Navy recruits, 17–21 years of age, the estimates for U.S. regions ranged from 1.6 to 2.9% over the period 1961–1968.[87] Among males of similar age, the average prevalence of infected persons was slightly less than 40% in the Bangalore district of south India in the same period[70] and slightly more than 40% in the East Central State of Nigeria in 1971.[79] In the Chingleput area, near Madras in south India, the prevalence of positive tuberculin reactors in 1968–1971 reached a plateau of about 80% among males at age 25 and among females of about 70% at age 35.[102]

The incidence of tuberculous *infection* is usually estimated from the change in prevalence of tuberculin reactors by age rather than from repeated testing of the same individuals.[72,100] This method minimizes errors in classification caused by technical variations in testing and reading and also those caused by the effects on the second test of the stimulus from the first test, the so-called booster effect (see Section 3.4.2). With few exceptions, the incidence of new

infections appears to have been decreasing, at least since the 1930s. Perhaps the most dramatic decrease occurred in the Bethel area of Alaska, where the estimated incidence in 1949–1951 was 25% per year, but was well under 0.1% per year in 1970, so low that there were not enough children to measure it accurately.[60] Extrapolation from published data indicates that recent incidence rates in Norway, Saskatchewan, the Netherlands, and most of the United States are likely to have been in the neighborhood of 10/100,000 person-years.[38,42,100,101,103] In south India and Nigeria, the incidence in the 1960s was between 1 and 2% per year.[70,79] Estimates of the incidence of tuberculous infection are also available from the prevalence of tuberculin reactors in the Chingleput district of south India during the period 1968–1971.[102] The average annual rates of infection among children during their lifetimes were 1.7% for the age group 1–4 years, 2.4% for the age group 5–9 years, and 4.0% for the age group 10–14 years. This trend is consistent with an increased risk of infection with increasing age or a decreased risk with the passage of time. In this area where little had been done to control tuberculosis prior to 1968, the former explanation appears more likely.

The frequency of tuberculous disease depends first on the probability of becoming infected and second on the ability of the infected person to withstand that infection. In most developed countries today, it is likely that fewer than 5–10% of newly infected individuals will develop demonstrable tuberculous disease during their lifetime. Only in extreme situations does the incidence of disease become so high that, if continued unabated, it would eventually result in nearly everyone becoming a victim of tuberculosis.

The prevalence of a disease depends on both the incidence of the disease and its average duration. In Muscogee County, Georgia, the prevalence of radiologically demonstrable tuberculosis, active and inactive, was 1700/100,000 among whites but only 1200/100,000 among blacks in 1946, whereas the subsequent incidence of new cases during the next 5 years was 34/100,000 per year among whites and 111/100,000 per year among blacks.[20] When the comparison of prevalence and incidence for the two ethnic groups is limited to bacteriologically positive cases, the ratio of incidence to prevalence remains lower for whites than for blacks. Prevalence of bacteriologically positive disease was 239/100,000 for whites and 385 for blacks, while the subsequent incidence was 14/100,000 per year for whites and 67 for blacks. Although a definite value for average duration of disease cannot be calculated because tuberculosis was not in a steady state during the observation period, the findings do indicate that duration for whites was longer than for blacks, largely because the case-fatality rate among blacks was nearly eight times that among whites.

In developing countries, both the prevalence and the incidence of bacteriologically positive cases are likely to be much higher than in Muscogee County. In East Central Nigeria, for example, a survey suggested that the prevalence of bacteriologically positive disease among persons over 10 years of age was approximately 500/100,000 in 1971.[79] Repeated surveys between 1961 and 1968 in south India showed that the prevalence of bacteriologically positive cases among persons over 15 years of age averaged 536/100,000 while the incidence in this area averaged 143/100,000 per year.[70] In the Chingleput area, tuberculosis cases with sputum positive for *M. tuberculosis* on culture were much more frequent among males than among females, increasing with age for both sexes and reaching levels of approximately 4% among males and 0.7% among females after age 50.[102]

5.2. Epidemic Behavior and Contagiousness

Tuberculosis can and sometimes does occur in sharply localized outbreaks. In nearly all such instances, these involve the exposure of previously uninfected persons to an infectious individual in crowded quarters, such as a schoolroom under wartime blacked-out conditions[56] or an air-conditioned naval vessel.[55] Perhaps the most remarkable aspect of these outbreaks is their relative rarity, given the frequency with which uninfected individuals are exposed to infectious cases under similar circumstances. A possible explanation is that some tuberculous patients are more effective spreaders than are others, as suggested by one experimental situation.[98] Another factor that may play a role is that tuberculosis is usually not highly communicable.[15] Secondary attack rates among 5- to 9-year-old household associates of cases of measles and mumps have been reported to be 81 and 86%, respectively; the infection rates, at least in mumps, are presumably even higher. In contrast, only 67% of 5- to 9-year-old household associates of active tuberculosis cases in Tennessee in the period 1933–1955 were positive tuberculin reactors, and only 48% of household associates of similar age were positive reactors in a large multicenter study in 1958. In 1985, 28.6% of close contacts of all ages reported to CDC were positive tuberculin reactors as were 15.6% of other contacts.[8] The "attack rate" of new infections among tuberculosis contacts is undoubtedly lower than these figures would suggest, since some contacts must have been infected prior to exposure to the index case. Because the communicability of measles or mumps is measured in days, while that of tuberculosis is

measured in weeks or months, the infectiousness of tuberculosis per day of exposure must be very low indeed.

The infectiousness of tuberculosis patients appears to be rapidly reduced by adequate chemotherapy. The most convincing study, because it was strictly controlled, came from the very useful series of chemotherapy trials in Madras, India.[59] Because there were too few hospital beds for all active cases of tuberculosis, cases that were not considered emergencies were randomly allocated to home and to hospital treatment. Both groups received the same chemotherapy. At the end of 5 years, there were actually fewer cases among contacts of patients treated at home than among contacts of those isolated in hospital. This result strongly suggests that chemotherapy was as effective as hospitalization in reducing the risk connected with being a close contact of an infectious patient.

5.3. Geographic Distribution

A recent study conducted within the European Community showed remarkable variation in tuberculosis death rates within the member nations (Fig. 1). The causes of this variation are under investigation.[50]

An earlier international study had shown that the spectrum of diagnosed and reported cases of tuberculosis differed greatly in various countries.[52] Among five European countries, one country in Southeast Asia, and two locations in the United States, there were significant differences in the proportion of cases confirmed bacteriologically and in the manner of their confirmation. The extent and nature of disease as shown by roentgenography also varied markedly. Consequently, geographic differences measured by official morbidity statistics may represent not only true differences in the frequency of disease but also diligence in searching for cases, criteria for diagnosis, and perhaps differing pathological responses of the populations.

Tuberculosis case rates for the United States during the period 1982–1984 are shown by county in Fig. 2.[9] The highest case rates are found along the South Atlantic coast, in the mid-South, in states along the Mexican border, and in Alaska and Hawaii. Case rates in 1984 were highest in cities with populations over 500,000 and lowest in rural areas.

The prevalence of positive reactors to tuberculin among white male Navy recruits aged 17–21 years who were lifetime residents of a single county is shown in Fig. 3.[38] In a sense, Fig. 3 also represents the relative risk of becoming infected with tubercle bacilli over the 19-year period (the average lifetime of the recruits) prior to the time of testing. There were high frequencies of tuberculin-positive recruits in the hard coal mining areas of Pennsylva-

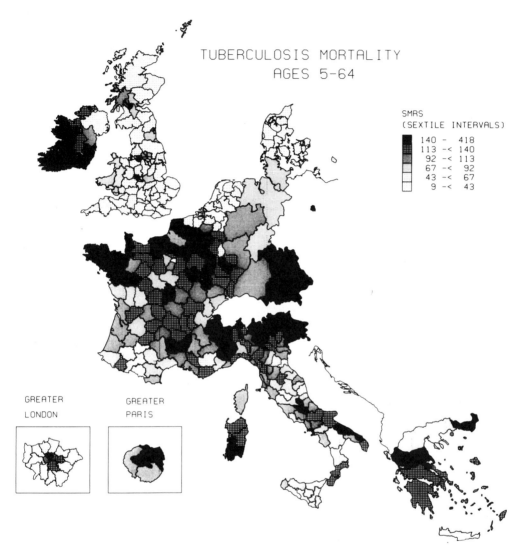

Figure 1. Standardized mortality ratios for tuberculosis by local geographic units, European Community, ages 5–64 years, 1974–1978.[50]

nia, around Chesapeake Bay, south of the lower Ohio River, and along the Mexican border. In at least two other areas, the high frequency of positively reacting recruits is known to have resulted from cross-reactions to tuberculin. The large section of northwestern Colorado owed its high reactor rate to cross-reactions produced by infections with *M. marinum* acquired in a popular swimming pool. The dark area in the center of the Georgia–Alabama border resulted from the high population of persons vaccinated with BCG in two controlled trials conducted in that area.

The causes of other discrepancies between Figs. 2 and 3 are not known. To some extent, they may result from the small numbers of cases now being reported from many counties. In 1984, 89% of U.S. counties, representing 39% of the national population, reported fewer than ten cases of tuberculosis.[9]

Residence abroad has often been considered to be a significant risk factor for acquiring tuberculous infection. Almost the only satisfactory evidence on this point comes from the study by Palmer and Edwards[65] of Navy recruits.

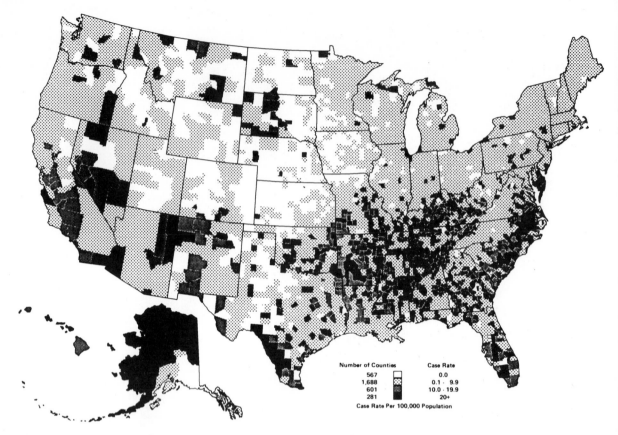

Figure 2. Average annual tuberculosis case rates per 100,000 population, United States, 1982–1984, by county.[9]

In that study population, there were 6817 white males who had lived abroad for at least 6 months. Their frequency of positive reactions was 4.7%, only slightly higher than the 3.9% found among recruits who had not been out of the country.

Little is known about geographic variation in the risk of developing disease following infection, and even less about the causes of variation. The 20-fold difference in incidence among tuberculin reactors in Alaska and Denmark, referred to in Section 5.1, might have resulted, at least in part, from the high dosage of infection associated with the extremely high infection rates and crowded living quarters of Alaskan Inuit only a few decades ago.[14]

5.4. Temporal Distribution

Tuberculosis case rates have been declining in the United States since the initiation of nationwide reporting in 1930. The annual rate of decrease was slight prior to 1950 but thereafter averaged close to 6% per year through 1984.[9] From 1975 to 1984, the rate of decline was similar for males and females. During this period, the rate of decline was more marked for persons over 25 years of age than among younger persons. Changes in diagnostic and reporting practices caused a temporary upturn in the number of cases reported in children during the early 1960s and among adults in many areas in the mid-1970s. In 1984, the reported case rate was 9.4/100,000; in 1988, it was 9.1/100,000. This is an unprecedented period of essentially no decline in the case rate since such records have been kept[10] (D. E. Snider, Jr., personal communication). Available evidence indicates that an important factor in this cessation of the decline in tuberculosis morbidity is the recrudescence of tuberculosis among persons infected with the human immunodeficiency virus (HIV).

Because any reaction to any dose of tuberculin was once considered to signify a previous infection with tubercle bacilli, information on temporal trends in the prevalence

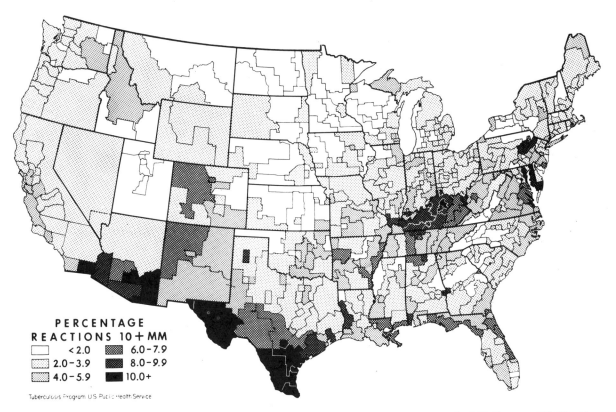

Figure 3. Frequency of positive reactors to 5 tuberculin units of a purified protein derivative of tuberculin (PPD-S) among 275,558 white male Navy recruits aged 17–21 years who were lifetime residents of a single county, 1958–1965, by state economic area.[38]

and incidence of tuberculous infection is limited. In the 1930s, the prevalence of positive reactors among persons 15–19 years of age, using a tuberculin and a definition of a positive reactor reasonably compatible with modern ideas, was 22 and 25% in Philadelphia and the rural South, respectively. The estimated incidence of infection was between 1.5 and 2.0% per year.[15]

In 1949–1951, the frequency of positive reactors to 5 TU of a purified protein derivative of tuberculin prepared from mammalian tubercle bacilli (PPD-S) was 6.6% among white male Navy recruits aged 17–21 years; in 1963–1964, this frequency was only 3.2%.[65] When the proportion of positive reactors becomes this low in a country in which cross-reactions from nontuberculous mycobacterial infections are common, it is probable that much if not most of the current tuberculin sensitivity results from cross-reactions. The proportion of young persons infected with tubercle bacilli in many parts of the United States is undoubtedly much lower than the proportion classified as positive tuberculin reactors. A number of considerations indicate that the

risk of becoming infected with tubercle bacilli in this country is now close to 10/100,000 per year.

There is no satisfactory information on changes with calendar time in the risk of disease following infection. There is some information, however, on the risk of disease among tuberculin-positive individuals by time after exposure to an infectious case, although there is some uncertainty because receipt of infection cannot be timed with accuracy. In the large study of tuberculosis contacts conducted by the PHS, it was found that the attack rate among tuberculin-positive contacts was 1000/100,000 during the first year after diagnosis of the index case.[44] Some 8–10 years later, their rate had fallen to 72/100,000 per year, not much higher than rates among tuberculin-positive individuals without a history of household exposure.

5.5. Age

Tuberculosis mortality rates, and presumably case rates also, show different patterns in areas and times with high and low risks of becoming infected with tubercle bacilli. When the risk is high, there is a peak in infancy, followed by a second peak in young adult life, and sometimes a third peak in old age. When the risk of becoming infected is low, tuberculosis case rates tend to increase steadily with age.[65]

The prevalence of positive tuberculin reactors usually increases at a fairly steady rate with age until about 40 to 50 years, when it tends to level off or even to fall somewhat. Determining the incidence of new infections with age is fraught with numerous problems. Most studies agree in finding an increase with age up to about 20 years; estimates of the incidence thereafter vary considerably.[81,100] When current risks of becoming infected are very low, it is likely that reversions from positive to negative may outnumber conversions, especially among older persons.

The probability of developing tuberculous disease among positive tuberculin reactors also varies with age (Fig. 4A,B).[15,24] There is a peak in infancy and early childhood, followed by a second peak in young adult life. The pattern among persons past the age of 45 is uncertain because studies of general populations have included only small numbers of infected persons this old. It seems likely that the peak in infancy largely reflects the effect of a recent infection since all infections among infants are of necessity recent. The reason for the increased incidence among infected persons in young adult life is not known.

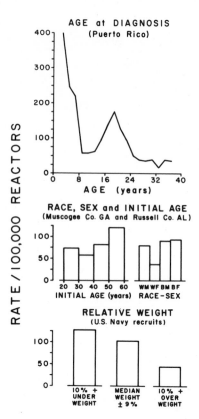

Figure 4. Average annual incidence of tuberculosis per 100,000 positive tuberculin reactors in three selected populations. (A) Children in Puerto Rico, 1949–1969. Rates by age at diagnosis. Adapted from Comstock et al.[24] (B) Adults in Muscogee County, Georgia, and Russell County, Alabama, 1950–1969. Rates by initial age adjusted for race and sex; rate by race–sex adjusted for initial age. Adapted from Comstock et al.[26] (C) U.S. Navy recruits tested in 1958–1967. Rates by relative weight during 4 years after enlistment. Adapted from Edwards et al.[39]

5.6. Sex

In the United States, tuberculosis death and case rates have been lower among females than among males at almost all ages.[9,65] The differences between the sexes are slight until 25 years of age, following which male rates increase with increasing age to a greater extent than do female rates.

The prevalence of positive tuberculin reactors, and presumably the incidence of tuberculous infections, is also lower among females.[15,65] There is conflicting evidence regarding the risk of disease among infected males and females. Among Danes and Alaskan Inuit, and young blacks and Puerto Ricans in the United States, rates were higher among females,[15,19,24,53] whereas among whites in the United States and persons in south India, rates were higher among males.[19,102]

5.7. Race

Both death and case rates have been higher among blacks, Indians, and Inuits than among whites in the United States.[65] Death rates have fallen somewhat more rapidly for nonwhites than for whites, while reported case rates have fallen somewhat more rapidly for whites.

The prevalence of positive tuberculin reactors in the United States is also generally higher among blacks, Indians, and Inuits.[15,37,65,84] Among men entering the Navy between 1958 and 1969, 3.8% of the whites were positive tuberculin reactors compared to 12.4% of the blacks and 60.2% of the Asians, who were mainly Filipinos.[25] The high percentage of positive reactions among the Asians may have resulted in part from BCG vaccination in their native countries.

The incidence of tuberculous disease among *infected* Navy recruits was 79/100,000 per year for whites, 93 for blacks, and 196 for Asians.[25] It is possible that special stresses accounted for the high rate among Asian reactors. In any case, their experience suggests that the BCG vaccination program in the Philippines had little effect on the subsequent tuberculosis experience of these recruits.

In a study of the nature of officially reported tuberculosis cases, several striking differences were found.[52] Alaskans (mostly Inuit and Indians) tended to have lesions that were not extensive and very rarely exudative in nature. Patients from Singapore and from Maryland had extensive disease and a high frequency of exudative and cavitary lesions. Patients from five European centers tended to fall between these extremes.

Among the subgroups with high rates of tuberculosis are refugee immigrants to the United States from Southeast Asia, Latin America, and Haiti.[76,77] During the late 1970s, their contribution to reported tuberculosis cases in the United States was responsible for a marked slowing in the annual rate of decline during that period. In subsequent years, 1981–1984, cases among Asians and Pacific Islanders decreased more rapidly than did those of other ethnic groups; cases among Hispanics declined at the same rates as for the United States as a whole.[9] In the United Kingdom, immigrants also accounted for a major portion of the tuberculosis problem, notably those from India, Pakistan, and Bangladesh.[68] There was evidence, however, that the high rates among immigrants were due to their poor socioeconomic status as well as to the high rates of infection acquired in their native countries.[46,76]

5.8. Occupation[65]

Little is known of the risks among various occupational groups of becoming infected or of developing disease following infection. Among hospital employees, there were only slight and nonsignificant differences in the frequency of positive tuberculin reactors by type of job or estimated exposure to patients after allowing for the fact that males, minority ethnic groups, and older persons all had higher rates of positive reactions.[94] Tuberculosis rates are often excessive in occupations with silica exposure. Because silica has been shown to lower host resistance to tuberculosis in experimental animals, it is presumed that persons with silicosis also have a lowered capability of controlling tuberculous infections.

5.9. Occurrence in Different Settings

In recent years, hospitalization of tuberculosis patients has shifted from tuberculosis sanatoriums to general hospitals as the need for hospital care has become less frequent and its duration shorter. With this change, some general hospitals have begun to institute periodic tuberculin testing programs for their employees. Rates of conversion from negative to positive have often been high, sometimes even among presumably unexposed personnel.[86] In the absence of two tuberculin tests given sequentially at the initial examination, however, it is likely that most of the reported conversions resulted from the booster effect and not from new infections.[94]

Tuberculosis can be a significant hazard in jails, particularly with the overcrowding that is virtually universal in American prisons. Screening of prisoners on admission by tuberculin tests, followed by periodic tuberculin testing of negative reactors and chest roentgenograms, and isoniazid prophylaxis for positive reactors have been shown to provide an effective means of control.[96]

Tuberculosis has also been shown to be a potential hazard in nursing homes, especially when the frequency of other cardiorespiratory illnesses and a reduced index of suspicion combine to make case detection unlikely.[97] Here, too, efforts to detect and treat new infections have been shown to be effective in preventing disease.

5.10. Socioeconomic Factors

Tuberculosis has long been known to be associated with poverty, crowding, and malnutrition.[36,65] Mortality, morbidity, and prevalence of tuberculosis all tend to be highest in the poorest areas. A group at particularly high risk of having tuberculosis consists of homeless persons living in large urban centers.[12,51] In Denmark, the incidence of tuberculosis was highest among divorced persons and lowest among married persons, the differences being marked for men and slight for women.

Relatively few studies, however, indicate whether the risk of disease associated with socioeconomic status results from the risk of becoming infected, of becoming diseased after infection, or both. One of these studies, a report of tuberculin testing of New York City school personnel in 1973–1974, showed that the frequency of tuberculous infection was indeed higher in the poorest areas, 22.4%, contrasted with 5.5% in areas with the highest socioeconomic rating, after adjustment for differences in composition by age, race, and sex (Fig. 5).[84]

Some of the individual factors that enter into the association of tuberculous infection with poverty are known from a study in Texas that related a number of personal and household characteristics to the probability that a contact would be infected, using a multiple regression method to

758 Part II • Acute Bacterial Infections

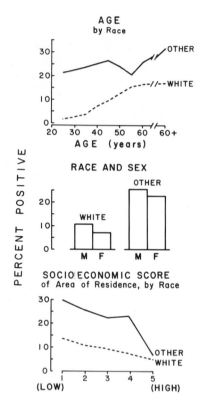

Figure 5. Percentage of positive reactors to 5 tuberculin units of PPD-S among New York City school employees, by age, sex, race, and socioeconomic rating of area of residence. All percentages are adjusted for the effects of the other characteristics shown in the figure. Adapted from information furnished by L. B. Reichman (see Reichman and O'Day[84]).

isolate insofar as possible the effect of each individual characteristic.[11] Infection of the contacts was most closely related to the extent of disease and sputum positivity of the source case. Crowding (measured as persons per room) and a subjective assessment of the intimacy of exposure were also related to the probability of infection but were not as important as the severity of disease in the source case. Household income *per se* was not important, but what the family had to show for its income in the way of household furnishings did seem to be a factor of considerable importance. Lack of household furnishings correlated as well with the probability of infection as did crowding or intimacy of exposure. In Washington County, Maryland, high-school children living in homes with one or more persons per room or in an inadequate dwelling as assessed by the absence of complete bathroom facilities were more than twice as likely

to be positive tuberculin reactors as were children living in less crowded, more adequate dwellings.[63]

Even less is known about the risk of developing disease after infection as related to socioeconomic status. In Muscogee County, Georgia, no significant association of the incidence of tuberculosis with adequacy of housing could be found, after controlling for the effects of initial tuberculin and BCG vaccination status.[15]

5.11. Nutritional Factors

Severe malnutrition has been shown to be associated with a diminution of tuberculin sensitivity following BCG vaccination.[61] There is no indication, however, that malnutrition protects against infection; rather, it appears that it masks our ability to detect the presence of infection.

For a long time, it has been observed that a variety of situations involving food deprivation are associated with increases in tuberculosis case and death rates.[36,65,88] Since the common factor in these situations is malnutrition, it is likely that the association is one of cause and effect. And since morbidity increases shortly after food shortages appear and decreases promptly when food supplies become adequate, it is likely that the effect of malnutrition is mediated primarily through a concomitant risk of disease among persons already infected.

Body build is related in part to nutrition. Studies among U.S. Navy recruits have demonstrated that there is no relationship of relative weight to the prevalence of positive reactions to tuberculin (see Fig. 4C).[39] Among positive reactors on initial examination, however, the subsequent case rate was nearly four times higher among men initially 10% or more underweight than among men initially 10% or more overweight. That fatness was the component of body weight likely to be responsible for this association was indicated by evidence from Muscogee County, Georgia.[15] This study population consisted of persons who had participated in tuberculosis surveys in 1946 and 1950 and whose chest roentgenograms were on each occasion considered by two readers to be negative for tuberculosis. The incidence of disease in the 14 years following 1950 was closely related to the thickness of subcutaneous fat measured over the trapezius ridges from photofluorograms of the chest taken in 1946. Tuberculosis was twice as high among persons with less than 5 mm of subcutaneous fat as among those with 10 mm or more.

The above-cited studies do not conclusively answer the questions about diet and tuberculosis. Although it is possible that undernutrition causes both leanness and susceptibility to tuberculosis, it is also possible that some other aspect of body build, such as hormonal or genetic factors, is the underlying cause of both. Two findings that favor the latter hypothesis are the impression that very few people in Muscogee County in 1946 could have been considered to be seriously undernourished and the observation among Navy recruits that tuberculosis contacts weighed less than men who had not lived in the same house with a tuberculosis case, even when the comparison was limited to tuberculin-negative persons in each group.[39]

5.12. Genetic Factors

That varying degrees of resistance to tuberculosis can be inherited was clearly shown by Lurie[66] in his work with inbred strains of rabbits. Whether or not this holds true for humans has been much less certain. While it is possible that there is inherent resistance to the acquisition of infection, it seems more likely that genetic factors are more important in keeping infection from progressing to disease. There have been numerous observations that the risk of tuberculosis among household contacts is greater for blood relatives than for others.[78] That there is a genetic component in this increased risk is indicated by studies of twins, in which concordance for tuberculosis is considerably greater among monozygotic twins than among dizygotic twins, even when other factors related to tuberculosis risk are taken into account.[17] An additional indication of inherited susceptibility is the report of higher case rates associated with blood groups B and AB among Inuit in Alaska.[73]

5.13. AIDS

Because of the importance of the cellular immune system in controlling infections with *M. tuberculosis*, it is not surprising that persons infected with HIV are at increased risk of reactivating dormant organisms.[99] In 1987, linking of registers for tuberculosis with those for AIDS indicated that nearly 5% of AIDS cases had tuberculosis, the association being most marked among populations at high risk of having been infected with *M. tuberculosis* and HIV (e.g., intravenous drug abusers in inner cities).[10] A prospective study of intravenous drug abusers showed that combined infections with *M. tuberculosis* and HIV resulted in an extremely high rate of clinical tuberculosis.[90] Active tuberculosis may precede or follow the development of AIDS. Further indication of depressed resistance in AIDS is the severe and unusual forms of pulmonary tuberculosis seen in these patients and the increased frequency of extrapulmonary and disseminated tuberculosis. AIDS is also associated

with a failure to react to tuberculin, increasing the difficulties of making a diagnosis of concurrent tuberculosis. For this reason, it has been recommended that a person who tests positive for HIV be tuberculin tested, and if a positive reactor, be given preventive therapy with isoniazid.[3]

5.14. Size of Tuberculin Reaction

Several studies have shown that persons who are most sensitive to tuberculin are also most likely to develop tuberculous disease later on.[15,40] Fifty years ago, attention was focused on whether allergy to tuberculo-protein was beneficial or harmful; now, at least in epidemiological circles, principal interest lies in the ability of the degree of hypersensitivity to indicate whether or not the infecting organism was one of the tubercle bacilli, *M. tuberculosis* or *M. bovis*, or one of the usually benign nontuberculous mycobacteria.

The prognostic importance of degree of sensitivity to tuberculin is clearly shown in Table 1, which was taken from a study of more than 1 million white Navy recruits.[40] On entry into the Navy, recruits routinely received a skin test with PPD-S (S) and also with a PPD prepared from a nontuberculous mycobacterium, either the so-called Battey (B) or Gause (G) strain, currently named *M. avium-intracellulare* or *M. scrofulaceum*, respectively. Cases of tuberculosis that developed among these men during their first 4 years of Navy service were identified. Numbers of cases and case rates according to their reaction to 5 TU of PPD-S

Table 1. Tuberculosis Morbidity According to Results of Dual Tests in 1,124,883 White Navy Recruits[a]

Dual test reactions (mm)[a]	Tuberculosis	
	Number	Rate per 100,000
PPD-S, 0–5	384	36
PPD-S, 6–11	36	110
S < B/G − 1	5	29
S = B/G ± 1	10	127
S > B/G + 1	21	272
PPD-S, 12–17	80	382
S < B/G − 1	5	216
S = B/G ± 1	12	297
S > B/G + 1	63	432
PPD-S, ≥ 18	49	372

[a]Data from Edwards *et al.*[40] The expression S < B/G − 1 denotes a reaction to PPD-S more than 1 mm smaller than that to the Battey (B) or Gause (G) antigen; similarly, S = B/G ± 1 and S > B/G + 1 denote, respectively, a reaction to PPD-S within 1 mm of and more than 1 mm larger than that to the B or G antigen.

on entry are shown in italic. Those with less than 6 mm on entry had a low rate of tuberculosis subsequently; those with intermediate reactions, an intermediate rate; and those with reactions of 12 mm or more, a high rate.

Both experimental and clinical evidence indicate that reactions to a homologous antigen are usually larger than cross-reactions to a heterologous antigen. Thus, in theory, the group of persons whose reactions to PPD-S are smaller than those to either PPD-B or PPD-G are not likely to have been infected with tubercle bacilli and should therefore have a low risk of tuberculosis. Although the numbers are small in the two subgroups whose reactions to S are smaller than those to B or G, the theory seems to hold well for persons with intermediate reactions to PPD-S, but not so well for persons whose reactions to PPD-S measure 12 mm or more in diameter.

These findings are not as neat as one might wish, possibly because of the bewildering variety of mycobacterial infections and the inability to test for more than a few of them. Furthermore, no one knows how to test for multiple infections in the same individual. Nevertheless, these and similar findings support the current belief that the larger the reaction to a small or intermediate dose of tuberculin, the more likely it is that an individual has been infected with tubercle bacilli, and consequently the more likely that tuberculous disease will develop at some time in the future.

6. Mechanisms and Routes of Transmission

For all practical purposes, tubercle bacilli are transmitted to humans in only two ways, by the ingestion of contaminated milk and by the inhalation of tubercle bacilli in droplet nuclei. The importance of spread by direct contact, sexual or otherwise, or by ingestion of organisms other than in infected dairy products is undetermined and probably slight. Tuberculin testing of dairy cattle and pasteurization of milk have nearly eliminated bovine tuberculosis in the United States and the possibility of its spread to man through dairy products.[69]

When an individual with tubercle bacilli in his sputum coughs, sneezes, talks, or sings, a spray of secretion may be expelled. The larger particles fall out of the air promptly and appear to be of little danger. Tiny droplets dry promptly when exposed to the air; the resultant droplet nuclei may float with the air currents for a long time and for long distances.[98] When inhaled, they usually are not trapped in the upper air passages or on the ciliated portions of the tracheobronchial tree, and pass directly to the alveoli. Cur-

rent evidence indicates that only droplet nuclei that carry tubercle bacilli and reach the alveoli are effective in infecting a susceptible host.

7. Pathogenesis and Immunity

The incubation period of tuberculosis might be defined as the time from receipt of infection to the development of hypersensitivity to tuberculin manifested by a positive reaction to the tuberculin test, since hypersensitivity apparently appears at about the time a focus of disease develops, even though this may be microscopic. In this case, the incubation period appears to vary from 3 to 8 weeks. More realistically, however, the incubation period as measured from the receipt of infection to the development of manifest disease may range from 3 weeks to the remainder of a lifetime. While some disease progresses inexorably from the very beginning, a period of latency, sometimes lasting for years, is usual. It is thus possible that disease in extreme old age may result from a childhood infection that has been latent in the interval. If events could be identified that were known to cause dormant tubercle bacilli to become active again, one might consider the time from those events to the development of manifest disease to be the incubation period of tuberculous *disease* as distinguished from the incubation period for tuberculous *infection,* which is the time from receipt of infection to the development of tuberculin hypersensitivity.

After tubercle bacilli are inhaled or ingested, they are engulfed by phagocytes and carried to the regional lymph nodes, occasionally passing into the bloodstream and then to many organs of the body. At first, they cause little or no reaction in the host tissues, but within 3 to 8 weeks, hypersensitivity to antigens elaborated by the organisms develops, along with some degree of acquired immunity. Phagocytes that contain tubercle bacilli and cells in the immediate neighborhood may then be killed, resulting in foci with central caseous necrosis and a peripheral zone of epithelioid cells, lymphocytes, and fibroblasts. The range of possible outcomes is extremely varied. In many organs and tissues, bloodborne tubercle bacilli show no evidence of becoming established. Bone marrow, liver, and spleen are usually involved, but infections in these organs are almost always controlled. More favorable sites for growth are the lungs, kidneys, meninges, and the epiphyseal portions of bone. Even in favorable sites, however, the majority of lesions heal as scar tissue surrounds the caseous foci and tubercle bacilli. Some lesions become partly or wholly calcified. Although the organisms can remain viable for years in these scarred areas, it is likely that most of them eventually die.

In a small proportion of persons, the balance tips against the host and in favor of the bacilli. Host resistance may be inadequate from the start, and the disease may progress to a fatal termination; or after an indefinite period of quiescence and apparent healing, the organisms may again start to grow and to destroy tissue. What factors are responsible for inability to control the infecting organisms at either time is uncertain. It is known, however, that resistance is lowered in diabetes, silicosis, diseases or therapy involving immunosuppression, and, as noted in Section 5.11, possibly by severe undernutrition.

Not all locations of disease are favorable for the transmission of infecting organisms, since organisms buried in most human tissues will never be excreted in the form of droplet nuclei small enough to be inhaled by another host. Only in the lungs is this likely to occur. Actively progressing caseous foci ultimately erode into a bronchus, the contents are expelled, and a cavity is formed. Tubercle bacilli flourish on the walls of a cavity and can readily pass with the expired air into the atmosphere, where a few, floating in droplet nuclei, may survive to be deposited in the lungs of another susceptible host.

For years there has been controversy regarding the role of endogenous or exogenous reinfection in causing reactivation on the initial tuberculous lesions after they had apparently healed. Endogenous reinfection is by far the more likely mechanism in countries where the likelihood of infection is now exceedingly low. However, exogenous reinfection (an apparent reactivation of disease from a second external source of infection) may occur under some circumstances.

8. Patterns of Host Response

The type of clinical disease that develops after infection depends to a considerable extent on the degree to which host resistance holds the multiplication of bacilli in check. Some lesions may be small and heal without ever producing symptoms or being recognizable by roentgenography or by pathological examination. Fortunately, many tuberculous lesions do tend to heal, even after reaching the symptomatic stage. Some, however, progress to a point where tissue destruction is incompatible with life. The nature of the disease that results from reactivation of an initial lesion or lesions depends most of all on the location of the lesion(s).

The manifestations of tuberculosis of various organs differ so markedly that it was not until Koch demonstrated the causative organisms that they were accepted as having a common etiology.

8.1. Clinical Features

Tuberculous disease is almost always symptomatic, although some patients may ignore their symptoms until they become extreme, particularly if the onset is asymptomatic and progression slow and insidious. With all forms of the disease, there may be symptoms of chronic infection—anorexia, weight loss, fatigue, and low-grade fever. The leukocyte count is usually normal or low.

Tuberculosis should always be suspected and ruled out in any continued febrile disease of unknown origin. The diagnosis should be especially suspected in middle-aged males in urban or lower socioeconomic settings and in immigrants from developing countries. A history of immunosuppression, alcoholism, diabetes, gastrectomy, pneumoconiosis, or social isolation increases the probability that tuberculosis is the cause.

Pulmonary tuberculosis is by far the most common form of the disease, accounting for 83% of the cases reported in the United States in 1985.[8] The most common symptom is chronic cough, usually productive of mucoid or mucopurulent sputum. Pleuritic pain or dull aching in the chest is sometimes reported. Hemoptysis, while common in advanced disease, is unusual as a presenting symptom. Occasionally, tuberculosis can present as an acute respiratory illness with symptoms resembling those of influenza or pneumonia. Pleurisy with effusion was once considered to be tuberculosis unless proven otherwise. This may still be a useful precept to keep in mind, even though in many areas tuberculosis is no longer a major cause of pleural effusion.

Miliary tuberculosis results from bloodborne dissemination of tubercle bacilli. With numerous lesions in many organs of the body, the manifestations are those of a cryptic fever because an untreated patient usually succumbs to the disease before any single organ is sufficiently involved to give localized symptoms. The one exception is tuberculous meningitis, which often accompanies miliary tuberculosis, although it may also be a separate entity. It occurs when a caseous nodule of the meninges ruptures into the subarachnoid space. The presenting symptoms are likely to be headache, abnormal behavior, clouded consciousness, or convulsions. The spinal fluid shows decreased sugar, increased protein, and a pleocytosis, polymorphonuclear at first and later lymphocytic.

Lymph node tuberculosis accounted for a quarter of the

extrapulmonary cases reported in 1984. The hilar and mediastinal nodes are most commonly involved, followed in order of frequency by cervical and supraclavicular nodes. Granulomatous lymphadenitis in adults, and multiple lymph node involvement at any age, are likely to have a tuberculous etiology. In children, on the other hand, granulomatous lymphadenitis of the cervical area is very likely to be caused by nontuberculous mycobacteria.

Pleural tuberculosis accounted for nearly as many cases as the lymphatic system. Genitourinary disease made up one eighth of the extrapulmonary cases. Since any portion of the genitourinary tract may be involved, symptoms may be those of chronic recurrent urinary tract infections, hematuria, nodular induration of prostate or vas deferens, pelvic inflammatory disease, amenorrhea, or infertility.

Fourteen percent of the extrapulmonary cases (2.3% of the total) were classified as miliary or meningeal. Bone and joint tuberculosis, 9% of the extrapulmonary cases, often occur together, with localized pain and swelling. Lower-spine and other weight-bearing joints are most commonly affected. All other sites, including the peritoneum, accounted for only 12% of the cases of extrapulmonary tuberculosis.

8.2. Diagnosis

The tuberculin skin test is the only feasible method for telling whether or not infection with tubercle bacilli has occurred. To be truly useful, it must be treated as a quantitative test, with attention to accurate administration of tuberculin and careful measurement of the diameter of any induration produced.[16] It is essential to use a well-standardized PPD, stabilized with a detergent and prepared from a large batch of material.[89] The dose should be 5 TU.

A positive reaction merely signifies that mycobacterial infection (or immunization) has occurred at some time in the past. The larger the reaction, the more likely it is to have resulted from tuberculous infection. Where the proportion of reactions due to tuberculous infection is high, the probability that any tuberculin reaction represents tuberculous infection is increased. In lifetime residents of Alaska, for example, induration of any size is likely to signify past infection with tubercle bacilli, because infections with other mycobacteria are exceedingly rare.[37] In the southeastern United States and most tropical areas, on the other hand, it is probable that most reactions under 10 mm result from nontuberculous mycobacterial infections, and probably a high proportion of those under 15 mm as well, because of the very high prevalence of such infections in such areas. Among household associates of active cases, in persons

with X-ray shadows suggestive of tuberculosis, or in older persons, small reactions are more likely to represent tuberculous infections than they are in other persons from the same area.[2]

Although a negative tuberculin test, properly given and interpreted, provides very strong evidence that a person does not have tuberculosis, there are important exceptions. From 2 to 5% of known tuberculous patients do not react to 5 TU of PPD.[106] In many such instances, failure to react is related to the severity of their disease—seriously ill patients, including those with tuberculosis, lose their skin sensitivity to tuberculin. Sensitivity may also be depressed by large doses of corticosteroids, by AIDS, and for a few weeks following measles, infectious mononucleosis, and vaccination with several viral antigens.[2]

The optimal dividing line between a positive and negative reaction to the test depends on a number of the preceding considerations, in addition to technical features related to administering and reading the tests. While a definition of a positive tuberculin reaction as one with 10 mm or more of induration following the administration of 5 TU of PPD is a reasonable compromise for much of the United States, it is probably best to determine this level by examining the frequency distribution of reaction sizes from the population with which one is working.[2,63] If local data are not available, findings from the Navy recruit study for that area can be used.[38]

Although tuberculosis of the lungs can produce roentgenographic findings similar to those of many different diseases, certain patterns are most common. If the initial infection produces a visible lesion, it is likely to involve the regional mediastinal nodes with or without a small infiltrate in the corresponding portions of the lungs, most commonly in the lower zones. Subsequent disease usually develops in the apical and posterior segments of the upper lobes or the superior segment of the lower lobes. Most commonly, the appearance is that of nodular infiltration, often with evidence of cavitation. No roentgenographic appearance, however, is pathognomonic.

A definitive diagnosis of tuberculosis can be made only by the isolation of *M. tuberculosis* from the involved tissues or secretions from the involved areas. Finding acid-fast bacilli is suggestive of a tuberculous etiology, but the ubiquitous occurrence of nontuberculous mycobacteria requires that definitive identification be made by cultures.

In making the diagnosis from specimens obtained at operation or autopsy, it is important to remember to place the suspected tissue in a container for specimens to be cultured. It is surprising how often such specimens are automatically put in formalin or other fixative, thus making cultures impossible.

9. Control and Prevention

9.1. General Concepts

Historians have noted that the decline in tuberculosis in many countries appears to have started before the discovery of the tubercle bacillus, and hence prior to any measures specifically designed to control the disease. Others have pointed out, however, that improved living and working conditions brought about by the sanitation and social reform movement of the 1800s might well have helped produce a decline in tuberculosis.[36] In particular, improved ventilation and daylight in homes and places of employment should have decreased the probability of becoming infected, while decreased working hours and improved nutrition should have increased resistance to disease. It seems likely that improvements along these lines have continued to contribute to the decline of tuberculosis to the present time.

When isolation of tuberculous patients is necessary, precautions should be aimed at the prevention of airborne spread.[1,7] The patient should be taught to cover the mouth and nose with disposable tissues when coughing or sneezing. There should be good ventilation of the room without recirculation of air; preferably, the air should be exhausted directly to the outside. Ultraviolet irradiation of the upper air or of exhaust ducts is also helpful. Masks need be worn by personnel only for patients who will not or cannot cover their mouths when coughing or sneezing. In the occasional instances when explanation and persuasion fail and a patient with infectious tuberculosis refuses to take the necessary steps to protect others, it is desirable to have legal powers and appropriate facilities for enforced isolation.

The major weapons in the control of bovine tuberculosis are periodic tuberculin testing of dairy cattle, slaughter of reactors, and pasteurization of milk. Although tuberculosis among cattle has been nearly eradicated from the United States and milkborne disease has become rare, this near success has led to diminished funding for the eradication program, laxity in tuberculin testing, and renewed interest in drinking raw milk, all of which could lead to the recrudescence of this potentially eradicable disease.

Tuberculosis-control measures among humans fall into three major categories: case-finding and chemotherapy, chemoprophylaxis, and vaccination. Each has its advantages and disadvantages, and each has a place under the appropriate circumstances. A simple model serves well to illustrate how each of these three control measures affects the tuberculosis problem.[43] The major elements of the model are shown in Fig. 6. While the numbers shown are for the United States in 1963, they can easily be changed to fit another situation. Missing from Fig. 6's portrayal of a 1-

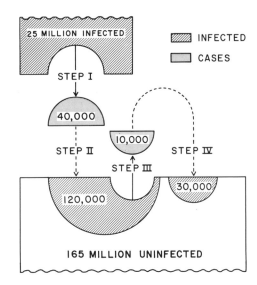

Figure 6. Schematic illustration of annual cycle of development of tuberculous infection and disease, United States, 1963.[43]

year cycle is the reduction of the uninfected and infected populations by deaths and the addition of the uninfected population by births.

In any given year, a certain number of cases develop from previously infected persons. Each of these cases infects others, some of whom develop tuberculosis during that year and others of whom are added to the infected group for the subsequent year. These new cases in turn infect others, who are also added to the infected group. For the United States in 1963, it was estimated that 80% (40,000) of the 50,000 cases came from the 25 million persons infected in previous years and 20% (10,000) from persons infected during that year. These numbers were based on the best estimates then available and reflect both the effect that the tuberculosis-control program was having at that time and the epidemiological characteristics of the disease in this country. It can be seen that *if* the current effectiveness of tuberculosis control could be maintained, tuberculosis would eventually disappear, although this would require many years.

9.2. Case-Finding and Chemotherapy

In an ideal but unfortunately imaginary world, case-finding endeavors would identify every case before it became infectious and chemotherapy would be completely effective in preventing future infectiousness. Such perfection would block the flow of tuberculosis at step II in the model shown in Fig. 6. Cases would continue to develop from the pool of infected persons until all had died, a process that would require approximately three generations.

In 1985 in the United States, 72% of the 22,201 reported cases had pulmonary tuberculosis with known positive sputum[8]; it is theoretically possible that with further examinations, all the pulmonary cases (83%) might be classified as communicable. Only 80% of the known cases at home had had a medical review within 3 months, and only 83% of those with two or more drugs recommended were known to be taking them. Although these figures show an improvement over 1976, much more needs to be done if this country hopes to eradicate tuberculosis by case-finding and chemotherapy before the end of the next century.

Case-finding in developed countries is now difficult because the prevalence of cases has become low enough to make mass screening procedures unproductive and to reduce the index of suspicion of most medical practitioners. In developing countries, where mass screening methods could be more useful but usually cannot be afforded, microscopic examination of stained specimens of sputum from persons with chronic cough has been shown to be productive. In both situations, the most appropriate combination of diagnostic modalities—medical history, skin testing, chest roentgenography, and bacteriology—will need to be selected after reviewing the local tuberculosis problem and the resources to combat it.[48]

Chemotherapy has become so effective that virtually every patient can now be cured if the necessary medication is taken conscientiously. Not only can the disease be cured, but patients are also quickly rendered noninfectious. Unfortunately, the expense of some drugs, the toxicity of others, and the duration of most chemotherapeutic regimens still make it difficult to achieve a high degree of patient compliance. Attention to administrative details, supervised intermittent regimens, and short-course combinations can all contribute to better patient acceptance of therapy.[1,3,4,28,45]

In this connection, it is worth noting that case-finding and chemotherapy can be remarkably effective if sufficient resources are made available. In 1953, Alaska was judged to have one of the worst tuberculosis problems in the world. Four years later, 1350 beds had been provided for Alaskan patients, roughly one for every 30 natives. In addition, an effective ambulatory chemotherapy program was started. After 20 years of active case-finding and treatment, there were so few tuberculosis patients that the last tuberculosis ward was closed, only a handful of active cases still remained in the tuberculosis case register, and new tuberculosis infections among children in what had been the worst tuberculosis area in the state had fallen from 8% per year in 1957 to less than 0.1% in 1970.[60]

9.3. Preventive Treatment

Following the introduction of isoniazid as a chemotherapeutic agent against tuberculosis, Edith Lincoln noted that children with primary tuberculosis treated with this drug showed a much lower incidence of serious tuberculous complications than had been noted with other medications and suggested that a controlled trial of the effectiveness of isoniazid in preventing these complications be undertaken.[44] The ensuing trial among 2750 children with asymptomatic primary tuberculosis or recent tuberculin conversions showed treatment with isoniazid to be remarkably effective, producing a 94% reduction in tuberculous complications during the year of preventive treatment and a 70% reduction over the subsequent 9-year period.

At least 20 controlled trials of preventive therapy with isoniazid involving more than 136,000 subjects have now been reported.[21] Among 14 trials with more than 1000 subjects, the median reduction in tuberculosis from preventive treatment was 60% during the periods of observation, which ranged from 1 to 13 years. The range of effectiveness in these 14 trials was 25 to 88%. The trials with low effectiveness included one that used small doses of isoniazid and one in which compliance was very poor. It should be noted, however, that these estimates are based on the total study populations regardless of how well medication was taken. Persons with high compliance tended to obtain greater protection than the preceding median values would indicate. Some degree of protection can be expected to be long-lasting. Any diminution caused by isoniazid in the numbers of tubercle bacilli harbored by the host increases the probability that host resistance can control any organisms that may remain. In addition, it has been shown that a treated infection in guinea pigs confers some resistance against subsequent reinfection.[75] Protection in humans has been shown to persist for at least 10–19 years.[27,44]

The generally accepted regimen for isoniazid preventive treatment is 5–10 mg isoniazid/kg body wt, not exceeding a total dose of 300 mg, given orally in a single dose for 6–12 months. A recent trial among persons with untreated inactive tuberculosis shows that some benefit is obtained from treatment lasting for 3 months and that the benefit from 12 months of treatment is slightly greater than that from 6 months.[57] Among persons with small lung lesions, the reduction in bacillary tuberculosis during a 5-year period among persons given isoniazid for 3 months was 20%; among those given isoniazid for 6 months, 66%; and among those on the 12-month regimen, 64%. However, persons who adhered well to their assigned regimens achieved a 69% reduction in risk with 6 months of treatment and a 93% reduction with 12 months of treatment.

The principal appeal of isoniazid preventive treatment lies in its ability to interrupt the chain of infection at step I in the model shown in Fig. 6. Universal application to reactors and perfect effectiveness of this preventive procedure could theoretically eradicate tuberculosis almost at once. While realism does not allow hope of even approaching such an outcome, whatever effectiveness preventive treatment may have affects every step in the model and not merely the later ones. This is particularly important in situations where the infection rate is low and the bulk of the tuberculosis cases occur in step I as a result of reactivation of latent infections.

There are several deterrents to widespread use of isoniazid in preventive treatment: toxicological, financial, and patient/provider noncompliance. Most side effects of isoniazid are usually not sufficient to cause its use to be discontinued and are largely restricted to adults.[44] In the large PHS trial among household contacts, a group composed largely of children and young adults, reactions that caused subjects to stop their medication were reported among 1.5% of persons taking placebo and 1.9% of those taking isoniazid, a difference of only 0.4% attributable to the drug. In the trial among persons with inactive lesions, a much older group, medication was discontinued because of side effects among 3.8% of the placebo group and 6.6% of those given isoniazid. The side effect of principal concern is hepatitis. Rare among children, its incidence increases with age, reaching a level of 2–4% among persons 50–64 years of age.[62] Careful explanation of the early symptoms of hepatitis and monthly monitoring for these symptoms among persons on preventive treatment appear to have markedly reduced the seriousness of this side effect.[31]

With increasing age, the lifetime risk of tuberculosis diminishes while the risk of developing isoniazid-associated hepatitis increases.[19] While some estimates suggest that there is net benefit from preventive treatment at almost all ages,[85] current recommendations are that tuberculin reactors over 35 years of age should not be given preventive treatment unless there are additional indications.[3] These include (1) household or other close association with persons who have infectious tuberculosis; (2) presence of roentgenographic findings consistent with nonprogressive pulmonary tuberculosis with neither positive bacteriological findings nor history of adequate chemotherapy; (3) skin-test evidence of new tuberculous infection; and (4) presence of special medical situations such as prolonged corticosteroid therapy, suppressed or depressed immune status, diabetes mellitus, silicosis, or gastrectomy.

Fears that the preventive use of isoniazid would lead to the emergence of isoniazid-resistant strains of tubercle bacilli have not been borne out.[44] Although the proportion of cases with resistant organisms may be higher among persons given isoniazid than among those given placebo, the incidence rate of resistant cases is not increased. If isoniazid were completely effective in preventing disease caused by foci of susceptible tubercle bacilli, 100% of the few cases that did develop would result from reactivation of organisms that were already resistant.

The cost of isoniazid preventive treatment, even with monthly monitoring of symptoms, is rarely a major consideration in developed countries in which the program is merely added to existing procedures in tuberculosis clinics. In countries with limited resources, however, it is reasonable to use scarce antituberculosis medications for prevention only after the needs of tuberculosis patients can be met.

Finally, noncompliance by physicians and patients is an impediment to preventive therapy. In 1985, only 63% of infected close contacts of tuberculosis patients—the group at greatest risk of developing disease—were given isoniazid by state and local tuberculosis control programs. And of the contacts who were started, less than 75% completed the recommended course.[8]

9.4. Immunization

Immunization against tuberculosis is currently limited to the use of BCG, an attenuated organism named for the two French investigators responsible for its development.[36] Working with *M. bovis* in 1908, they added bile to their culture media in an effort to obtain well-dispersed suspensions of the organisms. As an unexpected result, they noted that the organisms cultured in this way lost virulence for laboratory animals. After 13 years of subculturing and testing, they became convinced that they had developed a strain of organisms that would remain avirulent and could be used to immunize humans against tuberculosis.

BCG has probably had more, bigger, and possibly better-controlled trials of its usefulness and effectiveness than has almost any other preventive measure. Despite this, there is disagreement about its effectiveness. One group of trials, the best example of which is the one conducted by the British Medical Research Council,[49] showed that tuberculosis case rates were approximately 80% lower among vaccinated children for 15–20 years after vaccination than among comparable unvaccinated controls. Other trials, such as that by the PHS in Puerto Rico, showed a 29% reduction attributable to BCG, while a companion trial in the southeastern United States showed a reduction of only 6%.[23,26] An extremely large and well-conducted trial in south India showed no evidence that the two strains of BCG were effective.[102] Unfortunately, postvaccinal conversions of the tuberculin test from negative to positive, long used as an index of effectiveness, show essentially no correlation with effectiveness in the controlled trials for which this information is available.[18] Nor can animal testing be relied on, since various methods give markedly discrepant results[104] and none has been shown to correlate with results in humans.

The role that effective immunization might play in the control of tuberculosis is also indicated by the model in Fig. 6. As was the case for case-finding and chemotherapy (Section 9.2), the effect of immunization is on step II, namely, protecting the uninfected population against development of disease when exposed to infectious cases. While there is evidence that BCG vaccination does not harm persons who are already infected, there is also no reason to believe that it might help them.[80] Universal application of a vaccine with 100% efficacy would not eradicate tuberculosis until all infected reactors had died.

The major indication for BCG vaccination is a high risk among currently uninfected individuals of becoming infected *and*, from a practical programmatic point of view, a proportion of uninfected individuals that is large enough that protecting them would have a meaningful impact on the tuberculosis problem. Dealing with the first aspect of the problem involves a judgment regarding the costs and benefits of vaccination and the feasibility of alternative methods of tuberculosis control. The second indication can easily be met by directing the vaccination program toward infants and young children.

The financial costs of vaccination are low. The vaccine is inexpensive, its administration is simple, and vaccination probably does not have to be repeated. Preliminary tuberculin testing is not needed, though it may occasionally be useful for epidemiological purposes. The medical costs or side effects, with one exception, should not be troublesome. Most vaccines produce localized ulcerations that are limited in extent and duration and are unaccompanied by troublesome lymphadenopathy. More serious complications are very uncommon. The only potentially important side effect is the production of sensitivity to tuberculin. In areas with a high risk of infection, most persons will become tuberculin reactors in the course of time, and the premature production of tuberculin sensitivity by vaccination is rarely of any consequence. In areas with a low risk of infection, the help that the tuberculin test can give diagnostically and prognostically constitutes an added contraindication to BCG vaccination. A reasonable division point between high and low risks of infection may be 1% per year.[95]

The benefits of vaccination are at the heart of much contention about the role of this procedure in tuberculosis control. Characteristics of BCG vaccines can change with continued cultivation, and this seems a likely explanation for the marked differences observed among the results of various trials done around 1950 with different substrains of vaccines that were then more than 25 years removed from the original parent strain. With the lapse of nearly 40 more years since these trials, they do not provide reliable information on the effectiveness of currently available strains.

Case–control studies have been suggested as a means of assessing efficacy of current vaccines under ordinary field conditions.[93] A major problem with this approach is the possibility that the kinds of people who are vaccinated may have different tuberculosis risks than do those who are not vaccinated. One way of assessing the likelihood of such a bias is to compare vaccinated and unvaccinated persons with respect to demographic, social, and economic factors known to be related to tuberculosis risk.[74] An even better approach is possible in areas where a change has been made in the vaccine being used. Case–control estimates of each vaccine's efficacy should be subject to similar biases and their effects should be largely removed in the relative ranking of the two vaccines. A strong indication that one vaccine was appreciably better than another was made apparent in this way in a recent case–control study.[18,91]

Because of uncertainties regarding the efficacy of most vaccines, the decision on the use of vaccination must depend in part on the availability of other means of tuberculosis control. In much of the world, the decision is not difficult. In countries with a very low infection rate, such as the United States, there is very little need for the kind of protection that vaccination can give, considerable reason to protect the usefulness of the tuberculin test, and a readily available alternative program of tuberculosis control by case-finding, chemotherapy, and preventive therapy. In many other countries, there is clearly a high risk of infection and no prospect of really effective control through any procedure except BCG vaccination. In such situations, vaccination must be continued.

10. Unresolved Problems

Perhaps the major problem in tuberculosis control today is the uncertainty about the efficacy of BCG strains in current use. Almost none of them have been tested at any time in a controlled trial. The few that have been so tested have been subcultured for many years, giving reason to doubt that the previous relative ranking of tested strains still reflects their present effectiveness. As was the case with pertussis vaccines in the 1950s, the only reliable resolution of the present uncertainties about BCG strains seems to lie in setting up controlled trials of the currently available strains among humans in areas of the world where the risk of infection is still sufficiently high to indicate a need for BCG vaccination and also high enough to yield an answer in a reasonable length of time.

In such trials, vaccinated persons need not be compared with randomly allocated unvaccinated controls. While such a design is scientifically desirable, it does not seem ethically or politically feasible. For practical purposes, a much simpler scheme should be useful and would be more widely applicable. If several different BCG strains could be used in a country with high rates of infection and each strain were tested in a different region, a comparison of tuberculosis trends before and after vaccination with the trial strains could separate the highly potent strains from the weak if a reasonable effort were exerted to maintain similar levels of vaccination and case-finding in all regions. Alternatively, one vaccine could be used among newborn infants in odd years and a second in even years, with subsequent comparisons of case rates among children born in odd and even years. Less valid but more acceptable evaluations can be made by observational studies, case–control or prospective, in areas where the vaccine strain being used has changed in recent years. In such settings, the biases inherent in observational studies should affect the estimated efficacy of each strain similarly and thus have little effect on estimates of their relative potencies. Several such studies might allow a number of BCG vaccines to be ranked in the order of their potency, thereby providing material with which to identify reliable animal test systems. Once such a test system was found, objective ratings of the BCG vaccines could be done. Tuberculosis-control personnel working in areas of the world where protection by vaccination is still needed could then learn whether or not they were using an effective vaccine and would not have to proceed on faith alone, as they must do at present.

Another major need, though perhaps much more difficult of solution, is to develop a test that would identify infected persons who still harbor living tubercle bacilli. The present tuberculin skin test and serological tests fail on two counts: (1) positive reactions can be caused by mycobacteria other than *M. tuberculosis* or *M. bovis* and (2) reactions from a tuberculous infection may persist long after the infecting organisms have succumbed to the host's defenses. Improvement of the test on either count would make diagnosis and preventive therapy much more efficient.

Very little is known of factors that influence the probability that tuberculous infection will progress to manifest tuberculous disease either with or without a prolonged latent period. While repeated infections have been demonstrated to occur, their importance in causing tuberculous disease is uncertain; they are not likely to be important in developed countries where the risk of receiving any tuberculous infection is extremely low. The long-held belief that malnutrition and alcoholism are risk factors for tuberculous disease, while probably correct, is supported only by uncontrolled observations. Even the risk associated with diabetes is poorly established. From the point of view of local tuberculosis control, it would be very helpful to know much more about the characteristics of tuberculosis patients. What are their usual occupations? What about their diet and life-style? How many have had previous evidence of tuberculous infection or disease? What caused them to come to medical attention? Some of the simplest facts about tuberculosis cases are essentially unknown, but could be collected with attention to careful and consistent history-taking.

Although both chemotherapy and preventive therapy can be highly successful, the long duration of treatment required and the frequency of unpleasant side effects make it difficult to achieve high levels of compliance even with supervision by adequate numbers of dedicated personnel. Although the need for more rapidly effective and less toxic drugs is tremendous throughout the world, the inability of most persons who need these drugs to pay for them will require that the necessary pharmacological research be supported by public funds rather than by private capital.

A relatively neglected aspect of tuberculosis epidemiology concerns extrapulmonary tuberculosis. In 1962, extrapulmonary tuberculosis comprised 7.4% of reported active cases in the United States[6]; in 1985, it made up 16.9% of the total.[8] Another way of looking at this time trend is that pulmonary tuberculosis cases decreased by 65% over the 23-year interval while extrapulmonary tuberculosis cases decreased by only 5%. The relative lack of change in extrapulmonary disease seems paradoxical in that much of it was once thought to be the result of infections with *M. bovis,* which have diminished much more rapidly in the United States than have infections with human tubercle bacilli, and also in that extrapulmonary tuberculosis decreased least in persons under 25 years of age, the age group with the most marked decrease in pulmonary disease. There are geographic differences also. In 1985, only one state reported that fewer than 10% of the new cases were extrapulmonary; 20 reported this proportion to be over 20%; and the average for the five highest states was 33.7%.[8] The latter were mostly all Rocky Mountain or northwestern states; the five states with the lowest proportions were southern or midwestern. The reasons for the reported variations of extrapulmonary tuberculosis by time, place, and person remain a challenge to epidemiologists.

11. References

1. ADDINGTON, W. W., ALBERT, R. K., BASS, J. B., JR., CATLIN, B. J., LOUDON, R. G., SEGGERSON, J., AND SLUTKIN, G., Non-drug issues related to the treatment of tuberculosis, *Chest* **87**(2):125S–127S (1985).
2. American Thoracic Society, The tuberculin skin test, *Am. Rev. Respir. Dis.* **124**:356–363 (1981).
3. American Thoracic Society, Treatment of tuberculosis and tuberculosis infection in adults and children, *Am. Rev. Respir. Dis.* **134**:355–363 (1986).
4. ANDERSON, S., AND BANERJI, D., A sociological inquiry into an urban tuberculosis control programme in India, *Bull. WHO* **29**:685–700 (1963).
5. ARMSTRONG, D. B., Four years of the Framingham Demonstration, *Am. Rev. Tuberc.* **4**:908–919 (1921).
6. Centers for Disease Control, Tuberculosis Control Division, Extrapulmonary Tuberculosis in the United States, HEW Publ. (CDC) 78-8360 (1978).
7. Centers for Disease Control, Tuberculosis Control Division, Guidelines for Prevention of TB in Hospitals, Centers for Disease Control, Atlanta, 1983.
8. Centers for Disease Control, Division of Tuberculosis Control, 1985 Tuberculosis Statistics, States and Cities, HHS Publ. (CDC) 87-8249 (1986).
9. Centers for Disease Control, Division of Tuberculosis Control, Tuberculosis in the United States, 1981–1984, HHS Publ. (CDC) 86-8322 (1986).
10. Centers for Disease Control, Division of Tuberculosis Control, Tuberculosis final data—United States, 1986, *Morbid. Mortal. Weekly Rep.* **36**:817–820 (1988).
11. CHAPMAN, J. S., AND DYERLY, M. D., Social and other factors in intrafamilial transmission of tuberculosis, *Am. Rev. Respir. Dis.* **90**:48–60 (1964).
12. CHAVES, A. D., ROBINS, A. B., AND ABELES, H., Tuberculosis case finding among homeless men in New York City, *Am. Rev. Respir. Dis.* **84**:900–901 (1961).
13. COCHRANE, A. L., JARMAN, T. F., MIALL, W. E., AND CARPENTER, R. G., Factors influencing the attack rate of pulmonary tuberculosis, *Thorax* **11**:141–148 (1956).
14. COMSTOCK, G. W., Isoniazid prophylaxis in an undeveloped area, *Am. Rev. Respir. Dis.* **86**:810–822 (1962).
15. COMSTOCK, G. W., Frost revisited: The modern epidemiology of tuberculosis, *Am. J. Epidemiol.* **101**:363–382 (1975).
16. COMSTOCK, G. W., False tuberculin test results, *Chest* **68S**:465S–469S (1975).
17. COMSTOCK, G. W., Tuberculosis in twins: A re-analysis of the Prophit survey, *Am. Rev. Respir. Dis.* **117**:621–624 (1978).
18. COMSTOCK, G. W., Identification of an effective vaccine against tuberculosis, *Am. Rev. Respir. Dis.* **138**:479–480 (1988).
19. COMSTOCK, G. W., AND EDWARDS, P. Q., The competing risks of tuberculosis and hepatitis for adult tuberculin reactors, *Am. Rev. Respir. Dis.* **111**:573–577 (1975).
20. COMSTOCK, G. W., AND SARTWELL, P. E., Tuberculosis studies in Muscogee County, Georgia. IV. Evaluation of a community-wide X-ray survey on the basis of six years of observation, *Am. J. Hyg.* **61**:261–285 (1955).
21. COMSTOCK, G. W., AND WOOLPERT, S. F., Preventive therapy, in: *The Mycobacteria: A Sourcebook* (G. P. KUBICA AND L. W. WAYNE, eds.), pp. 1071–1082, Dekker, New York, 1984.
22. COMSTOCK, G. W., FEREBEE, S. H., AND HAMMES, L. M., A controlled trial of community-wide isoniazid prophylaxis in Alaska, *Am. Rev. Respir. Dis.* **95**:935–943 (1967).
23. COMSTOCK, G. W., LIVESAY, V. T., AND WOOLPERT, S. F., Evaluation of BCG vaccination among Puerto Rican children, *Am. J. Public Health,* **64**:283–291 (1974).
24. COMSTOCK, G. W., LIVESAY, V. T., AND WOOLPERT, S. F., The prognosis of a positive tuberculin reaction in childhood and adolescence, *Am. J. Epidemiol.* **99**:131–138 (1974).
25. COMSTOCK, G. W., EDWARDS, L. B., AND LIVESAY, V. T., Tuberculosis morbidity in the U.S. Navy: Its distribution and decline, *Am. Rev. Respir. Dis.* **110**:572–580 (1974).
26. COMSTOCK, G. W., WOOLPERT, S. F., AND LIVESAY, V. T., Tuberculosis studies in Muscogee County, Georgia. Twenty-year evaluation of a community trial of BCG vaccination, *Public Health Rep.* **91**:276–280 (1976).
27. COMSTOCK, G. W., BAUM, C., AND SNIDER, D. E., JR., Isoniazid prophylaxis among Alaskan Eskimos: A final report of the Bethel isoniazid studies, *Am. Rev. Respir. Dis.* **119**:827–830 (1979).
28. CURRY, F. J., District clinics for out-patient treatment of tuberculosis problem patients, *Dis. Chest* **46**:524–530 (1964).
29. DANIEL, T. M., New approaches to the rapid diagnosis of tuberculous meningitis, *J. Infect. Dis.* **155**:599–602 (1987).
30. DANIEL, T. M., AND DEBANNE, S. M., The serodiagnosis of tuberculosis and other mycobacterial diseases by enzyme-linked immunosorbent assay, *Am. Rev. Respir. Dis.* **135**:1137–1151 (1987).
31. DASH, L. A., COMSTOCK, G. W., AND FLYNN, J. P. G., Isoniazid preventive therapy. Retrospect and prospect, *Am. Rev. Respir. Dis.* **121**:1039–1044 (1980).
32. DAVID, H. L., Bacteriology of the Mycobacterioses, DHEW Publ. (CDC) 76-8316, U.S. Government Printing Office, Washington, D.C. (1976).
33. DE ABREU, M., AND DE PAULA, A., *Roentgenfotografia,* Livraria Ateneu, Rio de Janeiro, 1940.
34. DICKINSON, J. M., LEFFORD, M. J., LLOYD, J., AND MITCHISON, D. A., The virulence in the guinea-pig of tubercle bacilli from patients with pulmonary tuberculosis in Hong Kong, *Tubercle* **44**:446–451 (1963).

35. DONALDSON, J. C., AND ELLIOTT, R. C., A study of co-positivity of three multipuncture techniques with intradermal PPD tuberculin, *Am. Rev. Respir. Dis.* **118**:843–846 (1978).

36. DUBOS, R., AND DUBOS, J., *The White Plague: Tuberculosis, Man and Society,* Little, Brown, Boston, 1952.

37. EDWARDS, L. B., COMSTOCK, G. W., AND PALMER, C. E., Contributions of northern populations to the understanding of tuberculin sensitivity, *Arch. Environ. Health* **17**:507–516 (1968).

38. EDWARDS, L. B., ACQUAVIVA, F. A., LIVESAY, V. T., CROSS, F. W., AND PALMER, C. E., An atlas of sensitivity to tuberculin, PPD-B, and histoplasmin in the United States, *Am. Rev. Respir. Dis.* **99**(4):Part 2 (1969).

39. EDWARDS, L. B., LIVESAY, V. T., ACQUAVIVA, F. A., AND PALMER, C. E., Height, weight, tuberculous infection, and tuberculous disease, *Arch. Environ. Health* **22**:106–112 (1971).

40. EDWARDS, L. B., ACQUAVIVA, F. A., AND LIVESAY, V. T., Identification of tuberculous infected. Dual tests and density of reaction, *Am. Rev. Respir. Dis.* **108**:1334–1339 (1973).

41. ENTERLINE, P. E., AND KORDAN, B., A controlled evaluation of mass surveys for tuberculosis and heart disease, *Public Health Rep.* **73**:867–875 (1958).

42. FAYERS, P. M., AND BARNETT, G. D., The risk of tuberculous infection in Saskatchewan, *Bull. Int. Union Tuberc.* **50**:62–69 (1975).

43. FEREBEE, S. H., An epidemiological model of tuberculosis in the United States, *Bull. Natl. Tuberc. Assoc.* **53**:4–7 (1967).

44. FEREBEE, S. H., Controlled chemoprophylaxis trials in tuberculosis: A general review, *Adv. Tuberc. Res.* **17**:28–106 (1970).

45. FOX, W., The current status of short-course chemotherapy, *Tubercle* **60**:177–190 (1979).

46. FROGGETT, K., Tuberculosis: Spatial and demographic incidence in Bradford, 1980–2, *J. Epidemiol. Community Health* **39**:20–26 (1985).

47. FROST, W. H., How much control of tuberculosis? *Am. J. Public Health* **27**:759–766 (1937).

48. GRZYBOWSKI, S., Technical and operational appraisal of tuberculosis case-finding methods, in: *II. Regional Seminar on Tuberculosis,* Scientific Publ. 265, pp. 50–56, Pan American Health Organization, Washington, D.C., 1973.

49. HART, P. D., AND SUTHERLAND, I., BCG and vole bacillus vaccines in the prevention of tuberculosis in adolescence and early adult life, *Br. Med. J.* **2**:293–295 (1977).

50. HOLLAND, W. W., (ed.), *European Community Atlas of 'Avoidable Death,'* Oxford University Press, London, 1988.

51. HORWITZ, O., Tuberculosis risk and marital status, *Am. Rev. Respir. Dis.* **104**:22–31 (1971).

52. HORWITZ, O., AND COMSTOCK, G. W., What is a case of tuberculosis? The tuberculosis case spectrum in eight countries evaluated from 1235 case histories and roentgenograms, *Int. J. Epidemiol.* **2**:145–152 (1973).

53. HORWITZ, O., WILBEK, E., AND ERICKSON, P. A., Epidemiological basis of tuberculosis eradication. 10. Longitudinal studies on the risk of tuberculosis in the general population of a low-prevalence area, *Bull. WHO* **41**:95–113 (1969).

54. HORWITZ, O., EDWARDS, P. Q., AND LOWELL, A. M., National tuberculosis control program in Denmark and the United States, *Health Serv. Rep.* **88**:493–498 (1973).

55. HOUK, V. N., BAKER, J. H., SORENSEN, K., AND KENT, D. C., The epidemiology of tuberculosis infection in a closed environment, *Arch. Environ. Health* **16**:26–35 (1968).

56. HYGE, T. V., The efficacy of BCG vaccination, *Acta Tuberc. Scand.* **32**:89–107 (1956).

57. International Union Against Tuberculosis Committee on Prophylaxis, Efficacy of various durations of isoniazid preventive therapy for tuberculosis: Five years of follow-up in the IUAT trial, *Bull. WHO* **60**:555–564 (1982).

58. JARMAN, T. F., A follow-up tuberculin survey in the Rhondda Fach, *Br. Med. J.* **2**:1235–1239 (1955).

59. KAMAT, S. R., DAWSON, J. J. Y., DEVADATTA, S., FOX, W., JANARDHANAM, B., RADHAKRISHNA, S., RAMAKRISHNAN, C. V., SOMASUNDARAM, P. R., STOTT, H., AND VELU, S., A controlled study of the influence of segregation of tuberculous patients for one year on the attack rate of tuberculosis in a 5-year period in close family contacts in south India, *Bull. WHO* **34**:517–532 (1966).

60. KAPLAN, G. J., FRASER, R. I., AND COMSTOCK, G. W., Tuberculosis in Alaska, 1970. The continued decline of the tuberculosis epidemic, *Am. Rev. Respir. Dis.* **105**:920–926 (1972).

61. KIELMANN, A. A., OBEROI, I. S., CHANDRA, R. K., AND MEHRA, V. L., The effect of nutritional status on immune capacity and immune responses in preschool children in a rural community in India, *Bull. WHO* **54**:477–483 (1976).

62. KOPANOFF, D. E., SNIDER, D. E., JR., AND CARAS, G. J., Isoniazid-related hepatitis. A U.S. Public Health Service cooperative surveillance study, *Am. Rev. Respir. Dis.* **117**:991–1001 (1978).

63. KUEMMERER, J. M., AND COMSTOCK, G. W., Sociologic concomitants of tuberculin sensitivity, *Am. Rev. Respir. Dis.* **96**:885–892 (1967).

64. LOWELL, A. M., Tuberculosis in the World, HEW Publ. (CDC) 76-8317, U.S. Government Printing Office, Washington, D.C., 1976.

65. LOWELL, A. M., EDWARDS, L. B., AND PALMER, C. E., *Tuberculosis,* Harvard University Press, Cambridge, Mass., 1969.

66. LURIE, M. B., *Resistance to Tuberculosis: Experimental Studies in Native and Acquired Defensive Mechanisms,* pp. 115–180, Harvard University Press, Cambridge, Mass., 1984.

67. MAGNUS, K., Epidemiological basis of tuberculosis eradication. 6. Tuberculin sensitivity after human and bovine infection, *Bull. WHO* **36**:719–731 (1967).

68. Medical Research Council, Tuberculosis and Chest Diseases Unit, National survey of notifications of tuberculosis in England and Wales in 1983, *Br. Med. J.* **291**:658–661 (1985).

69. MYERS, J. A., *Tuberculosis: A Half Century of Study and Conquest,* pp. 222–241, Green, St. Louis, 1970.

70. National Tuberculosis Institute, Bangalore, Tuberculosis in a rural population in south India: A five-year epidemiological study, *Bull. WHO* **51**:473–488 (1974).

71. NISSEN MEYER, S., HOUGEN, A., AND EDWARDS, P., Experimental error in the determination of tuberculin sensitivity, *Public Health Rep.* **63**:561–569 (1951).

72. NYBOE, J., Interpretation of tuberculosis infection age curves, *Bull. WHO* **17**:319–339 (1957).

73. OVERFIELD, T., AND KLAUBER, M. R., Prevalence of tuberculosis in Eskimos having blood group B gene, *Hum. Biol.* **52**(1):87–92 (1980).

74. PADUNGCHAN, S., KONJANART, S., KASIRATTA, S., DARAMAS, S., AND TEN DAM, H. G., The effectiveness of BCG vaccination of the newborn against childhood tuberculosis in Bangkok, *Bull. WHO* **64**:247–258 (1986).

75. PALMER, C. E., FEREBEE, S. H., AND HOPWOOD, L., Studies on prevention of experimental tuberculosis with isoniazid. II. Effects of different dosage regimens, *Am. Rev. Respir. Dis.* **74**:917–939 (1956).

76. PEREZ-STABLE, E. J., SLUTKIN, G., PAX, E. A., AND HOPEWELL, P. C., Tuberculin reactivity in United States and foreign-born Latinos: Results of a community-based screening program. *Am. J. Public Health* **76**:643–646 (1986).

77. POWELL, K. E., BROWN, E. D., AND FARER, L. S., Tuberculosis among Indochinese refugees in the United States, *J. Am. Med. Assoc.* **249**:1455–1460 (1983).

78. PUFFER, R. R., *Familial Susceptibility to Tuberculosis,* Harvard University Press, Cambridge, Mass., 1944.

79. PUST, R. E., ONEJEME, S. E., AND OKAFOR, S. N., Tuberculosis survey in East Central State, Nigeria: Implications for tuberculosis programme development, *Trop. Geogr. Med.* **26**:51–57 (1974).

80. RAJ NARAIN, AND VALLISHAYEE, R. S., BCG vaccination of tuberculous patients and of strong reactors to tuberculin, *Bull. Int. Union Tuberc.* **51**:243–246 (1976).

81. RAJ NARAIN, NAIR, S. S., CHANDRASEKHAR, P., AND RAMANATHA RAO, G., Problems associated with estimating the incidence of tuberculosis infection, *Bull. WHO* **34**:605–622 (1966).

82. RAJ NARAIN, CHANDRASEKHAR, P., SATYANARAYANACHAR, R. A., AND LAL, P., Resistant and sensitive strains of *Mycobacterium tuberculosis* found in repeated surveys among a south Indian rural population, *Bull. WHO* **39**:681–699 (1968).

83. RAJ NARAIN, SUBBA RAO, M. S., CHANDRASEKHAR, P., AND PYARELAL, Microscopy positive and microscopy negative cases of pulmonary tuberculosis, *Am. Rev. Respir. Dis.* **103**:761–773 (1971).

84. REICHMAN, L. B., AND O'DAY, R., Tuberculous infection in a large urban population, *Am. Rev. Respir. Dis.* **117**:705–712 (1978).

85. ROSE, D. N., SCHECHTER, C. B., AND SILVER, A. L., The age threshold for isoniazid chemoprophylaxis: A decision analysis for low-risk tuberculin reactors, *J. Am. Med. Assoc.* **256**:2709–2713 (1986).

86. RUBEN, F. L., NORDEN, C. W., AND SCHUSTER, A., Analysis of a community hospital employee tuberculosis screening program 31 months after its inception, *Am. Rev. Respir. Dis.* **115**:23–28 (1977).

87. RUST, P., AND THOMAS, J., A method for estimating the prevalence of tuberculous infection, *Am. J. Epidemiol.* **101**:311–322 (1975).

88. SARTWELL, P. E., MOSELEY, C. H., AND LONG, E. R., Tuberculosis in the German population, United States Zone of Germany, *Am. Rev. Tuberc.* **59**:481–493 (1949).

89. SBARBARO, J., Skin test antigens: An evaluation whose time has come, *Am. Rev. Respir. Dis.* **118**:1–5 (1978).

90. SELWYN, P. A., HARTEL, D., LEWIS, V. A., SCHOENBAUM, E. E., VERMUND, S. H., KLEIN, R. S., WALKER, A. T., AND FRIEDLAND, G. H., A prospective study of the risk of tuberculosis among intravenous drug users with human immunodeficiency virus infection, *N. Engl. J. Med.* **320**:545–550 (1989).

91. SHAPIRO, C., COOK, N., EVANS, D., WILLETT, W., FAJARDO, I., KOCH-WESER, D., BERGONZOLI, G., BOLANOS, O., GUERRERO, R., AND HENNEKENS, C. H., A case–control study of BCG and childhood tuberculosis in Cali, Colombia, *Int. J. Epidemiol.* **14**:441–446 (1985).

92. SIDDIQI, S. H., HWANGBO, C. C., SILCOX, V., GOOD, R. C., SNIDER, D. E., JR., AND MIDDLEBROOK, G., Rapid radiometric methods to detect and differentiate *Mycobacterium tuberculosis/M. bovis* from other mycobacterial species, *Am. Rev. Respir. Dis.* **130**:634–640 (1984).

93. SMITH, P. G., Retrospective assessment of the effectiveness of BCG vaccination against tuberculosis using the case–control method, *Tubercle* **62**:23–35 (1982).

94. SNIDER, D. E., JR., AND CAUTHEN, G. M., Tuberculin skin testing of hospital employees: Infection, "boosting," and two-step testing, *Am. J. Infect. Control* **12**:305–311 (1984).

95. SPRINGETT, V. H., The value of BCG vaccination, *Tubercle* **46**:76–84 (1965).

96. STEAD, W. W., Undetected tuberculosis in prison, *J. Am. Med. Assoc.* **240**:2544–2547 (1978).

97. STEAD, W. W., LOFGREN, J. P., WARREN, E., AND THOMAS, C., Tuberculosis as an endemic and nosocomial infection among the elderly in nursing homes, *N. Engl. J. Med.* **312**:1483–1487 (1985).

98. SULTAN, L., NYKA, W., MILLS, C., O'GRADY, F., WELLS, W., AND RILEY, R. L., Tuberculosis disseminators. A study of the variability of aerial infectivity of tuberculous patients, *Am. Rev. Respir. Dis.* **82**:358–369 (1960).

99. SUNDERAM, G., MCDONALD, R. J., MANIATIS, T., OLESKE, J., KAPILA, R., AND REICHMAN, L. B., Tuberculosis as a manifestation of the acquired immunodeficiency syndrome, *J. Am. Med. Assoc.* **256**:362–366 (1986).

100. SUTHERLAND, I., AND FAYERS, P. M., The association of the

risk of tuberculous infection with age, *Bull. Int. Union Tuberc.* **50**:70–81 (1975).

101. SUTHERLAND, I., STYBLO, K., SAMPALIK, M., AND BLEIKER, M. A., Annual risks of tuberculous infection in 14 countries, derived from the results of tuberculin surveys in 1948–1952, *Bull. Int. Union Tuberc.* **45**:75–114 (1971).

102. Tuberculosis Prevention Trial, Madras, Trial of BCG vaccines in south India for tuberculosis prevention, *Indian J. Med. Res.* **72**(Suppl.):1–74 (1980).

103. WAALER, H., GALTUNG, O., AND MORDAL, K., The risk of tuberculous infection in Norway, *Bull. Int. Union Tuberc.* **50**:5–61 (1975).

104. WIEGESHAUS, E. H., HARDING, G., McMURRAY, D., GROVE, A. A., AND SMITH, D. W., A co-operative evaluation of test systems used to assay tuberculosis vaccines, *Bull. WHO* **45**:543–550 (1971).

105. WILSON, M. W., Fluorescence microscopy in examination of smears for *Mycobacterium tuberculosis, Am. Rev. Tuberc.* **65**:709–717 (1952).

106. World Health Organization, Tuberculosis Research Office, Further studies of geographic variation in naturally acquired tuberculin sensitivity, *Bull. WHO* **22**:63–83 (1955).

12. Suggested Reading

American Thoracic Society, Treatment of tuberculosis and tuberculosis infection in adults and children, *Am. Rev. Respir. Dis.* **134**:355–363 (1986).

COMSTOCK, G. W., Frost revisited: The modern epidemiology of tuberculosis, *Am. J. Epidemiol.* **101**:363–382 (1975).

DUBOS, R., AND DUBOS, J., *The White Plague: Tuberculosis, Man and Society,* Little, Brown, Boston, 1952.

EDWARDS, P. Q., AND EDWARDS, L. B., Story of the tuberculin test from an epidemiological viewpoint, *Am. Rev. Respir. Dis.* **81**(1):Part 2 (1960).

FEREBEE, S. H., Controlled chemoprophylaxis trials in tuberculosis: A general review, *Adv. Tuberc. Res.* **17**:28–106 (1970).

FROST, W. H., How much control of tuberculosis? *Am. J. Public Health* **27**:759–766 (1937).

Supplement on future research in tuberculosis. Prospects and priorities for elimination, *Am. Rev. Respir. Dis.* **134**:401–423 (1986).

THOMPSON, N. J., GLASSROTH, J. H., SNIDER, D. E., JR., AND FARER, L. S., The booster phenomenon in serial tuberculin testing, *Am. Rev. Respir. Dis.* **119**:587–597 (1979).

CHAPTER 37

Nontuberculous Mycobacterial Disease

Richard J. O'Brien and George W. Comstock

1. Introduction

Nomenclature for mycobacteria other than tuberculosis (MOTT) and leprosy and their associated diseases has not been entirely satisfactory and has varied considerably. The etiologic organisms have been called MOTT bacilli by mycobacteriologists and atypical mycobacteria by clinicians, with other designations such as anonymous, environmental, opportunistic, and unclassified also used. The diseases they cause have been given names such as nontuberculous mycobacteriosis, pseudotuberculosis, tuberculoidosis, and tuberculosis caused by a specified organism. To borrow a phrase from the review by Wolinsky,[79] "None of the proposed names is without criticism, but the most appropriate and least offensive, in my opinion, is nontuberculous mycobacteriosis." This designation appears to be gaining common acceptance and will be used in this chapter.

2. Historical Background

Tuberculosis in birds had been described several years prior to Robert Koch's report in 1882 on the isolation of the human tubercle bacillus, and many mycobacteria were iden-

tified in water, soil, vegetation, and a variety of other animals shortly thereafter. As these mycobacteria did not cause characteristic disease when inoculated into guinea pigs, they were recognized as distinct from *Mycobacterium tuberculosis* and were not believed to cause human disease. Because of the difficulties in isolation and identification by routine laboratory procedures and because of the much greater frequency of tuberculosis, little attention was paid to their pathogenic potential despite sporadic reports of human disease caused by a variety of nontuberculous mycobacteria during the first half of this century.[9,56] In the second half of the century, routine culturing for mycobacteria became commonplace and biochemical techniques for identification were developed, thus allowing the various species of mycobacteria to be more easily recognized. As tuberculosis in industrialized countries became much less common, the infrequent disease caused by nontuberculous mycobacteria came to comprise an increasingly larger proportion of illnesses caused by mycobacteria in developed countries.

In the 1950s, pulmonary disease due to nontuberculous mycobacteria became more commonly recognized and was found to comprise 1–2% of admissions to tuberculosis sanatoriums in the southeastern United States.[41] A paper by Timpe and Runyon[72] in 1954, classifying these "atypical" mycobacteria into four groups based on simple cultural characteristics, marked the upsurge in interest in nontuberculous mycobacteria. Although several other schemes for classifying these organisms have since been devised, the Runyon classification remains the most commonly used.[3] Those nontuberculous mycobacteria that have been associ-

Richard J. O'Brien · Clinical Research Branch, Division of Tuberculosis Control, Center for Prevention Services, Centers for Disease Control, Atlanta, Georgia 30333. **George W. Comstock** · School of Hygiene and Public Health, The Johns Hopkins University, Baltimore, Maryland 21205.

Table 1.   Nontuberculous Mycobacteria Causing Disease in Man

Species	Primary clinical presentations
Group I—photochromogens	
M. kansasii	Pulmonary disease, lymph node disease
M. marinum	Skin disease
M. simiae	Pulmonary disease
M. asiaticum	Pulmonary disease
Group II—scotochromogens	
M. scrofulaceum	Lymph node disease, pulmonary disease
M. xenopi	Pulmonary disease
M. szulgai	Pulmonary disease
M. gordonae	Nonpathogen[a]
Group III—nonchromogens	
M. avium complex	Pulmonary disease, disseminated disease,
(includes *M. intracellulare*)	lymph node disease
M. malmoense	Pulmonary disease
M. hemophilum	Pulmonary disease
M. terrae	Nonpathogen[a]
M. nonchromogenicum	Nonpathogen[a]
M. ulcerans	Skin ulcers
Group IV—rapid growers	
M. fortuitum complex	Soft-tissue and bone disease,
(includes *M. chelonae*)	pulmonary disease
M. thermoresistible	Nonpathogen[a]

[a]Usually a saprophyte but clinical disease has been reported.

ated with disease in man are listed in Table 1 by Runyon group; saprophytic mycobacteria that may be isolated from man but are not known to cause disease are not listed. Group I, the photochromogens, develop yellow or orange pigment when exposed to light; group II, the scotochromogens, form orange-yellow pigment in the dark; group III, the nonchromogens, are essentially unpigmented; group IV, the rapid growers, grow on artificial culture media within 1 week, as distinguished from the slow-growing mycobacteria, which usually take 3 to 6 weeks to appear.

The ability to recognize infections caused by nontuberculous mycobacteria by skin testing developed much later than their bacteriological identification and is still primarily a research tool. This capability and much of the ensuing information about these infections came almost entirely from the work of Carroll E. Palmer and his colleagues. The seed for this research was apparently planted in a conference called to discuss the differing results obtained from a variety of tuberculin skin test antigens and the poor correlation of two signs once thought to be pathognomonic of

tuberculous infection, tuberculin hypersensitivity and pulmonary calcification.[13] The first convincing evidence that infections other than those by *M. tuberculosis* or *M. bovis* caused tuberculin sensitivity came from a study of 10,058 student nurses in the United States conducted between 1943 and 1947.[53] Subsequent skin-testing studies with antigens from a variety of mycobacteria[24] in large numbers of subjects including over 600,000 Navy recruits,[43] and in locations from the tropics to the Arctic,[6,25] showed that infections with nontuberculous mycobacteria are very common, in marked contrast to the infrequency of disease.

More recently, there has been a resurgence of interest in nontuberculous mycobacterial diseases due to the finding of disseminated mycobacteriosis due to *M. avium* complex among large numbers of patients with the acquired immunodeficiency syndrome (AIDS).[82] This has occurred at a time when better understanding of the epidemiology of nontuberculous mycobacteria and advances in molecular biology and genetics have substantially increased our knowledge about these organisms.

3. Methodology

3.1. Sources of Mortality Data

Information on mortality has been available only since 1968, when nontuberculous mycobacterioses were first given a separate rubric in the eighth revision of the International Classification of Diseases. The classification does not permit listing the diseases by the infecting mycobacterial species and with the exception of pulmonary and cutaneous disease does not provide for coding the site of disease. Moreover, these diseases are seldom designated as an underlying cause of death, and thus information from death certificates is of limited usefulness.

3.2. Sources of Morbidity Data

These diseases are not reportable in most states. A rough estimate of their relative frequency may be obtained by comparing the relative frequency of isolations of *M. tuberculosis* and nontuberculous mycobacteria by large bacteriology laboratories, although, unlike tuberculosis, isolation of nontuberculous mycobacteria is not sufficient for the diagnosis of disease. There have been several reports from various states[37,50] and similar national reports of patients with nontuberculous mycobacterial disease.[49,76] While such reports are useful in better describing the occurrence of these diseases, they do not provide reliable information upon which to base estimates of disease incidence and prevalence.

3.3. Surveys

Skin-testing surveys with two or more antigens, one of which is almost always a standardized purified tuberculin prepared from *M. tuberculosis,* have been widely used. The results indicate the extent of infections with nontuberculous mycobacteria, but not which organism or organisms are responsible for the skin-test reactions (see Section 3.4.2 for interpretation of skin tests).

Very few sputum surveys have been done. They show the extent to which persons harbor these organisms in their oral or respiratory secretions, but do not indicate the frequency of persons with disease.

3.4. Laboratory Diagnosis

3.4.1. Isolation and Identification of the Organisms. Presumptive diagnosis of mycobacterial disease is often accomplished by acid-fast microscopy of body fluids or tissues. However, nontuberculous mycobacteria cannot be differentiated from *M. tuberculosis* by microscopy. The organisms can be isolated from body fluids and tissues by the same procedures used for the isolation of tubercle bacilli.[33] Biochemical tests are required to identify the various mycobacterial species and are generally performed by reference laboratories.[4] A convenient summary of cultural and biochemical characteristics of medically important species is published periodically by the American Lung Association.[3]

One deficiency of these procedures is the time required for isolation and identification of the infecting species of mycobacteria, up to 2 months in some cases. Radiometric methods (BACTEC) have decreased the isolation time to as short a period as 2 weeks and permit separation of nontuberculous mycobacteria from *M. tuberculosis* complex.[67] However, speciation by standard biochemical tests is still required to identify the organism.

A variety of other laboratory techniques have been described that might still shorten the time required for identification. Some of these techniques, such as DNA homology studies[5] and gas–liquid chromatography,[73] are relegated to the research laboratory. Other techniques, such as enzyme-linked immunosorbent assay (ELISA) of specific mycobacterial antigens,[81] may have wider applicability. Serotyping of isolates of the *M. avium–M. intracellulare–M. scrofulaceum* ("MAIS" complex), utilizing the agglutination method developed by Schaefer,[64] has been useful for epidemiological studies of these organisms.

Among the most promising of the newer rapid diagnostic techniques are genetic probes, which have proven to be highly specific. At present, two probes, both directed against ribosomal RNA, are being marketed for the identification of cultures of *M. avium* and *M. intracellulare*. In one report, these probes significantly reduced the time for identification of *M. avium* complex from patients with AIDS,[34] and preliminary information suggests that these probes may be as sensitive as microscopy for identifying *M. avium* complex in diagnostic specimens. It is likely that with improvement in techniques, the sensitivity of these probes will equal that of culture, rendering both culturing and biochemical identification of nontuberculous mycobacteria obsolete.

3.4.2. Serological and Immunological Diagnostic Methods. Although most patients with nontuberculous mycobacterial disease mount a serological response to the infection, no serological diagnostic tests have been described. There are several impediments to the development of a

useful diagnostic test. First, patients who have been infected but have not developed disease may have antibodies
against these organisms, and thus separation of persons with
and without disease may be difficult. Second, antibodies
produced by the immune response to infection tend to be
broadly reactive with a variety of antigens from many
strains of nontuberculous mycobacteria.

These same problems also apply to the use of skin-test
antigens for the diagnosis of infection and disease. Skin-
testing diagnostic procedures depend on the fact that cross-
reactions tend to be smaller than reactions to the homologous
antigen. If two properly standardized skin-test antigens are
administered simultaneously at separate sites, the smaller
reaction is likely to be a cross-reaction and the antigen that
causes this reaction is not likely to represent the mycobacterial species responsible for the infection. The larger reaction does not identify the responsible agent, however. Unless
all possible skin tests are used, one can never be sure that
another antigen might not cause an even larger reaction.

4. Biological Characteristics of the Organisms

Most nontuberculous mycobacteria are slowly growing, Gram-stain-neutral bacilli that require special nutrients
for growth on artificial media. They are distinguished by the
property of "acid fastness," being quite resistant to decolorization with acid–alcohol following staining with car-
bolfuchsin. Most of these organisms are much less virulent
than *M. tuberculosis,* both in man and in animals. The most
commonly used animal models for studying these organisms are strains of immunodeficient mice.

These organisms are, in general, resistant to most of
the commonly used antimycobacterial drugs. For *M. avium*
complex, this resistance has been attributed to the highly
lipophilic nature of the cell wall, creating a permeability
barrier to penetration by antibiotics.[58] However, some species such as *M. kansasii* are susceptible to agents such as
ethambutol and rifampin,[38] while others such as *M. fortuitum* are susceptible to antibiotics such as sulfonamides
and erythromycin.[70]

Nontuberculous mycobacteria are widely distributed in
nature. Some can be found in water and dairy products,
many reside in the soil, others are associated with plant
roots, and still others are found in insects, lower animals,
and man, usually without evidence of disease.[11,28,45,79]
Ongoing studies of the environmental epidemiology of
MAIS organisms by Falkinham and co-workers have greatly
increased our knowledge of these organisms.[29] These

strains have been found to grow well in brackish waters,
particularly in warmer climates such as estuaries and rivers
along the southeast coast of the United States. Strains that
are more commonly isolated from persons with disease tend
to be preferentially aerosolized from these waters, suggesting the possibility of airborne transmission of infection from
these sources.[54] Other studies have suggested that plas-
mid-carrying strains may be associated with virulence and
that such strains are more commonly aerosolized as
well.[46]

5. Descriptive Epidemiology

As with tuberculosis, it is helpful to consider the epidemiological characteristics associated with the risk of becoming infected with nontuberculous mycobacteria
separately from characteristics associated with the development of disease following infection. The characteristics associated with each event appear to differ considerably, although our knowledge is scanty. Moreover, epidemiological
characteristics of disease vary considerably with mycobacterial species. However, unlike tuberculosis, there is little
evidence bearing on the frequency with which nontuberculous mycobacterial disease arises from latent infection. In
addition, in contrast to tuberculosis, it is possible to harbor
nontuberculous mycobacteria in the respiratory secretions
without any evidence of disease, and some species may
appear as harmless commensals without causing infection.

5.1. Prevalence and Incidence

Evidence of past infection manifested by the results of
skin-testing surveys varies markedly. Skin-test reactivity is
virtually absent in some populations and as high as 80–90%
in others. In the latter, the incidence of infection may be as
high as 5% per year.[26,52] Skin tests given to U.S. Navy
recruits included 13 antigens from various mycobacteria in
addition to purified protein derivative of tuberculin prepared
from *M. tuberculosis* (PPD-S). Only about 5% reacted to an
antigen prepared from *M. fortuitum* (a rapid-growing mycobacterium), slightly more reacted to PPD-S, and over
40% reacted to PPD-G, an antigen prepared from *M.
scrofulaceum.*[52]

Because cross-reactions are very common in mycobacterial infections, the reactions to mycobacterial antigens are
not specific for the organisms from which they were prepared. A low prevalence of reactions to a particular antigen
indicates that infections with the corresponding organism

are uncommon; a high prevalence could be due to infections with the corresponding or a cross-reacting organism.

Information on the frequency of persons excreting these organisms, either as "carriers" or as diseased subjects, is scarce. Mycobacteria with the gross cultural characteristics of nontuberculous mycobacteria were found in the sputum of 15–30% of selected populations in Georgia who had no evidence of pulmonary disease.[18,21] In a similar survey of healthy men in tropical Australia, nontuberculous mycobacteria were isolated from the sputa of 7.5%,[36] and studies from other parts of the world have produced similar results. However, in these studies the mycobacteria were not well characterized, so that it is not known what proportion were potentially pathogenic organisms and what percentage were nonpathogens.

Because nontuberculous mycobacteria can be isolated from apparently normal persons, estimates of nontuberculous mycobacterial disease prevalence based upon reports of laboratory isolates are unreliable. While it is reasonable to expect that in most cases diagnostic specimens submitted for mycobacterial culture are from persons with clinical disease, the finding of mycobacteria in a specimen is not sufficient for the diagnosis. This is especially true for mycobacteria isolated from sputa. Nonetheless, laboratory surveillance data are helpful in describing the prevalent mycobacteria in an area and for following trends over time.

In a study in British Columbia, where skin-testing surveys indicated that about 20% of the population had been infected with nontuberculous mycobacteria, the average annual incidence of recognized disease was only 0.37/100,000, or approximately 2/100,000 infected individuals.[60] In most areas, however, the prevalence of excreters of nontuberculous mycobacteria can only be estimated from their frequency relative to tubercle bacilli in specimens submitted for bacteriological examination. This ratio depends on the frequency of both tuberculous and other mycobacterial diseases in the examined population. Nontuberculous mycobacteria accounted for 12% of all specimens positive for mycobacteria in a private hospital in Cleveland, Ohio,[19]·20% in West Irian, Indonesia,[30] and among tuberculosis contacts in Puerto Rico,[68] and slightly over 50% in South Carolina.[74] The relative frequency of persons with demonstrable disease due to tuberculous and nontuberculous mycobacteria is even more difficult to estimate because the latter cases are not reportable and the frequency of admission to treatment facilities is probably not the same for both types of disease. A summary of reports of the proportion of cases of nontuberculous mycobacterial disease shows a range of 0.5–30% with a median

value of 7% for the United States and Canada and a range of 0.5–15% with a median value of 4% overseas.[79]

Several recent national surveys have helped to define the prevalence of nontuberculous mycobacterial disease in the United States. Nationwide reporting by state mycobacterial laboratories indicated that nontuberculous mycobacteria accounted for approximately one-third of all mycobacterial isolates.[27] The most commonly isolated species of nontuberculous mycobacteria were *M. avium* complex (21%), *M. fortuitum–m. chelonae* (6%), *M. kansasii* (3%), and *M. scrofulaceum* (2%). Combining these laboratory data with results from a national survey that included clinical and epidemiological information on patients with suspected nontuberculous mycobacterial disease resulted in an estimated disease prevalence of 1.8/100,000 or approximately 20% that of tuberculosis.[49] Estimated disease prevalence by species from this survey is shown in Table 2, which also provides estimates of the probability of disease among persons from whom potentially pathogenic nontuberculous mycobacteria are isolated, ranging from 75% for persons with *M. kansasii* to 18% for those with *M. fortuitum.*

5.2. Epidemic Behavior and Contagiousness

While no epidemics of these diseases due to community-acquired infection have been reported, nosocomial outbreaks of disease have been recognized (see Section 5.9). Several reports have also suggested increases in respiratory colonization without disease due to nontuberculous mycobacteria in water supplies.[7,40] Available evidence suggests that person-to-person and animal-to-man transmission of nontuberculous mycobacteria is not an important factor in acquisition of infection. Most infections are believed to arise from environmental exposure to organisms in infected water, soil, dust, or aerosols.[11,16,29,79] Several skin-test studies have suggested that persons with disease excreting large numbers of organisms do not readily infect close contacts.[12,16] Because of the low virulence of these organisms, isolation of patients with disease is not indicated, although immunosuppressed patients at risk of disseminated nontuberculous mycobacterial disease (e.g., AIDS patients) should not be exposed to persons excreting large numbers of nontuberculous mycobacteria.

5.3. Geographic Distribution

Skin-testing surveys show that infections are most common in tropical and subtropical areas and at lower al-

Table 2.   Nontuberculous Mycobacterial Disease in the United States:
Estimates of Disease Prevalence from Surveillance Data

Species	Annual no. of isolates[a]	Disease (%)[b]	Estimated no. of cases	Estimated prevalence per 100,000
avium	6,229	47	2928	1.28
kansasii	1,016	75	762	0.33
fortuitum	1,423	18	256	0.11
scrofulaceum	680	22	150	0.07
chelonae	488	38	185	0.08
xenopi	71	25	18	0.01
simiae	71	21	15	0.01
marinum	142	88	125	0.05
szulgai	41	57	23	0.01
Total	10,161	40[c]	4064	1.78

[a]Estimated from 1980 laboratory surveillance data.[27]
[b]Estimated from epidemiology survey data, 1981–1983.[49]
[c]Includes a factor for overestimation of disease rate, so that next column does not add to total.

titudes and least common in the Arctic and at high elevations.[1,6,25,26,52,57] Within the United States, the prevalence of reactors to PPD-B and PPD-G, antigens prepared
from *M. intracellulare* and *M. scrofulaceum,* respectively,
was lowest in the Northwest and highest along the Gulf and
south Atlantic coasts.[52] In a study of over 250,000 naval
recruits who were lifelong single-county residents and who
were tested with PPD-B, the rate of sensitization was highest among residents of the southeastern United States (70%
and greater) and lowest among those from the North and
West (10 to 20%) (Fig. 1).[26,77] Moreover, there was no
correlation between rates of reactions to PPD-B and to PPD-
S (compare with Fig. 3 of Chapter 36). Unlike reactor rates
to tuberculin (PPD-S), those to PPD-B were higher among
persons living in rural areas than among residents of metropolitan areas.

A few efforts have been made to ascertain the mycobacterial species likely to have caused skin-test reactions.
This has been done by administering a battery of different
skin-test antigens (usually six) to population samples and
comparing the patterns of mean reaction sizes to the antigens with those obtained in guinea pigs infected by various
mycobacteria.[23] Such testing suggests that the only important source of mycobacterial infection among Alaskan
natives is *M. tuberculosis,*[25] that scotochromogens are
likely to be the major factor in infections in the United
States,[23] and that there may be considerable variation from
place to place in the nature of mycobacterial infections in a
country such as Norway.[7] However, such testing has gen-

erally utilized nonstandardized antigens, equivalent to PPD
tuberculin only on a protein weight basis. The assumed
relationship between the relative size of a skin-test reaction
and infection by (or lack of infection from) the homologous
mycobacterium has not been proven.

National reporting of clinical isolates of nontuberculous mycobacteria by state mycobacteriology laboratories
in 1979 and 1980 indicated that isolation rates for *M. avium*
were high in the Southeast,[27] similar to that noted by the
earlier skin-testing surveys. However, high rates were also
found among several states bordering Canada and among
other states such as Arizona and Kansas, a finding that
would not have been expected from the results of the skin-
test studies. Population mobility and geographic changes in
the environmental distribution of these organisms are
among the possible explanations for these differences. Rates
of isolation of *M. kansasii* were highest in the central portions of the United States.

In Georgia, the rates of admissions to Battey State
Hospital for nontuberculous mycobacterioses were much
higher from counties in the coastal plain below the "Fall
Line" than in the hilly areas to the north,[16] a pattern of
disease paralleling that for infections.[52] A careful study of
patients with pulmonary disease due to *M. avium* complex
and *M. kansasii* in Texas indicated that patients with *M.
avium* complex were twice as likely to be residents of rural
areas than cities.[2] However, the opposite was true for *M.
kansasii* disease patients, who were twice as likely to be
urban residents.

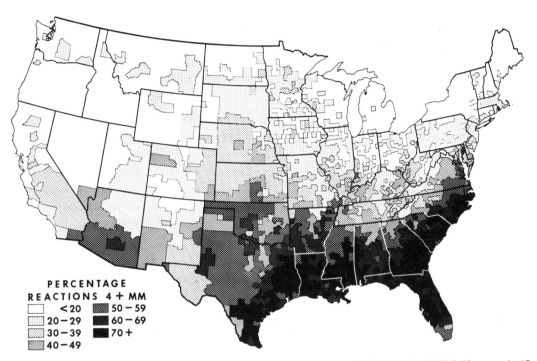

Figure 1. Geographic variations (1958 to 1964) in the frequency of reactors to 0.0001 mg PPD-B in 257,476 U.S. Navy recruits 17 to 21 years old, lifetime one-county residents.

5.4. Temporal Distribution

While some authors have noted an increase in the occurrence of nontuberculous mycobacterial disease,[2,48,61] others have noted no such change.[20,37,39] However, in countries that have experienced a significant decrease in tuberculosis and have laboratories that can speciate mycobacteria, there has been an increase in nontuberculous mycobacterial disease relative to tuberculosis. Given the opportunistic nature of these organisms, one might expect an increase in disease should there be a change in the host defenses of a population. This is certainly the case for disseminated *M. avium* complex disease, which had been rarely recognized before the 1980s and now may be the most common form of nontuberculous mycobacterial disease in North America because of its occurrence in significant numbers of AIDS patients.[82] Similarly, as the life expectancy of persons in the United States has increased and the incidence of chronic lung disease has increased, numbers of persons with nontuberculous mycobacterial pulmonary disease may be expected to increase.

5.5. Age

As with any condition that tends to persist, skin-test evidence of past infection increases with age.[22,42,77] Prevalence of sensitivity to PPD-B or PPD-G in the United States and Canada tends to reach a maximum at about the age of 55 years, but when the effects of cross-reactions from tuberculous infection are removed, there is little evidence of increasing frequency of sensitivity to PPD-B with age among adults.[22,60,77] It is not known whether this represents virtually universal infection with some organism(s) that is manifested only partially by reactions to PPD-B or PPD-G or whether sensitivity from nontuberculous mycobacteria is relatively short-lived so that an equilibrium is reached between new infections and loss of previous sensitivity.

Age distribution of persons with nontuberculous mycobacterial disease varies by mycobacterial species and site of disease.[16,42,60,79] Pulmonary disease is most commonly seen in older patients, and among such patients those with *M. avium* complex disease tend to be older than those with

M. kansasii disease.[2] With the exception of AIDS patients with disseminated mycobacteriosis, those with lymph node disease are children and commonly under 5 years of age. Skin disease due to *M. marinum* affects primarily younger and middle-aged persons, reflecting to an extent occupational exposure. Bone and soft-tissue infection from organisms in the *M. fortuitum* complex group are often nosocomially acquired during surgical procedures and thus affect a wider age spectrum of patients.

5.6. Sex

Scanty information indicates that males are more likely than females to react to nontuberculous mycobacterial antigens.[22,63,78] Cases of lymphadenitis in young children are slightly more common among females,[42] but in the past pulmonary disease in adults was considerably more common among males.[15,60] Male predominance is especially marked among those with pulmonary disease due to *M. kansasii* and less so among those with *M. avium* complex disease.[2] However, among older persons with *M. avium* complex pulmonary disease, women predominate, perhaps reflecting the presence of older numbers of women with underlying chronic lung disease.[49] Skin disease due to *M. marinum* is much more common among men.

5.7. Race

There appears to be little, if any, racial variation in infections with nontuberculous mycobacteria when place of residence is held constant.[26,66] Early reports from tuberculosis sanatoriums of patients with nontuberculous mycobacterial pulmonary disease noted the relative absence of nonwhite patients. However, more recent data suggest that there is no apparent racial susceptibility to disease.

5.8. Occupation

No information is available on infection status and occupation, except as workplaces are related to geography.

Sputum surveys of occupational groups in west central Georgia showed a marked association of exposure to agricultural dusts and the presence of nontuberculous mycobacteria in the sputum of well persons.[18,21] A very high frequency of these organisms was found in workers in a poultry-processing plant, but only among persons exposed to feathers. In Australia, 8 of 11 healthy workers exposed to pigs with lymphadenitis caused by *M. intracellulare* were found to harbor the same organisms.[59]

There is some evidence that patients with occupational pneumoconiosis, especially patients with silicosis, may be more likely to develop pulmonary disease due to nontuberculous mycobacteria.[65] However, other than workers with aquatic exposure, there is no known occupational association with nontuberculous mycobacterial disease.

5.9. Occurrence in Different Settings

Chronic granulomatous ulcers of the skin are caused by *M. marinum,* often following abrasions of the skin in infected water, notably fish tanks and swimming pools.[32] Nosocomial infections from *M. fortuitum* complex have been reported in a variety of settings, probably related to contamination during surgical procedures such as open-heart surgery and mammoplasty.[75] Disseminated infections from *M. chelonae* have also been noted among patients in a dialysis center.[8] Increases in respiratory colonization among hospitalized patients have been noted, on one occasion attributed to *M. xenopi* acquired presumably from contaminated hot-water systems[14] and on another to *M. fortuitum* from a contaminated ice machine.[40]

5.10. Socioeconomic Factors

There is no evidence that socioeconomic status is related to the development of infection or disease due to nontuberculous mycobacteria. Skin tests of male residents of Maryland who were Navy recruits or students of the University of Maryland showed no evidence of differences between these two groups in the prevalence of nontuberculous mycobacterial infections.[26,63]

5.11. Other Factors

Interference with local protective mechanisms (e.g., bronchopulmonary clearance) may be an important risk factor for the acquisition of pulmonary mycobacteriosis. Silicosis and malignancies are also reported to be risk factors for pulmonary disease.[51,79] The presence of immunodeficiency states, especially AIDS, and immunosuppressive therapy are risk factors for disseminated disease.[31,55,82] However, in many patients there is no apparent predisposing factor and usual tests of immune function are normal. Such patients may, however, have specific defects in cellular immunity, as has been recently demonstrated for patients with *M. marinum* disease.[17]

6. Mechanisms and Routes of Transmission

Although little is known about how infection is acquired, it is generally believed that the reservoirs and sources are environmental. Cutaneous ulcers are likely to be caused by direct implantation of infected material into skin cuts or abrasions. Nosocomial wound infections due to *M. fortuitum* complex organisms may be due to aerosols from tap water containing these organisms or from infected solutions or equipment used for surgical procedures.[75] In fection in dialysis patients has been attributed to contaminated hemodialysis equipment.[8] Lymphadenitis in children may result from close contact with the earth and the tendency of children to put things into their mouths.[42] Inhalation of aerosols containing *M. avium* complex may be the primary route of infection for persons with pulmonary disease due to this organism. Studies of the ecology of MAIS organisms in the Southeast have strengthened this hypothesis.[29,54]

Inhalation of infected dust and the ingestion of contaminated water, dairy products, or raw vegetables provide other possible sources of infection. Data on disseminated *M. avium* complex in AIDS patients suggest that infection is acquired via the oral route from a source such as water.

Despite the presence of *M. avium* disease in chicken flocks and swine herds, there are no data suggesting that animal-to-man transmission is an important source of infection.[45] Furthermore, no convincing evidence has yet been produced that persons who harbor these organisms are a significant hazard to their associates, although one skin-test study of household contacts of patients with pulmonary mycobacteriosis indicated higher reactor rates than among control subjects.[12] On the other hand, it would be exceedingly difficult to demonstrate such a risk when infection is widespread in the environment of most cases and when only a tiny fraction of infected individuals become ill.

7. Pathogenesis and Immunity

Relatively little is known about the pathogenesis of infection and disease with nontuberculous mycobacteria and about the development of immunity following infection. Most diagnosed infections in immunocompetent hosts are associated with a granulomatous response so that the model of pathogenesis developed for tuberculosis may be applicable to the majority of infections from nontuberculous mycobacteria. If the organisms gain entrance into the body through skin, mucous membranes, or the respiratory tract, it

is assumed that a granulomatous lesion develops that usually heals without becoming large enough to be noticeable. Disseminated disease may develop in the absence of the usual immune response. For example, among AIDS patients with disseminated *M. avium* complex disease, granulomas are conspicuously absent.[69] It is assumed that localized disease in the small intestine leads to bloodborne dissemination with widespread organ involvement. No information about the interval between the time of initial infection and the development of symptomatic disease (i.e., incubation period) is available. There is no evidence that, as is the case for tuberculosis, disease develops following a long period of asymptomatic infection.

8. Patterns of Host Response

It has already been emphasized that inapparent infections are very common in many geographic areas. These organisms can often be found in oral, respiratory, and genitourinary secretions without any evidence, other than positive skin tests, that they have invaded the body.

8.1. Clinical Features

8.1.1. Pulmonary Diseases. Chronic disease of the lungs is the major clinical problem associated with these organisms. It cannot be differentiated clinically from pulmonary tuberculosis and is usually diagnosed only when the results of sputum cultures are reported. Patients commonly present with respiratory symptoms, such as chronic cough and sputum production, abnormalities on chest radiograph, and AFB-positive sputum smears. Systemic signs and symptoms such as fever, malaise, and weight loss are generally less marked than for patients with tuberculosis. In addition, clinical progression seems to be much slower than for tuberculosis. Underlying lung diseases, such as COPD, cancer, bronchiectasis, or previous tuberculosis, are commonly associated. While the chest radiograph may simulate tuberculosis with upper lobe cavitary disease, scattered infiltrates throughout the lung fields and disease presenting as a solitary pulmonary nodule also occur. The most common etiological organisms are *M. kansasii* and *M. avium* complex. Other organisms occasionally associated with pulmonary disease are *M. fortuitum* complex and *M. scrofulaceum*.[49,79]

8.1.2. Lymphadenitis. The submaxillary and submandibular lymph nodes are characteristically involved, although any of the superficial lymph nodes may be affected. The involvement of only one or a few nodes, early suppuration, and associated salivary-gland disease point to nontuberculous mycobacterial disease rather than tuberculosis.[42] Almost all cases occur before the age of 5 years. The natural history of this disease is not well defined. It may be that many patients with undetected lymphadenopathy often have spontaneous regression of the disease. Recently, there has been an apparent change in the distribution of organisms causing disease, with *M. avium* complex predominating, and *M. scrofulaceum,* once the most commonly identified etiological organism, now much less frequent.[39,42,49] In a few areas, *M. kansasii* is also commonly identified.[42,79]

8.1.3. Soft-Tissue Lesions. Localized abscesses, usually caused by *M. fortuitum* complex, occur after injections, surgical wounds, or other trauma.[75,79] Chronic granulomas and ulcers follow cuts and abrasions that occur in swimming pools, fish tanks, or other marine environments harboring *M. marinum.* Indolent necrotic ulcers (Buruli or Bairnsdale ulcers) result from infections with *M. ulcerans,* most commonly found in central Africa and Australia.[10]

8.1.4. Other Sites of Localized Disease. Lesions at sites other than the above-named ones are uncommon. Other sites of disease are bones, joints, tendon sheaths, genitourinary tract, and the meninges.

8.1.5. Disseminated Disease. Until recently, disseminated mycobacteriosis was uncommon, occurring in persons with impaired immunity related to an underlying disease, such as leukemia or lymphoma or iatrogenically induced with immunosuppressive therapy.[31,79] However, the occurrence of disseminated mycobacteriosis, especially due to *M. avium* complex, among patients with AIDS has now resulted in the condition being commonly recognized in areas caring for AIDS patients. It is estimated that in some areas up to 50% of AIDS patients may have disseminated disease.[35] The clinical features of disease are quite variable; some patients with widely disseminated disease are asymptomatic while others have disabling fever, anemia, diarrhea, and wasting. Among these patients, gastrointestinal tract involvement with a histological picture resembling Whipple's disease is common.[62] Bloodstream infection and bone marrow involvement are also commonly recognized. Involvement of virtually every organ of the body in this disease has been described. However, CNS involvement is rare, and while organisms may be commonly isolated from bronchial secretions, respiratory disease due to *M. avium* complex is uncommon in AIDS.

8.2. Diagnosis

The diagnosis can sometimes be suspected from epidemiological and clinical information. The suspicion of nontuberculous mycobacterial disease should be raised by chronic infiltrative, fibrotic, or cavitary pulmonary disease in an older man; chronic lymphadenitis in a very young child; chronic ulcers of a vulnerable part of the body in persons exposed to marine environments; chronic necrotic ulcers in persons who have been in central Africa or Australia; and persistent undiagnosed fever and anemia in an AIDS patient. That suspicion should be heightened if there is little or no reaction to 5 tuberculin units of PPD-S and if the patient comes from an area where these infections are common. Finding tuberculin skin-test-negative household contacts of a patient with pulmonary disease and sputum containing acid-fast bacilli should also heighten suspicion of nontuberculous mycobacterial disease. However, the diagnosis can be made with reasonable certainty only when bacteriological examinations have isolated and identified the causative organism. In the case of patients with pulmonary disease, diagnosis requires the repeated isolation of the same organism in significant quantities and the exclusion of other disease that may be responsible for the radiographic abnormalities observed.[80]

There are problems, however, with the diagnosis of both past infection and present disease. Skin tests, like all medical tests, can yield false-negative and false-positive results. Skin sensitivity is often not demonstrable in severely ill or immunosuppressed patients. Cross-reactions to all mycobacterial antigens are common. When it is possible to obtain matched antigens from different mycobacteria, all that can be said from the results of giving two or more tests is that the smaller reaction may not represent the etiological agent. Multiple testing with a battery of mycobacterial antigens is unlikely to be useful in adults, but may be more reliable in very young children because interpretation of their skin-test reactions is not as likely to be confounded by multiple mycobacterial infections. However, while differential skin testing may be helpful in the presumptive diagnosis of children with lymphatic disease,[44] these products are not commercially available. Repeated testing of the same individuals may yield conversions from negative to positive that do not result from new infections but rather from the booster phenomenon[71] [see Chapter 36 (Section 3.4.2)].

Cultures of nontuberculous mycobacteria from body secretions may also fail to be definitive. False-negative results for *M. ulcerans* may be obtained if the cultures are incubated at 37°C, since this organism prefers cooler temperatures.[33] Isolation of mycobacteria from diseased lymph nodes, even those that are positive for acid-fast bacilli on microscopy, is sometimes difficult. False-positive results can occur as the result of contamination of laboratory water supplies or reagents,[47] or more often because the patient happens to be harboring nontuberculous mycobacteria that have nothing to do with his or her disease.

9. Control and Prevention

9.1. General Concepts

Because the disease appears to be nontransmissible, in general there is no need for reporting, isolation, or quarantine. However, immunodeficient patients such as those with AIDS should not be unnecessarily exposed to patients with pulmonary disease excreting large numbers of organisms. Measures taken to prevent infection from environmental sources are not indicated, because so little is known about factors that influence infection and, except for the immunocompromised host, serious consequences of infection are so rare.

9.2. Chemotherapeutic Prophylaxis

Chemotherapy for prophylaxis is rarely indicated because these organisms tend to be resistant to most antibiotics and because disease rarely follows infection. In the unusual instance in which a person with known nontuberculous mycobacterial disease must be given immunosuppressive treatment, combinations of antibiotics most likely to affect the particular organism can be given.[55] With the recent interest in disseminated *M. avium* complex in AIDS and drugs that demonstrate good *in vitro* activity against that organism, chemoprophylaxis of such patients may be of theoretical, though unproven, benefit.

9.3. Immunization

None is known.

10. Unresolved Problems

While our understanding of the environmental epidemiology of *M. avium* complex has advanced, we know very little about the epidemiology of other species of non-tuberculous mycobacteria. For all species, understanding the mechanisms of infection, pathogenesis, and immunity, and especially in knowing why some infected people develop illness and others do not is important. Improved diagnostic methods for differentiating persons with disease caused by these organisms from persons who merely harbor them would also be helpful. Finally, as satisfactory treatment is not available for the majority of persons with disease, improved drugs and treatment regimens are needed.

11. References

1. ABRAHAMS, E. W., AND SILVERSTONE, H., Epidemiological evidence of the presence of non-tuberculous sensitivity to tuberculin in Queensland, *Tubercle* **42:**487 (1961).
2. AHN, C. H., LOWELL, J. R., ONSTAD, G. D., SHUFORD, E. H., AND HURST, G. A., A demographic study of disease due to *Mycobacterium kansasii* or *M. intracellulare-avium* in Texas, *Chest* **75:**120–125 (1979).
3. American Thoracic Society, Diagnostic Standards and Classification of Tuberculosis and Other Mycobacterial Diseases, 14th ed., *Am. Rev. Respir. Dis.* **123:**343 (1981).
4. American Thoracic Society, Levels of laboratory services for mycobacterial diseases, *Am. Rev. Respir. Dis.* **128:**213 (1983).
5. BAESS, I., Deoxyribonucleic acid relatedness among species of slowly-growing mycobacteria, *Acta Pathol. Microbiol. Scand. Sect. B* **87:**221–226 (1979).
6. BATES, L. E., BUSK, T., AND PALMER, C. E., Research contributions of BCG vaccination programs. II. Tuberculin sensitivity at different altitudes of residence, *Public Health Rep.* **66:**1427 (1951).
7. BJERKEDAL, T., Mycobacterial infections in Norway: A preliminary note on determining their identity and frequency, *Am. J. Epidemiol.* **85:**157 (1967).
8. BOLAN, G., REINGOLD, A. L., CARSON, L. A., SILCOX, V. A., WOODLEY, C. L., HAYES, P. S., HIGHTOWER, A. W., McFARLAND, L., BROWN, J. W., III, PETERSEN, N. J., FAVERO, M. S., GOOD, R. C., AND BROOME, C. V., Infections with *Mycobacterium chelonei* in patients receiving dialysis and using processed hemodialyzers, *J. Infect. Dis.* **152:**1013–1019 (1985).
9. BRANCH, A., Avian tubercle bacillus infection, with special reference to mammals and to man: Its reported association with Hodgkin's disease, *Arch. Pathol.* **12:**253–274 (1931).
10. BURCHARD, G. D., AND BIERTHER, M., Buruli ulcer: Clinical pathological study of 23 patients in Lambaréné, Gabon, *Trop. Med. Parasitol.* **37:**1–8 (1986).
11. CHAPMAN, J. S., The ecology of the atypical mycobacteria, *Arch. Environ. Health* **22:**41 (1971).
12. CHAPMAN, J. S., DEWLETT, H. J., AND POTTS, W. E., Cu-

taneous reactions to unclassified mycobacterial antigens: A study of children in household contact with patients who excrete unclassified mycobacteria, *Am. Rev. Respir. Dis.* **86:**547–552 (1962).

13. COMSTOCK, G. W., The Hagerstown Tuberculosis Conference of 1938: A retrospective opinion, *Am. Rev. Respir. Dis.* **99:**119 (1969).

14. COSTRINI, A. M., MAHLER, D. A., GROSS, W. M., HAWKINS, J. E., YESNER, R., AND D'ESOPO, N. D., Clinical and roentgenographic features of nosocomial pulmonary disease due to *Mycobacterium xenopi, Am. Rev. Respir. Dis.* **123:**104 (1981).

15. CROW, H. E., KING, C. T., SMITH, C. E., CORPE, R. F., AND STERGUS, I., A limited clinical, pathologic, and epidemiologic study of patients with pulmonary lesions associated with atypical acid-fast bacilli in the sputum, *Am. Rev. Tuberc.* **75:**199 (1957).

16. CROW, H. E., CORPE, R. F., AND SMITH, C. E., Is serious pulmonary disease caused by nonphotochromogenic ("atypical") acid-fast mycobacteria communicable? *Dis. Chest* **39:**372–381 (1961).

17. DATTWYLER, R. J., THOMAS, J., AND HURST, L. C., Antigen-specific T-cell anergy in progressive *Mycobacterium marinum* infection in humans, *Ann. Intern. Med.* **107:**675–677 (1987).

18. DAVIS, S. D., AND COMSTOCK, G. W., Unpublished data.

19. DEMETER, S. L., AHMAD, M., AND TOMASHEFSKI, J., Epidemiological characteristics of mycobacterial infections in a referral clinic, *Am. Rev. Respir. Dis.* **119**(4) Part 2:399 (1979).

20. EDWARDS, F. G. B., Disease caused by 'atypical' (opportunist) mycobacteria: A whole population review, *Tubercle* **51:**285–295 (1970).

21. EDWARDS, L. B., AND PALMER, C. E., Isolation of "atypical" mycobacteria from healthy persons, *Am. Rev. Respir. Dis.* **80:**747 (1959).

22. EDWARDS, L. B., AND SMITH, D. T., Community-wide tuberculin testing study in Pamlico County, North Carolina, *Am. Rev. Respir. Dis.* **92:**43 (1965).

23. EDWARDS, L. B., HOPWOOD, L., AFFRONTI, L. F., AND PALMER, C. E., Sensitivity profiles of mycobacterial infection, *Bull. Int. Union Tuberc.* **32:**384 (1962).

24. EDWARDS, L. B., HOPWOOD, L., AND PALMER, C. E., Identification of mycobacterial infections, *Bull. WHO* **33:**405 (1965).

25. EDWARDS, L. B., COMSTOCK, G. W., AND PALMER, C. E., Contributions of northern populations to the understanding of tuberculin sensitivity, *Arch. Environ. Health* **17:**507 (1968).

26. EDWARDS, L. B., ACQUAVIVA, F. A., LIVESAY, V. T., CROSS, F. W., AND PALMER, C. E., An atlas of sensitivity to tuberculin, PPD-B, and histoplasmin in the United States, *Am. Rev. Respir. Dis.* 99(4) Part 2:1 (1969).

27. GOOD, R. C., AND SNIDER, D. E., JR., Isolation of nontuberculous mycobacteria in the United States, 1980, *J. Infect. Dis.* **146:**829–833 (1982).

28. GOSLEE, S., AND WOLINSKY, E., Water as a source of poten-

tially pathogenic mycobacteria, *Am. Rev. Respir. Dis.* **113:**287 (1976).

29. GRUFT, H., FALKINHAM, J. O., III, AND PARKER, B. C., Recent experience in the epidemiology of disease caused by atypical mycobacteria, *Rev. Infect. Dis.* **3:**990–996 (1981).

30. HANEGRAAF, T. A. C., AND WIJSMULLER, G., Atypical mycobacteria in New Guinea, *Sel. Pap. (R. Neth. Tuberc. Assoc.)* **8:**68 (1964).

31. HORSBURGH, C. R., JR., MASON, U. G., III, FARHI, D. C., AND ISEMAN, M. D., Disseminated infection with *Mycobacterium avium-intracellulare:* A report of 13 cases and a review of the literature, *Medicine* **64:**36–48 (1985).

32. JUDSON, F. N., AND FELDMAN, R. A., Mycobacterial skin tests in humans 12 years after infection with *Mycobacterium marinum, Am. Rev. Respir. Dis.* **109:**544 (1974).

33. KENT, P. T., AND KUBICA, G. P., Public health mycobacteriology: A guide for the level III laboratory, Centers for Disease Control, Atlanta, 1985.

34. KIEHN, T. E., AND EDWARDS, F. F., Rapid identification using a specific DNA probe of *Mycobacterium avium* complex from patients with acquired immunodeficiency syndrome, *J. Clin. Microbiol.* **25:**1551–1552 (1987).

35. KIEHN, T. E., EDWARDS, F. F., BRANNON, P., TSANG, A. Y., MAIO, M., GOLD, J. W. M., WHIMBEY, E., WONG, B., MCCLATCHY, J. K., AND ARMSTRONG, D., Infections caused by *Mycobacterium avium* complex in immunocompromised patients: Diagnosis by blood culture and fecal examination, antimicrobial susceptibility tests, and morphological and seroagglutination characteristics, *J. Clin. Microbiol.* **21:**168–173 (1985).

36. KIEWIET, A. A., AND THOMPSON, J. E., Isolation of 'atypical' mycobacteria from healthy individuals in tropical Australia, *Tubercle* **51:**296–299 (1970).

37. KRAJNACK, M. A., AND DOWDA, H., Non-tuberculous mycobacteria in South Carolina, 1971 to 1980, *J. S.C. Med. Assoc.* **77:**551–555 (1981).

38. KUZE, F., KURASAWA, T., BANDO, K., LEE, Y., AND MAEKAWA, N., *In vitro* and *in vivo* susceptibility of atypical mycobacteria to various drugs, *Rev. Infect. Dis.* **3:**885–897 (1981).

39. LAI, K. K., STOTTMEIER, K. D., SHERMAN, I. H., AND MCCABE, W. R., Mycobacterial cervical lymphadenopathy: Relation of etiologic agents to age, *J. Am. Med. Assoc.* **251:**1286–1288 (1984).

40. LAUSSUCQ, S., BALTCH, A., SMITH, R. P., SMITHWICK, R. W., DAVIS, B. J., DESJARDIN, E. K., SILCOX, B. A., SPELLACY, A., ZEIMIS, R., GRUFT, H., GOOD, R. C., AND COHEN, M. L., Nosocomial *Mycobacterium fortuitum* colonization from a contaminated ice machine, *Am. Rev. Respir. Dis.* **138:**891–894 (1988).

41. LEWIS, A. G., JR., LASCHÉ, E. M., ARMSTRONG, A. L., AND DUNBAR, F. P., A clinical study of the chronic lung disease due to nonphotochromogenic acid-fast bacilli, *Ann. Intern. Med.* **53:**273–285 (1960).

42. LINCOLN, E. M., AND GILBERT, L. A., Disease in children

due to mycobacteria other than *Mycobacterium tuberculosis,* *Am. Rev. Respir. Dis.* **105:**683 (1972).

43. LOWELL, A. M., EDWARDS, L. B., AND PALMER, C. E., *Tuberculosis,* Harvard University Press, Cambridge, Mass., 1969.

44. MARGILETH, A. M., CHANDRA, R., AND ALTMAN, P., Chronic lymphadenopathy due to mycobacterial infection: Clinical features, diagnosis, histopathology, and management, *Am. J. Dis. Child.* **138:**917–922 (1984).

45. MEISSNER, G., AND ANZ, W., Sources of *Mycobacterium avium* complex infection resulting in human diseases, *Am. Rev. Respir. Dis.* **116:**1057 (1977).

46. MEISSNER, P. S., AND FALKINHAM, J. O., III, Plasmid DNA profiles as epidemiological markers for clinical and environmental isolates of *Mycobacterium avium, Mycobacterium intracellulare,* and *Mycobacterium scrofulaceum, J. Infect. Dis.* **153:**325–331 (1986).

47. MURRAY, P. R., False-positive acid-fast smears, *Lancet* **2:**377 (1978).

48. Mycobacteriosis Research Group of the Japanese National Chest Hospitals, Rapid increase of the incidence of lung disease due to *Mycobacterium kansasii* in Japan, *Chest* **83:**890–892 (1983).

49. O'BRIEN, R. J., GEITER, L. J., AND SNIDER, D. E., JR., The epidemiology of nontuberculous mycobacterial diseases in the United States: Results from a national survey, *Am. Rev. Respir. Dis.* **135:**1007–1014 (1987).

50. OMONDI, P. P. G., ASAL, N. R., MUCHMORE, H. G., AND FLOURNOY, D. J., Epidemiology of nontuberculous mycobacteria in Oklahoma, *J. Okla. State Med. Assoc.* **78:**304–312 (1985).

51. ORTBALS, D. W., AND MARR, J. J., A comparative study of tuberculous and other mycobacterial infections and their associations with malignancy, *Am. Rev. Respir. Dis.* **117:**39 (1978).

52. PALMER, C. E., AND EDWARDS, L. B., Tuberculin test in retrospect and prospect, *Arch. Environ. Health* **15:**792 (1967).

53. PALMER, C. E., FEREBEE, S. H., AND STRANGE PETERSEN, O., Studies of pulmonary findings and antigen sensitivity among student nurses. VI. Geographic differences in sensitivity to tuberculin as evidence of nonspecific allergy, *Public Health Rep.* **65:**1111 (1950).

54. PARKER, B. C., FORD, M. A., GRUFT, H., AND FALKINHAM, J. O., III, Epidemiology of infection by nontuberculous mycobacteria. IV. Preferential aerosolization of *Mycobacterium intracellulare* from natural waters, *Am. Rev. Respir. Dis.* **128:**652–656 (1983).

55. PETTY, T. L., *Mycobacterium intracellulare-avium* complex infection (questions and answers), *J. Am. Med. Assoc.* **241:**1053 (1979).

56. PINNER, M., Atypical acid-fast microorganisms. III. Chromogenic acid-fast bacilli from human beings, *Am. Rev. Tuberc.* **32:**424 (1935).

57. RAJ NARAIN, ANANTHARAMAN, D. S., AND DIWAKARA, A. M., Prevalence of nonspecific tuberculin sensitivity in certain parts of India, *Bull. WHO* **51:**273 (1974).

58. RASTOGI, N., FREHEL, C., RYTER, A., OHAYON, H., LESOURD, M., AND DAVID, H. L., Multiple drug resistance in *Mycobacterium avium:* Is the wall architecture responsible for the exclusion of antimicrobial agents? *Antimicrob. Agents Chemother.* **20:**666–677 (1981).

59. REZNIKOV, M., AND ROBINSON, E., Serologically identical Battey mycobacteria from sputa of healthy piggery workers and lesions of pigs, *Aust. Vet. J.* **46:**606 (1970).

60. ROBAKIEWICZ, M., AND GRZYBOWSKI, S., Epidemiologic aspects of nontuberculous mycobacterial disease and of tuberculosis in British Columbia, *Am. Rev. Respir. Dis.* **109:**613 (1974).

61. ROSENZWEIG, D. Y., AND SCHLUETER, D. P., Spectrum of clinical disease in pulmonary infection with *Mycobacterium avium-intracellulare, Rev. Infect. Dis.* **3:**1046–1051 (1981).

62. ROTH, R. I., OWEN, R. L., KEREN, D. F., AND VOLBERDING, P. A., Intestinal infection with *Mycobacterium avium* in acquired immune deficiency syndrome (AIDS): Histological and clinical comparison with Whipple's disease, *Digest. Dis. Sci.* **30:**497–504 (1985).

63. SARTWELL, P. E., AND DYKE, L. M., Comparative sensitivity of college students to tuberculins PPD-S and PPD-B, *Am. J. Hyg.* **71:**204 (1960).

64. SCHAEFER, W. B., Serologic identification and classification of the atypical mycobacteria by their agglutination, *Am. Rev. Respir. Dis.* **92**(6) Part 2:85 (1965).

65. SCHAEFER, W. B., BIRN, K. J., JENKINS, P. A., AND MARKS, J., Infection with the Avian–Battey group of mycobacteria in England and Wales, *Br. Med. J.* **2:**412–415 (1969).

66. SHAW, L. W., Field studies on immunization against tuberculosis. I. Tuberculin allergy following BCG vaccination of school children in Muscogee County, Georgia, *Public Health Rep.* **66:**1415 (1951).

67. SIDDIQI, S. H., HWANGBO, C. C., SILCOX, V., GOOD, R. C., SNIDER, D. E., JR., AND MIDDLEBROOK, G., Rapid radiometric methods to detect and differentiate *Mycobacterium tuberculosis/M. bovis* from other mycobacterial species, *Am. Rev. Respir. Dis.* **130:**634–640 (1984).

68. SIFONTES, J. E., ALVAREZ, F. R., AND DE LA ROSA, J. C., The mycobacterioses in Puerto Rico, *Bol. Assoc. Med. Puerto Rico* **57:**135 (1965).

69. SOHN, C. C., SCHROFF, R. W., KLIEWER, K. E., LEBEL, D. M., AND FLIGIEL, S., Disseminated *Mycobacterium avium-intracellulare* infection in homosexual men with acquired cell-mediated immunodeficiency: A histologic and immunologic study of two cases, *Am. J. Clin. Pathol.* **79:**247–252 (1983).

70. SWENSON, J. M., WALLACE, R. J., SILCOX, V. A., AND THORNSBERRY, C., Antimicrobial susceptibility of five subgroups of *Mycobacterium fortuitum* and *Mycobacterium chelonae, Antimicrob. Agents Chemother.* **28:**807–811 (1985).

71. THOMPSON, N. J., GLASSROTH, J. L., SNIDER, D. E., JR., AND FARER, L. S., The booster phenomenon in serial tuberculin testing, *Am. Rev. Respir. Dis.* **119:**587 (1979).

72. TIMPE, A., AND RUNYON, E. H., The relationship of

"atypical" acid-fast bacteria to human disease: A preliminary report, *J. Lab. Clin. Med.* **44:**202 (1954).

73. TISDALL, P. A., ROBERTS, G. D., AND ANHALT, J. P., Identification of clinical isolates of mycobacteria with gas–liquid chromatography alone, *J. Clin. Microbiol.* **10:**506–514 (1979).

74. TOWNSEND, E. W., GEIGER, F. L., GREGG, D. B., AND FICKLING, A. M., An analysis of "atypical" mycobacteria as reported by the South Carolina State Board of Health Laboratory, *J. S.C. Med. Assoc.* **61:**267 (1965).

75. WALLACE, R. J., JR., SWENSON, J. M., SILCOX, V. A., GOOD, R. C., TSCHEN, J. A., AND STONE, M. S., Spectrum of disease due to rapidly growing mycobacteria, *Rev. Infect. Dis.* **5:**657–679 (1983).

76. WICKMAN, K., Clinical significance of nontuberculous mycobacteria. A bacteriological survey of Swedish strains isolated between 1973 and 1981, *Scand. J. Infect. Dis.* **18:**337–345 (1986).

77. WIJSMULLER, G., AND ERICKSON, P., The reaction to PPD-Battey: A new look, *Am. Rev. Respir. Dis.* **109:**29 (1974).

78. WIJSMULLER, G., RAJ NARAIN, MAYURNATH, S., AND PALMER, C. E., On the nature of tuberculin sensitivity in south India, *Am. Rev. Respir. Dis.* **97:**429 (1968).

79. WOLINSKY, E., Nontuberculous mycobacteria and associated diseases, *Am. Rev. Respir. Dis.* **119:**107 (1979).

80. WOLINSKY, E., When is an infection disease? *Rev. Infect. Dis.* **3:**1025–1027 (1981).

81. YANAGIHARA, D. L., BARR, V. L., KNISLEY, C. V., TSANG, A. Y., MCCLATCHY, J. K., AND BRENNAN, P. J., Enzyme-linked immunosorbent assay of glycolipid antigens for identification of mycobacteria, *J. Clin. Microbiol.* **21:**569–574 (1985).

82. ZAKOWSKI, P., FLIGIEL, S., BERLIN, O. G. W., AND JOHNSON, B. L., Disseminated *Mycobacterium avium-intracellulare* infection in homosexual men dying of acquired immunodeficiency, *J. Am. Med. Assoc.* **248:**2980–2982 (1982).

12. Suggested Reading

CHAPMAN, J. S., The ecology of the atypical mycobacteria, *Arch. Environ. Health* **22:**41 (1971).

EDWARDS, P. Q., AND EDWARDS, L. B., Story of the tuberculin test from an epidemiologic viewpoint, *Am. Rev. Respir. Dis.* **81**(1):Part 2 (1960).

LINCOLN, E. M., AND GILBERT, L. A., Disease in children due to mycobacteria other than *Mycobacterium tuberculosis, Am. Rev. Respir. Dis.* **105:**683 (1972).

WOLINSKY, E., Nontuberculous mycobacteria and associated diseases, *Am. Rev. Respir. Dis.* **119:**107 (1979).

CHAPTER 38

Tularemia

Richard B. Hornick

1. Introduction

Tularemia is a rare infectious disease caused by a small pleomorphic, gram-negative rod, *Francisella tularensis*. Patients who acquire the disease have symptoms and signs that relate to the portals of entry of the bacteria: oculoglandular, ulceroglandular, pneumonic, and typhoidal. This infectious disease has been thoroughly studied through induced infections in volunteers; hence, a considerable body of data has been accumulated in a quantitative fashion about the pathogenicity of tularemia bacilli in humans. Man appears to be one of the most susceptible mammalian hosts studied: fewer than 50 organisms can cause disease whether administered intradermally or by the respiratory route.[45] The usual sources of infections are animals, especially cottontail rabbits, voles, and muskrats. Humans acquire the disease by direct contact or by bites of the ticks, mosquitoes, deerflies, and other insects that infest such animals. An effective vaccine, unique for bacterial infections because it consists of a live attenuated strain, has been developed.[10]

2. Historical Background

Tularemia is one of the first human infectious diseases named by and carefully studied by United States scientists. The disease is named after Tulare County, California, where the organism was isolated. Following the great San Francisco earthquake and fire in 1910, Dr. George W. McCoy[27] of the U.S. Public Health Service was sent to the area to investigate a possible outbreak of bubonic plague. His studies uncovered a "plaguelike" disease among ground squirrels in Tulare County. The disease was characterized by pathological lesions similar to those of plague, but caused by a small pleomorphic, gram-negative rod he was able to isolate from the infected animals. He named it *Bacterium tularense*. The organism was later classified with *Pasteurella,* as *P. tularensis,* but subsequent differences in growth characteristics and DNA homology studies dictated the removal from that genus, and it is now called *Francisella tularensis* to honor Dr. Edward Francis, who described much of the early bacteriological and immunological information about tularemia. The initial reasons for distinguishing this newly found bacterium from plague were the apparent absence of organisms in stained smears of infected organs of guinea pigs and failure to isolate *P. pestis* on plain agar and in bouillon inoculated with infected tissues. The failure to stain organisms in infected tissues was a characteristic that persisted until fluorescent-antibody conjugate staining was developed in the 1950s.[41] In 1912, McCoy and Chapin[28] isolated the organism on coagulated egg-yolk media. The first human cases proven by isolation of the organism were reported in 1914 by Vail[52] from a patient with oculoglandular disease and also in 1914 by Wherry,[54] who additionally described transmission of the bacterium from rodent to man. The name *tularemia* was coined by Dr. Francis, who studied the plaguelike disease both in rodents in Tulare County and in patients with deerfly fever in Utah in 1919 and 1920. He concluded that since both diseases were manifestations of the same bacterium and were frequently bacteremic, the name should reflect these facts, i.e., tularemia.[14–16] He also implicated the deerfly, ticks, and other ectoparasites of animals in the transmission of disease.

Richard B. Hornick · Medical Education Administration, Orlando Regional Medical Center, Orlando, Florida 32806.

It is now recognized that the disease had been identified in Japan[33] and Norway[19] in the 19th century. In Japan, Soken had written a perfect description of glandular tularemia in 1818 and attributed the disease to "ingestion of poisonous hare meat."[33]

A disease of ill lemmings was studied in 1890 by Horne[19] in Norway, who isolated a bacterium from these animals. This was probably the first isolation of *F. tularensis,* but Horne has not been credited for this discovery in the literature.

In 1924, the first scientific article on tularemia was published in Japan describing a mild systemic febrile disease acquired from skinning a dead rabbit.[33] Ohara, who described this disease, also conducted the first volunteer study with tularemia when he rubbed heart blood from a dead rabbit onto the skin of his wife, who shortly thereafter developed self-limiting ulceroglandular disease. Dr. Francis recognized this description of the infection to be the same as tularemia, and he called the Japanese disease Ohara's disease, while Dr. Ohara named it yato-byo (wild hare disease).

Subsequent studies have demonstrated infection in over 100 species of wild and domestic animals as well as in ticks and deerflies. Furthermore, because of the highly contagious characteristics of this organism, man was frequently infected through laboratory-acquired infections. Epizootics among experimental animals also occurred.[36] It is obvious from these statements that this organism must be carefully handled when it is brought into a laboratory. Despite its reputation as a highly infectious agent, no person-to-person transmission has been reported. Reasons for this are unclear.

3. Methodology

Tularemia was made a disease reportable to the Public Health Service in 1927. Cases and deaths are regularly recorded in the United States in the *Morbidity and Mortality Weekly Report* of the Centers for Disease Control (CDC). Worldwide, the *Weekly Epidemiological Record* and the *Annual Statistical Report* of the World Health Organization (WHO) summarize the reported cases.

3.1. Sources of Mortality Data

The mortality rates for tularemia are based on small series of cases from around the world and are clouded by

antibiotic treatment and failure to discriminate which of the strains of tularemia is etiologically implicated. Two strains of tularemia differing in virulence have been characterized.[24] These strains will be referred to in this chapter as Jellison type A and type B. Type A is more virulent than type B.

The mortality rate from type B infections has not been clearly differentiated from that from type A infections because the proportion of cases caused by each strain in this country has not been ascertained. Some workers postulate that there are more cases caused by type B in this country, but that because of their mild nature they do not reach the reporting network or if seen by a physician may be misdiagnosed. Death caused by this strain is probably a very unusual event, unless the patient develops pneumonia. On the other hand, the more virulent form of disease caused by type A will usually be reported because the patient is more likely to seek medical help. Furthermore, since these strains are carried by the almost ubiquitous cottontail rabbit, there would appear to be greater opportunities for more people to come in contact with the organism from this source than from waterborne rodent-associated sources (type B), i.e., muskrats, voles, and the like. For these reasons, type A disease will appear to be the more common type of infection. Ulceroglandular disease caused by either strain should not be associated with any mortality in a normal human host, especially if appropriate antibiotic therapy is administered. In the preantibiotic era, the mortality rate was around 5% for this form of disease, but whether this rate was due to infections caused only by type A strains is not clear. It would appear that the mortality rates in European and Asian countries (type B strains) were low and that death was a rare occurrence. In the preantibiotic era, the mortality rate in patients with pleuropneumonic disease was 30–60%. The mortality rate for patients with tularemic pneumonia treated with streptomycin appears to be less than 1%. In a series of 29 cases collected over a 20-year period (1949–1969) in Arkansas, no deaths occurred in the 28 patients receiving streptomycin.[30] No deaths were reported in 20 of 34 persons who developed laboratory-acquired tularemic pneumonitis and were treated with broad-spectrum antibiotics.[35] In an early study in 1946, 12 patients with tularemic pneumonia were treated with streptomycin.[22] One died on day 7 after apparent recovery. The cause of death was thought to be a massive pulmonary embolus. These three series provide strong evidence that although tularemic pneumonia can be a life-threatening disease, early and appropriate antibiotic therapy can control the infectious process so that death from infection should not occur.

3.2. Sources of Morbidity Data

All diagnosed cases of tularemia in the United States must be reported to state health departments and from them to the CDC. It is likely that many undiagnosed cases occur because of the self-limiting nature of the tularemic infection, especially cases caused by type B strains. The difficulty (and risk) in isolating the causative organism—it requires a selective medium not routinely employed in microbiology laboratories (see Section 3.4.1)—and the spontaneous recovery of many cases of ulceroglandular tularemia compound the diagnostic difficulties. Many individual cases will not be diagnosed. Surveys are done only when a miniepidemic or an epizootic has been identified.[26] Otherwise, only the single diagnosed cases are reported, and the true incidence of the disease is unknown. Because of the seemingly huge reservoir of infection in animals, the potential for continued outbreaks in man is great.

3.3. Surveys

In addition to clinical histories, surveys have been made using various serological and skin tests. However, such surveys have been done largely when epidemics have occurred.[6] Because of the varied methods of transmission and potential sources of infection, surveys need to be generalized to include occupational and recreational activities in order to determine a common source and pattern of spread. Human-to-human transmission has not been shown, so appropriate histories will suggest populations to be surveyed who have had similar occupational or recreational exposures. Familial outbreaks occur from common sources, not by direct contact.

3.4. Laboratory Diagnosis

3.4.1. Isolation and Identification of the Organism. *F. tularensis* can be isolated from pus taken from ulcers or aspirated from a bubo, sputum, pharyngeal washes, or gastric aspirations from a patient with pneumonitis or typhoidal disease. Blood cultures are rarely positive but the readily available radiometric methods of detecting bacterial growth could change this concept. These blood culture techniques may be more sensitive than other methods in detecting the presence of tularemia bacilli. Indeed, some seriously ill patients with infections of unknown etiology have been fortuitously diagnosed in this manner.[25] The clinical specimens should be inoculated intraperitoneally into guinea pigs if the necessary animal-isolation facilities are available. The presence of one to five viable cells of *F. tularensis* will cause death within 5–10 days. The pathology in the spleen in these animals is pathognomonic of tularemia. Direct isolation of the organism can be undertaken in a laboratory with an effective hood or an adequate isolation lab that will prevent accidental aerogenic spread. The acceptable media used to grow the organisms are: glucose cysteine blood agar, cystine heart agar (Difco), eugon agar, and glucose cysteine agar (BBL). Potential contaminants in clinical specimens can be suppressed by the addition of 0.1 mg cycloheximide and 20 U penicillin/ml basal menstruum. Tularemia bacilli are small (0.2–0.7 μm), as are the colonies that appear on solid media after 48–72 h of incubation at 37 °C. Staining of infected tissues with the usual stains will not demonstrate this bacterium. Either fluorescent staining or a modified Dieterle stain must be used.[18]

3.4.2. Serological and Skin Tests. The skin test is a reliable method of detecting past infections.[6] Both skin tests and serological tests are useful for diagnostic and epidemiological investigations. The skin test is now performed with an antigen derived by ether extraction of *F. tularensis*. This material is prepared by the Rocky Mountain Laboratory, National Institute of Allergy and Infectious Diseases. A 0.1-ml dose of the antigen is injected intradermally into the volar surface of the forearm. A 48-h reading is performed and should be positive in most infected individuals at that time, rarely at 72 h. Induration of 5-mm diameter indicates a positive test. It appears to be the most reliable skin-test antigen, with excellent reproducibility; unfortunately, it is not readily available. Earlier preparations, i.e., Foshay antigen, a phenolized solution of killed bacteria diluted 1 : 1000, also gave good results, but were more reactive. The advantages of the skin test are that it is positive earlier than the agglutination test and also appears to be more sensitive in persons infected more than 2 years previously. The antibody titers may be undetectable or at low levels several years after infection, but the skin test remains positive. There are no known antigens cross-reactive with the skin-test antigens. The larger the infected dose of organisms, the more rapid the skin test converts; e.g., doses of vaccine organisms (attenuated or live attenuated vaccine strains) in the range of 5000–500,000 organisms produced conversions in 37% of recipients at 10 days and 75% conversion at 30 days.[17] Twenty million organisms produced conversions in 80% after 5 days.

The skin test is reproducible, i.e., persistently negative, in nonimmune individuals. A small number of immune persons may lack skin-test reproducibility—4% had intermittently positive tests; reasons for this are unknown, but in the case of the vaccinated person, this could represent a failure of the vaccine to colonize.[6]

There is no stimulation of agglutinins in persons who had negative antibody titers prior to skin testing. Persons with positive titers may demonstrate a boost in titer. Buchanan *et al.*[6] tested serum specimens from 33 persons who had had tularemia or had received vaccine. The paired serum specimens were tested on the same day; 3 (9.1%) demonstrated a fourfold or greater rise in titer.[6]

Various antibodies to the tularemia organisms can be tested, but the primary serological test has been the measurement of agglutinating antibodies. This has been the standard test because it is reliable and reproducible; a titer of 1 : 160 or greater is strong evidence of recent infection, but the fourfold rise in titer of paired specimens is the definitive serological confirmation of infection or disease or both. The titer will often begin to rise in the 2nd week of illness and peak during the 3rd and 4th weeks. Antibiotic therapy does not appear to modify the antibody response. Antibody titers may remain elevated for 6–8 months before declining to low or undetectable levels by 18–24 months. The antigen used in the agglutination test is a suspension of formalin-killed bacteria.[42] The serum—bacteria mixture is incubated overnight at 37 °C in a water bath before being read. The titers are recorded as the highest serum dilution showing a 2^+ agglutination. A microagglutination test has been developed to facilitate the test and uses less serum and reagents. The IgM antibodies appear to be highly effective in promoting the agglutination process.[8] As the IgG antibodies appear in the serum and replace IgM, there is a general fall in agglutinating titer. The agglutination test is known to cross-react with *Brucella* and *Proteus* OX-19 antigens.[43] Recent studies have suggested cross-reactivity with mycoplasma and legionella antigens. These cross-reacting antibodies occur in the first few weeks after exposure of the host to tularemia antigen. The studies of Saslaw and Carlisle[43] clarified the dynamics of the cross-reacting *Brucella* antibodies. Of volunteers receiving live vaccine or exposed to low doses of viable organisms, 25% developed *Brucella* agglutinins. The titer was not as high as the homologous tularemia titer. The *Brucella* antibodies frequently fell to undetectable levels after 6 months, and there was no rebound phenomenon when a viable challenge was administered to vaccinated volunteers. At the time of this study, measurements of IgM and IgG antibodies were not done. From subsequent data, it would appear that the cross-reacting antibodies may be primarily IgM and could be expected to be less specific in their antigen binding than the later-appearing, more specific IgG antibodies. This cross-reactivity may be confusing when a differentiation of etiological causes of a febrile illness is being considered and the serological data provide the discriminating diagnostic evidence.

Other antibody tests have been used to detect tularemia infection, but have not supplanted the agglutinin test. The hemagglutination test utilizing tularemia polysaccharide as the antigen attached to erythrocytes is more sensitive than the agglutination test in that the titers appear slightly earlier, i.e., 1 week, attain a higher titer, and appear to persist as long as the agglutinin titers.[42] There does not appear to be any cross-reactivity with *Brucella* antigens in this test system.[1]

Complement-fixation antibody tests usually respond later than the agglutination or hemagglutination test. The titers fail to reach the same dilution as do these two antibody tests, and there is also a more rapid decline in titers.

Specialized tests developed to study the pathogenesis of tularemia could possibly be adapted for rapid serological diagnosis. One sophisticated but promising test measures opsonizing antibodies by a radiometabolic assay.[8] The sensitive system detects opsonizing antibodies in monkey serum 3 days after immunization with live vaccine and obviously much earlier than agglutinating or hemagglutinating antibodies are detected. In human sera, similar antibodies could be found 1 month to 13 years after immunization, whereas nondiagnostic agglutinating antibody titers were present in these same specimens.

4. Biological Characteristics of the Organism

There are two strains of tularemia. Jellison type A is lethal for domestic rabbits (*Oryctolagus*), can ferment glycerol, and contains citrulline ureidase. This strain has been found only in North America, especially in cottontail rabbits. One suggestion has been to term this the "nearctic" strain.[3] Strain B is less virulent for the rabbit, lacks the biochemical characteristics listed for type A, and is found in Europe, Asia, and North America. Usually, it has been associated with rodents and waterborne disease. "Palearctic" has been suggested for this strain. However, this term is too restrictive, since there have been no differences shown between the type B strains isolated in Europe and Asia and the fresh isolates in North America.[3] Thus, the classification of Jellison type A and type B seems most appropriate at present.

F. tularensis can persist in at least 100 animal species without causing death of the host, e.g., pigs.[5] It is highly virulent (type A) for cottontail rabbits and has caused epizootics in nature in these animals. Indeed, this species is a common source of infection for man.

What offensive weapons these bacteria have to establish infection and disease with so few organisms is unknown. Within the host, they establish an intracellular habitat that may protect them from host defenses. They contain an endotoxin that has properties similar to those of the endotoxins of other gram-negative rods, e.g., pyrogenicity. They withstand freezing in nature so as to maintain their infectivity. However, there is a dichotomy between their infectivity and their viability when aerosolized: the ability to infect man or monkey declines as the aerosol ages, even though viability (ability to produce a colony on solid media) persists. A tenfold decrease in infectivity occurs after 3 h.[46] Reasons for this disassociation are unknown. The particle size in the aerosol is of great importance; the smaller the particle, the more likely it is that disease will result. Large particles containing many organisms may cause glandular enlargement of cervical nodes and fever because the initial site of entry presumably is the oral pharyngeal area and not the lower respiratory tract. Large particles are also swallowed, and unless there is a huge concentration of organisms, no enteric, typhoidal-type disease will develop.[21]

The biological characteristics of *F. tularensis* that are associated with the lack of person-to-person transmission are unknown. A simple experiment designed to optimally challenge the concept of no human-to-human transmission was conducted. Organisms collected from pharyngeal washes of volunteers immediately after inhalation of large quantities of virulent tularemia bacilli were shown to be viable, since they grew readily in large numbers on supportive media. Aliquots of these pharyngeal specimens containing organisms, when reaerosolized, failed to infect susceptible volunteers. The organisms in the washings had aged for about 2–3 h prior to instillation, and the particle size was variable (mostly > 5 μm). This experiment attempted to duplicate what might happen in nature when an infected patient creates an aerosol by sneezing or coughing. Similarly, large numbers of organisms could be grown from cough plates obtained from patients with pneumonia, but no disease in hospital personnel has been reported following this method of aerosolization of *F. tularensis*. Reasons for this failure of expelled bacteria to transmit tularemia to other susceptible humans may be related to particle size, but other unknown factors must also be involved. This lack of person-to-person transmission indicates that the disease dead-ends in the human host, preventing additional cases.

The biological properties responsible for the variation in virulence of the two strains of tularemia are also un-

known. Neither of these strains can penetrate through gloves, which should be worn when handling rabbits or other suspected hosts.

It must be clearly understood that a high risk of acquiring the disease exists when a clinical specimen is brought into a diagnostic laboratory. The laboratory personnel must be aware of the possible diagnosis of tularemia so that they are alerted to work with the specimens in efficient, protective hoods. The inoculation of animals is dangerous because of the risk not only of human disease but also of starting an epizootic among other animals. The spread from cage to cage occurs by exchange of ectoparasites and presumably aerosolization and from animal to animal by cannibalization.[36]

5. Descriptive Epidemiology

5.1. Prevalence and Incidence

In the United States, the number of reported cases peaked at 2291 in 1939 for a rate of 1.85 cases/100,000 population. Since that year, there has been a steady decline in reported cases, although isolated epidemics have occurred. The annual average number of cases for the years 1965–1969 were 164; 1970–1974, 165 cases; 1975–1979, 157 cases; 1980–1984, 227 cases; and 1985–1987, 187 cases. Reasons for the increase in the early 1980s are unknown. Figure 1 depicts the incidence curve in the United States since 1955.

Serological and skin-test surveys in various countries have provided evidence of the prevalence of infection. In Alaska, Philip *et al.*[38] in 1962 found that in some parts of that state, as many as 62% of native men had positive skin tests, and serological tests corroborated the specificity of the skin-test reactions. The lack of clinical cases in this population suggested that avirulent strains of tularemia may have been involved. Subsequent evaluations of strains of *F. tularensis* isolated from ticks of ptarmigan and snowshoe hares revealed the former to be relatively avirulent (Jellison type B), while the hare strain was virulent (type A).[3] Which strain is involved predominantly in the animal populations of Alaska is unknown. Nonetheless, it is conceivable that many undiagnosed human cases of tularemia occur in that state and are not reported.

5.2. Epidemic Behavior and Contagiousness

Some epidemics are directly related to epizootics in wild animals. However, the sporadic nature of human epi-

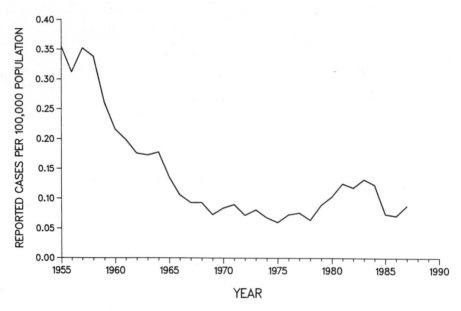

Figure 1. Tularemia—by year, United States, 1955–1987.

demics and the few known epizootics without spread to humans indicate that wild animals remain a potential infectious source, but only rarely has man entered the epizootic cycle. An example of this occurred in Vermont in 1967–1969 when an epidemic of tularemia involved trappers and "skinners" exposed to muskrats.[57] No tularemia had been reported from this state previously. It was shown in this study that infection was produced by the relatively avirulent strain of tularemia (Jellison type B). This organism is usually associated with waterborne disease of rodents. Indeed, the organism was isolated from samples of water, mud, and from muskrats. Despite the relatively benign nature of the clinical illnesses, there were 4 clinical cases to each inapparent infection. These cases were diagnosed by serological techniques. In the second phase of the study, skin testing was also performed, and an additional 4 cases of the 1968 epidemic were uncovered.[6] Furthermore, 16 cases originating in 1969 and 7 cases that could have had their onset in either 1968 or 1969 were discovered. The conclusion reached by this study was that the skin test provides the epidemiologist with the most sensitive tool for charting the incidence of tularemia over the past 40 years. It may also save the clinician valuable time in diagnosing tularemia because it becomes positive within the 1st or 2nd week of illness, while the agglutination titer may be negative in that period.

This epidemic in Vermont[57] is a good example of the

exceptional and fortuitous epidemiological circumstances that coincide with man's association with the epizootic. The muskrats were plentiful and may have been ill, since they were easy to trap, and there was evidence of cannibalism and fighting because many pelts were marred by rips or tears. This epizootic occurred during a very limited time when man could be exposed, the trapping and shooting season. Other epidemics in this country involved exposure to infected deerflies and ticks. In Utah, 30 laborers developed ulceroglandular disease acquired when they were working without shirts. They were bitten by deerflies, which apparently transmitted the disease from infected hares.[7] The illness was mild, probably caused by type B strain. In 1946, 50 men on military maneuvers in Tennessee were bitten by ticks and developed ulceroglandular disease; the reservoir in this epidemic was not uncovered.[53]

A unique miniepidemic occurred in 1978 in 7 persons staying in a cottage on Martha's Vineyard.[51] Of the 7, 5 developed pneumonia and 2 had typhoidal tularemia. An additional 8 cases, found on serosurveys and by reports from physicians of other states, had also been on the island during the same summer period as the initial 7 cases. The route of infection in many of the patients was presumed to be by aerosols. The source is uncertain, although several isolates were made from dead cottontail rabbits found on the island. It is suspected that other cases could have occurred but were not diagnosed. These 15 cases represented 11% of the 141 cases reported in the United States in 1978. Four sporadic cases were year-round residents of Martha's Vineyard, representing an annual attack rate of 0.66 case/100,000 inhabitants.

In Sweden, where tularemia was first diagnosed in 1931, five outbreaks subsequently occurred in 1937, 1953, 1960, 1962, and 1966–1967.[9] Most cases were rodent-associated. The last was an extensive outbreak involving 676 cases, of whom 444 were located in one county, Jämtland.[9] Voles were noted to have multiplied in the northern area of Sweden. These animals invaded the stored hay supplies of the farms in this area. The farmers who used this hay in the winter first had to shake out the spoiled hay, which included dead voles and heavy contamination with vole feces. Presumably, most farmers inhaled infected aerosols, since there was a larger number of patients with pneumonia than with ulceroglandular disease. Serological surveys revealed many subclinical cases—32% of the surveyed population in one area and another 16% in another area. Other farmers handled the voles directly and were more likely to develop ulceroglandular disease. Infected hares also caused 23 cases of tularemia, the majority of whom had ulceroglandular disease.

Voles and other rodents have apparently been responsible for contaminating sugar beets. When the beets are washed in the sugar factory, the tularemia organisms are aerosolized as small droplets and infect the factory workers.[40] Several outbreaks occurred in Austria and the Soviet Union. Some geographic areas of the Soviet Union appear to have been heavily contaminated, especially during World War II. For example, Rostov had 14,000 cases in January 1942.[47] Many of these patients had angioglandular disease secondary to the consumption of contaminated water (due to type B organisms).

In all the epidemics and outbreaks discussed, no mention of human-to-human transmission was made. This is an unexpected finding, since tularemia is highly infectious when man comes in contact with even small numbers of organisms derived from animals or vectors.

5.3. Geographic Distribution

Most areas of the world north of the 30th parallel have been identified as having tularemia. This includes the northern United States and Alaska,[38] Japan,[33] Norway,[19] Sweden,[9] Austria, and the Soviet Union.[47] The distribution depends on the range of the reservoir animals. Figure 2 depicts the reported cases by county in the United States in 1987. In North America, the main reservoirs are rabbits and, second, rodents. The cottontail rabbits (*Sylvilagus*)

range throughout the United States, with the U.S.–Canadian border being the northern limit.[23] There are only a few cottontails in Maine. These animals are very susceptible to tularemia and die within a week when infected. Their presence is highly pertinent to the epidemiology of tularemia in North America. In all states where tularemia has been endemic, the cottontail has been the only or the predominant rabbit species in that state. The cottontail ranges southward into Mexico and Central and South America. Tularemia has not been reported from Mexico, and reports of tularemia from others of these countries have been minimal.

The snowshoe rabbit (*Lepus americanus*) has been found infected in nature, but it is not an important source of human infections,[23] since it is relatively resistant to tularemia infection. On the other hand, jackrabbits (*Lepus* spp.), which occupy most of the area west of the Mississippi and extend into Canada and Mexico,[23] have been the source for many cases in the United States because they not only transmit disease directly to man when being skinned or eviscerated but also serve as important hosts for ticks and deerflies. These two ectoparasites are significant carriers of *F. tularensis* to man. Jackrabbits are not hunted as extensively as cottontails and in general inhabit areas with sparse human populations compared to regions where cottontails thrive.

The geographic distribution throughout the rest of the world is probably related to the rodent population as distinct from rabbits. These species are infected with the type B strain of tularemia. The number of reported cases is quite small compared to the number reported in the United States. For example, in 1976, there were 157 cases reported in the United States and 61 in Czechoslovakia, but no other European country reported more than 6 cases, and none were reported in Australia or Japan.[56]

The transmission of tularemia by ticks and deerflies helps to explain how at least 100 other species of animals can become infected. These animals have varying degrees of resistance to disease. Hunting dogs that frequently retrieve sick or dying rabbits may become infected; they demonstrate a serological response, but they do not die. Other carnivores may also eat infected rabbits and develop a nonfatal infection. Man may become infected from these sources, such as the bite or scratch of an animal (dog, cat,[18] skunk, coyote, fox, bull snake, wild hog) that has contaminated saliva or teeth from recently eating a diseased rabbit. Animals resistant to disease caused by *F. tularensis* may be temporary carriers with bacteremia and serve as a source of contamination for ticks and deerflies. The following species of ticks have been associated with the transmission of this organism: *Dermacentor andersoni* (Rocky

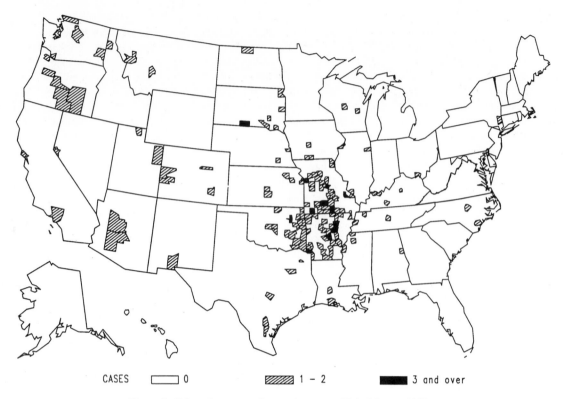

Figure 2. Tularemia—reported cases, by county, United States, 1987.

Mountain wood tick), *D. variabilis* (American dog tick), *D. occidentalis* (Pacific coast dog tick), and *D. americanum* (lonestar tick).

5.4. Temporal Distribution

The peak incidence of tularemia in the United States depends on the source of the infection. In the summer months, when ticks and deerflies are abundant, especially west of the Mississippi, the risk of acquiring tularemia is greatest. During the fall hunting season in the eastern United States, cases of tularemia contracted from captured game, especially cottontail rabbits, sporadically occur. The types of clinical presentations in the miniepidemic in late summer of 1978 on Martha's Vineyard suggest that tick bites or aerosols or both were responsible for the observed cases, but only 1 of the 15 had a history of a tick bite.[51] Ticks have been responsible for over half the cases reported in reviews of cases occurring in endemic states. Some tick bites may go unnoticed, and if this is the portal of entry of the tularemia organisms, an ulcer does not necessarily de-

velop or the lesion may be so small as to be ignored. Because of the importance of tick bites in the spread of tularemia, many cases occur in the spring and summer months.

5.5. Age

Susceptibility to tularemia does not vary with age. In most epidemics, the age of the patients reflects their exposure. Trappers in the Vermont epidemic ranged in age from 11 to 82.[56] There is no evidence to suggest that persons at the extremes of age are more susceptible or that they respond less quickly to antibiotic therapy than do young adults.

5.6. Sex

Both sexes develop tularemia after equal exposure. The incidence of the disease was higher in men than women in many epidemics because men were associated with trapping animals or heavy farming jobs. In sporadic cases, either sex may be involved. It has been suggested that women may have been at greater risk in some epidemics caused by ticks and deerflies because their clothing exposed axillary and inguinal areas to bites by these arthropods. However, since both sexes now commonly wear slacks and long-sleeved garments outdoors, they probably have equal opportunities, but fewer opportunities than before, to have their skin attacked by biting or bloodsucking insects.

5.7. Race

Stuart and Pullen[48] reported a higher incidence of pneumonia and a much higher mortality rate among black patients with tularemia than among white patients with tularemia studied in the same hospital. This racial susceptibility to more virulent illness did not appear in the many hundreds of volunteers challenged by various routes with *F. tularensis*.[20,44,45] The validity of the observations in Stuart and Pullen's study has not been confirmed. The question of equal opportunity for prompt medical attention for the patients in their study was not addressed.

5.8. Occupation

Occupation is a crucial epidemiological factor in the acquisition of tularemia. Hunters, trappers, farmers, laboratory workers, forest rangers, game wardens, hikers, campers, and others exposed to aerosolized or direct skin contact with the bacilli or to ticks, deerflies, and wild animals are at greatest risk to infection. Chapin and an assistant, unaware of the infectious threat of the organism they were the first to isolate, were the first to develop laboratory-acquired disease.[3] In one other laboratory accident, petri dishes containing the organism were dropped, resulting in tularemia in five persons.[2] The workup of any patient with suspected ulceroglandular or typhoidal tularemia should include a comprehensive and detailed history of possible occupational and recreational exposures to sources of *F. tularensis*.

5.9. Occurrence in Different Settings

A variety of settings may be involved in outbreaks of tularemia, each of which must include exposure to arthropods or wild animals. While some urban settings may appear less likely than rural or suburban areas for exposure to the organism, the reservoirs of this infection do not necessarily follow this geographic distribution. Cottontail rabbits have become well adapted to city life and range widely through urban neighborhoods. Three cases of tularemic

pneumonia were reported in Washington, D.C., in 1978 without any source being uncovered. Thus, while the usual setting for tularemia is in the rural areas, suburban and urban areas may also be involved.

As noted in Section 5.2, factory workers washing contaminated sugar beets (voles) developed tularemia[40] in an unusual epidemic that illustrates the viability and virulence of tularemia bacteria.

5.10. Socioeconomic Factors

The best evidence relates to the marked increase in tularemia during World War II, especially in Russia.[47] This increase was thought to be due to the breakdown of public-health and sanitation measures. Some of the cases reported in children implied that they were living in substandard rural housing with several dogs and cats living in the same house. Several sources of exposure can be anticipated under these circumstances, such as ticks, deerflies, dead or sick animals brought home by the dogs and cats, and the drinking of contaminated water. Lack of knowledge about the risk of handling diseased rodents and rabbits will lead to greater risk of tularemia.

6. Mechanisms and Routes of Transmission

Tularemia is a sporadic disease that humans acquire when they are bitten by an infected tick or deerfly or when they handle an infected animal. In the process of field-dressing a rabbit or skinning a muskrat, the hands may become contaminated because of infected blood or subcutaneous abscesses or from the liver and spleen, which contain millions of organisms. This act of eviscerating the animal can also create an aerosol, and humans become infected by the respiratory route. Rarely is ingestion of contaminated water or food a source of human infection. Increased awareness of the risk of handling sick or dying wild animals, especially rabbits, and the prohibition of selling wild rabbits in meat markets have been largely responsible for the decline in incidence of this disease. The main mechanisms of transmission are through contact of the organism with the skin, eye, oropharynx, or respiratory tract. Tularemia bacilli establish contact with these surfaces by direct contamination of hands, as when an infected animal is being skinned or eviscerated. As few as 50 bacteria can cause ulceroglandular disease in volunteers.[45] The bacterium is purported to be able to penetrate unbroken skin, but whether this is true has not been tested. There are numerous anatomical openings, e.g., hair follicles, through which the organism can gain entrance to the dermis. Minute defects in the epidermis, especially of the hands, due to trivial trauma are common. Entrance into the dermis and lymphatics through such openings could, in retrospect, be conceived as penetration through intact skin. The nail fold is an apparent portal of entry; the mantle area commonly has small tears in the region adjacent to the nail. Presumably, this is a common access route, since ulcers occur frequently in this area. The tick deposits the organisms on the skin adjacent to its bite wound, and rubbing this area could lead to contamination of that wound. Patients have been described in whom rubbing of an eye following apparent contamination of the fingers has led to oculoglandular manifestations of tularemia. Swallowing a large inoculum of tularemia usually results in angioglandular tularemia with few or no signs of gastrointestinal disease.[21] The respiratory tract is readily infected by small-particle aerosols containing as few as 10–50 bacteria.[45] Aerosols are created as an animal is skinned or eviscerated, since there are many organisms in liver (> 10^7/g tissue) and spleen and the usual rough extraction of these organs during field-dressing could easily cause aerosolization of an infectious dose of *F. tularensis* as well as contaminate the uncovered skin. Bites and scratches of animals have caused tularemia microorganisms to be inoculated directly into the skin.

7. Pathogenesis and Immunity

7.1. Pathogenesis

The incubation period of tularemia varies inversely with the dose of organisms received by the host. Ulceroglandular disease has an incubation of about 2–6 days.[44] In volunteers, injection of a large inoculum, i.e., 2500 minimal infectious doses, into the superficial layers of the skin results in 48 h in a macular erythematous lesion not unlike a positive tuberculin test.[20] This lesion becomes papular and pruritic and slowly enlarges. As it increases in size, the overlying skin becomes taut, thin, and shiny, and rarely is the papule fluctuant. At about 96 h, ulceration occurs; the resulting lesion is depressed with sharply demarcated edges. The base is frequently black and dry. Fever occurs as the papule is forming. In untreated patients infected with type A organisms, the draining lymph nodes enlarge and become caseous, i.e., buboes. These lesions rarely drain spontaneously. A similar sequence of events occurs with type B infections, but there is less systemic

reaction. If untreated, the lesion and lymph nodes may persist for months before completely resolving. After inoculation, an immune individual will not develop an ulcer, but rather will demonstrate a small indurated papule similar to a positive tularemia skin test. This is the histopathological process initiated by both live and inactivated antigens. Biopsy of skin lesions induced by killed *F. tularensis* or by live attenuated vaccine (LVS) strains reveals mononuclear perivascular infiltrates. In monkeys, studies have carefully quantitated the local and systemic bacteriological events and correlated these events to histological and immunological findings.[11] The LVS multiplied in the skin of monkeys, reaching at 3 days peak numbers that persisted for 10 days. By day 14, the count began to taper. Isolations from regional lymph nodes were made only on day 28. All tissues cultured were free of the strain by day 90. Similar but more extensive findings would be expected with the virulent strains. It is not known how long the organisms remain viable in human skin, but it is probably only for a relatively short time after antibiotic therapy is started. Residual antigen persists at the site of initial skin penetrance, as deduced from volunteer studies. The initial site flared as a positive skin test when viable organisms were inoculated into another area of skin, i.e., the opposite arm. As noted, the new site may also simulate a positive skin test. In the monkey studies, antitularensis γ-globulin appeared in plasma-cell precursors in regional lymph nodes by day 3, in the spleen on day 5, and at the site of dermal inoculation on day 14.[29] The antibody γ-globulin persisted in the spleen and regional nodes through the 90th day. In addition to this evidence of antitularensis γ-globulin appearing in the infected animals, other models, especially mouse and rat, have been employed to demonstrate development of cellular immunity. It is known that man develops delayed-type hypersensitivity during the first week of disease.[6]

Aerogenic infection accounts for primary pneumonic tularemia, the most serious form of disease. Pneumonia is probably initiated by terminal bronchial and/or alveolar localization of the inhaled small particles (< 5-μm diameter) containing *F. tularensis*.[11,55] The inflammatory reaction is acute and progressive in the animals infected with the virulent strain of tularemia. This results in necrosis of alveolar walls and evolves into small areas of pneumonitis. In the monkey models (small-particle challenge), the virulent organisms multiplied rapidly in the lung starting at first sampling, i.e., 20 min until 72 h. Microscopic findings were apparent at 24 and 48 h, with organisms demonstrated by fluorescent staining inside macrophages by 20 min after inhalation. These macrophages were in the lumina of the bronchioles. By 24 h bronchiolitis developed consisting of neutrophils and macrophages that involved the peribronchiolar tissues. This inflammatory reaction extended at 48 h, with evidence of necrosis and extension into the alveoli. A peribronchiolar and perivascular lymphangitis was evident. Tracheobronchial lymph nodes had definite microscopic changes by 48 h. Some had cortical foci of necrosis surrounded by neutrophils and histiocytes. At 72 and 96 h, the normal architecture of the lymph nodes was replaced by necrosis. Of interest is that no lesions were found in the nasal or nasopharyngeal areas of these aerogenically infected monkeys. The livers and spleens, however, had small focal lesions of necrosis with neutrophils and macrophages by 24 h. *F. tularensis* was found at these sites. The pneumonic process in man is presumed to be similar. Lesions appear on X rays as ill-defined, difficult-to-see, small oval infiltrates. Rarely does lobar consolidation occur. Occasionally, the necrosis progresses to a lung abscess.

7.2. Immunity

The immunity following tularemia in humans is probably lifelong and will prevent reinfection. Volunteers with acquired immunity after experimental infection resist even large challenge doses of virulent organisms introduced by the intradermal or respiratory routes.[20] Measurement of circulating agglutinating antibody in experimental animals as well as in volunteers shows no association between the level of antibody titer and resistance to disease.

Several studies have been reported by Swedish workers in which lymphocyte dynamics were evaluated following administration of tularemia vaccine or the disease itself.[49,50] It is clear from these studies that it was possible to demonstrate the presence of specifically sensitized circulating T lymphocytes that were completely macrophage- or monocyte-dependent. The time of appearance of these T cells correlates with the skin-testing data; i.e., 2–4 weeks after vaccination with the LVS, the tularemia-specific T lymphocytes were present. The presence of these T lymphocytes did not correlate with the agglutinin titers. These studies employed cellular membranes of the vaccine strain as the stimulating antigen. Other antigens may give different results. In this system, sensitized T lymphocytes could be detected up to 2 years after vaccine administration. The skin test detected infection that occurred more than 2 years previously. It is apparent that a more sensitive *in vitro* test is needed to detect the tularemia-sensitive T lymphocytes. Presumably, these cells indicate that the host is resistant to disease.

8. Patterns of Host Response

When tularemia is acquired from animals or arthropods by a healthy, active human host, several clinical responses may occur. The type of clinical presentation is determined by the portal of entry and the virulence of the infecting strain. Man is highly susceptible so that trivial exposure can lead to a mild or inapparent infection or progress to a systemic illness of moderate intensity. Inapparent infections appear to be common and may result in immunity in the host. Patients with serious underlying illnesses and those who delay seeking medical care or do not receive appropriate antibiotic therapy have greater mortality and morbidity than do patients with tularemia but without these implicating features. Patients with poor outcomes in one series had electrolyte or renal function abnormalities, pneumonia and pleural effusions, elevated serum creatine phosphokinase, and *F. tularensis* bacteremia.[37]

8.1. Clinical Features

The clinical picture is determined by the route of infection. Ticks frequently attach to the lower extremities and often obtain their blood meal in the inguinal area; thus, hosts who acquire tularemia by this route will have significant inguinal adenopathy. Hunters or trappers handling diseased animals may develop ulcers on fingers, around nail folds, or on hands, and buboes develop in axillary nodes. These types of illness are usually mild, but leave the patient too ill to work for several days to a week. Antibiotic therapy brings about a prompt recession of symptoms and signs. The buboes should not be drained during the initial days of the disease because this can lead to chronic draining sinus. These nodes will heal without draining.

Most patients with ulceroglandular disease will not have evidence of secondary spread. Secondary tularemic pneumonia due to bacteremia has been reported, but is unusual. The spleen may be enlarged during the latter stages of the infection. A rare patient may have generalized adenopathy without any evidence of skin ulcer.

Patients with oculoglandular tularemia may acquire the disease by rubbing the organism into the conjunctival sac. Conceivably, the eyes may be contaminated by aerosol exposure. This was not observed in the many volunteer subjects, but has been noted in monkeys exposed to extremely high doses of aerosolized tularemia particles. The conjunctivas become infected, with the formation of small yellowish nodules that resolve readily with appropriate antibiotic therapy.

Tularemic pneumonia has been thought to be more prevalent than cases reported. While this diagnosis should be considered in patients with suggestive exposure histories, there is little clinical or epidemiological evidence to indicate that many patients are being misdiagnosed. In epidemics, there does occur inapparent pneumonia that is diagnosed by reason of chest films taken as a routine procedure, not because of symptoms. The aerogenic infection of man creates substernal discomfort, a dry, paroxysmal cough, fever, and headache.[20] There may be cervical lymph-node enlargement. The more prominent the nodes in the neck, the more likely it is that large-particle aerosols were ingested. Patients with pneumonia have been described as having small oval densities on X ray as a classic finding.[34] Subsequent reviews have failed to confirm this finding, since a wide variety of X-ray findings have been described.[30] Pleural effusions, lung abscess, mediastinal adenopathy, and even tracheal compression have been noted. The clinical course of patients with tularemic pneumonia is one of rapid resolution when appropriate antibiotics are given. Prior to antibiotic utilization, the mortality rate was reported to be from 30 to 60%.

Rarely, patients develop pericarditis or meningitis as part of their disease.[13]

8.2. Diagnosis

Tularemia presenting as a typhoidal illness with no localizing signs other than adenopathy is a difficult diagnostic problem. A careful history of possible contact in the previous few days to a week or more with ticks, deerflies, cottontail rabbits, or other animals will provide significant leads for definitive diagnostic tests. Occupational history should be thorough, seeking similar links to such exposures. Serological studies will be helpful, but only after the first 10 days or so after contact with the organism. The initiation of treatment with streptomycin or gentamicin will bring about a prompt therapeutic response. In 24–48 h, the patient should be less febrile and symptomatically improved. This form of illness may be confused with infectious mononucleosis, toxoplasmosis, cytomegalovirus disease, psittacosis, and rarely with typhoid fever.

Ulceroglandular disease has to be differentiated from sporotrichosis, cat scratch fever, *Mycobacterium marinum* infection, and cutaneous anthrax. In all these diseases, the clue to diagnosis will be obtained from a thorough history and confirmed by appropriate serological studies and culture of material from the lesions on selective media.

9. Control and Prevention

9.1. General Concepts

Education about the risks of handling rodents and rabbits that appear ill should continue to limit the spread of illness from these animals to man. The prohibition of the sale of wild rabbits in markets has been an important public-health measure proven to be effective in preventing the spread of tularemia. A simple and useful means of preventing infection is to be aware of the hazards associated with tick attachment and feeding. Protective clothing is helpful, but search for and removal of ticks before retiring when camping or working in tick-infested areas will eliminate any possible chance of infection. Ticks usually feed by attaching to body hairs and feeding when the host is quiet (i.e., asleep).

All cases should be reported to the appropriate public-health officials so that a thorough epidemiological study can be made and control measures established to prevent additional exposure. Quarantine is not necessary.

9.2. Antibiotic and Chemotherapeutic Approaches to Prophylaxis

Volunteer studies have shown that streptomycin administered 24 h after intradermal inoculation of virulent organisms will prevent disease from developing. This is impractical except in unusual circumstances, e.g., when a laboratory worker is exposed by needle-stick or to accidental aerosolization of tularemia bacilli. In this instance, an unvaccinated person would benefit from initiation of gentamicin or streptomycin treatment for a period of 5–7 days. Under no circumstances should antibiotics be given routinely to persons known to have been bitten by a tick or deerfly. The administration of an antibiotic may cause drug fever, delay the incubation period, or fail to prevent tularemia or other infections, i.e., Rocky Mountain spotted fever, and the risk of infection is too low following the bites of most ticks and deerflies to justify antibiotic prophylaxis.

9.3. Immunization

A killed vaccine introduced by Foshay was the initial effort to induce resistance to *F. tularensis* invasion. This was a phenolized killed suspension of organisms. Studies in animals and in man indicated that this vaccine did not induce effective resistance to disease. An LVS was developed by Eigelsbach and Downs.[10] They selected one of the two attenuated strains employed earlier by Russian investigators. From this isolate, they evolved a standardized, stable, and effective vaccine strain. LVS has been extensively studied in animals and man, and its effectiveness has been quantitated by means of induced infections in volunteers. The recommended method of administration is by the acupuncture route, similar to smallpox vaccination, which creates excellent immunity against low-dose intradermal and aerogenic (200–2000 organisms) virulent challenges.[20] High doses (25,000 by aerosol) can overcome this immunity, although the illness is modified compared to controls. However, the magnitude of these challenge levels is much greater than what would be expected in nature or under less controlled conditions. For instance, at Fort Detrick, where tularemia was being studied in many laboratories, 10–12 cases of laboratory-acquired disease occurred each year. Since 1959, when all workers were routinely given LVS, no cases of typhoidal tularemia have occurred. The incidence of ulceroglandular disease remained the same, but the illnesses were mild and recovery occurred in a few days without antibiotic treatment. Since agglutinin titers and skin-test reactivity appear to diminish after 2 years, revaccination may be needed at some interval, probably 10–15 years, but data are not available to permit a firm recommendation.

LVS is an effective vaccine and should be administered to all persons considered at high risk: selected laboratory workers, forest rangers, game wardens, and others exposed during an outbreak. The vaccine is not generally available, but is produced commercially for the Army by the National Drug Co. The physician who wishes to obtain vaccine should direct an application for its release to the Commander, U.S. Army Medical Research Institute of Infectious Diseases, Frederick, Maryland 21701.

The mechanism of immunity following recovery from disease or induced by vaccine appears to be mediated by cellular means rather than antibody. This has been well studied in various animal models.[12,31,39] In the mouse model, transference of spleen cells from immune to nonimmune mice established excellent protection. These immune cells were collected on day 12 following a secondary immunization with a virulent strain in mice that had been previously immunized with the LVS. *In vitro* studies, employing alveolar macrophages from immune animals, demonstrated remarkable intracellular inhibitory power of these cells as well as their ability to survive when in contact with virulent *F. tularensis*.[32] This effect was demonstrated without the aid of "immune" serum, indicating the primary role played by the cellular defenses of the lung in resisting tularemic disease.

LVS has been experimentally administered by the aerogenic and oral routes.[20,21] The aerogenic route was investigated to ascertain whether the local immune mechanisms in the respiratory tract could be specifically stimulated. The rationale was to gain greater protection against respiratory challenge than could be induced by the intracutaneously administered vaccine. An aerosol dose of 10^4 LVS organisms induced immunity to subsequent small challenges of virulent organisms. When 10^6 or 10^8 LVS organisms were given, the recipients experienced mild flulike illness with headache, coryza, chest pain, and malaise. Of 42 men who received the 10^8 dose, 3 were given streptomycin to control symptoms. The men in the 10^6 and 10^8 dose groups developed increased resistance to challenge with 25,000 virulent organisms. That is, they did not require antibiotic treatment to control their illness, whereas 46% of those who were vaccinated by the intracutaneous route received antibiotic treatment. Measurement of IgA antibodies in sputum was not performed in this study. However, nasal agglutinating antibodies have been detected in patients following intradermal inoculation of LVS as well as in volunteers recovering from aerogenic exposure.[4] It appears that the vaccine can be given by the aerogenic method, but currently, equipment that would deliver a safe reproducible dose and with uniform particle size is not available. At present, the acupuncture method induces excellent protection for naturally acquired disease whether exposure is to the type A or the type B strain.

Massive doses of LVS have been swallowed without significant reactions.[21] Doses of 10^{10} LVS bacilli taken orally as a suspension caused a mild, self-limited febrile illness characterized by cervical adenopathy but no pharyngeal lesions. Serum agglutinating antibodies appeared later than expected, but peaked at 3–4 weeks. Challenge of these volunteers with a small aerosol dose demonstrated excellent protection. The oral route could be a safe and effective method of administering this vaccine strain.

10. Unresolved Problems

Tularemia has been well studied; however, additional investigations are needed to assess the range of susceptibility of animals to this disease. Where do cottontails acquire their disease? Presumably, they acquire it from infected ticks and then transmit it to other ticks. Ticks can transmit the organism transovarially, so that their offspring become infected. Additional studies of ticks feeding on cottontail rabbits are needed.

The duration of immunity induced by LVS requires further study. Skin-testing materials needed to be made readily available for more widespread use.

One fascinating problem remains: to explain adequately and clearly why human-to-human transmission does not occur with this organism. Why does a highly infectious agent like *F. tularensis* fail to cause disease in contacts of patients? There are organisms in pharyngeal washes and saliva; why are these organisms not infectious for man?

11. References

1. ALEXANDER, M. M., WRIGHT, G. G., AND BALDWIN, A. C., Observations on the agglutination of polysaccharide-treated erythrocytes by tularemia antisera, *J. Exp. Med.* **91**:561–566 (1950).
2. BARBEITO, M. S., ALG, R. L., AND WEDUM, A. G., Infectious bacterial aerosol from dropped petri dish cultures, *Am. J. Med. Technol.* **27**:318–322 (1961).
3. BELL, J. F., Ecology of tularemia in North America, *J. Jinsen Med.* **11**:33–44 (1965).
4. BELLANTI, J. A., BEUSCHER, E. L., BRANDT, W. E., DANGERFIELD, H. G., AND CROZIER, D., Characterization of human serum and nasal hemagglutinating antibody to *Francisella tularensis*, *J. Immunol.* **98**:171–178 (1967).
5. BIVIN, W. S., AND HOGGE, A. L., JR., Quantitation of susceptibility of swine to infection with *Pasteurella tularensis*, *Am. J. Vet. Res.* **28**:1619–1621 (1967).
6. BUCHANAN, T. M., BROOKS, G. F., AND BRACHMAN, P. S., The tularemia skin test—325 skin tests in 210 persons: Serologic correlation and review of the literature, *Ann. Intern. Med.* **74**:336–343 (1971).
7. BURNETT, T. W., Tularemia in a Rocky Mountain sector of the western front, *Mil. Surg.* **78**:193–199 (1936).
8. CANONICO, P. G., MCMANUS, A. T., MANGIAFICO, J. A., SAMMONS, L. S., MCGANN, V. G., AND DANGERFIELD, H. G., Temporal appearance of opsonizing antibody to *Francisella tularensis*: Detection by a radiometabolic assay, *Infect. Immun.* **11**:466–469 (1975).
9. DAHLSTRAND, S., RINGERTZ, O., AND ZETTERBERG, B., Airborne tularemia in Sweden, *Scand. J. Infect. Dis.* **3**:7–16 (1971).
10. EIGELSBACH, H. T., AND DOWNS, C. M., Prophylactic effectiveness of live and killed tularemia vaccines. I. Production of vaccine and evaluation in the white mouse and guinea pig, *J. Immunol.* **87**:415–425 (1961).
11. EIGELSBACH, H. T., TULIS, J. J., MCGAVRAN, M. H., AND WHITE, J. D., Live tularemia vaccine. I. Host–parasite relationship in monkeys vaccinated intracutaneously or aerogenically, *J. Bacteriol.* **84**:1020–1027 (1962).
12. EIGELSBACH, H. T., HUNTER, D. H., JANSSEN, W. A., DANGERFIELD, H. G., AND RABINOWITZ, S. G., Murine model for study of cell-mediated immunity: Protection against death from fully virulent *Francisella tularensis* infection, *Infect. Immun.* **12**:999–1005 (1975).
13. EVANS, M. E., GREGORY, D. W., SCHAFFNER, W., AND MCGEE, Z., Tularemia: A 30-year experience with 88 cases, *Medicine* **64**:251–269 (1985).
14. FRANCIS, E., Deer-fly fever: A disease of man of hitherto unknown etiology, *Public Health Rep.* **34**:2061–2062 (1919).
15. FRANCIS, E., The occurrence of tularemia in nature, as a disease of man, *Public Health Rep.* **36**:1731 (1921).
16. FRANCIS, E., AND MAYNE, B., Experimental transmission of tularemia by flies of the species *Chryops discalis*, *Public Health Rep.* **36**:1738–1746 (1921).
17. GAISKII, N. A., ALTAREVA, N. D., AND LENNIK, T. G., Rapidity of the appearance and length of persistence of immunity after vaccination with tularemia vaccine, in: *History and Incidence of Tularemia in the Soviet Union—A Review* (R. POLLITZER, ed.), pp. 125–136, Institute of Contemporary Russian Studies, Fordham University, New York, 1967.
18. GALLIVAN, M. V. E., DAVIS, W. A., III, GARAGUSI, V. F., PARIS, A. L., AND LACK, E. E., Fatal cat-transmitted tularemia: Demonstration of the organism in tissue, *South. Med. J.* **73**:240–242 (1980).
19. HORNE, H., En lemeng og marsvintest, *Nor. Vet. Tidsskr.* **23**:16 (1911).
20. HORNICK, R.B., AND EIGELSBACH, H. T., Aerogenic immunization of man with live tularemia vaccine, *Bacteriol. Rev.* **30**:532–538 (1966).
21. HORNICK, R. B., DAWKINS, A. T., EIGELSBACH, H. T., AND TULIS, J. J., Oral tularemia vaccine in man, *Antimicrob. Agents Chemother. 1966* pp. 11–14 (1967).
22. HUNT, J. S., Pleuropulmonary tularemia: Observations on 12 cases treated with streptomycin, *Ann. Intern. Med.* **26**:263–276 (1947).
23. JELLISON, W. L., AND PARKER, R. R., Rodents, rabbits and tularemia in North America: Some zoological and epidemiological considerations, *Am. J. Trop. Med.* **25**:349–362 (1945).
24. JELLISON, W. L., OWEN, C. R., BELL, J. F., AND KOHLS, G. M., Tularemia and animal populations: Ecology and epizootiology, *Wildl. Dis.* **17** (1961).
25. KLOTZ, S. A., PENN, R. L., AND PROVENZA, J. M., The unusual presentations of tularemia. Bacteremia, pneumonia and rhabdomyolysis, *Arch. Intern. Med.* **147**:214 1987).
26. MCCAHAN, G. R., MOODY, M. D., AND HAYES, F. A., An epizootic of tularemia among rabbits in northwestern South Carolina, *Am. J. Hyg.* **75**:335–338 (1962).

27. McCoy, G. W., A plague-like disease of rodents, *Public Health Bull*. No. 43 (1911).
28. McCoy, G. W., AND CHAPIN, C. W., *Bacterium tularense, the cause of a plague-like disease of rodents, Public Health Bull*. No. 53 (1912).
29. McGAVRAN, M. H., WHITE, J. D., EIGELSBACH, H. T., AND KERPSACK, R. W., Morphologic and immunohistochemical studies of the pathogenesis of infection and antibody formation subsequent to vaccination of *Macaca irus* with an attenuated strain of *Pasteurella tularensis*. I. Intracutaneous vaccination, *Am. J. Pathol*. **41:**259–271 (1962).
30. MILLER, R. P., AND BATES, J. H., Pleuropulmonary tularemia: A review of 29 patients, *Am. Rev. Respir. Dis*. **99:**31–41 (1969).
31. MOE, J. B., CANONICO, P. G., STOOKEY, J. L., POWANDA, M. C., AND COCKERELL, G. L., Pathogenesis of tularemia in immune and nonimmune rats, *Am. J. Vet. Res*. **36:**1505–1510 (1975).
32. NUTTER, J. E., AND MYRVIK, W. N., *In vitro* interactions between rabbit alveolar macrophages and *Pasteurella tularensis, J. Bacteriol*. **92:**645–651 (1966).
33. OHARA, S., *The Story of Yato-Byo (Tularemia in Japan)*, Obama, Fukushima City, 1955.
34. OVERHOLT, E. L., AND TIGERTT, W. D., Roentgenographic manifestations of pulmonary tularemia, *Radiology* **74:**758–765 (1960).
35. OVERHOLT, E. L., TIGERTT, W. D., KADULL, P. J., WARD, M. K., CHARKES, N. D., RENE, R. M., SALTZMAN, T. E., AND STEPHENS, M., An analysis of forty-two cases of laboratory-acquired tularemia: Treatment with broad-spectrum antibiotics, *Am. J. Med*. **30:**785 (1961).
36. OWEN, C. R., AND BUKER, E. O., Factors involved in the transmission of *Pasteurella tularensis* from inoculated animals to healthy cage mates, *J. Infect. Dis*. **99:**227–233 (1956).
37. PENN, R. L., AND KINSEWITZ, G. T., Factors associated with a poor outcome in tularemia, *Arch. Intern. Med*. **147:**265–268 (1987).
38. PHILIP, R. N., HUNTLEY, B., LACKMAN, D. B., AND COMSTOCK, G. W., Serologic and skin test evidence of tularemia infection among Alaskan Eskimos, Indians and Aleuts, *J. Infect. Dis*. **110:**220–230 (1962).
39. PROCTOR, R. A., WHITE, J. D., AYALA, E., AND CANONICO, P. G., Phagocytosis of *Francisella tularensis* by rhesus monkey peripheral leukocytes, *Infect. Immun*. **11:**145–151 (1975).
40. PUNTIGAM, F., Thorakale Formen in Seuchengeschehen der Tularämie in Österreich, *Wien. Klin. Wochenschr*. **72:**813–816 (1960).
41. RIGGS, J. L., SEIWALD, R. J., BURCKHALTER, J. H., DOWNS, C. M., AND METCALF, T. G., Isothiocyanate compounds as fluorescent labeling agents for immune serum, *Am. J. Pathol*. **34:**1081–1097 (1958).
42. SASLAW, S., AND CARHART, S., Studies with tularemia vaccines in volunteers. III. Serologic aspects following intracutaneous or respiratory challenge in both vaccinated and nonvaccinated volunteers, *Am. J. Med. Sci*. **241:**689–699 (1961).
43. SASLAW, S., AND CARLISLE, H. N., Studies with tularemia vaccines in volunteers. IV. Brucella agglutinins in vaccinated and nonvaccinated volunteers challenged with *Pasteurella tularensis, Am. J. Med. Sci*. **242:**166–172 (1961).
44. SASLAW, S., EIGELSBACH, H. T., WILSON, H. E., PRIOR, J. A., AND CARHART, S., Tularemia vaccine study. I. Intracutaneous challenge. *Arch. Inter. Med*. **107:**689–701 (1961).
45. SASLAW, S., EIGELSBACH, H. T., PRIOR, J. A., WILSON, H. E., AND CARHART, S., Tularemia vaccine study. II. Respiratory challenge, *Arch. Intern. Med*. **107:**702–714 (1961).
46. SAWYER, W. D., JEMSKI, J. V., HOGGE, A. L., JR., EIGELSBACH, H. T., WOLFE, E. K. DANGERFIELD, H. G., GOCHENOUR, W. S., JR., AND CROZIER, D., Effect of aerosol age on the infectivity of airborne *Pasteurella tularensis* for *Macaca mulatta* and man, *J. Bacteriol*. **91:**2180–2184 (1966).
47. SIL'CHENKO, V. S., Epidemiological and clinical features of tularemia caused by waterborne infection, *Zh. Mikrobiol. Epidemiol. Immunobiol*. **28:**788–795 (1957).
48. STUART, B. M., AND PULLEN, R. L., Tularemic pneumonia: Review of American literature and report of 15 additional cases, *Am. J. Med. Sci*. **210:**223–236 (1945).
49. TÄRNVIK, A., AND LÖFGREN, S., Stimulation of human lymphocytes by a vaccine strain of *Francisella tularensis, Infect. Immun*. **12:**951–957 (1975).
50. TÄRNVIK, A., SANDSTRÖM, G., AND LÖFGREN, S., Time of lymphocyte response after onset of tularemia and after tularemia vaccination, *J. Clin. Microbiol*. **10:**854–860 (1979).
51. TEUTSCH, S. M., MARTONE, W. J., BRINK, E. W., POTTER, M. E., ELIOT, G., HOXSIE, R., CRAVEN, R. B., AND KAUFMANN, A. F., Pneumonic tularemia on Martha's Vineyard, *N. Engl. J. Med*. **301:**826–828 (1979).
52. VAIL, D. T., *Bacillus tularense* infection of the eye, *Ophthalmol. Res*. **23:**487 (1914).
53. WARING, W. B., AND RUFFIN, J. J., A tick-borne epidemic of tularemia, *N. Engl. J. Med*. **234:**137 (1946).
54. WHERRY, W. B., A new bacterial disease of rodents transmissible to man, *Public Health Rep*. **29:**3387 (1914).
55. WHITE, J. D., McGAVRAN, M. H., PRICKETT, P. A., TULIS, J. J., AND EIGELSBACH, H. T., Morphologic and immunohistochemical studies of the pathogenesis of infection and antibody formation subsequent to vaccination of *Macaca irus* with an attenuated strain of *Pasteurella tularensis*. II. Aerogenic vaccination, *Am. J. Pathol*. **41:**405–413 (1962).
56. WHO, *Annual Statistics, Infectious Diseases: Cases and Deaths* **2:**1–204 (1978).
57. YOUNG, L. S., BICKNELL, D. S., ARCHER, B. G., CLINTON, J. M., LEAVENS, L. J., FEELEY, J. C., AND BRACHMAN, P. S., Tularemia epidemic: Vermont, 1968: Forty-seven cases linked

to contact with muskrats, *N. Engl. J. Med.* **280:**1253–1260 (1969).

12. Suggested Reading

BOYCE, J. M., Recent trends in the epidemiology of tularemia in the United States, *J. Infect. Dis.* **131:**197–199 (1975).

BROOKS, G. F., AND BUCHANAN, T. M., Tularemia in the United States: Epidemiologic aspects in the 1960's and followup of the outbreak of tularemia in Vermont, *J. Infect. Dis.* **121:**357–359 (1970).

BUTLER, T., Plague and tularemia, *Pediatr. Clin. North Am.* **26:**355–366 (1979).

JELLISON, W. L., OWEN, C. R., BELL, J. F., AND KOHLS, G. M., Tularemia and animal populations: Ecology and epizootiology, *Wildl. Dis.* **17** (1961).

CHAPTER 39

Typhoid Fever

Richard B. Hornick

1. Introduction

Typhoid fever is a uniquely human systemic infection caused primarily by *Salmonella typhi* (a few other strains of *Salmonella* also can cause typhoid fever or enteric fever). A protracted, debilitating febrile illness characterizes the clinical course in untreated patients. The mental cloudiness or stupor associated with this type of chronic illness accounts for the name *typhoid,* meaning stuporlike. The disease is acquired by ingestion of food or water that has been contaminated by a human who has acute disease, is recently convalescent, or is an asymptomatic chronic fecal shedder of typhoid bacilli. In areas of the world where safe water supplies and good sewage control are not available, typhoid fever remains an endemic disease. The disease is no longer common in the United States; this low prevalence has created a potential public-health problem, i.e., a large population that has become highly susceptible to infection. Thus, travelers to endemic areas account for over half the cases of typhoid fever reported in this country. And as long as some carriers exist, this disease will remain a threat to cause outbreaks when sanitation measures break down and water contamination results. Patients' illnesses can be easily controlled by appropriate and early institution of antibiotic therapy. Since the disease is rare and becoming more so, delays in diagnosis due to unfamiliarity with the clinical presentation have produced and will continue to produce unnecessary morbidity.[52]

Richard B. Hornick · Medical Education Administration, Orlando Regional Medical Center, Orlando, Florida 32806.

2. Historical Background

Much of the development of the science of microbiology was associated with the description and isolation of *S. typhi.* Detailed descriptive clinical and pathological information was published early in the 19th century by French clinicians. Bretonneau[7] and Chomel defined the anatomical features and described the disease as a severe enteric infection in young Parisians in 1829. They coined the term "boil of the intestine" (dothoienenterite) to illustrate the lesion that can lead to intestinal perforation. Pierre Louis studied and recorded the clinical and pathological findings in 158 patients in 1836. He carefully catalogued the abnormal lesions in the intestine, lymph nodes, spleen, and skin (rose spots), and hemorrhage and perforation in the gut. During this period, the pathogenesis of the intestinal lesions was thought to be a complication or unusual extension of typhus fever. Clarification of the differences between typhoid and typhus is credited to Gerhard[20] in 1836. By studying the clinical and pathological features of six patients, he separated the characteristic pathological features found in typhoid patients from those associated with typhus. Later, Budd surmised that typhoid must be contagious and that spread may occur through fecal contamination. Eberth[14] in 1880 described rodlike bacteria presumed to be typhoid bacilli in mesenteric lymph nodes and spleen obtained at autopsy of patients with typhoid fever. He described their intracellular location. Two other early microbiologists contributed significantly to the final confirmation of causation of typhoid fever. Gaffky[18] in 1884 isolated the organism from mesenteric nodes and Pfeiffer from feces. During the Spanish–American War, typhoid fever was the most common military casualty—one of every five soldiers developed the disease.[51] An Army commission headed by Walter Reed[51] (Reed, Vaughan, and Shakespeare Commission) studied this problem, and their evidence established the epidemiological importance of feces from cases of typhoid fever, but the significance of the carrier was not recognized. Further stressing the anal–oral route of spread quickly led to the supplying and education for use of toilet paper and provision of pure water. These measures effected a dramatic drop in the incidence of typhoid fever in the military by the time World War I began. Similar efforts to provide pure water to civilians and to control the occupations of carriers resulted in a dramatic decline of the disease. Typhoid vaccine, which was first employed experimentally in 1896,[60] has subsequently undergone many large-scale field evaluations. These have demonstrated some efficacy. However, the vaccine has had no significant influence on the control of typhoid fever in this country.

3. Methodology

Typhoid fever is a disease that has continued to receive great attention by public-health officials. For each case identified, extensive investigative efforts are conducted to discover the person, usually an asymptomatic carrier, who has served as a source of the outbreak. Carriers are carefully identified and regularly followed by city or county health departments. This monitoring is done to ensure that carriers do not become involved in occupations that would permit food or water contamination.

3.1. Sources of Mortality Data

Many published series of patients with typhoid fever admitted to infectious-disease hospitals in the years prior to the availability of antibiotic therapy indicated a mortality rate from 12 to 30%. Most deaths were reported to be due to hemorrhage or intestinal perforation. Some patients died of other complications rarely seen today: meningitis, myocarditis, and pneumonia. Since typhoid fever has long been a reportable disease to the Centers for Disease Control (CDC) in Atlanta, a reliable statement on mortality is available. Indeed, Mary Mallon, the infamous cook known as "Typhoid Mary"[48] because of the numerous cases of typhoid traced to her, was a major factor in the restructuring and increasing of the authority of the New York City Department of Health. The need to have the regulating authority to be able to investigate outbreaks of typhoid fever and other

contagious diseases strengthened the concept of centralized health-control administration.

The CDC formerly collected from states only minimal data on individual cases through the *Morbidity and Mortality Weekly Report* (MMWR) surveillance system. There was a national cumulative tally, and the CDC carried out investigations of outbreaks. However, beginning in 1975, additional data were collected from all bacteriologically confirmed cases by means of questionnaires that elicited more complete epidemiological information.[42] From 50 to 75% of the questionnaires are filled out on cases reported through the MMWR surveillance system.

There are many mild undiagnosed cases of typhoid fever among populations living in endemic areas who do not enter into any reporting system; thus, mortality rates do not reflect the true incidence of the disease. A mortality rate of less than 1% is obtained from records kept at large municipal hospitals in endemic areas. These statistics accurately reflect the mortality rate of those groups of patients who have been hospitalized and diagnosed as having typhoid fever. Many patients are not hospitalized because the infection is naturally attenuated or because of erratic, self-administered antibiotic therapy.

3.2. Sources of Morbidity Data

The overwhelming majority of diagnosed cases of typhoid fever that occur in the United States are reported to public-health departments because of two mechanisms. There are cases reported directly by physicians, and in addition, all positive stool, blood, or other cultures that yield *S. typhi* are reported by the laboratories making the isolations. The same two reporting systems mentioned above are used for collecting morbidity data.

In many endemic areas, there are less-reliable data on incidence. Many "fever" hospitals record the number of patients admitted with the clinical diagnosis of typhoid fever, while others report just the number of confirmed cases. The true incidence in many of these countries is not known because of difficulties in confirming suspected cases, suppression of disease by self-medication with antibiotics, and incomplete reporting. Furthermore, many mild cases occur, and these patients do not get reported. The number of carriers is largely unknown in these areas.

3.3. Surveys

Surveys of family members and persons known to be associated with an outbreak of typhoid fever are usually done by means of culturing at least three successive stool specimens from asymptomatic subjects. One or more of these three specimens will yield the organism in most carriers (> 90%), carriers being persons who shed *S. typhi* in the stool for more than 1 year. Persons exposed and in the incubation period before illness will often have positive stool cultures.

Serological studies are less helpful. The prevalence of O (somatic antigen) and H (flagellar antigen) antibodies is quite high in endemic areas, and the individual serum titers of these antibodies may also be high, i.e., O titers higher than 1:160 and H titers higher than 1:320. These antibodies are becoming less common in citizens of the United States. In endemic areas, there is obviously a greater opportunity to be exposed to typhoid bacilli antigens, and hence the Widal test (see Section 3.4.2) will more accurately detect exposure to the organism—when the exposure occurred cannot be predicted with certainty by a single titer. Paired specimens 2 weeks apart must demonstrate a fourfold or greater rise in titer to be diagnostic. The O and H antibodies peak during the 3rd week of illness and gradually decline in most patients during the ensuing 5 months to the pre-illness level. An additional weakness of the Widal test as a reliable epidemiological tool is the significant percentage of patients with bacteriologically proven typhoid fever who do not develop diagnostic titer increases. As many as 30% of patients will have insignificant titers or no fourfold rise in one or both of the major antigens, O and H.[59] Finally, patients with cirrhosis and hepatitis[40] have been shown to develop antibodies that agglutinate with the Widal antigens, giving false-positive results that may cause diagnostic confusion. There is a need for more specific serological tests to be developed.

3.4. Laboratory Diagnosis

3.4.1. Isolation and Identification of the Organism. Typhoid bacilli can be readily isolated from blood and feces using various media, e.g., *Salmonella–Shigella* (SS), and MacConkey's, as well as nutrient broth. The organism does not ferment sucrose or lactose, while the fermentation of glucose produces acid; these biochemical reactions help select the organism from other species of gram-negative rods in the fecal flora. These tests will give a tentative identification in 24–48 h. Confirmation is achieved by serological identification using the O and H antigens. Many strains contain virulence (Vi) antigen, a heat-labile envelope antigen, which may prevent the O antigen–antibody agglutination. Heating will destroy the Vi antigen and allow the heat-stable O antigen to persist and agglutination to

occur in O antisera. The Vi antigen is an important epidemiological aid, since its susceptibility to lysis by bacteriophages has allowed for the classification of 80 definite and stable varieties of typhoid bacilli. This test can help identify the source and spread of a specific strain. The CDC is the principal source of phage typing in this country.

3.4.2. Serological Diagnostic Methods. The Widal test, which has been in use since 1898,[57] is an agglutination test that measures O and H antibodies. The antigens used in the test consist of heat-killed and formalin-preserved whole bacteria. The typhoid bacillus O antigen consists of type 9 and type 12 O antigens. Cross-reacting salmonellae contain either 9 or 12 plus other of the 60-odd O antigen types contained in the genus *Salmonella*. These cross-reacting antigens dilute the specificity of the Widal test when it is used to measure antibodies in a population with little exposure to typhoid bacilli but with more opportunities to be infected with numerous other *Salmonella* strains. Similar comments can be made about H antigens.

The Vi antibodies are measured by hemagglutination techniques. These antibodies have been used in some studies as a means of detecting carriers serologically.[45] Persistence of Vi antibodies in serum specimens from carriers was thought to be due to the low-grade infection in the gallbladder caused by the typhoid bacillus. However, some carriers (30%) lack circulating Vi antibodies, and 6–8% of noncarriers may have detectable Vi antibody levels.[17] Isolation of the typhoid bacillus from fecal specimens is the most reliable means of detecting and following the shedding status of carriers.

Recent serological tests have been introduced that give much more specific information regarding exposure to *S. typhi*. The enzyme-linked immunosorbent assay (ELISA) is reported to be more specific and sensitive than the agglutination test.

4. Biological Characteristics of the Organism

Several biological characteristics of *S. typhi* have already been mentioned above, but their significance needs further emphasis. Strains may or may not contain the Vi antigen. Vi-containing strains are more virulent for man and experimental animals. The Vi-containing strains inhibit phagocytosis by decreasing the ability of serum to fix C3 to the surface of *S. typhi*. This results in defective opsonification and a slow uptake of the organisms by polymorphonuclear leukocytes. As a consequence, a lower oxidative burst occurs than that measured following the more rapid ingestion of non-Vi containing strains.[32] Vi antigen also increases resistance to the cytolytic effect of hydrogen peroxide, allowing typhoid bacilli to persist in resting macrophages. These cells are less dependent upon complement fixation for phagocytosis.

Typhoid bacilli are able to achieve an intracellular habitat promptly after oral ingestion. This property may account for the prolonged duration of disease in untreated patients and the slow response to antibiotic therapy. Inside the cell, the organism appears to be protected from the host's attempts to eliminate it, through specific immune mechanisms, circulating antibiotics, or constrained intracellular cytolytic processes.

The cell wall of the typhoid bacillus is a thick and complex structure. Like that of other gram-negative rods, the outer portion of the cell wall consists of lipopolysaccharide (LPS) or endotoxin. This substance has many biological properties that are important in the pathogenesis of typhoid fever. It consists of three layers, the outer being made up of a repeating sequence of sugars that determine the specificity of the O antigen. For typhoid, there are two major O antigens—9 and 12—in this surface complex. The middle layer of the LPS is the R-core. Rough or mutant strains that lack the outer layer of LPS are nonpathogenic. However, antibodies against this R-core have been found by some investigators to protect against infections caused by a wide variety of gram-negative bacteria. The inner or basal layer of LPS is the lipid moiety, which appears to bind the endotoxin molecule to the rest of the cell-wall structure. Endotoxin is pyrogenic, triggers the complement and clotting cascades, and may be responsible for septic shock. Its role in the pathogenesis of typhoid fever is discussed in Section 7.1.

The treatment of typhoid fever patients with effective antibiotics began in 1948.[59] Chloramphenicol was the first drug used, and it remains an important therapeutic agent. Despite the acquisition of resistance to chloramphenicol by many gram-negative bacteria within 10–12 years after its widespread use, no patient was found to have resistant typhoid strains in blood cultures until 1972.[54] In the next 2 years, strains similar to those found first in Mexico were isolated from the Middle East, India, and Southeast Asia. The plasmid [resistance (R) factor] responsible for the development of resistance to chloramphenicol (and other antibiotics not useful for treating typhoid fever) was prevalent in and around Mexico City for 2 years and then largely disappeared. There was a general impression from those who studied these patients that the resistant strain induced illnesses with more complications and severity than previous strains. The reasons for its sudden appearance and regression have not been explained. Initially, it was thought that this plasmid was transferred from *Shigella dysenteriae* strains that had earlier caused a large outbreak of severe bacilliary dysentery in Central America including southern Mexico.[19] Subsequent studies clearly showed that two different plasmids were involved. Why such chloramphenicol-resistant strains of *S. typhi* had not appeared earlier in endemic areas where the drug was used indiscriminately is not known. There had been occasional reports of strains isolated from stool cultures that had developed resistance, but none of these isolates was found in the blood of those patients. Presumably, during chloramphenicol treatment, resistant Enterobacteriacae were selected out of the patient's gut flora and transferred the R factor to the surviving *S. typhi*. These organisms, located in the colon, apparently did not penetrate the mucosa, and the patient continued the expected convalescence without a recurrence with the resistant strain.

One other important biological property of this bacterium is its ability to survive in the environment, such as in snow, water, and food. In some instances, this survival may be as long as several months. The hardy nature of the organism has permitted it to cause epidemics[3] that are unexpected because no apparent recent cause for the contamination was found. In one instance, the organisms had persisted through the winter, and when spring thawing occurred, spread was apparent.

5. Descriptive Epidemiology

5.1. Prevalence and Incidence

Figure 1 illustrates the rate of reported cases of typhoid fever in the United States since 1955. There has been a leveling off of the curve in the past 22 years (1965–1986) at about 0.2 case/100,000 population. In 1987, there were 188 cases reported with positive cultures and 32 carriers, and there were an additional 384 unspecified isolations of *S. typhi*. These figures are representative of the status of typhoid fever in the United States for the past two decades except for the large outbreak that occurred in 1973 in Dade County, Florida. In that outbreak (discussed in greater detail in Section 5.2), the water supply in a migrant-labor camp became contaminated, and 222 cases of mild to severe typhoid fever were induced. This was the largest single outbreak in over 30 years.

Between 1975 and 1984, 4641 cases were reported

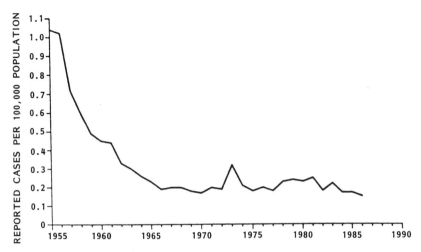

Figure 1. Typhoid fever—by year, United States, 1955–1986.

through the MMWR system.[41] Among these, more specific epidemiological data were collected by the special questionnaire forms from 2666 (57%) cases. Twenty-nine deaths were reported, 21 among domestically acquired cases and 8 among returned travelers. Mortality was five times higher for domestically acquired cases than for foreign travel-acquired cases (2.5 versus 0.5%). In the United States, the majority of cases are single case reports. However, 28% (266 of 934) of domestically acquired cases were outbreak related. There were three major outbreaks, all foodborne.

Travel-related cases have been increasing since 1967. During 1975 through 1984, 1653 of the 2666 reported cases (62%) were acquired during foreign travel. The median age for 1371 of the travel-related cases was 23 years, whereas the median age of 857 cases acquired in the United States was 20 years. Among the travel-related cases, the greatest single occupational group was students [365 of 1216 (30%) cases]. Travel within the Western Hemisphere accounted for 59% of the travel-related cases and travel to the Indian subcontinent (India, Burma, Sri Lanka, Bangladesh) was associated with 17%. Mexico-associated cases accounted for 39% of the total, with India associated with 14%.

Among the domestically acquired cases, 9% (81 of 905) were related to contact with a previously diagnosed typhoid carrier and 21% (168 of 800) were related to contact with a newly diagnosed carrier.

The WHO records the incidences sent to it by cooperating countries. These figures indicate that typhoid remains a major public-health problem in Central and South America, Africa, and Southeast Asia, and less so in Europe. In 1986, there were 5089 isolations reported from 35 countries. This figure appears to be a gross underestimation and indicates incomplete reporting and insufficient bacteriological data.

5.1.1. Prevalence of Carriers. The total number of typhoid carriers in the United States is not certain. In 1962, the number was estimated to be 3637 and in 1978 more than 2000.[38] In Arkansas, the rate of carriers was 3–4/100,000 in 1978.[38] However, in 1986, the CDC reported a total of 541 *S. typhi* isolations, with 115 from patients, 14 from carriers, and the remaining 412 of unknown status.[10]

Many of the known carriers are elderly, and with the low incidence of typhoid fever in this country, it seems logical to assume that very few new carriers will appear to replace those who will die in the next decade. In the preantibiotic era, similar predictions were made about the decline in numbers of carriers, and these predictions have come true. In one such predictive exercise,[1] the number of carriers was calculated as the number of survivors of typhoid fever multiplied by 2.9%. Furthermore, the number of survivors of typhoid fever was obtained by multiplying the reported deaths from the disease by 9, the assumption being that the mortality rate was 10%. Thus, the estimated carrier rates in 1935 for Massachusetts and Mississippi were 48 and 288/100,000, respectively. In New York there were an estimated 2490 carriers in 1940 for a rate of 41.8/100,000 population. These figures and methods for estimating the carrier prevalence were published in March 1943 by Ames and Robins[1] of the New York State Department of Health. These authors also calculated that by January 1, 1980, the number of carriers in New York would have fallen from 2490 to about 190. Their assumptions in arriving at these figures did not and could not consider the effect antibiotic therapy would have on the development of the carrier state. One of their considerations was that no carrier was cured of the chronic infection. It is now clear that some carriers can be cured with appropriate treatment. Nonetheless, the total number of carriers for New York in 1980 that they predicted 37 years earlier appears to have been only very slightly inflated: there actually were 175 known carriers in the state in 1980. The importance of the Ames and Robins study is that they correctly assessed the effectiveness of surveillance of carriers and the maintenance of good water supply and sewage disposal in decreasing the incidence of typhoid fever and, as a favorable consequence, the decline in prevalence of chronic carriers.

5.1.2. Prevalence of Antibody. Prevalence of antibodies to O, H, and Vi antigens in United States citizens in the late 1960s and early 1970s can be estimated from extensive serological data accumulated in a unique series of investigations. Volunteer studies were conducted to evaluate vaccine efficacy.[29] Baseline antibody titers (obtained at time of entry into the study) revealed that older men had higher geometric mean H antibody titers than those 15–20 years their junior.[59] The earlier the year of birth, the more likely a volunteer was to show an elevated titer of H antibody at the time of participation in the study, and if birth occurred after 1935, a period when the disease was rapidly disappearing in this country, the influence of age disappeared. These values held whether or not there was a military history, i.e., an opportunity to have received vaccine. Since these studies investigated persons living in a nonendemic area, the percentages of volunteers lacking detectable O, H, and Vi (envelope antigen) give an estimate of the lack of past exposure to *S. typhi* antigens, whether by previous disease, vaccine administration, or exposure to other salmonellae-containing common and cross-reacting O, H, or Vi antigens. Thus, of 331 men, 52% had no detectable H, 74% no detectable O, and 42% no detectable Vi serum antibodies.[59] The majority of the younger volunteers participating in the later phases of the study fall into these groups. Of those men who had demonstrable circulating-antibody titers, only a small percentage had elevated values. The presence of what have been assumed to be titers of diagnostic significance was as follows: 10% had H antibody titers of 1:320 or greater, 7% had O antibody titers of 1:80 or greater, and 6% had Vi antibody titers of 1:120 or great-

er.[59] If the trend noted in this study continues, it would appear that an increasing number of United States citizens will have no detectable antibodies in the next several decades as opportunities for exposure to typhoid antigens in the United States continue to diminish. Such a trend will make agglutinin titers more important as diagnostic aids for assessing patients with suspected infection as well as improve the reliability of these tests for survey purposes. This hypothesis is predicated on the assumptions that: (1) the sources of acquired disease will continue to decline, i.e., fewer carriers will develop and the present ones will die off; (2) there will be continued minimal utilization of typhoid vaccine in this country; and (3) there will be better control over other sources of salmonellae that may have cross-reacting antigens. There are 140 strains of salmonellae, many of which commonly cause gastroenteritis, that have O antigens that cross-react with typhoid bacillus antigens in the Widal agglutination test. Similarly, there are 61 strains with cross-reacting H antigens. Presumably, these antigens are most likely to be the source of O and H antibodies detected by the Widal test in most United States citizens today.

5.2. Epidemic Behavior and Contagiousness

In this country, scattered outbreaks of typhoid fever occur when a carrier contaminates food or a water supply. The epidemic mentioned in Section 5.1 that occurred in Dade County, Florida, illustrates how a segment of our society may become infected when sewage disposal and water supply are improperly controlled.[16] The index case in this outbreak was thought to be a mentally retarded child, who appeared to have acquired the infection from an asymptomatic carrier living in a neighboring house. Subsequent contamination of the flawed water supply in the migrant-labor camp resulted in 222 cases occurring in the camp population; 184 of these patients were hospitalized. As noted, this was the largest single outbreak in the past 40 years. Other large epidemics have occurred in the past 24 years in Scotland (504 cases)[3] and Zermatt, Switzerland (280 cases),[5] in which contaminated water was the source of *S. typhi*. In Scotland, the source of the organisms was canned corned beef shipped from Argentina. The meat did not contain typhoid bacilli (no raw meat has ever been found to be contaminated with this organism, attesting to the unique adaptation of typhoid bacilli to humans). After the canning process, the cans were heat-sterilized and then placed in contaminated river water to cool. As the cans cooled, the water was drawn into the cans through minute leaks in the seams. Those who handled the meat from the cans became potential cases as well as possible disseminators of the bacteria. Furthermore, when the meat was cut by machines, the blades became contaminated, and other meats cut subsequently on these machines also acquired typhoid bacilli, which was then spread to other consumers.

The epidemic in Zermatt occurred from contamination of the town water supply. The contamination lasted for at least a month before the epidemic was recognized and chlorination and other measures could be instituted to clean the water.

One other large epidemic mentioned earlier (Section 4) was related to contaminated water. In Mexico City from 1972 to 1974, a severe epidemic was caused by chloramphenicol-resistant S. typhi.[23,54] The disease is endemic in this city, but the marked increase in number of patients with disease admitted to hospitals quickly focused attention on the fact that this new strain was responsible for two thirds of the increased incidence. The strain may have been disseminated by soft drinks made with contaminated water. The Mexican strain was found to be responsible for typhoid fever in Switzerland, the United Kingdom, the United States, and other parts of the world. Travelers to Mexico acquired the disease and brought it back to this country and the others. In Los Angeles in 1972, the incidence of the disease doubled, due mainly to imported cases from Mexico.[39] Fortunately, very few secondary cases of typhoid fever occurred in this country as a result of the importation of the antibiotic-resistant Mexican strain.

One other water source of infection that has been documented involves oysters harvested from polluted water, in which typhoid and other enteric pathogens can be concentrated from the water strained by the bivalves. Flies have been shown to transmit typhoid bacilli by contamination of their feet as they feed on feces and subsequent carrying of the organisms to food.

Most single cases are produced by ingesting contaminated food. Rarely, there is direct person-to-person transmission through anal–oral spread, as may occur in children who transmit the organisms during the course of play or in homosexuals.

A distressing and preventable means of acquiring disease has been in hospital diagnostic bacteriology laboratories. The handling of specimens containing S. typhi has caused numerous cases of typhoid fever.[28,39] In the Los Angeles epidemic noted above, three cases were reported from laboratory personnel working with the isolation of the Mexican strain.[39] Holmes et al.[28] reported in 1980 that four cases of typhoid fever occurred in Massachusetts as a

consequence of the state's proficiency-testing program. Three of the laboratories in which cases occurred had not achieved a passing grade in these quality-control tests, and indeed three of the four laboratories involved failed to identify S. typhi in the unknown organisms submitted as part of the testing. This group also noted that nationwide, 25 cases of laboratory-acquired typhoid fever were reported to the CDC from 1977 to 1979. Of these cases, 14 were part of a proficiency-testing program. These data indicate the need for a good training program in order to upgrade the skills and techniques of microbiology technicians. The organism can be handled safely in hospital diagnostic laboratories, but great care mut be taken to avoid contaminating fingers, pens, pencils, and laboratory paraphernalia. These may serve as vectors to transmit the bacteria to the mouth.

Typhoid fever has a low risk of contagion. Person-to-person transmission can occur by anal–oral spread such as changing the soiled bed linens of an undiagnosed patient. Under this set of circumstances, the hands may not be adequately washed and can carry the organisms to food or directly to the mouth. Aerosol spread has been speculated to have occurred when a lyophilized vial of S. typhi exploded into the face of a laboratory worker. He subsequently developed disease. Whether he actually inhaled the aerosolized bacteria through the mouth or inhaled them through the nose and eventually swallowed them is unknown. Small numbers of volunteers exposed to small-particle aerosols containing 100,000 typhoid bacilli failed to develop signs of infection. This dose given by mouth causes disease in about 38% of volunteers; thus, the respiratory tract does not appear to be more susceptible than or even as susceptible to infection as the gastrointestinal tract. Patients with typhoid fever shed the etiological agent by the gut and urinary tract. Aerosol dissemination from these sources would appear to be highly unlikely.

5.3. Geographic Distribution

Areas of the world where ample opportunities abound for fecal contamination of water and food continue to have high rates of all types of enteric infections. Typhoid fever remains common in Central and South America, several European countries, the Middle East, and throughout Africa and Southeast Asia. Ashcroft[4] presented his classification of epidemiological patterns of S. typhi as follows:

1. Hygiene and sanitation appalling; S. typhi probably prevalent; typhoid fever rare. Immunity acquired in infancy or early childhood, when infection is either symptomless or unrecognized.

2. Hygiene and sanitation poor; *S. typhi* common; typhoid fever particularly frequent in children. Most infections occur in childhood and are recognizable, although often mild.
3. Hygiene and sanitation a mixture of primitive and modern, often associated with urbanization. Outbreaks of typhoid fever may involve all age groups.
4. Hygiene excellent; *S. typhi* rare; typhoid fever rare. A situation existing in much of northern Europe and northern North America.

This classification is helpful in explaining many of the epidemiological factors associated with typhoid fever and serves as a rational foundation for understanding the geographic distribution of typhoid fever. Many large cities in which typhoid fever is still common fit in group 1 or 2 or perhaps partially overlap the two. Examples are Mexico City, Mexico; Santiago, Chile; Cairo, Egypt; and Bombay, India. The provision of safe water supplies to all parts of every society will result in a dramatic drop in all enteric infections.

5.4. Temporal Distribution

Most cases of typhoid fever reported from endemic areas occur during the summer months. The cases acquired by United States tourists usually occur in the summer, coinciding with the peak travel time. The remaining cases appear sporadically during the year.

5.5. Age

In endemic areas, the highest attack rate occurs in children ages 8–13. The preferential attack rate for children is similar to those of other enteric infections and suggests that the disease is acquired with the first exposure to an infectious inoculum. Older citizens appear to be relatively immune, presumably because of frequently reinforced acquired immunity, i.e., numerous subinfectious exposures to typhoid bacilli. In this country, those most likely to acquire the disease at home are adults under age 30.[41,42] Three-fourths of 857 patients reported between 1975 and 1984 were in this age range. Median age was 20.[41] The travel-associated cases had a median age of 23. Persons of these ages had no background immunity, having been born and raised in a country where the disease is no longer prevalent (0.2 cases/100,000 since 1966, 1 case/100,000 in 1955, and about 3 cases/100,000 in 1945). Having no opportunity to develop specific natural immunity, a steadily increasing susceptible population will evolve. When these persons travel to endemic areas or are exposed to accidental con-

tamination of food or water, increasing age will not have any protective value. Furthermore, vaccine-induced immunity (especially with inactivated vaccine) appears to be most effective when added to background naturally acquired immunity.[61] In volunteer studies, the live attenuated vaccine did induce excellent immunity while the killed vaccines induced very little protection in a population that had minimal prior exposure to *S. typhi*.

While the median age of persons with typhoid fever was 22 to 24 years in the period 1984 to 1986, the median age of carriers in those years was 71, 58, and 69 years, respectively.

5.6. Sex

There is no effect of sex on the incidence of typhoid fever; both sexes are equally susceptible. However, there is a threefold greater incidence of female carriers. Known clinical reasons for this difference include primarily the increased occurrence of gallbladder disease in women. The deleterious effect on gallbladder function consequent to pregnancies can lead to inadequate and incomplete emptying. When typhoid bacilli reach this organ, they are not readily cleared. A subclinical infection of the mucosal lining occurs and may lead to the formation of stones, with typhoid bacilli serving as the nidi of the stones. Whether there are immunological defects in carriers that contribute to the development of the carrier state remains to be proven. Such a defect has been proposed[11] (see Section 7.1) but there is no known immunological reason that this should be sex-linked.

5.7. Race

There are no data to support racial susceptibility to typhoid fever. While many series indicate that more blacks have typhoid fever, it is probable that the living conditions, e.g., poor sanitary conditions, are the precipitating factor, not race. In volunteer studies, no evidence of race-associated susceptibility could be detected.

5.8. Occupation

There is no occupation that has stood out as a special risk for acquiring typhoid fever. There have been groups of soldiers and students who have acquired the disease because of exposure to food prepared by cooks who were carriers. However, there should be less chance of these outbreaks as cooks are required to take more stringent preemployment health examinations that include examination of stool specimens. Cooks who are carriers obviously pose a great threat of causing outbreaks. However, cooks are not at any increased risk to become carriers. Their job does not expose them to a frequent source of *S. typhi*. Since the organism is a human pathogen, it should not be part of the flora on the surface of meats they prepare. One exception to this statement was the epidemic in Glasgow, Scotland, in which canned meats were contaminated by river water used to cool the cans after sterilization and *S. typhi* gained access to the meat via incompetent seams in the can[3] (for detailed discussion, see Section 5.2).

5.9. Occurrence in Different Settings

The propensity for typhoid to occur in varying settings is great. There are multiple unique opportunities for a carrier to be involved either directly or indirectly. Examples of such outbreaks include an epidemic in Germany at a picnic for United States servicemen and their families.[15] This outbreak involved 62 patients (14% of those ingesting the incriminated meal prepared by a carrier). At a fraternity house in Stanford University, 26 students became ill.[53] The food-preparation area was thought to be contaminated by a toilet leaking through the ceiling into the kitchen. The large epidemic noted earlier (Section 5.1) in Dade County, Florida, in a migrant-worker camp caused illness in 222 people.[16] The source was a carrier who probably inadvertently infected the water supply. Numerous accounts of outbreaks occurring after banquets prepared by volunteer workers, such as at church functions, have been reported.[35,43] In these affairs, unknown carriers help prepare large quantities of food. Given the likelihood of poor sanitary conditions in the facility where the food is prepared and improper refrigeration of large quantities of food plus an unknown carrier, typhoid will occur. In the outbreaks reported from various military camps, especially those that occurred in the Middle East in the last 1940s,[2,34] native cooks who were unscreened carriers were responsible for the presence of typhoid bacilli in the food. Similar outbreaks should be seen with less and less frequency in the future as the number of carriers declines.

5.10. Socioeconomic Factors

The association of poverty with inadequate sanitary facilities and questionable water supplies enhances the op-

portunity for this segment of the world's population to acquire every type of enteric infection, but especially typhoid fever. The unique adaptation of *S. typhi* to humans and the survival characteristics of this organism make it a particular threat to spread among a population living under substandard sanitary conditions. Prior to the availability of good water and sewer systems, all strata of society were at risk. The present endemic regions of the world exist primarily because the poorer segments of the population remain in areas underserved by adequate water and sewer services and lack of detection and restriction of carriers. Provision of clear water and good sewers will largely eliminate typhoid fever from endemic loci.

5.11. Other Factors

There is no reliable evidence indicating increased or decreased susceptibility of patients with malnutrition to typhoid fever. The untreated disease causes a severe metabolic drain, so illness in a host with undernutrition will create a double hazard. Patients with various parasitic infections such as roundworms or schistosomes are readily infected with *S. typhi*. In the first instance, typhoid fever in the host will cause the roundworms to migrate out through the mouth, anus, and, rarely, umbilicus. Reasons for this exodus from the gut are unknown. Schistosomiasis causes tissue-scarring and obstruction, especially in the genitourinary tract by *Schistosoma haematobium*, and *S. typhi* can remain indefinitely in the scar tissue or in the trematode itself.[25] Furthermore, salmonellae contain type I pili that allow adherence to the glycolipids on the surface of the worm.[36] This results in recurrent bacteremia in the host without any clinical evidence of typhoid fever.

6. Mechanisms and Routes of Transmission

The typhoid bacilli enter the host by the oral route. Transmission is usually mediated by food or water. The disease has been shown to be one of the several enteric infections that can be sexually transmitted.[13] Such transmission occurs in homosexual sexual partners.

Flies have been shown to be able to carry *S. typhi* on their legs and theoretically may be a means of food contamination. However, it is more likely that the feces of an asymptomatic carrier is the source of contamination of both the food and the flies.

7. Pathogenesis and Immunity

7.1. Pathogenesis

In natural disease, the incubation period ranges from 1 to 3 weeks. When ingested in food or water, typhoid bacilli probably do not penetrate the mucosal lining of the oral pharynx, but are swallowed. In the stomach, the gastric acid will inactivate many of the organisms, but when they are ingested in water, the exposure to acid is probably short, since there is little retention in the stomach as the water rapidly proceeds through the pylorus into the small bowel. Some foods may also serve as a buffer to reduce the effectiveness of the acid barrier. There is no evidence of penetration through gastric mucosa by S. typhi. Biopsies obtained from the duodenum and upper jejunum in the late stages of the incubation period or during disease in volunteers who ingested large inocula of typhi bacilli revealed an inflammatory response in the lamina propria.[49] This infiltrate consisted primarily of monocytic cells, and even in the one biopsy obtained just before clinical symptoms appeared, these same cells were seen. In addition, degenerative changes were noted in the epithelial-cell layer and in the crypt glands. Occasionally, a microulcer was seen. It was assumed that all these changes occurred as a consequence of the multiple yet random penetrations through the epithelial cells by the ingested typhoid bacilli. All the observed changes were reversible. These biopsies were obtained proximally to the lymph follicles and Peyer's patches; thus, no involvement of these structures could be documented. Other studies, mainly autopsy analyses, have amply confirmed the marked inflammatory responses that occur in the distal ileum where Peyer's patches and other lymphocytic-cell accumulations are common. Presumably, the intracellular location of the organism and the local concentration of endotoxin are responsible for these cellular changes.[29] It is from these lesions in the distal ileum and ascending colon that hemorrhage can occur. Gross bleeding comes from eroded vessels in or near the Peyer's patches. This complication occurs late in the 2nd week of about 5% of untreated patients and rarely in patients whose treatment with an appropriate antibiotic is begun late in their clinical course. Perforations of the bowel wall occur in the same sections of the gut as the hemorrhages. Presumably, both these complications occur as a consequence of local tissue concentrations of endotoxin accumulated as the typhoid bacilli multiply and die.[29]

S. typhi localized in the lamina propria area are phagocytized by leukocytes and monocytes. During this process, there is the release of endogenous pyrogen and the stimulus to trigger the fever-producing mechanisms located in the anterior hypothalamus. Even though the organisms are ingested by the leukocytes or monocytes, they can survive longer than many other bacteria. There appears to be eventual killing inside the phagocytes, but it is delayed. This may allow the organism to escape from the site of phagocytosis and be transmitted to the liver or other elements of the reticuloendothelial system. It is in the cells of this organ that further multiplication occurs during the incubation phase.

When the organisms break out into the bloodstream, the symptoms of typhoid fever appear. Blood cultures are often positive with the first symptoms of disease. The bacteremia will persist for 2 weeks if antibiotic therapy is not given, and the blood may be seeded from the liver as well as the lesions in the intestinal tract. The symptoms and signs of typhoid fever may not be due to circulating endotoxin. Most patients have no detectable serum concentrations by the limulus assay.[9] However, in those patients who present with septic shock syndrome, circulating endotoxin can be demonstrated.[27] These patients have a higher mortality rate and require combination therapy of steroids and antibiotics. As noted above, the local concentrations of endotoxin may be contributing to the fever by stimulating inflammatory responses, by causing vasoconstriction severe enough to produce ischemia, or by direct cell destruction.

The incubation period of typhoid fever is inversely related to the inoculum size. In the volunteer model, the figures shown in Table 1 were obtained. These figures applied to the volunteers who developed disease and were given antibiotic therapy. There were some who did not receive treatment because of mild infections. The mean incubation period for this group, which had received 100,000 organisms, was 13 days. Persons known to have received vaccine during military service or who were given vaccines as part of the volunteer program and who developed disease after ingesting 100,000 S. typhi bacilli had prolongation of their incubation periods. The combination of prior military history and vaccine administered as part of the study ex-

Table 1.   Incubation Periods of Typhoid Fever Related to Size of Infecting Dose

Dose	Attack rate	Mean incubation period
100,000	38%	13 days
10,000,000	50%	11 days
1,000,000,000	90%	5.8 days

tended the incubation period to an average of 19 days. It is apparent that prior vaccine administration will prolong the incubation period. This study also allowed an analysis of the incubation periods of those volunteers who underwent a relapse of their infection after receiving antibiotic treatment. There was a statistically significant difference between those who did and those who did not relapse after the 100,000 dose, 9.7 versus 13.2 days ($p < 0.02$). Whether this shortened incubation period indicates a defect in immune mechanisms that allows a relapse to occur is unknown. Relapses have been recorded in about 8% of patients suffering from typhoid fever in the preantibiotic era. The rate in patients treated with antibiotics ranges from 15 to 35%. The rate appears to increase with earlier institution of treatment and may indicate an interference with the development of effective immunity. The source of the organisms that initiate the relapse appears to be the elements of the reticuloendothelial system. Typhoid bacilli can be isolated from liver biopsies during the relapse, and also from bone marrow many months after the patient has fully recovered from the symptoms. However, relapses occur only about 3 weeks after the last febrile day or about 2 weeks after the antibiotic was stopped. Most relapses are milder than the symptoms of the initial illness and last for only a few days. Antibiotic therapy effects a quick resolution of symptoms and signs.

The pathogenesis of the carrier state has never been clearly defined. Suitable animal models to allow a better understanding have not been developed. It is known that three times as many females as males become carriers, as many as 3% following acute cases of typhoid fever. Many of these carriers have asymptomatic disease. One study has defined a defect in ability to produce IgM antibodies to Vi antigen in carriers.[11] It is apparent that gallstones or a nonfunctioning gallbladder predisposes to the carrier state. *S. typhi* can remain inside stones and not be affected by antibodies or antibiotics in the *in vivo* situation. *In vitro*, contaminated stones placed in test tubes filled with disinfectants will protect the bacilli from the chemical destruction. Carriers shed as many as 10^{11} organisms/g feces.[37] These organisms are propelled the length of the gastrointestinal tract without penetrating and causing disease in the host. There is a remarkably effective barrier that keeps the bacilli in the gut lumen. The nature of these immune processes requires specific elucidation.

7.2. Immunity

Mechanisms involved in the immunity of typhoid fever are unknown. Several investigations have shown *in vitro*

evidence of activation of various cellular immune functions during the disease.[3] Current thinking focuses on these mechanisms rather than humoral antibodies as the primary defense mechanism as well as elements needed to recover from the acute disease. There is no correlation between levels of antibodies to O, H, or Vi antigens and ability to resist infection by the volunteers in the studies previously mentioned.[29] Individuals who had received one or more previous doses of vaccine were more immune than controls, but this immunity could not be correlated with levels of circulating antibodies. How cellular immune mechanisms prevent disease is unknown. Conceivably, organisms are blocked from penetration into the circulation at the level of the epithelial surface or perhaps in the lamina propria in immune persons. A new oral vaccine, consisting of an attenuated strain of *S. typhi,* has induced excellent immunity in the volunteer model as well as in field trials.[24] This vaccine does induce increased bactericidal activity in the gut, since volunteers receiving this vaccine had very few positive stool cultures for the virulent challenge strain compared to controls. The cause of this bacterial killing has not been identified.

8. Patterns of Host Response

There is a wide spectrum of clinical syndromes associated with infection by *S. typhi*.[8,50,52] Many persons exposed to small numbers of bacteria will be asymptomatic and probably show no signs of infection. There is a small percentage of individuals who have been identified in various epidemics and in the volunteer studies who develop bacteremia but are symptom-free.[47] Perhaps it is from this population that many carriers have developed. As noted above, most carriers, when detected, do not recall having had the disease.[48] They are frequently aware of typhoid fever having been present in some other member of the family in the remote past. Those persons who develop disease may have a short-lived mild clinical course. However, the majority of patients with the disease have a relatively uniform course. Several papers have pointed out the atypical presentation of children who developed typhoid fever.[8,52] The unusual symptoms delayed diagnosis.

8.1. Clinical Features

The major signs and symptoms of typhoid fever are relatively nonspecific. There is fever and an associated moderately severe generalized headache. The temperature increases in a stepwise fashion over the course of 2–3 days, reaching a peak of 103–104°F. During this time, the patient also complains of abdominal pain and is constipated. Examination of the abdomen will reveal palpation tenderness in the lower quadrants. Often, one can palpate dilated loops of bowel and sense the displacement of air and fluid under the probing fingers. This indicates that an ileus is present, a probable consequence of the inflammatory process occurring in the lamina propria and Peyer's patches. Late in the 1st week, careful inspection of the skin may reveal a few rose spots. These are slightly raised erythematous, nontender lesions found in light-skinned persons in the anterior chest or abdominal areas. They initially will blanch with pressure, but gradually remain fixed as small cutaneous hemorrhages. These lesions are caused by *S. typhi* organisms infiltrating the endothelial cells of skin capillaries and inducing a perivascular infiltrate and subsequent leaking of blood. Biopsy of fresh rose spots will yield the organism.[22]

The course of the disease in untreated patients is characterized by a continuous fever with a relative bradycardia. The continuous fever will persist for 2 weeks or longer if no antibiotic is given, and defervescence occurs slowly over the ensuing 2–3 weeks. Such patients have a prolonged convalescence (3–4 months) because of the severe negative nitrogen balance that is a consequence of the prolonged infection. Patients who are receiving an appropriate antibiotic will respond with a gradual reduction in the fever over a 3- to 5-day period.

Complications are the significant prognostic indicators. Gastrointestinal hemorrhage[58] or perforation is responsible for almost all the fatalities with this disease. Both these events occur after about 2 weeks of untreated disease. The signs and symptoms of a perforated loop of intestine, presenting as an acute abdominal crisis, are well known. Failure to recognize its occurrence will almost surely lead to death of the patient.

8.2. Diagnosis

The diagnosis should be suspected in any patient with fever, abdominal pain, constipation, and headache. A prior history of travel to an endemic area will be an alerting epidemiological fact that should be followed up by appropriate blood and stool cultures. Because of the long incubation period—2 weeks or longer—a thorough epidemiological history should be taken, since the patient may be the index case of a local outbreak. It is important to notify local health authorities promptly.

Typhoid bacilli appear in the blood with the onset of fever, and in untreated patients bacteremia remains for about 2 weeks before abating. The number of organisms in the blood is low, usually less than $50/cm^3$ cultured blood. In most series and in the volunteer model,[29] only about 75–85% of patients can be shown to have positive blood cultures. Diagnosis is confirmed in the other patients by stool culture or serological evidence. Stool cultures become positive shortly after ingestion of the organism and may become negative with onset of disease, but may again yield the organism by the end of the 1st week of disease. Without therapy, stools may readily remain positive for *S. typhi* for as long as 4 months; beyond this period, continued presence indicates a greater than 90% chance of being a permanent carrier. Antibiotic treatment may cause temporary suppression of the isolation of typhoid bacilli from stools during the therapy. Few adequately treated patients (6% of volunteers) continued to shed organisms in stools beyond 1 month.

The antibodies to O and H antigens may appear during the end of the 1st week of illness and peak by the end of the 3rd week of illness. The Vi antibodies are slow to appear and may increase only fourfold in titer by 1 month. The O antibodies tend to fall in titer more rapidly than the H. It is unknown why as many as a third of patients with bacteriologically confirmed disease do not develop significant O and H titer rises. In some of the volunteers with induced disease, the baseline titers prior to challenge with virulent *S. typhi* were undetectable or low, e.g., 1:20 or 1:40 for O antibodies, yet no rise in titer occurred during the entire time of the prolonged follow-up. These men also had bacteremia and positive stool cultures, an obvious source of antigens. No ready explanation is apparent for the lack of a diagnostic antibody response.

The differential diagnosis will include other infectious agents that may cause an enteric-fever-like syndrome such as tularemia and other salmonellae. Brucellosis, infectious mononucleosis, and infectious hepatitis may initially be confused because of similar symptoms associated with these febrile illnesses. Leptospirosis may occur with significant abdominal findings and mimic typhoid.

9. Control and Prevention

9.1. General Concepts

Control of typhoid fever requires knowledge of carriers, control of their occupational activities, and, most important, safe water supplies and effective sewage systems. All patients with the disease must be reported to the local health department. Patients should have enteric precautions. There is no need to disinfect feces prior to flushing in a toilet in this country; the typhoid bacilli will be destroyed in the treatment plant. Linen soiled by feces should be handled with disposable gloves. Hands should be scrupulously washed following contact with the patient.

Carriers, when discovered, are frequently elderly, e.g., grandmothers, and not willing or able to undergo the rigorous treatment needed to cure the carrier state. The approach to treatment requires a careful assessment of the functioning of the gallbladder. If there is no demonstrable dysfunction and no stones present, therapy with large daily doses of ampicillin (6–10 g i.v.) or amoxicillin for 6–9 weeks will often effect a cure.[38] When stones are present, only cholecystectomy under the cover of ampicillin treatment offers any hope of cure. With the removal of the gallbladder, cure is achieved in about 80% of patients.[17]

Local health departments maintain variable levels of surveillance of carriers. In some areas, these patients are required to submit stool specimens once or twice a year to confirm the continued presence of *S. typhi;* in other areas, only a listing is maintained. Carriers are prevented from working in any position that could result in contamination of food or drinking water. This type of control is lacking in most endemic areas, and hence typhoid fever can remain as a common disease.

9.2. Antibiotic and Chemotherapeutic Approaches to Prophylaxis

There is no evidence to indicate the usefulness of prophylactic antibiotic treatment in preventing disease. There is other evidence to suggest that such treatment would not be practical. In tissue cultures, typhoid bacilli persist in the intracellular environment despite adequate concentrations of antibiotics in the solution containing the cells.[46] The organisms were found to be viable after 21 days of this experiment, indicating that the intracellular habitat protected them from the antibiotics. No multiplication occurred until the antibiotic was removed from the medium. As part of the volunteer study adduced throughout this chapter, four men were begun on chloramphenicol treatment 24 h after ingesting the 90% infective dose (ID_{90}) of *S. typhi.*[29] In the two who took the drug for 6 days, the incubation period was delayed by that same period compared to controls. Two men were maintained on chloramphenicol for 28 days, and no disease developed, although there were positive signs of infection, e.g., positive stool cultures and antibody titer rises. There is no justification for employing prophylactic antibiotics to prevent typhoid fever. The variable attack rate after known exposure makes it impractical to attempt pro-

phylaxis. If known exposure has occurred, as at a church supper, it is much more clinically prudent to follow the potential patients closely and treat at the first signs of illness, after obtaining blood and stool cultures. Under these circumstances, treatment with chloramphenicol or ampicillin (amoxicillin) or trimethoprim–sulfamethoxazole will prevent complications by limiting the progression of the disease, and the patient should have a satisfactory recovery. Some strains of *S. typhi* are resistant to these antibiotics. The third-generation cephalosporin antibiotics, such as cefaperazone, have been utilized in several field trials and the associated cure rates have been excellent.

9.3. Immunization

Typhoid vaccine is not required for travel to endemic areas. It will cause tenderness at the site of injection, febrile reactions are not uncommon, and general malaise may accompany the fever. These reactions are due to the endotoxin contained in the vaccine.

Typhoid vaccine was developed and first used in 1896 in England.[60] It consisted of a heat-killed suspension of the whole organism. Subsequently, the vaccine enjoyed wide use in military units. However, no well-controlled double-blind study of vaccine efficacy was carried out until the WHO established a multicountry evaluation in the mid-1950s.[4,12,26,61] These studies were conducted in endemic areas and thus involved persons previously exposed to *S. typhi*. Children and adults were involved and were to have received two doses of one of three vaccines. One was a heat-killed, phenol-fixed suspension of whole organisms (L). The second was an acetone-dried, killed suspension (K) This form of vaccine preparation preserved the antigenicity of the Vi antigen to a greater extent than the phenol treatment. The third vaccine was tetanus toxoid used as a placebo. In several areas of the world where the vaccines were tested, the K vaccine gave superior results compared to the L vaccine in both children and adults. Protection was also apparent in the group who received the L vaccine compared to the placebo group. This protection was present for at least 8 years, and in children it seems that one dose of vaccine induced resistance equal to that following two doses. In the volunteer model, these same vaccines were tested, but in a population not residing in an endemic area and hence a population with less background immunity. Also, only adults were investigated. These studies clearly showed that protection from disease was related to the challenge dose of organisms. No evidence of immunity was noted following the ID_{50} or ID_{90} challenge level. When 100,000 bacilli were used, protection from disease was 67%

for the K and 75% for the L vaccine, a statistically significant difference compared to the controls. Collectively, all evidence indicates that the killed parenteral vaccines reduce the attack rate of disease in an exposed population, but that protection can be overcome by large challenge doses of bacteria. In nature, waterborne disease is probably caused by fewer than 10^5 bacteria, but food could allow for multiplication and ingestion of 10^7 or more organisms. Vaccine K is now the standard for routine military use. It should not be given intradermally, since local reactions may result. The use of the intradermal route had been advocated by some authors for the phenol vaccine.[30,55] The advantage was to prevent systemic reactions by using a smaller dose, 0.1 versus 0.5 ml. The antigenic stimulation is similar. It should be noted that patients will occasionally develop foreign-body granulomas after receiving vaccine by this route.[44]

Finally, one epidemic occurred in Yugoslavia that emphasizes the need to use proper sanitary techniques to prevent disease and not rely solely on vaccine-induced immunity. A small town, Pristina, was part of the WHO double-blind study of typhoid vaccines.[61] A breakdown in the sewer pipes caused contamination of the water supply, resulting in an outbreak of typhoid fever. Analysis of the exposed population revealed the following: attack rates in the vaccine groups were 3.9/1000 for the K group, 5.9 for the L group, 12.9 for the tetanus toxoid control group, and an overall rate of 7.5/1000 for all those participating in the study. The attack rate in the nonparticipant group was astonishingly high, 81.8/1000, over six times the rate in the group that received "placebo" vaccine. These data indicate the importance of motivation in such a double-blind study. Presumably, those persons who were willing to be a part of the study informed themselves about the nature of the disease, including means of spread, and at the time of the high risk of disease took necessary steps to prevent ingestion of the organisms. They boiled water prior to use and were careful about hand-washing and the preparation of food. On the other hand, those persons not convinced to be a part of the study apparently took few or none of these precautions out of either ignorance or an unbelieving attitude. Planners at the WHO appreciate the need in future campaigns to get vaccine to this uninformed segment of the population.

A new vaccine is currently being field tested that promises to be more effective and free from postvaccine side effects.[24] It consists of a suspension of living attenuated *S. typhi* that is administered in large doses by mouth. The attenuation is due to the incomplete synthesis of the cell wall: essentially, the polysaccharide side chains in the outer coat are incomplete.[21] An enzyme epimerase, which is needed to synthesize these chains, is lacking in this strain.

The organism is osmotically destroyed in the gut lumen because of the incomplete cell wall. This feature adds to the safety of the vaccine. No evidence of reversion to a fully virulent form has been found. In the volunteer model, large doses of this strain induced protection against disease in 87% of the volunteers. The attack rates for disease were 7% for the vaccine group and 51% for the controls.[24] Protection appears to be mediated by stimulation of bactericidal systems in the gut. Stool cultures were rarely positive in those who received the vaccine compared to controls. In field trials conducted with children in endemic areas, preliminary reports indicate outstanding efficacy without any side effects.[56] Should these excellent results continue, a vaccine that not only prevents the host from developing disease but also markedly decreases the shedding of organisms will have been developed. Its use in endemic areas and for travelers will influence favorably the struggle to eliminate typhoid fever.

The Vi antigen has been tried in animals and man with mixed results.[29] Conceivably, this antigen could be an effective vaccine, since Vi antigens appear to enhance the virulence of *S. typhi*. Recent field trials using a highly purified Vi antigen as a vaccine have shown it to be both safe and as effective as other vaccines, both killed and oral attenuated.[31] Protection in children at 17 to 21 months was 64 to 75%.

10. Unresolved Problems

Several important elements of the immune mechanisms involved in the recovery from typhoid fever need to be identified. The role of cellular immune functions in this process is not well defined. Further delineation of intestinal resistance factors is necessary to understand why typhoid carriers do not reinfect themselves as billions of the causative agent pass through the gut. Also, this understanding is important in assessing the efficacy of the new oral vaccines. The major unresolved problem is to find the economic means to provide clean water supplies to all the world's population and thereby help to eliminate most enteric infections.

11. References

1. AMES, W. R., AND ROBINS, M., Age and sex as factors in the development of the typhoid carrier state, and a method for estimating carrier prevalence, *Am. J. Public Health* **33**:221–230 (1943).

2. ANDERSON, E. S., AND RICHARD, H. G. H., An outbreak of typhoid fever in the Middle East, *J. Hyg.* **46**:146 (1948).

3. ASH, I., MCKENDRICK, G. D. W., ROBERTSON, M. H., AND HUGHES, H. L., Outbreak of typhoid fever connected with corned beef, *Br. Med. J.* **1**:1474–1478 (1964).

4. ASHCROFT, M. T., Immunization against typhoid and paratyphoid fevers, *Clin. Pediatr.* **3**(7):385–393 (1964).

5. BERNARD, R. P., The Zermatt typhoid outbreak in 1963, *J. Hyg.* **63**:537–563 (1965).

6. BOKKENHEUSER, V., SMIT, P., AND RICHARDSON, N., A challenge to the validity of the Vi test for the detection of chronic typhoid carriers, *Am. J. Public Health* **54**:1507 (1964).

7. BRETONNEAU, P., Notice sur la contagion de la dothinentérie, *Arch. Gen. Med.* **21**:57 (1829).

8. BRIEDIS, D. J., AND ROBSON, H. G., Epidemiologic and clinical features of sporadic *Salmonella* enteric fever, *Can. Med. Assoc. J.* **119**:1183–1187 (1978).

9. BUTLER, T., BELL, W. R., LEVIN, J., LINN, N. N., AND ARNOLD, K., Typhoid fever: Studies of blood coagulation, bacteremia and endotoxemia, *Arch. Intern. Med.* **138**:407–410 (1978).

10. Centers for Disease Control, Surveillance Summaries, Salmonella isolates from humans in the United States, 1984–1986, *Morbid. Mortal. Weekly Rep.* **37**(SS-2):25–31 (1988).

11. CHERNOKHVOSTOVA, E., LUXEMBURG, K. I., STARSHINOVA, V., ANDREEVA, N., AND GERMAN, G., Study on the production of IgG-, IgA- and IgM-antibodies to somatic antigens of *Salmonella typhi* in humans, *Clin. Exp. Immunol.* **4**:407–421 (1969).

12. CVJETANOVIĆ, B., AND UEMURA, K., The present status of field and laboratory studies of typhoid and paratyphoid vaccines: With special reference to studies sponsored by the World Health Organization, *Bull. WHO* **32**:29–36 (1965).

13. DRITZ, S. K., AND BRAFF, E. H., Sexually transmitted typhoid fever, *N. Engl. J. Med.* **296**:1359 (1977).

14. EBERTH, C. J., Die Organismen in den Organen bei Typhus abdominalis, *Virchows Arch. Pathol. Anat. Physiol.* **81**:58–74 (1880).

15. EDWARDS, W. M., CRONE, R. I., AND HARRIS, J. F., Outbreak of typhoid fever in previously immunized persons traced to a common carrier, *N. Engl. J. Med.* **267**:742–751 (1962).

16. FELDMAN, R. E., BAINE, W. B., NITZKIN, J. L., SASLAW, M. S., AND POLLARD, R. A., JR., Epidemiology of *Salmonella typhi* infection in a migrant labor camp in Dade County, Florida, *J. Infect. Dis.* **130**:334–342 (1974).

17. FREITAG, J. L., Treatment of chronic typhoid carriers by cholecystectomy, *Public Health Rep.* **79**:567–570 (1964).

18. GAFFKY, G., Zur Aeatiologie der Abdominal Typhus, *Mitt. Gesundheitsamte* **2**:372–570 (1884).

19. GANGAROSA, E. J., BENNETT, J. V., WYATT, C., PIERCE, P. E., OLARTE, S., HERNANDES, P. M., VAZQUEZ, V., AND BESSUDO, D. M., An epidemic-associated episome? *J. Infect. Dis.* **126**:215–218 (1972).

20. GERHARD, W. W., On the typhus fever, which occurred at Philadelphia in the spring and summer of 1836, illustrated by clinical observations at the Philadelphia hospital showing the distinction between this form of disease and dothienteritis or the typhoid fever with alteration of the follicles of the small intestine, *Am. J. Med. Sci.* **19**:289 (1836), **20**:289 (1837).

21. GERMANIER, R., AND FURER, E., Isolation and characterization of *S. typhi* gal E mutant Ty 21a: A candidate strain for a live oral typhoid vaccine, *J. Infect. Dis.* **131**:553–558 (1975).

22. GILMAN, R. H., TERMINEL, M., LEVINE, M. M., HERNANDEZ-MENDOZA, P., AND HORNICK, R. B., Relative efficacy of blood, urine, rectal swab, bone-marrow, and rose-spot cultures for recovery of *Salmonella typhi* in typhoid fever, *Lancet* **1**:1211–1213 (1975).

23. GILMAN, R. H., TERMINEL, M., LEVINE, M. M., HERNANDEZ-MENDOZA, P., CALDERONE, E., VASQUEZ, V., MARTINEZ, E., SNYDER, M. J., AND HORNICK, R. B., Comparison of trimethoprim-sulfamethoxazole and amoxicillin in therapy of chloramphenicol-resistant and chloramphenicol-sensitive typhoid fever, *J. Infect. Dis.* **132**:630–636 (1975).

24. GILMAN, R. H., HORNICK, R. B., WOODWARD, W. E., DUPONT, H. L., SNYDER, M. J., LEVINE, M. M., AND LIBONATI, J. P., Evaluation of UDP-glucose-4-epimeraseless mutant of *Salmonella typhi* as a live oral vaccine, *J. Infect. Dis.* **136**:717 (1977).

25. HATHOUT, S. E., EL-GHAFFAR, Y. A., AWNY, A. Y., AND HASSAN, K., Relation between urinary schistosomiasis and chronic enteric urinary carrier state among Egyptians, *Am. J. Trop. Med.* **15**:156–161 (1966).

26. HEJFEC, L. B., Results of the study of typhoid vaccine in four controlled field trials in the USSR, *Bull. WHO* **32**:1–14 (1965).

27. HOFFMAN, S. L., PUNJABI, N. H., KUMALA, S., MOECHTAR, M. A., PULUNGSIK, S. P., RIVAI, A. R., ROCKHILL, R. C., WOODWARD, T. E., AND LOEDIN, A. A., Reduction of mortality in chloramphenicol-treated severe typhoid fever by high-dose dexamethasone, *N. Engl. J. Med.* **310**:82–88 (1984).

28. HOLMES, M. B., JOHNSON, D. L., FIUMARA, N. J., AND McCORMACK, W. M., Acquisition of typhoid fever from proficiency-testing specimens, *N. Engl. J. Med.* **303**:519–521 (1980).

29. HORNICK, R. B., GREISMAN, S. E., WOODWARD, T. E., DUPONT, H. L., DAWKINS, A. T., AND SNYDER, M. J., Typhoid fever: Pathogenesis and immunologic control, *N. Engl. J. Med.* **283**:686–691, 739–746 (1970).

30. IWARSON, S., AND LARSSON, P., Intradermal versus subcutaneous immunization with typhoid vaccine, *J. Hyg.* **84**:11–16 (1980).

31. KLUGMAN, K. P., KOORNOF, H. S., SCHNEERSON, R., CADOZ, M., GILBERTSON, I. T., ROBBINS, J. B., SCHULTZ, D., AND ARMAND, J., Protective activity of Vi capsular polysaccharide vaccine against typhoid fever, *Lancet* **2**:1165–1169 (1987).

32. LOONEY, R. J., AND STEIGBIGEL, R. T., Role of the Vi antigen of *Salmonella typhi* in resistance to host defense in vitro, *J. Lab. Clin. Med.* **108**:506–516 (1986).

33. MALAVIYA, K. A. N., MURPHY, R. G. S., VENKATARAMAN,

M., AND MOHAPATRA, L. N., Immunological study of typhoid: Immunoglobulins, C3, antibodies, and leukocyte migration inhibition in patients with typhoid fever and TAB-vaccinated individuals, *Infect. Immun.* **10**:1219–1225 (1974).

34. MARMION, D. E., NAYLOR, G. R. E., AND STEWART, I. O., Second attacks of typhoid fever, *J. Hyg.* **51**:260–267 (1953).

35. MEANS, J. H., Reflections on typhoid fever, *King's Coll. Hosp. Gaz.* **39**:270–278 (1960).

36. MELHAM, R. F., AND LoVERDE, P. T., Mechanism of interaction of Salmonellae and Schistosoma species, *Infect. Immun.* **44**:274–281 (1984).

37. MERSELIS, J. G., JR., KAYE, D., CONNOLLY, C. S., AND HOOK, E. W., Quantitative bacteriology of the typhoid carrier state, *Am. J. Trop. Med. Hyg.* **13**:425–429 (1964).

38. NOLAN, C. M., AND WHITE, P. C., JR., Treatment of typhoid carriers with amoxicillin, *J. Am. Med. Assoc.* **239**:2352–2354 (1978).

39. OVERTURF, G., MARTON, K. I., AND MATHIES, A. W., Antibiotic resistance in typhoid fever: Chloramphenicol resistance among clinical isolates of *Salmonella typhosa* in Los Angeles, 1972—Epidemiologic and bacteriologic characteristics, *N. Engl. J. Med.* **289**:463–465 (1973).

40. PROTELL, R. L., SOLOWAY, R. D., AND MARTIN, W. J., Antisalmonella agglutinins in chronic active liver disease, *Lancet* **2**:330–331 (1971).

41. RYAN, C. A., HARGRETT-BEAN, N. T., AND BLAKE, P. A., *Salmonella typhi* infections in the United States, 1975–1984: Increasing role of foreign travel, *Rev. Infect. Dis.* **11**:1–8 (1989).

42. RYDER, R. W., AND BLAKE, P. A., Typhoid fever in the United States, 1975 and 1976, *J. Infect. Dis.* **139**:124–126 (1979).

43. SAWYER, W. A., Ninety-three persons infected by a typhoid carrier at a public dinner, *J. Am. Med. Assoc.* **63**:1537 (1914).

44. SCHNEIDMAN, H. M., AND STEINBERG, J., Reactions to intradermal vaccinations: A report of three cases of foreign body granulomas, *Calif. Med.* **100**:287–289 (1964).

45. SCHUBERT, J. H., EDWARDS, P. R., AND RAMSEY, C. H., Detection of typhoid carriers by agglutination tests, *J. Bacteriol.* **77**:648–654 (1959).

46. SHOWACRE, J. L., HOPPS, H. E., DuBUY, H. G., AND SMODEL, J. E., Effect of antibiotics on intracellular *Salmonella typhosa*. I. Demonstration by phase microscopy of prompt inhibition of intracellular multiplication, *J. Immunol.* **87**:153–174 (1961).

47. SNYDER, M. J., HORNICK, R. G., McCRUMB, F. R., MORSE, L. S., AND WOODWARD, T. E., Asymptomatic typhoidal bacteremia in volunteers, *Antimicrob. Agents Chemother.* **3**:604–607 (1963).

48. SOPER, G. A., The curious career of Typhoid Mary, *Bull. N.Y. Acad. Med.* **15**:698–712 (1939).

49. SPRINTZ, H., GANGAROSA, E. J., WILLIAMS, H., HORNICK, R. B., AND WOODWARD, T. E., Histopathology of the upper small intestines in typhoid fever, *Am. J. Dig. Dis.* N. Ser. **11**:615 (1966).

50. STUART, B. M., AND PULLEN, R. L., Typhoid, *Arch. Intern. Med.* **78**:629–661 (1946).

51. TIGERTT, W. D., The initial effort to immunize American soldier volunteers with typhoid vaccine, *Mil. Med.* **124**:342–349 (1959).

52. TOLAYMAT, A., FAKHREDDINE, F., DAVID, C. B., AND WHITWORTH, J. M., Typhoid fever in children: A forgotten disease? *South. Med. J.* **72**:136–138 (1979).

53. TORIN, D. E., BETTS, S. L., McCLENAHAN, J. B., PHILLIPS, G. M., AND SHIKAMURA, M. J., A typhoid fever outbreak on a university campus, *Arch. Intern. Med.* **124**:606–610 (1969).

54. VÁZQUEZ, V., CALDERÓN, E., AND RODRÍGUEZ, R., Chloramphenicol-resistant strains of *Salmonella typhosa*, *N. Engl. J. Med.* **286**:1220 (1972).

55. VOGELSANG, T. M., WETTELAND, P., AND WORMINES, A., Intradermal versus subcutaneous immunization with typhoid–paratyphoid A and B vaccine in human adults. 1. Antibody response, *Acta Pathol. Microbiol. Scand.* **61**:109–116 (1964).

56. WAHDAN, M. H., SERIE, C., CERISIER, Y., SALLAM, S., AND GERMANIER, R., A controlled field trial of live *Salmonella typhi* strain Ty21a oral vaccine against typhoid fever: Three-year results, *J. Infect. Dis.* **145**:292–295 (1982).

57. WIDAL, F., Sérodiagnostic de la fièvre typhoïde, *Sem. Med.* **16**:259 (1896).

58. WONG, S. H., The emergency surgical management of massive and persistent intestinal haemorrhage due to typhoid fever: A report of 3 cases, *Br. J. Surg.* **65**:74 (1978).

59. WOODWARD, T. E., SMADEL, J. E., LEY, H. L., GREEN, R., AND MANKAKAN, D. S., Preliminary report on the beneficial effect of chloromycetin in the treatment of typhoid fever, *Ann. Intern. Med.* **29**:131–134 (1948).

60. WRIGHT, A. E., On the association of serious haemorrhages with conditions of defective blood-coagulability, *Lancet* **2**:807–809 (1896).

61. Yugoslav Typhoid Commission, A controlled field trial of the effectiveness of acetone-dried and inactivated and heat–phenol-inactivated typhoid vaccines in Yugoslavia: Report, *Bull. WHO* **30**:623–630 (1964).

12. Suggested Reading

HORNICK, R. B., GREISMAN, S. E., WOODWARD, T. E., DUPONT, H. L., DAWKINS, A. T., AND SNYDER, M. J., Typhoid fever: Pathogenesis and immunologic control, *N. Engl. J. Med.* **283**:686–691, 739–746 (1970).

HUCKSTEP, R. L., *Typhoid Fever and Other Salmonella Infections*, Livingstone, Edinburgh, 1962.

RYDER, R. W., AND BLAKE, P. A., Typhoid fever in the United States, 1975 and 1976, *J. Infect. Dis.* **139**:124–126 (1979).

STUART, B. M., AND PULLEN, R. L., Typhoid, *Arch. Intern. Med.* **78**:629–661 (1946).

CHAPTER 40

Yersinia enterocolitica Infections

Sally Bryna Slome and Robert E. Black

1. Introduction

Bacteria of the genus *Yersinia* have been recognized for
centuries as the cause of devastating human illness in the
form of plague caused by *Yersinia pestis* and epizootic disease in animals due to *Y. pseudotuberculosis*. In more recent
years, a third member of the genus, *Y. enterocolitica*, has
been reported with increasing frequency throughout the
world. This ubiquitous organism has been found in a number
of animal species, foods, and environmental sources, and
now joins the ranks of its fellow genus members as an
important human pathogen.

Members of the genus *Yersinia*, formerly classified in
the genus *Pasteurella*, belong to the family Enterobacteriaceae. These facultative gram-negative bacteria include
the well-recognized *Y. pestis*, *Y. enterocolitica*, and *Y.
pseudotuberculosis*, as well as the new species *Y. frederiksenii*, *Y. intermedia*, *Y. kristensenii*, *Y. aldovae*, and *Y.
ruckeri*, former biogroups of *Y. enterocolitica*. While these
new species have been occasionally recovered from cases of
illness in man, their role as human pathogens remains to be
defined. The present discussion will focus on *Y. entero-*

Sally Bryna Slome and Robert E. Black · Department of
International Health, School of Hygiene and Public Health, Department of Medicine, Division of Infectious Diseases, School of Medicine, The Johns Hopkins University, Baltimore, Maryland
21205.   *Present address of S. B. S.:* Kaiser Permanente Medical
Center, Oakland, California 94611.

colitica and its emerging role in a variety of clinical syndromes afflicting humans.

2. Historical Background

The first description of human illness caused by *Y.
enterocolitica* was made by Gilbert in 1933.[42] Ten years
later, Schleifstein and Coleman proposed the name "*Bacterium enterocoliticum*" to describe a collection of isolates
submitted to the New York State Department of Health.[98]

Following its initial identification, *Y. enterocolitica* remained a relatively obscure pathogen, with only 61 human
cases reported in the United States by 1976. In sharp contrast to the American experience, European investigators
reported frequent isolation of this species from a host of
animal reservoirs, including chinchilla, hare, and pig, and
from humans. These isolations, most originating in the
Scandinavian countries, were variably identified as *Pasteurella* X, *P. pseudotuberculosis* type B, *B. enterocolitica*,
and Les Germes X.

In 1963, the similarity between the American and European strains of *Y. enterocolitica* from both human and
animal sources was established.[54] Frederiksen, a Norwegian scientist, demonstrated that 55 strains from his collection were distinct from *Y. pseudotuberculosis*, but were
similar enough to one another biochemically to be designated as a separate species.[40] He suggested the name *Y.
enterocolitica*, selecting a genus previously named by Van

819

Loghem (1944) in honor of the French bacteriologist Yersin, who first isolated the plague bacillus in 1894. The genus was to include three distinct species: *Y. enterocolitica, Y. pestis,* and *Y. pseudotuberculosis.*

The decade of the 1970s heralded a new interest in *Yersinia* as reports from throughout the world emphasized its importance as a human pathogen. Improved methods of stool culture facilitated isolation of the organism worldwide. In 1971, Mollaret described 642 cases of yersiniosis diagnosed at the Institute of Pasteur in Paris over a 4-year period.[68] In 1974, the World Health Organization designated the Institute as an international referral center for *Y. enterocolitica* and by 1976 there were 5800 isolates on file.

Coincident with this heightened awareness of *Y. enterocolitica,* it became evident that the original biochemical criteria proposed for the species *Y. enterocolitica* did in fact circumscribe a heterogeneous group of bacteria. Many isolates were described as *Y. enterocolitica*-like organisms but differed substantially in their biochemical reactions. Several biotyping schemes were proposed and at least five different biotypes were recognized.[73,120] Later, subgroups 3A and 3B were added to biogroup 3.[11]

Winblad, in 1967, described eight serogroups of *Y. enterocolitica* based on differences in heat-stable O antigens.[125] This antigenic scheme was subsequently expanded to include greater than 50 antigenic factors in *Y. enterocolitica* and related species.[73,112,120,122,123]

With the advent of DNA hybridization techniques, the biochemically diverse group of bacteria, previously recognized as *Y. enterocolitica* species, was divided into four subgroups that coincided with their distinct biochemical profiles. These included: *Y. enterocolitica, Y. frederiksenii,*[115] *Y. kristensenii,*[12] and *Y. intermedia.*[18–20] More recently, taxonomic studies have defined two new species within the same genus: *Y. aldovae,*[13] a biotype found in water, and *Y. ruckeri,*[34] a fish pathogen. This advancement brought a new order to *Yersinia* taxonomy. Ascription of distinct species status to the variety of organisms formerly classified as *Y. enterocolitica* and lacking invasive potential, served to emphasize the pathogenic potential inherent in the designation *Y. enterocolitica.*

3. Methodology

3.1. Sources of Mortality Data

Limited information is available concerning the role of *Y. enterocolitica* as a cause of fatal disease. True mortality rates are not available because of incomplete investigation

and reporting of deaths due to diarrhea and "pseudoappendicitis." Furthermore, while *Y. enterocolitica* is mostly recognized as an agent of diarrhea and "pseudoappendicitis," the organism causes a spectrum of clinical syndromes that vary with the age, sex, and physical condition of the host.[16] In addition, conventional culture methods often fail to identify *Y. enterocolitica* in stool.[78]

Enterocolitis, which accounts for two-thirds of reported cases of yersiniosis and predominantly affects infants and young children, is rarely fatal in developed countries. Although *Yersinia* enterocolitis does not appear to be common in developing countries, fatal diarrhea has been reported.[21] Patients with mesenteric adenitis and/or terminal ileitis are generally older children or adults who present with symptoms indistinguishable from acute appendicitis. Perforation of the appendix is rare and fatal cases have been generally attributed to extensive intestinal ulceration and peritonitis. The true case-fatality rate for the more common clinical syndromes of enterocolitis and pseudoappendicitis is unknown but is likely to be very low. Most extraintestinal manifestations of *Yersinia* infection, including nonsuppurative arthritis, erythema nodosum, Reiter's syndrome, carditis, and acute glomerular nephritis, are usually mild and self-limited. Septicemia, on the other hand, is most often reported in children or adults compromised by severe anemia, hemochromatosis, cirrhosis, malignancy, malnutrition, or immunosuppressive therapy and is associated with a significant mortality. Rabson and others found a case-fatality ratio of approximately 50% in 13 patients with disseminated *Y. enterocolitica* infection and a universal mortality in those with underlying hemochromatosis.[90] The complications of disseminated infection, which include suppurative hepatic, renal, and splenic lesions, osteomyelitis, wound infection, or meningitis, also carry a significant risk of death.

3.2. Sources of Morbidity Data

Information regarding morbidity due to *Y. enterocolitica* is imprecise, at best. In the United States, positive cultures may be submitted to state laboratories or to the Centers for Disease Control for confirmation. Case reporting is required in five states in the United States and in some European countries. However, these surveillance systems underestimate the number of actual cases. The protean clinical manifestations of *Yersinia* infections puzzle even the most astute clinician and often result in a failure to pursue a bacteriologic diagnosis. The lack of universal application of laboratory techniques that favor its isolation, as well as incomplete reporting of *Y. enterocolitica* isolates to public health agencies, limits the effectiveness of laboratory-based surveillance.

3.3. Surveys

Reports of community, family, and hospital outbreaks as well as sporadic cases of yersiniosis have increased the awareness of the extent of disease due to *Y. enterocolitica*. Surveys of the relative frequency of *Yersinia* in populations with diarrhea have justified its inclusion as a bacterial enteric pathogen of importance, along with *Shigella, Salmonella,* and *Campylobacter*.

Serologic assays have been employed in the investigation of outbreaks in which the reference organism is used to determine a serologic response. Although of little immediate clinical value, this technique aids in epidemiologic investigations. Serologic surveys performed in Denmark and Finland have attempted to estimate the incidence of yersiniosis. Agner *et al.* tested sera from Danish adults from 1967 to 1978 and found that the prevalence of elevated antibody titers against *Y. enterocolitica* O:3 had increased from 1% in 1967 to 7.7% in 1978.[3] In Finland, Leino showed that elevated agglutinin titers against *Y. enterocolitica* O:3 or O:9 or against *Y. pseudotuberculosis* IA occurred in 6.1% of sera tested.[61] This suggests that yersiniosis is common and widespread among Scandinavians. However, as yet, population-based serologic surveys have not been conducted to elucidate the epidemiology of the organism.

3.4. Laboratory Diagnosis

3.4.1. Isolation and Identification of Organisms. Morphologically, *Y. enterocolitica* presents as a relatively large, facultatively anaerobic, gram-negative asporogenic rod that exhibits significant pleomorphism. Coccobacillary forms may be seen. Motility is a feature that is not present at 37°C, but at 22°C the cells develop peritrichous flagella and become motile.[119]

The isolation and identification of *Yersinia* from normally sterile sites is not difficult, according to standard bacteriologic procedures. Recovery of the organism from stool, on the other hand, is hampered by the lack of characteristic colonial morphology as well as the organism's slow growth and the resultant overgrowth of normal fecal flora. The laboratory diagnosis of *Yersinia* can be facilitated by an awareness of the unique temperature-related growth characteristics associated with the species, as well as the employment of selective media.

Yersiniae grow well on enteric media and, on initial isolation, strongly resemble several other common Enterobacteriacae. Several distinguishing features allow them to be recognized. They are lactose and oxidase-negative, do not produce hydrogen sulfide in triple sugar iron medium, but are urease-positive. Inoculation of duplicate sets of enteric media followed by incubation at both 25 and 37°C for a minimum of 48 h will increase the recovery of the organism from feces. While *Salmonella–Shigella* (SS) agar favors the growth of serotypes O:3 and O:9, the addition of MacConkey agar enables the recovery of other serotypes that may be inhibited by SS agar.

Several selective and differential media have been developed to enhance the recovery of *Y. enterocolitica* from stool specimens. The addition of novobiocin or carbenicillin to a broth used with the standard enteric plates has been reported to allow isolation of 100% of serotype O:3 and O:9 strains from infected patients.

Cefsulodin–irgasan–novobiocin (CIN) agar is a highly selective and differential plating medium for *Y. enterocolitica*. The medium requires 18–20 h incubation at 25°C to create a unique colonial morphology for presumptive identification. *Y. enterocolitica* appears as 0.5- to 1.0-mm-diameter colonies with a dark red "bull's eye" and transparent border. Schiemann demonstrated its utility in differentiating 63 *Y. enterocolitica* and *Y. enterocolitica*-like isolates that traversed the DNA homology groups of Brenner.[94]

Cold enrichment (4°C) of stool specimens in phosphate-buffered saline with weekly subcultures for 28 days has been used to enhance the recovery of *Y. enterocolitica* from clinical specimens.[33,44,78,117,124] This technique adds little to direct isolation in the recovery of "classic" *Y. enterocolitica* serotypes (O:3, O:5,27, O:8) from patients with acute gastroenteritis. When there are large numbers of organisms in the stool relative to other enteric pathogens, isolation is readily achieved by conventional methods. However, cold enrichment can be especially useful in detecting small numbers of organisms, which may be shed up to 4 weeks in the convalescent phase of illness or by asymptomatic individuals with a relatively small burden of organisms.[78]

Identification of strains other than the commonly recognized human pathogenic serotypes is also facilitated by cold enrichment. Pai *et al.*[78] and Van Noyen *et al.*[117] have demonstrated that most *Y. enterocolitica* isolates recovered after prolonged cold enrichment are a serologically heterogeneous group, primarily biotype 1 strains, the majority of which do not appear to be pathogenic in humans.

Yersinia species are differentiated from one another by several distinguishing biochemical and serologic reactions.

Unlike the biochemical homogeneity found among strains of *Y. pestis* and *Y. pseudotuberculosis,* strains of *Y. enterocolitica* differ substantially in their biochemical reactions.[53] It is this variability that resulted in the formation of several new species from the *Y. enterocolitica* subgroup and serves as the basis for biotyping of these isolates. Two biotyping systems have been developed. The five biotypes as defined by Wauters' system are based on eight biochemical reactions[119]; most human strains are biotype 4, although biotypes 1 and 2 are occasionally pathogenic for humans. Using a similar system with several additional biochemical reactions, five biotypes are described by Nilehn.[73]

Serotyping as determined by bacterial agglutination using rabbit anti-O antisera is used in conjunction with biotyping to define those strains of *Y. enterocolitica* that are potentially pathogenic for humans. Serotypes vary with geographic origin, the majority being nonhuman isolates. The serotypes that have the most clearly defined potential for human disease are O:3, O:9, and O:8. The significance of other strains is often uncertain and many cross-reacting O factors may occur in strains of other biogroups or species. For example, nonpathogenic strains cross-reacting with serum O:3 and O:8 are found in biogroup 3A, and some *Y. frederiksenii* share an antigen in common with O:3 or O:9. Thus, accurate identification of pathogenic strains necessitates consideration of both biochemical and antigenic characteristics. Flagellar antigens (H antigens) occur in very complex patterns and are presently not used for serotyping.[120] Only a few strains exhibit fimbrial K or envelope antigens.[8,120]

3.4.2. Serologic and Immunologic Diagnostic Methods. Infection with *Y. enterocolitica* elicits an immunologic response that can be measured by a variety of techniques, including tube agglutination, indirect hemagglutination, enzyme-linked immunosorbent assay (ELISA), and solid-phase radioimmunoassay. An indirect immunofluorescent-antibody assay has also been used.[22] Agglutinating antibodies appear soon after the onset of illness and persist from 2 to 6 months.

Some serotypes may be associated with illness without eliciting a detectable serologic response.[5,111] The serologic response of young infants appears to be less vigorous than that of adults.[64] Patients with systemic disease mount a greater antibody titer than do persons with disease restricted to the gastrointestinal tract.[17] The serologic diagnosis of *Yersinia* infection may be complicated by the existence of cross-reacting antigens within the genera *Y. enterocolitica* and *Y. pseudotuberculosis,* as well as with such organisms as *Brucella, Vibrio* species, *Escherichia coli,* and *Salmonella* species. The enhanced sensitivity of the ELISA technique has revealed previously unrecognized antigenic differences between *Y. enterocolitica* serotype O:9 and *Brucella* species.[23] Patients with thyroiditis on an immunologic basis also have an unexplained increased frequency of cross-reacting antibodies to *Y. enterocolitica.*[100]

Serologic testing has been used minimally as an adjunct to the diagnosis of *Yersinia* infection, which continues to rely on recovery of the organism. Serologic efforts to support the diagnosis of *Yersinia* infection are restricted by the need to determine agglutinating antibody to a specific serogroup of the organism. This makes the use of serology for diagnosis of individual cases impractical and limits the use to outbreaks in which the serogroup is known. In one outbreak, a positive titer (> 1:128) was found in 61% of ill persons infected with *Y. enterocolitica* and 11 of 23 hospitalized patients had a fourfold change in titer.[14] Bottone and Sheehan evaluated the serologic response among three groups of 3232 subjects (control, febrile, and infected) and found that the serologic response of the individuals was multifactorial. The authors concluded that agglutinin titers of 1:128 in a previously healthy individual are suggestive of infection; however, negative titers do not rule out infection in infants or compromised hosts.[17] Interpretation may also be confounded by the prozone phenomenon as well as inadequate information on the prevalence of antibodies in the general population of interest.

The employment of serologic assays in the investigation of outbreaks of infection has provided a means of documenting the *Yersinia* type responsible for illness and the route of transmission. As further technologic advances allow improved specificity of the serologic assays, seroepidemiologic surveys may provide a useful measure of the extent of exposure of a given population to prevalent strains of *Yersinia.* Until that time, serologic diagnosis will remain an epidemiologic tool used primarily in the evaluation of outbreaks of yersiniosis.

4. Biological Characteristics of the Organism

Pathogenic and saprophytic strains of *Y. enterocolitica* have been differentiated according to biotype and serotype. Some serotypes present a uniform biotype and are always pathogenic (O:3, O:9, O:5,27, O:8, and O:13), whereas other serotypes include both nonpathogenic biotypes found in the environment and pathogenic biotypes isolated from humans (O:21 and O:4,32). There is a suggestion from one study that the clinical spectrum may differ even for the common pathogenic serotypes: O:8 strains were less frequently associated with diarrhea in comparison to O:3, O:5, and O:9 strains, but were more often found with serious extramesenteric manifestations.[48]

Human pathogenic strains of *Y. enterocolitica* are endowed with a number of bacterial properties that confer virulence to the organism. Several of these exhibit a marked temperature-dependent expression and have been shown to be mediated by a 41-mDa plasmid.[41,47,87,130] *Y. enterocolitica* was the first member of the Enterobacteriaceae in which a plasmid-mediated capacity to invade tissue was demonstrated, a property now known to be shared by other enteric pathogens. Animal studies confirm that strains harboring this plasmid create a purulent keratoconjunctivitis in the guinea pig eye(Sereny) model[95]; cause fetal infections in mice and gerbils[25,95]; and produce diarrhea in mice.[97] Other properties that appear to be plasmid-encoded include autoagglutination,[57] resistance to the bactericidal effect of human serum,[46,66,76] and synthesis of a unique outer-membrane antigen.[32]

Some properties endowed by the plasmid are also correlated with virulence in the plague bacillus, which shares with *Y. enterocolitica* tissue-invasive characteristics and a tropism for lymphoid tissue. Both organisms also manifest an ability to evade the primary immune response of the host. The shared plasmid properties recognized thus far include production of VW surface antigens[27,83] that enable the organism to resist phagocytosis by polymorphonuclear leukocytes, enhanced susceptibility to pesticin, and the capacity to bind hemin and Congo red dye.[89] The relationship between *Y. enterocolitica, Y. pseudotuberculosis,* and *Y. pestis* has been further elucidated with the isolation of plasmids in both *Y. pestis* and *Y. pseudotuberculosis* that share significant DNA homology with the plasmid isolated from *Y. enterocolitica*. It appears that a region of the plasmid encompassing 13.7 kb is particularly conserved among the genus *Yersinia,* and may encode a shared virulence mechanism.[15,43,59,86,88,104,127,128]

Other virulence properties harbored by *Y. enterocolitica* that are not plasmid encoded include an ability to attach to and invade animal cell lines in tissue cultures.[113] Only pathogenic *Y. enterocolitica* strains invade HeLa,[52,60,71,81,96,113] HEp-2,[63,87] and Henle intestinal epithelial cells.[66] This property, expressed after growth at low temperatures, is not dependent on the VW plasmid but is chromosomally mediated.

Many strains of *Y. enterocolitica* elaborate a heat-stable enterotoxin resembling that produced by enterotoxigenic *E. coli*. The two toxins share the property of stimulating guanylate cyclase, thus enhancing cellular fluid secretions, and are both positive in the suckling mouse assay.[35,77] While the toxin of *Y. enterocolitica* is more prevalent in virulent strains than in nonpathogenic strains, it is produced only at temperatures below 30°C and its role in the pathogenesis of yersiniosis remains uncertain.

One final intriguing feature of *Y. enterocolitica* relates to its iron dependency. Unlike most other aerobic bacteria, *Y. enterocolitica* fails to produce iron-binding compounds, or siderophores, and utilizes siderophores produced by other bacteria as well as exogenous siderophores such as therapeutic iron chelators. They are also able to use hemin as a source of iron, as demonstrated by Perry and Brubaker.[82] This property may explain the apparent increased susceptibility of patients with conditions of iron excess to yersiniosis. While there have been many speculations regarding the role of iron in enhancing *Yersinia* infections, the precise mechanism remains to be elucidated.

Among *Y. enterocolitica,* there exists a fair correlation between biogroup, antigenic pattern, ecology, and potential for pathogenicity. The *Y. enterocolitica*-related species, *Y. frederiksenii, Y. kristensenii,* and *Y. intermedia,* are primarily environmental strains. Although there have been reports of human illness due to these organisms, they lack virulence properties in standard laboratory assays and do not appear to be pathogenic. However, the persistence of nonpathogenic *Y. enterocolitica* strains and related species in the environment, as well as their unique geographic and host distribution is poorly understood.

Y. enterocolitica have been shown to be sensitive *in vitro* to aminoglycosides, chloramphenicol, tetracycline, trimethoprim–sulfamethoxazole, and third-generation cephalosporin antibiotics.[16,99] Isolates are frequently resistant to penicillin, ampicillin, and first-generation cephalosporins due to the elaboration of a β-lactamase.[29] Cornelis and co-workers have identified a plasmid of *Y. enterocolitica* that carries resistances to multiple antibiotics (chloramphenicol, streptomycin, sulfonamides, and tetracycline).[30] This plasmid could in turn be transferred to *E. coli* K12 and *Salmonella java,* thus establishing a potential reservoir of antibiotic resistance factors among distinct species. While these laboratory observations raise theoretical concerns regarding antibiotic resistance, intestinal infection with *Y. enterocolitica* is usually self-limited and is infrequently treated. Thus, information regarding the importance of antibiotic resistance in the spread of disease is not available.

5. Descriptive Epidemiology

5.1. Prevalence and Incidence

Reported cases of yersiniosis have increased dramatically in the last decade, coincident with a greater awareness of the organism and improved techniques for its isolation. The majority of isolates are reported from Europe and Canada.

Since *Y. enterocolitica* was first isolated in Belgium in 1963, the isolation rate has increased, with serotypes O:3 and O:9 accounting for up to 4% of routine stool cultures for enteric illnesses in recent years. The highest incidence is in children aged 1 to 4 years with a maximum of 2 per 1000 in children between ages 1 and 2.[109]

The incidence of *Yersinia* infection in patients with acute endemic enterocolitis ranges from 0 to 4%, depending on the geographic location, study method, and population (Table 1). In a prospective study of 6364 Canadian children with acute gastroenteritis by Marks *et al.*, *Y. enterocolitica* was isolated from 2.8%, *Salmonella* from 4.4%, and *Shigella* from 1.1%.[64] The highest incidence of *Yersinia* infection was found in Finland and accounted for 5% of acute enterocolitis among children.[6] In contrast, Carniel *et al.* found only two isolates of *Y. enterocolitica* from stools of 1450 children with fever and diarrhea in Bangladesh.[24] This apparent discrepancy in the incidence of *Yersinia* isolations from cases of enterocolitis has been attributed to the tropical climate of Bangladesh, which may not favor propagation of the organism.

Several studies of patients with the appendicitis-like syndrome have found *Y. enterocolitica* in up to 9% of patients (Table 2). In a report of 581 persons who underwent appendectomy for presumed appendicitis over a 1-year peri- od in Sweden, Nilehn and Sjostrom found 22 cases (3.8%) with bacteriologic evidence of *Yersinia* infection.[74] Of those found to have regional terminal ileitis at surgery, 80% were infected with *Y. enterocolitica;* 13% of those with mesenteric adenitis; and 0.5% of those with acute appendi- citis.

Although sometimes present in asymptomatic indi- viduals, several large surveys have found carriage rates of less than 1% in asymptomatic controls. There were no isola- tions of *Y. enterocolitica* among 918 asymptomatic indi- viduals serving as controls in three studies of *Yersinia* enterocolitis.[31,64,84]

5.2. Epidemic Behavior and Contagiousness

In addition to the usual sporadic cases of *Yersinia* in- fection, where the source of infection and mode of transmis- sion remain obscure, a number of outbreaks of yersiniosis in communities, families, and hospitals have served to empha- size the capacity of *Y. enterocolitica* to cause widespread disease (Table 3).

Epidemiologic investigations of outbreaks have served to identify vehicles of infection, such as foods, water, and domestic animals. In some instances, the mechanism of transmission from environmental sources to humans has

Table 1. Isolation of *Yersinia enterocolitica* from Patients with Endemic Diarrhea

Authors	Ref.	Year published	Location	Population	No. studied	Percentage with *Y. enterocolitica*
Ferrer *et al.*	36	1987	Spain	All	5199	0.8
Carniel *et al.*	24	1986	Bangladesh	Outpatient children	1450	0.7
Hoogkamp-Korstanje *et al.*	48	1986	Netherlands	All (< 40)	827	2.9
Poocharoen *et al.*	85	1986	Thailand	Hospitalized children	208	0
Figua and Rossolini	37	1985	Italy	Hospitalized children	188	3.7
Velasco *et al.*	118	1984	Spain	Hospitalized children	6970	0.2
DeMol *et al.*	31	1983	Zaire	Hospitalized and outpatient children	84	0
Agbonlahor *et al.*	2	1983	Nigeria	All	1082	1.3
Persson *et al.*	84	1982	Sweden	Hospitalized children	95	2.0
Samadi *et al.*	92	1982	Bangladesh	All	113	0
Marks *et al.*	64	1980	Canada	Hospitalized children	6364	2.8

Table 2. Isolation of *Yersinia enterocolitica* from Patients with Appendicitis-like Syndrome

Author(s)	Ref.	Year published	Location	Population	No. studied	Percentage with *Y. enterocolitica*
Megraud	67	1987	France	Appendectomy	600	3.0
Attwood *et al.*	10	1987	Ireland	Appendicitis	90	3.0
Butler *et al.*	21	1984	Bangladesh	Appendectomy	31	3.0
Pai *et al.*	79	1982	Canada	Appendectomy	363	1.4
				No appendectomy	441	2.3
Samadi *et al.*	92	1982	Bangladesh	Appendectomy	30	0
Jepsen *et al.*	50	1976	Denmark	Hospitalized	205	5.4
Ahvonen *et al.*	6	1972	Finland	Appendectomy	244	9.0
Nilehn and Sjostrom	74	1967	Sweden	Appendectomy	581	3.8
				No appendectomy	284	5.6

been elucidated. Questions regarding incubation period, the relationship of serotype to the clinical spectrum of *Y. enterocolitica* infection, and the potential for person-to-person transmission have been addressed.

In the United States, several major outbreaks of enteritis due to *Y. enterocolitica* have been investigated. The first of these occurred in 1972, in rural North Carolina, where 16 of 21 individuals from four families were affected.[45] The outbreak resulted in two exploratory laparotomies and two of the afflicted individuals died, one following surgery. Although the source was not culturally confirmed, five of nine newborn puppies died with diarrheal illness during the week prior to the first human illness. A serotype O:8 *Y. enterocolitica* was isolated from the human cases of enteritis.

A variety of foods have been implicated as vehicles of transmission in outbreaks of *Y. enterocolitica* infection. Several such outbreaks involved the distribution of contaminated milk, which probably became infected subsequent to the pasteurization process. The first of these occurred in 1976 in upstate New York.[14] Illness occurred in 222 school children and employees, 38 of whom had documented *Y. enterocolitica* serotype O:8 infection; 36 individuals were hospitalized and 16 appendectomies were performed. Illness was found to be associated with the consumption of chocolate milk purchased in the school cafeterias. Seroepidemiologic evaluation demonstrated that 61% of those infected had a titer greater than 1:160 OH agglutinin to serotype O:8 *Y. enterocolitica* and 48% of those hospitalized had a fourfold change in agglutinin titer. *Y. enterocolitica* was subsequently isolated from a carton of chocolate milk, which presumably was contaminated during the addition of chocolate syrup to pasteurized milk.

In 1982, a multistate outbreak of serotypes O:13 and O:18 caused illness in at least 172 persons; 17 individuals

underwent appendectomy and 24 cases of extraintestinal disease were documented.[107] Illness was associated with drinking pasteurized milk from a Memphis, Tennessee plant, but samples from the incriminated lots of milk were not available for culture. A survey revealed that 8.3% of those who drank the milk became ill; the attack rate was 22.2% in children 0–4 years old and 38.5% in children 5–9 years old. In a third outbreak, 53% of persons at a camp experienced illness and the investigation showed that illness was associated with consumption of reconstituted powdered milk and/or chow mein.[72] The organism appeared to have been introduced by a food handler during preparation.

Epidemiologic investigations have demonstrated that some products incriminated in foodborne outbreaks may become contaminated during processing with infected environmental water sources. An outbreak of 50 *Y. enterocolitica* infections occurred in Washington between December 15, 1981 and February 22, 1982.[108] Disease was associated with the ingestion of contaminated tofu (soybean curd) and *Y. enterocolitica* serotype O:8 was isolated from afflicted individuals. Culture of the tofu, as well as the untreated spring water used in the tofu manufacturing plant, yielded the same serotype, O:8. A second outbreak involved 16 of 33 (48%) members of a Brownie troop who were infected following the ingestion of bean sprouts that had been grown in refrigerated water from a well that was shown to be contaminated with *Y. enterocolitica*[1]; 15 of the children manifested gastrointestinal symptoms an average of 6 days following exposure and three underwent appendectomy.

While a number of additional well-defined outbreaks of yersiniosis have been reported, isolation of *Y. enterocolitica* from implicated vehicles is unusual. In Japan, epidemic *Y. enterocolitica* enteritis has been described in both

Table 3.   Outbreaks Due to *Yersinia enterocolitica*

Author(s)	Ref.	Year published	Location	Ill	At risk	Mode of transmission or vehicle	Serotype
Kondracki and Gallo	56	1987	New York (four-infant cluster)	4	4	Unknown No obvious common exposure	O:3 Biotype 4
Tacket *et al.*	108	1985	Washington	44		Tofu-plant spring water source contaminated	O:8
Morse *et al.*	72	1984	New York State (summer diet camp)	239	455	Reconstituted powdered milk milk dispenser or chow mein	O:8
Aber *et al.*	1	1982	Pennsylvania (Brownie troop)	16	33	Bean sprouts grown in water from contaminated well	—
Ratnam *et al.*	91	1982	Newfoundland, Canada (hospital)	9		Nosocomial	O:5 Biotype 1
Martin *et al.*	65	1982	Canada (family outbreak)	3	4	Unknown River water?	O:21 Biotype 1
Black *et al.*	14	1978	New York	222	2193	Contaminated chocolate milk	O:8
Olsovsky *et al.*	75	1975	Karvina (two nursery schools)	75	142	Unknown Common food supplies to both nurseries	
Toivanen *et al.*	110	1973	Finland (hospital)	6		Nosocomial	O:9
Zen-Yoji *et al.*	129	1973	Japan (Jr. high school)	198	1086	Unknown Presumed common source	O:3 O:5 O:9
Asakawa *et al.*	9	1973	Japan (community outbreak)	189	441	Unknown	O:3
			Japan (community outbreak	544	1042	Unknown	O:3
Gutman *et al.*	45	1972	North Carolina (intrafamilial)	16	21	Sick puppies	O:8

communities and schools.[9] One such outbreak occurred in 1972 in a Japanese junior high school where acute abdominal pain and fever were present in 198 of 1086 pupils.[129] *Y. enterocolitica* serotype O:3 was isolated from the fecal specimens of the majority of ill children; however, a single source of contaminated food or water was not identified.

5.3. Geographic Distribution

Y. enterocolitica has a worldwide distribution and has been isolated from humans, a variety of domestic and wild animals, and food and water sources. Little is known about the epizoology of *Y. enterocolitica* infection among reservoir hosts such as mammals, birds, and rodents. Strains of *Y. enterocolitica* associated with illness in man, particularly serotype 3, have been isolated from swine, dogs, and cats in Europe, Canada, and the United States.[49]

The incidence is highest in Scandinavia and Europe, but infections have been documented in North and South America, Africa, and Asia. In North America there appear to be more infections in Canada and the northern United States. The majority of isolates from Scandinavia and Europe are serotypes O:3 and O:9, while Canadian and United States isolates are of serotype O:3 and O:8, respectively. As the country with the highest reported incidence of yersiniosis, Belgium serves as a valuable source of information regarding the epidemiology and ecology of *Y. enterocolitica.* The laboratory of Vandepitte and Wauters has served as an unofficial reference center for identification and serotyping of most strains of *Y. enterocolitica* isolated in Belgium between 1963 and 1975. In Belgium, 89% of isolates were serotype O:3 and only 9% were O:9.[116] A phage type of serotype O:3 found in Canada is different from that found in Japan and South Africa.

Yersinia infections in the United States have a tendency to occur in rural communities. Snyder and co-workers reported that 30% of all *Y. enterocolitica* isolates were from counties in Wisconsin with less than 30,000 inhabitants, whereas only 13% of all specimens submitted came from these small counties.[101] It has been suggested that this increase in rural rates of infection may reflect an increased exposure to environmental or animal reservoirs of the organisms. Conversely, the infrequent occurrence of *Y. enterocolitica* in some areas of the world may be due in part to avoidance of certain environmental risk factors, such as eating pork in Muslim countries.

5.4. Temporal Distribution

In the United States, there are no clear seasonal patterns of disease due to *Y. enterocolitica,* although a summer peak has been suggested in a study in Wisconsin.[101] Surveillance of *Yersinia* isolations in Belgium from 1963 to 1975 demonstrated a steep rise in frequency during late summer and autumn, followed by a steady decline during the winter and spring seasons.[116] Mollaret emphasized the peak incidence of yersiniosis in Europe during autumn and winter months.[68] The seasonality of human illness can also be correlated with the isolation of *Yersinia* from domestic swine in these regions. The association of *Y. enterocolitica* with cooler seasons and the temperate climates of Scandinavia, Europe, the United States, Japan, and Canada

has been linked to the unique temperature-dependent properties of the organism, which grows optimally at 22–29°C.[70] Thus, the organism may survive in the environment after it is passed in the feces of the mammalian host. This biologic growth property provides *Y. enterocolitica* with a competitive advantage over other bacteria for propagation in environmental reservoirs. An infrequent isolation of *Yersinia* from tropical climates has been noted and seasonality in these locations is unknown.

5.5. Age

Although *Y. enterocolitica* causes a number of clinical syndromes that vary with the age, sex, and health of the host, children appear to be preferentially affected.[14,55,72,108] Of 359 infected patients reported by Mollaret, 47% were between 1 and 5 years of age.[68] Vandepitte and Wauters reported 1711 cases of *Yersinia* infection occurring in persons less than 1 month to 85 years old; approximately 20% of all cases occurred within the first year of life.[116] Nearly 80% of patients were less than 10 years old. This propensity of infection for childhood may relate to the presumed fecal–oral route of transmission and the less hygienic habits of young children. It is notable that infection in infants less than 3 months old is rare, perhaps due to transplacentally acquired antibody. Enhanced immunity to infection with increased age may also explain the age-specific differences in rates of *Yersinia* infection. It is notable that in a foodborne outbreak, 43% of children who ate the incriminated food developed yersiniosis and had a positive culture, compared with 14% of adults who ate the food (33% were culture positive).[108] Likewise, in milkborne outbreaks, children had the highest attack rates.[14]

A dramatic difference in age-specific incidence was noted when patients with enteritis were compared with those with the appendicitis-like syndrome.[105] While 80% of all patients with enteritis were less than 5 years old those with a pseudoappendicitis syndrome were most frequently older children and adults. The illness most commonly associated with *Y. enterocolitica* in children less than 5 years old is a mild diarrheal illness, indistinguishable from that caused by other enteric pathogens. Children over 5 years old are more likely to develop symptoms that mimic those of acute appendicitis. Most extraintestinal manifestations of *Yersinia* infection, including Reiter's syndrome, erythema nodosum, meningitis, hepatitis, and focal suppurative processes in bone, liver, spleen, kidney, and lung, are more frequently found in adults than in children. In hospital outbreaks, it has been noted that the old and the very young were more often infected, and may be predisposed by age and physical condition including immune status.[91]

5.6. Sex

Males have outnumbered females slightly in all age groups of patients with *Yersinia* diarrhea in most studies; however, the sexes were equally affected in outbreaks of mesenteric adenitis. Erythema nodosum is seen more commonly in females.

5.7. Occupation

Both sporadic cases and outbreaks of yersiniosis have been linked to exposure to animal and environmental reservoirs of infection. The organism has been found frequently in samples from swine in slaughterhouses, where it may readily be transferred to animal handlers.

5.8. Occurrence in Different Settings

Y. enterocolitica among hospital populations exhibits both sporadic and outbreak forms of infection (Table 3). The first nosocomial outbreak of *Y. enterocolitica* was reported from Finland in 1973 and involved six hospital employees who became ill approximately 10 days after a schoolgirl with *Y. enterocolitica* enteritis was admitted to their hospital. Spread of the infection, in this and other hospital outbreaks, appeared to be from the index patient to the staff and, subsequently, from person to person.[110]

Outbreaks have been reported among children attending nursery schools in eastern Europe and it is presumed that similar outbreaks are possible in day-care settings with poor hygiene.[75] As mentioned previously, outbreaks have occurred in schools.[14]

6. Mechanisms and Routes of Transmission

The precise mechanism of acquisition of *Y. enterocolitica* from its natural reservoir has yet to be determined. In most sporadic cases, the source of infection and mode of transmission remain obscure. *Yersinia* have been found in lakes, streams, and drinking water; however, most isolates from water sources have not been associated with human illness.[93]

Yersinia are frequently isolated from a variety of wild and domestic animals, including pigs, dogs, cats, hares, birds, rodents, and fish. In the United States, several small family outbreaks have apparently resulted from contact with infected dogs. Contact with swine or infected meat has been associated with human illness in a number of countries. In a case–control study of endemic yersiniosis, diarrhea in children was strongly associated with eating raw meat 2 weeks before illness.[109] Further analysis suggested that eating raw pork accounted for the increased risk. A frequent association of *Y. enterocolitica* with *Salmonella* has been noted by Vandepitte and Wauters.[116] Whereas only 4.3% of routine stool cultures were positive for *Salmonella* in 1976, 8.5% of those infected with *Y. enterocolitica* had concurrent *Salmonella* infection. The common source of these enteric pathogens seems to be related to their shared porcine origin.[121]

The ability of *Yersinia* to grow at low temperatures also makes it a potential source of food contamination. *Y. enterocolitica* has been isolated from a number of foods including meat, mussels, poultry, oysters, cheese, ice cream, and milk.[69,111] Foodborne transmission has been well documented in investigations of outbreaks related to a common infected food source. In the United States, the largest outbreak of yersiniosis was traced to contaminated pasteurized milk.[14] Although pasteurization will kill the organism, contamination of milk may occur with faulty pasteurization, or may follow the pasteurization. Refrigerated cows' milk is an excellent growth medium for *Y. enterocolitica*.

Person-to-person transmission has been implicated in hospital outbreaks of yersiniosis, as well as in an interfamilial outbreak. Person-to-person transmission may also be responsible for nursery outbreaks. Evidence for transmission to household contacts has been conflicting. In one milkborne outbreak, transmission by school children to household contacts could not be documented.[14] Likewise, person-to-person transmission was thought not to occur in large school outbreaks in Japan.[9] However, in a recent prospective study of *Y. enterocolitica*-related gastroenteritis in Canada, spread to others in the family occurred in 47% of the cases.[64] Although pharyngeal infection is not uncommon in yersiniosis, respiratory transmission is unlikely.[106]

7. Pathogenesis and Immunity

Human infection due to *Y. enterocolitica* is acquired predominantly by the oral route. The minimal infectious dose required to cause disease in humans is unknown. In one volunteer, ingestion of 3.5×10^9 organisms was sufficient to produce illness.[105]

The incubation period of *Yersinia* infection is uncertain; however, it has been estimated to be 2 to 11 days, based on two outbreaks in which personnel became ill after the hospital admission of patients with *Y. enterocolitica*.[91,110] An outbreak in a Brownie troop was reported to have a mean incubation period of 6 days,[1] while in a foodborne outbreak, the median was 4 days (range 1–9 days) following ingestion of the incriminated food.[108]

Enteric infection leads to proliferation of *Y. enterocolitica* in the lumen of the bowel and in the lymphoid tissue of the intestine. The mucosal surface of the lower gastrointestinal tract develops diffuse hyperemia, neutrophil infiltration, and ulceration. Necrosis may occur at the site of lymphoid follicles with resultant abscess formation.

The findings in patients with terminal ileitis at surgery are quite unique to *Yersinia* infection and include extensive mesenteric adenopathy with matted lymph nodes. Cellular infiltrates include lymphoid hyperplasia, epithelioid granulomas, and necrotic suppurative lesions in which the gram-negative organisms are easily demonstrated. Hematogenous dissemination from the gastrointestinal tract is transmitted through the portal system to produce metastatic lesions throughout the body.

Syndromes of inflammatory arthritis and erythema nodosum appear to be delayed immunologic sequelae of the original intestinal infection.

Human infection with pathogenic strains of *Y. enterocolitica* stimulates development of specific antibodies that can be detected by direct or indirect agglutination. It is not known whether specific serum antibody protects against reinfection with *Y. enterocolitica* organisms of the same or different serotypes. Immunization of mice with heat-killed *Yersinia* was found to produce an effective immune response to subsequent "intravenous challenge."[26] The challenge dose was quickly cleared in the immunized mice and no organisms were detectable in the liver or spleen 24 h after challenge. Corbel demonstrated that a formalin-killed suspension of *Y. enterocolitica* serotype O:9 was active in evoking protective immunity in mice against challenge with virulent *Salmonella*.[28] Thus, adults who have been exposed to a variety of gram-negative bacterial infections theoretically may have a degree of cross-protective immunity against *Yersinia* infection. The observation that diarrheal disease secondary to *Yersinia* is rare in infants less than 3 months old suggests that transplacentally derived maternal antibody to the organism may be protective, although lack of exposure to the pathogen in the first few months of life could also account for the low incidence. Although there is considerable evidence that both natural and experimental infection can confer some degree of immunity, the precise extent and duration of such immunity remain to be determined.

8. Patterns of Host Response

Inapparent infection with *Y. enterocolitica* is infrequent, occurring in less than 1% of individuals in large surveys.[74] Clearly, in outbreak settings, opportunities for acquisition of infection are enhanced. Studies by Marks *et al.*[64] found that 34 of 158 (21.5%) family contacts of 57 children with *Y. enterocolitica* enteritis were infected. Two-thirds of infected contacts were without symptoms. Colonization with a different serotype of *Y. enterocolitica* was noted in two index cases after clinical and microbiologic recovery from infection with *Y. enterocolitica* biotype 4, serotype O:3. In the investigation of an outbreak of yersiniosis caused by contaminated tofu (soybean curd), Tacket *et al.*[108] reported that 6 of 50 infected individuals were asymptomatic. However, each of these 6 family contacts of index cases also ingested the implicated vehicle, tofu. Thus, it appears that transient carriage and excretion of both pathogenic and nonpathogenic *Y. enterocolitica* may occur following exposure to *Y. enterocolitica*. The frequency of this phenomenon and its impact on transmission are not clear.

8.1. Clinical Features

The protean clinical manifestations produced by *Y. enterocolitica* vary with different serotypes of the organism and with host factors.[16] Several organ systems may be involved with *Y. enterocolitica* infection, by direct or immunologically mediated mechanisms, and the clinical manifestations frequently mimic those of other diseases. Patients may present with enterocolitis, mesenteric adenitis, terminal ileitis, reactive polyarthritis, erythema nodosum, exudative pharyngitis, or septicemia and coincident complications. Metastatic foci present as osteomyelitis, meningitis, and pulmonary and intraabdominal abscesses. Other less frequently reported symptoms include carditis, ophthalmitis, glomerulonephritis, hepatitis, pancreatitis, and hemolytic anemia. Infectious endocarditis due to *Y. enterocolitica* has been reported by Urbano-Márquez *et al.*[114]

Acute enteritis is the most common clinical form of *Y. enterocolitica* infection and affects primarily young children less than 5 years old and infants. In a prospective study of children with acute gastroenteritis, illness was mild in most cases and medical consultation was sought after an average of 1 week of diarrhea (range 1–43 days).[64] The symptoms most frequently noted were diarrhea (98%), fever (68%), abdominal pain (64.5%), and vomiting (38.5%). Blood was found in the stools of 26% of the children. The syndrome is indistinguishable from that caused by other enteric pathogens. However, the duration of illness, in an otherwise well individual, often exceeds that of other acute diarrheal diseases and lasts on average 2–3 weeks. The organism may be recovered from the stool for 14 to 97 days after clinical recovery, with a mean of 42 days.

Chronic diarrhea is less frequently reported but appears most common in childhood. Failure to thrive and malnutrition may accompany symptoms of colicky abdominal pain and diarrhea that persist for weeks to months. Radiologic and endoscopic evaluations show a variety of findings, some of which may suggest a diagnosis of idiopathic inflammatory bowel disease. There is no evidence that *Y. enterocolitica* is a primary cause of idiopathic inflammatory bowel disease.

The syndromes of mesenteric adenitis, terminal ileitis, or both occur in older children more than 5 years old and in adults. In these patients, diarrhea is infrequent; findings of fever, right lower quadrant pain, and leukocytosis often mimic those of acute appendicitis. While most cases are probably self-limited, severe intestinal disease, small-bowel gangrene, and death have been reported. Patients who undergo laparotomy for presumed appendicitis are at risk of surgical complications, including *Y. enterocolitica* wound infections.

A variety of extraintestinal manifestations may accompany enteric infection with *Y. enterocolitica*. Since intestinal symptoms may be mild or asymptomatic, many patients present with syndromes that mimic a host of other nonenteric diseases, and thus present a diagnostic challenge to the physician. The most common extraintestinal form of *Y. enterocolitica* infection is "reactive" arthritis. A polyarticular nonsuppurative arthritis has been reported most frequently in persons of northern European descent. In Scandinavia, 10–30% of adults with *Y. enterocolitica* infection develop inflammation of the knees, wrists, or ankles a few days to 1 month after the onset of diarrhea.[126] Symptoms are commonly accompanied by an elevated erythrocyte sedimentation rate, C-reactive protein, white blood cell count, and a stool culture positive for the organism. Synovial fluid cultures are generally negative. Symptoms usually persist for 4–6 months but may become chronic in some patients.[51] Ahvonen et al.[4] have demonstrated a predilection of individuals with the HLA B27 antigen for developing arthritis as a complication of *Yersinia* infection. They found HLA B27 antigen in 9 of 11 females and all 11 males

with *Yersinia* arthritis. Reiter's syndrome (conjunctivitis, urethritis, arthritis) and ankylosing spondylitis have also been described in individuals with the HLA B27 antigen following *Yersinia* infection.[58,102]

Erythema nodosum occurs in up to 30% of Scandinavian cases, most of whom are females. Ahvonen reported 106 cases of erythema nodosum in which females outnumbered males, 92 to 14; the female-to-male distribution of the group of infected patients was approximately 2 to 1.[6] In the majority of cases, erythema nodosum resolves spontaneously within a month. Some patients with erythema nodosum have histories of previous episodes of erythema nodosum, suggesting that *Yersinia* infection provokes an underlying predisposition to develop this inflammatory reaction.

Yersinia infection may also present with a syndrome indistinguishable from that of acute rheumatic fever.[7] Ahvonen et al.[4] described transient prolonged PR intervals or T-wave inversions in 5 of 25 patients with *Yersinia* arthritis. The clinical findings of fever, arthritis, and myocarditis raised the diagnosis of rheumatic fever in these patients who were without evidence of antecedent streptococcal infection. Leino and Kalliomaki observed myocarditis in 4 of 60 patients with *Yersinia* infection.[62] Electrocardiograms demonstrated characteristic ST segment elevation and T-wave inversion. A further analogy with poststreptococcal syndromes is suggested by the association of *Yersinia* gastroenteritis and arthritis with glomerulonephritis. Forsstrom et al.[39] reported one case of glomerulonephritis, which occurred 2 weeks following an episode of *Yersinia* gastroenteritis and arthritis. The renal biopsy demonstrated deposits of immunoglobulin and complement.

Exudative pharyngitis caused by *Y. enterocolitica* has also been documented. In one large outbreak reported by Tacket et al., 8% of patients presented with pharyngitis and fever, without accompanying gastrointestinal symptoms.[106]

Septicemia due to *Y. enterocolitica* is seen almost exclusively in individuals with underlying disease.[103] Those with cirrhosis and disorders of iron excess are particularly predisposed to infection and increased mortality. Two forms of generalized *Yersinia* infection have been noted.[90] The acute septicemic form is usually without an apparent focus of infection. Patients present with fever, abdominal pain, jaundice, and leukocytosis, but without localizing findings. In the subacute localized form of disseminated *Yersinia*, the accompanying gastrointestinal manifestations may be inapparent. A variety of metastatic foci of infection have been reported including osteomyelitis, meningitis, mycotic aneurysms, hepatic, renal, and splenic abscesses, pulmonary empyema, septic arthritis, peritonitis, and sinusitis. These forms of disease are quite rare and often portend a grave prognosis.

8.2. Diagnosis

The diagnosis of *Yersinia* infection requires a heightened awareness of the great diversity of clinical syndromes caused by *Y. enterocolitica* and the need for routine employment of isolation techniques that favor its recovery. Depending on the clinical syndrome, *Yersinia* can be easily isolated from otherwise sterile sites, including blood, peritoneal fluid, and mesenteric lymph nodes. Recovery from feces requires selective media that inhibit the growth of competing enteric organisms. A 28-day cold enrichment of fecal specimens facilitates recovery of *Y. enterocolitica* but is generally not necessary to recover the pathogen during the acute illness; more than 80% of these specimens are positive after direct plating. Even with cold enrichment, recovery of the organism during illness is not universal. In one outbreak, 59% of persons cultured during the first 2 weeks of illness were positive compared with 36% of persons cultured 3–4 weeks and only 10% of persons cultured 1–2 months after onset of illness.[14]

A method to detect coproantibody IgA in fecal samples of patients with *Y. enterocolitica* and *Y. frederiksenii* has been established. Fletcher and Noble found that of 28 strains of *yersiniae* isolated from symptomatic patients, those with coproantibody IgA at an agglutinating titer of 1:100 correlated positively with mouse virulence.[38] They therefore recommend the coproantibody IgA test for detection of pathogenic *Yersinia* species in humans. Serologic methods are infrequently employed to diagnose infection, although seroepidemiology has been a useful tool for the investigation of outbreaks due to *Y. enterocolitica*.

9. Control and Prevention

9.1. General Concepts

Most sporadic *Y. enterocolitica* cases appear to be acquired by the fecal–oral route. Consequently, enteric precautions for prevention of spread of the pathogens should be observed. Hand-washing and proper stool disposal must be employed in household, day-care, and hospital settings. Furthermore, food handlers should maintain strict personal hygiene and should not work when ill.

Numerous epidemics traced to contaminated foods indicate the need for careful attention to hygienic food-handling practices, especially with products of animal origin.

Furthermore, the incrimination of specific foods in transmission emphasizes the need to adhere to preventive measures such as pasteurization of milk and avoidance of contamination after treatment. Improved processing of pork to preclude contamination with *Y. enterocolitica,* and discouraging the ingestion of raw pork are useful public health measures. Avoidance of contact with excreta from domestic pets or animal reservoirs may reduce transmission. Although *Y. enterocolitica* isolated from water are not usually among the types pathogenic for humans, a potential risk of transmission through water is present. Therefore, because *Y. enterocolitica* is sensitive to chlorination, proper treatment of drinking water should eliminate the risk of infection from this source.

9.2. Antibiotic and Chemotherapeutic Approaches to Prophylaxis

The value of antimicrobial agents in the treatment of *Y. enterocolitica* diarrhea or mesenteric adentis has not been established. Intestinal infection is usually self-limited and there have been few clinical studies of efficacy. Black *et al.* in a retrospective evaluation of a *Y. enterocolitica* outbreak found that patients treated with a variety of antibiotics had a duration of illness similar to that of untreated children.[14] Pai *et al.* compared trimethoprim–sulfamethoxazole to placebo in 34 children with *Y. enterocolitica* enteritis.[80] Their study failed to demonstrate a shorter clinical course among the treated group of children. Although the latter children had negative cultures more often at the end of treatment, half of them had a bacteriologic relapse after therapy.

Therapy of extraintestinal disease or complications should be based on *in vitro* susceptibility testing of a given isolate. Most isolates are sensitive to aminoglycosides, tetracycline, trimethoprim–sulfamethoxazole, chloramphenicol, and the newer cephaolosporins. *Y. enterocolitica* frequently produces β-lactamase and isolates are often resistant to penicillin, ampicillin, and the first-generation cephalosporin agents. In the United States, the widest experience has been with aminoglycosides and trimethoprim–sulfamethoxazole. The duration of therapy for *Y. enterocolitica* infection is uncertain. Focal extraintestinal disease of the liver, bones, joints, and central nervous system may merit 3 or more weeks of therapy.

9.3. Immunization

Vaccines against *Y. enerocolitica* infections have not been developed.

10. Unresolved Problems

Over the last decade, *Y. enterocolitica* has emerged as an important pathogen, prevalent throughout the world, and endowed with virulence properties that mediate an ability to create a variety of clinical syndromes in humans. As we have enhanced our awareness of *Y. enterocolitica,* scientific efforts have refined our ability to recover and investigate this previously unrecognized pathogen. Despite an improved understanding of the biologic properties of the organism and its unique geographic and environmental distribution, a multitude of questions about the ecology, epidemiology, and pathogenicity of *Y. enterocolitica* remain unanswered.

Our understanding of the epidemiology of yersiniosis is in its infancy. The importance of *Y. enterocolitica* as the cause of a number of clinical syndromes is unknown in most areas of the world. Routes of transmission and risk factors for acquisition of disease remain to be defined. One important unresolved question relates to the role of ubiquitous environmental strains in human disease. It seems likely that the unique temperature-dependent growth and virulence properties of *Y. enterocolitica* provide a selective advantage to the organism and may facilitate its cycle between human host and environment.

Great strides have been made in our understanding, at the molecular level, of the mechanisms by which *Y. enterocolitica* causes disease. However, clarification of the role of enterotoxins, surface proteins, and other *Yersinia* antigens is needed. One recently explored avenue of investigation relates to the shared plasmid and virulence properties among the three species of *Yersinia* and serves to highlight global questions such as: Why do *Yersinia* invade host tissues? What accounts for their distinctive lymphoid tissue tropism? By what mechanism are they able to evade the immune response of the host? What are the critical virulence markers and what is the role of plasmids in the pathogenesis of disease?

In addition, several clinical puzzles of human yersiniosis need to be unraveled, such as the role of iron in enhancing disease, the relationship of *Y. enterocolitica* to the immune system in the creation of a diversity of autoimmune phenomena, and the nature, efficacy, and duration of immunity.

11. References

1. ABER, R. C., McCARTHY, M. A., BERMAN, R., DeMELLI, T., AND WHITE, E., An outbreak of *Yersinia enterocolitica* among members of a Brownie troop in Pennsylvania, *Program and Abstracts of the Twenty-Second Interscience Conference on Antimicrobial Agents and Chemotherapy,* Miami Beach, American Society for Microbiology, Washington, D.C., 1982.

2. AGBONLAHOR, D. E., ODUGBEMI, T. O., AND DOSUNMU-OGUNBI, O., Isolation of species of *Yersinia* from patients with gastroenteritis in Nigeria, *J. Med. Microbiol.* **16:**93–96 (1983).

3. AGNER, E., ERIKSEN, M., HOLLNAGEL, H., LARSEN, J. H., MORCK, H. I., AND SCHROLL, M., Prevalence of raised *Yersinia enterocolitica* antibody titre in unselected, adult populations in Denmark during 12 years, *Acta Med. Scand.* **209:**509–512 (1981).

4. AHO, K., AHVONEN, P., LASSUS, A., SIEVERS, K., AND TIILIKAINEN, A., HL-A antigen and reactive arthritis, *Lancet* **2:**157 (1973).

5. AHVONEN, P., Human yersiniosis in Finland. I. Bacteriology and serology, *Ann. Clin. Res.* **4:**30 (1972).

6. AHVONEN, P., Human yersiniosis in Finland. II. Clinical features, *Ann. Clin. Res.* **4:**39 (1972).

7. AHVONEN, P., HIISI-BRUMMER, L., AND AHO, K., Electrocardiographic abnormalities and arthritis in patients with *Yersinia enterocolitica* infection, *Ann. Clin. Res.* **3:**69–75 (1971).

8. ALEKSIC, S., ROHDE, R., MÜLLER, G., AND WOHLERS, B., Examination of the envelope antigen K1 in *Yersinia enterocolitica* which was identified as fimbriae, *Zentralbl. Bakteriol. Hyg. A* **234:**513–520 (1976).

9. ASAKAWA, Y., AKAHANE, S., KAGATA, N., NOGUCHI, M., SAKAZAKI, R., AND TAMURA, K., Two community outbreaks of human infection with *Yersinia enterocolitica, J. Hyg.* **71:**715–723 (1973).

10. ATTWOOD, S. E. A., MEALY, K., CAFFERKEY, M. T., BUCKLEY, T. F., WEST, A. B., BOYLE, N., HEALY, E., AND KEANE, F. B. V., *Yersinia* infection and acute abdominal pain, *Lancet* **1:**529–533 (1987).

11. BERCOVIER, H., BRAULT, J., BARRÉ, N., TREIGNIER, M., ALONSO, J. M., AND MOLLARET, H. H., Biochemical, serological, and phage typing characteristics of 459 *Yersinia* strains isolated from a terrestrial ecosystem, *Curr. Microbiol.* **1:**353–357 (1978).

12. BERCOVIER, H., MOLLARET, H. H., ALONSO, J. M., BRAULT, J., FANNING, G. R., STEIGERWALT, A. G., AND BRENNER, D. J., Intra- and interspecies relatedness of *Yersinia pestis* by DNA hybridization and its relationship to *Yersinia pseudotuberculosis, Curr. Microbiol.* **4:**225–229 (1980).

13. BERCOVIER, H., STEIGERWALT, A. G., GUIYOULE, A., HUNTLEY-CARTER, G., AND BRENNER, D. J., *Yersinia aldovae* (formerly *Yersinia enterocolitica*-like group X2): A new species of Enterobacteriaceae isolated from aquatic ecosystems, *Int. J. Syst. Bacteriol.* **34:**166–172 (1984).

14. BLACK, R. E., JACKSON, R. J., TSAI, T., MEDVESKY, M., SHAYEGANI, M., FEELEY, J. C., MACLEOD, K. I. E., AND WAKELEE, A. M., Epidemic *Yersinia enterocolitica* infection

due to contaminated chocolate milk, *N. Engl. J. Med.* **298:**76–79 (1978).

15. BÖLIN, I., AND WOLF-WATZ, H., Molecular cloning of the temperature-inducible outer membrane protein I of *Yersinia pseudotuberculosis, Infect. Immun.* **43:**72–78 (1984).

16. BOTTONE, E. J., *Yersinia enterocolitica:* A panoramic view of a charismatic microorganism, *CRC Crit. Rev. Microbiol.* **5:**211–241 (1977).

17. BOTTONE, E. J., AND SHEEHAN, D. J., *Yersinia enterocolitica:* Guidelines for serologic diagnosis of human infections, *Rev. Infect. Dis.* **5:**898–906 (1983).

18. BRENNER, D. J., Speciation in *Yersinia,* in: *Contributions in Microbiology and Immunology* (P. B. CARTER, L. LAFLEUR, AND S. TOMA, eds.), Karger, Basel, 1979.

19. BRENNER, D. J., STEIGERWALT, A. G. FALCAO, D. P., WEAVER, R. E., AND FANNING, G. R., Characterization of *Yersinia enterocolitica* and *Yersinia pseudotuberculosis* by deoxyribonucleic acid hybridization and by biochemical reactions, *Int. J. Syst. Bacteriol.* **26:**180–194 (1976).

20. BRENNER, D. J., URSING, J., BERCOVIER, H., STEIGERWALT, A. G., FANNING, G. R., ALONSO, J. M., AND MOLLARET, H. H., Deoxyribonucleic acid relatedness in *Yersinia enterocolitica* and *Yersinia enterocolitica*-like organisms, *Curr. Microbiol.* **4:**195–200 (1980).

21. BUTLER, T., ISLAM, M., ISLAM, M. R., AZAD, A. K., HUQ, M. I., SPEELMAN, P., AND ROY, K., Isolation of *Yersinia enterocolitica* and *Yersinia intermedia* from fatal cases of diarrhoeal illness in Bangladesh, *Trans. R. Soc. Trop. Med. Hyg.* **78:**449–450 (1984).

22. CAFFERKEY, M. T., AND BUCKLEY, T. F., Comparison of saline agglutination, antibody to human gammaglobulin, and immunofluorescence tests in the routine serological diagnosis of yersiniosis, *J. Infect. Dis.* **156:**845–848 (1987).

23. CARLSSON, H. E., HURVELL, B., AND LINDBERG, A. A., Enzyme-linked immunosorbent assay (ELISA) for titration of antibodies against *Brucella abortus* and *Yersinia enterocolitica, Acta Pathol. Microbiol. Scand. Sect. C* **84:**168 (1976).

24. CARNIEL, E., BUTLER, T., HOSSAIN, S., ALAM, N. H., AND MAZIGH, D., Infrequent detection of *Yersinia enterocolitica* in childhood diarrhea in Bangladesh, *Am. J. Trop. Med. Hyg.* **35:**370–371 (1986).

25. CARTER, P. B., VARGA, C. F., AND KEET, E. E., New strain of *Yersinia enterocolitica* pathogenic for rodents, *Appl. Microbiol.* **26:**1016 (1973).

26. CARTER, P. B., MACDONALD, T. T., AND COLLINS, F. M., Host responses to infection with *Yersinia enterocolitica, Contrib. Microbiol. Immunol.* **5:**346 (1979).

27. CARTER, P. B., ZAHORCHAK, R. J., AND BRUBAKER, R. R., Plague virulence antigens from *Yersinia enterocolitica, Infect. Immun.* **28:**638–640 (1980).

28. CORBEL, M. J., The serological relationship between Brucella spp, *Yersinia enterocolitica* serotype IX and Salmonella serotypes of Kauffman–White group, *J. Hyg.* **75:**151–171 (1975).

29. CORNELIS, G., AND ABRAHAM, E. P., Beta-lactamases from *Yersinia enterocolitica, J. Gen. Microbiol.* **87:**273–284 (1975).

30. CORNELIS, G., WAUTERS, G., AND BRUYNOGHE, G., Resistances transferables chez des souches sauvages de *Yersinia enterocolitica, Ann. Microbiol. (Paris)* **124A:**299–309 (1973).

31. DEMOL, P., HEMELHOF, W., BUTZLER, J. P., BRASSEUR, D., KALALA, T., AND VIS, H. L., Enteropathogenic agents in children with diarrhoea in rural Zaire, *Lancet* **1:**516–578 (1983).

32. DOYLE, M. P., HUGDAHL, M. B., CHANG, M. T., AND BARRY, J. T., Serological relatedness of mouse-virulent *Yersinia enterocolitica, Infect. Immun.* **37:**1234 (1982).

33. EISS, J., Selective culturing of *Yersinia enterocolitica* at a low temperature, *Scand. J. Infect. Dis.* **7:**249–251 (1975).

34. EWING, W. H., ROSS, A. J., BRENNER, D. J., AND FANNING, G. R., *Yersinia ruckeri* sp. nov., the Redmouth (RM) bacterium, *Int. J. Syst. Bacteriol.* **28:**37–44 (1978).

35. FEELEY, J. C., WELLS, J. G., TSAI, T. F., AND PUHR, N. D., Detection of enterotoxigenic and invasive strains of *Yersinia enterocolitica, Contrib. Microbiol. Immunol.* **5:**329–334 (1979).

36. FERRER, M. G., OTERO, B. M., FIGA, P. C., AND PRATS, G., *Yersinia enterocolitica* infections and pork, *Lancet* **2:**334 (1987).

37. FIGURA, N., AND ROSSOLINI, A., A prospective etiological and clinical study on gastroenteritis in Italian children, *Boll. Ist. Sieroter. Milan.* **64:**302–310 (1985).

38. FLETCHER, K. M., AND NOBLE, M. A., Detection of human coproantibody IgA as a marker of organism virulence in patients culture positive with *Yersinia* species, Abstracts of the 1987 ICAAC, University of British Columbia, Vancouver (1987).

39. FORSSTROM, J., VIANDER, M., LEHTONEN, A., AND EKFORS, T., *Yersinia enterocolitica* infection complicated by glomerulonephritis, *Scand. J. Infect. Dis.* **9:**253–256 (1977).

40. FREDERIKSEN, W., A study of some *Yersinia pseudotuberculosis*-like bacteria ("Bacterium enterocoliticum" and "Pasteurella X"), Proceedings of the XIV Scandinavian Congress of Pathology and Microbiology, Oslo, pp. 103–104 (1964).

41. GEMSKI, P., LAZERE, J. R., AND CASEY, T., Plasmid associated with pathogenicity and calcium dependency of *Yersinia enterocolitica, Infect. Immun.* **27:**682–685 (1980).

42. GILBERT, R., Interesting cases and unusual specimens, Annual Report of the Division of Laboratories and Research, Albany, p. 57 (1933).

43. GOGUEN, J. D., YOTHER, J., AND STRALEY, S. C., Genetic analysis of the low calcium response in *Yersinia pestis* Mu dl (Ap *lac*) insertion mutants, *J. Bacteriol.* **160:**842–848 (1984).

44. GREENWOOD, J. R., FLANIGAN, S. M., PICKETT, M. J., AND MARTIN, W. J., Clinical isolation of *Yersinia enterocolitica:*

Cold temperature enrichment, *J. Clin. Microbiol.* **2**:559–560 (1975).

45. GUTMAN, L. T., OTTESEN, E. A., QUAN, T. J., NOCE, P. S., AND KATZ, S. L., An inter-familial outbreak of *Yersinia enterocolitica* enteritis, *N. Engl. J. Med.* **288**:1372–1377 (1973).

46. HEESEMANN, J., KELLER, C., MORAWA, R., SCHMIDT, N., SIEMENS, H. J., AND LAUFS, R., Plasmids of human strains of *Yersinia enterocolitica:* Molecular relatedness and possible importance for pathogenesis, *J. Infect. Dis.* **147**:107–115 (1983).

47. HIGUCHI, K., AND SMITH, J. L., Studies on the nutrition and physiology of *Pasteurella pestis.* VI. A differential plating medium for the estimation of the mutation rate to avirulence, *J. Bacteriol.* **81**:605–608 (1961).

48. HOOGKAMP-KORSTANJE, J. A. A., DEKONING, J., AND SAMSOM, J. P., Incidence of human infection with *Yersinia enterocolitica* serotypes O3, O8, and O9 and the use of indirect immunofluorescence in diagnosis, *J. Infect. Dis.* **153**:138–141 (1986).

49. HUBBERT, W. T., Yersiniosis in mammals and birds in the United States, *Am. J. Trop. Med. Hyg.* **21**:458–463 (1972).

50. JEPSEN, O. B., KORNER, B., LAURITSEN, K. B., HANCKE, A.-B., ANDERSEN, L., HENRICHSEN, S., BRENOE, E., CHRISTIANSEN, P. M., AND JOHANSEN, A., *Yersinia enterocolitica* infection in patients with acute surgical abdominal disease, *Scand. J. Infect. Dis.* **8**:189–194 (1976).

51. KALLIOMAKI, J. L., AND LEINO, R., Follow-up studies of joint complications in yersiniosis, *Acta Med. Scand.* **205**:521 (1979).

52. KANDOLO, K., AND WAUTERS, G., Pyrazinamidase activity in *Yersinia enterocolitica* and related organisms, *J. Clin. Microbiol.* **21**:980–982 (1985).

53. KELLY, M. T., BRENNER, D. J., AND FARMER, J. J., III, Enterobacteriaceae, in: *Manual of Clinical Microbiology,* 4th ed. (E. H. LENNETTE, ed.), pp. 273–274, American Society for Microbiology, Washington, D.C., 1985.

54. KNAPP, W., AND THAL, E., Untersuchungen über die kulturell biochemischen serologischen, tierexperimentallen und immunologischen Eigenschaften einer vorlaufig "Pasteurella X" benannten Bakterienart, *Zentralbl. Bakteriol. Orig. A* **190**:472 (1963).

55. KOHL, S., *Yersinia enterocolitica* infection in children, *Pediatr. Clin. North Am.* **26**:433–443 (1979).

56. KONDRACKI, S., AND GALLO, R., Letter to the Editor: Unusual cluster of yersiniosis in four infants due to a rare serogroup, *Diagn. Microbiol. Infect. Dis.* **6**:183–184 (1987).

57. LAIRD, W. J., AND CAVANAUGH, D. C., Correlation of autoagglutination and virulence in yersiniae, *J. Clin. Microbiol.* **11**:430 (1980).

58. LAITINEN, O., LEIRISALO, M., AND SKYLV, G., Relation between HLA-B27 and clinical features in patients with *Yersinia* arthritis, *Arthritis Rheum.* **20**:1121 (1977).

59. LAROCHE, Y., VAN BOUCHAUTE, M., AND CORNELIS, G., A restriction map of virulence plasmid pVYE439-80 from a serogroup 9 *Yersinia enterocolitica* strain, *Plasmid* **12**:67–70 (1984).

60. LEE, W. H., MCGRATH, P. P., CARTER, P. H., AND EIDE, E. L., The ability of some *Yersinia enterocolitica* strains to invade HeLa cells, *Can. J. Microbiol.* **23**:1714–1722 (1977).

61. LEINO, R., Incidence of yersiniosis in Finland, *Scand. J. Infect. Dis.* **13**:309–310 (1981).

62. LEINO, R., AND KALLIOMAKI, J. L., Yersiniosis as an internal disease, *Ann. Intern. Med.* **81**:458–461 (1974).

63. MÄKI, M., GRÖNROOS, P., AND VESIKARI, T., In vitro invasiveness of *Yersinia enterocolitica* isolated from children with diarrhea, *J. Infect. Dis.* **138**:677–680 (1978).

64. MARKS, M. I., PAI, C. H., LAFLEUR, L., LACKMAN, L., AND HAMMERBERG, O., *Yersinia enterocolitica* gastroenteritis: A prospective study of clinical bacteriologic and epidemiologic features, *J. Pediatr.* **96**:26 (1980).

65. MARTIN, T., KASIAN, G. F., AND STEAD, S., Family outbreak of yersiniosis, *J. Clin. Microbiol.* **16**:622–626 (1982).

66. MARTINEZ, R. J., Plasmid-mediated and temperature-regulated surface properties of *Yersinia enterocolitica, Infect. Immun.* **41**:921–930 (1983).

67. MEGRAUD, F., *Yersinia* infection and acute abdominal pain, *Lancet* **1**:1147 (1987).

68. MOLLARET, H. H., L'infection humaine à *Yersinia enterocolitica* en 1970 à la lumière de 642 cas récents, *Pathol. Biol.* **19**:189–205 (1971).

69. MOLLARET, H. H., BERCOVIER, H., AND ALONSO, J. M., Summary of the data received at the WHO Reference Center for *Yersinia enterocolitica, Contrib. Microbiol. Immunol.* **5**:174–184 (1979).

70. MORRIS, G. K., AND FEELEY, J. C., *Yersinia enterocolitica:* A review of its role in food hygiene, *Bull. WHO* **54**:79–85 (1976).

71. MORS, V., AND PAI, C. H., Pathogenic properties of *Yersinia enterocolitica, Infect. Immun.* **28**:292–294 (1980).

72. MORSE, D. L., SHAYEGANI, M., AND GALLO, R. J., Epidemiologic investigation of a *Yersinia* camp outbreak linked to a food handler, *Am. J. Public Health* **74**:589–592 (1984).

73. NILEHN, B., Studies on *Yersinia enterocolitica* with special reference to bacterial diagnosis and occurrence in human acute enteric disease, *Acta Pathol. Microbiol. Scand. Suppl.* **206**:1–48 (1969).

74. NILEHN, B., AND SJOSTROM, B., Studies on *Yersinia enterocolitica:* Occurrence in various groups of acute abdominal disease, *Acta Pathol. Microbiol. Scand.* **71**:612 (1967).

75. OLSOVSKY, Z., OLSAKOVA, V., CHOBOT, S., AND SVIRIDOV, V., Mass occurrence of *Yersinia enterocolitica* in two establishments of collective care of children, *J. Hyg. Epidemiol. Microbiol. Immunol.* **19**:22–29 (1975).

76. PAI, C. H., AND DESTEPHANO, L., Serum resistance associated with virulence in *Yersinia enterocolitica, Infect. Immun.* **35**:605–611 (1982).

77. PAI, C. H., AND MORS, V., Production of enterotoxin by *Yersinia enterocolitica, Infect. Immun.* **19**:908–911 (1978).

78. PAI, C. H., SORGER, S., LAFLEUR, L., LACKMAN, L., AND MARKS, M., Efficacy of cold enrichment techniques for recovery of *Yersinia enterocolitica* from human stools, *J. Clin. Microbiol.* **9**:712–715 (1979).

79. PAI, C. H., GILLIS, F., AND MARKS, M. I., Infection due to *Yersinia enterocolitica* in children with abdominal pain, *J. Infect. Dis.* **146**:705 (1982).

80. PAI, C. H., GILLIS, F., TUOMANEN, E., AND MARKS, M. I., Placebo-controlled double-blind evaluation of trimethoprim-sulfamethoxazole treatment of *Yersinia enterocolitica* gastroenteritis, *J. Pediatr.* **104**:308–311 (1984).

81. PEDERSEN, K. B., WINBLAD, S., AND BITSCH, V., Studies on the interaction between different O-serotypes of *Yersinia enterocolitica* and HeLa cells, *Acta Pathol. Microbiol. Scand. Sect. B* **87**:141–145 (1979).

82. PERRY, R. D., AND BRUBAKER, R. R., Accumulation of iron by yersiniae, *J. Bacteriol.* **137**:1290–1298 (1979).

83. PERRY, R. D., AND BRUBAKER, R. R., Vwa+ phenotype of *Yersinia enterocolitica*, *Infect. Immun.* **40**:166–171 (1983).

84. PERSSON, B. L., THORÉN, A., TUFVESSON, B., AND WALDER, M., Diarrhoea in Swedish infants, *Acta Paediatr. Scand.* **71**:909–913 (1982).

85. POOCHAROEN, L., BRUIN, C. W., SIRISANTHANA, V., VANNAREUMOL, P., LEECHANACHAI, P., AND SUKHAVAT, K., The relative importance of various enteropathogens as a cause of diarrhoea in hospitalized children in Chiang Mai, Thailand, *J. Diarrhoeal Dis. Res.* **4**:10–15 (1986).

86. PORTNOY, D. A., AND FALKOW, S., Virulence-associated plasmids from *Yersinia enterocolitica* and *Yersinia pestis*, *J. Bacteriol.* **148**:877–883 (1981).

87. PORTNOY, D. A., MOSELEY, S. L., AND FALKOW, S., Characterization of plasmids and plasmid-associated determinants of *Yersinia enterocolitica* pathogenesis, *Infect. Immun.* **31**:775–782 (1981).

88. PORTNOY, D. A., WOLF-WATZ, H., BÖLIN, I., BEEDER, A. B., AND FALKOW, S., Characterization of common virulence plasmids in *Yersinia* species and their role in the expression of outer membrane proteins, *Infect. Immun.* **43**:108–114 (1984).

89. PRPIC, J. K., ROBINS-BROWNE, R. M., AND DAVEY, R. B., Differentiation between virulent and avirulent *Yersinia enterocolitica* isolates by using Congo red agar, *J. Clin. Microbiol.* **18**:486–490 (1983).

90. RABSON, A. R., HALLETT, A. F., AND KOORNHOF, H. J., Generalized *Yersinia enterocolitica* infection, *J. Infect. Dis.* **131**:447–451 (1975).

91. RATNAM, S., MERCER, E., PICCO, B., AND BUTLER, R., A nosocomial outbreak of diarrheal disease due to *Yersinia enterocolitica* serotype O:5, biotype I, *J. Infect. Dis.* **145**:242–247 (1982).

92. SAMADI, A. R., WACHSMUTH, K., HUQ, M. I., MAHBUB, M., AND AGBONLAHOR, D. E., An attempt to detect *Yersinia enterocolitica* infection in Dacca, Bangladesh, *Trop. Geogr. Med.* **34**:151–154 (1982).

93. SCHIEMANN, D. A., Isolation of *Yersinia enterocolitica* from surface and well waters in Ontario, *Can. J. Microbiol.* **24**:1048–1052 (1978).

94. SCHIEMANN, D. A., Synthesis of selective agar medium for isolation of *Yersinia enterocolitica*, *Can. J. Microbiol.* **25**:1298–1304 (1979).

95. SCHIEMANN, D. A., AND DEVENISH, J. A., Virulence of *Yersinia enterocolitica* determined by lethality in Mongolian gerbils and by the Sereny test, *Infect. Immun.* **29**:500 (1980).

96. SCHIEMANN, D. A., AND DEVENISH, J. A., Relationship of HeLa cell infectivity to biochemical, serological, and virulence characteristics of *Yersinia enterocolitica*, *Infect. Immun.* **35**:497–506 (1982).

97. SCHIEMANN, D. A., DEVENISH, J. A., AND TOMA, S., Characteristics of virulence in human isolates of *Yersinia enterocolitica*, *Infect. Immun.* **32**:400 (1981).

98. SCHLEIFSTEIN, J., AND COLEMAN, M., *Bacterium enterocoliticum*, Annual Report of the Division of Laboratories and Research, p. 56, New York State Department of Health (1943).

99. SCRIBNER, R. K., MARKS, M. I., WEBER, A., AND PAI, C. H., *Yersinia enterocolitica*: Comparative in vitro activities of seven new beta-lactam antibiotics, *Antimicrob. Agents Chemother.* **22**:140 (1982).

100. SHENKMAN, L., AND BOTTONE, E. J., Antibodies to *Yersinia enterocolitica* in thyroid disease, *Ann. Intern. Med.* **85**:735–739 (1976).

101. SNYDER, J. D., CHRISTENSON, E., AND FELDMAN, R. A., Human *Yersinia enterocolitica* infections in Wisconsin: Clinical laboratory, and epidemiologic features, *Am. J. Med.* **72**:768–774 (1982).

102. SOLEM, J. H., AND LASSEN, J., Reiter's disease following *Yersinia enterocolitica* infection, *Scand. J. Infect. Dis.* **3**:83–85 (1971).

103. SPIRA, T. J., AND KABINS, S. A., *Yersinia enterocolitica* septicemia with septic arthritis, *Arch. Intern. Med.* **136**:1305 (1976).

104. STRALEY, S. C., AND BOWMER, W. S., Virulence genes regulated at the transcriptional level by Ca^{2+} in *Yersinia pestis* include structural genes for outer membrane proteins, *Infect. Immun.* **51**:445–454 (1986).

105. SZITA, M. I., KÁLI, M., AND RÉDEY, B., Incidence of *Yersinia enterocolitica* infection in Hungary, *Contrib. Microbiol. Immunol.* **2**:106 (1973).

106. TACKET, C. O., DAVIS, B. R., CARTER, G. P., RANDOLPH, J. F., AND COHEN, M. L., *Yersinia enterocolitica* pharyngitis, *Ann. Intern. Med.* **99**:40 (1983).

107. TACKET, C. O., NARAIN, J. P., SATTIN, R., LOFGREN, J. P., KONIGSBERG, C., RENDTORFF, R. C., RAUSA, A., DAVIS, B. R., AND COHEN, M. L., A multistate outbreak of infections caused by *Yersinia enterocolitica* transmitted by pasteurized milk, *J. Am. Med. Assoc.* **251**:483–486 (1984).

108. TACKET, C. O., BALLARD, J., HARRIS, N., ALLARD, J., NOLAN, C., QUAN, T., AND COHEN, M. L., An outbreak of *Yersinia enterocolitica* infections caused by contaminated tofu (soybean curd), *Am. J. Epidemiol.* **121**:705–711 (1985).

109. TAUXE, R. V., WAUTERS, G., GOOSSENS, V., VAN NOYEN, R., VANDEPITTE, J., MARTIN, S. M., DE NOL, P., AND THIERS, G., *Yersinia enterocolitica* infections and pork: The missing link, *Lancet* **1**:1129–1132 (1987).

110. TOIVANEN, P., TOIVANEN, A., OLKKONEN, L., AND AANTAA, S., Hospital outbreak of *Yersinia enterocolitica* infection, *Lancet* **1**:801–803 (1973).

111. TOMA, S., Survey on the incidence of *Yersinia enterocolitica* in the province of Ontario, *Can. J. Public Health* **64**:477 (1973).

112. TOMA, S., WAUTERS, G., McCLURE, H. M., MORRIS, G. K., AND WEISSFELD, A. S., O:13a, 13b a new pathogenic serotype of *Yersinia enterocolitica*, *J. Clin. Microbiol.* **20**:843–845 (1984).

113. UNE, T., Studies on the pathogenicity of *Yersinia enterocolitica*. II. Interactions with cultured cells in vitro, *Microbiol. Immunol.* **21**:365–377 (1977).

114. URBANO-MÁRQUEZ, A., ESTRUCH, R., AGUSTÍ, A., JIMENEZ DE ANTA, M. T., RIBALTA, T., GRAU, J. M., AND ROZMAN, C., Infectious endocarditis due to *Yersinia enterocolitica*, *J. Infect. Dis.* **148**:940 (1983).

115. URSING, J., BRENNER, D. J., BERCOVIER, H., FANNING, G. R., STEIGERWALT, A. G., BRANDT, J., AND MOLLARET, H. H., *Yersinia frederiksenii*: A new species of Enterobacteriaceae composed of rhamnose-positive strains (formerly called atypical *Yersinia enterocolitica* or *Yersinia enterocolitica*-like), *Curr. Microbiol.* **4**:213–217 (1980).

116. VANDEPITTE, J., AND WAUTERS, G., Epidemiological and clinical aspects of human *Yersinia enterocolitica* infections in Belgium, *Contrib. Microbiol. Immunol.* **5**:150–158 (1979).

117. VAN NOYEN, R., VANDEPITTE, J., AND WAUTERS, G., Nonvalue of cold enrichment of stools for isolation of *Yersinia enterocolitica* serotypes 3 and 9 from patients, *J. Clin. Microbiol.* **11**:127–131 (1980).

118. VELASCO, A. C., MATEOS, M. L., MÁS, G., PEDRAZA, A., DÍEZ, M., AND GUTIÉRREZ, A., Three-year prospective study of intestinal pathogens in Madrid, Spain, *J. Clin. Microbiol.* **20**:290–292 (1984).

119. WAUTERS, G., Contribution à l'étude de *Yersinia enterocolitica*, Thesis, Vander, Louvain, Belgium, 1970.

120. WAUTERS, G., Antigens of *Yersinia enterocolitica*, in: *Yersinia enterocolitica* (E. J. Bottone, ed.), pp. 41–53, CRC Press, Boca Raton, 1981.

121. WAUTERS, G., AND JANSSENS, M., Portage de *Yersinia enterocolitica* par le porc de boucherie. II. Recherche de *Yersinia enterocolitica* sur les langues de porc achetées en boucherie, *Med. Mal. Infect.* **6**:517–519 (1976).

122. WAUTERS, G., LeMINOR, L., AND CHALON, A. M., Antigènes somatiques et flagellaires des *Yersinia enterocolitica*, Annales des *Yersinia enterocolitica*, *Ann. Inst. Pasteur Paris* **120**:631–642 (1971).

123. WAUTERS, G., LeMINOR, L., CHALON, A. M., AND LASSEN, J., Supplément au schéme antigénique de '*Yersinia enterocolitica*,' *Ann. Inst. Pasteur Paris* **122**:951–956 (1972).

124. WEISSFELD, A. S., AND SONNENWIRTH, A. C., *Yersinia enterocolitica* in adults with gastrointestinal disturbances: Need for cold enrichment, *J. Clin. Microbiol.* **11**:196–197 (1980).

125. WINBLAD, S., Studies on serological typing of *Yersinia enterocolitica*, *Acta Pathol. Microbiol. Scand. Suppl.* **187**:115 (1967).

126. WINBLAD, S., Arthritis associated with *Yersinia enterocolitica* infections, *Scand. J. Infect. Dis.* **7**:191 (1975).

127. YOTHER, J., AND GOGUEN, J. D., Isolation and characterization of Ca^{2+} blind mutants of *Yersinia pestis*, *J. Bacteriol.* **164**:704–711 (1985).

128. YOTHER, J., CHAMNESS, T. W., AND GOGUEN, J. D., Temperature-controlled plasmid regulon associated with low calcium response in *Yersinia pestis*, *J. Bacteriol.* **165**:443–447 (1986).

129. ZEN-YOJI, H., MARUYAMA, T., SAKAI, S., KIMURA, S., MIZUNO, T., AND MOMOSE, T., An outbreak of enteritis due to *Yersinia enterocolitica* occurring at a junior high school, *Jpn. J. Microbiol.* **17**:220–222 (1973).

130. ZINK, D. L., FEELEY, J. C., WELLS, J. G., VANDERZANT, C., VICKERY, J. C., ROOF, W. D., AND O'DONOVAN, G. A., Plasmid-mediated tissue invasiveness in *Yersinia enterocolitica*, *Nature* **283**:224–226 (1980).

12. Suggested Reading

AHVONEN, P., Human yersiniosis in Finland. I. Bacteriology and serology, *Ann. Clin. Res.* **4**:30 (1972).

AHVONEN, P., Human yersiniosis in Finland. II. Clinical features, *Ann. Clin. Res.* **4**:39 (1972).

BOTTONE, E. J., *Yersinia enterocolitica*: A panoramic view of a charismatic microorganism, *CRC Crit. Rev. Microbiol.* **5**:211–241 (1977).

CORNELIS, G., LAROCHE, Y., BALLIGAND, G., SORY, M. P., AND WAUTERS, G., *Yersinia enterocolitica*, a primary model for bacterial invasiveness, *Rev. Infect. Dis.* **9**:64–76 (1987).

KOHL, S., *Yersinia enterocolitica* infection in children, *Pediatr. Clin. North Am.* **26**:433–443 (1979).

VANDEPITTE, J., AND WAUTÉRS, G., Epidemiological and clinical aspects of human *Yersinia enterocolitica* infections in Belgium, *Contrib. Microbiol. Immunol.* **5**:150–158 (1979).

Index

Corynebacterium diphtheriae (*cont.*)
lysogenization and, 118
toxin of, 17
transmission mechanism and routes,
232–233
Cost-benefit evaluation, acute nosocomial
infection control, 488
Counseling, gonococcal infection and,
269–270
Coxiella burnetti
biological characteristics of, 550–551
described, 547
infection caused by: *see* Q fever
isolation of, 549
CPHA: *see* Commission on Professional and Hospital Activities
(CPHA)
Cranial neuritis, in Lyme disease, 416
Cross-sectional study, in epidemiological
investigation, 8–9
Croup, diphtheritic, 233–234
CSF: *see* Cerebrospinal fluid (CSF)
CSF shunt infection, staphylococcal, 630
Culture screening, gonococcal infection
and, 269
Cutaneous anthrax
clinical features of, 83
epidemic behavior and contagiousness
of, 78–79
incidence of, 78
pathogenesis of, 82
Cutaneous diphtheria, 234
Cutaneous infection, nosocomial, 478
clinical features, 484
"Cutter Incident" in vaccine-related poliomyelitis, 60
CYE: *see* Charcoal-yeast extract (CYE)
agar
Cytokines, role in immune response, 27
Cytotoxic activity
antibody-dependent, 30
of cells, 27
cell-mediated immunity and, 29

Danish typing system, for *Streptococcus
pneumoniae*, 645
Dapsone, leprosy treatment and prevention with, 359–360
Data, from surveillance studies
analysis of, 67–70
reporting of: *see* Reporting, of surveillance data
sources of, 60–63
Day-care centers
H. influenzae occurrence in, 290–291

Day-care centers (*cont.*)
H. influenzae secondary disease risk
in, 285–287
Shigella incidence in, 600
Deer: *see under Odocoileus*
Deerflies, tularemia via, 787
Delores, cholera carrier, 219
Demographics, surveillance and, 63
Dental caries
incidence of, 653
organism causing: *see Streptococcus
mutans*
vaccines against, 666
Deoxyribonucleases (DNases), *Strep-
tococcus pyogenes* and, 648
Dermacentor andersoni
as infection vector
for *R. diaporica*, 547
for *R. rickettsia*, 561
as vector for *R. rickettsia*, 564
Dermacentor variabilis, as vector for *R.
rickettsia*, 564
Dermal transmission route, for bacterial
infection, 22
Developing countries
Campylobacter infections in, 157
nosocomial infections in, 489
Shigella prevalence in, 598–599
Device-related nosocomial infections,
481–482
control and prevention of, 487
DFA: *see* Direct fluorescent antibody
smear (DFA)
Diagnosis, of bacterial infections, 39–40
specimen collection, 40
testing and: *see* Tests
Diarrhea
caused by *Campylobacter* spp.: *see
Campylobacter* infections
in cholera, 218, 219
Escherichia coli type: *see Escherichia
coli* diarrhea
WHO Diarrhea Treatment Solution,
220
Yersinia enterocolitica infection and
clinical features, 830
organism isolation, 824
Diethyltoluamide, for tick control, 570
Dilution-sensitivity tests, in bacteriological diagnosis, 41
Dimethylphthalate, for tick control, 570
Dimorphous leprosy, 358
Diphtheria
cases reported (1920–1987), 230
clinical features of, 233–234

Diphtheria (*cont.*)
control and prevention of, 235–236
described, 227
diagnosis of, 234
differential, 234
laboratory methods, 228–229
in different settings, 232
distribution of
by age, sex, and race, 231, 232
geographic, 230–231
by occupation, 231–232
temporal, 231
epidemic behavior and contagiousness,
230
historical background to, 227
incidence of, 68
morbidity/mortality data sources for,
228
organism isolation and identification,
228–229; *see also Corynebacterium diphtheriae*
pathogenesis and immunity, 233
prevalence and incidence of, 230,
231
socioeconomic and other factors involved in, 232
surveys on, 228
therapy for, 234–235
unresolved problems, 236
Diphtheria–pertussis–tetanus (DPT) vaccine, 48, 50
combinations with, 720
against diphtheria, 236
improved forms, 507–508
against pertussis, 506
safety concerns, 506–507
against tetanus, 715, 716
Diphtheria surveillance, 228
Diphtheria–tetanus (Td) antigen, adult
use of, 236
Diphtheritic croup, 233–234
Diplococcus pneumoniae Weichselbaum,
525
Direct fluorescent antibody smear (DFA),
in chlamydial infection diagnosis, 183–184
Disease
development of, 18
organisms causing, 15–17; *see also individually named organisms*
Disease intervention
in epidemiological process, 268–269
gonococcal infection priority criteria,
270
Disease surveillance: *see* Surveillance